WOLFSON INSTITUTE OF PREVENTIVE MEDICINE

OXFORD MEDICAL PUBLICATIONS

INTERNATIONAL SMOKING STATISTICS

A collection of historical data from 30 economically developed countries

This book is dedicated to the memory of Geoff Todd,
without whom it would never have been produced

INTERNATIONAL SMOKING STATISTICS

A collection of historical data from 30 economically developed countries

Second edition

Edited by

Barbara Forey, Jan Hamling and Peter Lee
P.N. Lee Statistics and Computing Limited
Sutton, Surrey

Nicholas Wald
Wolfson Institute of Preventive Medicine
Barts and The London Queen Mary's School of Medicine and Dentistry

Wolfson Institute of Preventive Medicine
London

OXFORD
UNIVERSITY PRESS

2002

Wolfson Institute of Preventive Medicine, Charterhouse Square, London EC1M 6BQ

OXFORD
UNIVERSITY PRESS

Great Clarendon Street, Oxford OX2 6DP

Oxford University Press is a department of the University of Oxford.
It furthers the University's objective of excellence in research, scholarship,
and education by publishing worldwide in

Oxford New York

Athens Auckland Bangkok Bogotá Bombay Buenos Aires
Cape Town Dar es Salaam Delhi Florence Hong Kong Istanbul
Karachi Kolkata Kuala Lumpur Madrid Melbourne Mexico City Mumbai
Nairobi Paris São Paulo Shanghai Singapore Taipei Tokyo Toronto Warsaw

and associated companies in Berlin Ibadan

Oxford is a registered trade mark of Oxford University Press
in the UK and in certain other countries

Published in the United States
by Oxford University Press Inc., New York

First published 1993
Second edition published 2002

British Library Cataloguing in Publication Data

Data available

Library of Congress Cataloging in Publication Data

ISBN 0 19 850856 5

10 9 8 7 6 5 4 3 2 1

Typeset by P.N. Lee Statistics and Computing Ltd, Sutton
Printed in Great Britain
on acid-free paper by Bookcraft Limited, Midsomer Norton

Preface to second edition

This book is a collection of smoking data relating to 30 economically developed countries. In a number of countries attempts have been made to relate national trends in mortality rates from various smoking-associated diseases to corresponding national trends in the consumption of cigarettes and other tobacco products. While comprehensive data on age- and sex-specific mortality rates are generally available, we are not aware of any other document which presents corresponding historical smoking data for a wide range of countries. The Tobacco Research Council provided historical data on tobacco consumption until 1973, but these were based on sales and provided no information classified according to age and sex, which is needed for more precise comparisons with mortality trends. The first edition of this book provided the necessary survey data on smoking habits classified according to age and sex for 22 countries up to 1985. This edition extends the coverage mainly to include Eastern Europe, and years up to 1995. The information for the 30 countries now included is presented in as consistent a format as possible for the various countries considered.

Data on sales of cigarettes and all tobacco products are presented from about 1920 to 1995, including estimates of the consumption of hand-rolled cigarettes. The Tobacco Research Council provided the sales data until 1973, while later sales data were obtained from government and industry sources. Smoking data by age and sex were obtained from a wide variety of surveys. A few data are available for the early part of this century, but for most countries these data are available from the 1950s or 1960s onwards. With a few exceptions, survey-based data are given up to 1995.

The figures are intended to provide an easily interpretable summary of the data presented in the tables and the commentary has been deliberately kept to a minimum.

Many of the data for the first edition of this monograph were collected by the late Mr. G.F. Todd, past director of the Tobacco Research Council, who had a life-long interest in smoking statistics. Shortly before he died in 1988 he had prepared a draft report summarizing relevant information for a number of countries. This work has been supplemented by contacts with government statistical services and industry organizations, and by literature and internet searches for further sources of information and this volume is based on the combined material.

April 2001
The Editors

Acknowledgements

We would like to acknowledge the help given by the tobacco industry and by the many government and research organizations and individuals who supplied much of the information in this book. We thank John Hamling for help in preparing the tables and figures, Yvonne Cooper for text processing, Yvonne Cooper, Pauline Wassell and Diane Morris for maintenance of our references database, and Jan Mackie for editorial assistance.

Contents

Tables

The title of each table is given together with the population to which the table applies. The sources of the data are presented in short form in the *Notes* for each country and in full in the *References* for each country.

Figures

Methods

Countries considered

The countries included in this study are shown in the list below. Countries were chosen for the first edition on the expectation that sufficient age- and sex-specific smoking data could be collected to enable a useful study of the relationship with mortality statistics, and in this edition, coverage has been extended to most of Europe. Chapters relate to political boundaries as they existed pre-1990, with the exception of Germany where the former Democratic and Federal Republics are presented in a single chapter.

1	Australia	16	Italy
2	Austria	17	Japan
3	Belgium	18	Netherlands
4	Bulgaria	19	New Zealand
5	Canada	20	Norway
6	Czechoslovakia	21	Poland
7	Denmark	22	Portugal
8	Finland	23	Romania
9	France	24	Spain
10	Germany	25	Sweden
11	Greece	26	Switzerland
12	Hungary	27	UK (United Kingdom)
13	Iceland	28	USA (United States of America)
14	Ireland	29	USSR (Union of Soviet Socialist Republics)
15	Israel	30	Yugoslavia

Further data for the United Kingdom are available in our earlier book[1], which includes more detailed information on smoking in the UK.

Main sources of data

The two main types of data presented in this book are sales data and survey data. Sales data give the total national consumption of tobacco. Survey data provide information on the prevalence and amount of smoking according to age and sex. We give the results of the original authors as closely as possible, whilst presenting them in a uniform format. In additional tables, we calculate further statistics by combining the sales and survey data using certain standardized assumptions. Each chapter contains the following tables for a specified country, unless otherwise stated (a few tables are missing because of lack of data).

Sales data

(1.1) Total annual sales of tobacco products before 1974
(1.2) Total annual sales of tobacco products for 1974 onwards
(1.3) Characteristics of manufactured cigarettes sold (filter, tar, nicotine)
(2) Consumption of cigarettes and of all tobacco products including estimated consumption of hand-rolled cigarettes (total and per adult)
(3) Percentage sales of tobacco in different forms (by weight)

Survey data
(4) Prevalence of smoking according to age and sex
(5) Number of cigarettes smoked per smoker per day according to age and sex

Additional survey-based data
(6) Number of cigarettes smoked per person per day according to age and sex
(7) Number of cigarettes smoked per person per day (sales-adjusted), according to age and sex
(8) Summary of adult smoking according to sex

Further explanation of the tables is given below.

Sales data

Consumption of tobacco products
Up to 1973 sales data on tobacco consumption were obtained from the Tobacco Research Council Research Paper 6 (RP6)[2-4] unless otherwise stated. Later data, and data for countries not represented in that report, were obtained from government or industry sources. Full citations of the sources are given in the *References* for each country.

Tables 1.1 and 1.2 show the total national consumption of all types of tobacco known to be used in each country. Factors such as smuggling, cross-border sales or stocks held by retailers are treated differently in the different countries and are described in the *Notes* for each country.

Tobacco products such as cigarettes and cigars are shown by both number and weight; in most countries the weights have been estimated by us for 1974 onwards. This estimation was made to allow calculation of an estimate for total tobacco consumption, which is a useful measure in comparing consumption between different countries as the market share of the various products can differ considerably. For a few countries, this estimation was based on data on the average weight of a cigarette. However, there has generally been little such information available and therefore we have used a constant weight per cigarette, cigar, etc. to convert numbers to weight, derived from the average weights of the products between 1970 and 1973 for each country as given in RP6, or 1 g per cigarette for countries not represented in RP6. A drawback of this method is that it cannot reflect certain changes in the cigarette market. Changes such as the switch from plain to filter cigarettes, variation in the weight of standard cigarettes and the varying market share of king size cigarettes will have had an effect on the weight of an 'average' cigarette. Estimates of total tobacco consumption are only presented if we are reasonably confident that data on all relevant types of tobacco are available.

Data are included on smokeless tobacco, which takes various forms in different countries. Chewing tobacco, chewed or held in the cheek or lower lip, is available in three main types—loose leaf, plug, and twist. Snuff has a much finer consistency and is held in the mouth without chewing; it may be moist or dry. Dry snuff may also be taken nasally, but this practice is now very limited. Snuff in small pouches the size of tea bags was introduced in some countries, and subsequently banned in many of them.

Data describing some characteristics of manufactured cigarettes sold are shown in Table 1.3. This includes the percentage of manufactured cigarettes sold as filter cigarettes, and the sales-weighted average yields of tar and nicotine. For some countries, additional tables are included to cover other aspects of tobacco consumption, such as sales of cigarette papers.

Table 2 provides sales-based information relevant to manufactured and hand-rolled cigarettes, and to total tobacco; the data are shown as total national consumption for the year and daily consumption per adult (aged 15 years and over). The consumption of manufactured cigarettes and total tobacco consumption by weight are taken from Tables 1.1 and 1.2 (see also comments above). When no data on hand-rolled cigarettes are available from other sources, we have estimated hand-rolled cigarette consumption where possible from 1950 onwards (see also *Notes* for each country and Appendix II, p. 785) and hence the total number of cigarettes smoked.

Table 3 is based on the data by weight in Tables 1.1 and 1.2, and includes data for selected years only. Tables 2 and 3 are also presented graphically as Figures 1 and 2 respectively.

In Tables 1-3, blank indicates that data are not available.

Survey data

Prevalence of smoking and cigarette consumption per smoker

These data have been obtained from a variety of sources. Nationally representative surveys have been used where possible. Other sources are included when nationally representative surveys do not exist (or are not available from trade sources) for some countries or for all years, or they provide little detail. Sources providing international comparisons are also included. Some surveys are based on specific regions or racial groups. Surveys of teenagers are frequently based on pupils at school, who may not be representative of teenagers who have left school. Control populations from case-control studies have sometimes been used where no other data are available. Studies of occupational groups have generally not been used. Even surveys based on large regions cannot necessarily be regarded as typical of the country, since the region may have been selected for study for reasons related to smoking habits.

While we have tried to include all survey data of value, choices are inevitably arbitrary and there may be omissions. Readers aware of other data are welcome to contact the authors, so that the data can be considered for inclusion in any future editions.

The prevalence of smoking (the percentage of the population who currently smoke cigarettes or any tobacco products) is given in Table 4. Cigarette consumption per smoker is given in Table 5. These data are presented according to sex and, if available, according to age group. Estimates of the prevalence of smoking are presented to the nearest whole number, and of cigarette consumption per smoker to two significant figures (if available).

Each row of Tables 4 and 5 includes age-specific data from one survey. Results for males and females are presented on facing pages. A blank row indicates that the survey did not report that sex. At the beginning of the row we have given the year in which the survey was carried out, the source number assigned to that source, and codes both for the tobacco products used and for the frequency of smoking, thus:

Frequency Product Source Year	Age group																					
	12	13	14	15	16	17	18	19	20 - 24	25 - 29	30 - 34	35 - 39	40 - 44	45 - 49	50 - 54	55 - 59	60 - 64	65 - 69	70 - 74	75 - 79	80+	All ages

Further explanation is given in the following sections.

a. Year

The year of each survey, or mid-point year if carried out over a longer period, is shown in the tables.

b. Source

Each source of survey data—either an individual survey or a series of surveys repeated over a number of years—is cited by a source number. This number is shown in the tables for cross-reference to the accompanying *Notes*, where details of the source publication are given, together with a brief description of the survey scope and methodology if available. Full citations of the sources are given in the *References* for each country.

c. Product

The definitions of smoking used in different surveys vary so much that comparisons are not straightforward. A 'product code' has been used to identify the smoking habits considered by the survey:

MC	manufactured cigarettes
TC	total cigarettes (manufactured and hand-rolled)
UC	cigarettes (type unspecified)
A	any product
U	product unspecified

The definition of cigarette smokers includes those who smoke either cigarettes only or cigarettes and other products (pipe, cigars, etc.). Smokers of any product include all cigarette smokers and also those who smoke other products but not cigarettes.

'Product unspecified' may mean that the questionnaire did not specify the product, leaving it to be self-defined by the respondent, for example in reply to the question 'Do you smoke?', or that the description available to us was not specific.

No attempt has been made to include data on smokers of hand-rolled cigarettes only, or of other products only, or by type of manufactured cigarette (e.g. filter/plain, high/low tar, dark/blond tobacco), although brief mention of such results is sometimes made in the *Notes*.

Where necessary, further details of the product definition are given in the *Notes*.

d. Frequency

Definitions of the frequency of smoking also vary; some are limited to regular or daily smokers (which can generally be regarded as synonymous for adult smokers), some relate to smoking the day before the survey, and some are self-defined. In the tables providing data on the prevalence of smoking (Table 4), a 'frequency code' has been used as follows:

R	regular smokers
A	all smokers (regular and occasional)
U	frequency unspecified

Where estimates for both regular and all smokers are available, both are presented. Further details of the frequency definition are given in the *Notes* for teenage surveys (if available), and where necessary for adult surveys.

e. Age group

The age groups used in Tables 4 and 5 are single years of age from 12 to 19, 5-year age groups from 20-24 to 75-79, and 80+. The overall age range covered by each survey, and the breakdown into age groups are indicated by the boundaries in the row. For ages 20 or over, original authors usually provide data by intervals of 5 years or more and there is then no problem in fitting the estimated prevalence of smoking or cigarette consumption into the available space. Exceptionally, data are provided for narrower age ranges, necessitating averaging of estimates and/or widening of boundaries. This is indicated in the *Notes* where it applies, as are cases where the lowest age group also includes persons below the age of 12.

Some surveys provide data relevant to the whole age group studied as well as for each age group. These estimates are included, where applicable, in the column under 'all ages'. The age range to which they are applicable is indicated by the boundaries to the results by age. (For estimates relevant to all adults' ages, see *Summary of adult smoking* on p. xxxvi).

Consumption category estimation

In many studies, information is not presented directly on the numbers of cigarettes smoked per smoker per day. Instead, the distribution of smokers according to various groupings of number smoked (e.g. 1-9, 10-19, 20-29, 30+) is given. Todd[5] introduced a method for estimating the mean consumption level for each consumption category and hence estimating the average consumption per smoker. We have used a modification of this method, described in Appendix III, p. 789. In the tables on cigarette consumption per smoker, the code E indicates that this estimation has been used. Details of the different consumption categories used are given in the *Notes* to the tables. This estimation will be less reliable when based on few categories, and cases where only two categories were available are indicated in Table 5 by the code *.

This method has also been applied to some surveys of teenage smoking and to surveys of weekly (rather than daily) consumption, where its validity is unproven.

Additional survey-based data

Cigarette consumption per person

The cigarette consumption per person (the number of cigarettes smoked per person per day averaged over both smokers and non-smokers) is given in Table 6. These estimates have generally been calculated by Todd or by us, by multiplying the percentage of cigarette smokers by the cigarette consumption per smoker, although in a few cases these data were given by the original author.

For some surveys, the prevalence of smoking is not available on an exactly equivalent base to the consumption per smoker, but the estimate has been presented as the best available. Such problems are indicated by the code *. For instance, we may have combined the prevalence of smoking *of any product* with the cigarette consumption *per cigarette smoker* to estimate the cigarette consumption per person. This estimate will be reasonable provided that the percentage of other smokers is small; otherwise it gives an overestimate. The extent to which this is a problem varies with both country and sex—in many countries more men than women smoke other products.

It is well known that the total consumption of cigarettes, when grossed up from survey findings, is almost invariably substantially lower than the total sales of cigarettes. The degree of this understatement is indicated in the column under '% Total sales' in Table 6, where the consumption implied by the survey is given as a percentage of the total sales. The method of calculating this percentage is described in the next section 'Adjustment for understatement'. The estimates for cigarette consumption per person, adjusted to match total sales are provided in Table 7. This method assumes that the degree of understatement is uniform over both sexes and all age groups. This assumption may not always be justifiable, but in general adjusted figures probably give a more realistic picture of consumption than unadjusted figures.

The year, source number, product code and the age groups shown in the tables on cigarette consumption per person, are all as described for Tables 4 and 5 (see pp. xxxiii-xxxiv). A frequency code is not generally needed (calculations were based on regular smokers if possible; if otherwise, this is mentioned in the *Notes*).

Adjustment for understatement

This method was applied only to surveys which covered both sexes and an age range of at least 21-64. The method was applied regardless of whether surveys were representative of the general population or of the whole country.

We filled gaps in the consumption per person data for ages 15-20 or 65 years and over, by assumed extensions to the age distribution which are shown in the *Notes* for each country. This process is unlikely to cause any bias, since the assumed extensions apply only to a relatively small proportion of the population. Smoking by persons aged under 15 was ignored in calculating the total consumption implied by the survey, except where the lowest age group 'overlapped' the age of 15. Such data have little effect on the total consumption. If a survey provided data both by age and on an overall basis, the data by age were used in the calculation.

Population data were taken from WHO 5-year age group data. Where population estimates for single years of age were required, they were assumed to be one-fifth of those for the 5-year age group.

The survey consumption data were combined with the population data to calculate the total national consumption by adults implied by the survey. This figure was compared with the sales estimate for the period of the survey and an under/overstatement (percentage total sales) was calculated. Consumption was then adjusted to match total sales, using percentage total sales as the adjustment factor. In some cases, there was a problem in aligning the type of product smoked, as recorded in the survey, with the available sales data. The product used is indicated by an adjustment code as follows.

Adjustment code	Explanation
M	Survey data relate (or probably relate) to manufactured cigarette consumption; adjustment was made to sales of manufactured cigarettes
T	Survey data (probably) relate to total cigarette consumption (manufactured and hand-rolled); adjustment was made to our estimate of total cigarette consumption
m	Survey data (probably) relate to total cigarette consumption; no estimate of hand-rolled cigarette consumption is available, but it is believed to be rare and so adjustment was made to sales of manufactured cigarettes
A	Survey data relate to consumption of all products (grams per person per day); adjustment was made to sales of all products; rarely used
---	Calculations previously made by Todd on a very similar basis, or by original authors, and not recalculated.

Summary of adult smoking

Table 8 presents a summary of adult smoking according to sex but not according to age. It gives estimates of the prevalence of smoking of cigarettes and of all products, and estimates of cigarette consumption per person, both original (unadjusted) and adjusted to match total sales.

All surveys in Tables 4, 6, and 7 covering an age range of at least 21-64 are included (required for both sexes in the sales-adjusted part of the table). The source number is given (see also p. xxxiii) so that the survey can be found in the age-specific tables and the *Notes* for each country. The product codes are also as shown in the age-specific tables (see also p. xxxiv), but the frequency of smoking is indicated by the type style (regular or daily smokers in normal type, all smokers in bold and unspecified in italics, see also p. xxxiv). The estimated percentage of total sales implied by the survey (used as adjustment factor) is given as provided in the tables on cigarette consumption per person (see also p. xxxv).

Any gaps in the cigarette consumption per person data for ages 15-20 or 65 years and over are filled in by assumed extensions to the age distribution as described in the above section 'Adjustment for understatement'. We used a similar procedure to extend the prevalence data. The age-specific data are then combined with the population data to calculate the average for the whole adult range (aged 15 years and over). The original 'all-ages' estimates (see also p. xxxiv) could transfer directly to Table 8, but our method uses age-specific data and WHO population data in preference if they are available. This can sometimes lead to an apparent anomaly, presumably because of a difference in population weighting.

For some surveys, no data on consumption per person were available in Table 6, but data on the percentage of cigarette smokers were specified in Table 4. Using the additional assumption that the consumption level per female smoker is 80% of that per male smoker, it was then possible to divide the total sales-based consumption figures into separate estimates for each sex. Such estimates are shown in parentheses. They have occasionally been included even if based on smoking of unspecified products, but only where it was reasonable to assume that they related to cigarettes.

Table 8 is also presented graphically in Figures 3-4.

In Appendix IV, p. 791, a method is described to estimate the prevalence of smoking from data presented in Table 4 of each country, according to a set of standard age groups. The different age groups used in Table 4 are often difficult to interpret and standardized data would facilitate comparison with, for instance, mortality trends, as these are commonly presented by 5-year age groups.

In Appendix V, p. 799, an indirect method of estimating past smoking habits is described. Indirect estimates are given for the UK and are compared with the direct estimates presented in Chapter 27, leading to the conclusion that indirect estimation represents a useful approach when direct estimates are not available. Appendix V also lists references to papers which have presented indirect estimates for countries in this book.

Population

Population data (see also Appendix I, p. 779) are taken from WHO estimates, usually for 1950 onwards. In earlier years, RP6 was used for total adult populations, and Alderson[6] for age- and sex-specific data.

Abbreviations

Abbreviations used in the *Notes* for each country are explained when first mentioned within each chapter, apart from RP6 (Research Paper 6 of the Tobacco Research Council, London, see Beese (1968,1972) and Lee (1975) in *References* below) and WHO (World Health Organization) which are used throughout.

References

Papers referred to in the *Notes* for each country are listed separately in the *References* for each country, where full citations of the sources are given. A paper marked with § indicates that we have not obtained the paper, but have taken information quoted by another author.

1. Wald N, Nicolaides-Bouman A, editors. *UK Smoking Statistics,* 2nd edition. London and Oxford: Wolfson Institute of Preventive Medicine and Oxford University Press; 1991.

2. Beese DH, editor. *Tobacco consumption in various countries,* 2nd edition. London: Tobacco Research Council; 1968. Research Paper 6.

3. Beese DH, editor. *Tobacco consumption in various countries,* 3rd edition. London: Tobacco Research Council; 1972. Research Paper 6.

4. Lee PN, editor. *Tobacco consumption in various countries,* 4th edition. London: Tobacco Research Council; 1975. Research Paper 6.

5. Todd GF. Cigarette consumption per adult of each sex in various countries. *J Epidemiol Community Health* 1978;**32**:289-93.

6. Alderson M. *International Mortality Statistics*. London: Macmillan; 1981.

Comparisons between countries

For the 30 countries included in this book, rank tables are presented for the consumption of cigarettes and all tobacco products per adult (Tables i and iii) and for the prevalence of smoking among adults (Table ii) at different time periods. The data are based on Tables 2 and 8 of each chapter. Tables iv and v give comparisons of some characteristics of manufactured cigarettes in the 30 countries.

Table vi presents data on the consumption of manufactured cigarettes and all tobacco products per adult for all 47 countries as given in RP6 for the years 1935, 1950, 1965, and 1973. Table vii gives a comparison of 121 countries, which include the countries listed in this book, for the consumption of manufactured cigarettes per adult in 1982-1983.

Table i Daily consumption of cigarettes and all tobacco products[1,2] per adult (sexes combined) at five time periods: 1931-1935, 1956-1960, 1971-1975, 1981-1985 and 1991-1995. Comparison of 30 countries, males and females aged 15 years and over

1931-1935

	Manufactured cigarettes Number/adult/day	Total cigarettes[3] Number/adult/day	All tobacco products[4] Grams/adult/day
10.0 or more			Netherlands
8.0-9.9			Belgium, USA
6.0-7.9			Denmark
4.0-5.9	UK	UK	Australia, Austria, Canada, Czechoslovakia, France, Germany, Ireland, New Zealand, Norway, Spain, Sweden, Switzerland, UK
2.0-3.9	Austria, Belgium, Czechoslovakia, Finland, Greece, Ireland, Japan, USA	Australia, Austria, Bulgaria, Finland, Germany, Greece, Japan	Bulgaria, Finland, Greece, Hungary, Iceland, Italy, Japan, Poland, Romania, Yugoslavia
Less than 2.0	Australia, Canada, Denmark, France, Germany, Hungary, Iceland, Italy, Netherlands, New Zealand, Norway, Poland, Romania, Spain, Sweden, Switzerland, Yugoslavia	Iceland, Norway	
No data	Bulgaria, Israel, Portugal, USSR	Belgium, Canada, Czechoslovakia, Denmark, France, Hungary, Ireland, Israel, Italy, Netherlands, New Zealand, Poland, Portugal, Romania, Spain, Sweden, Switzerland, USA, USSR, Yugoslavia	Israel, Portugal, USSR

1956-1960

	Manufactured cigarettes Number/adult/day	Total cigarettes[3] Number/adult/day	All tobacco products[4] Grams/adult/day
10.0 or more		USA	Canada, Netherlands, USA
8.0-9.9	Romania, USA	Australia, Canada, Romania	Australia, Belgium, Denmark, Ireland, New Zealand, Romania, Switzerland, UK
6.0-7.9	Canada, Ireland, Poland, UK	Belgium, Ireland, Netherlands, New Zealand, Poland, UK	Germany(W), Iceland, Poland
4.0-5.9	Australia, Austria, Belgium, Bulgaria, Czechoslovakia, Finland, Germany(W), Greece, Hungary, Iceland, Japan, Netherlands, New Zealand, Switzerland, Yugoslavia	Austria, Bulgaria, Denmark, Finland, France, Germany(W), Greece, Hungary, Iceland, Japan, Spain	Austria, Bulgaria, Finland, France, Greece, Hungary, Japan, Norway, Spain, Sweden, Yugoslavia
2.0-3.9	Denmark, France, Italy, Portugal, Spain, Sweden	Italy, Norway, Portugal, Sweden	Italy, Portugal
Less than 2.0	Norway		
No data	Israel, Germany(E), USSR	Czechoslovakia, Germany(E), Israel, Switzerland, USSR, Yugoslavia	Czechoslovakia, Germany(E), Israel, USSR

1971-1975

	Manufactured cigarettes Number/adult/day	Total cigarettes[3] Number/adult/day	All tobacco products[4] Grams/adult/day
10.0 or more	Romania, USA	Canada, Romania, USA	Belgium, Canada, Denmark, Netherlands, Romania, Switzerland, USA
8.0-9.9	Australia, Canada, Hungary, Ireland, Japan, Poland, Switzerland, UK	Australia, Belgium, Hungary, Ireland, Japan, Netherlands, New Zealand, Poland, UK	Australia, Germany(W), Hungary, Iceland, Ireland, Japan, New Zealand, Poland
6.0-7.9	Austria, Belgium, Germany(W), Greece, Israel, Netherlands, New Zealand, Spain, USSR, Yugoslavia	Austria, Denmark, France, Germany(W), Greece, Israel, Spain	Austria, France, Greece, Israel, Norway, Spain, UK, Yugoslavia
4.0-5.9	Bulgaria, Czechoslovakia, Denmark, Finland, France, Iceland, Italy, Portugal, Sweden	Bulgaria, Finland, Iceland, Italy, Norway, Portugal, Sweden	Bulgaria, Finland, Italy, Portugal, Sweden, USSR
2.0-3.9			
Less than 2.0	Norway		
No data	Germany(E)	Czechoslovakia, Germany(E), Switzerland, USSR, Yugoslavia	Czechoslovakia, Germany(E)

1981-1985

	Manufactured cigarettes Number/adult/day	Total cigarettes[3] Number/adult/day	All tobacco products[4] Grams/adult/day
10.0 or more	Romania	Romania	Romania
8.0-9.9	Australia, Canada, Greece, Hungary, Japan, Poland, Switzerland, USA, Yugoslavia	Australia, Canada, Greece, Hungary, Japan, Netherlands, Poland, USA	Belgium, Canada, Greece, Hungary, Iceland, Japan, Netherlands, New Zealand, Poland, Switzerland, USA, Yugoslavia
6.0-7.9	Austria, Czechoslovakia, Germany(W), Iceland, Ireland, Israel, Italy, New Zealand, Spain, UK	Austria, Belgium, Denmark, France, Germany(W), Iceland, Ireland, Israel, Italy, New Zealand, Spain, UK	Australia, Austria, Denmark, France, Germany(W), Ireland, Israel, Italy, Spain
4.0-5.9	Belgium, Bulgaria, Denmark, Finland, France, Netherlands, Portugal, Sweden, USSR	Bulgaria, Finland, Norway, Portugal, Sweden	Bulgaria, Norway, Portugal, Sweden, UK, USSR
2.0-3.9			Finland
Less than 2.0	Norway		
No data	Germany(E)	Czechoslovakia, Germany(E), Switzerland, USSR, Yugoslavia	Czechoslovakia, Germany(E)

1991-1995

	Manufactured cigarettes Number/adult/day	Total cigarettes[3] Number/adult/day	All tobacco products[4] Grams/adult/day
10.0 or more	Romania	Romania	Romania
8.0-9.9	Greece, Hungary, Japan, Poland	Greece, Hungary, Poland	Greece, Hungary, Japan, Poland
6.0-7.9	Australia, Bulgaria, Czechoslovakia, Ireland, Spain, USA, Yugoslavia	Australia, Belgium, Bulgaria, Canada, Germany, Ireland, Netherlands, USA	Belgium, Bulgaria, Denmark, France, Germany, Iceland, Netherlands, Spain, USA, Yugoslavia
4.0-5.9	Austria, Belgium, Canada, Denmark, Finland, France, Germany, Iceland, Italy, Portugal, UK, USSR	Austria, Denmark, Finland, France, Iceland, Italy, New Zealand, Norway, Portugal, UK	Australia, Austria, Canada, Ireland, Italy, New Zealand, Norway, Portugal, Sweden, UK
2.0-3.9	Netherlands, New Zealand, Norway, Sweden	Sweden	Finland, USSR
Less than 2.0			
No data	Israel, Switzerland	Czechoslovakia, Israel, Japan, Spain, Switzerland, USSR, Yugoslavia	Czechoslovakia, Israel, Switzerland

Note: countries are listed alphabetically in each category

1. Generally based on sales data, which for some countries may be distorted by factors such as inclusion of cross-border sales (e.g. Switzerland) or exclusion of clandestine sales (e.g. Italy), see *Notes on sources of sales data* of each chapter
2. 5-year averages
3. Including hand-rolled cigarettes; for methods of estimation of hand-rolled cigarette consumption, see *Notes on sources of sales data* of each chapter
4. Estimation of consumption of all tobacco products by weight in many countries incorporates assumptions about the average weight of tobacco in manufactured cigarettes. These assumptions may not adequately reflect changes in the cigarette market. See also Methods, p. xxxii, *Notes on sources of sales data* of each chapter, and Appendix II, p. 785

Source: calculated from Table 2 of each chapter

Table ii Estimated prevalence of smoking among adults by sex at four time periods: 1956-1960, 1971-1975, 1981-1985 and 1991-1995. Comparison of 30 countries, males and females aged 15 years and over

1956-1960

Percentage	Cigarettes[1], Males	All products, Males	Cigarettes[1,2], Females
80 or more		Netherlands	
70-79	Japan, Netherlands, USSR(Caucasus region)	France, Germany(W), Japan, Poland, UK, USA	
60-69	Belgium, Canada, Germany(W), Greece	Australia, Belgium, Denmark, Greece, Ireland, Italy, Norway	
50-59	Finland, France, Ireland, Italy, Norway, UK, USA	Finland	
40-49	Denmark	Sweden	UK
30-39	Sweden		Canada, Denmark, Ireland, Netherlands
20-29			Australia, France, Germany(W), Norway, Sweden, USA
Less than 20			Belgium, Finland, Italy, Japan, Poland, USSR(Caucasus region)
No data	Australia, Austria, Bulgaria, Czechoslovakia, Germany(E), Hungary, Iceland, Israel, New Zealand, Poland, Portugal, Romania, Spain, Switzerland, USSR(other), Yugoslavia	Austria, Bulgaria, Canada, Czechoslovakia, Germany(E), Hungary, Iceland, Israel, New Zealand, Portugal, Romania, Spain, Switzerland, USSR, Yugoslavia	Austria, Bulgaria, Czechoslovakia, Germany(E), Greece, Hungary, Iceland, Iceland, Israel, New Zealand, Portugal, Romania, Spain, Switzerland, USSR(other), Yugoslavia

1971-1975

Percentage	Cigarettes[1], Males	All products, Males	Cigarettes[1,2], Females
70-79	Japan	Japan	
60-69		Belgium, Denmark, France, Ireland, Netherlands, Poland, Spain, UK, USSR(Russia)	
50-59	Belgium, Czechoslovakia, France, Greece, Italy, Netherlands, Poland, Yugoslavia	Canada, Czechoslovakia, Germany(E,W), Greece, Italy, Norway, Sweden, Yugoslavia	
40-49	Australia, Canada, Denmark, Finland, Germany(E,W), Hungary, Ireland, Israel, New Zealand, Norway, UK, USA, USSR(Russia)	Australia, Finland, Israel, Romania, Switzerland	Netherlands, UK
30-39	Austria, Romania, Sweden, Switzerland	Austria	Canada, Denmark[2], Ireland, Israel, New Zealand, Norway, Sweden, Switzerland, USA
20-29			Australia, Belgium, France, Germany(E,W), Hungary, Poland
Less than 20			Austria, Czechoslovakia, Finland, Greece, Italy, Japan, Romania, Spain, USSR(Russia), Yugoslavia
No data	Bulgaria, Iceland, Portugal, Spain, USSR(other)	Bulgaria, Hungary, Iceland, New Zealand, Portugal, USA, USSR(other)	Bulgaria, Iceland, Portugal, USSR(other)

Table ii *(continued)*

1981-1985

Percentage	Cigarettes[1], Males	All products, Males	Cigarettes[1,2], Females
60-69	Greece, Japan, Poland	Greece, Japan, Poland	
50-59	Czechoslovakia, Hungary, Yugoslavia	Czechoslovakia, Denmark, France, Hungary, Spain, USSR(Russia), Yugoslavia	
40-49	Belgium, Denmark, France, Israel, Italy, Romania, UK	Belgium, Canada, Germany(W), Iceland, Ireland, Israel, Italy, Netherlands, Norway, Romania, Switzerland, UK	
30-39	Australia, Austria, Canada, Finland, Germany(W), Ireland, Netherlands, New Zealand, Portugal, Switzerland, USA	Australia, Austria, Finland, Portugal, Sweden, USA	Denmark[2], Canada, Iceland, Ireland, Israel, Netherlands, Norway, Poland, UK, Yugoslavia
20-29	Sweden		Australia, Austria, Belgium, France, Germany(W), Greece, Italy, Hungary, New Zealand, Spain, Sweden, Switzerland, USA
Less than 20			Czechoslovakia, Finland, Japan, Portugal, Romania, USSR(Russia)
No data	Bulgaria, Germany(E), Iceland, Norway, Spain, USSR	Bulgaria, Germany(E), New Zealand, USSR(other)	Bulgaria, Germany(E), USSR(other)

1991-1995

Percentage	Cigarettes[1], Males	All products, Males	Cigarettes[1,2], Females
60-69	USSR(Russia)	USSR(Russia, Latvia, Ukraine)	
50-59	Greece, Japan	Greece, Japan, USSR(Lithuania, Kazakhstan)	
40-49	Bulgaria, Czechoslovakia, Romania, USSR(Uzbekistan)	Bulgaria, Czechoslovakia, Denmark, France, Netherlands, Poland, Romania, Spain, USSR(Estonia, Moldova, Uzbekistan), Yugoslavia	
30-39	Austria, Denmark, France, Germany, Ireland, Italy, Portugal	Belgium, Germany, Hungary, Ireland, Israel, Italy, Norway, Portugal, Switzerland, UK	Denmark, Netherlands, Norway
20-29	Australia, Canada, New Zealand, UK, USA	Australia, Canada, Finland, Iceland, Sweden, USSR(Turkmenistan)	Australia, Austria, Belgium, Canada, Czechoslovakia, France, Greece, Hungary, Iceland, Ireland, Israel, Italy, Poland, New Zealand, Spain, Sweden, Switzerland, UK, USA, USSR(Estonia), Yugoslavia
Less than 20			Bulgaria, Finland, Germany, Japan, Portugal, Romania, USSR(Russia, Latvia, Lithuania, Ukraine, Moldova, Turkmenistan, Kazakhstan, Uzbekistan)
No data	Belgium, Finland, Hungary, Iceland, Israel, Netherlands, Norway, Poland, Spain, Sweden, Switzerland, USSR(other), Yugoslavia	Austria, New Zealand, USA, USSR(other)	USSR(other)

Note: countries are listed alphabetically in each category

1. Based where possible on regular smokers of all cigarettes (including hand-rolled)
2. For females, the prevalence of smoking of all tobacco products combined is similar to the prevalence of cigarette smoking in all the countries listed, except for Denmark in the periods 1971-1975 and 1981-1985, in which cases the prevalence of smoking of all tobacco products combined would be in the next higher category

Source: Estimated from Table 8 of each chapter

Table iii Estimated consumption[1] of cigarettes[2] per adult by sex at four time periods: 1956-1960, 1971-1975, 1981-1985 and 1991-1995. Comparison of 30 countries, males and females aged 15 years and over

1956-1960

Number/adult/day	Males	Females
12.0 or more	**Poland**, **USA**	
10.0-11.9	Belgium, Netherlands, **UK**	
8.0-9.9	France, **Germany(W)**, **Italy**, **Japan**	
6.0-7.9	*France*	
4.0-5.9	*Denmark*, **Sweden**	Netherlands, **UK**, **USA**
2.0-3.9		Belgium, *Denmark*, Germany(W), **Poland**, **Sweden**
Less than 2.0		**France**, *Germany(W)*, **Italy**, **Japan**
Not estimated for total cigarettes	Australia, Austria, Bulgaria, Canada, Czechoslovakia, Denmark, Finland, Germany(E), Greece, Hungary, Iceland, Ireland, Israel, New Zealand, Norway, Portugal, Romania, Spain, Switzerland, USSR, Yugoslavia	Australia, Austria, Bulgaria, Canada, Czechoslovakia, Denmark, Finland, Germany(E), Greece, Hungary, Iceland, Ireland, Israel, New Zealand, Norway, Portugal, Romania, Spain, Switzerland, USSR, Yugoslavia
Not estimated for manufactured cigarettes	Australia, Austria, Belgium, Bulgaria, Canada, Czechoslovakia, Finland, Germany(E), Greece, Hungary, Iceland, Ireland, Israel, Netherlands, New Zealand, Norway, Portugal, Romania, Spain, Switzerland, USSR, Yugoslavia	Australia, Austria, Belgium, Bulgaria, Canada, Czechoslovakia, Finland, Germany(E), Greece, Hungary, Iceland, Ireland, Israel, Netherlands, New Zealand, Norway, Portugal, Romania, Spain, Switzerland, USSR, Yugoslavia

1971-1975

Number/adult/day	Males	Females
12.0 or more	Belgium, Canada, **Greece**, **Hungary**, **Japan**, **Poland**, **Switzerland**, **USA**	
10.0-11.9	Australia, **Austria**, *Belgium*, *Czechoslovakia*, **Germany(W)**, **Ireland**, Netherlands, New Zealand, **Spain**, **UK**, *Yugoslavia*	
8.0-9.9	**Finland**, France, **Israel**, **Italy**, **Romania**, **USSR(Russia)**	**USA**
6.0-7.9	*France*, *Netherlands*, Norway	Australia, Canada, **Ireland**, Netherlands, New Zealand, **Switzerland**, **UK**
4.0-5.9	*Denmark*, **Sweden**	**Belgium**, *Denmark*, **Germany(W)**, **Hungary**, **Israel**, *Netherlands*, **Poland**
2.0-3.9		**Austria**, *Czechoslovakia*, **Finland**, **France**, **Greece**, **Italy**, Norway, **Sweden**
Less than 2.0		**Japan**, **Romania**, **Spain**, **USSR(Russia)** *Yugoslavia*
Not estimated for total cigarettes	Bulgaria, Czechoslovakia, Denmark, Germany(E), Iceland, Portugal, USSR(other), Yugoslavia	Bulgaria, Czechoslovakia, Denmark, Germany(E), Iceland, Portugal, USSR(other), Yugoslavia
Not estimated for manufactured cigarettes	Australia, Bulgaria, Canada, Germany(E), Iceland, New Zealand, Norway, Portugal, USSR(other)	Australia, Bulgaria, Canada, Germany(E), Iceland, New Zealand, Norway, Portugal, USSR(other)

Table iii *(continued)*

1981-1985

Number/adult/day	Males	Females
12.0 or more	**Greece**, **Hungary**, **Japan**, **Poland**	
10.0-11.9	**Austria**, Belgium, Canada, *Czechoslovakia*, Germany(W), **Ireland**, **Romania**, **Spain**, **Switzerland**, **USA**, *Yugoslavia*	
8.0-9.9	Australia, *Belgium*, **France**, **Israel**, **Italy**, **New Zealand**, **Portugal**, **USSR(Russia)**	Canada
6.0-7.9	**Finland**, *Germany(W)*, Norway, **UK**	Australia, **Hungary**, **Ireland**, **New Zealand**, **USA**
4.0-5.9	*Denmark*, *Netherlands*, **Sweden**	**Austria**, Belgium, *Denmark*, **Germany(W)**, **Greece**, **Israel**, **Italy**, *Netherlands*, **Poland**, **Sweden**, **Switzerland**, **UK**, *Yugoslavia*
2.0-3.9		*Belgium*, *Czechoslovakia*, **Finland**, **France**, **Japan**, Norway, **Spain**
Less than 2.0		**Portugal**, **Romania**, **USSR(Russia)**
Not estimated for total cigarettes	Bulgaria, Czechoslovakia, Denmark, Germany(E), Iceland, Netherlands, USSR(other), Yugoslavia	Bulgaria, Czechoslovakia, Denmark, Germany(E), Iceland, Netherlands, USSR(other), Yugoslavia
Not estimated for manufactured cigarettes	Australia, Bulgaria, Canada, Germany(E), Iceland, Norway, USSR(other)	Australia, Bulgaria, Canada, Germany(E), Iceland, Norway, USSR(other)

1991-1995

Number/adult/day	Males	Females
12.0 or more	**Hungary**, **Japan**, **Poland**, **USSR(Turkmenistan)**	
10.0-11.9	**Bulgaria**, **Greece**, *Switzerland*, *Yugoslavia*	
8.0-9.9	**Austria**, *Czechoslovakia*, Germany, Netherlands, **Portugal**, **Romania**, **Spain**, **USA**, **USSR(Russia, Latvia, Lithuania, Ukraine)**	
6.0-7.9	Australia, Belgium, Canada, Denmark, **France**, **Ireland**, **Italy**, Norway, UK, **USSR(Estonia, Moldova, Uzbekistan)**	**Hungary**, Netherlands
4.0-5.9	*Finland*, **Israel**, New Zealand, **USSR(Kazakhstan)**	Australia, Belgium, Canada, *Czechoslovakia*, Denmark, **France**, Germany, **Greece**, **Ireland**, Norway, **Poland**, **Spain**, *Switzerland*, UK, **USA**, *Yugoslavia*
2.0-3.9		**Austria**, **Bulgaria**, *Finland*, **Israel**, **Italy**, **Japan**, New Zealand, **Portugal**, **Romania**, **USSR(Estonia)**
Less than 2.0		**USSR(Russia, Latvia, Lithuania, Ukraine, Moldova, Turkmenistan, Uzbekistan, Kazakhstan)**
Not estimated for total cigarettes	Czechoslovakia, Denmark, Finland, Iceland, Sweden, Switzerland, USSR(other), Yugoslavia	Czechoslovakia, Denmark, Finland, Iceland, Sweden, Switzerland, USSR(other), Yugoslavia
Not estimated for manufactured cigarettes	Australia, Belgium, Canada, Germany, Iceland, Netherlands, New Zealand, Norway, Sweden, UK, USSR(other)	Australia, Belgium, Canada, Germany, Iceland, Netherlands, New Zealand, Norway, Sweden, UK, USSR(other)

Note: countries are listed alphabetically in each category

1. Sales-adjusted data, which for some countries may be distorted by factors such as inclusion of cross border sales (eg. Switzerland) or exclusion of clandestine sales (e.g. Italy), see *Notes on sources of sales data* for each chapter
2. Normal type indicates the appropriate category for total cigarette (including hand-rolled) consumption, italics indicates manufactured cigarette consumption, and bold indicates that the same category is appropriate for both product definitions

Source: Estimated from Table 8 of each chapter

Table iv Estimated percentage[1] of manufactured cigarettes which are filter cigarettes, at five time periods: 1951-1955, 1961-1965, 1971-1975, 1981-1985 and 1991-1995. Comparison of 30 countries

Percentage	1951-1955	1961-1965	1971-1975	1981-1985	1991-1995
90 or more		Australia	Australia, Canada, Finland, Japan, New Zealand	Australia[2], Austria, Bulgaria, Canada, Finland[2], Germany(W), Greece, Italy, Japan, New Zealand[2], Spain, Sweden, UK, USA, Yugoslavia	Australia[2], Austria[2], Belgium, Bulgaria, Canada[2], Czechoslovakia, Finland[2], Germany(W)[2], Greece[2], Hungary, Italy[2], Japan, New Zealand[2], Portugal, Spain[2], Sweden[2], UK[2], USA, Yugoslavia[2]
70-89		Germany(W)	Austria, Germany(W), Greece, Ireland, Italy, Sweden, UK, USA, Yugoslavia	Belgium, Czechoslovakia, Hungary, Ireland, Netherlands, Norway, Portugal	France, Netherlands, Poland
50-69		Finland, New Zealand, USA	Belgium, Czechoslovakia, Denmark, France, Hungary, Iceland, Norway, Portugal,Spain	Denmark, France	Romania
30-49		Austria, Belgium, Denmark, Italy, Norway, UK	Bulgaria, Netherlands	Poland, USSR[3]	
10 -29		France, Ireland, Japan, Netherlands, Portugal, Spain, Sweden	Poland, Romania, USSR[3]		
Less than 10	Australia, Austria[4], France[4], Greece[4], Hungary[4], Ireland[4], Japan[4], Poland[4], Spain[4], Sweden[4], UK, USSR[3,4], USA, Yugoslavia[4]	Bulgaria[4], Greece, Hungary, Poland[4], USSR[3], Yugoslavia[4]			
No data	Belgium, Bulgaria, Canada, Czechoslovakia, Denmark, Finland, Germany(W), Iceland, Israel, Italy, Netherlands, New Zealand, Norway, Portugal, Romania, Switzerland	Canada, Czechoslovakia , Iceland, Israel, Romania, Switzerland	Israel, Switzerland	Iceland, Israel, Romania, Switzerland	Denmark, Iceland, Ireland, Israel, Norway, Switzerland, USSR

1 5-year average if available, otherwise estimated from the available data
2 Assumed not to have decreased since most recent data
3 Excludes papyrosi
4 Assumed to have been at least as low as earliest data

Source: Estimated from Table 1.3 of each chapter

Table v Sales-weighted average[1] tar yield per cigarette (SWAT) at four time periods: 1961-1965, 1971-1975, 1981-1985 and 1991-1995. Comparison of 30 countries

mg per cigarette	1961-1965	1971-1975	1981-1985	1991-1995
More than 30	Austria, Sweden	Denmark, Hungary		
25-29	Denmark, France, Germany(W), UK	Norway		
20-24	USA	Belgium, Finland, France, Sweden , UK	Denmark, Poland	Hungary
15-19	Australia	Austria, Canada, Germany(W), Japan, USA	Belgium, France, Italy, Japan, UK	Belgium, Poland
10-14		Australia	Austria, Canada, Finland, Germany(W), Sweden, USA	Finland, France, Italy, Japan, New Zealand, Norway, UK, USA
No data	Belgium, Bulgaria, Canada, Czechoslovakia, Finland, Greece, Hungary, Iceland, Ireland, Israel, Italy, Japan, Netherlands, New Zealand, Norway, Poland, Portugal, Romania, Spain, Switzerland, USSR, Yugoslavia	Bulgaria, Czechoslovakia, Greece, Iceland, Ireland, Israel, Italy, Netherlands, New Zealand, Poland, Portugal, Romania, Spain, Switzerland, USSR, Yugoslavia	Australia, Bugaria, Czechoslovakia, Greece, Hungary, Iceland, Ireland, Israel, Netherlands, New Zealand, Norway, Portugal, Romania, Spain, Switzerland, USSR, Yugoslavia	Australia, Austria, Bulgaria, Canada, Czechoslovakia, Denmark, Germany, Greece, Iceland, Ireland, Israel, Netherlands, Portugal, Romania, Spain, Sweden, Switzerland, USSR, Yugoslavia

1 5-year average if available, otherwise estimated from the available data

Source: Estimated from Table 1.3 of each chapter

Table vi Consumption of manufactured cigarettes and of all tobacco products per adult (sexes combined) in 1935, 1950, 1965, and 1973. Comparison of 47 countries, males and females aged 15 years and over

Country	Manufactured cigarettes number/adult/day				All tobacco products grams/adult/day			
	1935	1950	1965	1973	1935	1950	1965	1973
Argentina	2.9	4.0	4.5	5.3	5.6	5.8	5.6	6.1
Australia	1.2	3.5	7.3	8.4	4.9	7.8	9.2	9.3
Austria	2.4	3.0	5.3	7.0	4.7	4.0	6.0	7.3
Barbados			3.0	4.4			3.2	4.6
Belgium	2.2	3.4	5.4	7.5	8.7	7.7	9.6	10.6
Brazil	1.6	3.1	3.3	4.1	6.8	7.1	5.7	5.6
Canada	1.9	4.9	9.1	9.5	6.1	9.5	12.6	12.4
Chile			3.3	3.6			3.1	3.1
Costa Rica			5.1	5.6			4.7	4.3
Denmark	1.3	3.5	4.1	5.1	8.1	10.1	10.2	10.0
El Salvador			2.1	2.8			4.6	4.1
Finland	3.7	4.5	5.3	5.6	3.4	4.5	5.6	6.5
France	1.5	2.5	4.1	5.3	4.7	5.1	6.5	7.3
Germany		1.7	5.8	7.2		5.1	7.7	8.5
Ghana			1.3	1.3			1.4	1.6
Greece	2.6	4.4	5.3	7.0	3.0	5.0	6.1	7.8
Hong Kong			9.1	7.6			8.6	6.8
Iceland	1.3	4.1	5.0	5.6	3.4	6.1	8.1	9.3
India	0.2	0.3	0.5	0.5	2.4	2.6	2.2	1.7
Indonesia				0.6				2.2
Ireland	3.3	6.9	7.4	9.2	5.6	8.6	8.2	8.5
Italy	1.2	1.8	4.2	5.3	2.4	2.5	4.6	5.5
Jamaica			3.5	3.7			3.6	3.7
Japan	2.4	3.3	6.4	8.9	3.7	3.9	6.5	9.0
Kenya			1.1	1.3			1.0	1.1
Malawi			0.4	0.5			0.4	0.6
Malaysia			3.9	4.4			3.9	4.2
Mauritius			4.4	5.3			3.5	4.1
Mexico	3.9	4.1	4.1	3.7	4.0	4.2	4.2	3.7
Morocco	0.7	1.4	1.6	1.9	1.1	1.7	2.0	2.2
Netherlands	1.9	3.1	5.5	6.5	10.4	9.3	11.6	12.2
New Zealand	1.5	3.9	6.2	6.9	5.6	9.0	9.5	8.8
Nicaragua			3.1	4.2			2.9	3.4
Norway	0.8	1.4	1.4	1.8	4.0	5.3	5.8	6.5
Pakistan			1.2	2.1			4.6	4.7
Portugal	0.7	1.7	3.1	4.1	1.7	2.4	3.4	4.2
Sierra Leone			0.8	1.2			1.9	1.6
Singapore			6.5	6.8			7.5	7.8
South Africa	1.4	3.2	3.0	3.8	4.0	6.1	5.7	6.3
Spain	1.1	1.2	4.8	6.2	4.4	3.8	5.6	7.0
Sweden	1.0	2.2	3.7	4.3	4.5	5.1	5.8	5.0
Switzerland	1.5	4.1	8.4	9.2	5.8	7.5	11.2	11.7
Turkey	2.6	3.3	5.0	5.6	3.4	3.9	5.5	6.0
UK	4.4	6.0	7.3	8.8	6.0	7.1	7.6	7.7
USA	4.0	8.9	10.4	10.5	9.7	12.6	13.3	11.4
Venezuela			5.2	6.1				

Notes
Data for other years up to 1973 are available in RP6 for all countries listed. For the 22 countries included in this book, the data, and for more years, are also presented in Table 2 of each chapter. Data were given in numbers and pounds per annum and have been converted to numbers and grams per day.

Source: Lee P.N. (ed) (1975). *Tobacco consumption in various countries,* 4th edition. Tobacco Research Council, London. Research Paper 6 (RP6).

Table vii Manufactured cigarette consumption[1] per adult[2] (sexes combined) in 1982-1983[3]. Comparison of 121 countries, males and females aged 15 years and over

Number/day	Africa	America	Asia	Australasia	Europe
10.0 or more		Cuba			Cyprus
8.0-9.9	Libya	Canada USA	Japan Kuwait Lebanon		Greece + Hungary Iceland Poland Switzerland -
6.0-7.9		Surinam -	Brunei China (Taiwan) Israel Korea South Macau Singapore	Australia + New Zealand + Philippines	Austria Belgium * Bulgaria + Czechoslovakia Germany East Germany West Ireland Italy Spain + UK Yugoslavia +
4.0-5.9	Algeria Mauritius South Africa Tunisia -	Argentina Belize Brazil Martinique Neth. Antilles Nicaragua Trinidad/Tobago Uruguay Venezuela	Egypt - Hong Kong + Jordan Malaysia Saudi Arabia Syria Yemen South	Fiji	Denmark Finland - France Netherlands Portugal Romania Sweden Turkey USSR +
2.0-3.9	Benin Congo Morocco Reunion Sierra Leone -	Barbados Chile Columbia Costa Rica Dominican Rep. Ecuador El Salvador Guyana Honduras Jamaica Mexico Panama	Cambodia China Indonesia Iraq Korea North Pakistan - Thailand		Albania Malta
Less than 2.0	Angola Cameroon Cape Verde Ethiopia Ghana Ivory Coast + Kenya Malawi Mozambique Nigeria Senegal + Sudan Tanzania Uganda Zaire Zambia Zimbabwe	Bolivia Guatemala Haiti Paraguay + Peru	Bangladesh Burma India Iran Laos Nepal Sri Lanka Vietnam +		Norway

See footnotes on next page

Table vi *(continued)*

Note: countries are listed alphabetically in each category.
+, -, * : see note 3 below.

1. Comparable with the first column of Table i, 1981-1985. We have not attempted to collect data on consumption of other tobacco products in countries not included as chapters in this book. However, it should be noted that consumption of products other than manufactured cigarettes may form a major proportion of consumption in some countries
2. Derived from tables of per capita consumption, using population data from World health statistics annual 1985. This ignores any smoking by persons aged under 15, and averages consumption over all adults. Although the level of smoking among young people is unknown, per adult estimates are likely to give a better indication of smoking levels in the population than per capita estimates. This markedly alters the ranking of countries compared with the source tables, since the proportion of the population aged under 15 varies considerably (between 20 and 50 per cent)
3. Based on source A for 1983. Data for additional countries also taken from source B for 1982; of the 86 countries given in both tables, 65 would have been allocated to the same category, 12 marked + would have been allocated to the next higher category, and 7 marked - would have been allocated to the next lower category had source B been used. Belgium (marked *) is the only country allocated to a different category compared with Table i, 1981-1985

Source: (A) World Smoking and Health, 1985. Manufactured cigarette consumption per capita in 130 countries, 1983. In: Tobacco in Australia, a summary of related statistics. Australian Government Publication Service, Canberra, 1990
(B) US Department of Agriculture, Foreign Agricultural Service, Washington, DC, FT-7-83, July 1983

Australia 1

Sales data

See Tables 1.1-1.3.

From 1920 until about 1945 the consumption of manufactured cigarettes per adult remained fairly stable, varying between 1 and 2 per day. Thereafter consumption rose steadily until the late 1970s when it peaked at 9 cigarettes per day. During the same period, there was a rapid switch to filter cigarettes, from 2% in 1950 to 90% in the mid-1960s. Consumption decreased to 6 cigarettes per adult per day by 1995. Although consumption per adult of loose tobacco remained fairly stable, estimates suggest that consumption of hand-rolled cigarettes per adult rose from 1 cigarette per day in 1925 to nearly 4 in the1950s. There was then a large reduction in consumption to about 0.3 cigarettes per day by1995. Between 1930 and 1950 more hand-rolled cigarettes were consumed than manufactured cigarettes. After 1955 this trend was reversed.

The consumption of all tobacco products combined per adult varied between 5 and 6 g per day from 1920 to 1945, when it started to rise, at first rapidly and then more slowly, peaking at nearly 10 g in 1961. It fell to around 5 g in 1994. From 1925 to 1945 about 30% of all tobacco was consumed in manufactured cigarettes. This proportion increased after the Second World War and has exceeded 80% since 1965. In recent decades, only about 1% of consumption has been in cigars, and consumption of smokeless tobacco has been negligible. Chewing tobacco and oral snuff were banned in 1991.

There have been notable trends in the weight and packaging of cigarettes. On average a cigarette contained approximately a gram of tobacco in the mid 1960s, and this had reduced to 0.7 g by the early 1990s. During the same period, the average number of cigarettes in a pack has been increasing. In 1991-1992, only 4% of cigarettes were sold in packs of 20 in Australia (packs of 25s: 37%; 30s: 16.2%; 35s: 11.3%; 40s:14.4%; 50s: 17.1%) (Chapman (1992)).

Survey data

See Tables 1.4-1.8

In 1945, the prevalence of tobacco smoking among those aged 15 years and over was about 70% in men and 25% in women. This difference has decreased since 1945. By 1995 the prevalence among men had fallen to about 28%. The prevalence among women remained around 30% from the 1960s to the 1980s but has reduced to 20-25% during the last decade.

No data on adult smoking by age are available before the 1970s. In general, more men smoked than women at all ages but from the 1980s onwards many surveys show that more young women smoked than young men. A lower prevalence of smoking in older age groups was more marked in women than in men.

Around 2-5% of men and 1% of women smoked other products but not cigarettes, with the prevalence somewhat higher for older men. There are few data on prevalence by type of cigarette, but smoking of hand-rolled cigarettes appears to be negligible among women and concentrated among older men.

The prevalence of teenage smoking among girls was much lower than among boys when first surveyed in 1968, but subsequently increased more rapidly. From the 1980s most surveys indicated that the prevalence among girls was similar to that among boys for regular smoking, but higher than among boys when occasional smoking was included. Definitions of regular smoking vary considerably in surveys of teenagers, and comparisons should be made with caution.

Comparison of survey and sales data suggests that surveys under-reported consumption by 20-40%; one recent survey, conducted in a medical screening setting, under-reported by over 50%. Since first estimated in 1972, the estimated number of cigarettes smoked per person per day (sales-adjusted) decreased steadily for men from about 12 to 8, while for women it remained fairly stable around 6-7 until the early 1990s when it fell to about 5.

Table 1.1.1 Total annual sales of tobacco products, 1920-1973

Year	Cigarettes		Cigars		Pipe & HR[1] tobacco	All tobacco products
	tonnes	millions	tonnes	millions	tonnes	tonnes
1920	2220	2204	320	64	5260	7800
1921	2360	2376	270	58	4810	7440
1922	2270	2267	270	53	5720	8260
1923	2130	2124	270	54	5670	8070
1924	2270	2286	230	50	5900	8390
1925	2360	2372	270	54	6030	8660
1926	2540	2542	230	50	6210	8980
1927	2720	2706	230	51	6260	9210
1928	2860	2851	230	48	6260	9340
1929	2900	2890	180	44	6400	9480
1930	2770	2783	180	44	6530	9480
1931	2090	2079	140	39	6120	8350
1932	1860	1858	90	23	6170	8120
1933	2040	2040	90	25	6260	8390
1934	2090	2072	140	29	6300	8530
1935	2180	2189	140	30	6400	8710
1936	2400	2417	90	26	6670	9160
1937	2630	2630	140	31	6800	9570
1938	2860	2869	140	33	7080	10070
1939	3180	3180	90	33	7170	10430
1940	3400	3384	90	27	7300	10800
1941	3130	3154	90	31	7030	10250
1942	3580	3585	140	35	7620	11340
1943	3630	3619	90	22	7940	11660
1944	3630	3627	50	17	7570	11250
1945	3360	3370	50	15	6890	10300
1946	3580	3618	50	15	7530	11160
1947	4350	4424	90	16	8800	13240
1948	5580	5575	90	20	8940	14610
1949	6670	6555	90	22	8710	15470

Table 1.1.1 *(continued)*

Year	Cigarettes		Cigars		Pipe & HR[1] tobacco	All tobacco products
	tonnes	millions	tonnes	millions	tonnes	tonnes
1950	7850	7665	90	25	9210	17150
1951	9480	9219	90	28	9660	19230
1952	9710	9420	90	29	9660	19460
1953	9070	8976	90	21	10250	19410
1954	10480	10487	90	25	10250	20820
1955	11570	11515	90	25	9620	21270
1956	12560	12616	90	27	8750	21410
1957	13830	13878	90	26	8620	22540
1958	14740	14699	90	32	8300	23130
1959	16010	15677	90	34	7620	23720
1960	17830	17101	90	38	7300	25220
1961	18910	18044	140	45	6890	25950
1962	19640	18824	140	60	6210	25990
1963	20500	19649	140	68	5670	26310
1964	21410	20572	180	84	5220	26810
1965	22040	21400	180	87	4720	26940
1966	22630	22644	180	83	4490	27310
1967	22140	22247	180	84	4220	26540
1968	23500	23667	230	93	4220	27940
1969	24630	24883	230	105	4170	29030
1970	25170	25938	230	118	4130	29530
1971	25810	26331	230	117	4040	30070
1972	26400	27321	270	133	4260	30930
1973	27580	28998	270	163	4040	31890

1 Tobacco for hand-rolled cigarettes

Source: see *Notes on sources of sales data*, p. 22

Table 1.1.2 Total annual sales of tobacco products, 1974-1995

Year	Cigarettes		Cigars tonnes	Loose tobacco tonnes	All tobacco products tonnes
	tonnes	millions			
1974	28350	31716	340	3890	32580
1975	29040	32178	330	3740	33110
1976	28360	30395	310	3910	32580
1977	28530	33672	360	3810	32700
1978	28520	33800	260	3480	32260
1979	27320	33850	240	3290	30850
1980	28080	35820	240	3180	31500
1981	28360	35587	230	2660	31250
1982	29010	35250	230	2770	32010
1983	27550	33680	200	2730	30480
1984	26930	33330	170	2730	29830
1985	26860	33870	170	2290	29320
1986	27080	34410	160	1940	29180
1987	26230	33670	140	1780	28150
1988	26340	34480		1570	27910
1989	25900	35000		1420	27320
1990	26490	36040		1410	27900
1991	24790	34670		1560	26350
1992	25220	35420		1460	26680
1993	22570	32991		1370	23940
1994	21870	32488		1750	23620
1995		32179			

Source : see *Notes on sources of sales data*, p. 22

Table 1.1.3 Manufactured cigarettes (i) percentage of total sales as filter cigarettes, 1951-1981, and (ii) sales-weighted average tar yield per cigarette (SWAT), 1969-1989

Year	% Filter	SWAT mg / cig
1951	2	
1960	59	
1961	71.0	
1962	78.0	
1963	82.5	
1964	83.0	
1965	87.7	
1966	90.0	
1967	89.4	
1968	90.5	
1969	91.7	19.6
1970	92.4	
1971	92.7	
1972	93.4	
1973	94.7	
1974	94.8	16.1
1975	95.2	
1976	95.4	
1977	96.0	
1978	96.4	
1979	96.9	
1980	97.3	
1981	98.7	12.7
1982		
1983		
1984		12.3
1985		
1986		
1987		10.8
1988		10.3
1989		9.3

Source : see *Notes on sources of sales data*, p. 22

Table 1.2 Consumption of (i) cigarettes and (ii) all tobacco products, 1920-1995 sales-based data, including estimated hand-rolled cigarette consumption. Males and females aged 15 years and over

Year	Manufactured cigarettes		Hand-rolled cigarettes		Total cigarettes		All tobacco products	
	Total annual in millions	Number/ adult/day	Total annual in millions	Number/ adult/day	Total annual in millions	Number/ adult/day	Total annual in tonnes	Grams/ adult/day
1920	2204	1.7					7800	5.9
1921	2376	1.8					7440	5.5
1922	2267	1.6					8260	6.0
1923	2124	1.5					8070	5.7
1924	2286	1.6					8390	5.7
1925	2372	1.6	1726	1.2	4098	2.7	8660	5.8
1926	2542	1.7					8980	5.9
1927	2706	1.7					9210	5.9
1928	2851	1.8					9340	5.8
1929	2890	1.7					9480	5.6
1930	2783	1.7	3312	2.0	6095	3.6	9480	5.6
1931	2079	1.2					8350	4.9
1932	1858	1.1					8120	4.7
1933	2040	1.2					8390	4.8
1934	2072	1.2					8530	4.8
1935	2189	1.2	4224	2.4	6413	3.6	8710	4.9
1936	2417	1.3					9160	5.0
1937	2630	1.4					9570	5.1
1938	2869	1.5					10070	5.3
1939	3180	1.7					10430	5.5

Table 1.2 *(continued)*

Year	Manufactured cigarettes		Hand-rolled cigarettes		Total cigarettes		All tobacco products	
	Total annual in millions	Number/ adult/day	Total annual in millions	Number/ adult/day	Total annual in millions	Number/ adult/day	Total annual in tonnes	Grams/ adult/day
1940	3384	1.7	5857	3.0	9241	4.8	10800	5.6
1941	3154	1.6					10250	5.2
1942	3585	1.8					11340	5.6
1943	3619	1.8					11660	5.8
1944	3627	1.8					11250	5.6
1945	3370	1.6	5858	2.9	9228	4.5	10300	5.0
1946	3618	1.8					11160	5.5
1947	4424	2.1					13240	6.4
1948	5575	2.7					14610	7.0
1949	6555	3.1					15470	7.3
1950	7665	3.5	8304	3.8	15969	7.3	17150	7.8
1951	9219	4.1					19230	8.6
1952	9420	4.1					19460	8.5
1953	8976	3.9					19410	8.4
1954	10487	4.5					20820	8.9
1955	11515	4.8	9120	3.8	20635	8.7	21270	8.9
1956	12616	5.2					21410	8.8
1957	13878	5.6	8208	3.3	22086	8.9	22540	9.1
1958	14699	5.8					23130	9.2
1959	15677	6.1					23720	9.2
1960	17101	6.5	6818	2.6	23919	9.1	25220	9.6
1961	18044	6.8	5856	2.2	23900	8.9	25950	9.7
1962	18824	6.9	5278	1.9	24102	8.8	25990	9.5
1963	19649	7.0	4820	1.7	24468	8.8	26310	9.4
1964	20572	7.2	4437	1.6	25009	8.8	26810	9.4
1965	21400	7.3	4012	1.4	25412	8.7	26940	9.2
1966	22644	7.6	3816	1.3	26460	8.9	27310	9.2
1967	22247	7.3	3587	1.2	25834	8.5	26540	8.7
1968	23667	7.6	3587	1.2	27254	8.8	27940	9.0
1969	24883	7.8	3544	1.1	28428	8.9	29030	9.1
1970	25938	8.0	3510	1.1	29448	9.1	29530	9.1
1971	26331	7.9	3434	1.0	29765	9.0	30070	9.1
1972	27321	8.1	3621	1.1	30942	9.2	30930	9.2
1973	28998	8.4	3434	1.0	32432	9.5	31890	9.3
1974	31716	9.1	3306	0.9	35022	10.0	32580	9.3
1975	32178	8.8	3179	0.9	35357	9.7	33110	9.1
1976	30395	8.2	3324	0.9	33718	9.1	32580	8.8
1977	33672	8.9	3238	0.9	36910	9.8	32700	8.7
1978	33800	8.8	2958	0.8	36758	9.6	32260	8.4
1979	33850	8.7	2796	0.7	36646	9.4	30850	7.9
1980	35820	9.0	2703	0.7	38523	9.7	31500	7.9
1981	35587	8.7	2261	0.6	37848	9.3	31250	7.6
1982	35250	8.4	2354	0.6	37604	9.0	32010	7.7
1983	33680	7.9	2320	0.5	36000	8.5	30480	7.2
1984	33330	7.7	2320	0.5	35650	8.3	29830	6.9
1985	33870	7.7	1946	0.4	35816	8.1	29320	6.7
1986	34410	7.7	1649	0.4	36059	8.0	29180	6.5
1987	33670	7.3	1513	0.3	35183	7.7	28150	6.1
1988	34480	7.4	1334	0.3	35814	7.6	27910	6.0
1989	35000	7.3	1207	0.3	36207	7.6	27320	5.7
1990	36040	7.4	1198	0.2	37238	7.7	27900	5.7
1991	34670	7.0	1326	0.3	35996	7.3	26350	5.3
1992	35420	7.1	1241	0.2	36661	7.3	26680	5.3
1993	32991	6.5	1164	0.2	34156	6.8	23940	4.7
1994	32488	6.4	1488	0.3	33976	6.7	23620	4.6
1995	32179	6.2						

Source : see *Notes on sources of sales data*, p. 22

Figure 1.1 Daily consumption of (i) manufactured and total number of cigarettes, and (ii) all tobacco products, 1920-1995.
Males and females aged 15 years and over. *Source:* see Table 1.2

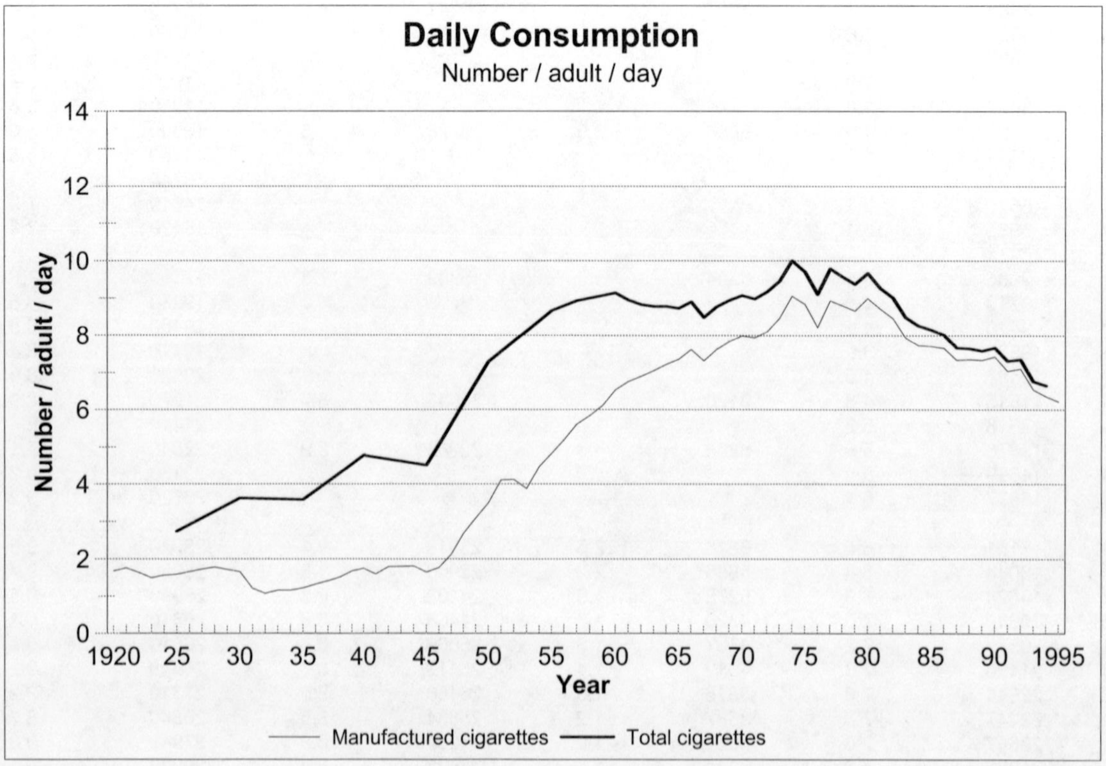

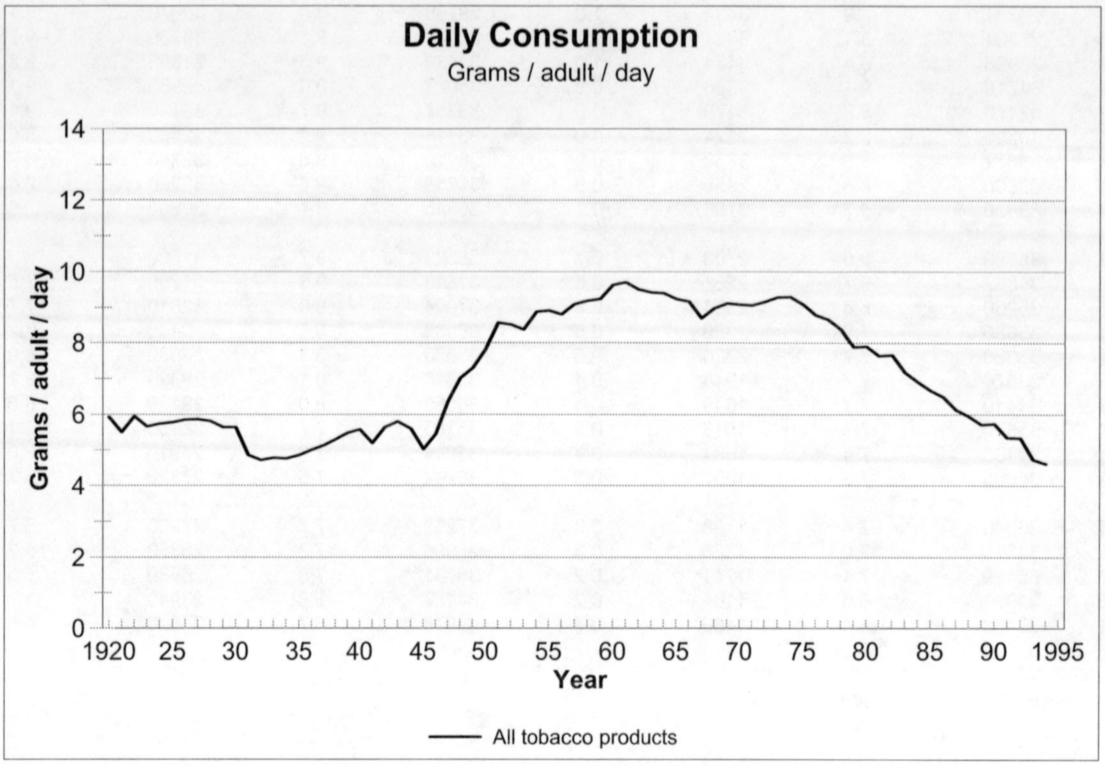

Table 1.3 Percentage sales of tobacco in different forms (by weight), selected years 1925-1994

Year	Cigarettes (%)	Cigars(%)	Loose tobacco(%)
1925	27.3	3.1	69.6
1935	25.0	1.6	73.5
1945	32.6	0.5	66.9
1955	54.4	0.4	45.2
1965	81.8	0.7	17.5
1975	87.7	1.0	11.3
1985	91.6	0.6	7.8
1994	92.6	0.0	7.4

Source : calculated from Tables 1.1.1 & 1.1.2

Figure 1.2 Percentage sales of tobacco in different forms (by weight), selected years 1925-1994
Source: see Table 1.3

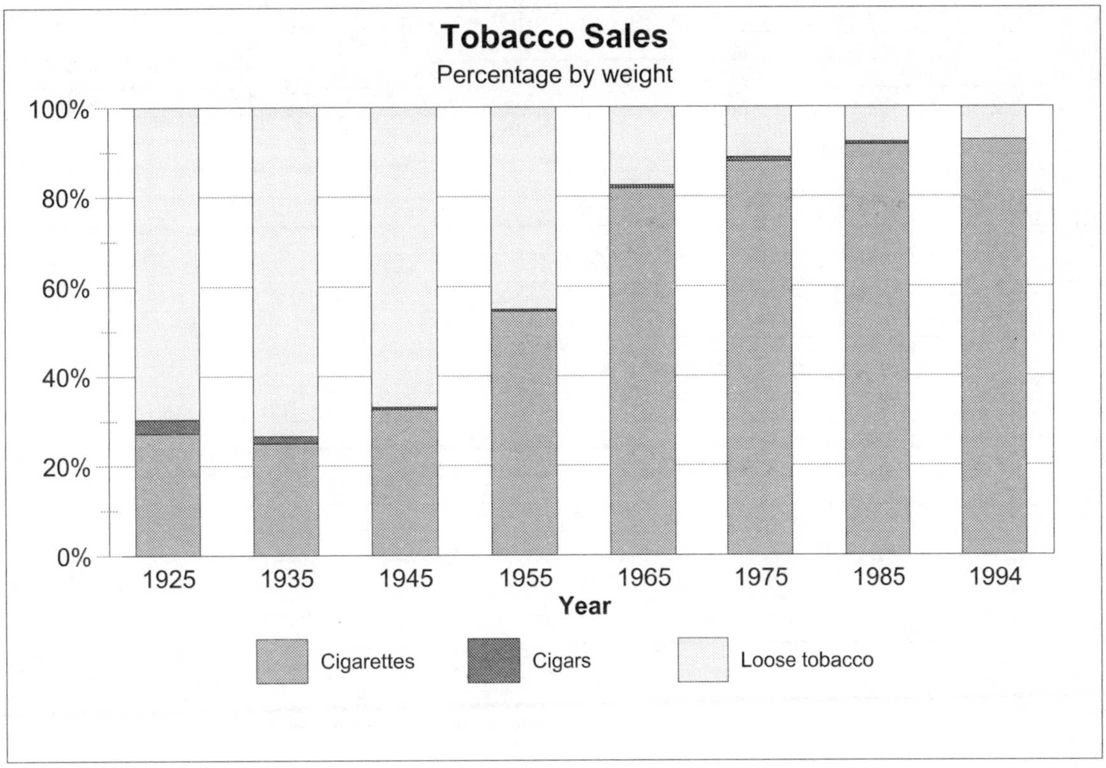

Table 1.4M Prevalence of smoking, males: some selected Australian surveys by age, 1945-1995 *(continues on p. 10)*

<table>
<tr><th rowspan="2">Frequency
Product
Source
Year</th><th colspan="21">Age group</th><th rowspan="2">All ages</th></tr>
<tr><th>12</th><th>13</th><th>14</th><th>15</th><th>16</th><th>17</th><th>18</th><th>19</th><th>20-24</th><th>25-29</th><th>30-34</th><th>35-39</th><th>40-44</th><th>45-49</th><th>50-54</th><th>55-59</th><th>60-64</th><th>65-69</th><th>70-74</th><th>75-79</th><th>80+</th></tr>
<tr><td>45 1 U U</td><td colspan="4"></td><td colspan="17">72</td><td></td></tr>
<tr><td>64 1 U U</td><td colspan="4"></td><td colspan="17">58</td><td></td></tr>
<tr><td>68 11 UC R</td><td>21</td><td>26</td><td>30</td><td>37</td><td>41</td><td colspan="16"></td><td></td></tr>
<tr><td>68 11 UC A</td><td>23</td><td>28</td><td>31</td><td>38</td><td>43</td><td colspan="16"></td><td></td></tr>
<tr><td>69 1 U U</td><td colspan="4"></td><td colspan="17">45</td><td></td></tr>
<tr><td>69 15 UC R</td><td colspan="3"></td><td>10</td><td colspan="17"></td><td></td></tr>
<tr><td>69 15 UC U</td><td colspan="3"></td><td>37</td><td colspan="17"></td><td></td></tr>
<tr><td>72 5 TC R</td><td></td><td colspan="5">20</td><td colspan="3">50</td><td colspan="3">52</td><td colspan="3">50</td><td colspan="6">38</td><td>44</td></tr>
<tr><td>73 5 TC R</td><td></td><td colspan="5">19</td><td colspan="3">48</td><td colspan="3">47</td><td colspan="3">46</td><td colspan="6">37</td><td>41</td></tr>
<tr><td>73 11 U R</td><td>26</td><td>32</td><td>38</td><td>45</td><td>56</td><td colspan="16"></td><td></td></tr>
<tr><td>73 11 U A</td><td>27</td><td>33</td><td>38</td><td>45</td><td>56</td><td colspan="16"></td><td></td></tr>
<tr><td>74 2 UC U</td><td colspan="4"></td><td colspan="4">36</td><td>49</td><td>44</td><td>46</td><td>44</td><td>39</td><td>43</td><td>43</td><td>35</td><td colspan="2">32</td><td colspan="3">28</td><td>41</td></tr>
<tr><td>74 2 A U</td><td colspan="4"></td><td colspan="4">38</td><td>52</td><td>49</td><td>52</td><td>48</td><td>46</td><td>47</td><td>47</td><td>41</td><td colspan="2">36</td><td colspan="3">31</td><td>45</td></tr>
<tr><td>74 5 TC R</td><td></td><td colspan="5">25</td><td colspan="3">46</td><td colspan="3">46</td><td colspan="3">45</td><td colspan="6">32</td><td>40</td></tr>
<tr><td>75 5 TC R</td><td></td><td colspan="5">23</td><td colspan="3">47</td><td colspan="3">46</td><td colspan="3">46</td><td colspan="6">31</td><td>40</td></tr>
<tr><td>76 2 UC U</td><td colspan="4"></td><td colspan="4">36</td><td>46</td><td>45</td><td>40</td><td>42</td><td>40</td><td>37</td><td>48</td><td>37</td><td colspan="2">32</td><td colspan="3">27</td><td>40</td></tr>
<tr><td>76 2 A U</td><td colspan="4"></td><td colspan="4">37</td><td>48</td><td>47</td><td>46</td><td>47</td><td>43</td><td>41</td><td>54</td><td>40</td><td colspan="2">36</td><td colspan="3">35</td><td>43</td></tr>
<tr><td>76 5 TC R</td><td></td><td colspan="5">23</td><td colspan="3">48</td><td colspan="3">44</td><td colspan="3">42</td><td colspan="6">32</td><td>39</td></tr>
<tr><td>77 3 MC U</td><td colspan="6"></td><td colspan="3">38</td><td colspan="4">41</td><td colspan="4">34</td><td colspan="4">18</td><td>36</td></tr>
<tr><td>77 3 TC U</td><td colspan="6"></td><td colspan="3">42</td><td colspan="4">46</td><td colspan="4">44</td><td colspan="4">29</td><td>43</td></tr>
<tr><td>77 5 TC R</td><td></td><td colspan="5">21</td><td colspan="3">47</td><td colspan="3">41</td><td colspan="3">42</td><td colspan="6">30</td><td>37</td></tr>
<tr><td>78 5 TC R</td><td></td><td colspan="5">21</td><td colspan="3">47</td><td colspan="3">45</td><td colspan="3">42</td><td colspan="6">28</td><td>38</td></tr>
<tr><td>80 2 UC U</td><td colspan="4"></td><td colspan="4">35</td><td>56</td><td>48</td><td>39</td><td>41</td><td>41</td><td>46</td><td>46</td><td>39</td><td colspan="2">25</td><td colspan="3">18</td><td>40</td></tr>
<tr><td>80 2 A U</td><td colspan="4"></td><td colspan="4">36</td><td>57</td><td>49</td><td>40</td><td>42</td><td>43</td><td>47</td><td>47</td><td>40</td><td colspan="2">27</td><td colspan="3">19</td><td>41</td></tr>
<tr><td>80 6 TC U</td><td colspan="9"></td><td>43</td><td>30</td><td>36</td><td>40</td><td>41</td><td>32</td><td>32</td><td>25</td><td colspan="4"></td><td>35</td></tr>
<tr><td>80 6 A U</td><td colspan="9"></td><td>44</td><td>36</td><td>39</td><td>45</td><td>45</td><td>35</td><td>36</td><td>30</td><td colspan="4"></td><td>39</td></tr>
<tr><td>83 2 UC U</td><td colspan="4"></td><td colspan="4">31</td><td>43</td><td>47</td><td>40</td><td>40</td><td>41</td><td>40</td><td>33</td><td>35</td><td colspan="2">28</td><td colspan="3">23</td><td>37</td></tr>
<tr><td>83 2 A U</td><td colspan="4"></td><td colspan="4">32</td><td>45</td><td>49</td><td>44</td><td>42</td><td>43</td><td>43</td><td>38</td><td>38</td><td colspan="2">34</td><td colspan="3">27</td><td>40</td></tr>
<tr><td>83 6 TC U</td><td colspan="9"></td><td>39</td><td>32</td><td>32</td><td>29</td><td>31</td><td>33</td><td>31</td><td>25</td><td colspan="4"></td><td>32</td></tr>
<tr><td>83 6 A U</td><td colspan="9"></td><td>41</td><td>33</td><td>36</td><td>30</td><td>33</td><td>35</td><td>34</td><td>30</td><td colspan="4"></td><td>35</td></tr>
<tr><td>83 7 UC R</td><td colspan="9"></td><td colspan="2">36</td><td colspan="2">35</td><td colspan="2">33</td><td colspan="2">30</td><td colspan="4"></td><td>33</td></tr>
<tr><td>83 7 A A</td><td colspan="9"></td><td colspan="2">38</td><td colspan="2">37</td><td colspan="2">37</td><td colspan="2">34</td><td colspan="4"></td><td>36</td></tr>
<tr><td>83 8 UC R</td><td colspan="11"></td><td colspan="2">32</td><td colspan="2">35</td><td colspan="2">32</td><td colspan="4"></td><td>33</td></tr>
<tr><td>83 8 A A</td><td colspan="11"></td><td colspan="2">33</td><td colspan="2">38</td><td colspan="2">34</td><td colspan="4"></td><td>35</td></tr>
<tr><td>83 9 U U</td><td colspan="2"></td><td colspan="19">39</td><td></td></tr>
<tr><td>84 9 U U</td><td colspan="2"></td><td colspan="19">36</td><td></td></tr>
<tr><td>84 10 UC R</td><td>2</td><td>4</td><td>7</td><td>13</td><td>13</td><td>12</td><td colspan="15"></td><td></td></tr>
<tr><td>84 10 UC A</td><td>10</td><td>17</td><td>24</td><td>29</td><td>29</td><td>27</td><td colspan="15"></td><td></td></tr>
<tr><td>85 4 A U</td><td colspan="6"></td><td colspan="15">34</td><td></td></tr>
<tr><td>85 12 UC *</td><td>6</td><td>12</td><td>17</td><td>27</td><td colspan="17"></td><td></td></tr>
<tr><td>85 12 UC R</td><td>12</td><td>17</td><td>19</td><td>30</td><td colspan="17"></td><td></td></tr>
<tr><td>85 14 U R</td><td colspan="2"></td><td colspan="6">23</td><td colspan="4">41</td><td colspan="9">31</td><td>33</td></tr>
<tr><td>85 14 U A</td><td colspan="2"></td><td colspan="6">32</td><td colspan="4">45</td><td colspan="9">31</td><td>36</td></tr>
<tr><td>85 16 UC A</td><td>5</td><td>12</td><td>17</td><td>26</td><td colspan="17"></td><td></td></tr>
<tr><td>86 2 UC U</td><td colspan="4"></td><td colspan="17">32</td><td></td></tr>
<tr><td>86 2 A U</td><td colspan="4"></td><td colspan="4">31</td><td>41</td><td>39</td><td>35</td><td>35</td><td>37</td><td>29</td><td>36</td><td>35</td><td colspan="2">29</td><td colspan="3">16</td><td>33</td></tr>
</table>

Table 1.4F Prevalence of smoking, females: some selected Australian surveys by age, 1945-1995 *(continues on p. 11)*

<table>
<tr><th rowspan="2">Frequency
Product
Source
Year</th><th colspan="21">Age group</th><th rowspan="2">All ages</th></tr>
<tr><th>12</th><th>13</th><th>14</th><th>15</th><th>16</th><th>17</th><th>18</th><th>19</th><th>20-24</th><th>25-29</th><th>30-34</th><th>35-39</th><th>40-44</th><th>45-49</th><th>50-54</th><th>55-59</th><th>60-64</th><th>65-69</th><th>70-74</th><th>75-79</th><th>80+</th></tr>
<tr><td>45 1 U U</td><td colspan="4"></td><td colspan="17">26</td><td></td></tr>
<tr><td>64 1 U U</td><td colspan="4"></td><td colspan="17">28</td><td></td></tr>
<tr><td>68 11 UC R</td><td>4</td><td>7</td><td>12</td><td>15</td><td>23</td><td colspan="16"></td><td></td></tr>
<tr><td>68 11 UC A</td><td>6</td><td>9</td><td>13</td><td>16</td><td>23</td><td colspan="16"></td><td></td></tr>
<tr><td>69 1 U U</td><td colspan="4"></td><td colspan="17">28</td><td></td></tr>
<tr><td>69 15 UC R</td><td colspan="3"></td><td>2</td><td colspan="17"></td><td></td></tr>
<tr><td>69 15 UC U</td><td colspan="3"></td><td>15</td><td colspan="17"></td><td></td></tr>
<tr><td>72 5 TC R</td><td></td><td colspan="5">14</td><td colspan="3">37</td><td colspan="3">36</td><td colspan="3">35</td><td colspan="6">20</td><td>29</td></tr>
<tr><td>73 5 TC R</td><td></td><td colspan="5">15</td><td colspan="3">35</td><td colspan="3">34</td><td colspan="3">33</td><td colspan="6">21</td><td>29</td></tr>
<tr><td>73 11 U R</td><td>13</td><td>24</td><td>31</td><td>31</td><td>32</td><td colspan="16"></td><td></td></tr>
<tr><td>73 11 U A</td><td>13</td><td>25</td><td>32</td><td>32</td><td>32</td><td colspan="16"></td><td></td></tr>
<tr><td>74 2 UC U</td><td colspan="4"></td><td colspan="4">29</td><td>38</td><td>37</td><td>30</td><td>29</td><td>27</td><td>33</td><td>37</td><td>25</td><td colspan="2">16</td><td colspan="3">10</td><td>29</td></tr>
<tr><td>74 2 A U</td><td colspan="4"></td><td colspan="4">30</td><td>38</td><td>37</td><td>30</td><td>29</td><td>28</td><td>33</td><td>37</td><td>25</td><td colspan="2">16</td><td colspan="3">10</td><td>30</td></tr>
<tr><td>74 5 TC R</td><td></td><td colspan="5">17</td><td colspan="3">39</td><td colspan="3">36</td><td colspan="3">34</td><td colspan="6">18</td><td>30</td></tr>
<tr><td>75 5 TC R</td><td></td><td colspan="5">20</td><td colspan="3">36</td><td colspan="3">35</td><td colspan="3">31</td><td colspan="6">18</td><td>29</td></tr>
<tr><td>76 2 UC U</td><td colspan="4"></td><td colspan="4">32</td><td>43</td><td>42</td><td>36</td><td>26</td><td>34</td><td>35</td><td>37</td><td>17</td><td colspan="2">18</td><td colspan="3">11</td><td>31</td></tr>
<tr><td>76 2 A U</td><td colspan="4"></td><td colspan="4">32</td><td>44</td><td>44</td><td>38</td><td>28</td><td>34</td><td>36</td><td>38</td><td>18</td><td colspan="2">19</td><td colspan="3">11</td><td>33</td></tr>
<tr><td>76 5 TC R</td><td></td><td colspan="5">21</td><td colspan="3">40</td><td colspan="3">35</td><td colspan="3">29</td><td colspan="6">18</td><td>29</td></tr>
<tr><td>77 3 MC U</td><td colspan="6"></td><td colspan="3">37</td><td colspan="4">33</td><td colspan="4">27</td><td colspan="4">12</td><td>29</td></tr>
<tr><td>77 3 TC U</td><td colspan="6"></td><td colspan="3">37</td><td colspan="4">33</td><td colspan="4">27</td><td colspan="4">12</td><td>29</td></tr>
<tr><td>77 5 TC R</td><td></td><td colspan="5">19</td><td colspan="3">41</td><td colspan="3">35</td><td colspan="3">33</td><td colspan="6">18</td><td>29</td></tr>
<tr><td>78 5 TC R</td><td></td><td colspan="5">20</td><td colspan="3">42</td><td colspan="3">33</td><td colspan="3">29</td><td colspan="6">21</td><td>29</td></tr>
<tr><td>80 2 UC U</td><td colspan="4"></td><td colspan="4">37</td><td>40</td><td>39</td><td>35</td><td>33</td><td>28</td><td>19</td><td>31</td><td>26</td><td colspan="2">23</td><td colspan="3">10</td><td>31</td></tr>
<tr><td>80 2 A U</td><td colspan="4"></td><td colspan="4">37</td><td>40</td><td>41</td><td>36</td><td>33</td><td>30</td><td>20</td><td>31</td><td>26</td><td colspan="2">23</td><td colspan="3">10</td><td>31</td></tr>
<tr><td>80 6 TC U</td><td colspan="9"></td><td>26</td><td>30</td><td>28</td><td>26</td><td>26</td><td>25</td><td>23</td><td>23</td><td colspan="4"></td><td>26</td></tr>
<tr><td>80 6 A U</td><td colspan="9"></td><td>26</td><td>30</td><td>28</td><td>26</td><td>26</td><td>25</td><td>23</td><td>23</td><td colspan="4"></td><td>26</td></tr>
<tr><td>83 2 UC U</td><td colspan="4"></td><td colspan="4">43</td><td>43</td><td>34</td><td>31</td><td>28</td><td>28</td><td>37</td><td>25</td><td>28</td><td colspan="2">22</td><td colspan="3">8</td><td>30</td></tr>
<tr><td>83 2 A U</td><td colspan="4"></td><td colspan="4">45</td><td>45</td><td>35</td><td>32</td><td>29</td><td>28</td><td>39</td><td>26</td><td>29</td><td colspan="2">22</td><td colspan="3">8</td><td>31</td></tr>
<tr><td>83 6 TC U</td><td colspan="9"></td><td>36</td><td>21</td><td>27</td><td>25</td><td>23</td><td>25</td><td>21</td><td>19</td><td colspan="4"></td><td>25</td></tr>
<tr><td>83 6 A U</td><td colspan="9"></td><td>36</td><td>21</td><td>27</td><td>25</td><td>23</td><td>25</td><td>21</td><td>19</td><td colspan="4"></td><td>25</td></tr>
<tr><td>83 7 UC R</td><td colspan="9"></td><td colspan="2">23</td><td colspan="2">20</td><td colspan="2">26</td><td colspan="2">19</td><td colspan="4"></td><td>22</td></tr>
<tr><td>83 7 A A</td><td colspan="9"></td><td colspan="2">25</td><td colspan="2">21</td><td colspan="2">26</td><td colspan="2">19</td><td colspan="4"></td><td>23</td></tr>
<tr><td>83 8 UC R</td><td colspan="11"></td><td colspan="2">28</td><td colspan="2">22</td><td colspan="2">18</td><td colspan="4"></td><td>23</td></tr>
<tr><td>83 8 A A</td><td colspan="11"></td><td colspan="2">28</td><td colspan="2">22</td><td colspan="2">18</td><td colspan="4"></td><td>23</td></tr>
<tr><td>83 9 U U</td><td colspan="2"></td><td colspan="19">29</td><td></td></tr>
<tr><td>84 9 U U</td><td colspan="2"></td><td colspan="19">29</td><td></td></tr>
<tr><td>84 10 UC R</td><td>1</td><td>3</td><td>8</td><td>12</td><td>14</td><td>13</td><td colspan="15"></td><td></td></tr>
<tr><td>84 10 UC A</td><td>8</td><td>18</td><td>29</td><td>34</td><td>34</td><td>30</td><td colspan="15"></td><td></td></tr>
<tr><td>85 4 A U</td><td colspan="6"></td><td colspan="15">27</td><td></td></tr>
<tr><td>85 12 UC *</td><td>7</td><td>17</td><td>24</td><td>32</td><td colspan="17"></td><td></td></tr>
<tr><td>85 12 UC R</td><td>10</td><td>20</td><td>27</td><td>35</td><td colspan="17"></td><td></td></tr>
<tr><td>85 14 U R</td><td colspan="2"></td><td colspan="6">27</td><td colspan="4">35</td><td colspan="9">21</td><td>26</td></tr>
<tr><td>85 14 U A</td><td colspan="2"></td><td colspan="6">40</td><td colspan="4">38</td><td colspan="9">22</td><td>30</td></tr>
<tr><td>85 16 UC A</td><td>8</td><td>16</td><td>24</td><td>32</td><td colspan="17"></td><td></td></tr>
<tr><td>86 2 UC U</td><td colspan="4"></td><td colspan="17">29</td><td></td></tr>
<tr><td>86 2 A U</td><td colspan="4"></td><td colspan="4">28</td><td>41</td><td>39</td><td>31</td><td>29</td><td>30</td><td>25</td><td>28</td><td>24</td><td colspan="2">21</td><td colspan="3">12</td><td>29</td></tr>
</table>

Table 1.4M *(continued from p. 8)*
Prevalence of smoking, males

<table>
<tr><th rowspan="2">Frequency
Product
Source
Year</th><th colspan="21">Age group</th><th rowspan="2">All ages</th></tr>
<tr><th>12</th><th>13</th><th>14</th><th>15</th><th>16</th><th>17</th><th>18</th><th>19</th><th>20-24</th><th>25-29</th><th>30-34</th><th>35-39</th><th>40-44</th><th>45-49</th><th>50-54</th><th>55-59</th><th>60-64</th><th>65-69</th><th>70-74</th><th>75-79</th><th>80+</th></tr>
<tr><td>87 10 UC R</td><td>1</td><td>2</td><td>6</td><td>12</td><td>13</td><td>11</td><td colspan="15"></td><td></td></tr>
<tr><td>87 10 UC A</td><td>5</td><td>10</td><td>19</td><td>25</td><td>27</td><td>25</td><td colspan="15"></td><td></td></tr>
<tr><td>89 2 A U</td><td colspan="4"></td><td colspan="4">20</td><td>41</td><td>39</td><td>37</td><td>35</td><td>32</td><td>26</td><td>22</td><td>26</td><td colspan="2">21</td><td colspan="3">21</td><td>30</td></tr>
<tr><td>89 6 TC U</td><td colspan="8"></td><td>25</td><td>34</td><td>25</td><td>23</td><td>22</td><td>25</td><td>23</td><td>21</td><td>17</td><td>17</td><td colspan="3"></td><td>24</td></tr>
<tr><td>89 6 A U</td><td colspan="8"></td><td>25</td><td>34</td><td>26</td><td>26</td><td>23</td><td>26</td><td>25</td><td>23</td><td>19</td><td>20</td><td colspan="3"></td><td>26</td></tr>
<tr><td>90 10 UC R</td><td>1</td><td>3</td><td>6</td><td>10</td><td>12</td><td>12</td><td colspan="15"></td><td></td></tr>
<tr><td>90 10 UC A</td><td>6</td><td>11</td><td>17</td><td>22</td><td>25</td><td>24</td><td colspan="15"></td><td></td></tr>
<tr><td>90 13 MC R</td><td colspan="6"></td><td colspan="3">35</td><td colspan="2">35</td><td colspan="2">31</td><td colspan="2">28</td><td colspan="2">22</td><td colspan="2">14</td><td colspan="2">6</td><td>28</td></tr>
<tr><td>90 13 TC R</td><td colspan="6"></td><td colspan="3">36</td><td colspan="2">38</td><td colspan="2">33</td><td colspan="2">31</td><td colspan="2">27</td><td colspan="2">18</td><td colspan="2">9</td><td>31</td></tr>
<tr><td>90 13 A R</td><td colspan="6"></td><td colspan="3">36</td><td colspan="2">38</td><td colspan="2">34</td><td colspan="2">32</td><td colspan="2">28</td><td colspan="2">20</td><td colspan="2">11</td><td>32</td></tr>
<tr><td>91 14 UC R</td><td colspan="2"></td><td colspan="6">28</td><td colspan="4">38</td><td colspan="9">28</td><td>32</td></tr>
<tr><td>91 14 UC A</td><td colspan="2"></td><td colspan="6">37</td><td colspan="4">48</td><td colspan="9">32</td><td>39</td></tr>
<tr><td>92 2 UC U</td><td colspan="4"></td><td colspan="17">26</td><td></td></tr>
<tr><td>92 2 A U</td><td colspan="4"></td><td colspan="4">21</td><td>37</td><td>37</td><td>34</td><td>30</td><td>35</td><td>30</td><td>27</td><td>27</td><td colspan="2">20</td><td colspan="3">11</td><td>28</td></tr>
<tr><td>93 10 UC R</td><td>1</td><td>3</td><td>6</td><td>11</td><td>12</td><td>15</td><td colspan="15"></td><td></td></tr>
<tr><td>93 10 UC A</td><td>8</td><td>13</td><td>20</td><td>24</td><td>27</td><td>28</td><td colspan="15"></td><td></td></tr>
<tr><td>93 14 UC R</td><td colspan="2"></td><td colspan="6">16</td><td colspan="2">36</td><td colspan="5">35</td><td colspan="6">17</td><td>29</td></tr>
<tr><td>93 14 UC A</td><td colspan="2"></td><td colspan="6">21</td><td colspan="2">45</td><td colspan="5">37</td><td colspan="6">19</td><td>33</td></tr>
<tr><td>95 2 A U</td><td colspan="4"></td><td colspan="4">29</td><td>33</td><td>35</td><td>34</td><td>30</td><td>30</td><td>27</td><td>30</td><td>28</td><td colspan="2">18</td><td colspan="3">14</td><td>27</td></tr>
<tr><td>95 13 A R</td><td colspan="6"></td><td colspan="15">27</td><td></td></tr>
<tr><td>95 14 UC A</td><td colspan="2"></td><td colspan="6">19</td><td>39</td><td colspan="2">36</td><td colspan="4">31</td><td colspan="6">18</td><td>28</td></tr>
</table>

Source: see *Notes on sources of survey data*, p. 23

Product:
MC = manufactured cigarettes
TC = total cigarettes (including hand-rolled)
UC = cigarettes (type unspecified)
A = all products

Frequency:
A = all smokers (including occasional)
R = regular or daily smokers

All ages: relevant to ages used and as given in original source

U = unspecified

* = refer to *Notes on sources of survey data*, p. 23

Table 1.4F *(continued from p. 9)*
Prevalence of smoking, females

Frequency / Product / Source / Year	12	13	14	15	16	17	18	19	20-24	25-29	30-34	35-39	40-44	45-49	50-54	55-59	60-64	65-69	70-74	75-79	80+	All ages
87 10 UC R	1	2	6	10	12	11																
87 10 UC A	5	13	22	28	30	29																
89 2 A U					31				38	37	30	26	24	29	28	18	20		11			27
89 6 TC U									32	25	22	21	18	23	19	16	15	11				21
89 6 A U									32	25	22	21	18	23	19	16	15	11				21
90 10 UC R	1	2	6	11	11	11																
90 10 UC A	5	13	20	29	28	28																
90 13 MC R							36			31		25		23		19		13		6		24
90 13 TC R							36			31		25		23		19		14		6		25
90 13 A R							36			31		25		23		19		14		6		25
91 14 UC R		29							36			26										31
91 14 UC A		46							43			30										39
92 2 UC U	23																					
92 2 A U					25				36	33	29	28	26	27	18	17	18		6			24
93 10 UC R	1	2	6	9	10	13																
93 10 UC A	7	14	23	28	28	31																
93 14 UC R		16							36		23					11						21
93 14 UC A		27							43		27					13						26
95 2 A U					31				34	35	33	25	27	15	21	18	15		8			23
95 13 A R							20															
95 14 UC A		19							41	34		21				16						24

Source: see *Notes on sources of survey data*, p. 23
Product: MC = manufactured cigarettes
TC = total cigarettes (including hand-rolled)
UC = cigarettes (type unspecified)
A = all products

Frequency: A = all smokers (including occasional)
R = regular or daily smokers
All ages: relevant to ages used and as given in original source
U = unspecified
* = refer to *Notes on sources of survey data*, p. 23

Table 1.5M Number of cigarettes smoked per smoker per day, males: some selected Australian surveys by age, 1968-1995

<table>
<tr><th rowspan="2">Product
Source
Year</th><th colspan="21">Age group</th><th rowspan="2">All ages</th></tr>
<tr><th>12</th><th>13</th><th>14</th><th>15</th><th>16</th><th>17</th><th>18</th><th>19</th><th>20-24</th><th>25-29</th><th>30-34</th><th>35-39</th><th>40-44</th><th>45-49</th><th>50-54</th><th>55-59</th><th>60-64</th><th>65-69</th><th>70-74</th><th>75-79</th><th>80+</th></tr>
<tr><td>68 11 UCE</td><td>0.9</td><td>1.1</td><td>1.5</td><td>1.7</td><td>2.0</td><td colspan="16"></td><td></td></tr>
<tr><td>72 5 TC</td><td></td><td colspan="5">12</td><td colspan="3">19</td><td colspan="3">21</td><td colspan="3">22</td><td colspan="6">20</td><td>19</td></tr>
<tr><td>73 5 TC</td><td></td><td colspan="5">10</td><td colspan="3">20</td><td colspan="3">21</td><td colspan="3">21</td><td colspan="6">19</td><td></td></tr>
<tr><td>73 11 UCE</td><td>1.3</td><td>1.9</td><td>2.3</td><td>2.6</td><td>2.4</td><td colspan="16"></td><td></td></tr>
<tr><td>74 2 UCE</td><td colspan="4"></td><td colspan="6">18</td><td colspan="2">20</td><td colspan="2">21</td><td colspan="2">21</td><td colspan="5">18</td><td>19</td></tr>
<tr><td>74 5 TC</td><td></td><td colspan="5">13</td><td colspan="3">20</td><td colspan="3">21</td><td colspan="3">22</td><td colspan="6">19</td><td></td></tr>
<tr><td>75 5 TC</td><td></td><td colspan="5">14</td><td colspan="3">19</td><td colspan="3">21</td><td colspan="3">22</td><td colspan="6">20</td><td></td></tr>
<tr><td>76 2 UCE</td><td colspan="4"></td><td colspan="4">14</td><td colspan="2">18</td><td colspan="2">22</td><td colspan="2">22</td><td colspan="2">21</td><td colspan="5">17</td><td>20</td></tr>
<tr><td>76 5 TC</td><td></td><td colspan="5">14</td><td colspan="3">19</td><td colspan="3">21</td><td colspan="3">22</td><td colspan="6">20</td><td></td></tr>
<tr><td>77 3 MCE</td><td colspan="6"></td><td colspan="3">16</td><td colspan="4">21</td><td colspan="4">21</td><td colspan="4">14</td><td>20</td></tr>
<tr><td>77 5 TC</td><td></td><td colspan="5">14</td><td colspan="3">18</td><td colspan="3">21</td><td colspan="3">22</td><td colspan="6">20</td><td></td></tr>
<tr><td>78 5 TC</td><td></td><td colspan="5">14</td><td colspan="3">19</td><td colspan="3">21</td><td colspan="3">22</td><td colspan="6">21</td><td></td></tr>
<tr><td>80 2 UC</td><td colspan="4"></td><td colspan="4">16</td><td>17</td><td>20</td><td>22</td><td>25</td><td>24</td><td>24</td><td>23</td><td>19</td><td colspan="2">16</td><td colspan="3">21</td><td>22</td></tr>
<tr><td>80 6 MC</td><td colspan="9"></td><td>18</td><td>18</td><td>21</td><td>28</td><td>21</td><td>21</td><td>21</td><td>23</td><td colspan="4"></td><td>21</td></tr>
<tr><td>83 2 UC</td><td colspan="4"></td><td colspan="17">18</td><td></td></tr>
<tr><td>83 6 MC</td><td colspan="9"></td><td>18</td><td>22</td><td>21</td><td>20</td><td>25</td><td>23</td><td>23</td><td>21</td><td colspan="4"></td><td>21</td></tr>
<tr><td>83 7 UC</td><td colspan="11"></td><td colspan="4">21</td><td colspan="6"></td><td></td></tr>
<tr><td>83 8 UC</td><td colspan="11"></td><td colspan="4">22</td><td colspan="6"></td><td></td></tr>
<tr><td>83 9 UC</td><td colspan="2"></td><td colspan="19">20</td><td></td></tr>
<tr><td>84 9 UC</td><td colspan="2"></td><td colspan="19">21</td><td></td></tr>
<tr><td>84 10 UC</td><td>2.0</td><td>2.6</td><td>3.3</td><td>4.9</td><td>5.0</td><td>6.0</td><td colspan="15"></td><td></td></tr>
<tr><td>85 12 UCE</td><td>1.0</td><td>1.7</td><td>2.3</td><td>3.2</td><td colspan="17"></td><td></td></tr>
<tr><td>85 14 UCE</td><td colspan="2"></td><td colspan="6">16</td><td colspan="4">22</td><td colspan="9">21</td><td>21</td></tr>
<tr><td>85 16 UC</td><td>0.9</td><td>3.6</td><td>2.9</td><td>5.1</td><td colspan="17"></td><td></td></tr>
<tr><td>87 10 UC</td><td>1.6</td><td>2.1</td><td>3.9</td><td>5.1</td><td>5.3</td><td>5.4</td><td colspan="15"></td><td></td></tr>
<tr><td>89 2 MC</td><td colspan="4"></td><td colspan="17">22</td><td></td></tr>
<tr><td>89 6 MC</td><td colspan="8"></td><td>15</td><td>14</td><td>17</td><td>19</td><td>21</td><td>23</td><td>22</td><td>15</td><td>15</td><td>15</td><td colspan="3"></td><td>18</td></tr>
<tr><td>90 10 UC</td><td>1.3</td><td>2.7</td><td>3.1</td><td>4.7</td><td>5.4</td><td>6.1</td><td colspan="15"></td><td></td></tr>
<tr><td>90 13 MCE</td><td colspan="6"></td><td colspan="3">17</td><td colspan="2">20</td><td colspan="2">23</td><td colspan="2">24</td><td colspan="2">22</td><td colspan="2">19</td><td colspan="2">15</td><td>21</td></tr>
<tr><td>91 14 UCE</td><td colspan="2"></td><td colspan="6">15</td><td colspan="4">21</td><td colspan="9">24</td><td>21</td></tr>
<tr><td>92 2 UC</td><td colspan="4"></td><td colspan="17">22</td><td></td></tr>
<tr><td>93 10 UC</td><td>1.2</td><td>1.8</td><td>2.8</td><td>4.1</td><td>5.3</td><td>6.3</td><td colspan="15"></td><td></td></tr>
<tr><td>95 2 UC</td><td colspan="4"></td><td colspan="17">20</td><td></td></tr>
</table>

Source: see *Notes on sources of survey data*, p.23

Product:
MC = manufactured cigarettes
TC = total cigarettes (including hand-rolled)
UC = cigarettes (type unspecified)
A = all products
U = unspecified

Product (cont): E indicates mean estimated from percentage distribution (see also *Consumption category estimation*, p. xxxiv, and Appendix III, p. 789)

All ages: relevant to ages used and as given in original source

* = refer to *Notes on sources of survey data*, p. 23

Table 1.5F Number of cigarettes smoked per smoker per day, females: some selected Australian surveys by age, 1968-1995

Product Source Year	12	13	14	15	16	17	18	19	20-24	25-29	30-34	35-39	40-44	45-49	50-54	55-59	60-64	65-69	70-74	75-79	80+	All ages
68 11 UCE	0.6	0.7	0.9	1.1	1.4																	
72 5 TC		10					15			16			18			16						16
73 5 TC		10					15			18			18			16						
73 11 UCE	0.9	1.3	1.7	2.0	2.4																	
74 2 UCE					15						15		17		17		14					16
74 5 TC		13					15			16			18			16						
75 5 TC		11					16			17			18			17						
76 2 UCE					13				16		17		17		17		16					16
76 5 TC		12					17			17			17			17						
77 3 MCE							13			15				15				11				15
77 5 TC		13					15			17			18			17						
78 5 TC		11					16			18			19			17						
80 2 UC					14				16	18	20	20	21	20	19	17	19		13			18
80 6 MC										13	19	13	18	16	15	15	13					15
83 2 UC					17																	
83 6 MC										13	15	19	18	15	16	19	16					16
83 7 UC												15										
83 8 UC												17										
83 9 UC			18																			
84 9 UC			17																			
84 10 UC	1.0	1.7	2.4	3.7	4.9	4.9																
85 12 UCE	1.4	1.7	2.6	3.0																		
85 14 UCE			15						19				19									18
85 16 UC	2.6	3.3	4.6	5.0																		
87 10 UC	1.4	1.7	2.9	3.7	4.3	4.3																
89 2 MC					19																	
89 6 MC									11	16	14	17	16	17	19	22	15	16				15
90 10 UC	1.1	1.9	3.1	3.9	4.0	4.3																
90 13 MCE							15			17		19		18		19		16		12		17
91 14 UCE			13						21				20									20
92 2 UC					19																	
93 10 UC	1.0	1.8	2.7	3.4	4.5	4.6																
95 2 UC					18																	

Source: see *Notes on sources of survey data*, p.23

Product:
MC = manufactured cigarettes
TC = total cigarettes (including hand-rolled)
UC = cigarettes (type unspecified)
A = all products
U = unspecified

Product (cont): E indicates mean estimated from percentage distribution (see also *Consumption category estimation*, p. xxxiv, and Appendix III, p. 789)

All ages: relevant to ages used and as given in original source

* = refer to *Notes on sources of survey data*, p. 23

Table 1.6M Number of cigarettes smoked per person per day, males: some selected Australian surveys by age, 1968-1995, with percentage total sales

<table>
<tr><th rowspan="2">Product
Source
Year</th><th colspan="21">Age group</th><th rowspan="2">All ages</th><th rowspan="2">% Total sales</th></tr>
<tr><th>12</th><th>13</th><th>14</th><th>15</th><th>16</th><th>17</th><th>18</th><th>19</th><th>20-24</th><th>25-29</th><th>30-34</th><th>35-39</th><th>40-44</th><th>45-49</th><th>50-54</th><th>55-59</th><th>60-64</th><th>65-69</th><th>70-74</th><th>75-79</th><th>80+</th></tr>
<tr><td>68 11 UC</td><td>0.2</td><td>0.3</td><td>0.4</td><td>0.6</td><td>0.8</td><td colspan="16"></td><td></td><td>**</td></tr>
<tr><td>72 5 TC</td><td></td><td colspan="5">2.4</td><td colspan="3">9.4</td><td colspan="3">11</td><td colspan="3">11</td><td colspan="6">7.4</td><td>8.5</td><td>78%T</td></tr>
<tr><td>73 5 TC</td><td></td><td colspan="5">1.9</td><td colspan="3">9.6</td><td colspan="3">9.9</td><td colspan="3">9.6</td><td colspan="6">7.1</td><td>8.2</td><td>72%T</td></tr>
<tr><td>73 11 UC</td><td>0.3</td><td>0.6</td><td>0.9</td><td>1.2</td><td>1.4</td><td colspan="16"></td><td></td><td>**</td></tr>
<tr><td>74 2 UC</td><td colspan="4"></td><td colspan="4">5.9</td><td>8.6</td><td>8.1</td><td>9.2</td><td>8.8</td><td>8.3</td><td>9.1</td><td>9.2</td><td>7.5</td><td colspan="2">5.7</td><td colspan="3">5.0</td><td>7.9</td><td>60%T</td></tr>
<tr><td>74 5 TC</td><td></td><td colspan="5">3.3</td><td colspan="3">8.9</td><td colspan="3">9.7</td><td colspan="3">9.4</td><td colspan="6">6.1</td><td>8.0</td><td>67%T</td></tr>
<tr><td>75 5 TC</td><td></td><td colspan="5">3.1</td><td colspan="3">9.0</td><td colspan="3">9.9</td><td colspan="3">10</td><td colspan="6">6.1</td><td>8.2</td><td>70%T</td></tr>
<tr><td>76 2 UC</td><td colspan="4"></td><td colspan="4">5.1</td><td>8.5</td><td>8.3</td><td>8.6</td><td>9.0</td><td>8.8</td><td>8.1</td><td>9.9</td><td>7.7</td><td colspan="2">5.5</td><td colspan="3">4.7</td><td>7.9</td><td>68%T</td></tr>
<tr><td>76 5 TC</td><td></td><td colspan="5">3.2</td><td colspan="3">9.2</td><td colspan="3">9.3</td><td colspan="3">9.1</td><td colspan="6">6.3</td><td>7.9</td><td>73%T</td></tr>
<tr><td>77 3 MC</td><td colspan="6"></td><td colspan="3">6.2</td><td colspan="4">8.5</td><td colspan="4">7.1</td><td colspan="4">2.5</td><td>7.2</td><td>60%M</td></tr>
<tr><td>77 5 TC</td><td></td><td colspan="5">3.0</td><td colspan="3">7.5</td><td colspan="3">8.8</td><td colspan="3">9.2</td><td colspan="6">6.0</td><td>7.3</td><td>66%T</td></tr>
<tr><td>78 5 TC</td><td></td><td colspan="5">2.9</td><td colspan="3">9.1</td><td colspan="3">9.6</td><td colspan="3">9.2</td><td colspan="6">5.7</td><td>7.8</td><td>69%T</td></tr>
<tr><td>80 2 UC</td><td colspan="4"></td><td colspan="4">5.7</td><td>9.5</td><td>9.6</td><td>8.5</td><td>10</td><td>9.9</td><td>11</td><td>11</td><td>7.6</td><td colspan="2">3.9</td><td colspan="3">3.8</td><td>8.8</td><td>69%T</td></tr>
<tr><td>80 6 TC *</td><td colspan="9"></td><td>7.7</td><td>5.4</td><td>7.5</td><td>11</td><td>8.6</td><td>6.6</td><td>6.7</td><td>5.6</td><td colspan="4"></td><td>7.4</td><td>**</td></tr>
<tr><td>83 2 UC</td><td colspan="4"></td><td colspan="17">6.8</td><td></td><td>70%T</td></tr>
<tr><td>83 6 TC *</td><td colspan="9"></td><td>7.1</td><td>7.1</td><td>6.7</td><td>5.8</td><td>7.8</td><td>7.5</td><td>7.7</td><td>5.3</td><td colspan="4"></td><td>6.8</td><td>**</td></tr>
<tr><td>83 7 UC *</td><td colspan="11"></td><td colspan="4">6.9</td><td colspan="6"></td><td></td><td>**</td></tr>
<tr><td>83 8 UC *</td><td colspan="11"></td><td colspan="4">7.2</td><td colspan="6"></td><td></td><td>**</td></tr>
<tr><td>83 9 UC</td><td colspan="2"></td><td colspan="19">8.0</td><td></td><td>85%T</td></tr>
<tr><td>84 9 UC</td><td colspan="2"></td><td colspan="19">7.4</td><td></td><td>81%T</td></tr>
<tr><td>84 10 UC</td><td>0.2</td><td>0.4</td><td>0.8</td><td>1.4</td><td>1.5</td><td>1.6</td><td colspan="15"></td><td></td><td>**</td></tr>
<tr><td>85 12 UC</td><td>0.1</td><td>0.2</td><td>0.3</td><td>0.8</td><td colspan="17"></td><td></td><td>**</td></tr>
<tr><td>85 14 UC</td><td colspan="2"></td><td colspan="6">3.6</td><td colspan="4">9.2</td><td colspan="9">6.7</td><td>7.0</td><td>77%T</td></tr>
<tr><td>85 16 UC</td><td>0.0</td><td>0.4</td><td>0.5</td><td>1.3</td><td colspan="17"></td><td></td><td>**</td></tr>
<tr><td>87 10 UC</td><td>0.1</td><td>0.2</td><td>0.7</td><td>1.3</td><td>1.4</td><td>1.4</td><td colspan="15"></td><td></td><td>**</td></tr>
<tr><td>89 2 MC</td><td colspan="4"></td><td colspan="17">6.6</td><td></td><td>79%M</td></tr>
<tr><td>89 6 TC *</td><td colspan="8"></td><td>3.8</td><td>4.7</td><td>4.2</td><td>4.4</td><td>4.5</td><td>5.6</td><td>5.0</td><td>3.2</td><td>2.5</td><td>2.6</td><td colspan="3"></td><td>4.4</td><td>45%T</td></tr>
<tr><td>90 10 UC</td><td>0.1</td><td>0.3</td><td>0.5</td><td>1.0</td><td>1.4</td><td>1.5</td><td colspan="15"></td><td></td><td>**</td></tr>
<tr><td>90 13 MC</td><td colspan="6"></td><td colspan="3">5.8</td><td colspan="2">7.0</td><td colspan="2">7.0</td><td colspan="2">6.6</td><td colspan="2">4.8</td><td colspan="2">2.6</td><td colspan="2">0.9</td><td>5.8</td><td>64%M</td></tr>
<tr><td>91 14 UC</td><td colspan="2"></td><td colspan="6">4.1</td><td colspan="4">7.9</td><td colspan="9">6.5</td><td>6.7</td><td>90%T</td></tr>
<tr><td>92 2 UC</td><td colspan="4"></td><td colspan="17">5.8</td><td></td><td>71%T</td></tr>
<tr><td>93 10 UC</td><td>0.1</td><td>0.2</td><td>0.6</td><td>1.0</td><td>1.4</td><td>1.8</td><td colspan="15"></td><td></td><td>**</td></tr>
<tr><td>95 2 UC *</td><td colspan="4"></td><td colspan="17">5.3</td><td></td><td>72%T</td></tr>
</table>

Source: see *Notes on sources of survey data*, p.23
Product: MC = manufactured cigarettes
TC = total cigarettes (including hand-rolled)
UC = cigarettes (type unspecified)
A = all products
U = unspecified

All ages: relevant to ages used and as given in original source
% Total sales: estimated % of total sales of M = manufactured or T = total cigarette consumption implied by survey, sexes combined
** = cannot be calculated
--- = adjusted by original author
* = refer to *Notes on sources of survey data*, p. 23

Table 1.6F Number of cigarettes smoked per person per day, females: some selected Australian surveys by age, 1968-1995, with percentage total sales

Product Source Year	12	13	14	15	16	17	18	19	20-24	25-29	30-34	35-39	40-44	45-49	50-54	55-59	60-64	65-69	70-74	75-79	80+	All ages	% Total sales
68 11 UC	0.0	0.0	0.1	0.2	0.3																		**
72 5 TC		1.4					5.4			5.8			6.2			3.1						4.7	78%T
73 5 TC		1.6					5.3			6.2			6.1			3.3						4.8	72%T
73 11 UC	0.1	0.3	0.5	0.6	0.8																		**
74 2 UC					4.1				5.9	5.8	4.6	4.4	4.5	5.5	6.1	4.2	2.2		1.4			4.5	60%T
74 5 TC		2.2					5.8			6.1			5.8			3.0						4.8	67%T
75 5 TC		2.3					5.8			6.0			5.7			3.1						4.8	70%T
76 2 UC					4.2				6.8	6.6	6.2	4.5	5.8	6.0	6.1	2.8	2.9		1.8			5.1	68%T
76 5 TC		2.5					6.6			5.9			5.1			3.0						4.7	73%T
77 3 MC							4.9			4.9				4.0				1.3				4.3	60%M
77 5 TC		2.5					6.3			6.1			6.0			3.1						4.9	66%T
78 5 TC		2.2					6.7			5.8			5.4			3.6						4.9	69%T
80 2 UC					5.0				6.5	6.9	6.9	6.7	5.7	3.8	5.9	4.4	4.3		1.3			5.6	69%T
80 6 TC *										3.3	5.7	3.6	4.6	4.2	3.8	3.5	3.0					3.9	**
83 2 UC					5.2																		70%T
83 6 TC *										4.6	3.1	5.1	4.4	3.4	4.0	4.0	3.0					4.0	**
83 7 UC *												3.3											**
83 8 UC *												4.0											**
83 9 UC			6.2																				85%T
84 9 UC			5.7																				81%T
84 10 UC	0.1	0.3	0.7	1.3	1.4	1.3																	**
85 12 UC	0.1	0.3	0.6	0.9																			**
85 14 UC			4.0						6.5				3.9									4.6	77%T
85 16 UC	0.2	0.5	1.1	1.6																			**
87 10 UC	0.1	0.2	0.6	1.0	1.3	1.2																	**
89 2 MC					5.1																		79%M
89 6 TC *									3.5	4.0	3.1	3.6	2.8	3.9	3.5	3.6	2.2	1.8				3.2	45%T
90 10 UC	0.1	0.2	0.6	1.1	1.1	1.2																	**
90 13 MC							5.2			5.2		4.6		4.2		3.5		2.1		0.7		4.1	64%M
91 14 UC			3.8						7.5				5.4									6.0	90%T
92 2 UC					4.9																		71%T
93 10 UC	0.1	0.3	0.6	0.9	1.3	1.4																	**
95 2 UC *					4.2																		72%T

Source: see *Notes on sources of survey data*, p.23

Product:
MC = manufactured cigarettes
TC = total cigarettes (including hand-rolled)
UC = cigarettes (type unspecified)
A = all products
U = unspecified

All ages: relevant to ages used and as given in original source

% Total sales: estimated % of total sales of M = manufactured or T = total cigarette consumption implied by survey, sexes combined
** = cannot be calculated
--- = adjusted by original author
* = refer to *Notes on sources of survey data*, p. 23

Table 1.7M Number of cigarettes smoked per person per day, sales-adjusted, males: some selected Australian surveys[1] by age, 1972-1995, with percentage total sales

<table>
<tr><th rowspan="2">Product
Source
Year</th><th colspan="21">Age group</th><th rowspan="2">All ages</th><th rowspan="2">% Total sales</th></tr>
<tr><th>12</th><th>13</th><th>14</th><th>15</th><th>16</th><th>17</th><th>18</th><th>19</th><th>20-24</th><th>25-29</th><th>30-34</th><th>35-39</th><th>40-44</th><th>45-49</th><th>50-54</th><th>55-59</th><th>60-64</th><th>65-69</th><th>70-74</th><th>75-79</th><th>80+</th></tr>
<tr><td>72 5 TC</td><td></td><td colspan="5">3.1</td><td colspan="3">12</td><td colspan="3">14</td><td colspan="3">14</td><td colspan="6">9.5</td><td>11</td><td>78%T</td></tr>
<tr><td>73 5 TC</td><td></td><td colspan="5">2.6</td><td colspan="3">13</td><td colspan="3">14</td><td colspan="3">13</td><td colspan="6">9.8</td><td>11</td><td>72%T</td></tr>
<tr><td>74 2 UC</td><td colspan="4"></td><td colspan="4">9.8</td><td>14</td><td>13</td><td>15</td><td>15</td><td>14</td><td>15</td><td>15</td><td>12</td><td colspan="2">9.5</td><td colspan="3">8.3</td><td>13</td><td>60%T</td></tr>
<tr><td>74 5 TC</td><td></td><td colspan="5">4.9</td><td colspan="3">13</td><td colspan="3">14</td><td colspan="3">14</td><td colspan="6">9.1</td><td>12</td><td>67%T</td></tr>
<tr><td>75 5 TC</td><td></td><td colspan="5">4.4</td><td colspan="3">13</td><td colspan="3">14</td><td colspan="3">14</td><td colspan="6">8.7</td><td>12</td><td>70%T</td></tr>
<tr><td>76 2 UC</td><td colspan="4"></td><td colspan="4">7.5</td><td>12</td><td>12</td><td>13</td><td>13</td><td>13</td><td>12</td><td>15</td><td>11</td><td colspan="2">8.1</td><td colspan="3">6.9</td><td>12</td><td>68%T</td></tr>
<tr><td>76 5 TC</td><td></td><td colspan="5">4.4</td><td colspan="3">13</td><td colspan="3">13</td><td colspan="3">13</td><td colspan="6">8.7</td><td>11</td><td>73%T</td></tr>
<tr><td>77 3 MC</td><td colspan="6"></td><td colspan="3">10</td><td colspan="4">14</td><td colspan="4">12</td><td colspan="4">4.2</td><td>12</td><td>60%M</td></tr>
<tr><td>77 5 TC</td><td></td><td colspan="5">4.5</td><td colspan="3">11</td><td colspan="3">13</td><td colspan="3">14</td><td colspan="6">9.1</td><td>11</td><td>66%T</td></tr>
<tr><td>78 5 TC</td><td></td><td colspan="5">4.2</td><td colspan="3">13</td><td colspan="3">14</td><td colspan="3">13</td><td colspan="6">8.2</td><td>11</td><td>69%T</td></tr>
<tr><td>80 2 UC</td><td colspan="4"></td><td colspan="4">8.3</td><td>14</td><td>14</td><td>12</td><td>15</td><td>14</td><td>16</td><td>15</td><td>11</td><td colspan="2">5.7</td><td colspan="3">5.5</td><td>13</td><td>69%T</td></tr>
<tr><td>83 2 UC</td><td colspan="4"></td><td colspan="17">9.8</td><td></td><td>70%T</td></tr>
<tr><td>83 9 UC</td><td colspan="2"></td><td colspan="19">9.3</td><td></td><td>85%T</td></tr>
<tr><td>84 9 UC</td><td colspan="2"></td><td colspan="19">9.1</td><td></td><td>81%T</td></tr>
<tr><td>85 14 UC</td><td colspan="2"></td><td colspan="6">4.6</td><td colspan="4">12</td><td colspan="9">8.6</td><td>9.1</td><td>77%T</td></tr>
<tr><td>89 2 MC</td><td colspan="4"></td><td colspan="17">8.4</td><td></td><td>79%M</td></tr>
<tr><td>89 6 TC *</td><td colspan="8"></td><td>8.5</td><td>10</td><td>9.3</td><td>9.8</td><td>10</td><td>12</td><td>11</td><td>7.1</td><td>5.6</td><td>5.8</td><td colspan="3"></td><td>9.8</td><td>45%T</td></tr>
<tr><td>90 13 MC</td><td colspan="6"></td><td colspan="3">9.1</td><td colspan="2">11</td><td colspan="2">11</td><td colspan="2">10</td><td colspan="2">7.4</td><td colspan="2">4.0</td><td colspan="2">1.5</td><td>9.1</td><td>64%M</td></tr>
<tr><td>91 14 UC</td><td colspan="2"></td><td colspan="6">4.6</td><td colspan="4">8.8</td><td colspan="9">7.3</td><td>7.5</td><td>90%T</td></tr>
<tr><td>92 2 UC</td><td colspan="4"></td><td colspan="17">8.0</td><td></td><td>71%T</td></tr>
<tr><td>95 2 UC *</td><td colspan="4"></td><td colspan="17">7.4</td><td></td><td>72%T</td></tr>
</table>

1 Based on those surveys in Table 1.6 with data for both sexes and age range at least 21-64 (see *Cigarette consumption per person*, p. xxxv)

Source: See *Notes on sources of survey data*, p. 23

Product: MC = manufactured cigarettes
TC = total cigarettes (including hand-rolled)
UC = cigarettes (type unspecified)
A = all products
U = unspecified

All ages: relevant to ages used and as given in original source

% Total sales: Adjustment factor used, estimated % of total sales of M = manufactured or T = total cigarette consumption implied by survey, sexes combined

--- = adjusted by original author

* = refer to *Notes on sources of survey data*, p. 23

Table 1.7F Number of cigarettes smoked per person per day, sales-adjusted, females: some selected Australian surveys[1] by age, 1972-1995, with percentage total sales

<table>
<tr><th rowspan="2">Product
Source
Year</th><th colspan="21">Age group</th><th rowspan="2">All ages</th><th rowspan="2">% Total sales</th></tr>
<tr><th>12</th><th>13</th><th>14</th><th>15</th><th>16</th><th>17</th><th>18</th><th>19</th><th>20-24</th><th>25-29</th><th>30-34</th><th>35-39</th><th>40-44</th><th>45-49</th><th>50-54</th><th>55-59</th><th>60-64</th><th>65-69</th><th>70-74</th><th>75-79</th><th>80+</th></tr>
<tr><td>72 5 TC</td><td></td><td colspan="5">1.8</td><td colspan="3">6.9</td><td colspan="3">7.5</td><td colspan="3">8.0</td><td colspan="6">4.0</td><td>6.0</td><td>78%T</td></tr>
<tr><td>73 5 TC</td><td></td><td colspan="5">2.2</td><td colspan="3">7.3</td><td colspan="3">8.6</td><td colspan="3">8.4</td><td colspan="6">4.6</td><td>6.6</td><td>72%T</td></tr>
<tr><td>74 2 UC</td><td colspan="4"></td><td colspan="4">6.8</td><td>9.8</td><td>9.6</td><td>7.6</td><td>7.3</td><td>7.5</td><td>9.1</td><td>10</td><td>7.0</td><td colspan="2">3.7</td><td colspan="3">2.3</td><td>7.5</td><td>60%T</td></tr>
<tr><td>74 5 TC</td><td></td><td colspan="5">3.3</td><td colspan="3">8.6</td><td colspan="3">9.1</td><td colspan="3">8.6</td><td colspan="6">4.5</td><td>7.2</td><td>67%T</td></tr>
<tr><td>75 5 TC</td><td></td><td colspan="5">3.3</td><td colspan="3">8.3</td><td colspan="3">8.6</td><td colspan="3">8.1</td><td colspan="6">4.4</td><td>6.9</td><td>70%T</td></tr>
<tr><td>76 2 UC</td><td colspan="4"></td><td colspan="4">6.2</td><td>10</td><td>9.7</td><td>9.1</td><td>6.6</td><td>8.5</td><td>8.8</td><td>9.0</td><td>4.1</td><td colspan="2">4.3</td><td colspan="3">2.6</td><td>7.5</td><td>68%T</td></tr>
<tr><td>76 5 TC</td><td></td><td colspan="5">3.4</td><td colspan="3">9.1</td><td colspan="3">8.1</td><td colspan="3">7.0</td><td colspan="6">4.1</td><td>6.5</td><td>73%T</td></tr>
<tr><td>77 3 MC</td><td colspan="6"></td><td colspan="3">8.2</td><td colspan="4">8.2</td><td colspan="4">6.7</td><td colspan="4">2.2</td><td>7.2</td><td>60%M</td></tr>
<tr><td>77 5 TC</td><td></td><td colspan="5">3.8</td><td colspan="3">9.5</td><td colspan="3">9.2</td><td colspan="3">9.1</td><td colspan="6">4.7</td><td>7.4</td><td>66%T</td></tr>
<tr><td>78 5 TC</td><td></td><td colspan="5">3.2</td><td colspan="3">9.7</td><td colspan="3">8.4</td><td colspan="3">7.8</td><td colspan="6">5.2</td><td>7.1</td><td>69%T</td></tr>
<tr><td>80 2 UC</td><td colspan="4"></td><td colspan="4">7.3</td><td>9.5</td><td>10</td><td>10</td><td>9.8</td><td>8.3</td><td>5.5</td><td>8.6</td><td>6.4</td><td colspan="2">6.3</td><td colspan="3">1.9</td><td>8.2</td><td>69%T</td></tr>
<tr><td>83 2 UC</td><td colspan="4"></td><td colspan="17">7.5</td><td></td><td>70%T</td></tr>
<tr><td>83 9 UC</td><td colspan="2"></td><td colspan="19">7.3</td><td></td><td>85%T</td></tr>
<tr><td>84 9 UC</td><td colspan="2"></td><td colspan="19">7.0</td><td></td><td>81%T</td></tr>
<tr><td>85 14 UC</td><td colspan="2"></td><td colspan="6">5.1</td><td colspan="4">8.5</td><td colspan="9">5.1</td><td>6.0</td><td>77%T</td></tr>
<tr><td>89 2 MC</td><td colspan="4"></td><td colspan="17">6.5</td><td></td><td>79%M</td></tr>
<tr><td>89 6 TC *</td><td colspan="8"></td><td>7.8</td><td>8.9</td><td>6.9</td><td>8.0</td><td>6.2</td><td>8.7</td><td>7.8</td><td>8.0</td><td>4.9</td><td>4.0</td><td colspan="3"></td><td>7.1</td><td>45%T</td></tr>
<tr><td>90 13 MC</td><td colspan="6"></td><td colspan="3">8.1</td><td colspan="2">8.1</td><td colspan="2">7.1</td><td colspan="2">6.6</td><td colspan="2">5.5</td><td colspan="2">3.2</td><td colspan="2">1.1</td><td>6.4</td><td>64%M</td></tr>
<tr><td>91 14 UC</td><td colspan="2"></td><td colspan="6">4.2</td><td colspan="4">8.4</td><td colspan="9">6.0</td><td>6.7</td><td>90%T</td></tr>
<tr><td>92 2 UC</td><td colspan="4"></td><td colspan="17">6.9</td><td></td><td>71%T</td></tr>
<tr><td>95 2 UC *</td><td colspan="4"></td><td colspan="17">5.8</td><td></td><td>72%T</td></tr>
</table>

1 Based on those surveys in Table 1.6 with data for both sexes and age range at least 21-64 (see *Cigarette consumption per person*, p. xxxv)

Source: See *Notes on sources of survey data*, p. 23

Product: MC = manufactured cigarettes
TC = total cigarettes (including hand-rolled)
UC = cigarettes (type unspecified)
A = all products
U = unspecified

All ages: relevant to ages used and as given in original source

% Total sales: Adjustment factor used, estimated % of total sales of M = manufactured or T = total cigarette consumption implied by survey, sexes combined
--- = adjusted by original author

* = refer to *Notes on sources of survey data*, p. 23

Table 1.8 Estimated[1] prevalence of smoking and estimated[1] number of cigarettes per person per day (unadjusted and sales-adjusted): summary of Tables 1.4, 1.6 and 1.7, 1945-1995. Males and females aged 15 years and over

Year	Source[2]	Product[3]	Prevalence[4]						Number of cigarettes						
									Unadjusted[7]			Sales-adjusted[8]			
			Manufactured cigarettes		Total cigarettes[5]		All products[6]		Number/ person/day		Total sales %	Manufactured cigarettes number/ person/day		Total cigarettes[9] number/ person/day	
			M	F	M	F	M	F	M	F		M	F	M	F
1945	1	*U*					71	26							
1964	1	*U*					57	28							
1969	1	*U*					44	28							
1972	5	TC			44	29			9.4	4.9	78			12.1	6.3
1973	5	TC			41	29			8.7	5.0	72			12.0	7.0
1974	2	*UC+A*			40	28	44	28	7.7	4.4	60			12.8	7.3
	5	TC			40	29			8.4	5.0	67			12.5	7.5
1975	5	TC			40	28			8.6	5.0	70			12.3	7.1
1976	2	*UC+A*			39	30	43	31	7.5	4.9	68			11.1	7.1
	5	TC			39	28			8.3	4.9	73			11.4	6.8
1977	3	*MC+TC*	35	28	41	28			6.7	4.0	60	11.2	6.7	(12.6	7.0)
	5	TC			37	29			7.8	5.2	66			11.8	7.8
1978	5	TC			38	29			8.2	5.1	69			11.8	7.4
1980	2	*UC+A*			40	29	41	30	8.1	5.2	69			11.8	7.6
1983	2	*UC+A*			37	29	40	30	6.7	5.1	70			9.6	7.4
	9	UC+*U*					39	29	8.2	6.4	85			9.5	7.4
1984	9	UC+*U*					36	29	7.5	5.8	81			9.4	7.2
1985	4	*A*					34	27							
	14	UC+U					34	27	7.5	5.1	77			9.7	6.6
	14	**U**					37	31							
1986	2	*UC+A*			32	29	33	28						(9.3	6.7)
1989	2	MC+*A*					30	26	6.5	5.0	79	8.3	6.4		
	6	*TC+A*			23	20	25	20	3.8	3.0	45			8.5	6.7
1990	13	MC+TC+A	28	24	30	24	31	24	5.6	4.0	64	8.7	6.2	(9.4	6.0)
1991	14	UC			32	30			6.9	6.2	89			7.7	6.9
	14	**UC**			39	37									
1992	2	*UC+A*			26	23	28	24	5.7	4.9	71			7.9	6.8
1993	14	UC			29	22								(8.5	5.1)
	14	**UC**			33	26								(8.2	5.3)
1995	2	UC+*A*					28	23	5.3	4.1	72			7.3	5.7
	14	**UC**			28	24								(7.8	5.2)
	13	A					27	20							

See next page for footnotes

Table 1.8 *(continued)*

1 Surveys covering an age range of at least 21-64 are included. Any gaps in the data for ages 15-20 and 65 years and over are filled in by assumed extensions to the age distribution, given in *Notes on sources of survey data*, p.23. Method: see *Summary of adult smoking*, p. xxxvi
2 See *Notes on sources of survey data*, p.23
3 Product: MC = manufactured cigarettes, TC = total cigarettes (including hand-rolled), UC = cigarettes (type unspecified), A = all products, U = unspecified. Frequency of smoking is indicated by: regular or daily smokers in normal type, all smokers (including occasional) in bold, unspecified in italics
4 From Table 1.4
5 This column includes prevalence of smoking classified as UC = cigarettes (type unspecified)
6 This column includes prevalence of smoking classified as U = unspecified product
7 From Table 1.6
8 From Table 1.7, except data in parentheses, which are derived from the prevalence of smoking from Table 1.4 as described in *Summary of adult smoking*, p. xxxvi
9 Number of cigarettes classified as UC = cigarettes (type unspecified) has been adjusted to total cigarette sales and included in this column. For 1995, adjustment to sales of total cigarettes is to 1994 sales

Figure 1.3 Estimated prevalence of smoking of (i) cigarettes and (ii) all tobacco products: by year of survey, 1945-1995.
Males and females aged 15 years and over. *Source:* see Table 1.8

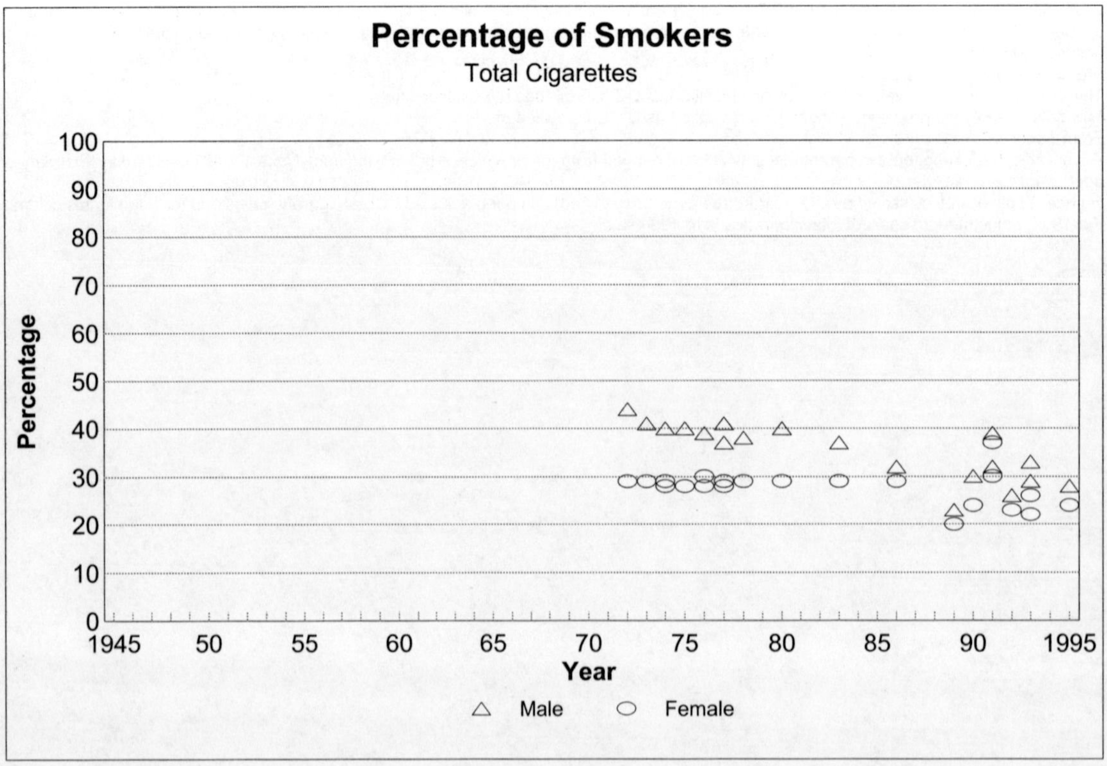

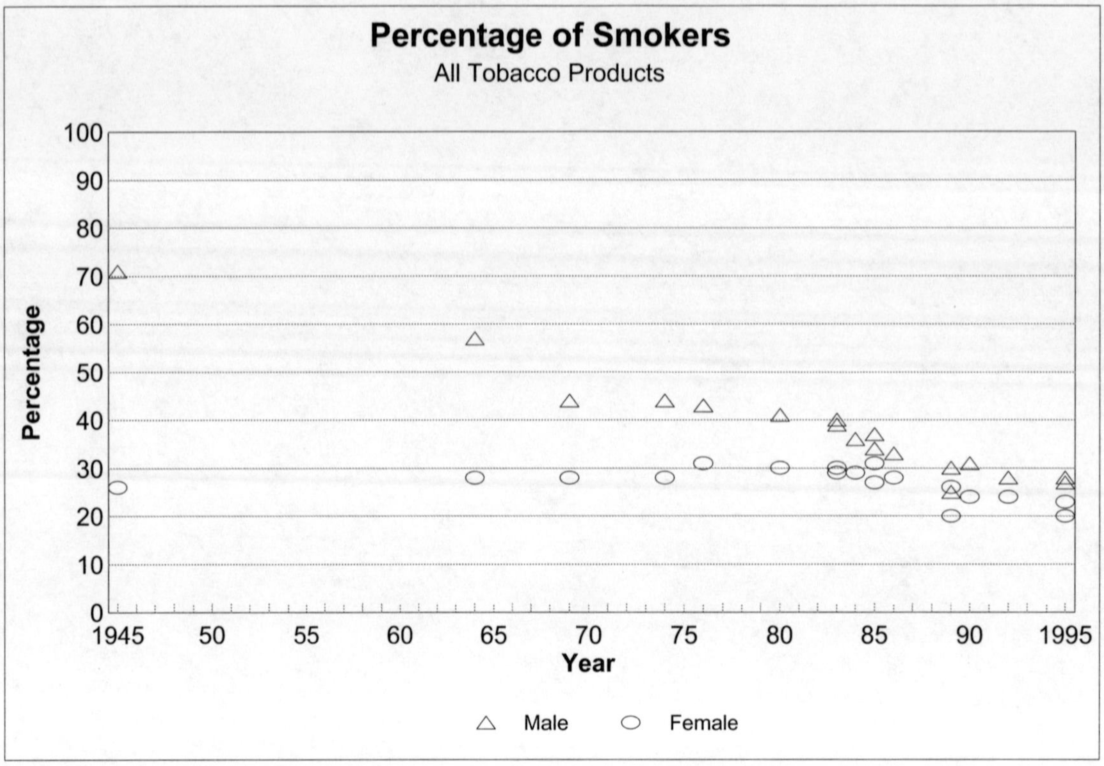

Figure 1.4 Estimated number of cigarettes smoked per person per day, sales-adjusted, 1945-1995.
Males and females aged 15 years and over. *Source:* see Table 1.8

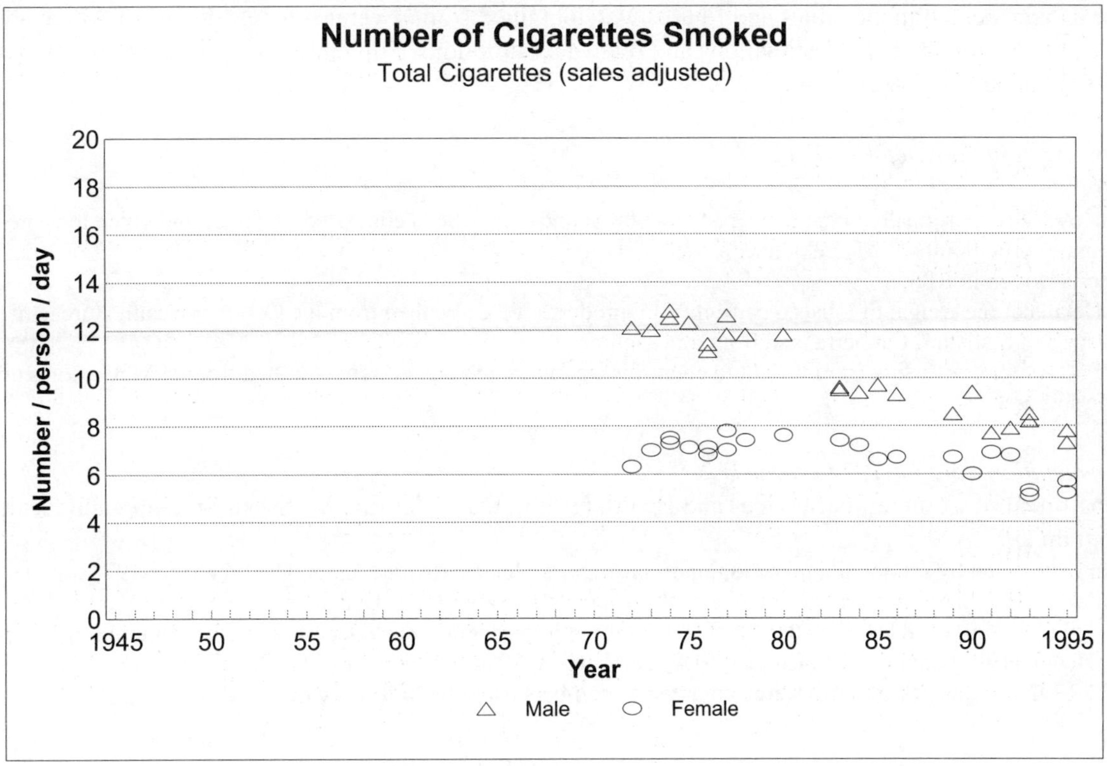

Notes on sources of sales data

The data presented in the tables and figures were obtained from several sources, details of which are given below, together with estimations and related assumptions. Full citations of the sources are given on p. 27 under *References*.

Consumption data before 1974
RP6
Data by weight, originally given to nearest 100 000 pounds, have been converted to tonnes and given to nearest 10 tonnes (100 000lbs = 45.359 tonnes).
Notes as given in RP6:
(a) Details of the weight of tobacco consumed by products were obtained from the Commonwealth Bureau of Census and Statistics, Canberra, and from trade sources.
(b) Factors for conversion from weight to count for cigarettes and cigars were obtained from H.M. Customs and trade sources.

Consumption data for 1974 onwards
Department of Community Services and Health (1990), Quit Victoria: Victorian Smoking and Health Program (1995)
Data were given by weight and relate to import clearances plus excise clearances. Data for 1965-1973 also available from this source are very similar to those shown in Table 1.1.1. Data on smokeless tobacco were not given, but it comprised less than 0.01% of consumption in recent decades (Department of Community Services and Health (1990)) and was banned in 1991 (Quit Victoria: Victorian Smoking and Health Program (1995)). For 1982-1992 weights of cigarettes were converted to numbers using the following data:

Year	Weight (g/1 000 cigarettes)
1982	823
1983	818
1984	808
1985	793
1986	787
1987	779
1988	764
1989	740
1990	735
1991	715
1992	712

Source: Quit Victoria: Victorian Smoking and Health Program (1995)

Numbers of cigarettes thus calculated were similar to those quoted by United States Department of Agriculture (USDA) Economic Research Service (1996) and that source has been used for the number of cigarettes for other years.

Plain/Filter cigarette consumption
1951-1961 Todd (1963)
1961-1981 Maxwell (successive years)

Tar yield of cigarettes
Quit Victoria: Victorian Smoking and Health Program (1995)
Alternative data are presented by Doyle (1985) quoting Thompson (1978) (no details of reference):

Years	SWAT
1961-1965	26.5
1966-1970	25.8
1971-1975	22.6

Hill *et al* (1998) gives the average tar per cigarette in 1995 as 8.2 mg for men, and 7.2 mg for women.

Estimates of hand-rolled cigarette consumption for 1925-1960
Dean (1962) quoting British Tobacco Company (Australia) Ltd.

Estimates of hand-rolled cigarette consumption for 1961 onwards
We have taken as our estimate of hand-rolled cigarette consumption 85% of loose tobacco sales, at 1 g per cigarette, on the following basis:
Hand-rolled cigarette consumption shows an increase from around 30% in 1925 to 95% in 1957 as the percentage of tobacco used in hand-rolled cigarettes rather than pipes (assuming 1 g per cigarette), then a slight fall to 93% in 1960 (Dean (1962)).
Estimates of hand-rolled cigarette consumption in the latest available year were also given in the introductions to successive editions of RP6:

Year	Annual (millions)	Number/ adult/day	Percentage of tobacco used in hand-rolled cigarettes
1966	3 456	1.2	77
1970	3 552	1.1	87
1973	3 292	1	82

Notes on sources of survey data

Each source of survey data—either an individual survey or a series of surveys repeated over a number of years—is cited by a source number. This number is shown in the tables and corresponds to the source numbers given below, where details of the source publication and of the survey methodology are given. Full citations of the sources are given on p. 27 under *References*.

Source number

1 **Woodward (1984)**
   a. Surveys by Australian Gallup Poll
   b. Presumed age 16 years and over
   c. Assumed extension to age distribution for prevalence, age 15: males (1945 and 1964) 25%, (1969) 20%; females (1945, 1964, and 1969) 10%

2 **Gray and Hill (1975, 1977), Hill and Gray (1982, 1984), Hill *et al* (1988, 1991), Hill and White (1995), Hill *et al* (1998)**
   a. National surveys of adults commissioned by the Anti-Cancer Council of Victoria. Part of 'omnibus' market research survey. Personal interviews, one interview per household

Year	Sample size	
	Males	Females
1974	3 316	3 037
1976	2 044	1 829
1980	2 137	2 172
1983	2 677	2 903
1986	4 537	4 903
1989	2 364	2 456
1992	2 983	3 063
1995	2 819	2 880

   b. Consumption per smoker based on broader age groups than prevalence of smoking for 1974 and 1976
   c. In 1992 7.9% of men and 2.3% of women smoked hand-rolled cigarettes, and in 1995 8% of men and 4% of women smoked them
   d. Non-respondents to the smoking questionnaires (<2% in each year) may have been included in the bases for calculations of prevalence in the reports published up to 1984, possibly understating prevalence, and where possible we have taken results from Hill *et al* (1988)

e. Consumption category estimation (1974 and 1976) based on 1-19, 20-24, and 25+ cigarettes/smoker/day

f. Assumed extension to age distribution for prevalence, age 15: males (1974, 1976, 1980, 1983, 1986 and 1989) 20%, (1992) 18%; females (1974 and 1976) 15%, (1980 ,1983, 1986 and 1989) 20%, (1992 and 1995) 18%. Number of cigarettes/person/day, males and females (1974, 1976, 1980, 1983) 2.0, (1989, 1992, 1995) 1.0

3 Australian Bureau of Statistics (1978)

a. Part of the Alcohol and Tobacco Consumption Patterns Survey: a multistage area sample of private and non-private dwellings, comprising about 0.66% of population of Australia. Members of armed forces and institutionalized populations excluded. Personal interviews: alcohol and tobacco consumption sample obtained in about a quarter of households

b. Assumed extension to age distribution for prevalence, age 15-17: 25%. Number of cigarettes/person/day, 3.0

4 Tobacco Institute of Australia

a. Assumed extension to age distribution for prevalence, age 15-17: 25%

5 Doyle (1985), quoting McNair Anderson Associates Pty Ltd (1972-1979)

a. 1972 represents 1972-1973, and similarly for other years

b. Consumption category estimation by Doyle, based on 1-10, 11-10, and 20+ cigarettes/smoker/day, using an earlier method by Todd

6 National Heart Foundation of Australia (1983), Department of Community Services and Health (1990) quoting National Heart Foundation of Australia (1980), Risk Factor Prevalence Study Management Committee (1990)

a. National Heart Foundation of Australia Risk Factor Prevalence Study. Surveys in Australian State capital cities. Sampling based on electoral rolls, resulting in under-representation of migrants, the young, and the more mobile. Results calculated by an estimation procedure designed to reduce bias arising from this source, and from non-response. Participants invited to take part in a risk factor prevalence study: self-completed questionnaire before physical examination.

Year	Sample size		
	Males	Females	Total
1980	—	—	5 617
1983	3 740	3 875	7 640
1989	4 552	4 727	9 279

b. Non-response rate around 25%

c. Calculation of consumption per person based on prevalence of all cigarette smokers and number of manufactured cigarettes per manufactured cigarette smoker—this assumes the same smoking level by hand-rolled cigarette smokers as by manufactured cigarette smokers. In 1983, there were 100 (2.7%) male and 10 (0.3%) female hand-rolled cigarette-only smokers

d. Assumed extension to age distribution (1989 only) for prevalence, age 15-17: 25%; age 70+: males, cigarettes 15%, all products 18%, females 8%. Number of cigarettes/person/day, age 15-17: males and females 3.0, age 70+: 1.0

7, 8 WHO (1989),WHO MONICA Project (1988)

a. Two regional surveys forming part of WHO MONICA Project:

	Region	Population size	Sample size	Participation rate (%)	Sample used*		Date
					Males	Females	
7	Perth	307 500	1 535	85	861	921	May 1983-Nov 1983
8	Newcastle	136 200	3 658	67	1 218	1 241	May 1983-Dec 1983

* Perth 'sample used' includes age 25-34, all other figures are for age 35-64 only

b. *All ages* column relates only to age 35-64 and is standardized to world population

c. Regular cigarette smokers: smoked cigarettes daily. All smokers: smoked cigarettes daily or occasionally, or smoked 1 g pipe tobacco or 1 cigar per week

d. Cigarettes per smoker refers to regular and occasional cigarette smokers. Calculation for cigarettes per person based on % regular cigarette smokers and cigarettes per regular or occasional cigarette smoker, so may underestimate.

9 Dwyer *et al* (1986)

a. Nationwide survey excluding Sydney. Control part of a study of anti-smoking campaign in Sydney. Sample size in 1983: 5 154; response rate 60%. Sample size in 1984: 4 318

10 Hill *et al* (1987, 1990, 1993, 1995)

a. A collaborative project between state member organizations of the Australian Cancer Society and other bodies—a series of three-yearly surveys of the prevalence of cigarette smoking among Australian secondary school students. Questionnaires completed anonymously, usually with teachers absent. All states and territories included except as shown below:

Year	Sample size		Excluded regions
	Males	Females	
1984	11 058	10 846	Australian Capital Territory (ACT)
1987	9 490	9 676	South Australia
1990	12 411	12 481	ACT
1993	11 194	11 502	ACT

b. Regular smokers: smoked daily in past week. All smokers: smoked in past week

c. Prevalence of regular smoking in 12-year-olds (represented as 1% in Table 1.1.4) is actually given as '<1%' for girls only (1987 survey) and for both boys and girls (1990 survey)

11 Department of Community Services and Health (1990) quoting National Health and Medical Research Council (1969, 1979)

a. National surveys of school children aged 9-16 by the National Health and Medical Research Council. 1968 represents 1967-1968.

Year	Sample size
1967-1968	26 000
1973	25 253

b. Both surveys used the same sample schools except that schools in Victoria were omitted in 1973. The Northern Territories were apparently excluded from both surveys

c. Regular smokers: smoked more than 10 cigarettes in their lifetime and considered themselves smokers at time of survey. Consumption per smoker: based on amount smoked in past week

d. Consumption category estimation based on weekly consumption of 0, 1-4, 5-10, 11-20, and 20+ cigarettes/smoker

12 Department of Community Services and Health (1990), quoting Australian Council for Health Physical Education and Recreation (1985)

a. Survey in all states and territories. Sample size 7 000 school students, age 9-15. Consent not obtained in 22.5% of initial sample, eventual sample 6 451

b. Regular smokers: smoked once or more per week. Data labelled UC* in Table 1.4, and data in Tables 1.5, 1.6, and 1.7 based on those who responded positively to number of cigarettes smoked in last 7 days, adjusted for non-respondents

c. Unexplained discrepancy with data presented by Gliksman *et al* (1989)

d. Consumption category estimation based on weekly consumption of 1-5, 6-10, 11-20, 21-30, and 31+ cigarettes/smoker

13 Castles (1992), Australian Bureau of Statistics (1996)

a. National Health Survey. Five-yearly national surveys. Personal interviews with all residents age 18+ of selected dwellings (except those too old or sick), personal or proxy interviews with those aged 15-17.

Year	Sample size (households)	Date
1989-1990	22 200	Oct 1989-Sep 1990
1995-1996	23 800	Feb 1995-Jan 1996

b. Castles (1992) states that the methodology was broadly similar to source 3 (Alcohol and Tobacco Consumption Patterns Survey)

c. Assumed extension to age distribution for prevalence, age 15-17: regular smoking 20%, all smokers (1990 only) 25%. Number of cigarettes/person/day, 2.0

14 Department of Community Services and Health (1990), Jones (1993), Commonwealth Department of Health and Family Services (1995)

a. National Campaign against Drug Abuse, later National Drug Strategy, Household Survey. Face-to face interviews. Random selection of households in all States and Territories. Estimates based on weighted combined samples.

	Sample size		
Year	**Males**	**Females**	**Total**
1985	—	—	2 791
1988	—	—	2 255
1991	—	—	2 850
1993	1 498	2 002	3 500
1995	1 786	2 064	3 850

b. Regular smoking: smokes daily/most days. Occasional smoking: smokes less often than daily/most days

15 Anonymous (1969)

a. National Health and Medical Research Council survey of children aged 9-16 years. Sample size 2 20 000 children

b Regular smokers: smoked more than 20 cigarettes a week

16 Gliksman *et al* (1989)

a. Health and Fitness Survey of Australian Schoolchildren. Age 9 to 15. Sample size 6 451

b. Smokers: smoked at least one cigarette in the last seven days

References

Anonymous (1969). Smoking habits of school children. *Health,* **19**, 16-8.

Australian Bureau of Statistics (1978). *Alcohol and tobacco consumption patterns, February 1977*. ABS, Canberra. ABS Catalogue no. 4312.0.

Australian Bureau of Statistics (1996). *1995 national health survey: first results*. ABS, Canberra. ABS Catalogue no. 4392.0.

Australian Council for Health Physical Education and Recreation (1985). *Australian health and fitness survey*. Australian Council for Health, Physical Education and Recreation.§

Beese D.H. (ed) (1968). *Tobacco consumption in various countries,* 2nd edition. Tobacco Research Council, London. Research Paper 6.

Beese D.H. (ed) (1972). *Tobacco consumption in various countries,* 3rd edition. Tobacco Research Council, London. Research Paper 6.

Castles I. (1992). *1989-90 National health survey, health risk factors, Australia*. Australian Bureau of Statistics, Canberra. ABS Catalogue no. 4380.0.

Chapman S. (1992). Changes in adult cigarette consumption per head in 128 countries, 1986-90. *Tob Control,* **1**, 281-4.

Commonwealth Department of Health and Family Services (1995). *National Drug Strategy Household Survey 1995*. Commonwealth Department of Health and Family Services, Canberra. http://www.health.gov.au/pubhlth/data/index.htm.

Dean G. (1962). Lung cancer in Australia. *Med J Aust,* 1003-6.

Department of Community Services and Health (1990). *Tobacco in Australia, a summary of related statistics*. Australian Government Publishing Service, Canberra. Catalogue no. 89.0765.7.

Doyle E. (1985). *A cohort analysis of smoking and lung cancer in Australia, Canada and the United Kingdom* [Thesis]. University of Newcastle, New South Wales.

Dwyer T., Pierce J.P., Hannam C.D. and Burke N. (1986). Evaluation of the Sydney 'Quit for life' anti-smoking campaign. Part 2. Changes in smoking prevalence. *Med J Aust,* **144**, 344-7.

Gliksman M.D., Dwyer T., Wlodarczyk J. and Pierce J.P. (1989). Cigarette smoking in Australian schoolchildren. *Med J Aust,* **150**, 81-4.

Gray N.J. and Hill D.J. (1975). Patterns of tobacco smoking in Australia. *Med J Aust,* **2**, 819-22.

Gray N.J. and Hill D.J. (1977). Patterns of tobacco smoking in Australia, 2. *Med J Aust,* **2**, 327-8.

Hill D. and Gray N. (1984). Australian patterns of tobacco smoking and related health beliefs in 1983. *Community Health Studies,* **VIII**, 307-16.

Hill D., White V. and Segan C. (1995). Prevalence of cigarette smoking among Australian secondary school students in 1993. *Aust J Public Health,* **19**, 445-9.

Hill D.J. and Gray N.J. (1982). Patterns of tobacco smoking in Australia. *Med J Aust,* 23-5.

Hill D.J. and White V.M. (1995). Australian adult smoking prevalence in 1992. *Aust J Public Health,* **19**, 305-8.

Hill D.J., White V.M. and Gray N.J. (1988). Measures of tobacco smoking in Australia 1974-1986 by means of a standard method. *Med J Aust,* **149**, 10-2.

Hill D.J., White V.M. and Gray N.J. (1991). Australian patterns of tobacco smoking in 1989. *Med J Aust,* **154**, 797-801.

Hill D.J., White V.M., Pain M.D. and Gardner G.J. (1990). Tobacco and alcohol use among Australian secondary schoolchildren in 1987. *Med J Aust,* **152**, 124-30.

Hill D.J., White V.M. and Scollo M.M. (1998). Smoking behaviours of Australian adults in 1995: trends and concerns. *Med J Aust,* **168**, 209-13.

Hill D.J., White V.M., Williams R.M. and Gardner G.J. (1993). Tobacco and alcohol use among Australian secondary school students in 1990. *Med J Aust,* **158**, 228-34.

Hill D.J., Willcox S., Gardner G. and Houston J. (1987). Tobacco and alcohol use among Australian secondary schoolchildren. *Med J Aust,* **146**, 125-30.

Jones R. (1993). *Drug use and exposure in the Australian community*. Commonwealth of Australia. (Australian National Campaign Against Drug Abuse, National Household Survey Report, Volume 1.)

Lee P.N. (ed) (1975). *Tobacco consumption in various countries,* 4th edition. Tobacco Research Council, London. Research Paper 6.

Maxwell J.C. (successive years). How the brands ranked, Maxwell international estimates. *World Tobacco.*

McNair Anderson Associates Pty Ltd (1972-1979). *Prime prospect profiles.*[§]

National Health and Medical Research Council (1969). Smoking habits and attitudes of Australian schoolchildren, 1967-1968. In: *Report of the 68th session of the NHMRC, Brisbane.*[§]

National Health and Medical Research Council (1979). *Smoking habits of Australian schoolchildren.* Australian Government Publishing Service, Canberra.

National Heart Foundation of Australia (1980). *Risk factor prevalence study, report 1.* NHF, Canberra.[§]

National Heart Foundation of Australia (1983). *Risk factor prevalence study, report 2.* NHF, Canberra.

Quit Victoria: Victorian Smoking and Health Program (1995). *Tobacco in Australia: facts and issues*. Quit Victoria, Carlton South, Victoria. http://www.peg.apc.org/~vshp/.

Risk Factor Prevalence Study Management Committee (1990). *Risk factor prevalence study. Survey No.3, 1989.* National Heart Foundation of Australia and Australian Institute of Health, Canberra.

RP6, See Beese (1968), Beese (1972), Lee (1975)

Todd G.F. (ed) (1963). *Cigarette smoking characteristics in the UK, South Africa and Australia.* Tobacco Research Council, London. Research Paper 5.

USDA Economic Research Service (1996). *Tobacco statistics*. Albert R. Mann Library, Cornell University, Ithaca, New York. ERS 94012. http://usda.mannlib.cornell.edu/data-sets/specialty/94012.

WHO (1989). The WHO MONICA project: a worldwide monitoring system for cardiovascular diseases. In: *World health statistics annual 1989.* WHO, Geneva; 25-149.

WHO MONICA Project (1988). Geographical variation in the major risk factors of coronary heart disease in men and women aged 35-64 years. *World Health Stat Q,* **41**, 115-40.

Woodward S.D. (1984). Trends in cigarette consumption in Australia. *Aust N Z J Med,* **14**, 405-7.

§ Original paper not obtained, but information taken as quoted by another author

Austria 2

Sales data

See Tables 2.1-2.3.

Sales data are available from 1923. In the 1920s and 1930s the consumption of manufactured cigarettes per adult remained fairly stable, varying around 2-3 cigarettes per day. After an increase around the beginning of the Second World War, consumption fell sharply to about 1 cigarette per day in 1946. Consumption then rose steadily until the late 1970s when it reached around 7 cigarettes per day, then fell, dropping below 6 cigarettes per day by the mid 1990s.

Our estimates of hand-rolled cigarette consumption, based on all sales of cigarette tobacco, show that consumption of hand-rolled cigarettes per adult fell from around 1 cigarette per day in 1923 to 0.3 in 1933, but rose again to the same level during the Second World War. Since then consumption has been very low. These estimates may be too high, since in Germany, comparison of sales of fine-cut (cigarette) tobacco with sales of cigarette paper suggest that only about 70% of cigarette tobacco was used for hand-rolled cigarettes (see also *Notes on sources of sales data*, p. 43).

The consumption of all tobacco products combined followed a similar trend to that of manufactured cigarettes, but the post-war increase was slower, so that the 1920s level of 6 g per adult per day was not reached again until the mid-1960s. Consumption exceeded 7 g per adult per day between the mid-1970s and mid-1980s and fell to below 6 g by 1995. In 1925, 37% of all tobacco consumed was in manufactured cigarettes, increasing steadily to over 95% by 1975, by which time 90% of manufactured cigarettes were filtered.

Survey data

See Tables 2.4-2.8

National data on adult smoking are only available from 1972. Between 1972-1995, the prevalence of regular smoking among men aged 15 years and over remained about 35-39%, while among women it increased from about 10% to over 20%. Another 6-10% of men and 4-7% of women smoked occasionally. Earlier data relate only to Vienna, where the smoking prevalence in 1954 was substantially higher than the later national results.

Comparing the census results of 1972-1986, the prevalence of smoking increased among women in all age groups, particularly for ages 16-49. A decrease was seen for men aged 50 years and over. When reported separately by the census, smoking prevalence among older teenage boys was much higher than among girls. However, school-based surveys show little difference between the sexes among younger teenagers. The most recent survey reported a steep rise (from about 20% in 1984-1990 to 30% in 1994) in weekly smokers at age 15.

Comparison of survey and sales data suggests that surveys under-reported consumption by about 40% in the 1970s, but as survey-based reports showed little signs of decline while sales were falling, this changed gradually to an over-reporting by 1995. Since 1972, the estimated number of cigarettes smoked per person per day (sales-adjusted) has fallen from about 12 to about 8 for men and increased from 2 to 4 for women.

Table 2.1.1 Total annual sales of tobacco products, 1923-1973

Year	Cigarettes		Cigars		Cigarette tobacco	Pipe tobacco	Chewing tobacco	Snuff	All tobacco products
	tonnes	millions	tonnes	millions	tonnes	tonnes	tonnes	tonnes	tonnes
1923	3180	2935	730	158	1680	3950	230	140	9890
1924	3860	3741	910	205	1410	3990	270	140	10570
1925	4040	3973	950	216	1360	3900	320	140	10700
1926	4450	4395	910	204	1320	3860	320	140	10980
1927	4540	4512	860	201	1410	3580	360	140	10890
1928	4760	4800	910	209	1450	3400	410	140	11070
1929	4760	4925	910	207	1540	3220	410	140	10980
1930	4670	4809	910	206	1590	3180	360	140	10840
1931	4810	4940	770	175	1180	3130	360	140	10390
1932	5170	5512	640	144	730	2990	360	90	9980
1933	4850	5102	540	122	640	3040	360	90	9530
1934	4450	4658	450	107	730	3220	320	90	9250
1935	4260	4452	450	104	860	3080	270	90	9030
1936	4170	4332	450	106	1090	3080	270	90	9160
1937	4040	4211	450	103	1090	3040	270	90	8980
1938	4810	5004	540	129	1180	2950	270	90	9840
1939	6400	6395	640	157	1180	2860	230	50	11340
1940	7800	7810	680	175	1410	2990	320	90	13290
1941	9250	9249	730	176	1680	3490	410	90	15650
1942	8570	8561	590	147	1540	3310	360	50	14420
1943	8160	8168	500	121	1860	2450	320	50	13340
1944	6530	6510	360	94	1450	2040	140	50	10570
1945	2540	2554	140	37	540	450	50	0	3720
1946	2220	2244	230	62	50	230	50	0	2770
1947	2860	3136	270	57	0	230	50	0	3400
1948	3860	3923	360	72	0	410	50	50	4720
1949	4760	4781	320	60	0	1270	90	50	6490
1950	5940	5953	270	58	90	1360	140	50	7850
1951	6620	6609	320	66	140	1320	140	50	8570
1952	6890	6913	320	72	180	1180	90	50	8710
1953	7120	7132	320	76	180	1130	90	0	8850
1954	6350	6329	320	77	180	1040	90	0	7980
1955	7170	7144	360	85	180	1000	90	0	8800
1956	7940	7918	410	89	180	910	90	0	9530
1957	8350	8349	360	94	180	860	50	0	9800
1958	8800	8899	360	98	180	820	50	0	10210
1959	9210	9295	360	98	180	770	50	0	10570
1960	9480	9451	360	96	180	730	50	0	10800
1961	9620	9284	360	101	180	730	50	0	10930
1962	9710	9719	590	103	180	680	50	0	11200
1963	10120	10101	450	91	180	640	50	0	11430
1964	10430	10436	410	86	180	640	50	0	11700
1965	10840	10827	410	85	180	590	50	0	12070
1966	11520	11507	410	83	180	640	50	0	12790
1967	11790	11771	410	82	180	640	50	0	13060
1968	12020	11982	410	80	180	590	0	0	13200
1969	12430	12379	410	84	140	500	0	0	13470
1970	13060	13037	410	80	140	450	0	0	14060
1971	13610	13603	410	77	90	410	0	0	14510
1972	13470	13451	410	69	90	320	0	0	14290
1973	14510	14499	360	68	90	320	0	0	15290

Source: see *Notes on sources of sales data*, p. 43

Table 2.1.2 Total annual sales of tobacco products, 1974-1995

Year	Cigarettes tonnes	Cigarettes millions	Cigars tonnes	Cigars millions	Fine-cut tobacco tonnes	Pipe tobacco tonnes	Chewing tobacco tonnes	Snuff tonnes	All tobacco products tonnes
1974	14419	14419	347	63	67	286	9	6	15134
1975	13975	13975	325	59	60	257	9	5	14631
1976	14415	14415	314	57	54	240	9	6	15038
1977	14705	14705	297	54	52	231	6	7	15298
1978	15127	15127	286	52	46	223	2	6	15690
1979	15670	15670	281	51	45	211	2	6	16215
1980	15515	15515	275	50	52	204	2	7	16055
1981	15721	15721	264	48	65	202	1	8	16261
1982	15540	15540	237	43	96	200	1	8	16082
1983	15878	15878	220	40	115	188	1	8	16410
1984	15550	15550	209	38	136	180	1	8	16084
1985	15645	15645	204	37	135	168	1	7	16160
1986	15645	15645	193	35	146	151		8	16143
1987	15233	15233	187	34	146	140		7	15713
1988	14496	14496	182	33	147	129		8	14962
1989	14079	14079	182	33	149	119		8	14537
1990	14401	14401	176	32	152	114		8	14851
1991	14737	14737	171	31	153	112		9	15182
1992	14319	14319	165	30	155	107		9	14755
1993	13782	13782	160	29	156	100		10	14208
1994	14077	14077	154	28	162	94		10	14497
1995	13245	13245	160	29	163	89		10	13667

Source : see *Notes on sources of sales data*, p. 43

Table 2.1.3 Manufactured cigarettes (i) percentage of total sales as filter cigarettes, 1960-1981, (ii) sales-weighted average tar yield per cigarette (SWAT), 1960-1984, and (iii) sales-weighted average nicotine yield per cigarette (SWAN), 1960-1983

Year	% Filter	SWAT mg / cig	SWAN mg / cig
1960	8.8	33.67	1.95
1961		36.51	1.73
1962	35.0	32.38	1.26
1963	41.0	30.91	1.85
1964	44.6	26.83	1.33
1965	47.5	27.32	1.34
1966	53.7	23.73	1.04
1967	60.0	21.57	1.06
1968	66.6	22.26	1.02
1969	71.4	22.25	0.96
1970	75.7	21.50	0.95
1971	79.2	19.50	0.93
1972	82.1	18.40	0.86
1973	84.9	18.10	0.83
1974	87.0	18.70	
1975	88.9	18.30	0.75
1976	90.9	16.30	
1977	92.6	15.30	
1978	93.6	14.60	
1979	94.4	14.10	
1980	95.1	14.40	0.70
1981	96.0	12.90	
1982		12.80	0.65
1983		12.70	0.65
1984		12.80	

Source : see *Notes on sources of sales data*, p. 43

Table 2.2 Consumption of (i) cigarettes and (ii) all tobacco products, 1923-1995 sales-based data, including estimated hand-rolled cigarette consumption. Males and females aged 15 years and over

Year	Manufactured cigarettes		Hand-rolled cigarettes		Total cigarettes		All tobacco products	
	Total annual in millions	Number/ adult/day	Total annual in millions	Number/ adult/day	Total annual in millions	Number/ adult/day	Total annual in tonnes	Grams/ adult/day
1923	2935	1.6	1680	0.9	4615	2.6	9890	5.5
1924	3741	2.1	1410	0.8	5151	2.9	10570	5.9
1925	3973	2.2	1360	0.8	5333	3.0	10700	6.0
1926	4395	2.4	1320	0.7	5715	3.1	10980	6.0
1927	4512	2.5	1410	0.8	5922	3.2	10890	6.0
1928	4800	2.6	1450	0.8	6250	3.4	11070	5.9
1929	4925	2.6	1540	0.8	6465	3.5	10980	5.9
1930	4809	2.6	1590	0.9	6399	3.4	10840	5.8
1931	4940	2.7	1180	0.6	6120	3.3	10390	5.6
1932	5512	3.0	730	0.4	6242	3.4	9980	5.4
1933	5102	2.7	640	0.3	5742	3.1	9530	5.1
1934	4658	2.5	730	0.4	5388	2.8	9250	4.9
1935	4452	2.3	860	0.5	5312	2.8	9030	4.8
1936	4332	2.2	1090	0.6	5422	2.8	9160	4.7
1937	4211	2.2	1090	0.6	5301	2.7	8980	4.6
1938	5004	2.6	1180	0.6	6184	3.2	9840	5.1
1939	6395	3.3	1180	0.6	7575	3.9	11340	5.9
1940	7810	4.0	1410	0.7	9220	4.8	13290	6.9
1941	9249	4.8	1680	0.9	10929	5.6	15650	8.1
1942	8561	4.4	1540	0.8	10101	5.2	14420	7.5
1943	8168	4.2	1860	1.0	10028	5.2	13340	6.9
1944	6510	3.4	1450	0.7	7960	4.1	10570	5.5
1945	2554	1.3	540	0.3	3094	1.6	3720	1.9
1946	2244	1.1	50	0.0	2294	1.1	2770	1.4
1947	3136	1.6	0	0.0	3136	1.6	3400	1.7
1948	3923	2.0	0	0.0	3923	2.0	4720	2.4
1949	4781	2.4	0	0.0	4781	2.4	6490	3.3
1950	5953	3.0	90	0.0	6043	3.1	7850	4.0
1951	6609	3.4	140	0.1	6749	3.5	8570	4.4
1952	6913	3.6	180	0.1	7093	3.6	8710	4.5
1953	7132	3.7	180	0.1	7312	3.8	8850	4.6
1954	6329	3.2	180	0.1	6509	3.3	7980	4.1
1955	7144	3.6	180	0.1	7324	3.7	8800	4.5
1956	7918	4.0	180	0.1	8098	4.1	9530	4.8
1957	8349	4.2	180	0.1	8529	4.3	9800	4.9
1958	8899	4.5	180	0.1	9079	4.6	10210	5.1
1959	9295	4.6	180	0.1	9475	4.7	10570	5.3
1960	9451	4.7	180	0.1	9631	4.8	10800	5.4
1961	9284	4.6	180	0.1	9464	4.7	10930	5.5
1962	9719	4.8	180	0.1	9899	4.9	11200	5.6
1963	10101	5.0	180	0.1	10281	5.1	11430	5.7
1964	10436	5.1	180	0.1	10616	5.2	11700	5.8
1965	10827	5.3	180	0.1	11007	5.4	12070	5.9
1966	11507	5.7	180	0.1	11687	5.7	12790	6.3
1967	11771	5.8	180	0.1	11951	5.9	13060	6.4
1968	11982	5.9	180	0.1	12162	6.0	13200	6.5
1969	12379	6.1	140	0.1	12519	6.2	13470	6.6

Table 2.2 *(continued)*

Year	Manufactured cigarettes		Hand-rolled cigarettes		Total cigarettes		All tobacco products	
	Total annual in millions	Number/ adult/day	Total annual in millions	Number/ adult/day	Total annual in millions	Number/ adult/day	Total annual in tonnes	Grams/ adult/day
1970	13037	6.4	140	0.1	13177	6.5	14060	6.9
1971	13603	6.6	90	0.0	13693	6.7	14510	7.1
1972	13451	6.5	90	0.0	13541	6.6	14290	6.9
1973	14499	7.0	90	0.0	14589	7.0	15290	7.4
1974	14419	6.9	67	0.0	14486	6.9	15134	7.2
1975	13975	6.6	60	0.0	14035	6.7	14631	7.0
1976	14415	6.8	54	0.0	14469	6.8	15038	7.1
1977	14705	6.9	52	0.0	14757	6.9	15298	7.2
1978	15127	7.0	46	0.0	15173	7.1	15690	7.3
1979	15670	7.2	45	0.0	15715	7.3	16215	7.5
1980	15515	7.1	52	0.0	15567	7.1	16055	7.4
1981	15721	7.2	65	0.0	15786	7.2	16261	7.4
1982	15540	7.1	96	0.0	15636	7.1	16082	7.3
1983	15878	7.1	115	0.1	15993	7.2	16410	7.4
1984	15550	6.9	136	0.1	15686	7.0	16084	7.2
1985	15645	6.9	135	0.1	15780	7.0	16160	7.2
1986	15645	6.9	146	0.1	15791	7.0	16143	7.1
1987	15233	6.7	146	0.1	15379	6.7	15713	6.9
1988	14496	6.3	147	0.1	14643	6.4	14962	6.5
1989	14079	6.1	149	0.1	14228	6.2	14537	6.3
1990	14401	6.2	152	0.1	14553	6.2	14851	6.4
1991	14737	6.3	153	0.1	14890	6.3	15182	6.4
1992	14319	6.0	155	0.1	14474	6.1	14755	6.2
1993	13782	5.7	156	0.1	13938	5.8	14208	5.9
1994	14077	5.8	162	0.1	14239	5.9	14497	6.0
1995	13245	5.5	163	0.1	13408	5.5	13667	5.6

Source : see *Notes on sources of sales data*, p. 43

Figure 2.1 Daily consumption of (i) manufactured and total number of cigarettes, and (ii) all tobacco products, 1923-1995.
Males and females aged 15 years and over. *Source:* see Table 2.2

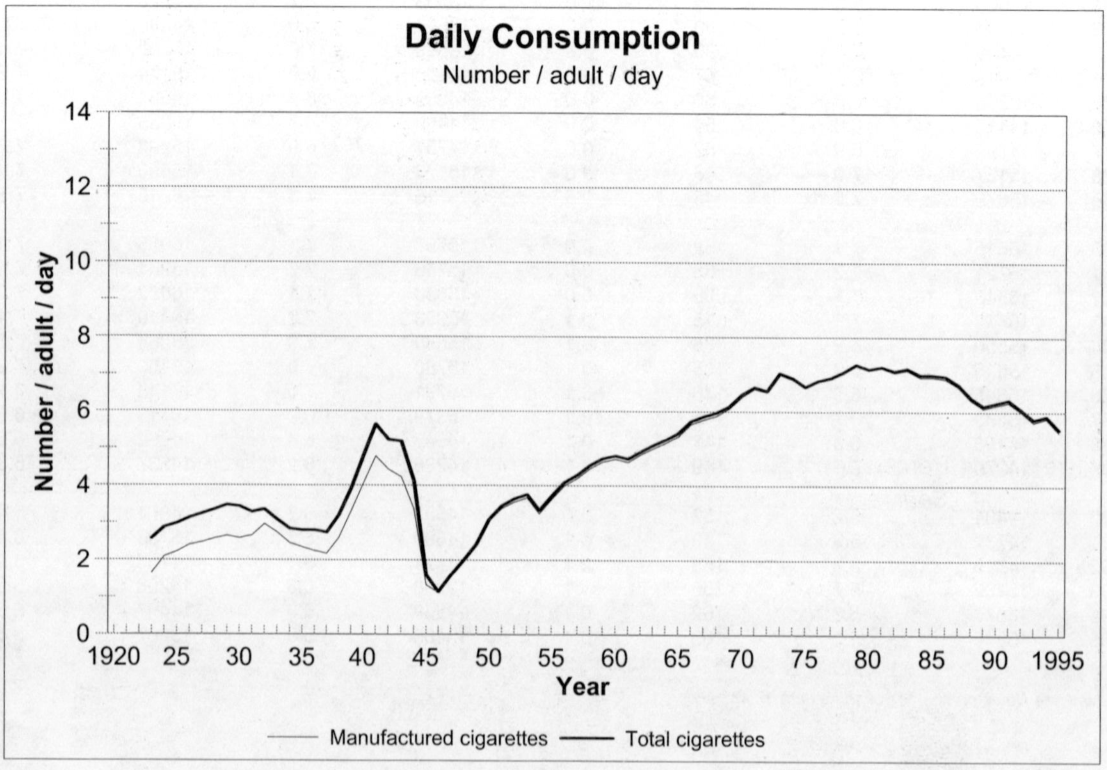

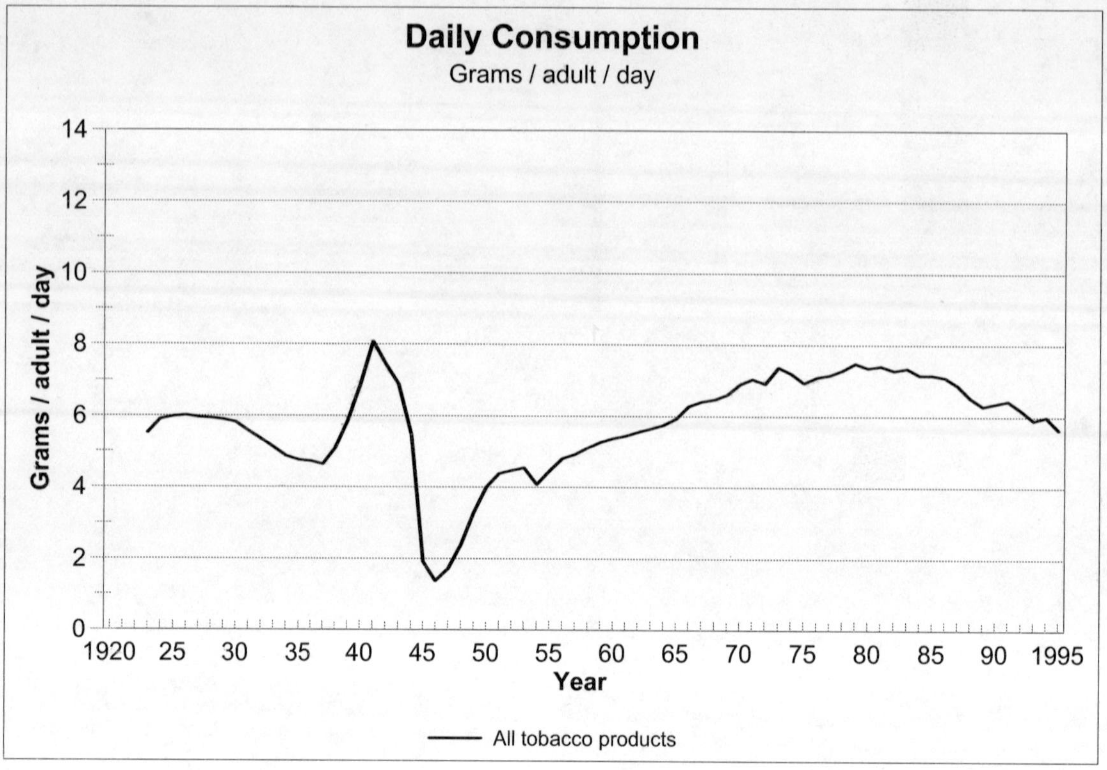

Table 2.3 Percentage sales of tobacco in different forms (by weight), selected years 1925-1995

Year	Cigarettes (%)	Cigars (%)	Cigarette / fine-cut tobacco (%)	Pipe tobacco (%)	Snuff and chewing tobacco (%)
1925	37.8	8.9	12.7	36.4	4.3
1935	47.2	5.0	9.5	34.1	4.0
1945	68.3	3.8	14.5	12.1	1.3
1955	81.5	4.1	2.0	11.4	1.0
1965	89.8	3.4	1.5	4.9	0.4
1975	95.5	2.2	0.4	1.8	0.1
1985	96.8	1.3	0.8	1.0	0.0
1995	96.9	1.2	1.2	0.7	0.1

Source : calculated from Tables 2.1.1 & 2.1.2

Figure 2.2 Percentage sales of tobacco in different forms (by weight), selected years 1925-1995
Source: see Table 2.3

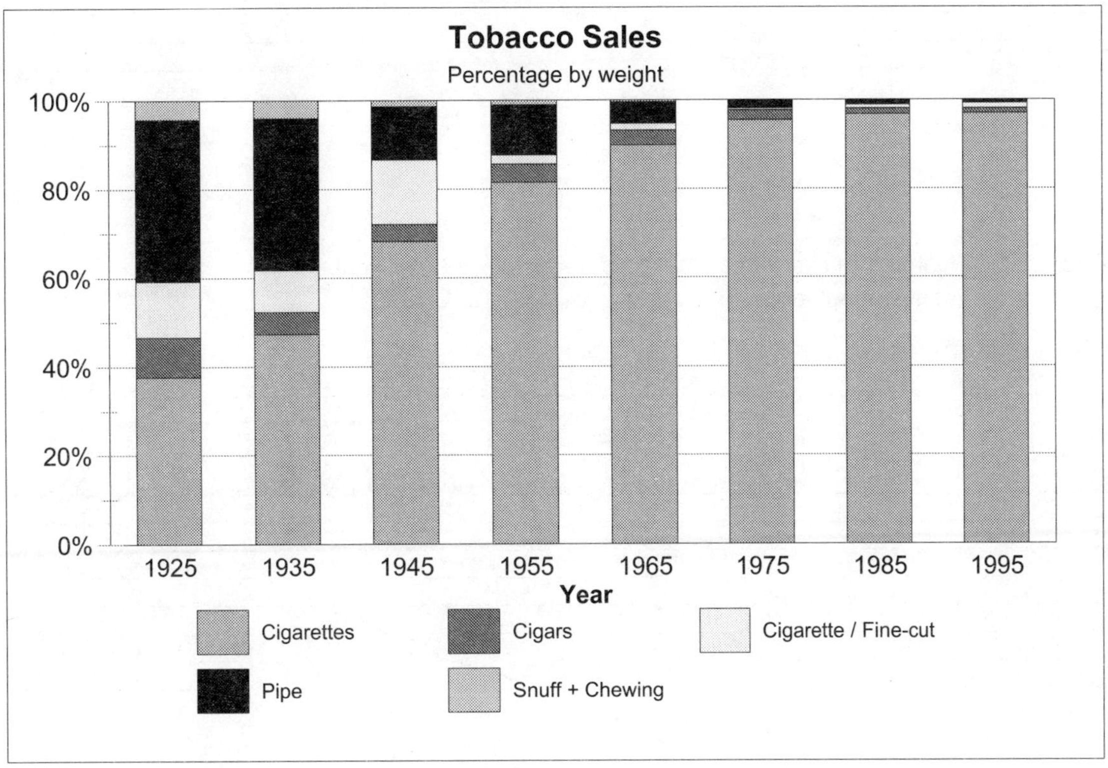

Table 2.4M Prevalence of smoking, males: some selected Austrian surveys by age, 1954-1995

Frequency / Product / Source / Year	12	13	14	15	16	17	18	19	20-24	25-29	30-34	35-39	40-44	45-49	50-54	55-59	60-64	65-69	70-74	75-79	80+	All ages
54 5 UC A				78																		
54 5 A A				83																		
72 1 UC R					36																	
72 1 A R					39																	
72 1 A A					43					56	49	44	49		46		42					45
77 3 A R				37							35				32							35
77 3 A A				51							46				39							45
78 2 UC R					41						36				39		36					38
78 2 UC A					60						42				44		39					47
79 1 UC R					34																	
79 1 A R					35																	
79 1 UC A					39																	
79 1 A A					25		43		51	53	51	46	40	40	42	38	33	33	34	25		41
81 4 UC U					39						33				29							33
83 6 U R		6		17																		
86 1 A R					35																	
86 1 UC A					38																	
86 1 A A					21		39		47	52	53	47	47	36	34	35	31	27	27	22		40
86 6 U *		3		12																		
86 6 U R		7		18																		
86 6 U A		19		29																		
90 6 UC R		5		23																		
90 6 UC A		11		29																		
91 1 UC R				40							46				33		23			12		36
94 6 UC R		8		29																		
95 7 UC R				34						45		44		45		34		23				39
95 7 UC A				44						53		54		47		36		27				46

Table 2.5M Number of cigarettes smoked per smoker per day, males: some selected Austrian surveys by age, 1972-1995

Product / Source / Year	12	13	14	15	16	17	18	19	20-24	25-29	30-34	35-39	40-44	45-49	50-54	55-59	60-64	65-69	70-74	75-79	80+	All ages
72 1 UCE					18																	
78 2 UCE					22																	
79 1 UCE					21																	
81 4 UCE					19						23				21							21
86 1 UCE					20																	
91 1 UCE				17							21			22			20			17		20
95 7 UC				24																		

Source see *Notes on sources of survey data*, p. 43
Frequency: A = all smokers (including occasional)
R = regular or daily smokers
All ages relevant to ages used and as given in original source
U = unspecified
* = refer to *Notes on sources of survey data*, p. 43

Product: MC = manufactured cigarettes
TC = total cigarettes (including hand-rolled)
UC = cigarettes (type unspecified)
A = all products
E indicates mean estimated from percentage distribution (see also *Consumption category estimation*, p. xxxiv, and Appendix III, p. 789)

Table 2.4F Prevalence of smoking, females: some selected Austrian surveys by age, 1954-1995

Year Source Product Frequency	12	13	14	15	16	17	18	19	20-24	25-29	30-34	35-39	40-44	45-49	50-54	55-59	60-64	65-69	70-74	75-79	80+	All ages
54 5 UC A				26																		
54 5 A A				26																		
72 1 UC R					10																	
72 1 A R					10																	
72 1 A A					21					28	20	15	14		12		5					13
77 3 A R				24							14				7							14
77 3 A A				40							21				9							22
78 2 UC R					16						16				12		6					14
78 2 UC A					31						26				17		8					23
79 1 UC R					14																	
79 1 A R					14																	
79 1 UC A					17																	
79 1 A A					14		26		35	32	34	22	17	12	15	13	9	6	5	2		17
81 4 UC U					31						24				15							22
83 6 U R		4		19																		
86 1 A R					18																	
86 1 UC A					21																	
86 1 A A					15		27		37	38	35	31	30	18	14	12	10	9	6	3		21
86 6 U *		3		11																		
86 6 U R		6		17																		
86 6 U A		13		27																		
90 6 UC R		4		20																		
90 6 UC A		9		26																		
91 1 UC R				28							32			18			8			3		21
94 6 UC R		7		31																		
95 7 UC R				30						36		34		22		9		9				24
95 7 UC A				38						44		40		29		12		10				30

Table 2.5F Number of cigarettes smoked per smoker per day, females: some selected Austrian surveys by age, 1972-1995

Year Source Product	12	13	14	15	16	17	18	19	20-24	25-29	30-34	35-39	40-44	45-49	50-54	55-59	60-64	65-69	70-74	75-79	80+	All ages
72 1 UCE					13																	
78 2 UCE					17																	
79 1 UCE					15																	
81 4 UCE					13						15				15							14
86 1 UCE					15																	
91 1 UCE				13							16			17			16			11		15
95 7 UC				19																		

Source: see *Notes on sources of survey data*, p. 43
Frequency: A = all smokers (including occasional)
R = regular or daily smokers
All ages: relevant to ages used and as given in original source
U = unspecified
* = refer to *Notes on sources of survey data*, p. 43

Product: MC = manufactured cigarettes
TC = total cigarettes (including hand-rolled)
UC = cigarettes (type unspecified)
A = all products
E indicates mean estimated from percentage distribution (see also *Consumption category estimation*, p. xxxiv, and Appendix III, p. 789)

Table 2.6M Number of cigarettes smoked per person per day, males: some selected Austrian surveys by age, 1972-1995, with percentage total sales

<table>
<tr><th rowspan="2">Product
Source
Year</th><th colspan="21">Age group</th><th rowspan="2">All ages</th><th rowspan="2">% Total sales</th></tr>
<tr><th>12</th><th>13</th><th>14</th><th>15</th><th>16</th><th>17</th><th>18</th><th>19</th><th>20-24</th><th>25-29</th><th>30-34</th><th>35-39</th><th>40-44</th><th>45-49</th><th>50-54</th><th>55-59</th><th>60-64</th><th>65-69</th><th>70-74</th><th>75-79</th><th>80+</th></tr>
<tr><td>72 1 UC</td><td colspan="4"></td><td colspan="17">6.6</td><td></td><td>56%T</td></tr>
<tr><td>78 2 UC</td><td colspan="4"></td><td colspan="14">8.3</td><td colspan="3"></td><td></td><td>65%T</td></tr>
<tr><td>79 1 UC</td><td colspan="4"></td><td colspan="17">7.1</td><td></td><td>59%T</td></tr>
<tr><td>81 4 UC</td><td colspan="4"></td><td colspan="6">7.6</td><td colspan="4">7.5</td><td colspan="4">6.0</td><td colspan="3"></td><td>6.9</td><td>64%T</td></tr>
<tr><td>86 1 UC</td><td colspan="4"></td><td colspan="17">7.0</td><td></td><td>67%T</td></tr>
<tr><td>91 1 UC</td><td colspan="3"></td><td colspan="7">7.0</td><td colspan="3">9.5</td><td colspan="3">7.3</td><td colspan="3">4.5</td><td colspan="2">2.0</td><td>7.1</td><td>80%T</td></tr>
<tr><td>95 7 UC</td><td colspan="3"></td><td colspan="18">9.4</td><td></td><td>124%T</td></tr>
</table>

Table 2.7M Number of cigarettes smoked per person per day, sales-adjusted, males: some selected Austrian surveys[1] by age, 1972-1995, with percentage total sales

<table>
<tr><th rowspan="2">Product
Source
Year</th><th colspan="21">Age group</th><th rowspan="2">All ages</th><th rowspan="2">% Total sales</th></tr>
<tr><th>12</th><th>13</th><th>14</th><th>15</th><th>16</th><th>17</th><th>18</th><th>19</th><th>20-24</th><th>25-29</th><th>30-34</th><th>35-39</th><th>40-44</th><th>45-49</th><th>50-54</th><th>55-59</th><th>60-64</th><th>65-69</th><th>70-74</th><th>75-79</th><th>80+</th></tr>
<tr><td>72 1 UC</td><td colspan="4"></td><td colspan="17">12</td><td></td><td>56%T</td></tr>
<tr><td>78 2 UC</td><td colspan="4"></td><td colspan="14">13</td><td colspan="3"></td><td></td><td>65%T</td></tr>
<tr><td>79 1 UC</td><td colspan="4"></td><td colspan="17">12</td><td></td><td>59%T</td></tr>
<tr><td>81 4 UC</td><td colspan="4"></td><td colspan="6">12</td><td colspan="4">12</td><td colspan="4">9.4</td><td colspan="3"></td><td>11</td><td>64%T</td></tr>
<tr><td>86 1 UC</td><td colspan="4"></td><td colspan="17">11</td><td></td><td>67%T</td></tr>
<tr><td>91 1 UC</td><td colspan="3"></td><td colspan="7">8.8</td><td colspan="3">12</td><td colspan="3">9.2</td><td colspan="3">5.7</td><td colspan="2">2.5</td><td>9.0</td><td>80%T</td></tr>
<tr><td>95 7 UC</td><td colspan="3"></td><td colspan="18">7.6</td><td></td><td>124%T</td></tr>
</table>

1 Based on those surveys in Table 2.6 with data for both sexes and age range at least 21-64 (see *Cigarette consumption per person*, p. xxxv)

Source: see *Notes on sources of survey data*, p. 43
All ages: relevant to ages used and as given in original source
% Total sales: estimated % of total sales of M = manufactured or T = total cigarette consumption implied by survey, sexes combined, used as adjustment factor in Table 2.7
** = cannot be calculated
--- = adjusted by original author

Product: MC = manufactured cigarettes
TC = total cigarettes (including hand-rolled)
UC = cigarettes (type unspecified)
A = all products
U = unspecified
* = refer to *Notes on sources of survey data*, p. 43

Table 2.6F Number of cigarettes smoked per person per day, females: some selected Austrian surveys by age, 1972-1995, with percentage total sales

Product Source Year	Age group 12	13	14	15	16	17	18	19	20-24	25-29	30-34	35-39	40-44	45-49	50-54	55-59	60-64	65-69	70-74	75-79	80+	All ages	% Total sales
72 1 UC					1.3																		56%T
78 2 UC					2.3																		65%T
79 1 UC					2.0																		59%T
81 4 UC					3.9						3.5				2.2							3.1	64%T
86 1 UC					2.7																		67%T
91 1 UC				3.8							5.1			3.0			1.2			0.4		3.1	80%T
95 7 UC				4.5																			124%T

Table 2.7F Number of cigarettes smoked per person per day, sales-adjusted, females: some selected Austrian surveys[1] by age, 1972-1995, with percentage total sales

Product Source Year	Age group 12	13	14	15	16	17	18	19	20-24	25-29	30-34	35-39	40-44	45-49	50-54	55-59	60-64	65-69	70-74	75-79	80+	All ages	% Total sales
72 1 UC					2.3																		56%T
78 2 UC					3.5																		65%T
79 1 UC					3.5																		59%T
81 4 UC					6.1						5.5				3.5							4.9	64%T
86 1 UC					4.0																		67%T
91 1 UC				4.7							6.4			3.8			1.6			0.5		3.9	80%T
95 7 UC				3.6																			124%T

1 Based on those surveys in Table 2.6 with data for both sexes and age range at least 21-64 (see *Cigarette consumption per person*, p. xxxv)

Source: see *Notes on sources of survey data*, p. 43
All ages: relevant to ages used and as given in original source
% Total sales: estimated % of total sales of M = manufactured or T = total cigarette consumption implied by survey, sexes combined, used as adjustment factor in Table 2.7
** = cannot be calculated
--- = adjusted by original author

Product: MC = manufactured cigarettes
TC = total cigarettes (including hand-rolled)
UC = cigarettes (type unspecified)
A = all products
U = unspecified
* = refer to *Notes on sources of survey data*, p. 43

Table 2.8 Estimated[1] prevalence of smoking and estimated[1] number of cigarettes per person per day (unadjusted and sales-adjusted): summary of Tables 2.4, 2.6 and 2.7, 1954-1995. Males and females aged 15 years and over

Year	Source[2]	Product[3]	Prevalence[4]						Number of cigarettes						
									Unadjusted[7]			Sales-adjusted[8]			
			Manufactured cigarettes		Total cigarettes[5]		All products[6]		Number/ person/day		Total sales %	Manufactured cigarettes number/ person/day		Total cigarettes[9] number/ person/day	
			M	F	M	F	M	F	M	F		M	F	M	F
1954	5	**UC+A**			77	26	83	26						(5.6	1.5)
1972	1	UC+A			36	10	38	10	6.5	1.3	56			11.7	2.3
	1	**A**					45	14							
1977	3	A					35	13							
	3	**A**					45	21							
1978	2	UC			37	12			7.6	2.1	65			11.6	3.2
	2	**UC**			45	20									
1979	1	UC+A			33	13	35	13	6.9	2.0	59			11.8	3.4
	1	**UC+A**			38	17	41	17							
1981	4	*UC*			33	20			6.6	2.8	64			10.4	4.4
1986	1	A					34	17							
	1	**UC+A**			37	21	39	21	6.9	2.6	67			10.3	4.0
1991	1	UC			36	21			7.2	3.1	80			9.0	3.9
1995	7	UC			39	23			9.4	4.5	124			7.6	3.6
	7	**UC**			45	29									

1 Surveys covering an age range of at least 21-64 are included. Any gaps in the data for ages 15-20 and 65 years and over are filled in by assumed extensions to the age distribution, given in Notes on sources of survey data, p. 43. Method: see Summary of adult smoking, p. xxxvi
2 See Notes on sources of survey data, p. 43
3 Product: MC = manufactured cigarettes, TC = total cigarettes (including hand-rolled), UC = cigarettes (type unspecified), A = all products, U = unspecified. Frequency of smoking is indicated by: regular or daily smokers in normal type, all smokers (including occasional) in bold, unspecified in italics
4 From Table 2.4
5 This column includes prevalence of smoking classified as UC = cigarettes (type unspecified)
6 This column includes prevalence of smoking classified as U = unspecified product
7 From Table 2.6
8 From Table 2.7, except data in parentheses, which are derived from the prevalence of smoking from Table 2.4 as described in Summary of adult smoking, p. xxxvi
9 Number of cigarettes classified as UC = cigarettes (type unspecified) has been adjusted to total cigarette sales and included in this column

Figure 2.3 Estimated prevalence of smoking of (i) cigarettes and (ii) all tobacco products: by year of survey, 1954-1995.
Males and females aged 15 years and over. *Source:* see Table 2.8

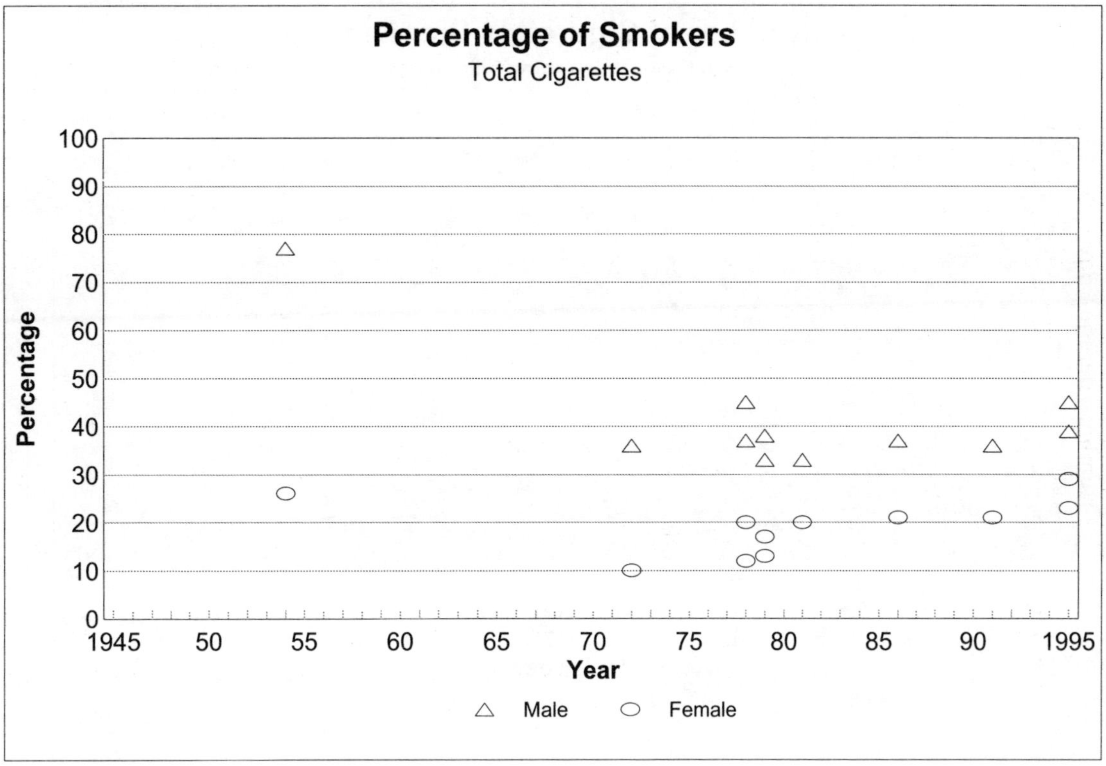

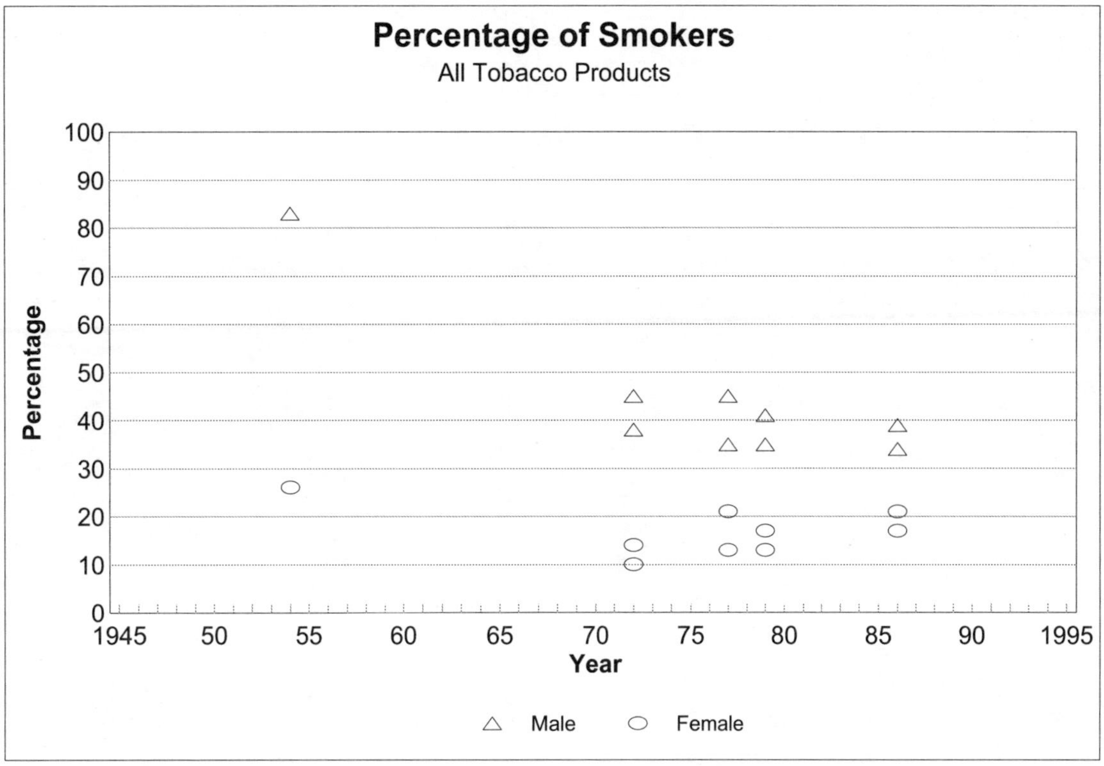

Figure 2.4 Estimated number of cigarettes smoked per person per day, sales-adjusted, 1954-1995.
Males and females aged 15 years and over. *Source:* see Table 2.8

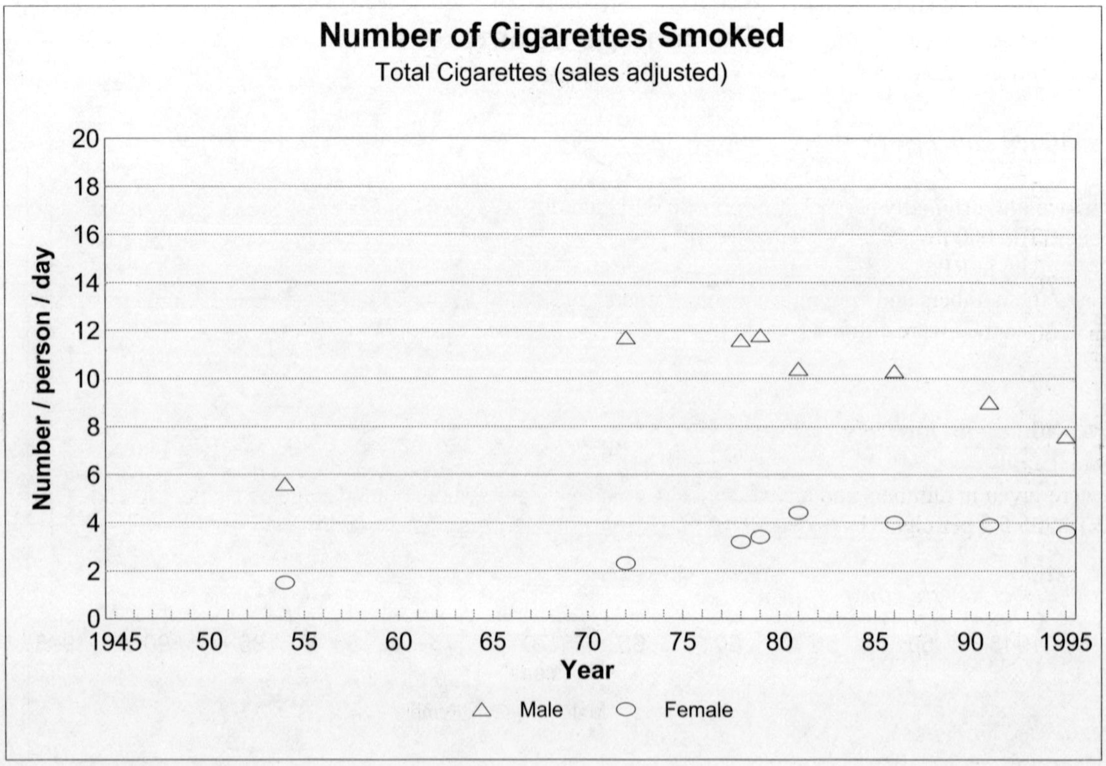

Notes

Notes on sources of sales data

The data presented in the tables and figures were obtained from several sources, details of which are given below, together with estimations and related assumptions. Full citations of the sources are given on p. 45 under *References*.

Consumption data before 1974
RP6
Data by weight, originally given to nearest 100 000 pounds, have been converted to tonnes and given to nearest 10 tonnes (100 000 lbs = 45.359 tonnes).
Notes as given in RP6:
Details of the numbers and weight of cigarettes and cigars and of the weight of other manufactured tobacco products consumed were either provided by the Austrian Tobacco Monopoly or obtained from the annual reports of the Monopoly.

Consumption data for 1974 onwards
Austria Tabak
Data were given in numbers and have been converted to weight assuming an average of 1 g per cigarette (Austria Tabak) and 5.5 g per cigar (based on 1970-1973 values in RP6).

Plain/Filter cigarette consumption
1960 Klus and Kuhn (1978)
1962-1981 Maxwell (successive years)

Tar yield of cigarettes
1960-1969 Flamm *et al* (1975)
1970-1984 Austria Tabak
The tar yield per cigarette is limited to 15 mg (Harkin *et al* (1997)).

Nicotine yield of cigarettes
1960-1973 Flamm *et al* (1975)
1975-1983 Klus (1986)

Estimates of hand-rolled cigarette consumption for 1923-1985
We have taken as our estimate of hand-rolled cigarette consumption all sales of cigarette tobacco, at 1 g per cigarette.
This may be an overestimate; in Germany, where sales of cigarette papers are also known, we have used 70% of fine-cut (cigarette) tobacco as our estimate of hand-rolled cigarette consumption.

Notes on sources of survey data

Each source of survey data—either an individual survey or a series of surveys repeated over a number of years—is cited by a source number. This number is shown in the tables and corresponds to the source numbers given below, where details of the source publication and of the survey methodology are given. Full citations of the sources are given on p. 45 under *References*.

Source number

1 **Friedl (1980a, 1980b, 1987), Österreichischen Statistischen Zentralamt (1996)**

a. Mikrozensus for Austrian Central Statistical Office

b. Consumption category estimation based on 1-10, 11-20, 21-40, and 41+ cigarettes/smoker/day

c. Assumed extension to age distribution for percentage smokers of all tobacco and of unspecified cigarettes, age 15: males 20% and females 10%. Number of cigarettes/person/day: males 1.0 and females (1972-1979) 0.5, (1986) 1.0

2 **Gredler *et al* (1981)**

a. Survey on behalf of the Austrian Heart Foundation. Sample size 2 002

b. Consumption category estimation based on 1-10, 11-20, 21-40, and 41+ cigarettes/smoker/day

c. Assumed extension to age distribution for percentage smokers, age 15: males 20% and females 10%. Number of cigarettes/person/day: males 1.0 and females 0.5. For age 70+: males 30% and females 4%. Number of cigarettes/person/day: males 3.0 and females 1.0

3 **Kunze *et al* (1980)**

a. Study for Bundesministeriums für Gesundheit und Umweltschutz. Lowest age limit not stated

b. 99% of smokers smoked cigarettes

4 **Gredler and Kunze (1981)**

a. Part of survey assessing public awareness and attitudes to a national anti-smoking campaign. Sample size 2 004, representative sample

b. Consumption category estimation based on 1-10, 11-20, and 21+ cigarettes/smoker/day

c. Assumed extension to age distribution for percentage smokers, age 15: males 20% and females 10%. Number of cigarettes/person/day: males and females 1.0. For age 70+: males 30% and females 4%. Number of cigarettes/person/day: males 3.0 and females 1.0

5 **Ossadnik (1955)**

a. Survey of smoking habits of adults in Vienna, partly by questionnaire, partly by interviews. Sample sizes, questionnaires (males) 2 883, (females) 3 643; interviews (males) 340, (females) 370

6 **Aarø *et al* (1986), Nutbeam and Aarø (1990), King and Coles (1992), King *et al* (1996)**

a. Part of the HBSC (Health Behaviour in School-Aged Children) Study, a collaborative cross-national research study sponsored by the WHO. School classes or schools were randomly selected, targeting age groups 11 (not presented here), 13 and 15. The target sample size was 1 300 in each age group.

Year	Mean age				Sample size		
	Target age 13		Target age 15		Target age 13	Target age 15	Total
	Boys	Girls	Boys	Girls			
1983-1984	13.0	12.9	14.8	14.8			3 083
1986-1987						857	
1990	13.3		15.2				2 984
1994	13.3		15.2		1 788	1 815	

b. Regular smokers: smoke once a week or more. Smokers marked as frequency *: smoked daily

7 **Haidinger *et al* (1998)**

a. Survey funded by the Austrian Cancer Society using a representative sample of Austrians. Sample size 2 065

References

Aarø L.E., Wold B., Kannas L. and Rimpelä M. (1986). Health behaviour in school children. A WHO cross-national survey. *Health Promotion,* **1**, 17-33.

Beese D.H. (ed) (1968). *Tobacco consumption in various countries,* 2nd edition. Tobacco Research Council, London. Research Paper 6.

Beese D.H. (ed) (1972). *Tobacco consumption in various countries,* 3rd edition. Tobacco Research Council, London. Research Paper 6.

Flamm H., Kunze M. and Kunze M.J. (1975). *Smoking and health in Austria. State of affairs in July 1975,* 2nd edition.

Friedl H.P. (1980a). Rauchgewohnheiten der Österreichischen Bevölkerung. *Statistische Nachrichten,* **35**, 508-9.

Friedl H.P. (1980b). Rauchgewohnheiten der Österreichischen Bevölkerung; Ergebnisse des Mikrozensus September 1979, Teil 2. *Statistische Nachrichten,* **35**, 584-6.

Friedl H.P. (1987). Rauchgewohnheiten der Österreichischen Bevölkerung; Ergebnisse des Mikrozensus September 1986. *Statistische Nachrichten,* **42**, 328-32.

Gredler B. and Kunze M. (1981). Impact of a national campaign on smoking attitudes and patterns in Austria. *International Journal of Health Education,* **24**, 271-9.

Gredler B., Vutuc Ch. and Kunze M. (1981). Rauchkondensat-Exposition der österreichischen Zigarettenraucher (Exposure to tar of Austrian cigarette smokers). *Praxis der Pneumologie Vereinigt mit der Tuberkulosearzt,* **35**, 76-8.

Haidinger G., Waldhoer T. and Vutuc C. (1998). The prevalence of smoking in Austria. *Prev Med,* **27** , 50-5.

Harkin A.M., Anderson P. and Goos C. (1997). *Smoking, drinking and drug taking in the European Region.* Alcohol, Drugs and Tobacco Programme, WHO Regional Office for Europe, Copenhagen.

King A., Wold B., Tudor-Smith C. and Harel Y. (1996). *The health of youth, a cross-national survey.* WHO Regional Publications, Europe, Copenhagen. European Series No. 69.

King A.J.C. and Coles B. (1992). *The health of Canada's youth. Views and behaviours of 11-, 13- and 15-year-olds from 11 countries*. Health and Welfare Canada, Ottawa.

Klus H. (1986). Low-tar cigarettes—possibilities and limitations. In: Zaridze D.G. and Peto R. (eds) *Tobacco, a major international health hazard. Proceedings of an international meeting organized by the IARC and co-sponsored by the All-Union Cancer Research Centre of the Academy of Medical Sciences of the USSR, held in Moscow, 4-6 June 1985*. IARC, Lyon; 265-81. Scientific Publication No.74.

Klus H. and Kuhn H. (1978). Die Reduktion der Rauchwerte von Zigaretten und ihre Annahme durch den Konsumenten in Österreich. *Fachliche Mitteilungen Tabakwerke,* **18**, 376-88.

Kunze M., Gredler B., Herberg D., Kunze M.J., Schoberberger R. and Vutuc Ch. (1980). Rauchen und Gesundheit in Österreich (Smoking and health in Austria), Teil 1: Epidemiologie des Tabakkonsums in Österreich. *Offentliche Gesundheitswesen,* **42**, 993-9.

Lee P.N. (ed) (1975). *Tobacco consumption in various countries,* 4th edition. Tobacco Research Council, London. Research Paper 6.

Maxwell J.C.Jr. (successive years). How the brands ranked. Maxwell International Estimates. *World Tobacco.*

Nutbeam D. and Aarø L.E. (1990). Smoking and alienation from school: the implications for health education with young people. Results from the WHO study of health behaviour in schoolchildren. In: Durston B. and Jamrozik K. (eds) *Tobacco & health 1990. The global war. Seventh World Conference on Tobacco and Health, Perth, Western Australia, 1-5 April 1990*. Organising Committee of the Seventh World Conference on Tobacco and Health, 189 Royal Street, East Perth, Western Australia 6004; 539-44.

Ossadnik W. (1955). Tabakkonsum und Erkrankungen der Atmungsorgane. II Teil: Die Rauchergewohnheiten der Wiener Bovölkerung. *Statistische Vierteljahresschrift,* **8**, 163-88.

Österreichischen Statistischen Zentralamt (1996). *Gesundheitszustand der österreichischen Bevölkerung. Mikrozensus—December 1991*. Österreichischen Statistischen Zentralamt, Vienna.

RP6, See Beese (ed) (1968), Beese (ed) (1972), Lee (ed) (1975)

Belgium 3

Sales data

See Tables 3.1-3.3.

From 1921 to 1940 the consumption of manufactured cigarettes per adult was about 2 cigarettes per day. During the Second World War it fell to about 1 cigarette per day, but rapidly jumped to exceed pre-war levels in the late 1940s. Thereafter consumption rose until 1973, when it peaked at 7 cigarettes per day. It decreased to 4 by 1995. Our estimates suggest that consumption of hand-rolled cigarettes per adult fell from over 3 per day in the 1950s to about 1.5 in the late 1970s, but later estimates may be distorted by cross-border sales.

Apart from a sharp decline during the Second World War, the consumption per adult of all tobacco products combined varied between 8 and 10 g per day in the period 1921-1985 then decreased to about 6 g by 1995. In 1925, about 20 % of all tobacco consumed was in manufactured cigarettes. This proportion increased to 70% in 1975, but fell again to about 60% in 1995. 90% of manufactured cigarettes were filtered by 1990. The proportion of cigars and cigarillos remained around 10% between 1925 and 1995. No breakdown is available of the remaining category covering pipe and hand-rolling tobacco, chewing tobacco, and snuff, which still accounted for over 30% of all tobacco sales in 1995, including cross-border sales.

Survey data

See Tables 3.4-3.8

Data on adult smoking are available since 1955. In 1955, the estimated prevalence of tobacco smoking among those aged 15 years and over was 74% in men and 19% in women. The difference in the percentage of men and women who smoke has decreased since then, mainly because of a decrease in the prevalence among men to 31-33% in the 1990s. The percentages of men smoking manufactured cigarettes decreased from about 50% in 1972 to 35% in 1984; in 1980 another 9% of men smoked hand-rolled cigarettes only. The prevalence of smoking among women was shown by most surveys to be decreasing from about 25% in the mid-1970s to 21% in 1984, but another series of surveys put the level higher at 26-28% in the 1980s (source 17, see Table 3.8). Smoking of products other than manufactured cigarettes was negligible among women.

No direct trends of the prevalence of smoking by age are available, but in general the percentages of men smoking decreased in all age groups, declining more markedly among men aged 65 years and over. A lower percentage of smokers in older age groups was clear in women from the earliest surveys, and is now also occurring among men. Most surveys of teenagers continue to show more boys smoking than girls.

Comparison of survey and sales data was only possible in one case, where consumption was under-reported by about 25% (see Table 3.6). Between 1972 and 1986, the estimated number of manufactured cigarettes smoked per person per day (sales-adjusted) decreased for men from about 10 to 7 with a further 3 hand-rolled cigarettes per day; for women it remained around 4 to 5 cigarettes, based on source 17.

Table 3.1.1 Total annual sales of tobacco products, 1921-1973

Year	Cigarettes		Cigars		Cigarillos		Other tobacco	All tobacco products
	tonnes	millions	tonnes	millions	tonnes	millions	tonnes	tonnes
1921	3420	3421	1140	240	480	192	11610	16660
1922	3550	3546	1410	297	520	210	12610	18100
1923	3780	3775	1500	314	630	252	12970	18870
1924	4160	4155	1430	301	650	259	12970	19210
1925	4210	4207	1320	277	750	301	12880	19160
1926	4460	4457	1120	235	650	262	13290	19520
1927	4830	4829	1300	274	700	279	13200	20030
1928	5540	5540	1310	275	710	286	12840	20400
1929	6110	6108	1380	289	830	331	12610	20920
1930	6800	6799	1350	283	870	347	12470	21490
1931	6840	6838	1310	275	830	334	12700	21680
1932	5980	5982	1090	228	800	321	12700	20570
1933	5530	5525	970	203	890	357	12470	19860
1934	4980	4981	850	178	1030	412	12790	19650
1935	4960	4955	920	193	1280	511	12930	20080
1936	5120	5116	940	197	1450	580	13340	20840
1937	5260	5258	910	192	1460	584	12930	20560
1938	5110	5108	920	194	1540	615	13200	20770
1939	5130	5128	850	179	1390	556	14330	21700
1940	4150	4150	830	175	1070	429	11570	17620
1941	3720	3723	670	140	610	243	10610	15610
1942	3280	3284	500	105	540	218	8750	13080
1943	1890	1889	480	101	520	208	4400	7290
1944	2070	2070	360	75	450	181	3950	6830
1945	2560	2563	510	107	620	250	6080	9780
1946	6390	6386	600	125	750	302	10120	17850
1947	8550	8549	450	94	590	238	9840	19440
1948	8900	8901	410	87	650	260	9840	19810
1949	8420	8414	400	85	650	261	9980	19450
1950	8400	8399	400	83	650	261	9800	19250
1951	8200	8197	430	91	710	285	9660	19010
1952	8120	8115	590	123	960	383	10480	20140
1953	8220	8217	620	131	1110	445	10020	19980
1954	8260	8263	710	149	1270	510	9840	20090
1955	8650	8652	750	158	1340	537	9210	19960
1956	9130	9132	820	173	1440	577	9300	20700
1957	9860	9859	900	190	1490	596	9070	21330
1958	10480	10480	920	193	1400	561	8850	21650
1959	10310	10308	1030	217	1490	597	8750	21590
1960	10970	10973	1100	232	1620	647	8390	22090
1961	11250	11253	1220	257	1650	661	8210	22340
1962	11870	11868	1340	282	1830	732	7980	23030
1963	12330	12325	1270	267	1700	681	7530	22830
1964	12790	12791	1440	303	2070	829	7300	23610
1965	14090	14083	1510	317	2030	814	7030	24660
1966	15150	15147	1510	316	1820	730	6620	25100
1967	15450	15448	1420	299	1860	746	7620	26360
1968	15820	15814	1350	284	2000	801	6580	25750
1969	16640	16633	1360	285	1970	790	5990	25950
1970	17630	17632	1260	265	1870	749	5400	26170
1971	18340	18334	1360	285	2150	859	5170	27010
1972	19170	19165	1400	295	2230	891	4900	27700
1973	20240	20236	1430	301	2110	845	4670	28460

Source: see *Notes on sources of sales data*, p. 65

Table 3.1.2 Total annual sales of tobacco products, Belgium 1974-1995

Year	Cigarettes		Cigars		Cigarillos		Other tobacco	All tobacco products
	tonnes	millions	tonnes	millions	tonnes	millions	tonnes	tonnes
1974	20179	20179	1350	281	1983	793	4583	28095
1975	18868	18868	1307	272	2131	852	4594	26900
1976	18370	18370	1227	256	2184	874	4873	26654
1977	17673	17673	1166	243	2070	828	4985	25894
1978	15590	15590	1074	224	2079	832	4779	23522
1979	16878	16878	982	204	1893	757	4548	24301
1980	16858	16858	937	195	1924	769	4421	24140
1981	16657	16657	736	153	1730	692	4792	23915
1982	17927	17927	669	139	1682	673	6042	26320
1983	17033	17033	633	132	1735	694	6692	26093
1984	17178	17178	620	129	1697	679	7151	26646
1985	15897	15897	554	116	1711	684	7046	25208
1986	15485	15485	472	98	1549	620	6425	23931
1987	14507	14507	450	94	1528	611	5846	22331
1988	14903	14903	407	85	1513	605	5585	22408
1989	14184	14184					5387	
1990	13687	13687					4904	
1991	13966	13966					4899	
1992	13543	13543					5181	
1993	12556	12556					5129	
1994	12058	12058					5616	
1995	12373	12373	255	53	1387	555	7294	21309

Source: see *Notes on sources of sales data*, p. 65

Table 3.1.3 Total annual sales of tobacco products, UEBL, 1974-1994

Year	Cigarettes millions	Cigars millions	Cigarillos millions	Other tobacco[1] tonnes
1974	21200			
1975	20600			
1976	20200			
1977	19800			
1978	17900			
1979	19300			
1980	19500	204	809	4547
1981	19800			
1982	21800			
1983	21300			
1984	20900			
1985	19600	122	717	7387
1986	18900	104	650	6738
1987	17900	99	641	6124
1988	18200	90	632	5852
1989	17600	82	599	5367
1990	17500	73	600	4904
1991	17900	73	565	4899
1992	17700	67	514	5181
1993	16700	56	507	5129
1994	16200	57	554	5616

[1] Other tobacco: smoking tobacco, chewing tobacco and snuff
Source : see *Notes on sources of sales data*, p. 65

Table 3.1.4 Manufactured cigarettes (i) percentage of total sales as filter cigarettes, 1960-1991, and (ii) sales-weighted average tar yield per cigarette (SWAT), 1973-1993

Year	% Filter	SWAT mg / cig
1960	30.0	
1961	35.0	
1962	38.0	
1963	40.0	
1964	42.0	
1965	50.0	
1966	49.0	
1967	52.0	
1968	56.0	
1969	58.2	
1970	61.8	
1971	64.0	
1972	66.9	
1973	68.0	23.2
1974	72.2	
1975	75.1	
1976	77.2	
1977	77.9	
1978	76.6	
1979	80.3	
1980	81.6	16.5
1982	84.0	
1983	85.0	
1985		15.0
1991	90.0	
1993		15.0

Source : see *Notes on sources of sales data*, p. 65

Table 3.2 Consumption of (i) cigarettes and (ii) all tobacco products, 1921-1995 sales-based data, including estimated hand-rolled cigarette consumption. Males and females aged 15 years and over.

Year	Manufactured cigarettes		Hand-rolled cigarettes		Total cigarettes		All tobacco products	
	Total annual in millions	Number/ adult/day	Total annual in millions	Number/ adult/day	Total annual in millions	Number/ adult/day	Total annual in tonnes	Grams/ adult/day
1921	3421	1.6					16660	8.0
1922	3546	1.7					18100	8.7
1923	3775	1.8					18870	8.9
1924	4155	2.0					19210	9.1
1925	4207	2.0					19160	8.9
1926	4457	2.1					19520	9.1
1927	4829	2.2					20030	9.1
1928	5540	2.5					20400	9.2
1929	6108	2.7					20920	9.4
1930	6799	3.0					21490	9.5
1931	6838	3.0					21680	9.6
1932	5982	2.6					20570	8.9
1933	5525	2.4					19860	8.6
1934	4981	2.2					19650	8.5
1935	4955	2.2					20080	8.7
1936	5116	2.2					20840	8.9
1937	5258	2.2					20560	8.7
1938	5108	2.2					20770	8.8
1939	5128	2.2					21700	9.1

Table 3.2 *(continued)*

Year	Manufactured cigarettes		Hand-rolled cigarettes		Total cigarettes		All tobacco products	
	Total annual in millions	Number/ adult/day	Total annual in millions	Number/ adult/day	Total annual in millions	Number/ adult/day	Total annual in tonnes	Grams/ adult/day
1940	4150	1.7					17620	7.4
1941	3723	1.6					15610	6.6
1942	3284	1.4					13080	5.5
1943	1889	0.8					7290	3.1
1944	2070	0.9					6830	2.9
1945	2563	1.1					9780	4.1
1946	6386	2.7					17850	7.4
1947	8549	3.5					19440	7.9
1948	8901	3.6					19810	8.0
1949	8414	3.4					19450	7.8
1950	8399	3.4	8820	3.5	17219	6.9	19250	7.7
1951	8197	3.3	8694	3.5	16891	6.8	19010	7.6
1952	8115	3.2	9432	3.8	17547	7.0	20140	8.0
1953	8217	3.3	9018	3.6	17235	6.8	19980	7.9
1954	8263	3.3	8856	3.5	17119	6.8	20090	8.0
1955	8652	3.4	8289	3.3	16941	6.7	19960	7.9
1956	9132	3.6	8370	3.3	17502	6.9	20700	8.2
1957	9859	3.9	8163	3.2	18022	7.1	21330	8.4
1958	10480	4.1	7965	3.1	18445	7.3	21650	8.5
1959	10308	4.0	7875	3.1	18183	7.1	21590	8.5
1960	10973	4.3	7551	3.0	18524	7.3	22090	8.7
1961	11253	4.4	7389	2.9	18642	7.3	22340	8.8
1962	11868	4.6	7182	2.8	19050	7.4	23030	9.0
1963	12325	4.8	6777	2.6	19102	7.4	22830	8.8
1964	12791	4.9	6570	2.5	19361	7.4	23610	9.1
1965	14083	5.4	6327	2.4	20410	7.8	24660	9.4
1966	15147	5.7	5958	2.3	21105	8.0	25100	9.5
1967	15448	5.8	6858	2.6	22306	8.4	26360	9.9
1968	15814	5.9	5922	2.2	21736	8.2	25750	9.7
1969	16633	6.2	5391	2.0	22024	8.2	25950	9.7
1970	17632	6.6	4860	1.8	22492	8.4	26170	9.7
1971	18334	6.8	4653	1.7	22987	8.5	27010	10.0
1972	19165	7.0	4410	1.6	23575	8.7	27700	10.2
1973	20236	7.4	4203	1.5	24439	8.9	28460	10.4
1974	20179	7.3	4125	1.5	24304	8.8	28095	10.2
1975	18868	6.8	4135	1.5	23003	8.3	26900	9.7
1976	18370	6.6	4386	1.6	22756	8.1	26654	9.5
1977	17673	6.3	4487	1.6	22160	7.9	25894	9.2
1978	15590	5.5	4301	1.5	19891	7.0	23522	8.3
1979	16878	5.9	4093	1.4	20971	7.3	24301	8.5
1980	16858	5.9	3979	1.4	20837	7.3	24140	8.4
1981	16657	5.8	4313	1.5	20970	7.3	23915	8.3
1982	17927	6.2	5438	1.9	23365	8.1	26320	9.1
1983	17033	5.9	6023	2.1	23056	8.0	26093	9.0
1984	17178	5.9	6436	2.2	23614	8.1	26646	9.2
1985	15897	5.4	6341	2.2	22238	7.6	25208	8.6
1986	15485	5.3	5783	2.0	21268	7.2	23931	8.1
1987	14507	4.9	5261	1.8	19768	6.7	22331	7.6
1988	14903	5.0	5027	1.7	19930	6.7	22408	7.6
1989	14184	4.8	4848	1.6	19032	6.4		
1990	13687	4.6	4414	1.5	18101	6.1		
1991	13966	4.7	4409	1.5	18375	6.1		
1992	13543	4.5	4663	1.6	18206	6.1		
1993	12556	4.2	4616	1.5	17172	5.7		
1994	12058	4.0	5054	1.7	17112	5.7		
1995	12373	4.1	6565	2.2	18938	6.3	21309	7.0

Source : see *Notes on sources of sales data*, p. 65

Figure 3.1 Daily consumption of (i) manufactured and total number of cigarettes, and (ii) all tobacco products, 1921-1995
Males and females aged 15 years and over. *Source:* see Table 3.2

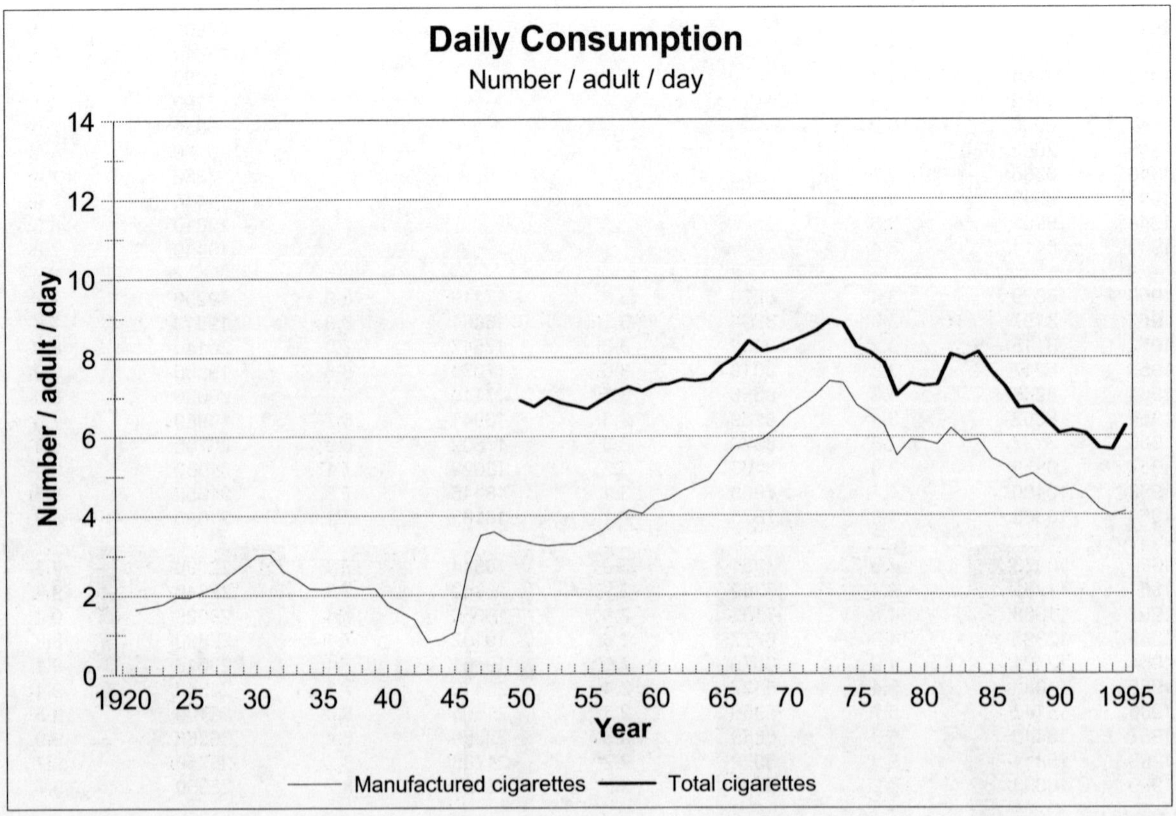

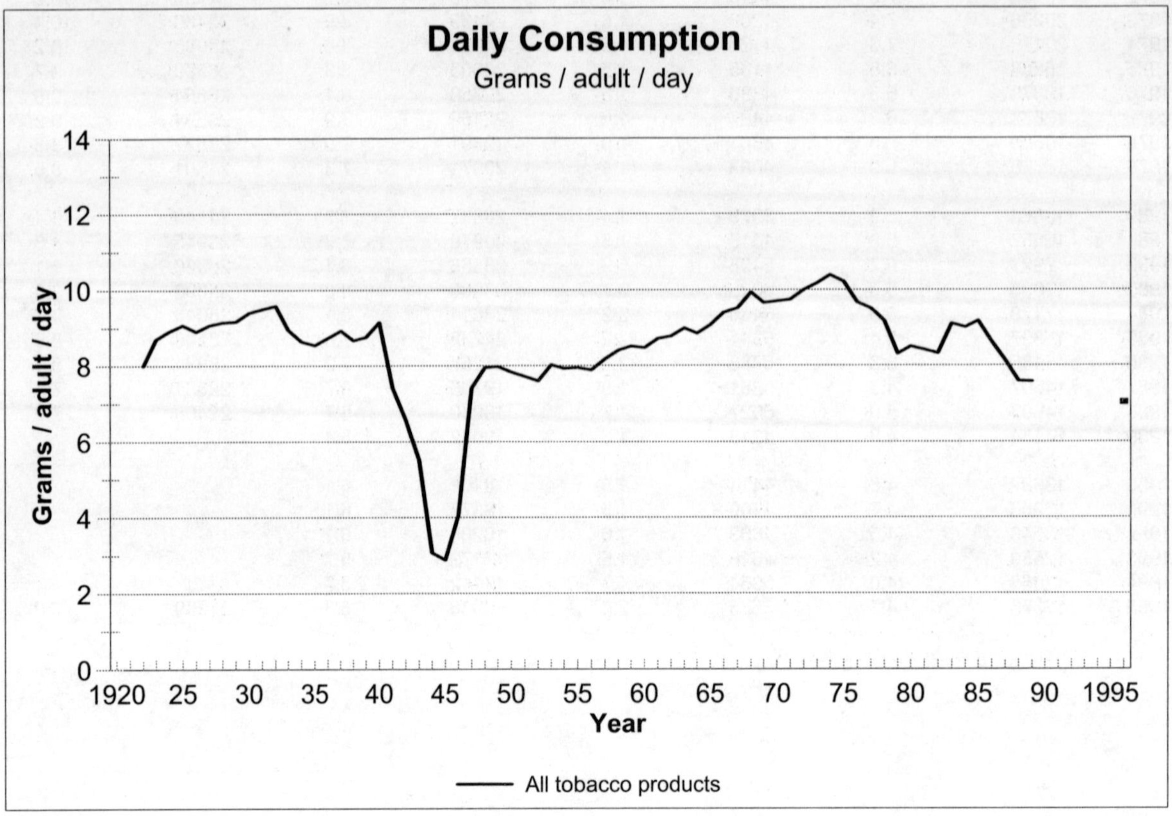

Table 3.3 Percentage sales of tobacco in different forms (by weight), selected years 1925-1995

Year	Cigarettes (%)	Cigars (%)	Cigarillos (%)	Other tobacco (%)
1925	22.0	6.9	3.9	67.2
1935	24.7	4.6	6.4	64.4
1945	26.2	5.2	6.3	62.2
1955	43.3	3.8	6.7	46.1
1965	57.1	6.1	8.2	28.5
1975	70.1	4.9	7.9	17.1
1985	63.1	2.2	6.8	28.0
1995	58.1	1.2	6.5	34.2

Source : calculated from Tables 3.1.1 & 3.1.2

Figure 3.2 Percentage sales of tobacco in different forms (by weight), selected years 1925-1995
Source: see Table 3.3

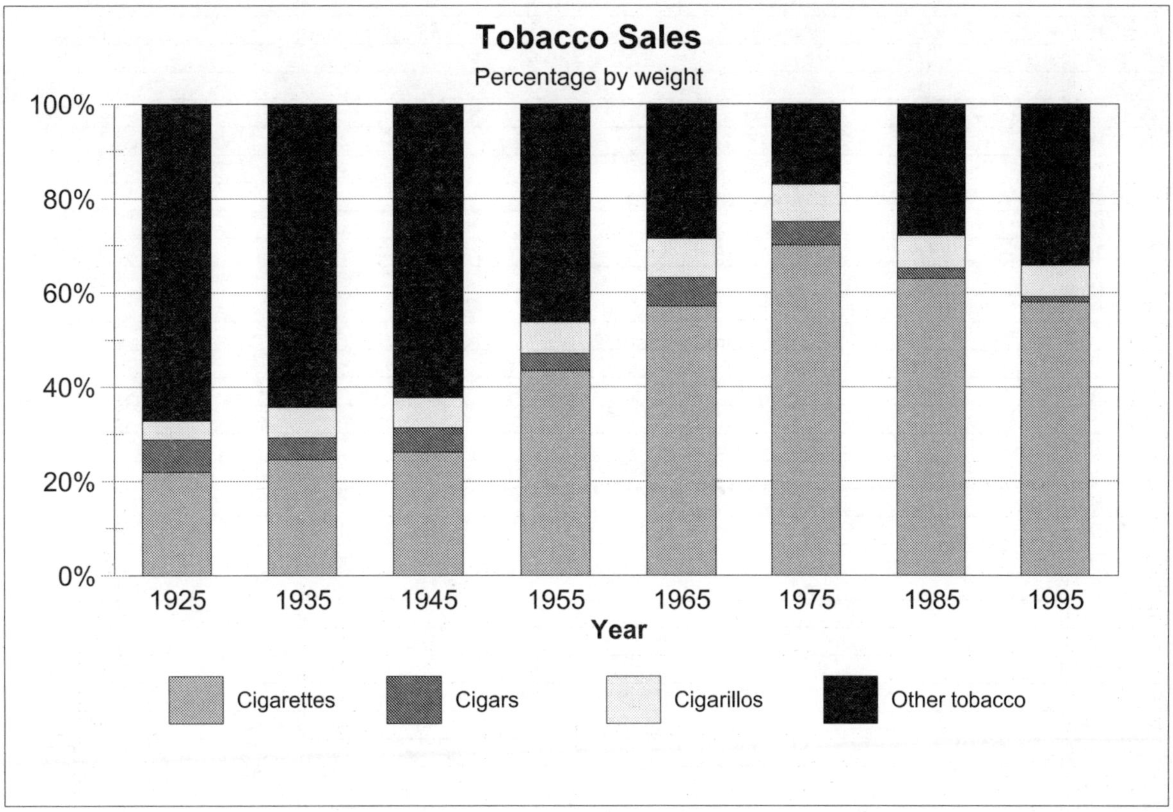

Table 3.4M Prevalence of smoking, males: some selected Belgian surveys by age, 1955-1995 *(continues on p. 56)*

Frequency / Product / Source / Year	Age group 12	13	14	15	16	17	18	19	20-24	25-29	30-34	35-39	40-44	45-49	50-54	55-59	60-64	65-69	70-74	75-79	80+	All ages
55 21 A A	5			54					73	77	79	79	83	79	84	83	81	81	78	75		79
60 22 U R				48																		
63 6 A U									80													
63 6 UC U									66													
63 7 A U									75	69				70				68				70
72 2 MC U				51																		
72 22 U R				45																		
73 4 A U			40																			
73 5 A R	1	10	8	24	29	35	35	45	53													
73 11 UC U	56																					
74 2 MC U				48																		
74 18 U U	11	30		50			65															
75 20 U U	24			44			82															
75 22 U R				43																		
76 3 A R				53						56				65				55				58
76 12 MC U				49					55	56		52		48		32		20				44
76 12 A U				62																		
76 13 A U				58																		
76 14 A U						59																
77 2 MC U				40																		
77 4 MC U				48																		
79 22 U R				42																		
80 1 MC R				35																		
80 1 TC R				46						54				40				27				44
80 1 A R				51						59				53				41				53
80 2 MC U				38																		
80 13 A U				53																		
80 15 U R							50															
81 2 MC U				37																		
82 17 U R							53															
82 19 U U						25																
83 17 U R							47															
84 2 MC U				35																		
84 10 UC R												44		40		45						43
84 10 A A												53		49		51						51
84 17 U R							47															
84 17* U R							45			50				48				42				47
85 8 UC R										45		47		42		38						43
85 8 A A										51		56		51		47						52
85 9 UC R										54		55		50		44						50
85 9 A A										58		59		54		53						56
85 17 U R							45															
86 2 MC U				32																		
86 2 U U				16			40		47	53		52		51		49		38				
86 17 U R							46															
86 23 U *		4		17																		
86 23 U R		7		22																		
86 23 U A		12		27																		

Table 3.4F Prevalence of smoking, females: some selected Belgian surveys by age, 1955-1995 *(continues on p. 57)*

Frequency / Product / Source / Year	12	13	14	15	16	17	18	19	20-24	25-29	30-34	35-39	40-44	45-49	50-54	55-59	60-64	65-69	70-74	75-79	80+	All ages
55 21 A A	5			15					26	31	32	29	27	21	18	15	12	8	6	3		19
60 22 U R																						
63 6 A U									15													
63 6 UC U									15													
63 7 A U									36	26				22				17				23
72 2 MC U				24																		
72 22 U R																						
73 4 A U			37																			
73 5 A R	1	5	10	16	26	28	34	33	29													
73 11 UC U	8																					
74 2 MC U				26																		
74 18 U U																						
75 20 U U	17			45			67															
75 22 U R																						
76 3 A R				34						29								3				22
76 12 MC U				39					48	43		25		24		13		5				25
76 12 A U				26																		
76 13 A U				22																		
76 14 A U																						
77 2 MC U				21																		
77 4 MC U				40																		
79 22 U R																						
80 1 MC R				21																		
80 1 TC R				21																		
80 1 A R				33						29				10				2				21
80 2 MC U				21																		
80 13 A U				21																		
80 15 U R																						
81 2 MC U				22																		
82 17 U R							28															
82 19 U U						32																
83 17 U R							28															
84 2 MC U				21																		
84 10 UC R												25		16		9						18
84 10 A A												26		16		9						18
84 17 U R							26															
84 17* U R							39			38				20				9				27
85 8 UC R										35		34		22		15						25
85 8 A A										35		35		22		15						25
85 9 UC R										42		26		22		22						24
85 9 A A										42		26		23		22						24
85 17 U R							27															
86 2 MC U				21																		
86 2 U U				10			27		40	40		30		20		17		9				
86 17 U R							26															
86 23 U *		3		14																		
86 23 U R		8		20																		
86 23 U A		13		25																		

Table 3.4M *(continued from p. 54)* Prevalence of smoking, males

Frequency / Product / Source / Year	12	13	14	15	16	17	18	19	20-24	25-29	30-34	35-39	40-44	45-49	50-54	55-59	60-64	65-69	70-74	75-79	80+	All ages
87 17 U R							31			46				42				36				42
88 17 U R							42															
89 17 U R							39															
90 17 U R							38															
90 23 UC R		7		15																		
90 23 UC A		12		20																		
90 27 U R			5	9																		
90 27 U A	2	8																				
91 17 U R							33															
92 17 U R							31															
92 26 U R				33						42		58		35				21				33
93 17 U R							31															
94 17 U R							33															
94 24 UC R		10		32																		
94 25 UC R		6		23																		
95 17 U R				25			35			42		32		35				15				33
95 17 U A				29			44			46		35		38				18				36

Source: see *Notes on sources of survey data*, p. 66

Product:
- MC = manufactured cigarettes
- TC = total cigarettes (including hand-rolled)
- UC = cigarettes (type unspecified)
- A = all products

Frequency:
- A = all smokers (including occasional)
- R = regular or daily smokers

All ages: relevant to ages used and as given in original source

U = unspecified

* = refer to *Notes on sources of survey data*, p. 66

Table 3.4F (continued from p. 55)
Prevalence of smoking, females

<table>
<tr><th rowspan="2">Frequency
Product
Source
Year</th><th colspan="21">Age group</th><th rowspan="2">All ages</th></tr>
<tr><th>12</th><th>13</th><th>14</th><th>15</th><th>16</th><th>17</th><th>18</th><th>19</th><th>20-24</th><th>25-29</th><th>30-34</th><th>35-39</th><th>40-44</th><th>45-49</th><th>50-54</th><th>55-59</th><th>60-64</th><th>65-69</th><th>70-74</th><th>75-79</th><th>80+</th></tr>
<tr><td>87 17 U R</td><td colspan="6"></td><td colspan="3">35</td><td colspan="4">34</td><td colspan="4">18</td><td colspan="4">6</td><td>26</td></tr>
<tr><td>88 17 U R</td><td colspan="6"></td><td colspan="15">24</td><td></td></tr>
<tr><td>89 17 U R</td><td colspan="6"></td><td colspan="15">26</td><td></td></tr>
<tr><td>90 17 U R</td><td colspan="6"></td><td colspan="15">26</td><td></td></tr>
<tr><td>90 23 UC R</td><td></td><td>5</td><td></td><td>17</td><td colspan="17"></td><td></td></tr>
<tr><td>90 23 UC A</td><td></td><td>8</td><td></td><td>23</td><td colspan="17"></td><td></td></tr>
<tr><td>90 27 U R</td><td colspan="2"></td><td>1</td><td>8</td><td colspan="17"></td><td></td></tr>
<tr><td>90 27 U A</td><td>0</td><td colspan="3">5</td><td colspan="17"></td><td></td></tr>
<tr><td>91 17 U R</td><td colspan="6"></td><td colspan="15">24</td><td></td></tr>
<tr><td>92 17 U R</td><td colspan="6"></td><td colspan="15">21</td><td></td></tr>
<tr><td>92 26 U R</td><td colspan="3"></td><td colspan="6">30</td><td colspan="2">35</td><td colspan="2">26</td><td colspan="4">22</td><td colspan="4">6</td><td>24</td></tr>
<tr><td>93 17 U R</td><td colspan="6"></td><td colspan="15">19</td><td></td></tr>
<tr><td>94 17 U R</td><td colspan="6"></td><td colspan="15">19</td><td></td></tr>
<tr><td>94 24 UC R</td><td></td><td>8</td><td></td><td>18</td><td colspan="17"></td><td></td></tr>
<tr><td>94 25 UC R</td><td></td><td>8</td><td></td><td>21</td><td colspan="17"></td><td></td></tr>
<tr><td>95 17 U R</td><td colspan="3"></td><td colspan="3">11</td><td colspan="3">35</td><td colspan="2">35</td><td colspan="2">26</td><td colspan="4">22</td><td colspan="4">6</td><td>24</td></tr>
<tr><td>95 17 U A</td><td colspan="3"></td><td colspan="3">11</td><td colspan="3">37</td><td colspan="2">37</td><td colspan="2">28</td><td colspan="4">24</td><td colspan="4">8</td><td>26</td></tr>
</table>

Source: see *Notes on sources of survey data*, p. 66
Product: MC = manufactured cigarettes
TC = total cigarettes (including hand-rolled)
UC = cigarettes (type unspecified)
A = all products

Frequency: A = all smokers (including occasional)
R = regular or daily smokers
All ages: relevant to ages used and as given in original source
U = unspecified
* = refer to *Notes on sources of survey data*, p. 66

Table 3.5M Number of cigarettes smoked per smoker per day, males: some selected Belgian surveys by age, 1980-1985

<table>
<tr><th rowspan="2">Product
Source
Year</th><th colspan="21">Age group</th><th rowspan="2">All ages</th></tr>
<tr><th>12</th><th>13</th><th>14</th><th>15</th><th>16</th><th>17</th><th>18</th><th>19</th><th>20-24</th><th>25-29</th><th>30-34</th><th>35-39</th><th>40-44</th><th>45-49</th><th>50-54</th><th>55-59</th><th>60-64</th><th>65-69</th><th>70-74</th><th>75-79</th><th>80+</th></tr>
<tr><td>80 1 MC</td><td colspan="3"></td><td colspan="6">17</td><td colspan="4">20</td><td colspan="4">20</td><td colspan="4">19</td><td>19</td></tr>
<tr><td>80 1 TC</td><td colspan="3"></td><td colspan="6">19</td><td colspan="4">20</td><td colspan="4">18</td><td colspan="4">17</td><td>19</td></tr>
<tr><td>85 8 UC</td><td colspan="11"></td><td colspan="6">22</td><td colspan="4"></td><td></td></tr>
<tr><td>85 9 UC</td><td colspan="11"></td><td colspan="6">21</td><td colspan="4"></td><td></td></tr>
</table>

Table 3.6M Number of cigarettes smoked per person per day, males: some selected Belgian surveys by age, 1980-1985, with percentage total sales

<table>
<tr><th rowspan="2">Product
Source
Year</th><th colspan="21">Age group</th><th rowspan="2">All ages</th><th rowspan="2">% Total sales</th></tr>
<tr><th>12</th><th>13</th><th>14</th><th>15</th><th>16</th><th>17</th><th>18</th><th>19</th><th>20-24</th><th>25-29</th><th>30-34</th><th>35-39</th><th>40-44</th><th>45-49</th><th>50-54</th><th>55-59</th><th>60-64</th><th>65-69</th><th>70-74</th><th>75-79</th><th>80+</th></tr>
<tr><td>80 1 TC</td><td colspan="3"></td><td colspan="6">8.6</td><td colspan="4">11</td><td colspan="4">7.2</td><td colspan="4">4.5</td><td>8.3</td><td>74%T</td></tr>
<tr><td>80 16 MC</td><td colspan="3"></td><td colspan="18">8.4</td><td></td><td>---M</td></tr>
<tr><td>85 8 UC *</td><td colspan="11"></td><td colspan="6">9.4</td><td colspan="4"></td><td></td><td>**</td></tr>
<tr><td>85 9 UC *</td><td colspan="11"></td><td colspan="6">11</td><td colspan="4"></td><td></td><td>**</td></tr>
</table>

Table 3.7M Number of cigarettes smoked per person per day, sales-adjusted, males: some selected Belgian surveys[1] by age, 1980, with percentage total sales

<table>
<tr><th rowspan="2">Product
Source
Year</th><th colspan="21">Age group</th><th rowspan="2">All ages</th><th rowspan="2">% Total sales</th></tr>
<tr><th>12</th><th>13</th><th>14</th><th>15</th><th>16</th><th>17</th><th>18</th><th>19</th><th>20-24</th><th>25-29</th><th>30-34</th><th>35-39</th><th>40-44</th><th>45-49</th><th>50-54</th><th>55-59</th><th>60-64</th><th>65-69</th><th>70-74</th><th>75-79</th><th>80+</th></tr>
<tr><td>80 1 TC</td><td colspan="3"></td><td colspan="6">12</td><td colspan="4">15</td><td colspan="4">9.8</td><td colspan="4">6.1</td><td>11</td><td>74%T</td></tr>
<tr><td>80 16 MC</td><td colspan="3"></td><td colspan="18">8.4</td><td></td><td>---M</td></tr>
</table>

1 Based on those surveys in Table 3.6 with data for both sexes and age range at least 21-64 (see *Cigarette consumption per person*, p. xxxv)

Source: see *Notes on sources of survey data*, p. 66
All ages: relevant to ages used and as given in original source
% Total sales: estimated % of total sales of M = manufactured or T = total cigarette consumption implied by survey, sexes combined, used as adjustment factor in Table 3.7
** = cannot be calculated
--- = adjusted by original author
* = refer to *Notes on sources of survey data*, p. 66

Product: MC = manufactured cigarettes
TC = total cigarettes (including hand-rolled)
UC = cigarettes (type unspecified)
A = all products
U = unspecified
E indicates mean estimated from percentage distribution (see also *Consumption category estimation*, p. xxxiv, and Appendix III, p. 789)

Table 3.5F Number of cigarettes smoked per smoker per day, females: some selected Belgian surveys by age, 1980-1995

<table>
<tr><th rowspan="2">Product
Source
Year</th><th colspan="21">Age group</th><th rowspan="2">All ages</th></tr>
<tr><th>12</th><th>13</th><th>14</th><th>15</th><th>16</th><th>17</th><th>18</th><th>19</th><th>20-24</th><th>25-29</th><th>30-34</th><th>35-39</th><th>40-44</th><th>45-49</th><th>50-54</th><th>55-59</th><th>60-64</th><th>65-69</th><th>70-74</th><th>75-79</th><th>80+</th></tr>
<tr><td>80 1 MC</td><td colspan="3"></td><td colspan="6">13</td><td colspan="3">15</td><td colspan="4">16</td><td colspan="4">12</td><td>14</td></tr>
<tr><td>80 1 TC</td><td colspan="3"></td><td colspan="6">13</td><td colspan="3">13</td><td colspan="4">17</td><td colspan="4">15</td><td>14</td></tr>
<tr><td>85 8 UC</td><td colspan="11"></td><td colspan="6">19</td><td colspan="4"></td><td></td></tr>
<tr><td>85 9 UC</td><td colspan="11"></td><td colspan="6">20</td><td colspan="4"></td><td></td></tr>
</table>

Table 3.6F Number of cigarettes smoked per person per day, females: some selected Belgian surveys by age, 1980-1985, with percentage total sales

<table>
<tr><th rowspan="2">Product
Source
Year</th><th colspan="21">Age group</th><th rowspan="2">All ages</th><th rowspan="2">% Total sales</th></tr>
<tr><th>12</th><th>13</th><th>14</th><th>15</th><th>16</th><th>17</th><th>18</th><th>19</th><th>20-24</th><th>25-29</th><th>30-34</th><th>35-39</th><th>40-44</th><th>45-49</th><th>50-54</th><th>55-59</th><th>60-64</th><th>65-69</th><th>70-74</th><th>75-79</th><th>80+</th></tr>
<tr><td>80 1 TC *</td><td colspan="3"></td><td colspan="6">4.2</td><td colspan="3">3.8</td><td colspan="4">1.7</td><td colspan="4">0.3</td><td>2.8</td><td>74%T</td></tr>
<tr><td>80 16 MC</td><td colspan="3"></td><td colspan="18">3.6</td><td></td><td>---M</td></tr>
<tr><td>85 8 UC *</td><td colspan="11"></td><td colspan="6">4.8</td><td colspan="4"></td><td></td><td>**</td></tr>
<tr><td>85 9 UC *</td><td colspan="11"></td><td colspan="6">4.7</td><td colspan="4"></td><td></td><td>**</td></tr>
</table>

Table 3.7F Number of cigarettes smoked per person per day, sales-adjusted, females: some selected Belgian surveys[1] by age, 1980, with percentage total sales

<table>
<tr><th rowspan="2">Product
Source
Year</th><th colspan="21">Age group</th><th rowspan="2">All ages</th><th rowspan="2">% Total sales</th></tr>
<tr><th>12</th><th>13</th><th>14</th><th>15</th><th>16</th><th>17</th><th>18</th><th>19</th><th>20-24</th><th>25-29</th><th>30-34</th><th>35-39</th><th>40-44</th><th>45-49</th><th>50-54</th><th>55-59</th><th>60-64</th><th>65-69</th><th>70-74</th><th>75-79</th><th>80+</th></tr>
<tr><td>80 1 TC *</td><td colspan="3"></td><td colspan="6">5.7</td><td colspan="3">5.1</td><td colspan="4">2.3</td><td colspan="4">0.4</td><td>3.8</td><td>74%T</td></tr>
<tr><td>80 16 MC</td><td colspan="3"></td><td colspan="18">3.6</td><td></td><td>---M</td></tr>
</table>

1 Based on those surveys in Table 3.6 with data for both sexes and age range at least 21-64 (see *Cigarette consumption per person*, p. xxxv)

Source: see *Notes on sources of survey data*, p. 66
All ages: relevant to ages used and as given in original source
% Total sales: estimated % of total sales of M = manufactured or T = total cigarette consumption implied by survey, sexes combined, used as adjustment factor in Table 3.7
** = cannot be calculated
--- = adjusted by original author
* = refer to *Notes on sources of survey data*, p. 66

Product: MC = manufactured cigarettes
TC = total cigarettes (including hand-rolled)
UC = cigarettes (type unspecified)
A = all products
U = unspecified
E indicates mean estimated from percentage distribution (see also *Consumption category estimation*, p. xxxiv, and Appendix III, p. 789)

Table 3.8 Estimated[1] prevalence of smoking and estimated[1] number of cigarettes per person per day (unadjusted and sales-adjusted): summary of Tables 3.4, 3.6 and 3.7, 1955-1995. Males and females aged 15 years and over

Year	Source[2]	Product[3]	Prevalence[4]						Number of cigarettes						
									Unadjusted[7]			Sales-adjusted[8]			
			Manufactured cigarettes		Total cigarettes[5]		All products[6]		Number/ person/day		Total sales %	Manufactured cigarettes number/ person/day		Total cigarettes[9] number/ person/day	
			M	F	M	F	M	F	M	F		M	F	M	F
1955	21	A					74	19							
1960	22	U					48								
1963	6	*UC+A*			63	15	75	15						(12.7	2.4)
	7	*A*					66	23							
1972	2	*MC*	51	24								(10.4	3.9)		
	22	U					45								
1973	11	*UC*			56	8								(16.5	1.9)
1974	2	*MC*	48	26								(10.4	4.5)		
1975	22	U					43								
1976	3	A					58	22							
	12	*MC+A*	45	26			62	26				(9.1	4.2)		
	13	*A*					58	22							
1977	2	*MC*	40	21								(8.9	3.8)		
1979	22	U					42								
1980	1	MC+TC+A	35	21	44	21	53	19	8.4	2.6	74	(8.0	3.9)	11.3	3.5
	2	*MC*	38	21								(8.3	3.7)		
	13	*A*					53	21							
	16	MC							8.4	3.6	---	8.4	3.6		
1981	2	*MC*	37	22								(8.0	3.8)		
1982	17	U					51	28						(11.3	5.0)
1983	17	U					46	27						(10.9	5.2)
1984	2	*MC*	35	21								(8.1	3.9)		
	17	U					46	26						(11.4	5.1)
1985	17	U					44	27						(10.3	5.1)
1986	2	*MC+U*	32	21			46	24				(7.0	3.7)		
	17	U					45	26						(10.0	4.6)
1987	17	U					40	23						(9.3	4.3)
1988	17	U					41	24						(9.4	4.3)
1989	17	U					38	26						(8.4	4.6)
1990	17	U					37	26						(7.9	4.4)

Table 3.8 *(continued)*

Year	Source[2]	Product[3]	Prevalence[4]						Number of cigarettes						
									Unadjusted[7]			Sales-adjusted[8]			
			Manufactured cigarettes		Total cigarettes[5]		All products[6]		Number/ person/day		Total sales %	Manufactured cigarettes number/ person/day		Total cigarettes[9] number/ person/day	
			M	F	M	F	M	F	M	F		M	F	M	F
1991	17	U					33	24						(7.8	4.6)
1992	17	U					31	21						(7.9	4.4)
	26	U					38	23						(8.3	4.0)
1993	17	U					31	19						(7.7	3.9)
1994	17	U					33	19						(7.8	3.7)
1995	17	U					32	22						(8.1	4.5)
	17	**U**					36	24							

1 Surveys covering an age range of at least 21-64 are included. Any gaps in the data for ages 15-20 and 65 years and over are filled in by assumed extensions to the age distribution, given in Notes on sources of survey data, p. 66. Method: see Summary of adult smoking, p. xxxvi
2 See Notes on sources of survey data, p. 66
3 Product: MC = manufactured cigarettes, TC = total cigarettes (including hand-rolled), UC = cigarettes (type unspecified), A = all products, U = unspecified. Frequency of smoking is indicated by: regular or daily smokers in normal type, all smokers (including occasional) in bold, unspecified in italics
4 From Table 3.4
5 This column includes prevalence of smoking classified as UC = cigarettes (type unspecified)
6 This column includes prevalence of smoking classified as U = unspecified product
7 From Table 3.6
8 From Table 3.7, except data in parentheses, which are derived from the prevalence of smoking from Table 3.4 as described in Summary of adult smoking, p. xxxvi
9 Number of cigarettes classified as UC = cigarettes (type unspecified), or U = product unspecified for recent years, has been adjusted to total cigarette sales and included in this column

Figure 3.3 Estimated prevalence of smoking of (i) manufactured cigarettes, (ii) total cigarettes and (iii) all tobacco products: by year of survey, 1955-1995. Males and females aged 15 years and over. Source: see Table 3.8

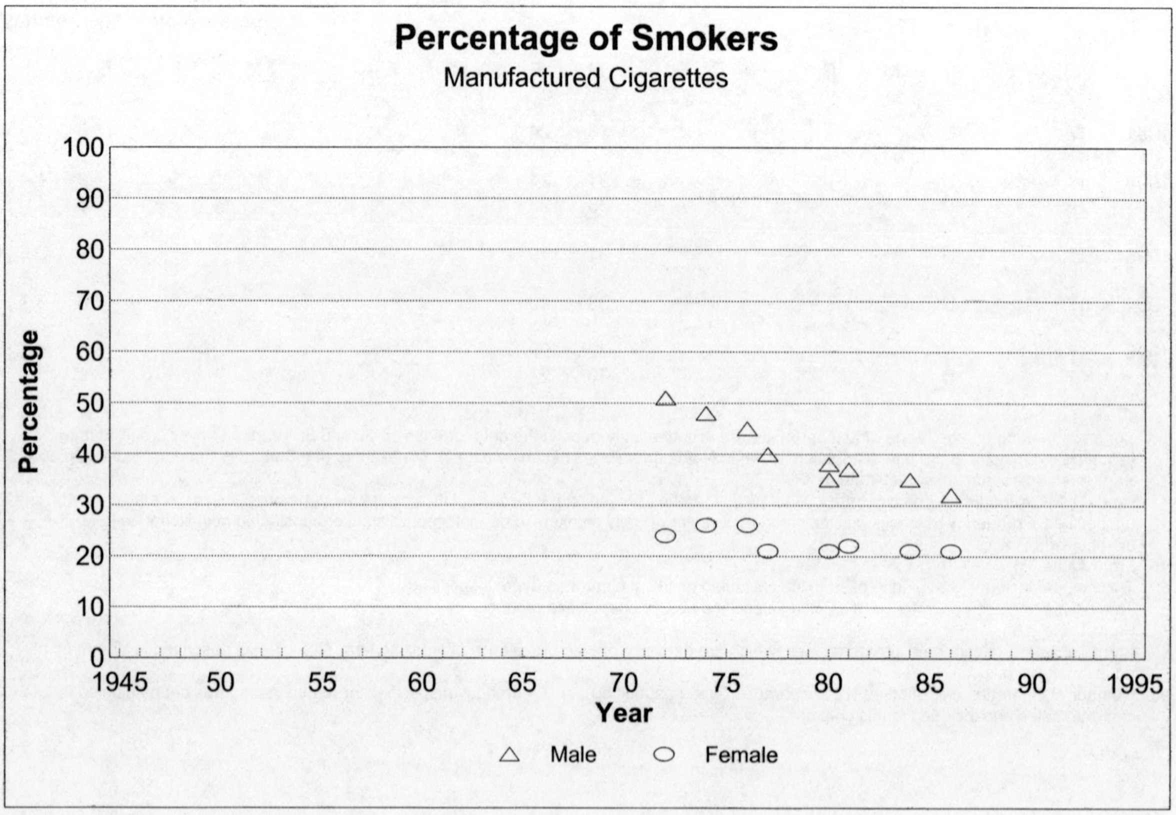

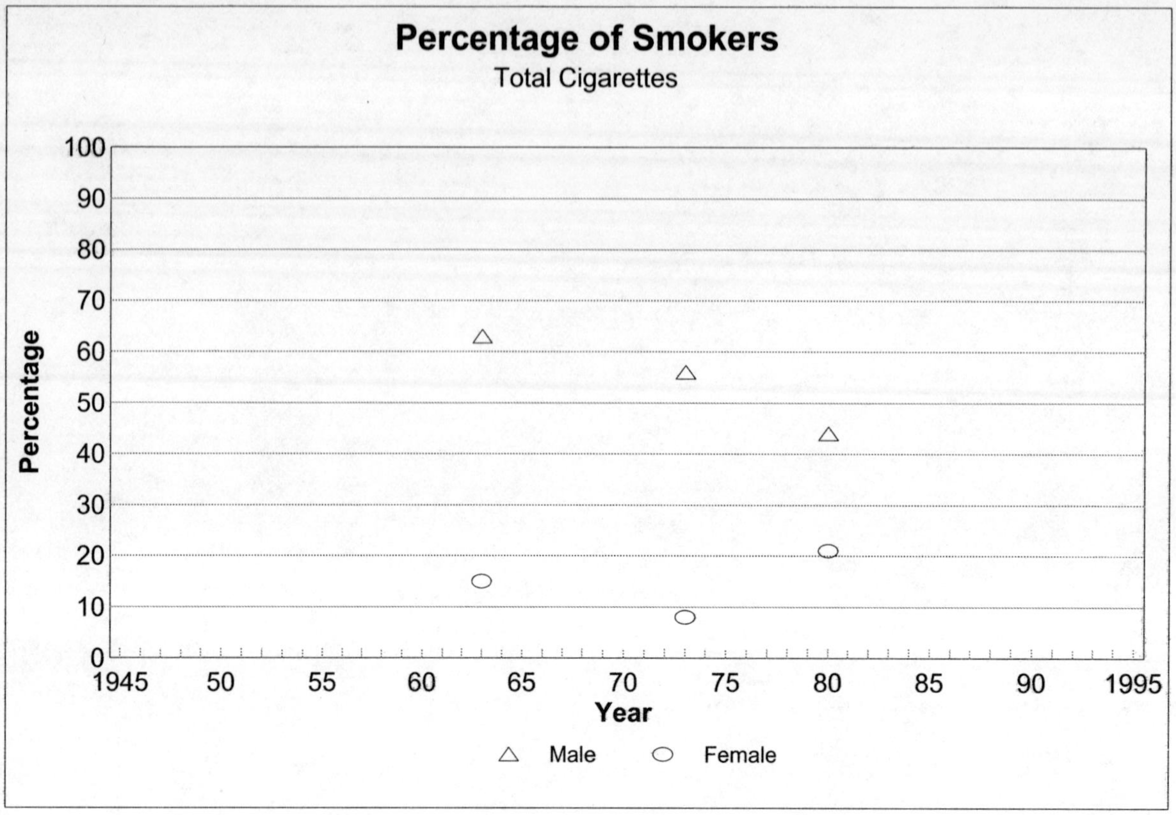

Figure 3.3 *(continued)*

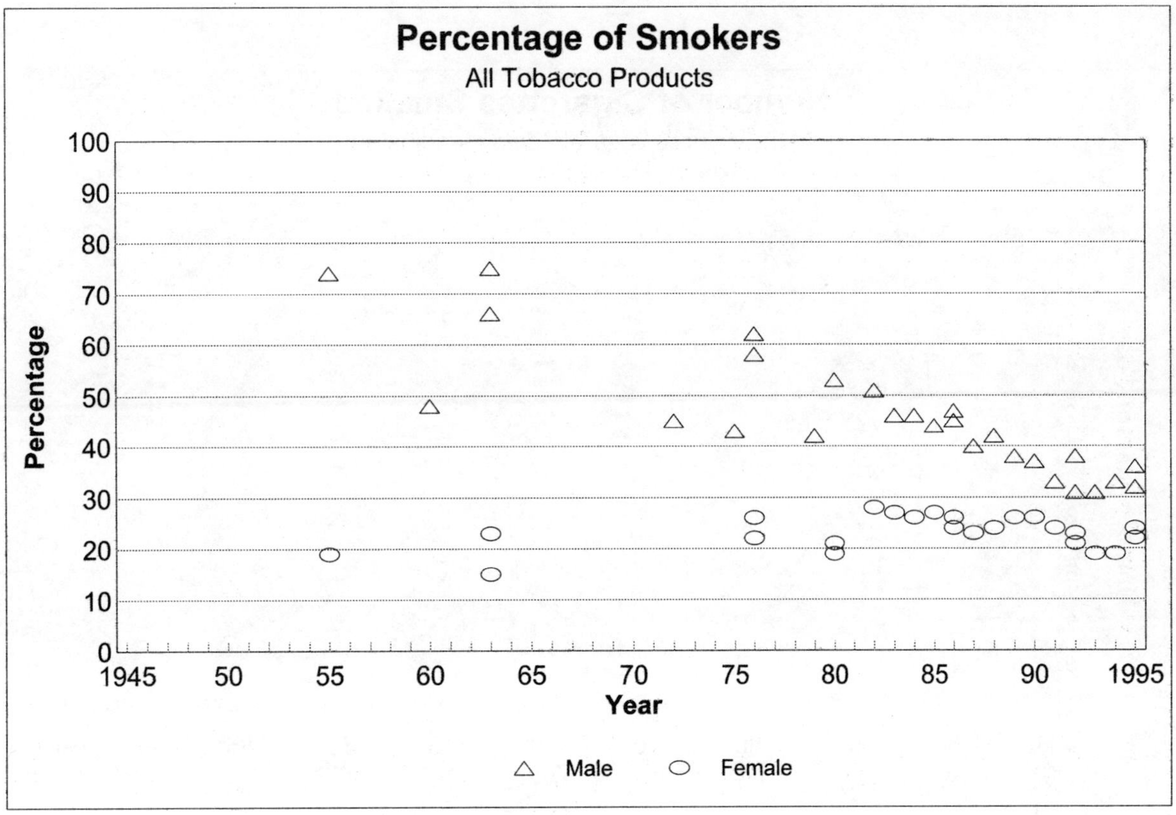

Figure 3.4 Estimated number of cigarettes smoked per person per day, sales-adjusted, 1963-1995.
Males and females aged 15 years and over. Source: see Table 3.8

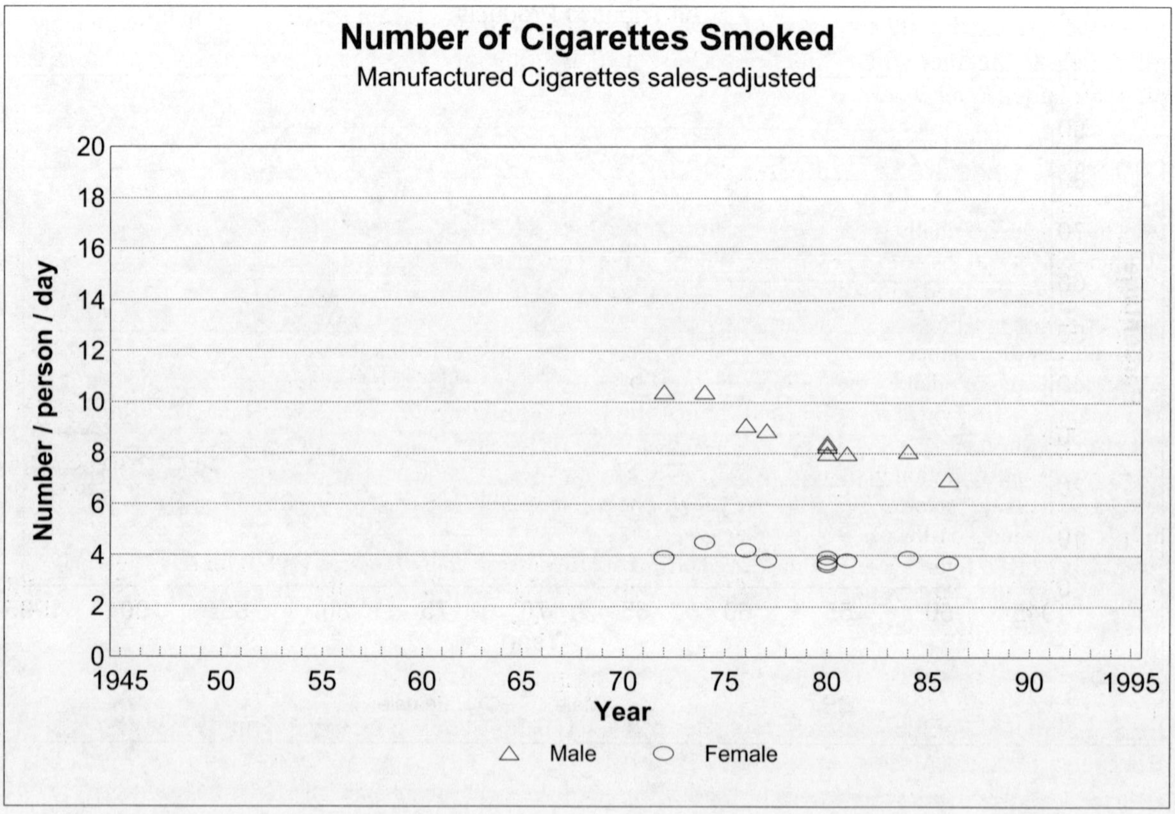

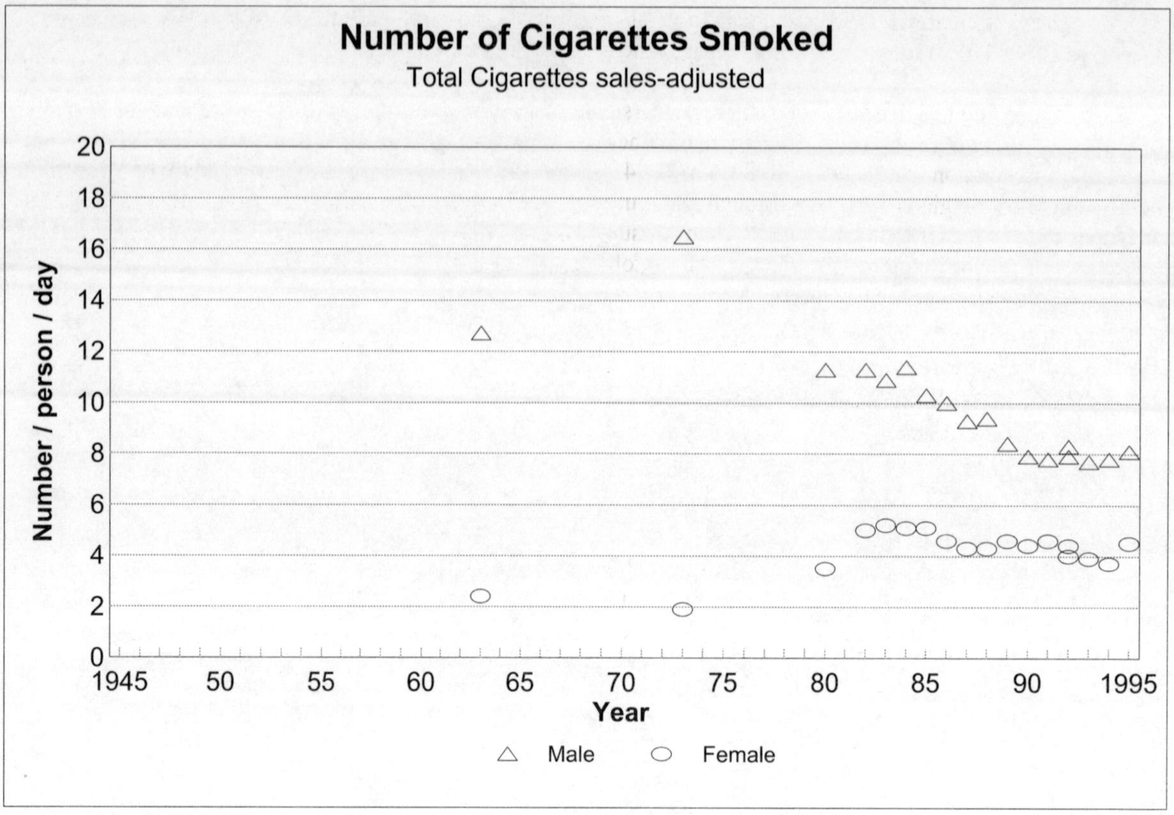

Notes on sources of sales data

The data presented in the tables and figures were obtained from several sources, details of which are given below, together with estimations and related assumptions. Full citations of the sources are given on p. 69 under *References*.

Consumption data before 1974
RP6
Data by weight, originally given to nearest 100 000 pounds, have been converted to tonnes and given to nearest 10 tonnes (100 000 lbs = 45.359 tonnes). Where weight conversion factors have been quoted in RP6, the weights have been re-calculated without rounding and then converted to tonnes.
Notes as given in RP6:
(a) Details of the numbers of cigarettes, cigars and cigarillos, and of the weight of other manufactured tobacco consumed were provided by the National Institute of Statistics of Belgium, Brussels, for the years up to 1950. The figures for 1951 onwards were obtained from trade sources and confirmed by the Belgian Federation of Tobacco Producers.
(b) Cigarette consumption in pounds weight has been estimated from the number of cigarettes consumed by using a conversion factor of 2.025 lbs per 1 000. The conversion factors used for cigars and cigarillos were 10.5 lbs per 1 000 and 5.51 lbs per 1 000 respectively.

The RP6 figures for 1951 onwards correspond to those given by Joossens (1989) for sales in UEBL (Union Economique Belgo-Luxembourgeoise) in selected years. Source: Fedetab (Fédération belgo-luxembourgeoise des industries du tabac)

Consumption data for 1974 onwards
Institut National de Statistique, Service des Renseignments et de la Documentation Generale, Bruxelles, Joossens (1996), Anonymous (1999)
Data used are based on excise bandelettes and stamps issued. Data were given in numbers and have been converted to weight assuming an average of 1 g per cigarette, 4.8 g per cigar, and 2.5 g per cigarillo (based on values in RP6). Quantities for tobacco reserved for use by growers and for moist chewing tobacco (negligible, to 1970 only) have been omitted.

Data for cigarette, cigar and cigarillo and loose tobacco sales in UEBL from 1974 to 1995 are also shown in Table 3.1.3. (Joossens (1989), Verbrugghen (1990) quoting Fedetab (1997) and personal communication).

According to Joossens (1989) there was a substantial rise in cross-border sales to the Federal Republic of Germany following substantial price increases there in June 1982. According to Joossens *et al* (1994) differences in taxation led, in 1993, to 80% of the 4.2 million cigarettes sold in the Grand Duchy of Luxembourg being bought by Belgians, Germans, French and Dutch. This results in sales figures for Belgium being lower, and sales figures for UEBL being higher, than consumption. According to Crescenti (1996) much of the fall in UK sales and rise in Belgian sales of hand-rolling tobacco during 1991-1995 was due to Britons travelling to Belgium to buy cheaper tobacco there.

Plain/Filter cigarette consumption
1960-1980 Maxwell (successive years)
1982-1983 Todd (1986)
1991 Bell (1992)

Tar and nicotine yield of cigarettes
1973-1985 Belgian Association for Smoking Prevention (1989)
1973 and 1980 figures are calculated on the 80 most important brands. The 1985 figure is calculated on the 10 best-selling brands which accounted for 60% of sales. The tar yield per cigarette was limited by EC directive (Directive 90/239/EEC) to 15 mg by the end of 1992, and to 12 mg by the end of 1997; nicotine yield is limited to 1.5 mg (Harkin *et al* (1997)).

Estimates of hand-rolled cigarette consumption for 1950-1995

We have estimated hand-rolled cigarette consumption as 90% of 'other' tobacco sales, at 1 g per cigarette.

This is the same estimate as used by Merzdorf *et al* (1982), although their figures for taxed sales of pipe and hand rolled tobacco are slightly different.

Notes on sources of survey data

Each source of survey data—either an individual survey or a series of surveys repeated over a number of years—is cited by a source number. This number is shown in the tables and corresponds to the source numbers given below, where details of the source publication and of the survey methodology are given. Full citations of the sources are given on p. 69 under *References*.

Source number

1 Joossens (1981) and personal communication

a. Survey by INUSOP (Institut Interuniversitaire de Sondage d'Opinion Publique, Bruxelles) for CRIOC (Centre de Recherche et d'Information des Organisations de Consommateurs, Bruxelles). Quota sample size 1 130, representative of the Flemish population (excluding Brussels)

b. For women, calculation of cigarettes per person is based on percentage smokers of any product, since percentage smokers of cigarettes is not given by age. Since cigarette smokers accounted for 20% of 21% total smokers, this is likely to have little effect

2 Joossens (1987)

a. Studies conducted by CIM (Centre d'Information des Media). Sample size 10 000

b. The percentage of hand-rolled cigarette smokers among men (with or without other products) was 22% in 1972, 20% in 1981, and 18% in 1986. Percentage of hand-rolled cigarette smokers among women was 4% in 1986

3 Joossens (1981)

a. Programme National de Recherches en sciences sociales, project Soins de Santé Primaires. Sample size 1 745, representative of the Flemish population (excluding Brussels)

b. Comparable with source 1 as identical questions were used

c. Female data for age 45-64 missing owing to apparent misprint in original report

4 Merzdorf *et al* (1982), quoting Joossens (1978)

a. Survey among Flemings

b. Not clear whether these data relate to the same surveys as source 2

5 Graffar and Decrucq (1976)

a. Sample size 3 037 young persons. Lowest age group 11-12

b. Regular smokers: smoked 1 cigarette, 1 cigar or 1 cigarillo, or 1 pipe at least once a day. 97% of smokers in sample smoked cigarettes

6-7 Readers Digest (1963), Joossens (1987)

a. Data given as source **6** taken from Readers Digest (1963). Series of surveys conducted in European countries using identical questionnaires. Belgian survey conducted by SOBEMAP. Random sample of about 2 000 people

b. It is also reported that 16% of men (9% age <40 and 20% age 40+) smoke a pipe, and that 35% of men (26% age <40 and 40% age 40+) smoke cigars

c. Data given as source **7** taken from Joossens (1987). Sample size 2 196. Age-specific data derived by Joossens directly from the data. The reason for the discrepancies between the two sources is unknown

d. Joossens presents a table showing the percentage of male smokers of cigarettes, pipe and cigars (reproduced below). It is unclear whether these results should be interpreted directly as the prevalence of cigarette (etc) smokers in the male population, or as the percentage of smokers who smoke cigarettes, in which case the prevalence of cigarette smoking in the male population would be estimated as shown in the final column.

Age group	Percentage of male smokers Joossens (1987)			Derived prevalence of cigarette smoking among men
	cigarettes	pipe	cigar	
21-25	73	8	19	55
26-44	63	8	26	43
45-64	58	10	33	41
65+	37	32	36	25
All ages	57	14	30	40

e. Assumed extension to age distribution for percentage smokers, age 15-20: males 40% and females 15%

8-10 WHO (1989), WHO MONICA Project (1988)

a. Three regional surveys forming part of WHO MONICA project:

	Region	Population size	Sample size	Participation rate (%)	Sample used*		Date
					Males	Females	
8	Ghent	85 500	1 437	72	703	651	Feb 1985-June 1987
9	Charleroi	78 500	1 391	54	89	565	Mar 1985-Aug 1987
10	Luxembourg Province	71 800	3 614	54	990	958	May 1983-Jan 1985

* Ghent and Charleroi 'sample used' includes age 25-34; all other figures are for age 35-64 only

b. *All ages* column in Table 3.4 only related to age 35-64 and is standardized to world population

c. Regular cigarette smokers: smoked cigarettes daily. All smokers: smoked cigarettes daily or occasionally, or smoked 1 g pipe tobacco or 1 cigar per week. Cigarettes per smoker refers to regular and occasional cigarette smokers

d. Calculation for cigarettes per person based on % regular cigarette smokers and cigarettes per regular or occasional cigarette smoker, so may underestimate

11 Merzdorf *et al* (1982), quoting Vuylsteek *et al* (unpublished)

a. Survey in Flanders, rural population. Lower age limit 11

12 Anonymous (1977)

a. EIU (Economist Intelligence Unit) estimates based on trade interviews

13 Merzdorf *et al* (1982), quoting personal communication

a. Survey in Flanders

14 Merzdorf *et al* (1982), quoting Vuylsteek (1979)

a. Survey among Flemish recruits

15 Vuylsteek *et al* (1985)

a. Average of two random samples of Flemish and French speaking military recruits. Sample size 2 008. Overall age range 17-30, but predominantly 18-19

16 Todd (1986)

a. Estimated by Todd from available data

17 Joossens (1987, 1989)

a. Surveys for CRIOC by INUSOP. Sample size 2 000

b. Age-specific figures given as 1984 are averages for five annual surveys, 1982-1986

c. Smoker: (1982-1986) regular smoker, (1987-1988) daily smoker

d. Assumed extension to age distribution for percentage smokers, age 15-17: males and females 25%

18 Benjamin (1978), quoting Free University of Brussels

a. Survey carried out in schools by The School of Public Health of the Free University of Brussels. Prevalence believed to be the same among girls, 'except that a reduction in smoking at the end of secondary studies is observed in one category of girls who do not proceed to higher studies'. Lowest age group 11-12

19 Geizerova and Masironi (1988)

a. No original source

20 Masironi and Roy (1982)

21 Tuyns (1956)

a. Survey of an urban community close to Brussels. Lower age limit not stated. Sample size (males) 7 438, (females) 8 501 women

b. Smokers: included those who answered 'a little', 'sometimes' or 'rarely'

22 Organisation for Economic Co-operation and Development (1993)

a. No original source

23-25 Nutbeam and Aarø (1990), King and Coles (1992), King *et al* (1996), Piette *et al* (1993)

a. Part of the HBSC (Health Behaviour in School-Aged Children) Study, a collaborative cross-national research study sponsored by the WHO School classes or schools were randomly selected, targeting age groups 11 (not presented here), 13 and 15. The target sample size was 1 300 in each age group

b. 1986 survey: carried out in Wallonia only. Sample size for 15-year-olds (males) 603, (females) 502

c. 1990 survey: sample size 3 007

Target age	Mean age
13	13.5
15	15.4

d. 1994 survey: the Flemish-speaking community and the French-speaking community were surveyed independently (shown as sources **24** and **25** respectively)

	Flemish-speaking		French-speaking	
Target age	Mean age	Sample size	Mean age	Sample size
13	13.5	1 424	13.5	1 585
15	15.6	1 349	15.5	1 676

e. Regular smokers: smoke once a week or more. Smokers marked as frequency *: smoked daily

26 Statistika Centralbyrån (1995)

a. Quoting Centre d'Information et de Documentation sur le Tabac / CRIOC. Sample size 1 904

27 van Reek *et al* (1992), van Reek and Adriaanse (1995)

a. A series of surveys of Young Europeans. About 800 children aged 11-15 years interviewed in each EC country except Luxembourg (where only 250 interviewed). Lowest age group 11-12. Interviews conducted at home, with parents absent

b. Regular smokers: smoked daily. All smokers: smoked at least once a week

References

Anonymous (1977). Cigarettes in Belgium. *Marketing in Europe,* **179**, 52-3.

Anonymous (1999). *Tabactualité.* Centre d'information et de documentation sur le tabac, Brussels.

Beese D.H. (ed) (1968). *Tobacco consumption in various countries,* 2nd edition. Tobacco Research Council, London. Research Paper 6.

Beese D.H. (ed) (1972). *Tobacco consumption in various countries,* 3rd edition. Tobacco Research Council, London. Research Paper 6.

Belgian Association for Smoking Prevention (1989). *Tobacco, health, economy and the tar-yield of cigarettes.* Belgian Association for Smoking Prevention, Brussels.

Bell J. (1992). Bastos and the irony of Belgium. *Tobacco International,* **194**, 35-6.

Benjamin B. (1978). *Tobacco smoking in the world. Report of the WHO Expert Committee on Smoking Control, Geneva 23-28 October 1978*

Crescenti M.G. (1996). RYO remains strong alternative for European smokers. *Tobacco Journal International,* **5**, 58-66.

Fedetab (1997). *Bulletin statistique.* 1996 No.12.

Geizerova H. and Masironi R. (1988). Cigarette smoking in children and adolescents: world review. In: Aoki M., Hisamichi S. and Tominaga S. (eds) *Smoking and health 1987. Proceedings of the 6th World Conference on Smoking and Health, Tokyo, 9-12 November 1987.* Elsevier Science Publishers B.V. (Biomedical Division), Amsterdam; 601-5. International Congress Series No. 780.

Graffar M. and Decrucq J. (1976). Etude sur la consommation de tabac dans un échantillon d'enfants et d'étudiants de la Ville de Bruxelles (Consumption of tobacco in a sample of children and students from Brussels). *Archives Belges de Medecine Sociale, Hygiene, Medecine du Travail et Medecine Legale,* **34**, 23-31.

Harkin A.M., Anderson P. and Goos C. (1997). *Smoking, drinking and drug taking in the European Region.* Alcohol, Drugs and Tobacco Programme, WHO Regional Office for Europe, Copenhagen.

Joossens L. (1978). *Le campagne anti-tabac en Belgique: sens et evaluation.* Unpublished.§

Joossens L. (1981). *Les comportements et les attitudes de la population Flamande face à la consommation du tabac.* CRIOC, Brussels.

Joossens L. (1987). *L'évolution du tabagisme en Belgique avant le 1 Septembre 1987.* CRIOC, Bruxelles. (Hilgers P. (ed) .) Série études sociologiques B11.

Joossens L. (1989). *Documentation Tabac.* CRIOC, Bruxelles. (Hilgers P. (ed) .)

Joossens L. (1996). *Stijging van het aantal rokers in Belgie in 1995: preventiecampagnes hebben dringend een tweede adem nodig! (Increase in the percentage of smokers in Belgium in 1995: prevention campaigns urgently need a second wind!). Press release.* CRIOC/OIVO.

Joossens L., Naett C., Howie C. and Muldoon A. (1994). *Tobacco and health in the European Union. An overview.* European Bureau for Action on Smoking Prevention (BASP), Brussels.

King A., Wold B., Tudor-Smith C. and Harel Y. (1996). *The health of youth, a cross-national survey.* WHO Regional Publications, Europe, Copenhagen. European Series No. 69.

King A.J.C. and Coles B. (1992). *The health of Canada's youth. Views and behaviours of 11-, 13- and 15-year-olds from 11 countries.* Health and Welfare Canada, Ottawa.

Lee P.N. (ed) (1975). *Tobacco consumption in various countries,* 4th edition. Tobacco Research Council, London. Research Paper 6.

Masironi R. and Roy L. (1982). Cigarettes smoking in young age groups. Geographic prevalence. In: Fontana F. (ed) *Tabacco e giovani (Tobacco and youth), International conference, Venice 9-11 November 1981 .* ATTI, Venice; 21-40.

Maxwell J.C.Jr. (successive years). How the brands ranked. Maxwell International Estimates. *World Tobacco.*

Merzdorf J., Reuter U. and Welsch G. (1982). *Daten und Fakten zur Entwicklung des Rauchens in Mitgliedsländern der Europäischen Gemeinschaften (Facts and figures on the development of smoking in the member states of the European Communities).* Kommission der Europäischen Gemeinschaften, Luxemburg. Medizin—EUR 7907 DE.

Nutbeam D. and Aarø L.E. (1990). Smoking and alienation from school: the implications for health education with young people. Results from the WHO study of health behaviour in schoolchildren. In: Durston B. and Jamrozik K. (eds) *Tobacco & health 1990. The global war. Seventh World Conference on Tobacco and Health, Perth, Western Australia, 1-5 April 1990.* Organising Committee of the Seventh World Conference on Tobacco and Health, 189 Royal Street, East Perth, Western Australia 6004; 539-44.

Organisation for Economic Co-operation and Development (1993). *OECD health systems. Facts and trends 1960-1991. Health policy studies no 3.* OECD, Paris. (Health policy studies, Volume 1.)

Piette D., Maes L., Peeters R., Prevost M., *et al* (1993). The WHO-collaborative study: health behaviour in school children in Belgium. Methodology and dissemination of data. *Archives of Public Health,* 387-405.

Readers Digest (1963). *Products and people. A digest of the marketing survey of the European Common Market and Britain, 1963* . Reader's Digest Association Limited, London.

RP6, See Beese (ed) (1968), Beese (ed) (1972), Lee (ed) (1975)

Statistika Centralbyrån (1995) *Tobacco consumption 1970-1994 in the member states of the European Union and in Norway and Iceland.* European Commission.

Todd G. (1986). *Medicine. Statistics of smoking in the Member States of the European Community.* Commission of the European Communities, Luxembourg.

Tuyns A. (1956). Fréquence de l'habitude de fumer, dans une population urbaine. *Archives Belges de Medecine Sociale, Hygiene, Medecine du Travail et Medecine Legale,* **14**, 275-8.

van Reek J. and Adriaanse H. (1995). Daily smoking among adolescents in the European Community. *Rev Epidemiol Sante Publique,* **43**, 281-2.

van Reek J., Adriaanse H. and Karaoglou A. (1992). Smoking among children in the European Community. *J Public Health Med,* **14**, 93-4.

Verbrugghen A. (1990). *Revue de secteurs belges; le tabac. (Review of the Belgian sectors; tobacco).* Banque Brusseles Lambert. Department Etudes. Division Analyse Financière.

Vuylsteek K. (1979). *Rookgewoonten bij vlaamstatige rekruten van de Belgische Krijgsmacht (Base-line studie voor de evaluatie van een kampagne tegen roken bij jongeren). Onderzoeksprojekt Nr 3.002-78.* Rijksuniversiteit Gent, Gent.§

Vuylsteek K., Everaert J.P. and Raveel E. (1985). Invloed van anti-tabakkampagne op het rookgedrag nagegaan bij rekruten van de Belgische krijgsmacht (lichting 1980). *Belgisch Archief van Sociale Geneeskunde en Hygiene, Arbeidsgeneeskunde en Gerechtelijke Geneeskunde,* **43**, 124-36.

Vuylsteek K., Hendrick A.M. and Depoorter A.M. *Evaluation in a rural population of a TV-program on smoking and health.* Dept of Hygiene and Social Medicine, University of Gent.§

WHO (1989). The WHO MONICA project: a worldwide monitoring system for cardiovascular diseases. In: *World health statistics annual 1989.* WHO, Geneva; 25-149.

WHO MONICA Project (1988). Geographical variation in the major risk factors of coronary heart disease in men and women aged 35-64 years. *World Health Stat Q,* **41**, 115-40.

§ Original paper not obtained, but information taken as quoted by another author

Bulgaria 4

Sales data

See Tables 4.1-4.3.

Between 1913 and 1923, the consumption of manufactured cigarettes per adult increased from 0.2 to 2 cigarettes per day. For the following decade, data are available only for manufactured cigarettes and cigarette tobacco (i.e. for hand-rolled cigarettes) combined. This implies that consumption of hand-rolled cigarettes per adult was about 1 cigarette per day around 1923. Consumption of all cigarettes was 3-4 cigarettes per day until 1930, and fell below 2 by 1934. No data are then available until 1960.

Consumption of manufactured cigarettes per adult increased from 4 cigarettes per day in 1960 to about 7 in the 1990s. Virtually no cigarettes were filtered until the late 1960s, but the proportion increased rapidly, reaching about 80% by 1980.

Between 1913 and 1923, the percentage of all tobacco consumed in cigarettes increased from 10% to 65%, with most of the remainder sold as smoking mixtures. A change in the categories reported for 1924 suggests that by that date virtually all smoking mixtures were used for hand-rolled cigarettes. Insignificant quantities of snuff were also used. No data are available on the consumption of other tobacco products after 1960, but it is believed to be low.

Survey data

See Tables 4.4-4.8

Very few surveys are available on the smoking situation in Bulgaria, and some data are presented beyond 1995 (the end of the period usually considered). The estimated prevalence of smoking among men aged 15 years and over was 40-50% in the 1990s. Among women, it was estimated as 17-19% by two surveys, although unofficial estimates by United States Department of Agriculture (USDA) put it much higher, almost equal to the prevalence among men.

Among both men and women, there is a markedly lower prevalence of smoking among older age groups. One source estimates that more teenage girls than boys smoke.

Comparison of sales and survey data was only possible in one case, where consumption was under-reported by about 40%. Between 1989 and 1997, the estimated number of manufactured cigarettes smoked per person per day (sales-adjusted) varied for men between 8-12 cigarettes, and for women between 2-6 cigarettes.

Table 4.1.1 Total annual sales of tobacco products, 1913-1934

Year	Cigarettes [1] tonnes	Cigarettes [1] millions	Smoking mixtures [2] tonnes	Snuff tonnes	All tobacco products tonnes
1913	245	245	2264	2	2511
1920	1059	1059	2348	3	3410
1921	1862	1862	2467	2	4331
1922	2667	2667	1785	2	4454
1923	3100	3100	1626	1	4727
1924	4169	4169	13	1	4183
1925	5196	5196	17	1	5214
1926	4663	4663	26	1	4690
1927	4574	4574	25	0	4599
1928	4999	4999	38	0	5037
1929	4875	4875	42	0	4917
1930	4477	4477	22	0	4499
1931	3850	3850	38	0	3888
1932	3433	3433	33	0	3466
1933	2932	2932	52	0	2984
1934	2720	2720	106	0	2826

1 Includes cigarette tobacco after 1923
2 Includes cigarette tobacco up to 1923

Source: see *Notes on sources of sales data*, p. 79

Table 4.1.3 Manufactured cigarettes, percentage of total sales as filter cigarettes, 1966-1995

Year	% Filter
1966	1.0
1967	10.8
1968	38.8
1969	40.0
1970	49.5
1971	50.3
1972	17.2
1973	27.0
1974	47.7
1975	56.4
1977	77.9
1978	76.6
1979	80.3
1984	94.0
1993	84.4
1994	90.7
1995	93.3

Source : see *Notes on sources of sales data*, p. 79

Table 4.2 Consumption of (i) cigarettes and (ii) all tobacco products, 1913-1997 sales-based data, including estimated hand-rolled cigarette consumption. Males and females aged 15 years and over.

Year	Manufactured cigarettes[1]		Hand-rolled cigarettes		Total cigarettes		All tobacco products	
	Total annual in millions	Number/ adult/day	Total annual in millions	Number/ adult/day	Total annual in millions	Number/ adult/day	Total annual in tonnes	Grams/ adult/day
1913	245	0.2					2511	2.1
1920	1059	0.8					3410	2.7
1921	1862	1.5					4331	3.4
1922	2667	2.0					4454	3.4
1923	3100	2.3					4727	3.6
1924	4169	3.1					4183	3.1
1925	5196	3.8					5214	3.8
1926	4663	3.3					4690	3.3
1927	4574	3.2					4599	3.2
1928	4999	3.4					5037	3.5
1929	4875	3.3					4917	3.3
1930	4477	3.0					4499	3.0
1931	3850	2.5					3888	2.6
1932	3433	2.2					3466	2.3
1933	2932	1.9					2984	1.9
1934	2720	1.7					2826	1.8
1960	8513	4.0					8513	4.0
1961	9208	4.3					9208	4.3
1962	9763	4.5					9763	4.5
1963	10755	4.9					10755	4.9
1964	10121	4.5					10121	4.5
1965	8899	3.9					8899	3.9
1966	11692	5.1					11692	5.1
1967	7932	3.4					7932	3.4
1968	11047	4.7					11047	4.7
1969	15006	6.3					15006	6.3
1970	9814	4.1					9814	4.1
1971	12350	5.1					12350	5.1
1972	12931	5.3					12931	5.3
1973	13341	5.5					13341	5.5
1974	16577	6.7					16577	6.7
1975	13221	5.3					13221	5.3
1976	14000	5.6					14000	5.6
1977	16643	6.7					16643	6.7
1978	13906	5.6					13906	5.6
1979	14000	5.6					14000	5.6
1980	13000	5.2					13000	5.2
1981	13000	5.1					13000	5.1
1982	13000	5.1					13000	5.1
1983	14400	5.7					14400	5.7
1984	16000	6.3					16000	6.3
1985	17000	6.6					17000	6.6
1986	18468	7.1					18468	7.1
1987	16000	6.2					16000	6.2
1988	13768	5.3					13768	5.3
1989	14000	5.4					14000	5.4
1990	12200	4.7					12200	4.7
1991	15726	6.0					15726	6.0
1992	17927	7.1					17927	7.1
1993	18774	7.5					18774	7.5
1994	15107	6.0					15107	6.0
1995	16000	6.4					16000	6.4
1996	19103	7.6					19103	7.6
1997	20390	8.1					20390	8.1

1 Includes hand-rolled cigarettes 1923-1934

Source : see *Notes on sources of sales data*, p. 79

Figure 4.1 Daily consumption of (i) manufactured cigarettes[1] and (ii) all tobacco products, 1920-1995
Males and females aged 15 years and over. *Source:* see Table 4.2

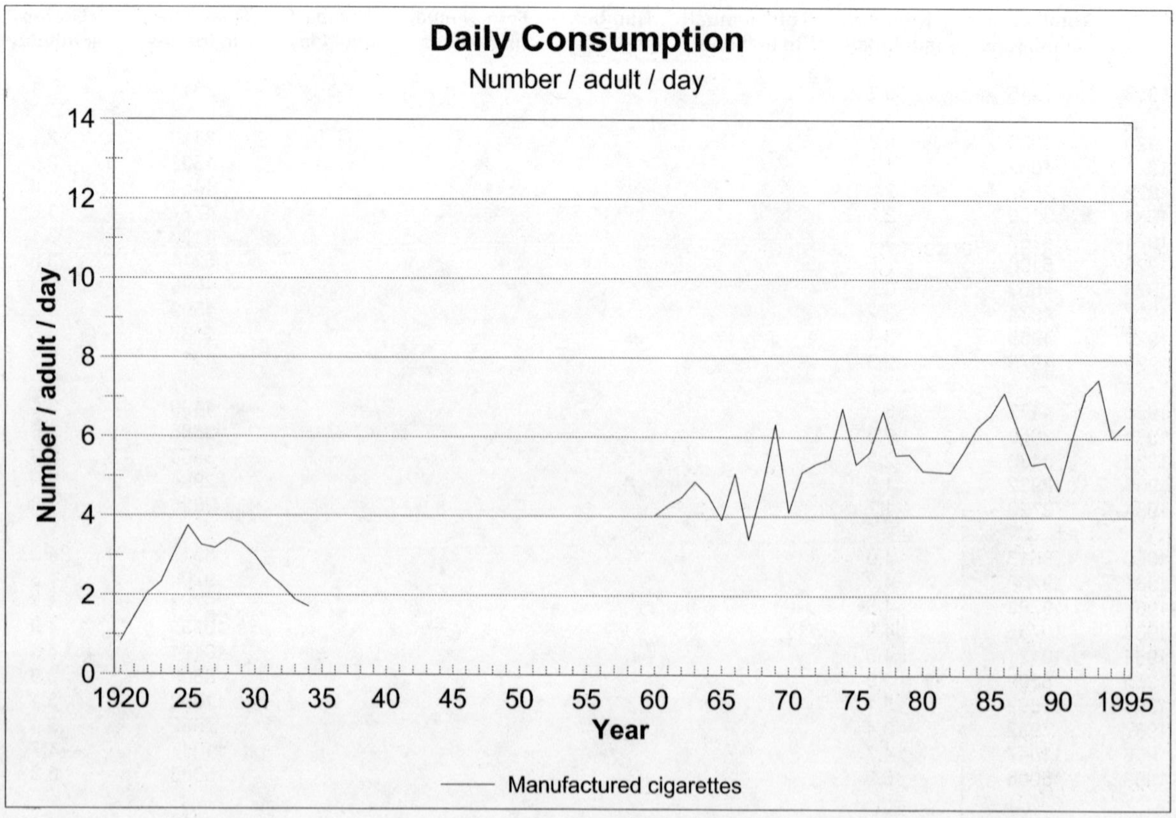

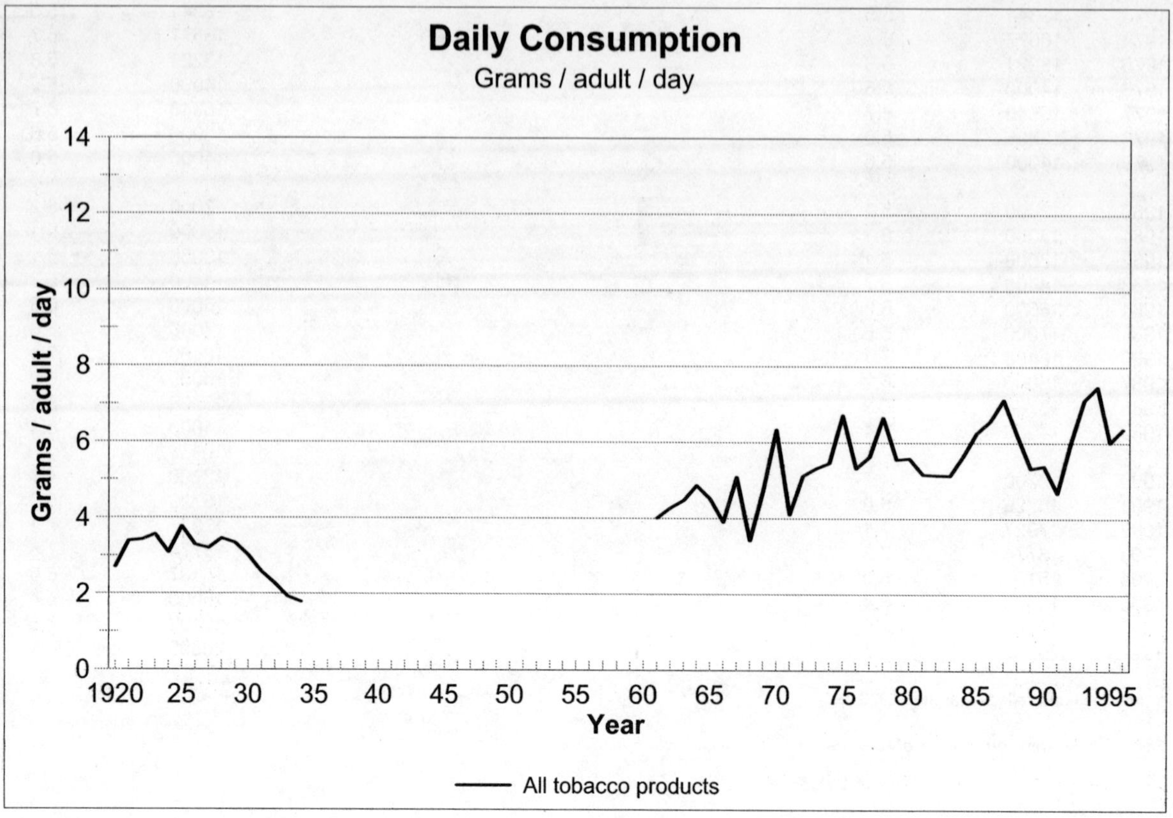

1 Includes hand-rolled cigarettes 1924-1934

Table 4.3 Percentage sales of tobacco in different forms (by weight), selected years 1913-1934

Year	Cigarettes[1] (%)	Smoking mixtures (%)	Snuff (%)
1913	9.8	90.2	0.1
1925	99.7	0.3	0.0
1934	96.2	3.8	0.0

1 Includes cigarette tobacco 1925-1934

Source : calculated from Table 4.1.1

Figure 4.2 Percentage sales of tobacco in different forms (by weight), selected years 1925-1934
Source: see Table 4.3

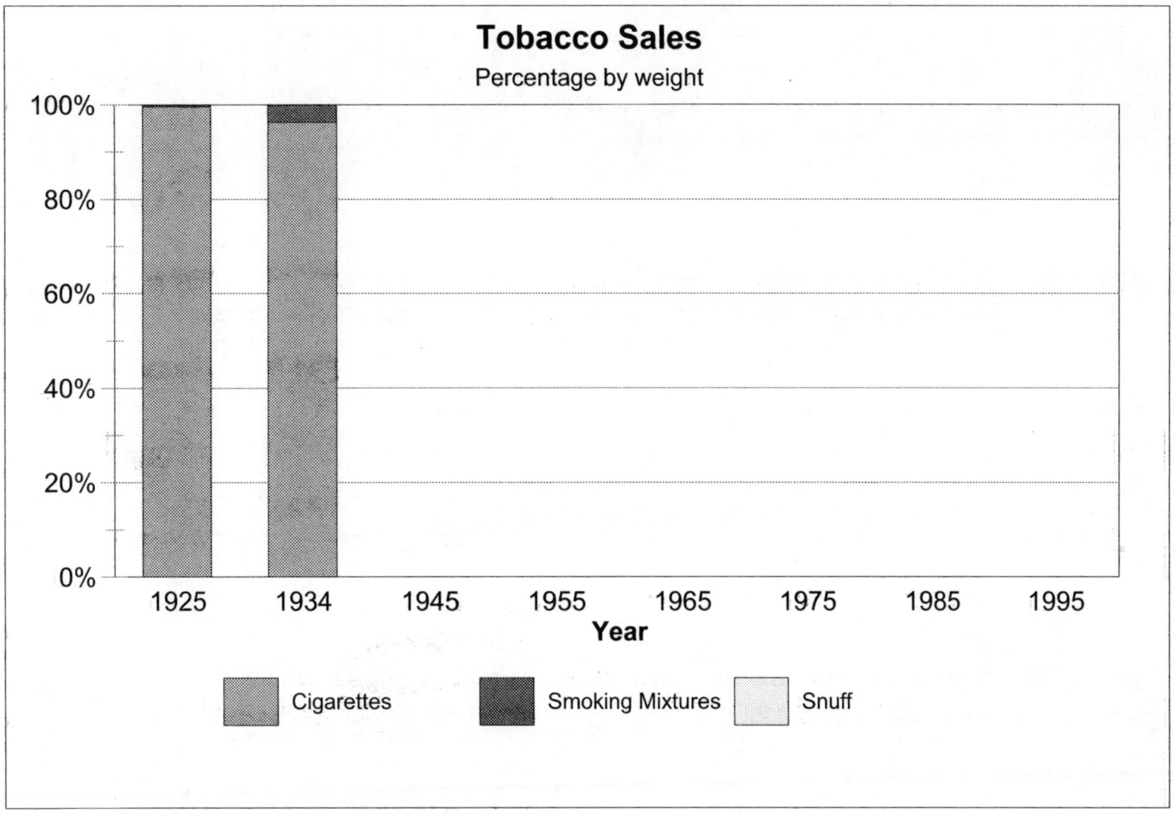

Table 4.4M Prevalence of smoking, males: some selected Bulgarian surveys by age, 1989-1997

Frequency / Product / Source / Year	12	13	14	15	16	17	18	19	20-24	25-29	30-34	35-39	40-44	45-49	50-54	55-59	60-64	65-69	70-74	75-79	80+	All ages
89 1 U A									65													49
96 3 U U				49																		
97 2 UC R							48.4				58.2		52.4		40.8		15.5		6.2			38.4
97 4 U R	49																					

Table 4.5M Number of cigarettes smoked per smoker per day, males: selected Bulgarian survey by age, 1997

Product / Source / Year	12	13	14	15	16	17	18	19	20-24	25-29	30-34	35-39	40-44	45-49	50-54	55-59	60-64	65-69	70-74	75-79	80+	All ages
97 2 UCE							19.9															

Table 4.6M Number of cigarettes smoked per person per day, males: selected Bulgarian survey by age, 1997, with percentage total sales

Product / Source / Year	12	13	14	15	16	17	18	19	20-24	25-29	30-34	35-39	40-44	45-49	50-54	55-59	60-64	65-69	70-74	75-79	80+	All ages	% Total sales
97 2 UC							7.6																59%m

Table 4.7M Number of cigarettes smoked per person per day, sales-adjusted, males: selected Bulgarian survey[1] by age, 1997, with percentage total sales

Product / Source / Year	12	13	14	15	16	17	18	19	20-24	25-29	30-34	35-39	40-44	45-49	50-54	55-59	60-64	65-69	70-74	75-79	80+	All ages	% Total sales
97 2 UC							12.9																59%m

1 Based on those surveys in Table 4.6 with data for both sexes and age range at least 21-64 (see *Cigarette consumption per person*, p. xxxv)

Source: see *Notes on sources of survey data*, p. 79
Frequency: A = all smokers (including occasional)
R = regular or daily smokers
All ages: relevant to ages used and as given in original source
% Total sales: estimated % of total sales of M = manufactured or T = total cigarette consumption implied by survey, sexes combined, used as adjustment factor in Table 4.7
** = cannot be calculated
--- = adjusted by original author

Product: MC = manufactured cigarettes
TC = total cigarettes (including hand-rolled)
UC = cigarettes (type unspecified)
A = all products
E indicates mean estimated from percentage distribution (see also *Consumption category estimation*, p. xxxiv, and Appendix III, p. 789)
U = unspecified
* = refer to *Notes on sources of survey data*, p. 79

Table 4.4F Prevalence of smoking, females: some selected Bulgarian surveys by age, 1989-1997

Frequency / Product / Source / Year	12	13	14	15	16	17	18	19	20-24	25-29	30-34	35-39	40-44	45-49	50-54	55-59	60-64	65-69	70-74	75-79	80+	All ages
89 1 U A									35													17
96 3 U U				47																		
97 2 UC R							37.1				30.2		20.6		9.1		1.5		0.0			16.7
97 4 U R	58																					

Table 4.5F Number of cigarettes smoked per smoker per day, females: selected Bulgarian survey by age, 1997

Product / Source / Year	12	13	14	15	16	17	18	19	20-24	25-29	30-34	35-39	40-44	45-49	50-54	55-59	60-64	65-69	70-74	75-79	80+	All ages
97 2 UCE							13.4															

Table 4.6F Number of cigarettes smoked per person per day, females: selected Bulgarian survey by age, 1997 with percentage total sales

Product / Source / Year	12	13	14	15	16	17	18	19	20-24	25-29	30-34	35-39	40-44	45-49	50-54	55-59	60-64	65-69	70-74	75-79	80+	All ages	% Total sales
97 2 UC							2.2																59%m

Table 4.7F Number of cigarettes smoked per person per day, sales-adjusted, females: selected Bulgarian survey[1] by age, 1997 with percentage total sales

Product / Source / Year	12	13	14	15	16	17	18	19	20-24	25-29	30-34	35-39	40-44	45-49	50-54	55-59	60-64	65-69	70-74	75-79	80+	All ages	% Total sales
97 2 UC							3.8																59%m

1 Based on those surveys in Table 4.6 with data for both sexes and age range at least 21-64 (see *Cigarette consumption per person*, p. xxxv)

Source: see *Notes on sources of survey data*, p. 79
Frequency: A = all smokers (including occasional)
R = regular or daily smokers
All ages: relevant to ages used and as given in original source
% Total sales: estimated % of total sales of M = manufactured or T = total cigarette consumption implied by survey, sexes combined, used as adjustment factor in Table 4.7
** = cannot be calculated
--- = adjusted by original author

Product: MC = manufactured cigarettes
TC = total cigarettes (including hand-rolled)
UC = cigarettes (type unspecified)
A = all products
E indicates mean estimated from percentage distribution (see also *Consumption category estimation*, p. xxxiv, and Appendix III, p. 789)
U = unspecified
* = refer to *Notes on sources of survey data*, p. 79

Table 4.8 Estimated[1] prevalence of smoking and estimated[1] number of cigarettes per person per day (unadjusted and sales-adjusted): summary of Tables 4.4, 4.6 and 4.7, 1989-1997 Males and females aged 15 years and over.

Year	Source[2]	Product[3]	Prevalence[4]						Number of cigarettes						
									Unadjusted[7]			Sales-adjusted[8]			
			Manufactured cigarettes		Total cigarettes[5]		All products[6]		Number/ person/day		Total sales %	Manufactured cigarettes[9] number/ person/day		Total cigarettes number/ person/day	
			M	F	M	F	M	F	M	F		M	F	M	F
1989	1	**U**					49	17				(8.5	2.4)		
1996	3	*U*					49	47				(8.6	6.6)		
1997	2	UC			40	19			7.4	2.3	59	12.5	3.9		

1 Surveys covering an age range of at least 21-64 are included. Any gaps in the data for ages 15-20 and 65 years and over are filled in by assumed extensions to the age distribution, given in *Notes on sources of survey data*, p. 79. Method: see *Summary of adult smoking*, p. xxxvi
2 See *Notes on sources of survey data*, p. 79
3 Product: MC = manufactured cigarettes, TC = total cigarettes (including hand-rolled), UC = cigarettes (type unspecified), A = all products, U = unspecified. Frequency of smoking is indicated by: regular or daily smokers in normal type, all smokers (including occasional) in bold, unspecified in italics
4 From Table 4.4
5 This column includes prevalence of smoking classified as UC = cigarettes (type unspecified)
6 This column includes prevalence of smoking classified as U = unspecified product
7 From Table 4.6
8 From Table 4.7, except data in parentheses, which are derived from the prevalence of smoking from Table 4.4 as described in *Summary of adult smoking*, p. xxxvi
9 Number of cigarettes classified as UC = cigarettes (type unspecified), or U = product unspecified has been adjusted to total cigarette sales and included in this column

Notes

Notes on sources of sales data

The data presented in the tables and figures were obtained from several sources, details of which are given below, together with estimations and related assumptions. Full citations of the sources are given on p. 80 under *References*.

Consumption data

1913-1935 Hutson (1937)

Data were originally given to the nearest 1 000 pounds. They have been converted to tonnes (1 000 lbs = 0.45359 tonnes) and given to the nearest tonne. For conversion from weights to numbers we assumed an average cigarette weight of 1 g. Cigarette tobacco was included with smoking mixtures for 1913-1922, and with cigarettes from 1923-1935. No consumption of cigars was reported. Actual consumption may exceed the figures given, since production was not entirely controlled, and home-grown tobacco may have been used avoiding excise tax.

1960-1995 United States Department of Agriculture (USDA) Economic Research Service (1996) *(Table 4.2)*

Data are available for cigarettes only. For conversion from numbers to weights we assumed an average cigarette weight of 1 g. Traditionally, tobacco is used primarily for cigarette production with very little processed for snuff or chewing tobacco. Despite high levels of imports, there was only one company that registered as an importer in 1994, leading to the assumption that 95% of imports were illegal.

For comparison, the following figures for sales of tobacco products were given by WHO (1975):

Year	Tonnes
1970	12 420
1971	12 608
1972	13 378
1973	14 220
1974	14 180

Since these figures are quite similar to our estimates for the sales of manufactured cigarettes, we have assumed that by this period, sales of other products were low. They have been ignored in the calculation of total sales from 1960 onwards.

Plain/Filter cigarette consumption

1966-1979 Maxwell (successive years)

1984 Boddewyn (1986)

1993-1996 USDA Economic Research Service (1996)

For 1993 onwards the data represent percentage of production rather than of sales.

Tar yield of cigarettes

No data available. The tar yield per cigarette was limited to 20 mg during the 1990s, and to 15 mg from 2001 (Harkin *et al* (1997)).

Estimates of hand-rolled cigarettes

Hand-rolled cigarette consumption is included with manufactured cigarettes for 1922-1934 (Table 4.2). It is assumed to have been negligible in recent decades.

Notes on sources of survey data

Each source of survey data—either an individual survey or a series of surveys repeated over a number of years—is cited by a source number. This number is shown in the tables and corresponds to the source numbers given below, where details of the source publication and of the survey methodology are given. Full citations of the sources are given on p. 80 under *References*.

Several surveys conducted after the period usually considered in this report have been included, since very few sex- or age-specific data are available for Bulgaria.

Notes *(continued)*

Source number

1 WHO (1997)

a. Overall age group not stated (adults)

b. Representativeness not stated. Balabanova *et al* (1998) state that in their study (see source 2) results from major cities only were similar to this study

2 Balabanova *et al* (1998)

a. Household survey, representative of general population (although ethnic minorities may have been under-represented). Sample size 1 550, response rate at least 70%

b. Consumption category estimation based on 1-9, 10-19, 20-29, 30-39 and 40+ cigarettes per day, taken from graph

c. Assumed extension to age distribution for percentage smokers, age 15-17: males and females 35%. Number of cigarettes/person/day: makes and females 4.0

3 USDA Economic Research Service (1996)

a. Unofficial data. Age group not stated

4 USDA Economic Research Service (1996)

a. Unofficial data. Age group not stated (teenagers). Year not stated

Additional information (not presented in tables)

Zatonski (1991) states that the prevalence of smoking was 28% (sexes combined) in 1987, which represented a considerable decline since 1980.

References

Boddewyn J.J. (ed) (1986). *Tobacco advertising bans and consumption in 16 countries*. International Advertising Association, New York.

Balabanova D., Bobak M. and McKee M. (1998). Patterns of smoking in Bulgaria. *Tob Control,* **7**, 383-5.

Hutson J.B. (1937). *Consumption and production of tobacco in Europe*. USDA, Washington DC. Technical bulletin No. 587.

Harkin A.M., Anderson P. and Goos C. (1997). *Smoking, drinking and drug taking in the European Region*. Alcohol, Drugs and Tobacco Programme, WHO Regional Office for Europe, Copenhagen.

Maxwell J.C.Jr. (successive years). How the brands ranked. Maxwell International Estimates. *World Tobacco.*

USDA Economic Research Service (1996). *Tobacco statistics*. Albert R. Mann Library, Cornell University, Ithaca, New York. ERS 94012. (With supplementary material from Tobacco Annual Reports.). http://usda.mannlib.cornell.edu/data-sets/specialty/94012.

WHO (1997). *Tobacco or health: A global status report*. WHO, Geneva. www.cdc.gov/nccdphp/osh/who/whoampro.htm.

WHO (1975). Survey on smoking and health in the European Region, 1974-75: preliminary data as at 1 May 1975. In: *Third World Conference on Smoking and Health, New York, 2-5 June 1975*. WHO; 1-55.

Zatonski W. (1991). Country reports. *World Smoking and Health,* **16**, 12-21.

Canada 5

Sales data

See Tables 5.1-5.3.

From 1920 to the early 1980s the consumption of manufactured cigarettes per adult increased steadily from 1 cigarette per day to nearly 10. By 1995 it had decreased again to 5 cigarettes per day. Legal sales were even lower in the early 1990s when smuggled cigarettes formed a major part of the market. Consumption of hand-rolled cigarettes per adult declined from 2 to about 0.6 cigarettes per day between 1955 and 1985.

The consumption of all tobacco products per adult was about 6 g per day between 1920 and 1935, after which it rose to about 12 g per day in the 1960s and early 1970s. It fell to 5 g per day by 1995. In 1925, 22% of all tobacco consumed was in manufactured cigarettes, increasing to 88% in 1995. Use of plug tobacco (for chewing) and snuff declined rapidly from 30% of all tobacco in 1925 to 2% in 1965. Sales of pipe and hand-rolling tobacco increased during the 1920s and 1930s, but declined thereafter. A change in the categories available implies that pipe tobacco accounted for only a small proportion of pipe and hand-rolling tobacco by 1974.

Three quarters of manufactured cigarettes sold in 1968 were filtered, and this proportion increased to 98% by the mid 1980s. The sales-weighted tar yield was 21 mg per cigarette in 1968, falling to 13 mg in 1981. Sales-weighted data are not available thereafter, but other data suggest tar yield may have fallen by about 2-3 mg between 1981 and 1995.

Survey data

See Tables 5.4-5.8

A comprehensive series of data is available from surveys conducted almost annually from 1964-1986 (source 1). However, it has been suggested that these data under-estimate the prevalence of smoking, particularly among teenagers, because of the use of proxy interviews (source 2, see *Notes on sources of survey data*, p. 103).

In the mid-1960s, the prevalence of regular cigarette smoking among those aged 15 years and over was about 55% in men and 30% in women. The difference between the percentages of men and women who smoke cigarettes has decreased since then owing almost entirely to a decrease in the prevalence among men, with estimates around 30% in the 1990s. The prevalence among women remained fairly level, just above 30% in the 1970s, then declining very gradually to below 30% in the 1990s. Another 3-4% of both sexes smoked cigarettes occasionally.

In general, more men than women smoked at all ages, but since the late 1970s some surveys have shown that there were more young women than young men who smoked. For all age groups there was a decrease in the percentages of men smoking. For women there was a rise in smoking prevalence at ages 15-19 from 20% in the mid 1960s to about 30% in the early 1970s, returning to about 20% by 1986, according to source 1. Source 2 gave higher estimates of prevalence but also showed a decrease between 1981-1986.

The prevalence of teenage smoking among girls was lower than among boys when first surveyed in 1960, but since 1978 most surveys have found that more girls than boys smoked. Definitions of a regular smoker vary considerably in surveys of teenagers, and comparisons should be made with caution.

Only very few women or men aged under 25 smoke other tobacco products but not cigarettes; for men, the prevalence increases with age to 6-9% at age 65 years and over. No data are available on prevalence by type of cigarette.

Comparison of survey and sales data suggests that surveys under-reported consumption by 25-40%. Between 1964 and 1995, the estimated number of cigarettes smoked per person per day (sales-adjusted) decreased for men from about 14 to 7. For women this increased somewhat from nearly 7 to 8.5 by about 1980, then decreased to 5 by 1990.

Table 5.1.1 Total annual sales of tobacco products, 1920-1973

Year	Cigarettes		Cigars		Pipe & HR[1] tobacco	Plug tobacco	Snuff	All tobacco products
	tonnes	millions	tonnes	millions	tonnes	tonnes	tonnes	tonnes
1920	2660	2441	1530	270	6400	2990	320	13900
1921	2660	2440	1210	214	5850	2810	320	12850
1922	2220	2043	1010	179	5130	4580	320	13260
1923	2490	2291	1090	193	5030	4130	360	13110
1924	2740	2515	960	169	5130	3760	360	12950
1925	3070	2823	1000	177	5530	3860	360	13830
1926	3510	3227	1000	177	5810	3630	360	14310
1927	4120	3781	1010	178	5990	3490	410	15010
1928	4830	4436	1060	187	6940	3220	450	16500
1929	5530	5081	1130	199	6580	2950	450	16640
1930	5480	5036	1040	183	7030	2680	450	16680
1931	4930	4533	860	152	7480	2400	410	16090
1932	4040	3713	750	133	7850	2090	360	15090
1933	4700	4317	650	115	7850	1910	320	15420
1934	5250	4822	680	120	8160	1910	360	16360
1935	5780	5305	710	125	8300	1770	360	16920
1936	6100	5600	690	122	8710	1680	360	17540
1937	7290	6698	740	130	9480	1630	360	19500
1938	7480	6872	750	132	9660	1450	360	19710
1939	7760	7126	750	133	10750	1450	360	21080
1940	8240	7572	940	166	11570	1410	360	22520
1941	9340	8582	1080	191	11340	1360	410	23530
1942	11150	10240	1140	201	11250	1590	410	25530
1943	12250	11257	1110	196	10800	1590	410	26160
1944	12700	11666	1120	198	10480	1450	450	26210
1945	15530	14265	1170	207	11480	1450	450	30080
1946	16180	14867	1250	221	11610	1320	450	30820
1947	16480	15143	1220	216	11290	1220	450	30680
1948	17260	15853	1190	210	11750	1040	450	31690
1949	18330	16836	1190	209	11430	1130	450	32530

Table 5.1.1 *(continued)*

Year	Cigarettes		Cigars		Pipe & HR[1] tobacco	Plug tobacco	Snuff tonnes	All tobacco products
	tonnes	millions	tonnes	millions	tonnes	tonnes		tonnes
1950	18690	17172	1130	199	11750	1040	410	33020
1951	17060	15672	960	169	12380	910	410	31720
1952	19430	17844	1130	200	14060	820	410	35850
1953	22860	21000	1330	235	11840	820	360	37210
1954	24080	22116	1390	245	11110	680	410	37670
1955	26750	24576	1430	253	10700	680	360	39940
1956	29390	27000	1450	256	9620	540	360	41370
1957	32820	30144	1660	293	9430	500	360	44770
1958	35280	32404	1830	323	9890	590	360	47950
1959	36820	33822	1760	311	10210	540	360	49700
1960	37330	34289	1880	332	10300	500	410	50410
1961	39950	36699	1910	337	10390	500	360	53110
1962	42110	38683	2000	352	10570	500	410	55580
1963	43410	39877	2190	387	10120	450	360	56540
1964	44240	40639	2230	491	9620	450	410	56950
1965	46820	43013	2220	489	9980	410	410	59840
1966	50380	46276	1980	437	8710	410	360	61840
1967	51020	46864	2020	445	8160	360	360	61930
1968	50370	46269	2100	462	8750	320	360	61900
1969	50710	46582	2310	509	8620	270	360	62270
1970	54240	49823	2540	560	8660	270	360	66080
1971	55370	50864	2830	624	8890	270	360	67730
1972	58010	53291	2590	570	8710	270	360	69940
1973	59720	54863	2760	609	8940	270	360	72060

1 Tobacco for hand-rolled cigarettes

Source: see *Notes on sources of sales data*, p. 102

Table 5.1.2 Total annual sales of tobacco products, 1974-1995

Year	Cigarettes			Cigars		Fine-cut tobacco[1]	Other-cut tobacco	Smokeless tobacco	All tobacco products
	tonnes	millions Legal	millions Smuggled	tonnes	millions	tonnes	tonnes	tonnes	tonnes
1974	51411	57123		2660	591	6706	600		6705
1975	51980	57756		2223	494	6759	953		6710
1976	54671	60745		2300	511	6577	524		6575
1977	55608	61787		2093	465	6313	865		6315
1978	49288	61610		1976	439	5660	856		5659
1979	51093	63866		1895	421	5227	813		5227
1980	51594	64492		1536	415	4785	691		4783
1981	53247	66559		1624	439	4765	721		4764
1982	53070	66338		1410	381	5552	309		5552
1983	50471	63089		1277	345	6023	292		6023
1984	49387	61734		1154	312	6166	250		6166
1985	47162	58953		1129	305	6866	192		6866
1986	44350	55437		1047	283	7413			9266
1987	42090	52613		969	262	7863			9829
1988	40842	51053		884	239	8027			10034
1989	38082	47602		821	222	7749		370	9686
1990	37750	45918	1270	703	190	6658		290	8323
1991	34700	38945	4430	1251	338	6360		285	7950
1992	35913	35061	9830	581	157	5080		260	6350
1993	35548	30225	14210	544	147	3829		310	4786
1994	39954	45743	4200	537	145	3964		325	4955
1995	36466	45582		492	133	3833		485	4791

1 Intended for hand-rolled cigarettes

Source : see *Notes on sources of sales data*, p. 102

Table 5.1.3 Manufactured cigarettes (i) percentage of total sales as filter cigarettes, 1966-1987, (ii) sales-weighted average tar yield per cigarette (SWAT), 1968-1981, (iii) tar, average of seven brands and (iv) nicotine, average of seven brands, 1968-1995

Year	% Filter	SWAT mg/cig	Tar mg/cig	Nicotine mg/cig
1966	75.0			
1967	77.0			
1968	80.6	21.1	21	1.59
1969	83.8	19.6	21	1.68
1970	86.1	18.7	21	1.59
1971	87.7	18.7	21	1.54
1972	89.1	18.6	20	1.53
1973	90.5	17.0	20	1.57
1974	91.6	16.9	20	1.51
1975	92.9	17.0		
1976	93.9	16.6	21	1.62
1977	94.8	15.8	21	1.46
1978	96.0	15.0	20	1.41
1979	96.1	14.2	18	1.42
1980	96.5	13.7	18	1.29
1981	96.8	13.2	17	1.29
1982			16	1.23
1983			17	1.40
1984			17	1.41
1985			16	1.43
1986	98.3		16	1.45
1987	98.4		16	1.31
1988			15	1.34
1989			17	1.49
1990			15	1.36
1991			14	1.32
1992			15	1.27
1993			14	1.27
1995			15	1.27

Source : see *Notes on sources of sales data*, p. 102

Table 5.2 Consumption of (i) cigarettes and (ii) all tobacco products, 1920-1995 sales-based data, including estimated hand-rolled cigarette consumption. Males and females aged 15 years and over

Year	Manufactured cigarettes		Hand-rolled cigarettes		Total cigarettes		All tobacco products	
	Total annual in millions	Number/ adult/day	Total annual in millions	Number/ adult/day	Total annual in millions	Number/ adult/day	Total annual in tonnes	Grams/ adult/day
1920	2441	1.2					13900	6.7
1921	2440	1.2					12850	6.1
1922	2043	0.9					13260	6.2
1923	2291	1.0					13110	6.0
1924	2515	1.1					12950	5.8
1925	2823	1.2					13830	6.1
1926	3227	1.4					14310	6.2
1927	3781	1.6					15010	6.3
1928	4436	1.8					16500	6.8
1929	5081	2.0					16640	6.7
1930	5036	2.0					16680	6.5
1931	4533	1.7					16090	6.2
1932	3713	1.4					15090	5.7
1933	4317	1.6					15420	5.7
1934	4822	1.8					16360	6.0
1935	5305	1.9					16920	6.1
1936	5600	2.0					17540	6.2
1937	6698	2.4					19500	6.8
1938	6872	2.4					19710	6.8
1939	7126	2.4					21080	7.2

Table 5.2 *(continued)*

Year	Manufactured cigarettes		Hand-rolled cigarettes		Total cigarettes		All tobacco products	
	Total annual in millions	Number/ adult/day	Total annual in millions	Number/ adult/day	Total annual in millions	Number/ adult/day	Total annual in tonnes	Grams/ adult/day
1940	7572	2.5					22520	7.5
1941	8582	2.8					23530	7.8
1942	10240	3.3					25530	8.3
1943	11257	3.6					26160	8.4
1944	11666	3.7					26210	8.3
1945	14265	4.5					30080	9.6
1946	14867	4.6					30820	9.6
1947	15143	4.7					30680	9.4
1948	15853	4.8					31690	9.5
1949	16836	4.9					32530	9.4
1950	17172	4.9					33020	9.4
1951	15672	4.4					31720	8.9
1952	17844	4.9					35850	9.8
1953	21000	5.7					37210	10.0
1954	22116	5.8					37670	9.9
1955	24576	6.4	8600	2.2	33176	8.6	39940	10.4
1956	27000	6.8	7800	2.0	34800	8.8	41370	10.4
1957	30144	7.4	7600	1.9	37744	9.3	44770	11.0
1958	32404	7.8	8000	1.9	40404	9.7	47950	11.5
1959	33822	8.0	8200	1.9	42022	9.9	49700	11.7
1960	34289	7.9	8300	1.9	42589	9.9	50410	11.7
1961	36699	8.3	8400	1.9	45099	10.3	53110	12.1
1962	38683	8.6	8600	1.9	47283	10.6	55580	12.4
1963	39877	8.7	8200	1.8	48077	10.5	56540	12.4
1964	40639	8.7	7800	1.7	48439	10.4	56950	12.2
1965	43013	9.0	8160	1.7	51173	10.7	59840	12.6
1966	46276	9.4	7000	1.4	53276	10.9	61840	12.6
1967	46864	9.3	6600	1.3	53464	10.6	61930	12.3
1968	46269	8.9	7021	1.4	53290	10.3	61900	12.0
1969	46582	8.8	6817	1.3	53399	10.1	62270	11.7
1970	49823	9.2	6922	1.3	56745	10.5	66080	12.2
1971	50864	9.2	7189	1.3	58053	10.5	67730	12.2
1972	53291	9.4	6974	1.2	60265	10.6	69940	12.3
1973	54863	9.5	7359	1.3	62222	10.7	72060	12.4
1974	57123	9.6	6705	1.1	63828	10.7	61377	10.3
1975	57756	9.5	6710	1.1	64466	10.6	61915	10.1
1976	60745	9.8	6575	1.1	67320	10.9	64072	10.4
1977	61787	9.7	6315	1.0	68102	10.7	64879	10.2
1978	61610	9.5	5659	0.9	67269	10.4	57780	8.9
1979	63866	9.7	5227	0.8	69093	10.5	59028	8.9
1980	64492	9.6	4783	0.7	69275	10.3	58606	8.7
1981	66559	9.7	4764	0.7	71323	10.4	60357	8.8
1982	66338	9.6	5552	0.8	71890	10.4	60341	8.7
1983	63089	8.9	6023	0.8	69112	9.7	58063	8.2
1984	61734	8.6	6166	0.9	67900	9.5	56957	7.9
1985	58953	8.1	6866	0.9	65819	9.1	55349	7.6
1986	55437	7.6	9266	1.3	64703	8.9	52810	7.3
1987	52613	7.1	9829	1.3	62442	8.5	50922	6.9
1988	51053	6.8	10034	1.3	61087	8.2	49753	6.7
1989	47602	6.3	9686	1.3	57288	7.6	47022	6.2
1990	47188	6.1	8323	1.1	55511	7.2	45401	5.9
1991	43375	5.5	7950	1.0	51325	6.5	42596	5.4
1992	44891	5.5	6350	0.8	51241	6.2	41834	5.1
1993	44435	5.3	4786	0.6	49221	5.9	40231	4.8
1994	49943	5.9	4955	0.6	54898	6.5	44780	5.3
1995	45582	5.3	4791	0.6	50373	5.8	41276	4.8

Source : see *Notes on sources of sales data*, p. 102

Figure 5.1 Daily consumption of (i) manufactured and total number of cigarettes, and (ii) all tobacco products, 1920-1995.
Males and females aged 15 years and over. *Source:* see Table 5.2

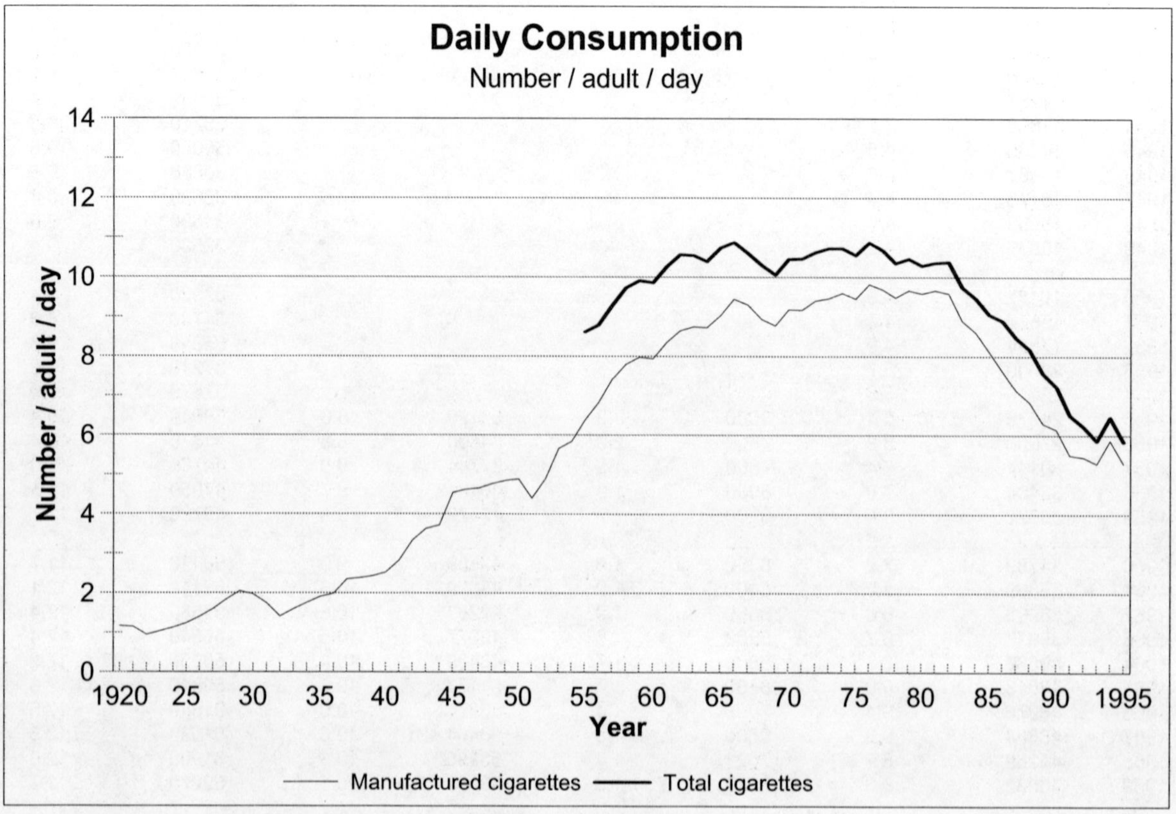

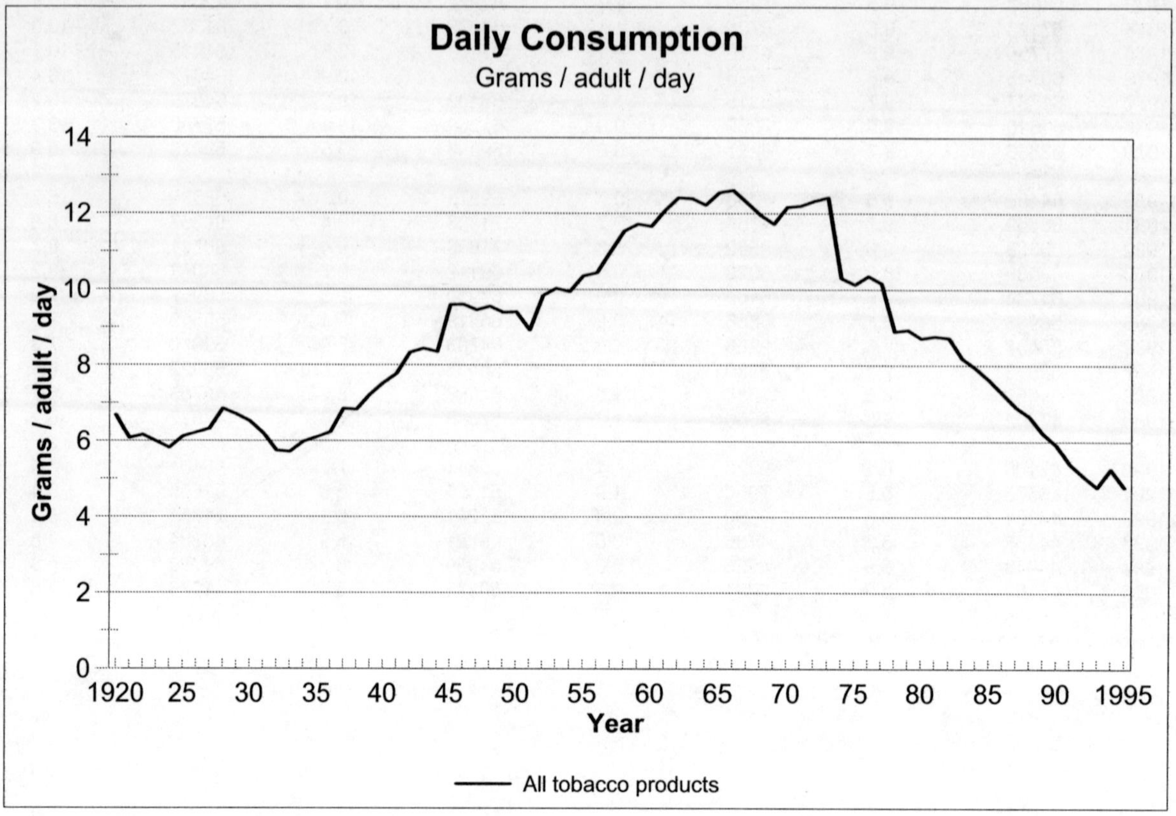

Table 5.3 Percentage sales of tobacco in different forms (by weight), selected years 1925-1995

Year	Cigarettes (%)	Cigars(%)	Other tobacco(%)
1925	22.2	7.2	70.5
1935	34.2	4.2	61.6
1945	51.6	3.9	44.5
1955	67.0	3.6	29.4
1965	78.2	3.7	18.0
1975	84.0	3.6	12.5
1985	85.2	2.0	12.8
1995	88.3	1.2	1.2

Source : calculated from Tables 5.1.1 & 5.1.2

Figure 5.2 Percentage sales of tobacco in different forms (by weight), selected years 1925-1995
Source: see Table 5.3

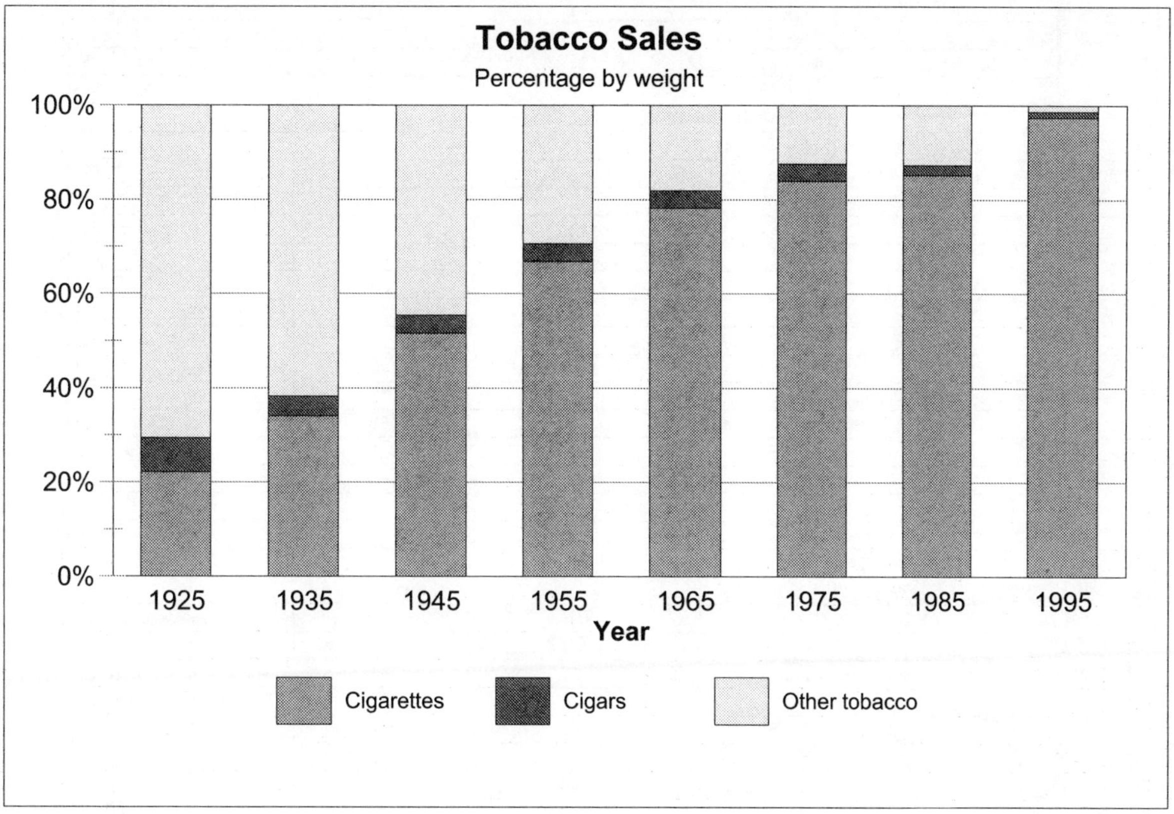

Table 5.4M Prevalence of smoking, males: some selected Canadian surveys by age, 1956-1995 *(continues on p. 90)*

Frequency Product Source Year	Age group 12	13	14	15	16	17	18	19	20-24	25-29	30-34	35-39	40-44	45-49	50-54	55-59	60-64	65-69	70-74	75-79	80+	All ages
56 5 UC U										83	80	79	80	82	83	75	70	68	63	59	43	
60 6 UC R	6	14	24	37	47	50	55	56														
60 6 UC R		25			44																	
63 6 UC R		29			41																	
64 1 TC R						36			59		62					58				32		54
65 1 TC R						35			62		63					59				32		55
65 1 TC A						39			66		66					62				36		58
66 1 TC R						35			60		62					58				32		54
67 1 TC R						36			59		62					56				33		53
67 6 U R	13	22	30	45	50	49	52	67														
67 7 U R	16	21	37	42	51	49	50	50														
68 1 TC R						35			58		59					55				33		52
69 1 TC R						34			55		56					53				32		50
70 1 TC R						36			54		56					51				31		49
70 1 TC A						39			58		58					54				34		52
71 1 TC R						34			56		54					52				32		48
71 1 U R			8	16	25	40	41	48														
71 8 U *	6	12	24	35	42	44	48															
71 8 U *		16				41																25
71 8 U R	15	24	37	46	52	53	58	56														
71 8 U A	21	30	44	51	57	57	62															
71 9 U R	6	12	24	35	42	44	48	47														
72 1 TC R						35			53		53					50				30		47
72 1 U R			9	17	28	38	43	50														
73 1 TC R						34			53		53					51				32		48
74 1 TC R						32			52		51					47				29		45
74 1 TC A						38			56		54					50				31		49
75 1 TC R						30			48		48					47				29		43
75 1 TC A						35			53		52					50				34		48
77 1 TC R						27			45		47					42				28		41
77 1 TC A						32			50		51					45				31		45
77 1 A A						32			50		51					51				40		49
78 8 U *		9				24																17
78 10 UC R						35			51		47					45				33		44
78 10 UC A						39			54		50					47				35		47
78 10 A A						39			56		54					51				42		50
78 11 U R	4	8	15	19	24	27	27	30														
78 11 U A	21	27	34	38	41	42	44	50														
79 1 TC R						27			42		44					41				25		39
79 1 TC A						31			46		47					44				28		42
79 1 A A						31			46		52					50				37		46
81 1 TC R						23			40		43					39				21		37
81 1 TC A						27			44		46					43				24		40
81 1 A R						27			44		50					48				31		
81 2 TC R						41			44		44					42				24		40
81 2 TC A						45			48		48					46				27		44
81 12 U *		4				30																21
82 4 U *		6				30																20
83 1 TC R						20			37		39					36				22		34
83 1 TC A						25			41		43					38				25		37
83 1 A A						25			41		46					42				31		41
83 2 TC R						34			40		40					38				24		37
83 2 TC A						38			44		44					41				27		41
83 4 U *		7				30																23
83 4 U U																						
84 4 U *		9				32																23
84 4 U U																						

Table 5.4F Prevalence of smoking, females: some selected Canadian surveys by age, 1956-1995 *(continues on p. 91)*

Year	Frequency	Product	Source	12	13	14	15	16	17	18	19	20-24	25-29	30-34	35-39	40-44	45-49	50-54	55-59	60-64	65-69	70-74	75-79	80+	All ages
56	5	UC	U																						
60	6	UC	R	3	8	18	25	33	33	30	23														
60	6	UC	R	15			29																		
63	6	UC	R	20			29																		
64	1	TC	R				19					41	40				28				8				31
65	1	TC	R				19					41	41				30				9				31
65	1	TC	A				22					46	44				34				11				35
66	1	TC	R				20					43	41				32				8				32
67	1	TC	R				21					42	41				32				10				32
67	6	U	R	11	24	32	38	44	44	45	39														
67	7	U	R	8	15	25	36	37	41	41	37														
68	1	TC	R				21					43	41				32				9				32
69	1	TC	R				23					39	40				32				11				32
70	1	TC	R				25					41	40				32				11				32
70	1	TC	A				29					46	43				34				12				36
71	1	TC	R				25					40	39				32				10				32
71	1	U	R			6	12	20	26	35	35														
71	8	U	*	4	12	22	31	34	33	33															
71	8	U	*	12			24																		18
71	8	U	R	12	25	37	45	46	45	46	48														
71	8	U	A	17	33	43	51	52	52	51															
71	9	U	R	4	12	22	31	34	33	33	38														
72	1	TC	R				28					41	39				32				10				32
72	1	U	R			7	15	20	29	38	43														
73	1	TC	R				29					41	38				32				11				32
74	1	TC	R				28					40	37				30				11				32
74	1	TC	A				33					44	41				33				13				35
75	1	TC	R				27					38	37				32				11				31
75	1	TC	A				33					43	41				36				13				36
77	1	TC	R				27					41	37				31				12				31
77	1	TC	A				32					45	40				34				15				35
77	1	A	A				32					45	40				34				15				35
78	8	U	*	11			29																		21
78	10	UC	R				36					47	39				35				16				36
78	10	UC	A				42					51	43				37				18				40
78	10	A	A				43					51	43				37				19				40
78	11	U	R	3	9	20	27	30	30	30	31														
78	11	U	A	17	28	40	45	46	45	48	44														
79	1	TC	R				26					40	36				29				11				30
79	1	TC	A				31					43	40				32				13				34
79	1	A	A				31					43	40				32				13				34
81	1	TC	R				23					41	33				29				11				29
81	1	TC	A				28					45	37				32				13				32
81	1	A	R				28					45	37				31				13				
81	2	TC	R				38					46	35				31				12				32
81	2	TC	A				42					50	38				33				14				35
81	12	U	*	10			36																		27
82	4	U	*	10			32																		24
83	1	TC	R				20					37	34				28				12				28
83	1	TC	A				24					41	37				31				14				32
83	1	A	A				24					41	37				31				14				32
83	2	TC	R				35					44	37				29				13				31
83	2	TC	A				39					48	40				32				15				34
83	4	U	*	12			33																		25
83	4	U	U	32																					
84	4	U	*	13			33																		24
84	4	U	U	36																					

Table 5.4M *(continued from p. 88)*
Prevalence of smoking, males

Frequency / Product / Source / Year	12	13	14	15	16	17	18	19	20-24	25-29	30-34	35-39	40-44	45-49	50-54	55-59	60-64	65-69	70-74	75-79	80+	All ages
85 3 U R				20					32	38				36				23				33
85 3 UC R				37										38		36		28	23	21	13	
85 3 TC A				27					40	42				37				22				36
85 4 UC *	35																					
85 13 TC R				24					34													
85 13 UC A				36																		
86 1 TC R				17					31	35				34				19				31
86 1 UC R				33										37		32		23	17			
86 1 TC A				21					36	39				36				20				34
86 1 A A				21					37	42				39				26				37
86 2 TC R				20					33	35				34				18				32
86 2 TC A				24					38	39				36				20				35
86 4 U U				33					42													
87 14 UC R										30		32		26		26						28
87 14 A R										32		35		28		30						32
88 15 UC R							33			35		32		31		22		16				30
88 15 UC A							37			40		36		33		25		20				34
88 15 A A							38			42		39		38		27		23				36
88 16 UC A				34																		
89 17 UC R				35										36		33		24	23	16	14	
89 17 UC A				22					37	38		38		36		33		22				33
90 13 UC A				22					35	34								18				31
90 16 UC A				33																		
90 18 UC R		8		17																		
90 18 UC A		14		22																		
90 19 UC A				21					35													31
91 3 UC R				12					28	33				25				18		9		26
91 3 UC A				20					44	37				29				21		11		32
91 16 UC A				29																		
91 22 U R									30					34								30
91 22 U A									30					35								30
92 16 UC A				31																		
92 22 U R									34					21								29
92 22 U A									35					21								30
93 16 UC A				30																		
93 18 UC R		11		21																		
93 22 U R									28					24								26
93 22 U A									31					25								28
94 16 UC A				30																		
94 19 UC R				17					31													
94 19 UC A				26					41	34								18				32
94 20 U R				19					27	34		31				19						28
94 20 U A				28					33	40		36				23						33
94 21 U R				13			23															
94 21 UC A	3	12		18			31															15
94 21 UC A				23																		
94 22 U R									28					20								25
94 22 U A									31					21								27
95 22 U R									32					32								29
95 22 U A									30					30								30

Source: see *Notes on sources of survey data*, p. 103

Product: MC = manufactured cigarettes
TC = total cigarettes (including hand-rolled)
UC = cigarettes (type unspecified)
A = all products

Frequency: A = all smokers (including occasional)
R = regular or daily smokers

All ages: relevant to ages used and as given in original source

U = unspecified

* = refer to *Notes on sources of survey data*, p. 103

Table 5.4F *(continued from p. 89)*
Prevalence of smoking, females

Frequency / Product / Source / Year	12	13	14	15	16	17	18	19	20-24	25-29	30-34	35-39	40-44	45-49	50-54	55-59	60-64	65-69	70-74	75-79	80+	All ages
85 3 U R				21					28	31				29				15				28
85 3 UC R				32										33		27		20	18	13	5	
85 3 TC A				28					43	36				31				18				32
85 4 UC *	39																					
85 13 TC R				21					38													
85 13 UC A				32																		
86 1 TC R				18					32	31				25				11				26
86 1 UC R				31										29		23		17	9			
86 1 TC A				21					37	34				28				13				29
86 1 A A				21					37	34				28				13				29
86 2 TC R				25					34	33				26				12				28
86 2 TC A				28					39	36				29				14				31
86 4 U U																						
87 14 UC R										30		26		30		24						27
87 14 A R										30		26		30		24						27
88 15 UC R							32			34		33		26		18		12				28
88 15 UC A							39			39		37		30		21		15				32
88 15 A A							39			39		37		30		21		15				32
88 16 UC A				31																		
89 17 UC R				34										33		29		19	19	15	9	
89 17 UC A				24					38	36		34		33		29		17				31
90 13 UC A				21					35	31								14				28
90 16 UC A				28																		
90 18 UC R		14		23																		
90 18 UC A		20		29																		
90 19 UC A				21					34													28
91 3 UC R				20					27	30				28				14		9		26
91 3 UC A				26					35	34				31				17		11		30
91 16 UC A				27																		
91 22 U R									32					28								28
91 22 U A									32					28								29
92 16 UC A				28																		
92 22 U R									23					20								22
92 22 U A									25					21								23
93 16 UC A				27																		
93 18 UC R		14		28																		
93 22 U R									23					14								19
93 22 U A									23					15								19
94 16 UC A				28																		
94 19 UC R				19					29													23
94 19 UC A				29					38	31								15				29
94 20 U R				21					30	30	26				15							24
94 20 U A				30					38	37	29				17							28
94 21 U R				17			22															
94 21 UC A	2	14		22			27															16
94 21 UC A				24																		
94 22 U R									26					17								23
94 22 U A									29					17								24
95 22 U R									31					23								25
95 22 U A									29					22								27

Source: see *Notes on sources of survey data*, p. 103
Product: MC = manufactured cigarettes
TC = total cigarettes (including hand-rolled)
UC = cigarettes (type unspecified)
A = all products

Frequency: A = all smokers (including occasional)
R = regular or daily smokers
All ages: relevant to ages used and as given in original source
U = unspecified
* = refer to *Notes on sources of survey data*, p. 103

Table 5.5M Number of cigarettes smoked per smoker per day, males: some selected Canadian surveys by age, 1960-1994

Product / Source / Year	Age group 12	13	14	15	16	17	18	19	20-24	25-29	30-34	35-39	40-44	45-49	50-54	55-59	60-64	65-69	70-74	75-79	80+	All ages
60 6 UCE	1.1	1.5	2.2	3.0	3.9	4.6	5.0	4.6														
64 1 TCE				13					17	19				19				16				18
65 1 TCE				13					18	19				19				16				18
66 1 TCE				14					18	19				19				16				18
67 1 TCE				13					17	19				19				16				18
68 1 TCE				13					17	19				19				16				18
69 1 TCE				13					17	20				19				16				18
70 1 TCE				13					18	20				20				17				19
71 1 TCE				13					18	20				20				17				19
72 1 TCE				13					18	20				20				17				19
73 1 TCE				14					18	20				20				17				19
74 1 TCE				14					18	20				20				17				19
75 1 TCE				15					18	20				20				17				19
77 1 TCE				14					18	20				21				18				20
78 10 UCE				14					20	23				23				16				21
79 1 TCE				17					18	21				21				18				20
81 1 TCE				15					18	20				21				17				20
81 2 TCE				16					19	21				21				18				20
83 1 TCE				14					18	21				21				17				20
83 2 TCE				17					19	21				21				17				21
85 3 UC				18					18	21				23				19				20
85 3 UCE				21														20				
85 4 UC	17																					
86 1 TCE				14					17	20				21				18				20
86 1 UCE				19														18				
86 2 TCE				15					17	20				21				16				20
88 15 UC							17			20		22		26		25		20				21
89 17 UCE				14					18	18		20		21		19		17				19
91 3 UCE				13					16	19				21				19				19
91 19 UC				13					17													
94 19 UC				15					17	22								18				21
94 20 UC				16					17	19		23				21						21
94 21 UC	7.0	7.3		9.6			13															10

Source: see *Notes on sources of survey data*, p. 103

Product: MC = manufactured cigarettes
TC = total cigarettes (including hand-rolled)
UC = cigarettes (type unspecified)
A = all products
U = unspecified

Product (cont): E indicates mean estimated from percentage distribution (see also *Consumption category estimation*, p. xxxiv, and Appendix III, p. 789)

All ages: relevant to ages used and as given in original source

* = refer to *Notes on sources of survey data*, p. 103

Table 5.5F Number of cigarettes smoked per smoker per day, females: some selected Canadian surveys by age, 1960-1994

<table>
<tr><th rowspan="2">Product
Source
Year</th><th colspan="21">Age group</th><th rowspan="2">All ages</th></tr>
<tr><th>12</th><th>13</th><th>14</th><th>15</th><th>16</th><th>17</th><th>18</th><th>19</th><th>20-24</th><th>25-29</th><th>30-34</th><th>35-39</th><th>40-44</th><th>45-49</th><th>50-54</th><th>55-59</th><th>60-64</th><th>65-69</th><th>70-74</th><th>75-79</th><th>80+</th></tr>
<tr><td>60 6 UCE</td><td colspan="21"></td><td></td></tr>
<tr><td>64 1 TCE</td><td colspan="3"></td><td colspan="5">12</td><td>14</td><td colspan="4">15</td><td colspan="4">15</td><td colspan="4">12</td><td>15</td></tr>
<tr><td>65 1 TCE</td><td colspan="3"></td><td colspan="5">12</td><td>14</td><td colspan="4">15</td><td colspan="4">15</td><td colspan="4">13</td><td>15</td></tr>
<tr><td>66 1 TCE</td><td colspan="3"></td><td colspan="5">12</td><td>15</td><td colspan="4">16</td><td colspan="4">15</td><td colspan="4">12</td><td>15</td></tr>
<tr><td>67 1 TCE</td><td colspan="3"></td><td colspan="5">12</td><td>15</td><td colspan="4">16</td><td colspan="4">15</td><td colspan="4">12</td><td>15</td></tr>
<tr><td>68 1 TCE</td><td colspan="3"></td><td colspan="5">12</td><td>15</td><td colspan="4">16</td><td colspan="4">15</td><td colspan="4">12</td><td>15</td></tr>
<tr><td>69 1 TCE</td><td colspan="3"></td><td colspan="5">12</td><td>15</td><td colspan="4">16</td><td colspan="4">16</td><td colspan="4">13</td><td>15</td></tr>
<tr><td>70 1 TCE</td><td colspan="3"></td><td colspan="5">12</td><td>16</td><td colspan="4">16</td><td colspan="4">16</td><td colspan="4">13</td><td>16</td></tr>
<tr><td>71 1 TCE</td><td colspan="3"></td><td colspan="5">12</td><td>16</td><td colspan="4">17</td><td colspan="4">16</td><td colspan="4">14</td><td>16</td></tr>
<tr><td>72 1 TCE</td><td colspan="3"></td><td colspan="5">12</td><td>16</td><td colspan="4">17</td><td colspan="4">16</td><td colspan="4">13</td><td>16</td></tr>
<tr><td>73 1 TCE</td><td colspan="3"></td><td colspan="5">13</td><td>16</td><td colspan="4">17</td><td colspan="4">16</td><td colspan="4">13</td><td>16</td></tr>
<tr><td>74 1 TCE</td><td colspan="3"></td><td colspan="5">13</td><td>16</td><td colspan="4">17</td><td colspan="4">17</td><td colspan="4">15</td><td>16</td></tr>
<tr><td>75 1 TCE</td><td colspan="3"></td><td colspan="5">13</td><td>16</td><td colspan="4">17</td><td colspan="4">16</td><td colspan="4">15</td><td>16</td></tr>
<tr><td>77 1 TCE</td><td colspan="3"></td><td colspan="5">14</td><td>17</td><td colspan="4">18</td><td colspan="4">17</td><td colspan="4">14</td><td>17</td></tr>
<tr><td>78 10 UCE</td><td colspan="3"></td><td colspan="5">14</td><td>16</td><td colspan="4">19</td><td colspan="4">18</td><td colspan="4">12</td><td>17</td></tr>
<tr><td>79 1 TCE</td><td colspan="3"></td><td colspan="5">14</td><td>17</td><td colspan="4">18</td><td colspan="4">18</td><td colspan="4">14</td><td>17</td></tr>
<tr><td>81 1 TCE</td><td colspan="3"></td><td colspan="5">15</td><td>17</td><td colspan="4">18</td><td colspan="4">18</td><td colspan="4">14</td><td>17</td></tr>
<tr><td>81 2 TCE</td><td colspan="3"></td><td colspan="5">16</td><td>18</td><td colspan="4">18</td><td colspan="4">18</td><td colspan="4">14</td><td>18</td></tr>
<tr><td>83 1 TCE</td><td colspan="3"></td><td colspan="5">13</td><td>17</td><td colspan="4">18</td><td colspan="4">18</td><td colspan="4">13</td><td>17</td></tr>
<tr><td>83 2 TCE</td><td colspan="3"></td><td colspan="5">15</td><td>16</td><td colspan="4">18</td><td colspan="4">18</td><td colspan="4">15</td><td>18</td></tr>
<tr><td>85 3 UC</td><td colspan="3"></td><td colspan="5">14</td><td>17</td><td colspan="4">18</td><td colspan="4">17</td><td colspan="4">16</td><td>17</td></tr>
<tr><td>85 3 UCE</td><td colspan="3"></td><td colspan="14">18</td><td colspan="4">15</td><td></td></tr>
<tr><td>85 4 UC</td><td colspan="10">17</td><td colspan="11"></td><td></td></tr>
<tr><td>86 1 TCE</td><td colspan="3"></td><td colspan="5">14</td><td>16</td><td colspan="4">18</td><td colspan="4">17</td><td colspan="4">15</td><td>17</td></tr>
<tr><td>86 1 UCE</td><td colspan="3"></td><td colspan="14">17</td><td colspan="4">15</td><td></td></tr>
<tr><td>86 2 TCE</td><td colspan="3"></td><td colspan="5">13</td><td>13</td><td colspan="4">15</td><td colspan="4">18</td><td colspan="4">17</td><td>14</td></tr>
<tr><td>88 15 UC</td><td colspan="6"></td><td colspan="3">16</td><td colspan="2">18</td><td colspan="2">21</td><td colspan="2">21</td><td colspan="2">18</td><td colspan="2">16</td><td colspan="2"></td><td>19</td></tr>
<tr><td>89 17 UCE</td><td colspan="3"></td><td colspan="5">11</td><td>13</td><td colspan="2">16</td><td colspan="2">17</td><td colspan="2">18</td><td colspan="2">15</td><td colspan="4">14</td><td>16</td></tr>
<tr><td>91 3 UCE</td><td colspan="3"></td><td colspan="5">14</td><td>14</td><td colspan="4">17</td><td colspan="4">18</td><td colspan="4">13</td><td>17</td></tr>
<tr><td>91 19 UC</td><td colspan="3"></td><td colspan="5">16</td><td>15</td><td colspan="8">19</td><td colspan="4">15</td><td></td></tr>
<tr><td>94 19 UC</td><td colspan="3"></td><td colspan="5">12</td><td>16</td><td colspan="8">18</td><td colspan="4">16</td><td>17</td></tr>
<tr><td>94 20 UC</td><td colspan="3"></td><td colspan="5">11</td><td>13</td><td colspan="2">16</td><td colspan="4">19</td><td colspan="6">17</td><td>17</td></tr>
<tr><td>94 21 UC</td><td>5.4</td><td colspan="2">5.8</td><td colspan="3">9.6</td><td colspan="2">11</td><td colspan="13"></td><td>9.4</td></tr>
</table>

Source: see *Notes on sources of survey data*, p. 103

Product:
MC = manufactured cigarettes
TC = total cigarettes (including hand-rolled)
UC = cigarettes (type unspecified)
A = all products
U = unspecified

Product (cont): E indicates mean estimated from percentage distribution (see also *Consumption category estimation*, p. xxxiv, and Appendix III, p. 789)

All ages: relevant to ages used and as given in original source

* = refer to *Notes on sources of survey data*, p. 103

Table 5.6M Number of cigarettes smoked per person per day, males: some selected Canadian surveys by age, 1964-1994, with percentage total sales

Product Source Year	12	13	14	15	16	17	18	19	20-24	25-29	30-34	35-39	40-44	45-49	50-54	55-59	60-64	65-69	70-74	75-79	80+	All ages	% Total sales
64 1 TC				4.8					10	12				11				5.1				9.7	67%T
65 1 TC				4.6					11	12				11				5.1				9.9	67%T
66 1 TC				4.8					11	12				11				5.2				9.8	67%T
67 1 TC				4.5					10	12				11				5.2				9.6	68%T
68 1 TC				4.5					10	11				10				5.2				9.4	69%T
69 1 TC				4.3					9.6	11				10				5.2				9.1	69%T
70 1 TC				4.8					9.5	11				10				5.2				9.1	67%T
71 1 TC				4.5					9.9	11				10				5.4				9.1	67%T
72 1 TC				4.7					9.2	11				10				5.2				8.8	65%T
73 1 TC				4.8					9.2	10				10				5.3				8.9	65%T
74 1 TC				4.6					9.3	10				9.3				4.9				8.6	63%T
75 1 TC				4.3					8.6	9.1	9.7	9.7	10	11	9.6	9.4	8.2	6.4	4.5	3.0			63%T
77 1 TC				3.9					8.2	9.6				8.8				4.8				8.0	61%T
78 10 UC				5.0					10	11				10				5.1				9.3	73%T
79 1 TC				4.5					7.7	9.1				8.5				4.3				7.6	61%T
81 1 TC				3.4					7.1	8.7				8.1				3.7				7.2	58%T
81 2 TC				6.5					8.2	9.3				8.8				4.3				8.1	66%T
83 1 TC				2.9					6.6	8.0				7.5				3.9				6.7	59%T
83 2 TC				5.7					7.5	8.6				8.2				4.2				7.6	67%T
85 3 UC				7.7														4.5					68%T
85 4 UC	6																						**
86 1 TC				2.5					5.4	7.2				7.0				3.4				6.1	58%T
86 1 UC	6.4																	3.3					58%T
86 2 TC				3.0					5.6	7.2				7.3				2.8				6.3	60%T
88 15 UC							6			7		7		8		5		3				6	65%T
89 17 UC				3.0					6.5	6.7		7.6		7.5		6.2		3.8				6.2	71%T
91 3 UC				1.6					4.4	6.2				5.1				2.9				4.8	69%T
94 19 UC				2.5					5.3														**
94 20 UC				2.9					4.5	6.4		7.0				4.0						5.6	73%T
94 21 UC	0.2	0.9		1.7			3.9															1.6	**

Source: see *Notes on sources of survey data*, p. 103

Product: MC = manufactured cigarettes
TC = total cigarettes (including hand-rolled)
UC = cigarettes (type unspecified)
A = all products
U = unspecified

All ages: relevant to ages used and as given in original source

% Total sales: estimated % of total sales of M = manufactured or T = total cigarette consumption implied by survey, sexes combined
** = cannot be calculated
--- = adjusted by original author
* = refer to *Notes on sources of survey data*, p. 103

Table 5.6F Number of cigarettes smoked per person per day, females: some selected Canadian surveys by age, 1964-1994 with percentage total sales

Year Source Product	12	13	14	15	16	17	18	19	20-24	25-29	30-34	35-39	40-44	45-49	50-54	55-59	60-64	65-69	70-74	75-79	80+	All ages	% Total sales
64 1 TC				2.2					5.7	6.0				4.2				0.9				4.5	67%T
65 1 TC				2.2					5.6	6.2				4.5				1.1				4.6	67%T
66 1 TC				2.4					6.3	6.5				4.8				1.0				4.9	67%T
67 1 TC				2.5					6.1	6.3				4.9				1.2				4.8	68%T
68 1 TC				2.6					6.5	6.6				4.8				1.1				4.9	69%T
69 1 TC				2.8					5.9	6.3				4.9				1.4				4.9	69%T
70 1 TC				3.0					6.5	6.6				5.0				1.4				5.0	67%T
71 1 TC				3.0					6.2	6.5				5.2				1.4				5.1	67%T
72 1 TC				3.5					6.4	6.5				5.0				1.3				5.1	65%T
73 1 TC				3.7					6.5	6.4				5.2				1.5				5.1	65%T
74 1 TC				3.6					6.5	6.4				5.0				1.6				5.1	63%T
75 1 TC				3.6					6.1	6.3	6.4	6.5	5.9	6.4	5.6	4.8	3.8	2.5	1.3	0.7			63%T
77 1 TC				3.6					6.8	6.5				5.2				1.6				5.3	61%T
78 10 UC				4.9					7.6	7.4				6.2				2.0				6.2	73%T
79 1 TC				3.7					6.8	6.5				5.1				1.4				5.2	61%T
81 1 TC				3.4					6.9	6.0				5.1				1.5				5.0	58%T
81 2 TC				5.9					8.0	6.3				5.5				1.7				5.6	66%T
83 1 TC				2.7					6.2	6.1				4.9				1.6				4.9	59%T
83 2 TC				5.5					7.2	6.7				5.1				1.8				5.5	67%T
85 3 UC				5.6														2.2					68%T
85 4 UC	7																						**
86 1 TC				2.5					5.1	5.6				4.2				1.7				4.3	58%T
86 1 UC				4.9														1.6					58%T
86 2 TC				3.3					5.2	5.9				4.3				1.7				4.7	60%T
88 15 UC							5			6		7		5		3		2				5	65%T
89 17 UC				2.7					4.8	5.7		5.5		5.8		4.3		2.2				4.8	71%T
91 3 UC				2.8					3.5	5.0				4.9				1.4				4.2	69%T
94 19 UC				2.3					4.6													3.9	**
94 20 UC				2.4					3.9	4.8		4.8				2.5						3.9	73%T
94 21 UC	0.1	0.8		2.1			3.0															1.5	**

Source: see *Notes on sources of survey data*, p. 103

Product: MC = manufactured cigarettes
TC = total cigarettes (including hand-rolled)
UC = cigarettes (type unspecified)
A = all products
U = unspecified

All ages: relevant to ages used and as given in original source

% Total sales: estimated % of total sales of M = manufactured or T = total cigarette consumption implied by survey, sexes combined
** = cannot be calculated
--- = adjusted by original author
* = refer to *Notes on sources of survey data*, p. 103

Table 5.7M Number of cigarettes smoked per person per day, sales-adjusted, males: some selected Canadian surveys[1] by age, 1964-1994, with percentage total sales

Product Source Year	12	13	14	15	16	17	18	19	20-24	25-29	30-34	35-39	40-44	45-49	50-54	55-59	60-64	65-69	70-74	75-79	80+	All ages	% Total sales
64 1 TC						7.0			15		17				16				7.5			14	67%T
65 1 TC						6.8			16		18				17				7.5			15	67%T
66 1 TC						7.1			16		18				16				7.7			15	67%T
67 1 TC						6.7			15		18				16				7.6			14	68%T
68 1 TC						6.5			15		17				15				7.6			14	69%T
69 1 TC						6.2			14		16				15				7.6			13	69%T
70 1 TC						7.1			14		16				15				7.7			14	67%T
71 1 TC						6.7			15		16				15				8.0			14	67%T
72 1 TC						7.2			14		16				15				8.0			14	65%T
73 1 TC						7.3			14		16				16				8.2			14	65%T
74 1 TC						7.3			15		16				15				7.7			14	63%T
75 1 TC						6.9			14	15	16	16	16	17	15	15	13	10	7.2	4.8			63%T
77 1 TC						6.3			13		16				14				7.9			13	61%T
78 10 UC						6.7			14		15				14				6.9			13	73%T
79 1 TC						7.3			13		15				14				7.1			13	61%T
81 1 TC						5.8			12		15				14				6.3			12	58%T
81 2 TC						9.8			12		14				13				6.5			12	66%T
83 1 TC						5.0			11		14				13				6.6			11	59%T
83 2 TC						8.5			11		13				12				6.3			11	67%T
85 3 UC										11									6.6				68%T
86 1 TC						4.3			9.3		13				12				5.9			10	58%T
86 1 UC										11									5.7				58%T
86 2 TC						5.0			9.4		12				12				4.8			11	60%T
88 15 UC								8		11		11		12			8	5				10	65%T
89 17 UC						4.2			9.2	9.4		11		11		8.8			5.3			8.8	71%T
91 3 UC						2.2			6.3		9.0				7.4				4.2			7.0	69%T
94 20 UC						4.0			6.1	8.7			9.6					5.5				7.7	73%T

1 Based on those surveys in Table 5.6 with data for both sexes and age range at least 21-64 (see *Cigarette consumption per person*, p. xxxv)

Source: See *Notes on sources of survey data*, p. 103

Product: MC = manufactured cigarettes
TC = total cigarettes (including hand-rolled)
UC = cigarettes (type unspecified)
A = all products
U = unspecified

All ages: relevant to ages used and as given in original source

% Total sales: Adjustment factor used, estimated % of total sales of M = manufactured or T = total cigarette consumption implied by survey, sexes combined

--- = adjusted by original author

* = refer to *Notes on sources of survey data*, p. 103

Table 5.7F Number of cigarettes smoked per person per day, sales-adjusted, females: some selected Canadian surveys[1] by age, 1964-1994, with percentage total sales

<table>
<tr><th rowspan="2">Product Source Year</th><th colspan="21">Age group</th><th rowspan="2">All ages</th><th rowspan="2">% Total sales</th></tr>
<tr><th>12</th><th>13</th><th>14</th><th>15</th><th>16</th><th>17</th><th>18</th><th>19</th><th>20-24</th><th>25-29</th><th>30-34</th><th>35-39</th><th>40-44</th><th>45-49</th><th>50-54</th><th>55-59</th><th>60-64</th><th>65-69</th><th>70-74</th><th>75-79</th><th>80+</th></tr>
<tr><td>64 1 TC</td><td colspan="3"></td><td colspan="5">3.3</td><td>8.4</td><td colspan="4">8.9</td><td colspan="4">6.3</td><td colspan="4">1.4</td><td>6.7</td><td>67%T</td></tr>
<tr><td>65 1 TC</td><td colspan="3"></td><td colspan="5">3.3</td><td>8.4</td><td colspan="4">9.3</td><td colspan="4">6.7</td><td colspan="4">1.6</td><td>6.9</td><td>67%T</td></tr>
<tr><td>66 1 TC</td><td colspan="3"></td><td colspan="5">3.5</td><td>9.3</td><td colspan="4">9.7</td><td colspan="4">7.2</td><td colspan="4">1.5</td><td>7.3</td><td>67%T</td></tr>
<tr><td>67 1 TC</td><td colspan="3"></td><td colspan="5">3.7</td><td>9.0</td><td colspan="4">9.3</td><td colspan="4">7.3</td><td colspan="4">1.7</td><td>7.2</td><td>68%T</td></tr>
<tr><td>68 1 TC</td><td colspan="3"></td><td colspan="5">3.7</td><td>9.5</td><td colspan="4">9.6</td><td colspan="4">6.9</td><td colspan="4">1.6</td><td>7.1</td><td>69%T</td></tr>
<tr><td>69 1 TC</td><td colspan="3"></td><td colspan="5">4.0</td><td>8.6</td><td colspan="4">9.2</td><td colspan="4">7.1</td><td colspan="4">2.0</td><td>7.1</td><td>69%T</td></tr>
<tr><td>70 1 TC</td><td colspan="3"></td><td colspan="5">4.5</td><td>9.7</td><td colspan="4">9.7</td><td colspan="4">7.4</td><td colspan="4">2.0</td><td>7.5</td><td>67%T</td></tr>
<tr><td>71 1 TC</td><td colspan="3"></td><td colspan="5">4.5</td><td>9.2</td><td colspan="4">9.7</td><td colspan="4">7.7</td><td colspan="4">2.1</td><td>7.6</td><td>67%T</td></tr>
<tr><td>72 1 TC</td><td colspan="3"></td><td colspan="5">5.4</td><td>9.9</td><td colspan="4">10</td><td colspan="4">7.7</td><td colspan="4">2.1</td><td>7.9</td><td>65%T</td></tr>
<tr><td>73 1 TC</td><td colspan="3"></td><td colspan="5">5.7</td><td>10</td><td colspan="4">9.9</td><td colspan="4">8.0</td><td colspan="4">2.3</td><td>7.9</td><td>65%T</td></tr>
<tr><td>74 1 TC</td><td colspan="3"></td><td colspan="5">5.7</td><td>10</td><td colspan="4">10</td><td colspan="4">7.9</td><td colspan="4">2.5</td><td>8.1</td><td>63%T</td></tr>
<tr><td>75 1 TC</td><td colspan="3"></td><td colspan="5">5.8</td><td>9.8</td><td>10</td><td>10</td><td>10</td><td>9.4</td><td>10</td><td>9.0</td><td>7.7</td><td>6.1</td><td>4.0</td><td>2.1</td><td colspan="2">1.1</td><td></td><td>63%T</td></tr>
<tr><td>77 1 TC</td><td colspan="3"></td><td colspan="5">5.9</td><td>11</td><td colspan="4">11</td><td colspan="4">8.4</td><td colspan="4">2.7</td><td>8.6</td><td>61%T</td></tr>
<tr><td>78 10 UC</td><td colspan="3"></td><td colspan="5">6.6</td><td>10</td><td colspan="4">10</td><td colspan="4">8.4</td><td colspan="4">2.7</td><td>8.5</td><td>73%T</td></tr>
<tr><td>79 1 TC</td><td colspan="3"></td><td colspan="5">6.1</td><td>11</td><td colspan="4">11</td><td colspan="4">8.4</td><td colspan="4">2.4</td><td>8.5</td><td>61%T</td></tr>
<tr><td>81 1 TC</td><td colspan="3"></td><td colspan="5">5.8</td><td>12</td><td colspan="4">10</td><td colspan="4">8.7</td><td colspan="4">2.6</td><td>8.6</td><td>58%T</td></tr>
<tr><td>81 2 TC</td><td colspan="3"></td><td colspan="5">8.9</td><td>12</td><td colspan="4">9.5</td><td colspan="4">8.3</td><td colspan="4">2.6</td><td>8.5</td><td>66%T</td></tr>
<tr><td>83 1 TC</td><td colspan="3"></td><td colspan="5">4.6</td><td>10</td><td colspan="4">10</td><td colspan="4">8.4</td><td colspan="4">2.7</td><td>8.3</td><td>59%T</td></tr>
<tr><td>83 2 TC</td><td colspan="3"></td><td colspan="5">8.2</td><td>11</td><td colspan="4">10</td><td colspan="4">7.6</td><td colspan="4">2.7</td><td>8.2</td><td>67%T</td></tr>
<tr><td>85 3 UC</td><td colspan="3"></td><td colspan="14">8.2</td><td colspan="4">3.2</td><td></td><td>68%T</td></tr>
<tr><td>86 1 TC</td><td colspan="3"></td><td colspan="5">4.3</td><td>8.7</td><td colspan="4">9.6</td><td colspan="4">7.3</td><td colspan="4">3.0</td><td>7.5</td><td>58%T</td></tr>
<tr><td>86 1 UC</td><td colspan="3"></td><td colspan="14">8.4</td><td colspan="4">2.7</td><td></td><td>58%T</td></tr>
<tr><td>86 2 TC</td><td colspan="3"></td><td colspan="5">5.5</td><td>8.8</td><td colspan="4">9.8</td><td colspan="4">7.3</td><td colspan="4">2.8</td><td>7.9</td><td>60%T</td></tr>
<tr><td>88 15 UC</td><td colspan="6"></td><td colspan="3">8</td><td colspan="2">10</td><td colspan="2">10</td><td colspan="2">8</td><td colspan="2">5</td><td colspan="2">3</td><td colspan="2"></td><td>8</td><td>65%T</td></tr>
<tr><td>89 17 UC</td><td colspan="3"></td><td colspan="5">3.8</td><td>6.7</td><td colspan="2">8.1</td><td colspan="2">7.8</td><td colspan="2">8.2</td><td colspan="2">6.0</td><td colspan="4">3.2</td><td>6.7</td><td>71%T</td></tr>
<tr><td>91 3 UC</td><td colspan="3"></td><td colspan="5">4.1</td><td>5.1</td><td colspan="4">7.2</td><td colspan="4">7.1</td><td colspan="4">2.1</td><td>6.1</td><td>69%T</td></tr>
<tr><td>94 20 UC</td><td colspan="3"></td><td colspan="5">3.2</td><td>5.3</td><td colspan="2">6.5</td><td colspan="4">6.6</td><td colspan="6">3.4</td><td>5.3</td><td>73%T</td></tr>
</table>

1 Based on those surveys in Table 5.6 with data for both sexes and age range at least 21-64 (see *Cigarette consumption per person*, p. xxxv)

Source: See *Notes on sources of survey data*, p. 103
Product: MC = manufactured cigarettes
TC = total cigarettes (including hand-rolled)
UC = cigarettes (type unspecified)
A = all products
U = unspecified

All ages: relevant to ages used and as given in original source
% Total sales: Adjustment factor used, estimated % of total sales of M = manufactured or T = total cigarette consumption implied by survey, sexes combined
--- = adjusted by original author
* = refer to *Notes on sources of survey data*, p. 103

Table 5.8 Estimated[1] prevalence of smoking and estimated[1] number of cigarettes per person per day (unadjusted and sales-adjusted): summary of Tables 5.4, 5.6 and 5.7, 1964-1995. Males and females aged 15 years and over

Year	Source[2]	Product[3]	Prevalence[4]						Number of cigarettes						
									Unadjusted[7]			Sales-adjusted[8]			
			Manufactured cigarettes		Total cigarettes[5]		All products[6]		Number/ person/day		Total sales %	Manufactured cigarettes number/ person/day		Total cigarettes[9] number/ person/day	
			M	F	M	F	M	F	M	F		M	F	M	F
1964	1	TC			54	30			9.6	4.4	67			14.2	6.5
1965	1	TC			55	31			9.9	4.6	67			14.7	6.8
	1	**TC**			58	35									
1966	1	TC			54	32			9.8	4.8	67			14.6	7.2
1967	1	TC			53	32			9.6	4.8	68			14.2	7.1
1968	1	TC			52	32			9.3	4.9	69			13.5	7.1
1969	1	TC			50	32			9.1	4.8	69			13.2	7.0
1970	1	TC			49	32			9.1	5.0	67			13.5	7.5
	1	**TC**			52	35									
1971	1	TC			48	32			9.1	5.0	67			13.5	7.5
1972	1	TC			47	32			8.8	5.0	65			13.6	7.8
1973	1	TC			48	32			8.9	5.1	65			13.6	7.9
1974	1	TC			45	31			8.5	5.1	63			13.5	8.0
	1	**TC**			49	35									
1975	1	TC			43	31			8.2	5.0	63			13.1	8.0
	1	**TC**			47	35									
1977	1	TC			41	31			7.9	5.2	61			12.9	8.5
	1	**TC+A**			45	35	47	35							
1978	10	UC			44	35			9.2	6.1	73			12.5	8.3
	10	**UC+A**			47	39	50	39							
1979	1	TC			39	30			7.6	5.2	61			12.5	8.5
	1	**TC+A**			42	33	46	33							
1981	1	TC+A			37	29	44	32	7.1	5.0	58			12.2	8.5
	1	**TC**			40	32									
	2	TC			41	32			8.1	5.6	66			12.3	8.5
	2	**TC**			45	35									
1983	1	TC			34	28			6.7	4.8	59			11.4	8.2
	1	**TC+A**			37	31	40	31							
	2	TC			37	32			7.5	5.5	67			11.3	8.3
	2	**TC**			41	35									
1985	3	UC+U			35	29	33	27	7.3	5.1	68			10.7	7.5
	3	**TC**			37	32									
	13	**UC**			36	32								(10.5	7.6)
1986	1	UC			32	26			6.0	4.4	58			10.3	7.5
	1	TC			31	26									
	1	**TC+A**			34	29	37	29							
	2	TC			31	28			6.1	4.5	60			10.3	7.6
	2	**TC**			34	31									

Year	Source[2]	Product[3]	Prevalence[4]						Number of cigarettes						
									Unadjusted[7]			Sales-adjusted[8]			
			Manufactured cigarettes		Total cigarettes[5]		All products[6]		Number/ person/day		Total sales %	Manufactured cigarettes number/ person/day		Total cigarettes[9] number/ person/day	
			M	F	M	F	M	F	M	F		M	F	M	F
1988	15	UC			28	26			5.9	4.7	65			9.1	7.3
	15	**UC+A**			32	30	35	30							
	16	**UC**			34	31								(9.5	6.9)
1989	17	UC			33	30			6.2	4.6	71			8.7	6.5
	17	**UC**			33	30									
1990	13	**UC**			31	28								(8.4	6.1)
	16	**UC**			33	28								(8.7	5.9)
	19	**UC**			31	28								(8.4	6.1)
1991	3	UC			26	25			4.9	4.1	76			7.1	5.9
	3	**UC**			32	29									
	16	**UC**			29	27								(7.5	5.6)
	22	U					27	24							
	22	**U**					28	26							
1992	16	**UC**			31	28								(7.2	5.2)
	22	U					27	20							
	22	**U**					28	21							
1993	16	**UC**			30	27								(6.8	4.9)
	22	U					24	17							
	22	**U**					26	18							
1994	16	**UC**			30	28								(7.4	5.5)
	19	**UC**			32	29								(7.5	5.5)
	20	UC+U					27	24	5.6	3.9	79			7.6	5.3
	20	**U**					33	28							
	22	U					23	20							
	22	**U**					25	22							
1995	22	U					27	22							
	22	**U**					28	24							

1 Surveys covering an age range of at least 21-64 are included. Any gaps in the data for ages 15-20 and 65 years and over are filled in by assumed extensions to the age distribution, given in *Notes on sources of survey data*, p. 103. Method: see *Summary of adult smoking*, p. xxxvi
2 See *Notes on sources of survey data*, p. 103
3 Product: MC = manufactured cigarettes, TC = total cigarettes (including hand-rolled), UC = cigarettes (type unspecified), A = all products, U = unspecified. Frequency of smoking is indicated by: regular or daily smokers in normal type, all smokers (including occasional) in bold, unspecified in italics
4 From Table 5.4
5 This column includes prevalence of smoking classified as UC = cigarettes (type unspecified)
6 This column includes prevalence of smoking classified as U = unspecified product
7 From Table 5.6
8 From Table 5.7, except data in parentheses, which are derived from the prevalence of smoking from Table 5.4 as described in *Summary of adult smoking*, p. xxxvi
9 Number of cigarettes classified as UC = cigarettes (type unspecified) has been adjusted to total cigarette sales and included in this column

Figure 5.3 Estimated prevalence of smoking of (i) cigarette and (ii) all tobacco products: by year of survey, 1964-1995.
Males and females aged 15 years and over. *Source:* see Table 5.8

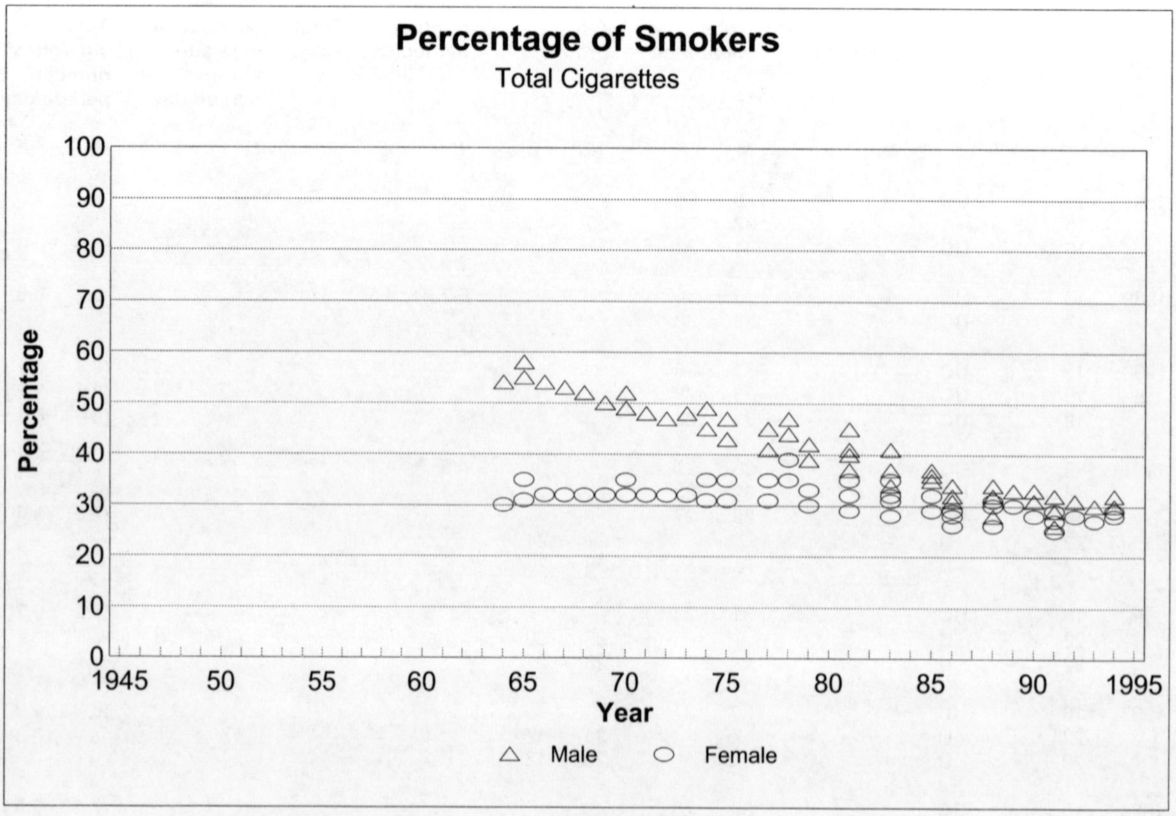

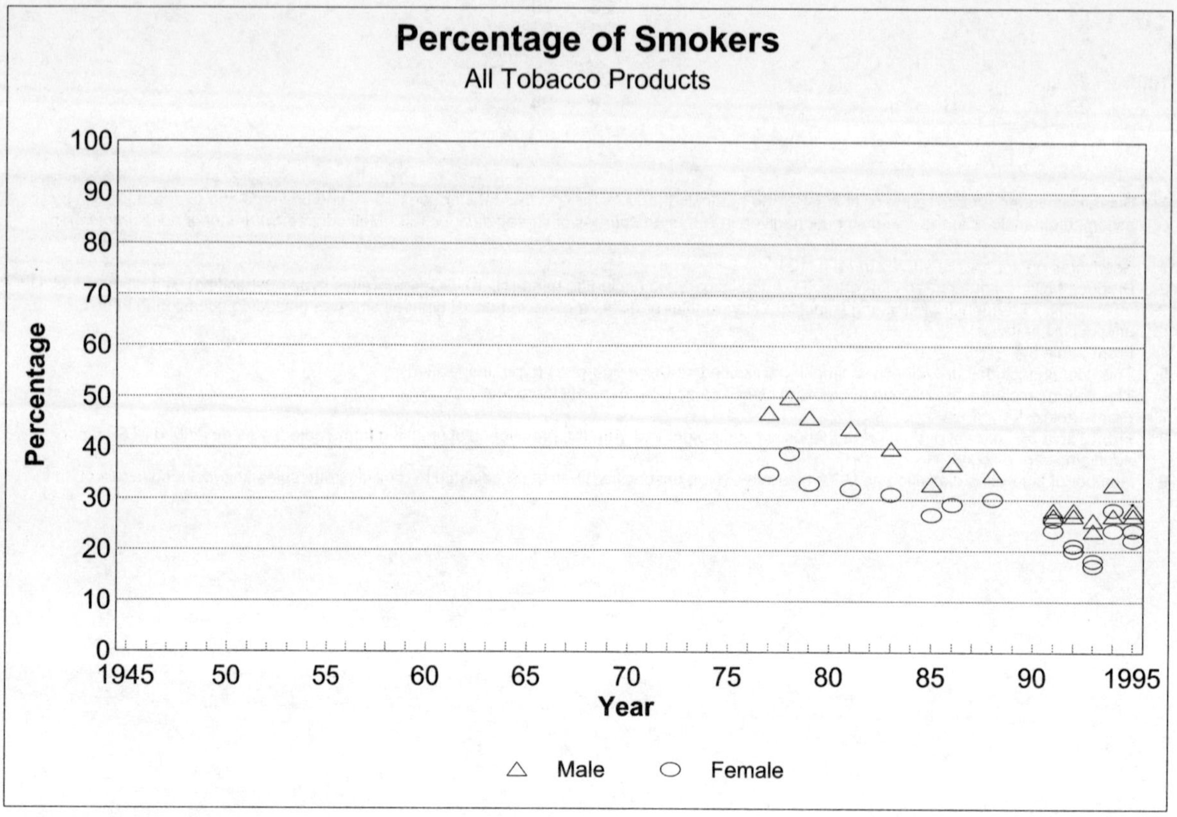

Figure 5.4 Estimated number of cigarettes smoked per person per day, sales-adjusted, 1964-1994.
Males and females aged 15 years and over. *Source:* see Table 5.8

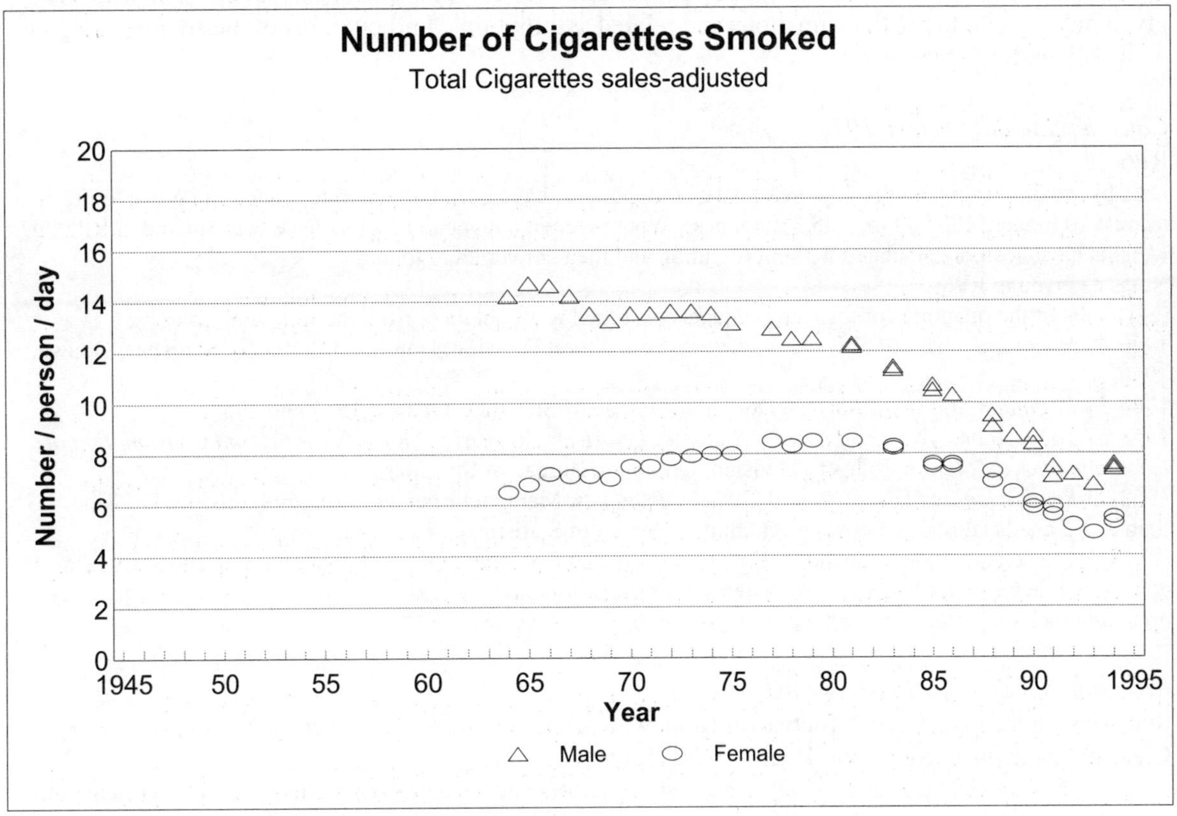

Notes on sources of sales data

The data presented in the tables and figures were obtained from several sources, details of which are given below, together with estimations and related assumptions. Full citations of the sources are given on p. 108 under *References*.

Consumption data before 1974

RP6

Data by weight, originally given to nearest 100 000 pounds, have been converted to tonnes and given to the nearest 10 tonnes (100 000 lbs =45.359 tonnes). Where weight conversion factors have been quoted in RP6, the weights have been re-calculated without rounding and then converted to tonnes.

Notes as given in RP6:

(a) Details of the quantities of tobacco products consumed were obtained from the following sources:

1920-48 *Historical Series of Tobacco Statistics*, Agricultural Division, Dominion Bureau of Statistics, Ottawa, 1950.

1949-57 *Canadian Statistical Review*, Dominion Bureau of Statistics, Ottawa, 1957 and 1958.

1958-67 *Tobacco and Tobacco Products Statistics Quarterly*, formerly *Quarterly Stocks and Consumption of Unmanufactured Tobacco*, Industry Division, Dominion Bureau of Statistics.

1968-73 *Production and Disposition of Tobacco Products*, Manufacturing and Primary Industries Division, Statistics Canada (formerly known as Dominion Bureau of Statistics).

(b) Cigarette consumption in pounds weight was estimated from the number of cigarettes consumed by using a conversion factor of 2.4 lbs per 1 000. The conversion factor used for cigars was 12.5 lbs per 1 000 for the years up to and including 1963, thereafter a figure of 10 lbs per 1 000 was used.

Consumption data for 1974 onwards

Statistics Canada—Canadian Statistical Review, Kaiserman and Rogers (1992), National Clearinghouse on Tobacco and Health (NCTH) (1996).

Data for cigarettes and cigars were given in numbers and have been converted to weight. For cigarettes we have used a conversion factor of 0.9 g per cigarette for 1974-1977 and 0.8 g for 1978-1990, as given by NCTH (1996). We have assumed 0.8 g for 1991-1995. For cigars we have assumed an average of 4.5 g per cigar for 1974-1979 (based on RP6) and 3.7 g per cigar for 1980-1995 (as in Anonymous (1990)).

Smuggled cigarettes: Stephens (1995)

In recent years smuggling of cigarettes into Canada became a problem. There is little evidence of organized smuggling before 1986 but by 1993 some sources estimate that smuggled cigarettes constituted almost 40% of the cigarette market. Following increases in federal and provincial taxes (1989-1992) there was a large difference in cigarette retail prices between Canada and the USA. It is thought that Canadian-blend cigarettes were being exported to the USA and then re-imported illegally—between 1990 and 1992 exports of tobacco products increased by 384%. There is also evidence of increasing smuggling of US-blend cigarettes into Canada. In February 1994 anti-smuggling measures were implemented and the federal tobacco tax was cut by $5.00 a carton in an effort to reduce the scale of illegal importation. In that year exports of cigarettes decreased by 90%. The export figure for 1996 is said to be in line with the US domestic market for Canadian cigarettes (Kondro (1994), Crichton (1998), Galbraith and Kaiserman (1997)). No figure was available for the number of smuggled cigarettes in 1995 and so our sales figure for that year is likely to be low.

Smokeless tobacco: Wyckham (1999)

Smokeless tobacco production in Canada ceased in 1987 when manufacturing was moved to the United States. Sales data are not available. The data quoted are import figures and so are subject to variations due to increasing and decreasing stock levels.

Plain/Filter cigarette consumption

1966-1981 Maxwell (successive years)

Tar and nicotine yield of cigarettes

1968-1981 Millar (1983), Rickert and Robinson (1981) and Canadian Tobacco Manufacturers' Council

1968-1995 Rickert (1995)

The data from Rickert (1995) (under the headings 'Tar' and 'Nicotine') are the result of analyses on seven popular brands of Canadian cigarettes which, together, make up approximately 25% of sales. The data are not sales-weighted and values are not available in some years for each of the seven brands. However, these figures provide a reasonably consistent measure of the changes over time.

Delarue (1961) reported that the tar yield was in the range 10-47 mg per cigarette in 1960.

Kaiserman and Rickert (1992) reported that the mean values (and ranges) per cigarette for 31 brands of hand-rolling cigarette tobacco, bought during December 1989, were 15.47 mg tar (range 14.64-16.29 mg), 1.14 mg nicotine (range 0.96-1.44 mg) and 17.69 mg carbon dioxide (range 16.53-18.79 mg). These were prepared and smoked under standard conditions. It was also found that yields varied considerably when a standard blend of tobacco was tested using various brands of tubes and filters.

Estimates of hand-rolled cigarette consumption for 1955-1995

Millar (1983), Todd (1987), Stephens (1995), NCTH (1996)

For years up to 1973 Todd / Millar estimated hand-rolled cigarette consumption as 81% of pipe and hand-rolling tobacco sales, at 1 g per cigarette.

Estimates of hand-rolled cigarette consumption in the latest available year were also given in the introductions to successive editions of RP6:

Year	Annual (millions)	Number/ adult/day	As percentage of Millar/Todd estimate
1966	6 160	1.3	88
1970	6 120	1.1	88
1973	6 723	1.2	91

For 1973-1995 onwards Todd / Millar estimated hand-rolled cigarette consumption as all fine-cut tobacco sales intended for hand-rolled cigarettes, at 1 g per cigarette. (The sales data for 1973 include 7 363 tonnes of fine-cut tobacco intended for hand-rolled cigarettes and 638 tonnes of other cut tobacco. These data are taken from the Canadian Statistical Review, but have not been included in Table 5.1.2.)

For 1986-1995 NCTH (1996) calculated hand-rolled cigarette consumption as all fine cut sales at 1 g per cigarette and we use their estimates for 1986-1989. However, for 1990 onwards we follow Stephens (1995) in using 0.8 g as the weight of one hand-rolled cigarette.

Notes on sources of survey data

Each source of survey data—either an individual survey or a series of surveys repeated over a number of years—is cited by a source number. This number is shown in the tables and corresponds to the source numbers given below, where details of the source publication and of the survey methodology are given. Full citations of the sources are given on p. 103 under *References*.

Source number

1,2 Health and Welfare Canada (successive editions), Thomson (1984), Stephens (1988), Maxwell and Hirdes (1993)

a. Labour Force Survey Supplements. Conducted annually (in December), using one-third of panel from monthly Labour Force Survey. Sample size around 17 000 (except 30 799 in 1986). Representative of 97-98% of population, excluding those in institutions, Indian reserves, and the Northern Territories. Sampling based on households and telephone interviews with extensive use of proxy respondents

b. Data given as source **2** are by Stephens (1988) using self-respondents only. (Proxy interviews excluded were 47% (1981), 50% (1983) and 26% (1986) of interviews.) The prevalence of smoking, particularly by teenagers, may be underestimated by proxy interviews, which could not be distinguished in earlier years
c. Regular cigarette smokers: smoked cigarettes usually daily
d. The percentage specifying hand-rolled cigarettes as their main brand type smoked was consistently 7-8% for males and 4-5% for females in the period 1977-1983. In 1986 the age/sex distribution was:

	15-19	**20-24**	**25-44**	**45-64**	**65+**	**15+**
Males	6.1	6.2	6.9	14.8	16.1	9.6
Females	5.7	7.3	7.2	9.6	9.3	7.8

e. Consumption category estimation based on 1-10, 11-25, and 26+ cigarettes/smoker/day
f. In calculations (i.e. combining smokers of cigarettes and other products, consumption category estimation) percentages indicated as being based on too small numbers to be reliable have been taken as zero

3 Stephens (1988), Maxwell and Hirdes (1993), Statistics Canada (1994)

a. General Social Survey. Questionnaire and population very similar to source 1, but only one respondent per household. Telephone interviews for persons age under 65, face-to-face interviews for persons age 65 years and over. Sample size (1985) 11 200, (1991) 11 924. Response rate (1985) 84%, (1991) 80%
b. Consumption category estimation based on 1-10, 11-25 and 26+ cigarettes/smoker/day (Stephens (1988), Statistics Canada (1994)), and 1-9, 10-19, 20-29 and 30+ cigarettes/smoker/day (Maxwell and Hirdes (1993))

4 Canadian Gallup Poll, cited by Canadian Gallup Poll Limited (1985), Millar (1985), Stephens (1988)

a. Conducted annually (in February) for the Health Promotion Directorate, primarily to assess reaction to the Directorate's media campaigns. Self-completed questionnaire at home. Parent's consent sought for participants under 16 years; parent invited to leave the interview room. Sample size about 2 000, over-weighted to the 12-19 age group, response rate about 65%.
b. Smokers marked as frequency *: smoked daily

5 Best and Walker (1964)

a. Baseline of prospective study among Department of Veterans Affairs pensioners, excluding those in hospital. Conducted September 1955-June 1956. Mailed questionnaire, 57% response, of which 59% (69 891) were males with adequate smoking data. Not representative of the Canadian population
b. Age distribution of sample reflects ages of enlisted men in the two World Wars and the Korean War. Ages 35-39 and 60-64 most heavily represented

6 Morison and Medovy (1961), Morison *et al* (1964) and Hanley and Robinson (1976), quoting Morison (1968) (no details of reference)

a. Surveys in Winnipeg, 1960, 1963 and year unknown (assumed 1967). Broader age bands are approximate, corresponding to school grades 7-9 and 10-12
b. Sample size (1960) 17 329, (1963) 14 140, (1967) unknown
c. Regular smokers: smoked more than one cigarette a week/'serious smokers'
d. Consumption category estimation based on weekly consumption of 1-4, 5-9, 10-19, 20-39 and 40+ cigarettes/smoker

7 Hanley and Robinson (1976), quoting Playfair (1968) (no details of reference)

a. Survey in Kenora, year not stated
b. Regular smokers: 'serious smokers'

8 Hanley and Robinson (1976), Millar (1985)

a. National studies carried out in 1971-1972 and 1978. Not a probability sample—distributed to schools through Home and School and Parent-Teacher Federation members, representing rural/urban and social structure. Sample size of 12-19-year-olds (1971) 52 129, (1978) 71 770

b. Smokers marked as frequency *: smoked daily. Regular smokers: smoked 1 or more cigarettes weekly. All smokers: smoked 1 or more cigarettes weekly or had smoked in the last 4 weeks

9 Hanley (1973)

a. Waterloo School Survey. Year not stated

10 Canada Health Survey (1981)

a. Canada Health Survey. A national household survey using a self-completed questionnaire for persons aged 15+. Sample size 5 662, response rate 86%

b. Regular smokers: smoked cigarettes daily

c. Consumption category estimation based on 1-12, 13-22, 23-32 and 33+ cigarettes/smoker/day.

11 Health and Welfare Canada (successive editions)

a. Public school students. Sample size (males) 53 539, (females) 51 610. Age 8-20

b. Regular smokers: smoked daily in the last 4 weeks. All smokers: smoked in the last 4 weeks, or had smoked at some time but whose current status is unknown

c. Results from this survey have also been published by Brown *et al* (1978) using imputed estimates, which assign subjects with incomplete data

12 Millar (1985)

a. Canada Fitness Survey. A national household survey using a self-completed questionnaire. Sample size of 12-19-year-olds 2 934

b. Smokers marked as frequency *: smoked daily

13 Stephens (1988), Health Canada (1999a, 2000)

a. Health Promotion Survey. Questionnaire and population very similar to source 1, but only one respondent per household. Telephone interviews. Sample size (1985) 11 164, (1990) 13 778

14 WHO (1989)

a. Regional survey forming part of WHO MONICA project:

Region	Population size	Sample size	Participation rate (%)	Sample used*		Date
				Male	Female	
Halifax County	98 800	1 190	64	459	458	Sep 1985-Nov 1988

* age 25-64, all other figures relate to age 35-64

b. *All ages* column relates to age 35-64 and is standardized to world population

c. Regular smokers: smoked cigarettes daily. All smokers: smoked cigarettes daily or occasionally, or 1 g pipe tobacco or 1 cigar per week

15 Stachenko *et al* (1992)

a. Canadian Heart Health Surveys Research Group surveys of non-institutionalized people aged 18-74 in nine provinces. Probability sample. Questions on smoking were a subset of those used by the Labour Force Survey. Sample size 20 585, response rate 78%

b. Results presented are average of surveys conducted in nine provinces between 1986 and 1990, age-standardized to the 1986 population of Canada

c. Assumed extension to age distribution for percentage smokers, age 15-17: males and females (cigarettes, regular) 15%, (cigarettes and all products, all smokers) 18%. For age 75+: males (cigarettes, regular) 10%, (cigarettes, all smokers) 13%, (all products) 15%, females (cigarettes, regular) 8%, (cigarettes and all products, all smokers) 10%. Number of cigarettes/person/day, age 15-17: males and females 2.0. For age 75+: males 2.0, females 1.0

16 Health Canada (1994a)

a. Canada Health Monitor surveys of people aged 15+. Sample size approximately 2 500

b. Smokers: 'smoke cigarettes now'

17 Eliany and Courtemanche (1992), Maxwell and Hirdes (1993)

a. National Alcohol and Other Drugs Survey. Survey of non-institutionalized people aged 15+. Sample size 11 634

b. Consumption category estimation based on 1-10, 11-25 and 26+ cigarettes/smoker/day (Eliany and Courtemanche (1992)). Calculation of cigarettes per person based on percentage of current smokers (daily and occasional) and number of cigarettes per daily smoker but, as only 1% of people surveyed were occasional smokers this makes little difference

18 King and Coles (1992), King *et al* (1996)

a. Part of the HBSC (Health Behaviour in School-Aged Children) Study, a collaborative cross-national research study sponsored by the WHO. School classes or schools were randomly selected, targeting age groups 11 (not presented here), 13 and 15. The target sample size was 1 300 in each age group

b. The Canadian part of the 1989-1990 survey was carried out during February-May 1990. The sample size was 5 565

Target age	Mean age
13	14.1
15	16

c. The Canadian part of the 1993-1994 survey was carried out during October1993-January 1994

Target age	Mean age	Sample size
13	13.5	2 250
15	15.5	2 219

d. Regular smokers: smoke once a week or more

19 Health Canada (1994b, 1999a)

a. The Survey on Smoking in Canada Cycle 1. One of the initiatives of the federal Tobacco Demand Reduction Strategy (TDRS). The purpose of the survey was to measure levels and changes in cigarette-smoking behaviour over the 1994-95 fiscal year, subsequent to the reduction in tobacco taxes early in 1994. Cycle 1 was the baseline survey

b. Telephone survey of non-institutionalized people aged 15+ in the provinces. One person per household, no proxy responses. Sample size 15 804, response rate 84%

c. Smoker: smoked cigarettes daily or non-daily

d. Prevalence of regular smoking estimated from overall proportions of daily and non-daily smokers

20 Health Canada (1999b)

a. National Population Health Survey. A longitudinal household-based survey conducted every two years by Statistics Canada. 1994 survey is the baseline. Sample size 22 622. Response rate 85-95%

b. Regular smokers: smoked daily. All smokers: smoked at the time of the interview

21 Stephens *et al* (1996), WHO (1997)

a. Youth Smoking Survey. National survey of 10-19-year-olds. 10-14-year-olds surveyed at school, 15-19-year-olds interviewed at home by telephone. The telephone sample includes residents of institutions such as group homes and hotels. Sample size 23 800, response rate 80-81%

b. Regular smokers: smoked at least one cigarette per day for the 30 days preceding the survey. Smokers: had smoked at least 100 cigarettes in lifetime and had smoked during the past 30 days

c. Stephens *et al* (1996) gives prevalence of use of other tobacco independent of cigarette smoking in the past week by people aged 10-19 in 1994 as follows:

	Cigars or Pipes (%)	Chewing tobacco (%)	Snuff (%)
Male	4	2	1
Female	2	0.3	1

d. Calculation of cigarettes per person based on prevalence of current smoking (daily and non-daily) and number of cigarettes per daily smoker, so may overestimate

22 Bondy and Ialomiteanu (1997) quoting Addiction Research Foundation

a. Telephone surveys in Ontario. Although regional, these surveys are widely quoted as they are consistent and cover a period when few national surveys were conducted.

Survey and Year	Sample size	Response rate (%)
Adult Drug Use Survey, 1991	1 047	67
OADOS 1992	1 058	63
OADOS 1993	1 034	65
OADOS 1994	2 022	63
OADOS 1995	994	63

OADOS: Ontario Alcohol and Other Drugs Opinion Survey

b. Regular smokers: smoke daily. Smokers: smoke cigarettes daily or occasionally, or have quit for less than one month

c. Data shown in the *All ages* column in Table 5.4 relate to ages 18+

d. There are slight discrepancies between the results resented here (all ages prevalence) and those reported by Health Canada (1994a) for some years

e. Assumed extension to age distribution for percentage smokers, age 15-17: males and females (regular) 15%, (all smokers) 18%. For age 65+: males (regular) 15%, (all smokers) 18%, females (regular 10%, (all smokers) 13%

References

Anonymous (1990). Trends in Canadian tobacco consumption, 1980-89. *Can Med Assoc J,* **143**, 905-6.

Beese D.H. (ed) (1968). *Tobacco consumption in various countries,* 2nd edition. Tobacco Research Council, London. Research Paper 6.

Beese D.H. (ed) (1972). *Tobacco consumption in various countries,* 3rd edition. Tobacco Research Council, London. Research Paper 6.

Best E.W.R. and Walker C.B. (1964). A Canadian study of smoking and health, second report. *Can J Public Health,* **55**, 1-11.

Bondy S.J. and Ialomiteanu A.R. (1997). Smoking in Ontario, 1991 to 1996. *Can J Public Health,* **88** , 225-9.

Brown K.S., Cherry W.H. and Forbes W.F. (1978). *The 1978 National Survey of smoking habits of Canadian schoolchildren.* University of Waterloo, Waterloo, Ontario.

Canada Health Survey (1981). *The Health of Canadians. Report of the Canada Health Survey.* Minister of Supply and Services Canada, Ottawa.

Canadian Gallup Poll Limited (1985). *A summary report on tobacco, alcohol & marijuana use and norms among young people in Canada—year 3 and study on parents and marijuana.* Health promotion directorate.

Crichton M. (1998). Annex 13. Tobacco and alcohol smuggling in Canada. In: *Report of the Alcohol and Tobacco Fraud Review.* H.M. Customs and Excise, UK; 4pp http://www.hmce.gov.uk/bus/excise/atfr-a10.htm.

Delarue N.C. (1961). A review of some important problems concerning lung cancer. Part I: considerations of epidemiology, etiology and pathogenesis. *Can Med Assoc J,* **84**, 1374-85.

Eliany M. and Courtemanche J.-R. (1992). *Smoking behaviour of Canadians. A national alcohol and other drugs survey report, 1989.* Health and Welfare Canada.

Galbraith J.W. and Kaiserman M. (1997). Taxation, smuggling and demand for cigarettes in Canada: evidence from time-series data. *Journal of Health Economics,* **16**, 287-301.

Hanley J.A. (1973). *Quantitative Studies in Cigarette Smoking Behaviour* [Thesis]. University of Waterloo.[§]

Hanley J.A. and Robinson J.C. (1976). Cigarette smoking and the young: a national survey. *Can Med Assoc J,* **114**, 511-7.

Health and Welfare Canada (successive editions). *Smoking habits of Canadians (or Smoking behaviour of Canadians).* Health and Welfare Canada, Canada.

Health Canada (1994b). *Survey on smoking in Canada.* Health Canada. Cycle 1.

Health Canada (1994a). *Trends in the prevalence of smoking, 1991-1994. Report of a workshop.* Health Canada.

Health Canada (1999b). *Smoking behaviour of Canadians,* January 1999 No 1. Health Canada. (National population health survey highlights.) http://www.hc-sc.gc.ca/hpb/lcdc/bc/nphs/nphs11_e.html.

Health Canada (1999a). *Smoking in Canada during the past 16 years.* Health Canada. Wired Health Jan 99. http://www.hc-sc.gc.ca/hppb/wired/smoking.htm .

Health Canada (2000). *Canadian tobacco use monitoring survey. List of Fact Sheets.* Health Canada. Wave 1, February-June 1999.

Kaiserman M.J. and Rickert W.S. (1992). Handmade cigaretes: it's the tube that counts. *Am J Public Health,* **82**, 107-9.

Kaiserman M.J. and Rogers B. (1992). Forty year trends in Canadian tobacco sales. *Can J Public Health,* **83**, 404-6.

King A., Wold B., Tudor-Smith C. and Harel Y. (1996). *The health of youth, a cross-national survey.* WHO Regional Publications, Europe, Copenhagen. European Series No. 69.

King A.J.C. and Coles B. (1992). *The health of Canada's youth. Views and behaviours of 11-, 13- and 15-year-olds from 11 countries.* Health and Welfare Canada, Ottawa.

Kondro W. (1994). Cuts in Canadian tobacco taxes [Abstract]. *Lancet,* **343**, 470.

Lee P.N. (ed) (1975). *Tobacco consumption in various countries,* 4th edition. Tobacco Research Council, London. Research Paper 6.

Maxwell C.J. and Hirdes J.P. (1993). The prevalence of smoking and implications for quality of life among the community-based elderly. *Am J Prev Med,* **9**, 338-45.

Maxwell J.C.Jr. (successive years). How the brands ranked. Maxwell International Estimates. *World Tobacco.*

Millar W.J. (1983). *Smoking behaviour of Canadians 1981.* Health and Welfare Canada, Canada.

Millar W.J. (1985). Smoking prevalence among Canadian adolescents. A comparison of survey estimates. *Can J Public Health,* **76**, 33-7.

Morison J.B. and Medovy H. (1961). Smoking habits of Winnipeg school children. *Can Med Assoc J,* **84**, 1006-12.

Morison J.B., Medovy H. and MacDonell G.T. (1964). Health education and cigarette smoking: a report of a three-year program in the Winnpeg School Division, 1960-1963. *Can Med Assoc J,* **91**, 49-56.

National Clearinghouse on Tobacco and Health (NCTH) (1996). *NCTH statistics.* Canadian Council for Tobacco Control. http://www.cctc.ca/ncth/stats/index.html.

Rickert W.S. (1995). *A historical study of nicotine yields of Canadian cigarettes in relation to the composition and nicotine content of cigarette tobacco (1968-1995) and associated press releases.* Health Canada, Ottawa.

Rickert W.S. and Robinson J.C. (1981). Estimating the hazards of less hazardous cigarettes. II. Study of cigarette yields of nicotine, carbon monoxide, and hydrogen cyanide in relation to levels of cotinine, carboxyhemoglobin, and thiocyanate in smokers. *J Toxicol Environ Health,* **7**, 391-403.

RP6, See Beese (ed) (1968), Beese (ed) (1972), Lee (ed) (1975)

Stachenko S.J., Reeder B.A., Lindsay E., Donovan C., Lessard R. and Balram C. (1992). Smoking prevalence and associated risk factors in Canadian adults. *Can Med Assoc J,* **146**, 1989-96.

Statistics Canada (1994). *Health status of Canadians: Report of the 1991 general social survey.* Statistics Canada, Ottawa. (General Social Survey Analysis.) Catalogue no. 11-612E, No 8.

Stephens T. (1988). *A critical review of Canadian survey data on tobacco use, attitudes and knowledge. Report prepared for Tobacco Programs Unit, Health Promotion Directorate, Health and Welfare Canada.* Health and Welfare Canada, Ottawa.

Stephens T. (1995). Trends in the prevalence of smoking, 1991-1994. *Chronic Diseases in Canada,* **16**, 27-32.

Stephens T., Morin M., Adlaf E.M., Bondy S.J., *et al* (1996). *Youth smoking survey 1994. Technical report.* Health Canada, Ottawa. http://www.hc-sc.gc.ca/ehp/ehd/tobacco/research/index.htm then choose Technical Report (1996) 1994.

Thomson M.E. (1984). *Statistics of smoking in Canada, 5th World Conference on Smoking and Health, Winnipeg, Canada, July 10th-15th, 1983.* Canadian Council on Smoking and Health, Ottawa.

Todd G.F. (1987). *Cigarette consumption in Canada by sex,age and birth cohort 1921-85.* P.N.Lee Statistics and Computing Ltd, Sutton.

WHO (1989). The WHO MONICA project: a worldwide monitoring system for cardiovascular diseases. In: *World health statistics annual 1989.* WHO, Geneva; 25-149.

WHO (1997). *Tobacco or health: A global status report.* WHO, Geneva. www.cdc.gov/nccdphp/osh/who/whoampro.htm.

Wyckham R.G. (1999). Smokeless tobacco in Canada: deterring market development. *Tob Control,* **8**, 411-20.

§ Original paper not obtained, but information taken as quoted by another author

Czechoslovakia 6

Czechoslovakia came into being in 1918. The Second World War split the two nations but after the war Czechs and Slovaks were again united as republics within the Czechoslovak state. At the start of 1993 Czechoslovakia split into the Czech Republic and the Republic of Slovakia.

Sales data

See Tables 6.1-6.3.

Although no data are available for the war years, consumption of manufactured cigarettes per adult increased fairly steadily from 2 cigarettes per day in 1923 to about 7 in the mid 1980s, after which it decreased slightly. When separate data are available for both republics, consumption per adult in the Czech Republic was higher than in Slovakia. The proportion of cigarettes which were filtered rose rapidly from about 20% in the mid 1960s to 80% in the mid 1970s, and had reached 94% by 1995 in the Czech Republic.

Between 1923 and 1934 about half of all tobacco was consumed as manufactured cigarettes, with most of the remainder accounted for by smoking mixtures. The proportion used as cigars declined from 10% to 5%, and insignificant quantities of snuff were also used. No data are available on the consumption of tobacco products other than cigarettes for later years, but production data suggest that it was very low compared with cigarettes in recent decades.

Survey data

See Tables 6.4-6.8

Few nationally representative surveys are available, and much of the survey data presented comes from individual regional epidemiological studies. It is difficult to draw conclusions from such disparate data, particularly as the few studies which report separately for regular and occasional smokers show a high proportion of occasional smokers, both among men and women. Estimates of the prevalence of smoking among men varied between 40% and 60% before 1990, and between 30% and 55% in the 1990s. For women, some regional surveys gave very low estimates, below 5%, but more generally estimates varied between 10% and 35%.

The prevalence of smoking was higher among men than among women at all ages, the decline in prevalence with age being more marked among women than among men. Only one study has reported the prevalence of smoking among younger teenagers, about 5-7% among boys and 2-4% among girls at age 13. Among older pupils, the prevalence of smoking was about 20% among boys and 10% among girls at age 15-16. The prevalence among apprentices was more than double that among students.

It was not possible to assess under-statement of smoking by comparison of survey and sales data. The estimated number of cigarettes smoked per person per day (based on sales data and prevalence) appears to have fallen from about 11 to 7-9 for men between the 1970s and the 1990s and risen from about 2 to 3-5 for women in the same period.

Table 6.1.1 Total annual sales of tobacco products, 1923-1934

Year	Cigarettes tonnes	Cigarettes millions	Cigars tonnes	Smoking mixtures tonnes	Snuff tonnes	All tobacco products tonnes
1923	7997	7997	1875	8998	84	18954
1924	8905	8905	1851	9044	93	19893
1925	9492	9492	1865	8509	97	19963
1926	10244	10244	1759	8833	95	20931
1927	10813	10813	1684	9013	90	21600
1928	11536	11536	1696	8816	93	22141
1929	11922	11922	1671	8492	92	22177
1930	12120	12120	1629	8173	89	22011
1931	12249	12249	1409	7965	85	21708
1932	11365	11365	1090	8573	79	21107
1933	10667	10667	919	8395	68	20049
1934	10951	10951	826	8238	61	20076

Source : see *Notes on sources of sales data*, p. 128

Table 6.1.3 Manufactured cigarettes, percentage of total sales as filter cigarettes, 1966-1995

	Year	% Filter
Czechoslovakia		
	1966	18.0
	1967	26.0
	1968	24.0
	1969	30.4
	1970	36.5
	1971	46.4
	1972	55.6
	1973	65.9
	1974	75.0
	1975	81.3
	1984	86.0
Czech Republic		
	1993	92.0
	1994	94.0
	1995	94.0

Source : see *Notes on sources of sales data*, p. 128

Table 6.2.1 Consumption of (i) cigarettes and (ii) all tobacco products, 1923-1992 sales-based data, including estimates of consumption of hand-rolled. Males and females aged 15 years and over

Year	Manufactured cigarettes		Hand-rolled cigarettes		Total cigarettes		All tobacco products	
	Total annual in millions	Number/ adult/day	Total annual in millions	Number/ adult/day	Total annual in millions	Number/ adult/day	Total annual in tonnes	Grams/ adult/day
1923	7997	2.2					18954	5.3
1924	8905	2.5					19893	5.5
1925	9492	2.6					19963	5.6
1926	10244	2.7					20931	5.6
1927	10813	2.9					21600	5.7
1928	11536	3.1					22141	5.9
1929	11922	3.2					22177	5.9
1930	12120	3.2					22011	5.9
1931	12249	3.0					21708	5.3
1932	11365	2.8					21107	5.2
1933	10667	2.6					20049	4.9
1934	10951	2.7					20076	4.9
1937	11565	2.7						

Table 6.2.1 *(continued)*

Year	Manufactured cigarettes		Hand-rolled cigarettes		Total cigarettes		All tobacco products	
	Total annual in millions	Number/ adult/day	Total annual in millions	Number/ adult/day	Total annual in millions	Number/ adult/day	Total annual in tonnes	Grams/ adult/day
1948	12984	3.9						
1950	14304	4.3						
1953	16246	4.7						
1955	16136	4.7						
1960	18620	5.1						
1961	19407	5.3						
1962	18389	4.9						
1963	18688	5.0						
1964	17640	4.6						
1965	19320	5.0						
1966	20100	5.1						
1967	20058	5.1						
1968	21370	5.4						
1969	18500	4.6						
1970	20472	5.1						
1971	21190	5.2						
1972	21058	5.1						
1973	21200	5.2						
1974	21790	5.3						
1975	22955	5.5						
1976	23300	5.6						
1977	24000	5.7						
1978	23300	5.6						
1979	24000	5.7						
1980	24000	5.7						
1981	28330	6.7						
1982	28406	6.7						
1983	28416	6.7						
1984	29400	6.9						
1985	27940	6.5						
1986	27700	6.5						
1987	27765	6.4						
1988	27902	6.4						
1989	26828	6.1						
1990	29108	6.6						
1991	26640	6.0						
1992	29150	6.5						

Source : see *Notes on sources of sales data,* p. 128

Table 6.2.2 Consumption of manufactured cigarettes, Czech Republic and Slovakia 1975-1995 sales-based data.
Males and females aged 15 years and over

Year	Czech Republic		Slovakia	
	Total annual in millions	Number/ adult/day	Total annual in millions	Number/ adult/day
1975	18950	6.8	7274	5.3
1980	19588	6.9	8868	6.3
1981	19809	7.0	9114	6.5
1982	19117	6.7	9279	6.6
1983	19699	6.9	8775	6.3
1984	19255	6.7	8469	6.0
1985	19424	6.8	8520	6.0
1986	19601	6.8	8491	6.0
1987	18961	6.5	8542	6.0
1988	18129	6.2	8229	5.7
1989	18407	6.2	8114	5.6
1993	16000	5.3		
1994	20500	6.7		
1995	21000	6.8		

Source : see *Notes on sources of sales data,* p. 128

Figure 6.1 Daily consumption of manufactured cigarettes, 1923-1995.
Males and females aged 15 years and over. *Source:* see Table 6.2.1 and 6.2.2

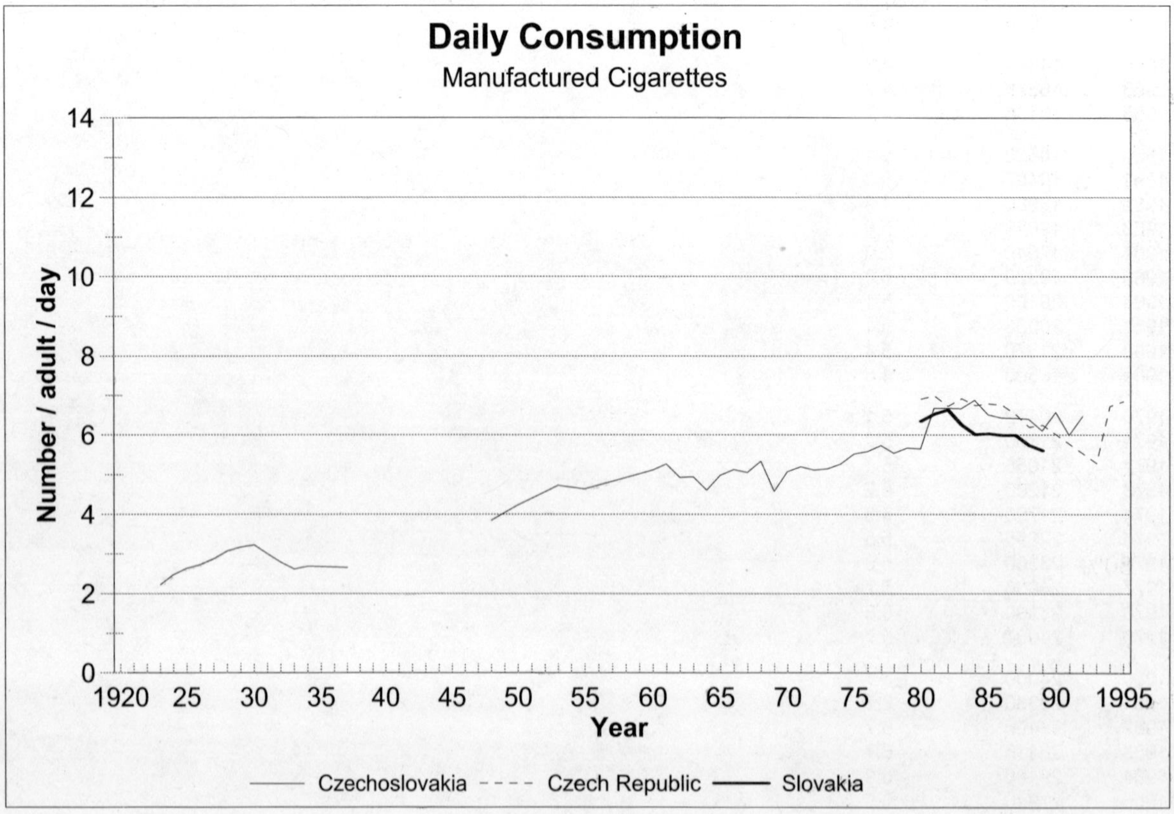

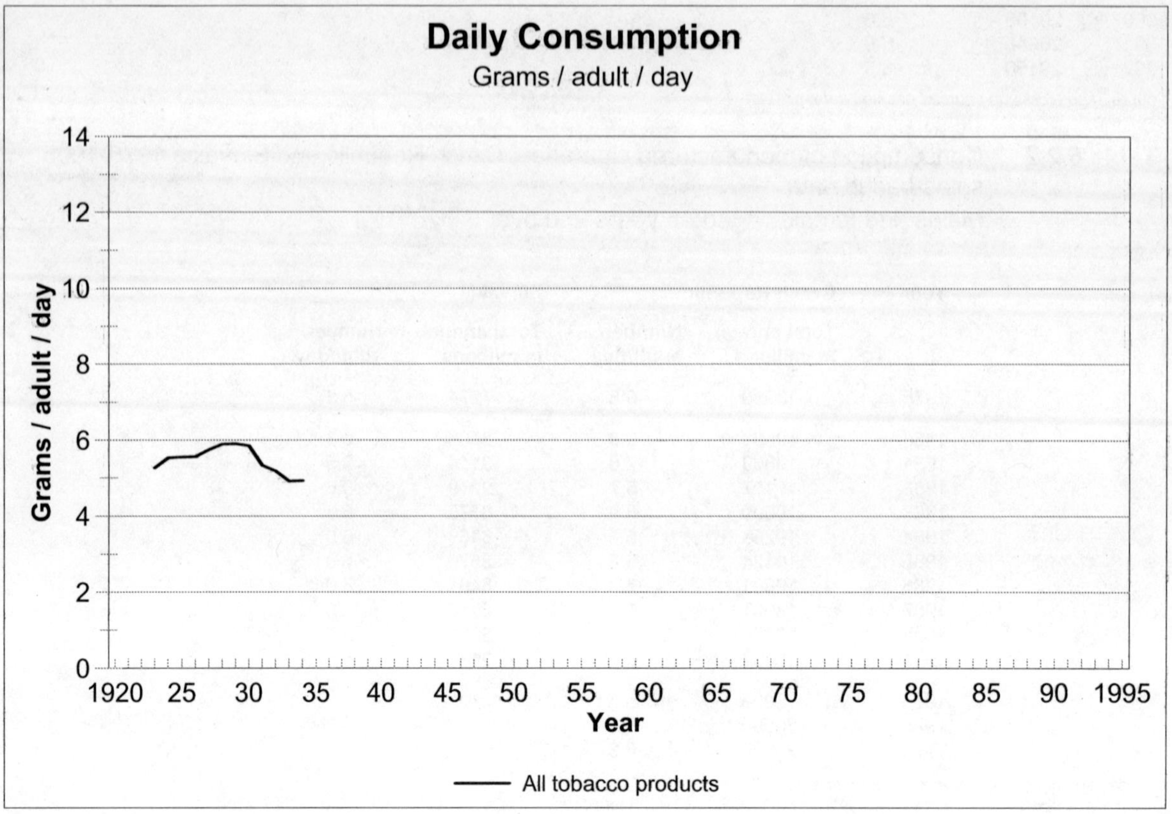

Table 6.3 Percentage sales of tobacco in different forms (by weight), selected years 1925-1934

Year	Cigarettes (%)	Cigars (%)	Smoking mixtures (%)	Snuff (%)
1925	47.5	9.3	42.6	0.5
1934	54.5	4.1	41.0	0.3

Source : calculated from Table 6.1.1

Figure 6.2 Percentage sales of tobacco in different forms (by weight), selected years 1925-1934
Source: see Table 6.3

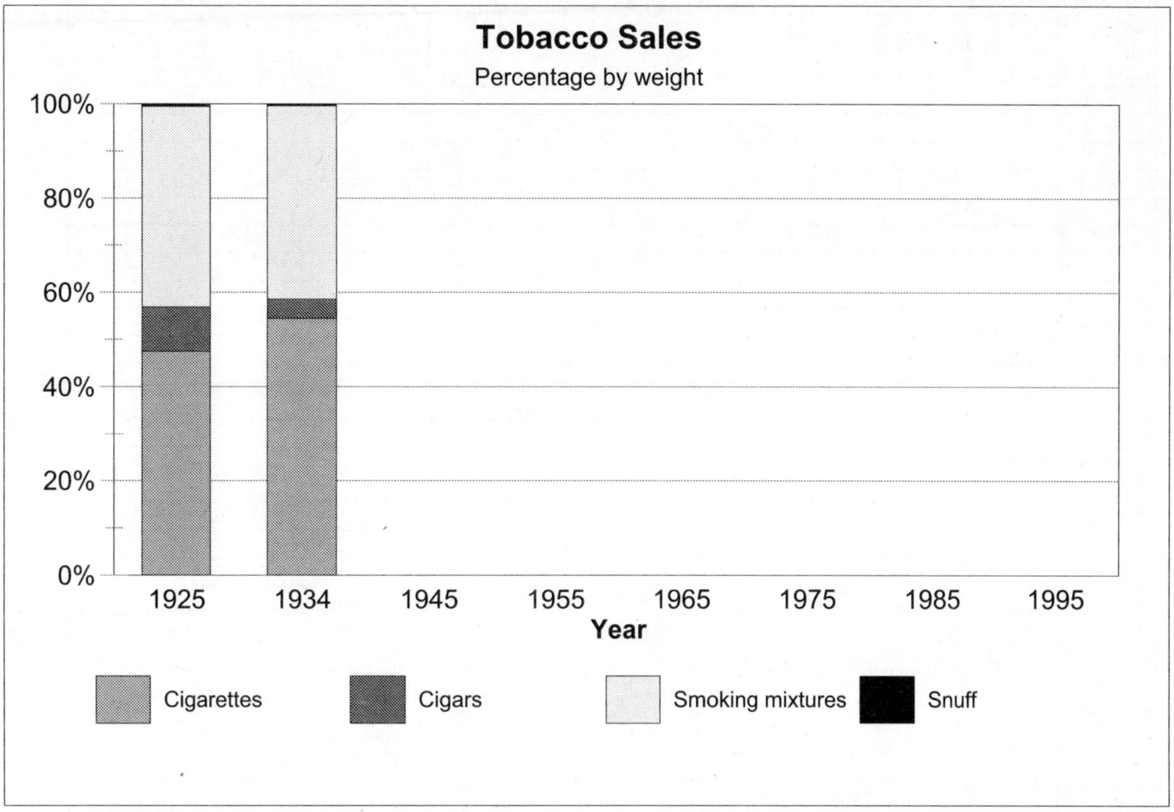

Table 6.4M Prevalence of smoking, males: some selected Czech and Slovak surveys by age, 1965-1996 *(continues on p.118)*

Czechoslovakia

<table>
<tr><th rowspan="2">Year</th><th rowspan="2">Source</th><th rowspan="2">Product</th><th rowspan="2">Frequency</th><th colspan="21">Age group</th><th rowspan="2">All ages</th></tr>
<tr><th>12</th><th>13</th><th>14</th><th>15</th><th>16</th><th>17</th><th>18</th><th>19</th><th>20-24</th><th>25-29</th><th>30-34</th><th>35-39</th><th>40-44</th><th>45-49</th><th>50-54</th><th>55-59</th><th>60-64</th><th>65-69</th><th>70-74</th><th>75-79</th><th>80+</th></tr>
<tr><td>73</td><td>1</td><td>U</td><td>R</td><td colspan="3"></td><td colspan="18">44</td><td></td></tr>
<tr><td>73</td><td>1</td><td>U</td><td>A</td><td colspan="3"></td><td colspan="18">61</td><td></td></tr>
<tr><td>82</td><td>2</td><td>U</td><td>U</td><td colspan="3"></td><td>33</td><td colspan="17"></td><td></td></tr>
<tr><td>84</td><td>3</td><td>U</td><td>U</td><td colspan="3"></td><td colspan="18">57</td><td></td></tr>
<tr><td>90</td><td>4</td><td>U</td><td>U</td><td colspan="3"></td><td colspan="18">50</td><td></td></tr>
</table>

Czech Republic

<table>
<tr><th rowspan="2">Year</th><th rowspan="2">Source</th><th rowspan="2">Product</th><th rowspan="2">Frequency</th><th colspan="21">Age group</th><th rowspan="2">All ages</th></tr>
<tr><th>12</th><th>13</th><th>14</th><th>15</th><th>16</th><th>17</th><th>18</th><th>19</th><th>20-24</th><th>25-29</th><th>30-34</th><th>35-39</th><th>40-44</th><th>45-49</th><th>50-54</th><th>55-59</th><th>60-64</th><th>65-69</th><th>70-74</th><th>75-79</th><th>80+</th></tr>
<tr><td>65</td><td>9</td><td>UC</td><td>U</td><td colspan="14"></td><td colspan="3">46</td><td colspan="4"></td><td></td></tr>
<tr><td>65</td><td>9</td><td>A</td><td>U</td><td colspan="14"></td><td colspan="3">49</td><td colspan="4"></td><td></td></tr>
<tr><td>66</td><td>10</td><td>UC</td><td>*</td><td colspan="12"></td><td>56</td><td>55</td><td>50</td><td>47</td><td>51</td><td colspan="4"></td><td>51</td></tr>
<tr><td>66</td><td>10</td><td>A</td><td>*</td><td colspan="12"></td><td>57</td><td>56</td><td>52</td><td>49</td><td>54</td><td colspan="4"></td><td>53</td></tr>
<tr><td>66</td><td>11</td><td>U</td><td>U</td><td colspan="12"></td><td colspan="5">54</td><td colspan="4"></td><td></td></tr>
<tr><td>66</td><td>12</td><td>U</td><td>U</td><td colspan="17"></td><td colspan="2">41</td><td colspan="2"></td><td></td></tr>
<tr><td>69</td><td>13</td><td>U</td><td>U</td><td colspan="3"></td><td colspan="14">43</td><td colspan="4"></td><td></td></tr>
<tr><td>71</td><td>14</td><td>U</td><td>U</td><td colspan="4"></td><td colspan="15">52</td><td colspan="2"></td><td></td></tr>
<tr><td>71</td><td>15</td><td>U</td><td>U</td><td colspan="4"></td><td colspan="15">59</td><td colspan="2"></td><td></td></tr>
<tr><td>72</td><td>16</td><td>U</td><td>U</td><td colspan="12"></td><td colspan="4">64</td><td colspan="5"></td><td></td></tr>
<tr><td>72</td><td>19</td><td>UC</td><td>*</td><td colspan="3"></td><td colspan="6">58</td><td colspan="2">70</td><td colspan="2">63</td><td colspan="2">57</td><td colspan="2">49</td><td colspan="4">40</td><td>57</td></tr>
<tr><td>72</td><td>19</td><td>A</td><td>*</td><td colspan="3"></td><td colspan="6">58</td><td colspan="2">71</td><td colspan="2">64</td><td colspan="2">58</td><td colspan="2">51</td><td colspan="4">46</td><td>59</td></tr>
<tr><td>73</td><td>17</td><td>U</td><td>U</td><td colspan="3"></td><td colspan="14">40</td><td colspan="4"></td><td></td></tr>
<tr><td>73</td><td>18</td><td>U</td><td>U</td><td colspan="10"></td><td colspan="6">63</td><td colspan="5"></td><td></td></tr>
<tr><td>78</td><td>20</td><td>UC</td><td>U</td><td colspan="11"></td><td colspan="2">23</td><td colspan="5"></td><td colspan="2">8</td><td>6</td><td></td></tr>
<tr><td>83</td><td>21</td><td>UC</td><td>U</td><td colspan="9"></td><td colspan="3">55</td><td colspan="3">50</td><td>32</td><td colspan="5"></td><td></td></tr>
<tr><td>85</td><td>22</td><td>UC</td><td>R</td><td colspan="9"></td><td colspan="2">52</td><td colspan="2">55</td><td colspan="2">41</td><td colspan="2">33</td><td colspan="4"></td><td>44</td></tr>
<tr><td>85</td><td>22</td><td>A</td><td>A</td><td colspan="9"></td><td colspan="2">58</td><td colspan="2">60</td><td colspan="2">44</td><td colspan="2">36</td><td colspan="4"></td><td>48</td></tr>
<tr><td>85</td><td>23</td><td>UC</td><td>R</td><td colspan="9"></td><td colspan="2">52</td><td colspan="2">55</td><td colspan="2">41</td><td colspan="2">33</td><td colspan="4"></td><td>46</td></tr>
<tr><td>85</td><td>24</td><td>U</td><td>A</td><td colspan="3"></td><td colspan="6">37</td><td colspan="12"></td><td></td></tr>
<tr><td>87</td><td>25</td><td>U</td><td>U</td><td colspan="6"></td><td>23</td><td colspan="14"></td><td></td></tr>
<tr><td>87</td><td>26</td><td>U</td><td>U</td><td colspan="6"></td><td>59</td><td colspan="14"></td><td></td></tr>
<tr><td>88</td><td>23</td><td>UC</td><td>R</td><td colspan="9"></td><td colspan="2">50</td><td colspan="2">47</td><td colspan="2">43</td><td colspan="2">26</td><td colspan="4"></td><td>42</td></tr>
<tr><td>92</td><td>23</td><td>UC</td><td>R</td><td colspan="9"></td><td colspan="2">41</td><td colspan="2">46</td><td colspan="2">43</td><td colspan="2">25</td><td colspan="4"></td><td>40</td></tr>
<tr><td>92</td><td>27</td><td>U</td><td>U</td><td colspan="3"></td><td colspan="18">49</td><td></td></tr>
<tr><td>92</td><td>28</td><td>UC</td><td>R</td><td colspan="6"></td><td colspan="15">47</td><td></td></tr>
<tr><td>92</td><td>29</td><td>UC</td><td>R</td><td colspan="6"></td><td colspan="15">38</td><td></td></tr>
<tr><td>93</td><td>24</td><td>U</td><td>A</td><td colspan="3"></td><td colspan="18">38</td><td></td></tr>
<tr><td>94</td><td>5</td><td>UC</td><td>R</td><td></td><td>7</td><td></td><td>16</td><td colspan="17"></td><td></td></tr>
<tr><td>94</td><td>24</td><td>U</td><td>A</td><td colspan="3"></td><td colspan="6">51</td><td colspan="12"></td><td>43</td></tr>
<tr><td>94</td><td>30</td><td>U</td><td>U</td><td colspan="3"></td><td colspan="18">31</td><td></td></tr>
<tr><td>94</td><td>31</td><td>U</td><td>A</td><td colspan="3"></td><td colspan="18">43</td><td></td></tr>
<tr><td>95</td><td>7</td><td>UC</td><td>R</td><td colspan="3"></td><td colspan="2">27</td><td colspan="16"></td><td></td></tr>
<tr><td>95</td><td>7</td><td>UC</td><td>A</td><td colspan="3"></td><td colspan="2">37</td><td colspan="16"></td><td></td></tr>
<tr><td>95</td><td>32</td><td>U</td><td>U</td><td colspan="3"></td><td>18</td><td colspan="17">43</td><td></td></tr>
</table>

Table 6.4F Prevalence of smoking, females: some selected Czech and Slovak surveys by age, 1965-1996 *(continues on p. 119)*

Czechoslovakia

<table>
<tr><th rowspan="2">Frequency
Product
Source
Year</th><th colspan="21">Age group</th><th rowspan="2">All ages</th></tr>
<tr><th>12</th><th>13</th><th>14</th><th>15</th><th>16</th><th>17</th><th>18</th><th>19</th><th>20-24</th><th>25-29</th><th>30-34</th><th>35-39</th><th>40-44</th><th>45-49</th><th>50-54</th><th>55-59</th><th>60-64</th><th>65-69</th><th>70-74</th><th>75-79</th><th>80+</th></tr>
<tr><td>73 1 U R</td><td colspan="3"></td><td colspan="18">11</td><td></td></tr>
<tr><td>73 1 U A</td><td colspan="3"></td><td colspan="18">29</td><td></td></tr>
<tr><td>82 2 U U</td><td colspan="3"></td><td>17</td><td colspan="17"></td><td></td></tr>
<tr><td>84 3 U U</td><td colspan="3"></td><td colspan="18">14</td><td></td></tr>
<tr><td>90 4 U U</td><td colspan="3"></td><td colspan="18">34</td><td></td></tr>
</table>

Czech Republic

<table>
<tr><th rowspan="2">Frequency
Product
Source
Year</th><th colspan="21">Age group</th><th rowspan="2">All ages</th></tr>
<tr><th>12</th><th>13</th><th>14</th><th>15</th><th>16</th><th>17</th><th>18</th><th>19</th><th>20-24</th><th>25-29</th><th>30-34</th><th>35-39</th><th>40-44</th><th>45-49</th><th>50-54</th><th>55-59</th><th>60-64</th><th>65-69</th><th>70-74</th><th>75-79</th><th>80+</th></tr>
<tr><td>65 9 UC U</td><td colspan="21"></td><td></td></tr>
<tr><td>65 9 A U</td><td colspan="21"></td><td></td></tr>
<tr><td>66 10 UC *</td><td colspan="21"></td><td></td></tr>
<tr><td>66 10 A *</td><td colspan="21"></td><td></td></tr>
<tr><td>66 11 U U</td><td colspan="21"></td><td></td></tr>
<tr><td>66 12 U U</td><td colspan="12"></td><td colspan="7">9</td><td colspan="2"></td><td></td></tr>
<tr><td>69 13 U U</td><td colspan="3"></td><td colspan="14">1</td><td colspan="4"></td><td></td></tr>
<tr><td>71 14 U U</td><td colspan="21"></td><td></td></tr>
<tr><td>71 15 U U</td><td colspan="21"></td><td></td></tr>
<tr><td>72 16 U U</td><td colspan="12"></td><td colspan="4">18</td><td colspan="5"></td><td></td></tr>
<tr><td>72 19 UC *</td><td colspan="3"></td><td colspan="6">22</td><td colspan="2">26</td><td colspan="2">17</td><td colspan="2">13</td><td colspan="2">5</td><td colspan="4">1</td><td>14</td></tr>
<tr><td>72 19 A *</td><td colspan="3"></td><td colspan="6">22</td><td colspan="2">26</td><td colspan="2">17</td><td colspan="2">13</td><td colspan="2">5</td><td colspan="4">1</td><td>14</td></tr>
<tr><td>73 17 U U</td><td colspan="3"></td><td colspan="14">4</td><td colspan="4"></td><td></td></tr>
<tr><td>73 18 U U</td><td colspan="21"></td><td></td></tr>
<tr><td>78 20 UC U</td><td colspan="13"></td><td colspan="2">21</td><td colspan="3"></td><td colspan="2">0</td><td>0</td><td></td></tr>
<tr><td>83 21 UC U</td><td colspan="9"></td><td colspan="3">42</td><td colspan="3">25</td><td>12</td><td colspan="5"></td><td></td></tr>
<tr><td>85 22 UC R</td><td colspan="9"></td><td colspan="2">37</td><td colspan="2">35</td><td colspan="2">17</td><td colspan="2">10</td><td colspan="4"></td><td>22</td></tr>
<tr><td>85 22 A A</td><td colspan="9"></td><td colspan="2">43</td><td colspan="2">39</td><td colspan="2">20</td><td colspan="2">10</td><td colspan="4"></td><td>23</td></tr>
<tr><td>85 23 UC R</td><td colspan="9"></td><td colspan="2">37</td><td colspan="2">35</td><td colspan="2">17</td><td colspan="2">10</td><td colspan="4"></td><td>26</td></tr>
<tr><td>85 24 U A</td><td colspan="3"></td><td colspan="6">24</td><td colspan="12"></td><td></td></tr>
<tr><td>87 25 U U</td><td colspan="6"></td><td>22</td><td colspan="14"></td><td></td></tr>
<tr><td>87 26 U U</td><td colspan="6"></td><td>47</td><td colspan="14"></td><td></td></tr>
<tr><td>88 23 UC R</td><td colspan="9"></td><td colspan="2">30</td><td colspan="2">35</td><td colspan="2">19</td><td colspan="2">12</td><td colspan="4"></td><td>25</td></tr>
<tr><td>92 23 UC R</td><td colspan="9"></td><td colspan="2">28</td><td colspan="2">30</td><td colspan="2">25</td><td colspan="2">9</td><td colspan="4"></td><td>24</td></tr>
<tr><td>92 27 U U</td><td colspan="3"></td><td colspan="18">28</td><td></td></tr>
<tr><td>92 28 UC R</td><td colspan="6"></td><td colspan="15">18</td><td></td></tr>
<tr><td>92 29 UC R</td><td colspan="6"></td><td colspan="15">26</td><td></td></tr>
<tr><td>93 24 U A</td><td colspan="3"></td><td colspan="18">29</td><td></td></tr>
<tr><td>94 5 UC R</td><td></td><td>4</td><td></td><td>12</td><td colspan="17"></td><td></td></tr>
<tr><td>94 24 U A</td><td colspan="3"></td><td colspan="6">34</td><td colspan="12"></td><td>31</td></tr>
<tr><td>94 30 U U</td><td colspan="3"></td><td colspan="18">19</td><td></td></tr>
<tr><td>94 31 U A</td><td colspan="3"></td><td colspan="18">31</td><td></td></tr>
<tr><td>95 7 UC R</td><td colspan="3"></td><td colspan="2">18</td><td colspan="16"></td><td></td></tr>
<tr><td>95 7 UC A</td><td colspan="3"></td><td colspan="2">31</td><td colspan="16"></td><td></td></tr>
<tr><td>95 32 U U</td><td colspan="3"></td><td>15</td><td colspan="17">31</td><td></td></tr>
</table>

Table 6.4M *(continued from p. 116)* Prevalence of smoking, males

Slovakia

<table>
<tr><td rowspan="2">Frequency
Product
Source
Year</td><td colspan="21">Age group</td><td rowspan="2">All ages</td></tr>
<tr><td>12</td><td>13</td><td>14</td><td>15</td><td>16</td><td>17</td><td>18</td><td>19</td><td>20-24</td><td>25-29</td><td>30-34</td><td>35-39</td><td>40-44</td><td>45-49</td><td>50-54</td><td>55-59</td><td>60-64</td><td>65-69</td><td>70-74</td><td>75-79</td><td>80+</td></tr>
<tr><td>72 33 UC U</td><td></td><td></td><td></td><td colspan="18">54</td><td></td></tr>
<tr><td>72 33 A U</td><td></td><td></td><td></td><td colspan="18">56</td><td></td></tr>
<tr><td>79 34 U R</td><td colspan="21"></td><td></td></tr>
<tr><td>79 34 U A</td><td colspan="21"></td><td></td></tr>
<tr><td>81 35 UC R</td><td>1</td><td></td><td></td><td>2</td><td colspan="17"></td><td></td></tr>
<tr><td>81 35 UC A</td><td>1</td><td></td><td></td><td>2</td><td colspan="17"></td><td></td></tr>
<tr><td>81 36 UC R</td><td></td><td></td><td></td><td>20</td><td colspan="17"></td><td></td></tr>
<tr><td>81 36 UC A</td><td></td><td></td><td></td><td>22</td><td colspan="17"></td><td></td></tr>
<tr><td>83 37 UC U</td><td></td><td></td><td></td><td colspan="6">54</td><td colspan="12"></td><td>54</td></tr>
<tr><td>83 37 A U</td><td></td><td></td><td></td><td colspan="18">56</td><td></td></tr>
<tr><td>86 38 UC R</td><td></td><td></td><td></td><td colspan="18">43</td><td></td></tr>
<tr><td>91 34 U R</td><td></td><td></td><td></td><td colspan="18">33</td><td></td></tr>
<tr><td>91 34 U A</td><td></td><td></td><td></td><td colspan="5">31</td><td colspan="2">61</td><td colspan="11"></td><td>43</td></tr>
<tr><td>92 39 U R</td><td></td><td></td><td></td><td colspan="18">43</td><td></td></tr>
<tr><td>93 6 UC R</td><td></td><td>5</td><td></td><td>19</td><td colspan="17"></td><td></td></tr>
<tr><td>95 8 UC R</td><td></td><td></td><td></td><td colspan="2">22</td><td colspan="16"></td><td></td></tr>
<tr><td>95 8 UC A</td><td></td><td></td><td></td><td colspan="2">34</td><td colspan="16"></td><td></td></tr>
<tr><td>95 34 U U</td><td></td><td></td><td></td><td colspan="5">39</td><td colspan="13"></td><td></td></tr>
<tr><td>96 38 UC R</td><td></td><td></td><td></td><td colspan="3">45</td><td colspan="3">59</td><td>67</td><td colspan="2">58</td><td colspan="2">54</td><td colspan="2">49</td><td colspan="5">48</td><td>55</td></tr>
</table>

Table 6.5M Number of cigarettes smoked per smoker per day, males: some selected Czech and Slovak surveys by age, 1981-1995

Czech Republic

<table>
<tr><td rowspan="2">Product
Source
Year</td><td colspan="21">Age group</td><td rowspan="2">All ages</td></tr>
<tr><td>12</td><td>13</td><td>14</td><td>15</td><td>16</td><td>17</td><td>18</td><td>19</td><td>20-24</td><td>25-29</td><td>30-34</td><td>35-39</td><td>40-44</td><td>45-49</td><td>50-54</td><td>55-59</td><td>60-64</td><td>65-69</td><td>70-74</td><td>75-79</td><td>80+</td></tr>
<tr><td>83 21 UCE</td><td colspan="9"></td><td colspan="3">15</td><td colspan="3">17</td><td>17</td><td colspan="5"></td><td></td></tr>
<tr><td>85 22 UC</td><td colspan="11"></td><td colspan="6">17</td><td colspan="4"></td><td></td></tr>
<tr><td>85 23 UC</td><td colspan="9"></td><td colspan="2">16</td><td colspan="2">19</td><td colspan="2">19</td><td colspan="2">18</td><td colspan="4"></td><td>18</td></tr>
<tr><td>88 23 UC</td><td colspan="9"></td><td colspan="2">14</td><td colspan="2">16</td><td colspan="2">17</td><td colspan="2">13</td><td colspan="4"></td><td>15</td></tr>
<tr><td>95 7 UCE</td><td></td><td></td><td></td><td colspan="2">9.9</td><td colspan="16"></td><td></td></tr>
</table>

Slovakia

<table>
<tr><td rowspan="2">Product
Source
Year</td><td colspan="21">Age group</td><td rowspan="2">All ages</td></tr>
<tr><td>12</td><td>13</td><td>14</td><td>15</td><td>16</td><td>17</td><td>18</td><td>19</td><td>20-24</td><td>25-29</td><td>30-34</td><td>35-39</td><td>40-44</td><td>45-49</td><td>50-54</td><td>55-59</td><td>60-64</td><td>65-69</td><td>70-74</td><td>75-79</td><td>80+</td></tr>
<tr><td>81 36 UCE</td><td></td><td></td><td></td><td>8.3</td><td colspan="17"></td><td></td></tr>
<tr><td>82 37 UCE</td><td></td><td></td><td></td><td colspan="18">23</td><td></td></tr>
<tr><td>95 8 UCE</td><td></td><td></td><td></td><td colspan="2">13</td><td colspan="16"></td><td></td></tr>
<tr><td>96 38 UCE</td><td></td><td></td><td></td><td colspan="18">13</td><td></td></tr>
</table>

Source: see *Notes on sources of survey data*, p. 129
Frequency: A = all smokers (including occasional)
R = regular or daily smokers
All ages: relevant to ages used and as given in original source
U = unspecified
* = refer to *Notes on sources of survey data*, p. 129

Product: MC = manufactured cigarettes
TC = total cigarettes (including hand-rolled)
UC = cigarettes (type unspecified)
A = all products
E indicates mean estimated from percentage distribution (see also *Consumption category estimation*, p. xxxiv, and Appendix III, p. 789)

Table 6.4F *(continued from p. 117)* Prevalence of smoking, females

Slovakia

Frequency / Product / Source / Year	12	13	14	15	16	17	18	19	20-24	25-29	30-34	35-39	40-44	45-49	50-54	55-59	60-64	65-69	70-74	75-79	80+	All ages
72 33 UC U																						
72 33 A U																						
79 34 U R				18																		
79 34 U A				33																		
81 35 UC R	0			1																		
81 35 UC A	1			1																		
81 36 UC R				9																		
81 36 UC A				12																		
83 37 UC U																						
83 37 A U																						
86 38 UC R				28																		
91 34 U R				16																		
91 34 U A				21					31		33											26
92 39 U R				26																		
93 6 UC R		2		5																		
95 8 UC R				10																		
95 8 UC A				20																		
95 34 U U				16						25		27		17								
96 38 UC R				29			33			32	42		36		29		11					30

Table 6.5F Number of cigarettes smoked per smoker per day, females: some selected Czech and Slovak surveys by age, 1981-1995

Czech Republic

Product / Source / Year	12	13	14	15	16	17	18	19	20-24	25-29	30-34	35-39	40-44	45-49	50-54	55-59	60-64	65-69	70-74	75-79	80+	All ages
83 21 UCE										9.4			11			11						
85 22 UC												10										
85 23 UC										10		12		12		12						11
88 23 UC										9.6		11		9.9		10						10
95 7 UCE				8.3																		

Slovakia

Product / Source / Year	12	13	14	15	16	17	18	19	20-24	25-29	30-34	35-39	40-44	45-49	50-54	55-59	60-64	65-69	70-74	75-79	80+	All ages
81 36 UCE				5.1																		
82 37 UCE																						
95 8 UCE				9.6																		
96 38 UCE				9.3																		

Source: see *Notes on sources of survey data*, p. 129
Frequency: A = all smokers (including occasional)
R = regular or daily smokers
All ages: relevant to ages used and as given in original source
U = unspecified
* = refer to *Notes on sources of survey data*, p. 129

Product: MC = manufactured cigarettes
TC = total cigarettes (including hand-rolled)
UC = cigarettes (type unspecified)
A = all products
E indicates mean estimated from percentage distribution (see also *Consumption category estimation*, p. xxxiv, and Appendix III, p. 789)

Table 6.6M Number of cigarettes smoked per person per day, males: some selected Czech and Slovak surveys by age, 1981-1995, with percentage total sales

Czech Republic

<table>
<tr><th rowspan="2">Product Source Year</th><th colspan="21">Age group</th><th rowspan="2">All ages</th><th rowspan="2">% Total sales</th></tr>
<tr><th>12</th><th>13</th><th>14</th><th>15</th><th>16</th><th>17</th><th>18</th><th>19</th><th>20-24</th><th>25-29</th><th>30-34</th><th>35-39</th><th>40-44</th><th>45-49</th><th>50-54</th><th>55-59</th><th>60-64</th><th>65-69</th><th>70-74</th><th>75-79</th><th>80+</th></tr>
<tr><td>83 21 UC</td><td colspan="9"></td><td colspan="3">8.0</td><td colspan="3">8.6</td><td>5.5</td><td colspan="5"></td><td></td><td>**</td></tr>
<tr><td>85 22 UC</td><td colspan="11"></td><td colspan="6">7.5</td><td colspan="4"></td><td></td><td>**</td></tr>
<tr><td>85 23 UC</td><td colspan="9"></td><td colspan="2">8.1</td><td colspan="2">11</td><td colspan="2">7.8</td><td colspan="2">5.9</td><td colspan="4"></td><td>8.2</td><td>**</td></tr>
<tr><td>88 23 UC</td><td colspan="9"></td><td colspan="2">7.1</td><td colspan="2">7.6</td><td colspan="2">7.0</td><td colspan="2">3.4</td><td colspan="4"></td><td>6.3</td><td>**</td></tr>
<tr><td>95 7 UC</td><td colspan="3"></td><td colspan="2">2.7</td><td colspan="16"></td><td></td><td>**</td></tr>
</table>

Slovakia

<table>
<tr><th rowspan="2">Product Source Year</th><th colspan="21">Age group</th><th rowspan="2">All ages</th><th rowspan="2">% Total sales</th></tr>
<tr><th>12</th><th>13</th><th>14</th><th>15</th><th>16</th><th>17</th><th>18</th><th>19</th><th>20-24</th><th>25-29</th><th>30-34</th><th>35-39</th><th>40-44</th><th>45-49</th><th>50-54</th><th>55-59</th><th>60-64</th><th>65-69</th><th>70-74</th><th>75-79</th><th>80+</th></tr>
<tr><td>81 36 UC</td><td colspan="3"></td><td>1.7</td><td colspan="17"></td><td></td><td>**</td></tr>
<tr><td>82 37 UC</td><td colspan="21">12</td><td></td><td>**</td></tr>
<tr><td>95 8 UC</td><td colspan="3"></td><td colspan="2">2.9</td><td colspan="16"></td><td></td><td>**</td></tr>
<tr><td>96 38 UC</td><td colspan="3"></td><td colspan="18">7.3</td><td></td><td>**</td></tr>
</table>

Table 6.6F Number of cigarettes smoked per person per day, females: some selected Czech and Slovak surveys by age, 1981-1995, with percentage total sales

Czech Republic

<table>
<tr><th rowspan="2">Product Source Year</th><th colspan="21">Age group</th><th rowspan="2">All ages</th><th rowspan="2">% Total sales</th></tr>
<tr><th>12</th><th>13</th><th>14</th><th>15</th><th>16</th><th>17</th><th>18</th><th>19</th><th>20-24</th><th>25-29</th><th>30-34</th><th>35-39</th><th>40-44</th><th>45-49</th><th>50-54</th><th>55-59</th><th>60-64</th><th>65-69</th><th>70-74</th><th>75-79</th><th>80+</th></tr>
<tr><td>83 21 UC</td><td colspan="9"></td><td colspan="3">3.9</td><td colspan="3">2.6</td><td>1.3</td><td colspan="5"></td><td></td><td>**</td></tr>
<tr><td>85 22 UC</td><td colspan="11"></td><td colspan="6">2.2</td><td colspan="4"></td><td></td><td>**</td></tr>
<tr><td>85 23 UC</td><td colspan="9"></td><td colspan="2">3.7</td><td colspan="2">4.0</td><td colspan="2">2.0</td><td colspan="2">1.1</td><td colspan="4"></td><td>2.9</td><td>**</td></tr>
<tr><td>88 23 UC</td><td colspan="9"></td><td colspan="2">2.9</td><td colspan="2">3.8</td><td colspan="2">1.9</td><td colspan="2">1.2</td><td colspan="4"></td><td>2.6</td><td>**</td></tr>
<tr><td>95 7 UC</td><td colspan="3"></td><td colspan="2">1.5</td><td colspan="16"></td><td></td><td>**</td></tr>
</table>

Slovakia

<table>
<tr><th rowspan="2">Product Source Year</th><th colspan="21">Age group</th><th rowspan="2">All ages</th><th rowspan="2">% Total sales</th></tr>
<tr><th>12</th><th>13</th><th>14</th><th>15</th><th>16</th><th>17</th><th>18</th><th>19</th><th>20-24</th><th>25-29</th><th>30-34</th><th>35-39</th><th>40-44</th><th>45-49</th><th>50-54</th><th>55-59</th><th>60-64</th><th>65-69</th><th>70-74</th><th>75-79</th><th>80+</th></tr>
<tr><td>81 36 UC</td><td colspan="3"></td><td>0.5</td><td colspan="17"></td><td></td><td>**</td></tr>
<tr><td>82 37 UC</td><td colspan="21"></td><td></td><td>**</td></tr>
<tr><td>95 8 UC</td><td colspan="3"></td><td colspan="2">1.0</td><td colspan="16"></td><td></td><td>**</td></tr>
<tr><td>96 38 UC</td><td colspan="3"></td><td colspan="18">2.8</td><td></td><td>**</td></tr>
</table>

Table 6.7 is omitted because no sales-adjustment was possible

Source: see *Notes on sources of survey data*, p. 129

Product:
MC = manufactured cigarettes
TC = total cigarettes (including hand-rolled)
UC = cigarettes (type unspecified)
A = all products
U = unspecified

All ages: relevant to ages used and as given in original source

% Total sales: estimated % of total sales of M = manufactured or T = total cigarette consumption implied by survey, sexes combined
** = cannot be calculated
--- = adjusted by original author
* = refer to *Notes on sources of survey data*, p. 129

Table 6.8 Estimated[1] prevalence of smoking and estimated[1] number of cigarettes per person per day (unadjusted and sales-adjusted): summary of Tables 6.4 and 6.6, 1969-1996. Males and females aged 15 years and over

Year	Source[2]	Product[3]	Prevalence[4]						Number of cigarettes						
									Unadjusted[7]			Sales-adjusted[8]			
			Manufactured cigarettes		Total cigarettes[5]		All products[6]		Number/ person/day		Total sales %	Manufactured cigarettes[9] number/ person/day		Total cigarettes number/ person/day	
			M	F	M	F	M	F	M	F		M	F	M	F
Czechoslovakia															
1973	1	U					44	11				(8.8	1.8)		
	1	**U**					61	29							
1984	3	*U*					57	14				(11.9	2.3)		
1990	4	*U*					50	34				(8.6	4.7)		
Czech Republic															
1969	13	*U*					43	1							
1971	14	*U*					51								
	15	*U*					57								
1972	19	UC+A			57	15	59	15				(11.7	2.4)		
1973	17	*U*					40	4							
1992	27	*U*					49	28				(7.4	3.4)		
	28	UC			45	18						(8.2	2.7)		
	29	UC			37	26						(6.9	3.9)		
1993	24	**U**					38	29				(6.6	4.0)		
1994	24	**U**					43	31				(8.6	5.0)		
	30	*U*					31	19				(9.1	4.5)		
	31	**U**					43	31				(8.6	5.0)		
1995	32	*U*					42	31				(8.8	5.1)		
Slovakia															
1972	33	*UC+A*			54		56								
1979	34	U						18							
	34	**U**						33							
1982	37	UC							12.7						
1983	37	*UC*+A			54		56								
1986	38	UC			43	28						(8.0	4.2)		
1991	34	U					33	16				(8.2	3.2)		
	34	**U**					43	26							
1992	39	U					43	26				(7.5	3.6)		
1996	38	UC			55	29			7.3	2.8					

See next page for footnotes

Table 6.8 *(continued)*

1 Surveys covering an age range of at least 21-64 are included. Any gaps in the data for ages 15-20 and 65 years and over are filled in by assumed extensions to the age distribution, given in *Notes on sources of survey data*, p. 129. Method: see *Summary of adult smoking*, p. xxxvi
2 See *Notes on sources of survey data*, p. 129
3 Product: MC = manufactured cigarettes, TC = total cigarettes (including hand-rolled), UC = cigarettes (type unspecified), A = all products, U = unspecified. Frequency of smoking is indicated by: regular or daily smokers in normal type, all smokers (including occasional) in bold, unspecified in italics
4 From Table 6.4
5 This column includes prevalence of smoking classified as UC = cigarettes (type unspecified)
6 This column includes prevalence of smoking classified as U = unspecified product
7 From Table 6.6
8 Data in parentheses are derived from the prevalence of smoking from Table 6.4 as described in *Summary of adult smoking*, p. xxxvi
9 Number of cigarettes classified as UC = cigarettes (type unspecified) or U = unspecified product has been adjusted to manufactured cigarette sales and included in this column. For 1972 and 1992, Czech Republic, adjustment is to 1975 and 1993 sales respectively; for 1991 and 1992, Slovakia, adjustment is to 1989 sales; for 1996, Slovakia, no adjustment has been done due to lack of suitable sales data

Figure 6.3 Estimated prevalence of smoking of cigarettes (i) Czech Republic, (ii) Slovakia, of all tobacco products (iii) Czechoslovakia, (iv) Czech Republic and (v) Slovakia: by year of survey, 1969-1995.
Males and females aged 15 years and over. *Source:* see Table 6.8

Czech Republic

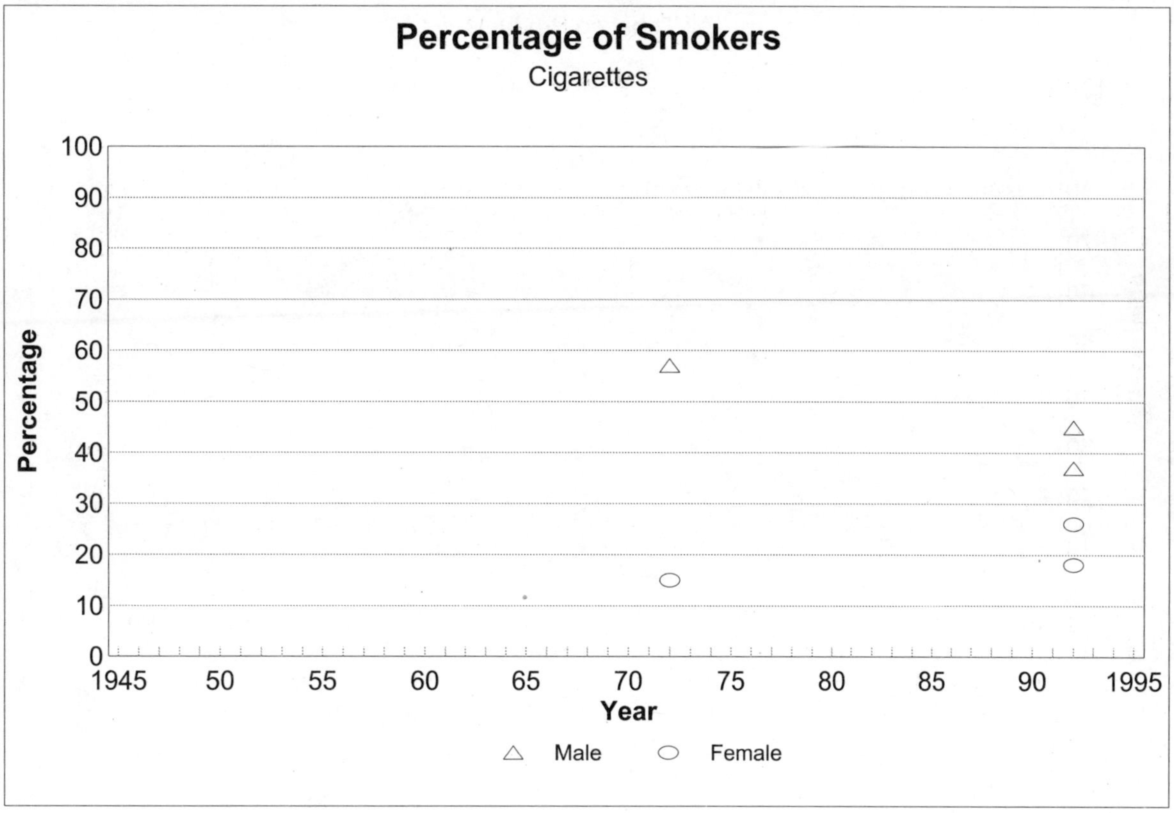

Slovakia

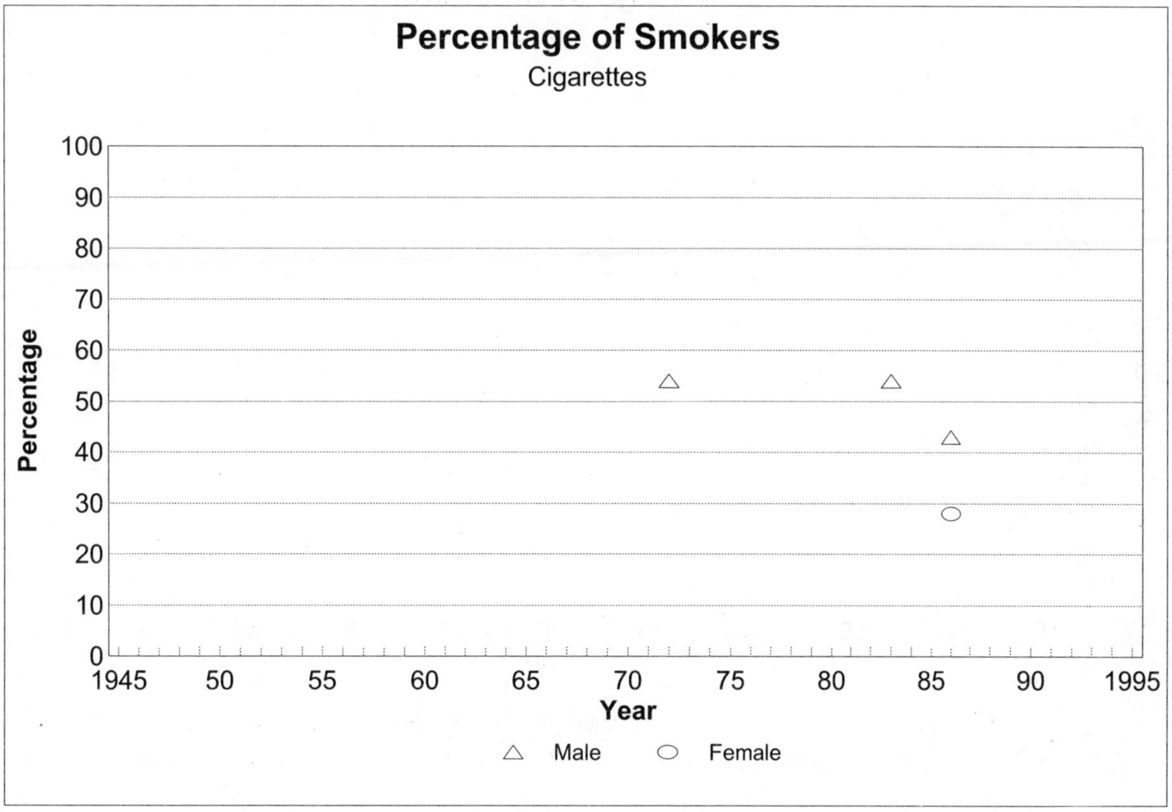

Czechoslovakia

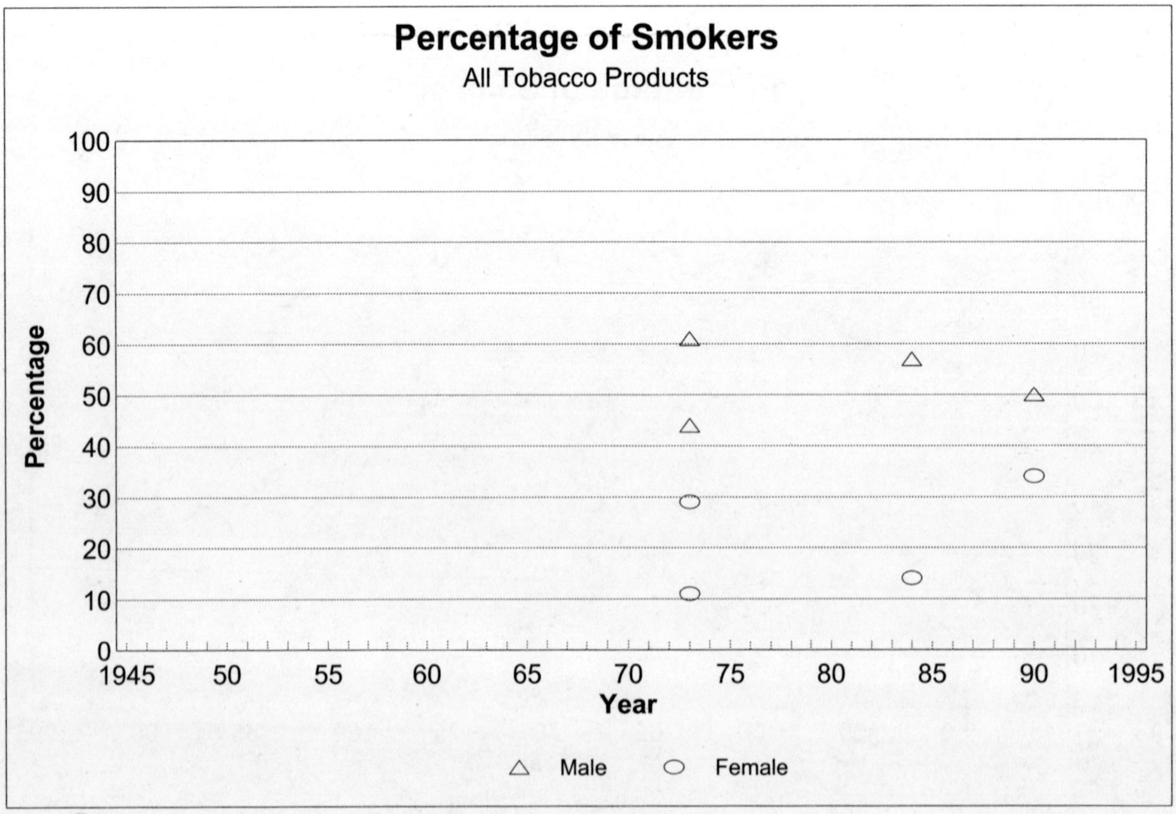

Czech Republic

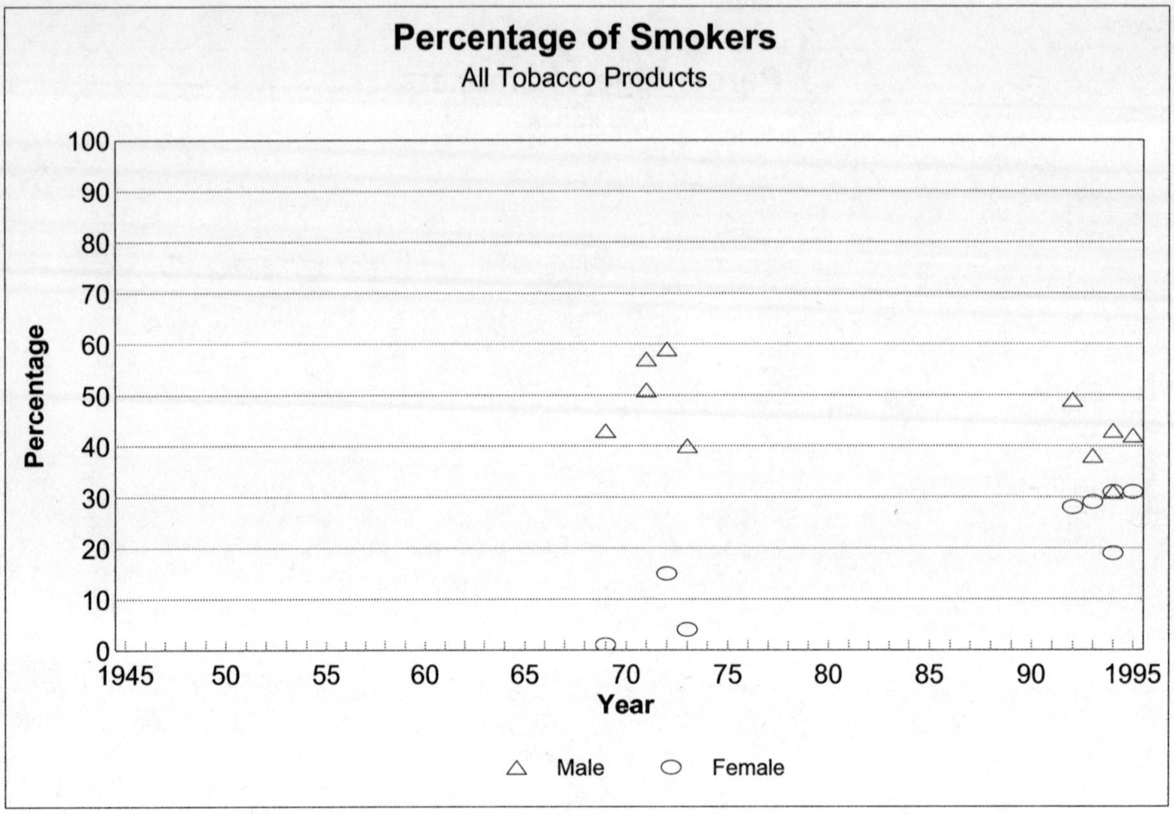

Figure 6.3 *(continued/2)*

Slovakia

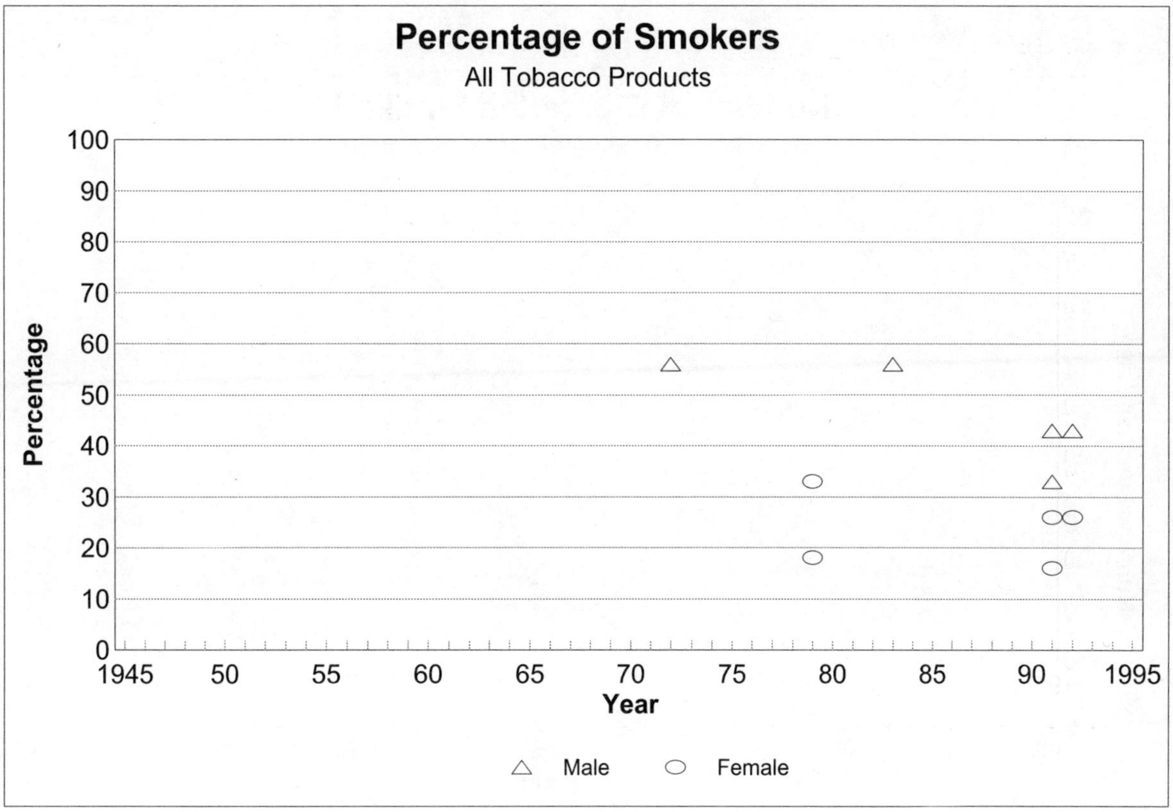

Figure 6.4 Estimated number of cigarettes smoked per person per day (i) Czechoslovakia, (ii) Czech Republic and (iii) Slovakia, sales-adjusted, 1972-1995. Males and females aged 15 years and over. *Source:* see Table 6.8

Czechoslovakia

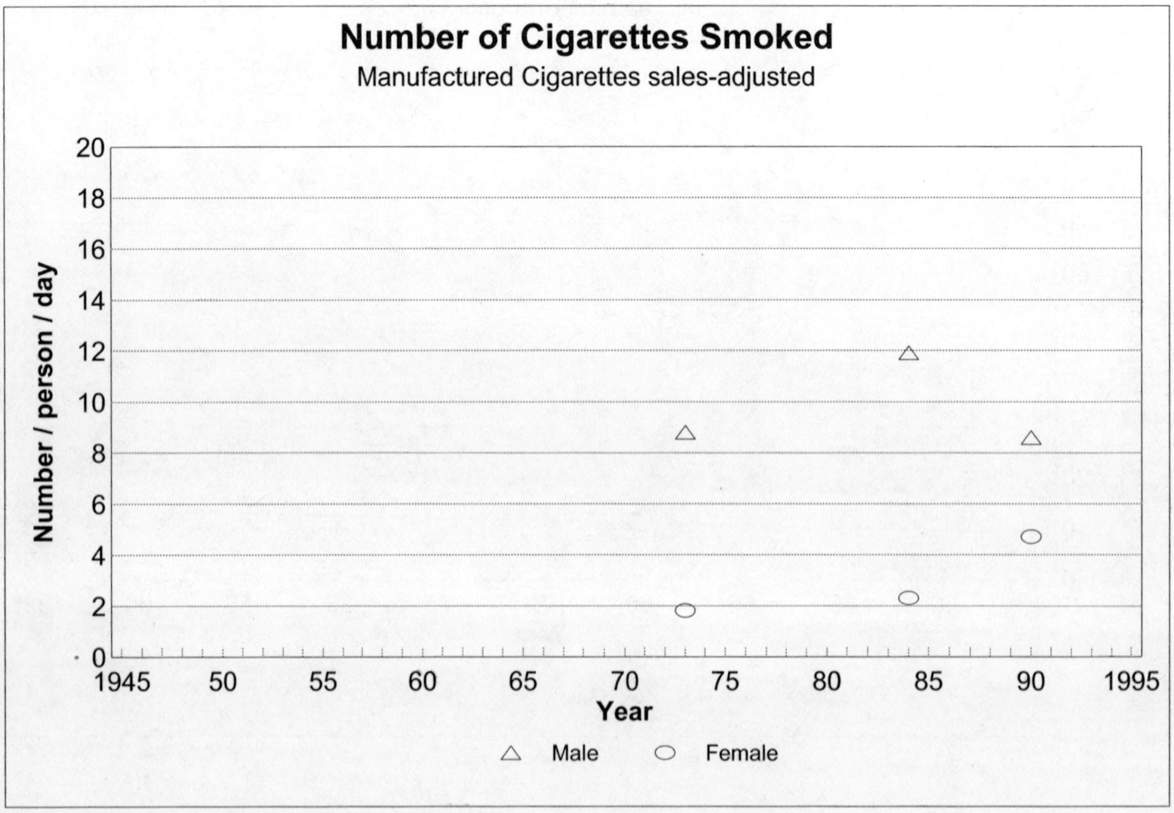

Czech Republic

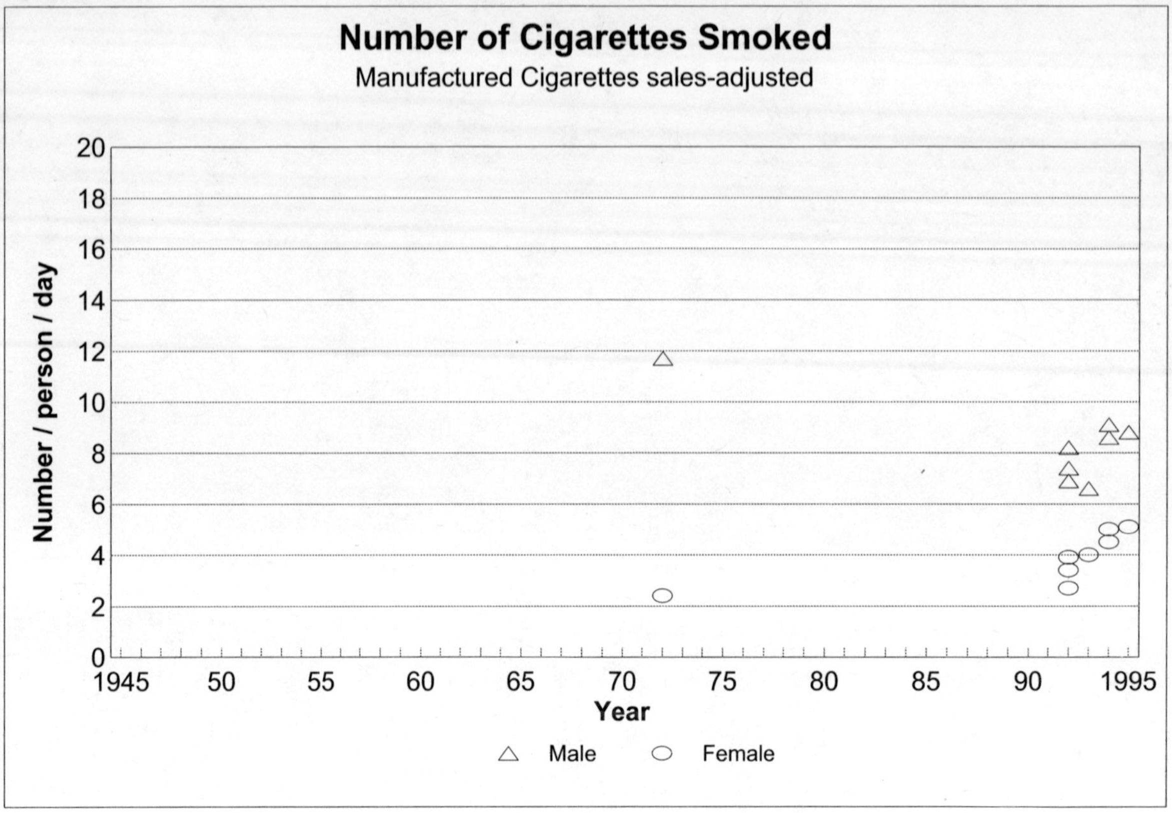

Figure 6.4 *(continued)*

Slovakia

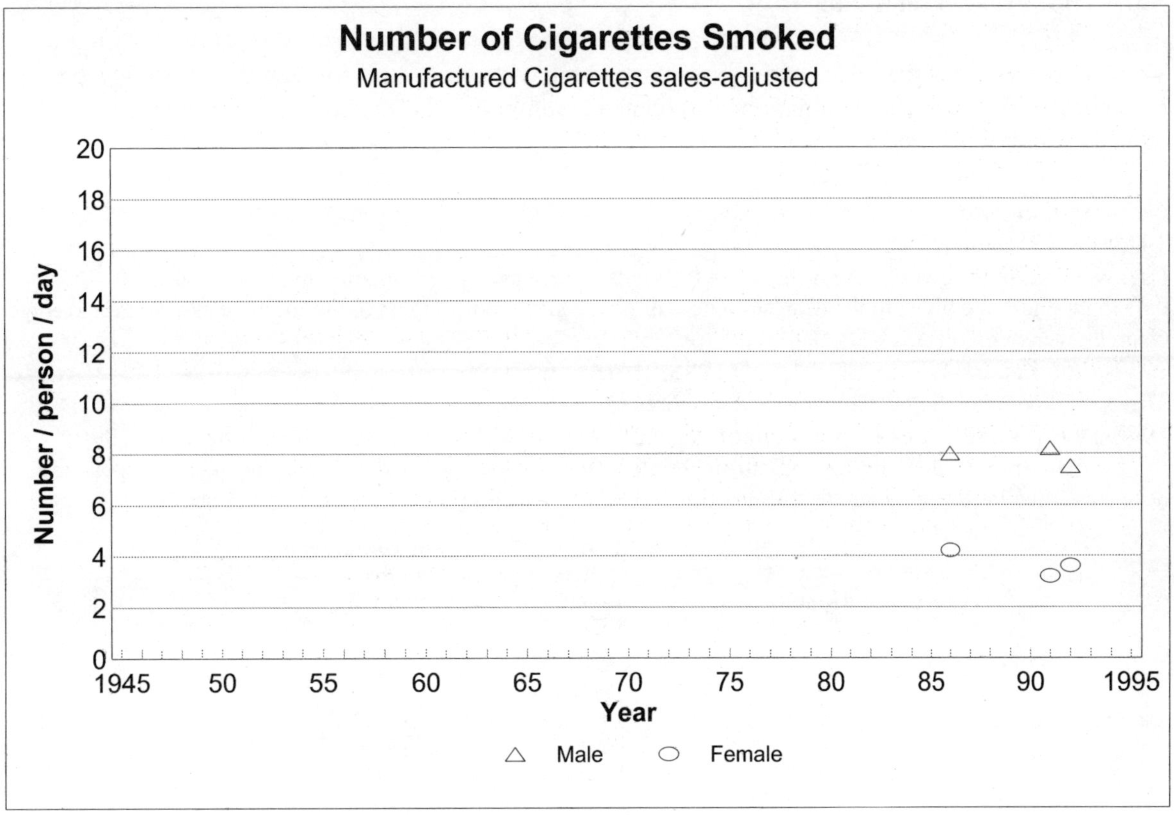

Notes on sources of sales data

The data presented in the tables and figures were obtained from several sources, details of which are given below, together with estimations and related assumptions. Full citations of the sources are given on p. 133 under *References*.

Consumption data

1923-1934 Hutson (1937)

Data were originally given to the nearest 1 000 pounds. They have been converted to tonnes (1 000 lbs = 0.45359 tonnes) and given to the nearest tonne. For conversion from weights to numbers we assumed an average cigarette weight of 1 g.

1937-1955 Federální Statistický Úřad (1985, 1990)

These are production figures, rather than consumption.

1960-1995 United States Department of Agriculture (USDA) Economic Research Service (1996)

Data provided by the Czech Statistical Office, and by Honzatkova (1995) for Slovakia, on a per capita basis imply the following cigarette consumption, given here for comparison with the USDA series:

	Year	Cigarette consumption, millions
Czech Republic	1988	18 124
	1989	18 403
	1990	22 290
	1991	20 875
	1992	20 120
	1993	19 752
	1994	21 086
	1995	22 573
Slovakia	1990	8 626

Honzatkova (1995) states that for Slovakia it is possible to assume that cigarette consumption is much higher [than 1 600 pieces per capita per year] due to uncontrolled imports of cheap high-tar cigarettes from other countries.

Franceschi and Naett (1995) gives cigarette sales in 1993 as 18 000 million in Czech Republic and 10 000 million in Slovakia.

Sales data for products other than cigarettes not available after 1934. Production figures for Czechoslovakia quoted by Federální Statistický Úřad (1985, 1990) are as follows:

Year	Cigars millions	Hand-rolled tonnes	Pipe tobacco tonnes
1983	34	12	293
1984	31	9	315
1988	20	6	257
1989	18	4	246

Due to the lack of sufficient data on sales of other products, (and the lack of any data on the average weight of cigarettes other than our usual assumption of 1 g per cigarette) we have not included estimates of the consumption of all tobacco products in Table 6.2.1. No information on smoking of hand-rolled cigarettes is available.

Plain/Filter cigarette consumption

1966-1975 Maxwell (successive years)

1984 Boddewyn (1986)

1993-1995 USDA Economic Research Service (1996)

For 1993 onwards the data represent percentage of production rather than of sales.

Tar yield of cigarettes
Kubík *et al* (1993) quotes the Czech Tobacco Industry (1991) giving the range of tar yields of 14 types of cigarettes as 16-27 mg (mean 20.8 mg).
Franceschi and Naett (1995) states that in the Czech Republic, in the previous 2 years (presumably 1993 and 1994), the tar levels in full flavour cigarettes had dropped from between 22 and 23 mg to 16 mg and light products had between 10 and 12 mg of tar.

Notes on sources of survey data

Each source of survey data—either an individual survey or a series of surveys repeated over a number of years—is cited by a source number. This number is shown in the tables and corresponds to the source numbers given below, where details of the source publication and of the survey methodology are given. Full citations of the sources are given on p. 133 under *References*.

One survey conducted in Slovakia after the period usually considered in this report has been included, since few age-specific data are available.

Source number

1 Svobodová (1975) quoting J Vrchota (no details)

a. Representative study of Czechoslovak population, carried out in 1963 and then at 5-yearly intervals. Only results from latest (1973) available

2 Geizerova and Masironi (1988)

a. Czechoslovakia. No original source given

3 Masironi and Rothwell (1988)

a. Czechoslovakia. No original source, age group not stated

4 Zatonski (1991)

a. Estimates for Czechoslovakia by Institute of Health Education, Prague. Age group not stated. Year not stated

5-6 King *et al* (1996)

a. Part of the HBSC (Health Behaviour in School-Aged Children) Study, a collaborative cross-national research study sponsored by the WHO. School classes or schools were randomly selected, targeting age groups 11 (not presented here), 13 and 15. The target sample size was 1 300 in each age group.

	5		6	
	Czech Republic		Slovakia	
Target age	Mean age	Sample size	Mean age	Sample size
13	14	1 290	13.7	1 352
15	16	1 201	15.6	934

b. Regular smokers: smoke once a week or more

7-8 Hibell *et al* (1997)

a. Nationally representative surveys forming part of ESPAD (European School Survey Project on Alcohol and Other Drugs). Target was pupils born in 1979, thus age 15-16 at time of survey in April 1995. Approximately 90% (Czech Republic) and 98% (Slovak Republic) of this group still in school. Anonymous questionnaire completed and sealed in envelope by pupil, in class. Teachers absent.

		Sample size		Response rate (%)	
		Male	Female	Male	Female
7	Czech Republic	1 626	1 336	91	93
8	Slovak Republic	1 262	1 114	94	97

b. Regular smokers: smoked 1 or more cigarettes per day in last 30 days. All smokers: smoked in last 30 days

c. Consumption category estimation based on 1-5, 6-10, 11-20, 21+ cigarettes/smoker/day

9 Boudik *et al* (1970)

a. Study of all men (excluding those with active pulmonary tuberculosis) aged 50-65 on election list of Prague 2, a district in central Prague with predominantly manual workers. Nov 1964-July 1965. Sample size 8 292, response rate 73%

10 Kubík *et al* (1970)

a. Baseline of prospective study of lung cancer, in Kolín, an industrial and agricultural district 50 kms east of Prague. Sept 1965-Jan 1967. Results are restricted to those with normal photofluorogram

b. Cigarette smokers (shown as UC *) : current regular cigarette smokers who have smoked at least 1 000 cigarettes, including the 'very few' mixed smokers (cigarette + pipe/cigar), and those who had given up less than 6 months ago. Smokers (shown as A *) : additionally includes all smokers (current and ex) of pipe/cigars only

11-18 Novák *et al* (1975)

a. Review of regional studies of chronic bronchitis over 10 years. The studies covered the whole population or representative samples:

	Location	Period	Sample size	
			Males	Females
11	Brno (urban)	1966	2 736	
12	Brno (urban)	1966-1967	801	4 491
13	Blansko	1969-1970	4 968	5 671
14	Prague 7	1970-1972	3 520	
15	Zatec	1970-1972	1 296	
16	Kutná Hora (urban)	1972-1973	1 783	1 947
17	Brno (rural)	1973-1974	2 221	2 506
18	Ostrava	1973-1974	2 097	

b. Assumed extensions to age distribution for percentage of smokers. Sources 13 and 17, age 66+: males 40%, females 1%. Sources 14 and 15, males only, age 15: 15%, age 76+: 30%

19 Kubík (1984)

a. Study in Kolín. Results are restricted to those with normal photofluorogram

b. Cigarette smokers (shown as UC *) : current regular cigarette smokers who have smoked at least 3 cigarettes per day for at least a year (i.e. 1 000 cigarettes), and those who had given up less than 6 months ago. Smokers (shown as A *) : additionally includes all smokers (current and ex) of pipe/cigars only

20 Ždichynec (1980)

a. Study conducted in Semily, Eastern Bohemia, a mountainous industrial-agricultural area with a high population of very elderly people. Sampling based on Social Security and Municipal records.

Age	Target (% of population)	Sample size		Response rate (%)
		Males	Females	
70-79	12.5	253	327	77
80-89	33.3	283	651	82
90+	100	24	68	66

Sample sizes not available for the younger groups. Year not stated

b. Results shown in the *80+* column in Table 6.4 are for 80-89-year-olds. There were no smokers aged 90+

21 Kozák (1986)

a. A study carried out in seven districts representing the population of CSR (Czech Socialist Republic) within the framework of the Integrated Programme for the Prevention of Non-Infectious Diseases (IPP). Sample size (males) 1 054 and (females) 999

b. Consumption category estimation based on 1-10, 11-20, 21+ cigarettes/smoker/day

22-23 Škodová *et al* (1991, 1993), WHO (1989)

a. Studies forming part of WHO MONICA project. Carried out in 6 districts of the Czech Republic (Prague-East, Cheb, Chrudim, Jindřichův Hradec, Benešov and Pardubice).

Year	Sample size		Response rate (%)	
	Males	Females	Males	Females
1985	1 256	1 317	82	85
1988	1 357	1 412	86	88
1992	1 139	1 214	71	75

b. Results shown as source **23** taken from WHO (1989), *all ages* column relates only to age 35-64 and is standardized to world population. Results shown as source **24** taken from Škodová *et al* (1991), Škodová *et al* (1993), *all ages* column relates to age 25-64 and is standardized to the Czechoslovak (1985, 1988) or Czech (1992) population. There are also minor unexplained discrepancies with the results presented by Bobak *et al* (1997), Škodová *et al* (1988)

c. Regular cigarette smokers: smoked cigarettes daily. All smokers: smoked cigarettes daily or occasionally, or smoked 1 g pipe tobacco or 1 cigar per week

24 WHO (1997)

a. Czech Republic. No original source

25-26 Omelka *et al* (1988)

a. Questionnaire study as part of myocardial infarction and stroke prevention programme. Year not stated.

		Sample size	
		Males	Females
25	Students	81	102
26	Apprentices	68	43

27 Piha *et al* (1993)

a. WHO data for Czech Republic. Age group not stated (adults)

28-29 Vondra *et al* (1996)

a. Epidemiological study carried out in 2 districts of the Czech Republic.

		Sample size	
		Males	Females
28	Uherské Hradiste, South Moravia	284	338
29	Prague 8	2 618	3 384

b. Assumed extension to age distribution for percentage of smokers, age 15-17: males 20%, females 15%

30 Franceschi and Naett (1995)

a. Quoting 'most recent survey data' for Czech Republic, but no original reference. Age group and year not stated

31 Harkin *et al* (1997)

a. Czech Republic. Age group not stated (adults)

32 Kozák *et al* (1996)

a. Czech Republic. Year not stated

33 Bajan *et al* (1976)

a. Study in 1971-1973 in an area of Western Slovakia with population 20 000. Sample size 5 753

34 Honzatkova (1995, 2000)

a. Representative surveys of Slovak population by the Institute of Health Education, Bratislava

b. Results shown in *All ages* column of Table 6.4 relate to age 15+

35-36 Babál *et al* (1986)

a. Study in 1981-1982 of 12-year-olds (6th form pupils), 15-year-old students and 15-year-old apprentices

		Sample size	
		Males	**Females**
35	Pupils	203	190
35	Students	202	485
36	Apprentices	256	88

b. Regular smokers: smoked daily. Occasional smokers: smoked weekly

c. Consumption category estimation based on 1-5, 5-10 (assume 6-10), >10 cigarettes/smoker/day. Results only presented for apprentices as the number of smokers were very small for other groups

37 Kandráčová *et al* (1984)

a. Part of a clinical-epidemiolgical study of chronic bronchitis in the South Slovakia by Institute for Tuberculosis and Respiratory Diseases, Bratislava. Date uncertain. Sample size 5 753

b. Consumption category estimation based on <10, 10-14, 15-30, >30 cigarettes/smoker/day

38 Urban and Luha (2000), and personal communication

a. No source stated for 1986 estimates. Survey in Slovakia in 1996 including all regions and socioeconomic groups, by the Slovak Research Institute of Public Opinion. Sample size 1 322

b. Regular cigarette smoker: smoked 1 cigarette per day or 7 per week

c. Results after the period usually considered in this report have been included, since very few age-specific data are available for Slovakia

d. Consumption category estimation based on 1-5, 6-10, 11-20, 21-30, 31+ cigarette/smoker/day. The % total sales (Table 6.6) could not be calculated due to lack of suitable sales data

39 Harkin *et al* (1997)

a. Slovakia, 1991-1992. Age group not stated (adults)

b. A further 10% (sexes combined) are reported to be occasional smokers

References

Boddewyn J.J. (ed) (1986). *Tobacco advertising bans and consumption in 16 countries*. International Advertising Association, New York.

Babál M., Belicayová R., Košinárová V., Sány L. and Tamášová M. (1986). Fajčenie u dospievajúcej mládeže. *Studia Pneumologica et Phtiseologica Cechoslovaca,* **46**, 147-50.

Bajan A., Kandráčová Z. and Badalís L. (1976). Fajčiarsky návyk a jeho charakteristika v mužskej populácii na vybranom území Slovenskej socialistickej republiky. (The tobacco habit and its characteristics in the male population of a selected area in the Slovak Socialist Republic). *Studia Pneumologica et Phtiseologica Cechoslovaca,* **36**, 677-81.

Bobak M., Skodova Z., Pisa Z., Poledne R. and Marmot M. (1997). Political changes and trends in cardiovascular risk factors in the Czech Republic, 1985-92. *J Epidemiol Community Health,* **51**, 272-7.

Boudik F., Goldsmith J.R., Teichman V. and Kaufmann P.-C. (1970). Epidemiology of chronic bronchitis in Prague. *Bull World Health Organ,* **42**, 711-22.

Federální Statistický Úřad (1985). *Statistická ročenka (Statistical Yearbook of the Czech and Slovak Federal Republic)*. SNTL—Nakladatelství technické literatury, Praha.

Federální Statistický Úřad (1990). *Statistická ročenka (Statistical Yearbook of the Czech and Slovak Federal Republic)*. SNTL—Nakladatelství technické literatury, Praha.

Franceschi S. and Naett C. (1995). Trends in smoking in Europe. *Eur J Cancer Prev,* **4**, 271-84.

Geizerova H. and Masironi R. (1988). Cigarette smoking in children and adolescents: world review. In: Aoki M., Hisamichi S. and Tominaga S. (eds) *Smoking and health 1987. Proceedings of the 6th World Conference on Smoking and Health, Tokyo, 9-12 November 1987*. Elsevier Science Publishers B.V. (Biomedical Division), Amsterdam; 601-5. International Congress Series No. 780.

Harkin A.M., Anderson P. and Goos C. (1997). *Smoking, drinking and drug taking in the European Region.* Alcohol, Drugs and Tobacco Programme, WHO Regional Office for Europe, Copenhagen.

Hibell B., Andersson B., Bjarnason T., Kokkevi A., Morgan M. and Narusk A. (1997). *The 1995 ESPAD report. The European school survey project on alcohol and other drugs. Alcohol and other drug use among students in 26 European countries*. The Swedish Council for Information on Alcohol and Other Drugs. Council of Europe (Pompidou Group).

Honzatkova Z. (1995). Review of tobacco consumption in Slovakia. In: Slama K. (ed) *Tobacco and Health, Ninth World Conference on Tobacco and Health, Paris, Oct 10-14 1994*. Plenum Press, New York and London; 571-3.

Honzátková Z. (2000). Slovakia: evaluation of tobacco control initiatives. In: Lu R., Mackay J., Niu S. and Peto R. (eds) *Tobacco: The Growing Epidemic. Proceedings of the Tenth World Conference on Tobacco or Health, 24-28 August 1997, Beijing, China*. Springer-Verlag, London; 483-5.

Hutson J.B. (1937). *Consumption and production of tobacco in Europe*. USDA, Washington DC. Technical bulletin No. 587.

Kandráčová Z., Badalík L. and Virsík K. (1984). Epidemiology of smoking habit in the Danube river valley. In: *Symposium on Smoking and Health in the South European countries, Barcelona (March 22-24, 1984)*. Institut d'Estudis de la Salut, Barcelona; 5-6.

King A., Wold B., Tudor-Smith C. and Harel Y. (1996). *The health of youth, a cross-national survey*. WHO Regional Publications, Europe, Copenhagen. European Series No. 69.

Kozák J.T. (1986). Smoking and health in Czechoslovakia. *New York State Journal of Medicine,* **86**, 468-71.

Kozák J.T., Kralíková E. and Hora K. (1996). Anti-smoking legislation in the Czech Republic [Abstract]. Conference on global lung health and the 1996 annual meeting of the International Union Against Tubercluosis and Lung Disease (IUATLD) Paris, France 2-5 October 1996. *Tuber Lung Dis,* **77(Suppl 2)**, 40-1.

Kubík A. (1984). The influence of smoking and other etiopathogenetic factors on the incidence of bronchogenic carcinoma and chronic nonspecific respiratory diseases. *Czechoslovak Medicine,* **7**, 25-34.

Kubík A., Bonassi S., Filiberti R. and Reissigová J. (1993). Regional and national variation in lung cancer mortality in Italy and Czechoslovakia. *Eur J Cancer Prev,* **2**, 337-44.

Kubík A., Křivinka R., Stašek V., Švandová E., Křivánek J. and Neumann V. (1970). Screening for lung cancer high-risk groups. *Scandinavian Journal of Respiratory Diseases,* **51**, 290-300.

Masironi R. and Rothwell K. (1988). Tendances et effets du tabagisme dans le monde (Smoking trends and effects worldwide). *World Health Stat Q,* **41**, 228-41.

Maxwell J.C.Jr. (successive years). How the brands ranked. Maxwell International Estimates. *World Tobacco.*

Novák M., Olejníček M., Kubík F., Boudík F., *et al* (1975). Přehled epidemiologických studií o prevalenci chronické bronchitidy v ČSR (A review of epidemiological studies of chronic bronchitis prevalance in the Czech Socialist Republic). *Studia Pneumologica et Phtiseologica Cechoslovaca,* **35**, 696-708.

Omelka F., Horáčková E. and Bystrý J. (1988). Kouření u současné mládeže (Smoking in contemporary youth). *Ceskoslovenska pediatria,* **43**, 341-3.

Piha T., Besselink E. and Lopez A.D. (1993). Tobacco or health. *World Health Stat Q,* **46**, 188-94.

Škodová Z., Píša Z., Emrová R., Vorlíček J., *et al* (1991). Cardiovascular risk factors in the Czech population. *Cor et Vasa,* **33**, 114-22.

Škodová Z., Píša Z., Grafnetter D., Wiesner E., *et al* (1988). Prevalence kuřactiví v šesti okresech ČSR. *Prakticky Lekar,* **68**, 446-8.

Škodová Z., Píša Z., Pikhartová J., Cícha Z., *et al* (1993). Development of the cardiovascular risk in the population of the Czech Republic. *Cor et Vasa,* **35**, 178-82.

Svobodová A. (1975). Kouření mezi mládeží a dospělou populací. (Smoking habits of children and adult populations). *Studia Pneumologica et Phtiseologica Cechoslovaca,* **35**, 161-5.

USDA Economic Research Service (1996). *Tobacco statistics.* Albert R. Mann Library, Cornell University, Ithaca, New York. ERS 94012. (With supplementary material from Tobacco Annual Reports.). http://usda.mannlib.cornell.edu/data-sets/specialty/94012.

Urban S. and Luha J. (2000). Epidemiology of smoking in Slovakia. In: Lu R., Mackay J., Niu S. and Peto R. (eds) *Tobacco: The Growing Epidemic. Proceedings of the Tenth World Conference on Tobacco or Health, 24-28 August 1997, Beijing, China.* Springer-Verlag, London; 55-6.

Vondra V., Reisová M., Petřík P., Hlobil Z. and Kozák J. (1996). Výskyt kouřeni v jihomoravském okrese a srovnání s tímto zlozvykem v Praze 8 (Occurrence of smoking in the southern Moravian District in comparison with the Prague 8 District). *Vnitr Lek,* **42**, 331-5.

WHO (1989). The WHO MONICA project: a worldwide monitoring system for cardiovascular diseases. In: *World health statistics annual 1989.* WHO, Geneva; 25-149.

WHO (1997). *Tobacco or health: A global status report.* WHO, Geneva. www.cdc.gov/nccdphp/osh/who/whoampro.htm.

Zatonski W. (1991). Country reports. *World Smoking and Health,* **16**, 12-21.

Ždichynec B. (1980). Smoking among 70-105-year-olds. *World Smoking and Health,* **5**, 37-40.

Denmark 7

Sales data
See Tables 7.1-7.3.
From 1920 until 1945 the consumption of manufactured cigarettes per adult remained around 1.5 cigarettes per day. After the Second World War consumption rose, rapidly at first to 3 cigarettes per day around 1950, then gradually to about 5 cigarettes per day in the early 1970s. It remained at about this level until the mid 1980s, but then fell to about 4 cigarettes per day in 1995. Although there is conflicting information on hand-rolled cigarette consumption, our estimates suggest that consumption per adult has decreased from nearly 2 hand-rolled cigarettes per day about 1950 to 1 about 1980, then increased to 1.5 by 1995. Thus total cigarette consumption per adult has remained between 5 and 6 cigarettes per day since 1950.

There is some uncertainty in our estimates of the total weight of tobacco consumed, due to conflicting information on the average weight of cigarettes. The consumption of tobacco products per adult was about 8 g per day from 1920 until the beginning of the Second World War. After a decline during the war, consumption rose rapidly to about 10 g per day in 1950 and varied between 9 and 10 g per day in the remaining period until the mid 1970s, then decreased to 6 g in 1995. From 1925 to 1945, the tobacco consumed was divided fairly equally between manufactured cigarettes, cigars and cigarillos, pipe and hand-rolling tobacco, and chewing tobacco and snuff. After the war, the percentage of tobacco consumed as manufactured cigarettes rose steadily to about 65% since the mid 1980s; chewing tobacco and snuff declined rapidly to very low levels, cigars and cigarillos declining more slowly to 6% in 1995. Pipe and hand-rolling tobacco reversed their decline in the 1990s. The percentage of manufactured cigarettes sold as filtered increased slowly from 30% in 1960 to 70% in the mid 1980s. Sales-weighted average tar yields fell from 27 mg per cigarette in 1964 to 19 mg in 1990.

There is some evidence that consumption may be higher than the data presented due to cross border sales (see *Notes on sources of sales data*, p. 160).

Survey data
See Tables 7.4-7.8
From the late 1950s, two sources provided survey data almost annually (source 1, OBSERVA, and source 2, Gallup).

In 1953, the prevalence of tobacco smoking among those aged 15 years and over was 77% in men and nearly 40% in women. The difference between the percentages of men and women who smoke has decreased since then, mainly because of a decrease in the prevalence among men to about 43% in 1995. The prevalence among women has changed little, rising to about 45% in the late 1960s and declining again to below 40% by 1995. Exceptionally, one national source (source 6) reported in 1953-1954 that the prevalence of cigarette smoking was higher among women (32%) than among men (24%). This situation had reversed by the late 1950s and the prevalence of cigarette smoking has changed relatively little in either sex since then, although a slight increase among women since the mid-1960s virtually eliminated the difference in prevalence between the sexes by the mid-1980s. Denmark is unique among the countries in this book in that a substantial proportion of women smoked products other than cigarettes.

Data on adult smoking by age are available occasionally only from 1953 until 1970, and annually thereafter. In all age groups, there was a decrease in the prevalence of tobacco smoking among men. However, since 1970 the prevalence of cigarette smoking for both men and women has fallen among younger age groups, whilst rising among older age groups. The prevalence of smoking of other products but not cigarettes has always been higher in the old than the young. For instance, in 1953 around half the male smokers and very few female smokers aged under 30 smoked other products but not cigarettes, compared with nearly 90% of male smokers and about half of female smokers aged over 50; by the 1990s very few young people of either sex smoked other products but not cigarettes, but over age 60 other products continue to be smoked by 40% of male and about 15% of female smokers.

In 1959, the prevalence of smoking among teenage girls was lower than among teenage boys. In the 1980s and 1990s most surveys have reported higher prevalence of smoking among girls than boys.

Comparison of survey and sales data suggests that the regular surveys (source 2) under-reported consumption by 20-30% in the early 1970s, but this gradually reduced and since about 1985 under-reporting has been less than 10%. Other sources vary between under-reporting by 50% in the 1950s (source 6) to over-reporting by 20% (source 7, regional survey). This may to some extent be attributable to low estimates of sales and the uncertainty of estimates of hand-rolled cigarette consumption, as mentioned above. Between 1953 and 1995, the estimated number of cigarettes smoked per person per day (sales-adjusted) for men remained between 6 and 7, while for women it increased from about 4 to nearly 6 in the early 1980s, then decreased to about 5.

Table 7.1.1 Total annual sales of tobacco products, 1920-1973

Year	Cigarettes		Cigars		Cigarillos		Smoking tobacco	Chewing tobacco	Snuff	All tobacco products
	tonnes	millions	tonnes	millions	tonnes	millions	tonnes	tonnes	tonnes	tonnes
1920	1090	860	321	321	230	86	2490	1410	180	6990
1921	1090	868	284	284	180	72	2360	1130	230	6400
1922	1180	943	284	284	230	90	2310	910	180	6210
1923	1410	1109	292	292	320	126	2310	1180	270	6940
1924	1450	1159	285	285	320	125	2180	1130	270	6760
1925	1540	1219	258	258	360	139	2130	1130	270	6710
1926	1680	1325	251	251	410	155	2310	1090	320	7080
1927	1720	1373	233	233	410	167	2220	1040	320	6890
1928	1950	1544	222	222	500	196	2270	1000	320	7120
1929	1270	1017	278	278	500	195	2270	950	360	6760
1930	1630	1319	289	289	590	213	2310	950	360	7300
1931	1630	1332	284	284	630	262	2270	910	410	7260
1932	1450	1170	268	268	720	293	2540	820	410	7300
1933	1450	1142	314	314	820	333	2450	770	410	7480
1934	1540	1214	366	366	910	360	2450	730	410	7850
1935	1630	1307	406	406	950	379	2400	730	450	8210
1936	1770	1404	437	437	1000	393	2540	680	450	8620
1937	1910	1507	459	459	1000	402	2400	680	450	8750
1938	2000	1605	469	469	1000	407	2450	640	450	8890
1939	2180	1748	487	487	1040	425	2540	590	450	9250
1940	2090	1662	409	409	820	333	2590	590	500	8620
1941	2000	1577	227	227	680	269	2000	640	540	6990
1942	2220	1779	145	145	770	317	2590	640	500	7440
1943	1360	1094	116	116	720	284	1720	410	450	5260
1944	1630	1318	117	117	770	305	1860	410	540	5810
1945	1450	1163	137	137	820	335	1410	360	540	5260
1946	2680	2150	308	308	1180	474	2630	540	640	9210
1947	2990	2380	347	347	1090	441	2720	500	540	9570
1948	3310	2663	383	383	1180	479	3080	450	540	10480
1949	4350	3489	383	383	1000	402	2540	450	500	10750

Table 7.1.1 *(continued)*

Year	Cigarettes		Cigars		Cigarillos		Smoking tobacco tonnes	Chewing tobacco tonnes	Snuff tonnes	All tobacco products tonnes
	tonnes	millions	tonnes	millions	tonnes	millions				
1950	5030	4008	383	383	1000	400	2490	410	500	11340
1951	4350	3483	282	282	1040	423	2400	410	500	10120
1952	4850	3881	214	214	1360	542	2590	360	500	10750
1953	4900	3931	208	208	1500	597	2590	360	500	10890
1954	4810	3834	208	208	1540	621	2680	360	500	10930
1955	4760	3787	216	216	1540	612	2630	320	450	10800
1956	4850	3882	225	225	1540	615	2590	320	450	10890
1957	5030	4010	229	229	1540	621	2540	270	450	10980
1958	5400	4349	239	239	1630	657	2590	270	450	11520
1959	5900	4706	262	262	1720	683	2450	270	450	12110
1960	6170	4990	275	275	1720	699	2450	270	450	12430
1961	6350	5097	286	286	1770	705	2270	230	410	12470
1962	6760	5257	286	286	1810	722	2270	230	410	12930
1963	6800	5600	271	271	1810	720	2180	230	410	12790
1964	6530	5277	293	293	2130	854	2450	230	410	13200
1965	6890	5414	300	300	2040	851	2450	180	360	13430
1966	7080	5566	288	288	2000	808	2310	180	360	13380
1967	7120	5614	290	290	2000	809	2360	180	320	13430
1968	7350	5799	270	270	1900	784	2310	140	320	13380
1969	7940	6274	274	274	1900	782	2180	140	270	13790
1970	8070	6357	267	267	1810	762	2130	140	270	13740
1971	8210	6481	250	250	1720	718	2090	140	270	13650
1972	8800	6940	240	240	1680	702	1950	90	270	13970
1973	9160	7202	234	234	1590	670	1910	90	230	14110

Source: see *Notes on sources of sales data,* p. 160

Table 7.1.2 Total annual sales of tobacco products, 1974-1995

Year	Cigarettes		Cigars and cigarillos		Pipe and HR[1] tobacco tonnes	Chewing tobacco tonnes	Snuff tonnes	All tobacco products tonnes
	tonnes	millions	tonnes	millions				
1974	6909	6909	2775	881	2551	99	227	12561
1975	7295	7295	2756	875	2023	93	223	12390
1976	7690	7690	2674	849	1792	82	207	12445
1977	7610	7610	2655	843	1889	76	198	12428
1978	7435	7435	2460	781	1780	47	185	11907
1979	7431	7431	2331	740	1821	65	170	11818
1980	7151	7151	2192	696	2128	61	159	11691
1981	7299	7299	1991	632	2315	58	149	11812
1982	7989	7989	1792	569	2474	52	142	12449
1983	7411	7411	1673	531	2202	49	131	11466
1984	7720	7720	1566	497	2223	44	117	11670
1985	7787	7787	1487	472	2314	43	107	11738
1986	7502	7502	1452	461	2419	39	98	11510
1987	7183	7183	1367	434	2547	37	84	11218
1988	6939	6939	1232	391	2662	32	76	10941
1989	6776	6776	1153	366	2760	29	75	10793
1990	6584	6584	1033	328	2953	26	70	10666
1991	6517	6517	964	306	2931	25	62	10499
1992	6745	6745	891	283	2776	22	52	10486
1993	6382	6382	784	249	2899	19	48	10132
1994	6440	6440	709	225	2771	16	40	9976
1995	6429	6429	636	202	2718	14	37	9834

1 Tobacco for hand-rolled cigarettes

Source : see *Notes on sources of sales data,* p. 160

Table 7.1.3 Manufactured cigarettes (i) percentage of total sales as filter cigarettes, 1960-1984, and (ii) sales-weighted average tar yield per cigarette (SWAT), 1964-1990

Year	% Filter	SWAT mg / cig	Year	% Filter	SWAT mg / cig
1960	29.0		1980	62.1	25.0
1961	30.0		1981	63.2	25.0
1962	30.5		1982	66.0	24.0
1963	35.3		1983	67.0	24.0
1964	37.5	27.0	1984	68.0	23.0
1965	39.1	27.0	1985		23.0
1966	41.8	27.0	1986		21.8
1967	44.5	28.0	1987		21.0
1968	48.1	29.0	1988		20.3
1969	49.4	29.0	1989		18.9
1970	47.8	30.0	1990		18.6
1971	48.3	30.0			
1972	49.5	30.0			
1973	51.9	30.0			
1974	52.6	29.0			
1975	53.5	29.0			
1976	56.6	28.0			
1977	59.7	27.0			
1978	60.6	27.0			
1979	61.9	26.0			

Source : see *Notes on sources of sales data*, p. 160

Table 7.2 Consumption of (i) cigarettes and (ii) all tobacco products, 1920-1995 sales-based data, including estimated hand-rolled cigarette consumption. Males and females aged 15 years and over

Year	Manufactured cigarettes		Hand-rolled cigarettes		Total cigarettes		All tobacco products	
	Total annual in millions	Number/ adult/day	Total annual in millions	Number/ adult/day	Total annual in millions	Number/ adult/day	Total annual in tonnes	Grams/ adult/day
1920	860	1.1					6990	8.7
1921	868	1.1					6400	8.0
1922	943	1.1					6210	7.4
1923	1109	1.3					6940	7.9
1924	1159	1.3					6760	7.7
1925	1219	1.4					6710	7.7
1926	1325	1.5					7080	8.1
1927	1373	1.6					6890	7.9
1928	1544	1.7					7120	7.8
1929	1017	1.1					6760	7.4
1930	1319	1.4					7300	7.7
1931	1332	1.4					7260	7.7
1932	1170	1.2					7300	7.7
1933	1142	1.2					7480	7.6
1934	1214	1.2					7850	8.0
1935	1307	1.3					8210	8.0
1936	1404	1.4					8620	8.4
1937	1507	1.5					8750	8.6
1938	1605	1.5					8890	8.4
1939	1748	1.7					9250	8.7

Table 7.2 *(continued)*

Year	Manufactured cigarettes		Hand-rolled cigarettes		Total cigarettes		All tobacco products	
	Total annual in millions	Number/ adult/day	Total annual in millions	Number/ adult/day	Total annual in millions	Number/ adult/day	Total annual in tonnes	Grams/ adult/day
1940	1662	1.6					8620	8.1
1941	1577	1.5					6990	6.6
1942	1779	1.6					7440	6.8
1943	1094	1.0					5260	4.8
1944	1318	1.2					5810	5.3
1945	1163	1.1					5260	4.8
1946	2150	1.9					9210	8.1
1947	2380	2.1					9570	8.5
1948	2663	2.4					10480	9.3
1949	3489	3.1					10750	9.5
1950	4008	3.5	1992	1.7	6000	5.2	11340	9.9
1951	3483	3.0	1920	1.7	5403	4.7	10120	8.8
1952	3881	3.3	2072	1.8	5953	5.1	10750	9.2
1953	3931	3.4	2072	1.8	6003	5.1	10890	9.3
1954	3834	3.2	2144	1.8	5978	5.1	10930	9.3
1955	3787	3.2	2104	1.8	5891	5.0	10800	9.1
1956	3882	3.2	2072	1.7	5954	5.0	10890	9.1
1957	4010	3.3	2032	1.7	6042	5.0	10980	9.1
1958	4349	3.6	2072	1.7	6421	5.3	11520	9.5
1959	4706	3.8	1960	1.6	6666	5.4	12110	9.8
1960	4990	4.0	1960	1.6	6950	5.6	12430	9.9
1961	5097	4.0	1816	1.4	6913	5.4	12470	9.8
1962	5257	4.1	1816	1.4	7073	5.5	12930	10.1
1963	5600	4.3	1744	1.3	7344	5.7	12790	9.8
1964	5277	4.0	1960	1.5	7237	5.5	13200	10.1
1965	5414	4.1	1960	1.5	7374	5.6	13430	10.1
1966	5566	4.2	1848	1.4	7414	5.6	13380	10.0
1967	5614	4.2	1888	1.4	7502	5.6	13430	10.0
1968	5799	4.3	1848	1.4	7647	5.6	13380	9.9
1969	6274	4.6	1744	1.3	8018	5.9	13790	10.1
1970	6357	4.6	1704	1.2	8061	5.8	13740	10.0
1971	6481	4.7	1672	1.2	8153	5.9	13650	9.8
1972	6940	5.0	1560	1.1	8500	6.1	13970	10.0
1973	7202	5.1	1528	1.1	8730	6.2	14110	10.0
1974	6909	4.9	2041	1.4	8950	6.3	12561	8.8
1975	7295	5.1	1618	1.1	8913	6.2	12390	8.7
1976	7690	5.4	1434	1.0	9124	6.4	12445	8.7
1977	7610	5.3	1511	1.0	9121	6.3	12428	8.6
1978	7435	5.1	1424	1.0	8859	6.1	11907	8.2
1979	7431	5.1	1457	1.0	8888	6.0	11818	8.0
1980	7151	4.8	1702	1.1	8853	6.0	11691	7.9
1981	7299	4.9	1852	1.2	9151	6.1	11812	7.9
1982	7989	5.3	1979	1.3	9968	6.6	12449	8.3
1983	7411	4.9	1762	1.2	9173	6.1	11466	7.6
1984	7720	5.1	1778	1.2	9498	6.3	11670	7.7
1985	7787	5.1	1851	1.2	9638	6.3	11738	7.7
1986	7502	4.9	1935	1.3	9437	6.2	11510	7.5
1987	7183	4.7	2038	1.3	9221	6.0	11218	7.3
1988	6939	4.5	2130	1.4	9069	5.9	10941	7.1
1989	6776	4.4	2208	1.4	8984	5.8	10793	7.0
1990	6584	4.2	2362	1.5	8946	5.7	10666	6.9
1991	6517	4.2	2345	1.5	8862	5.7	10499	6.7
1992	6745	4.3	2221	1.4	8966	5.7	10486	6.7
1993	6382	4.1	2319	1.5	8701	5.5	10132	6.4
1994	6440	4.1	2217	1.4	8657	5.5	9976	6.3
1995	6429	4.1	2174	1.4	8603	5.5	9834	6.2

Source : see *Notes on sources of sales data*, p. 160

Figure 7.1 Daily consumption of (i) manufactured and total number of cigarettes, and (ii) all tobacco products, 1920-1995.
Males and females aged 15 years and over. *Source:* see Table 7.2

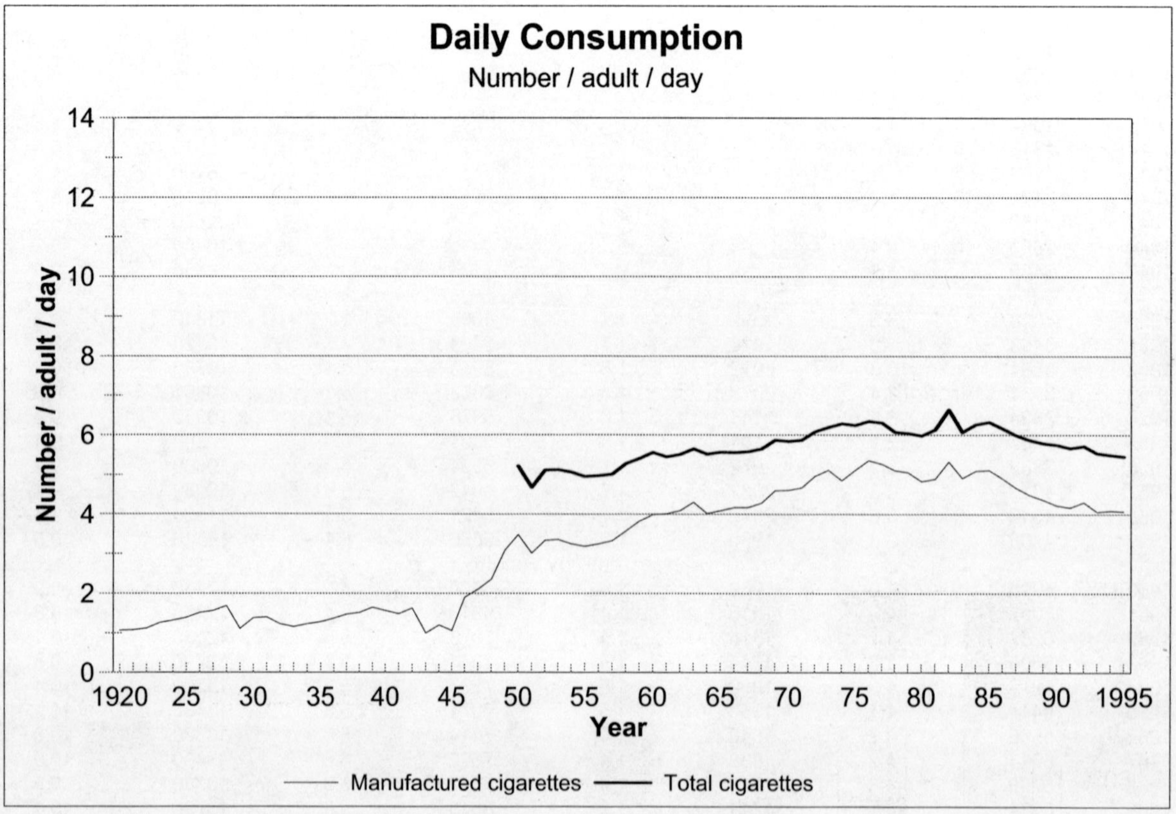

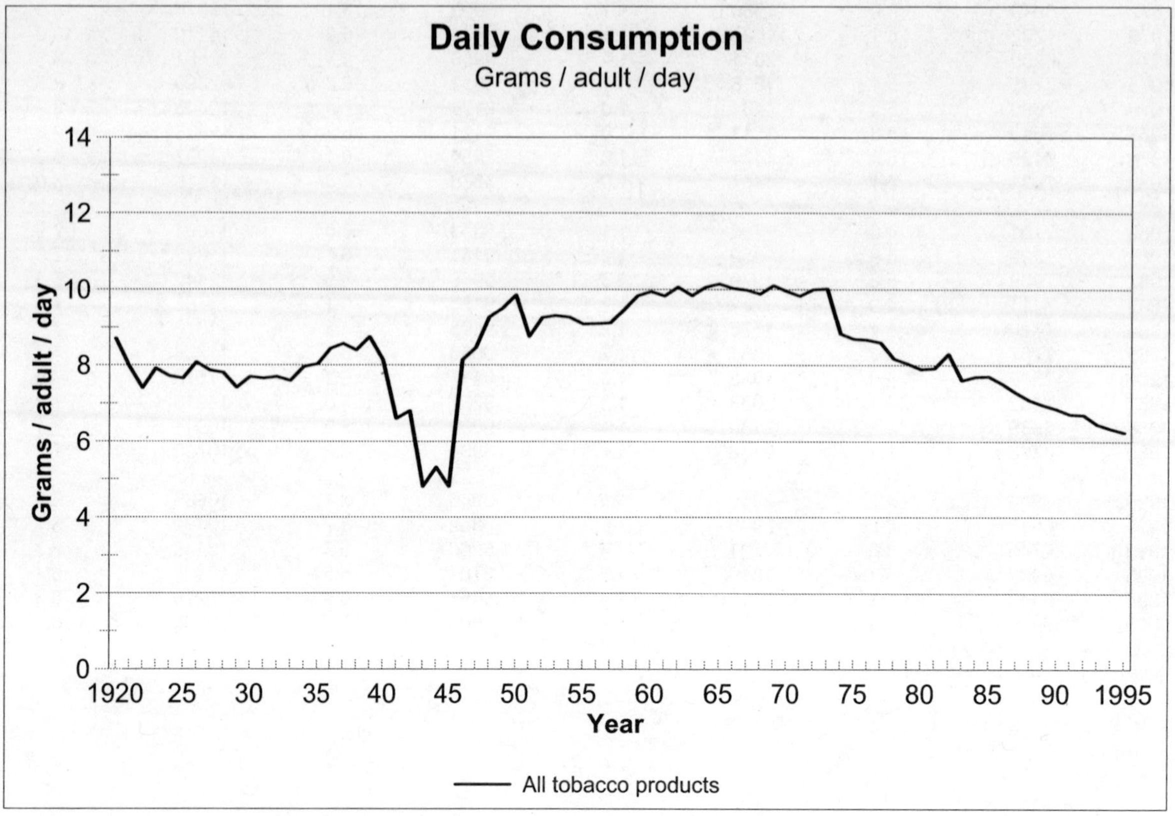

Table 7.3 Percentage sales of tobacco in different forms (by weight), selected years 1925-1995

Year	Cigarettes (%)	Cigars and cigarillos (%)	Pipe and hand-rolling tobacco (%)	Snuff and chewing tobacco (%)
1925	23.0	24.3	31.7	20.9
1935	19.9	36.4	29.2	14.4
1945	27.6	28.5	26.8	17.1
1955	44.1	24.4	24.4	7.1
1965	51.3	26.4	18.2	4.0
1975	58.9	22.2	16.3	2.6
1985	66.3	12.7	19.7	1.3
1995	65.4	6.5	27.6	0.5

Source : calculated from Tables 7.1.1 & 7.1.2

Figure 7.2 Percentage sales of tobacco in different forms (by weight), selected years 1925-1995
Source: see Table 7.3

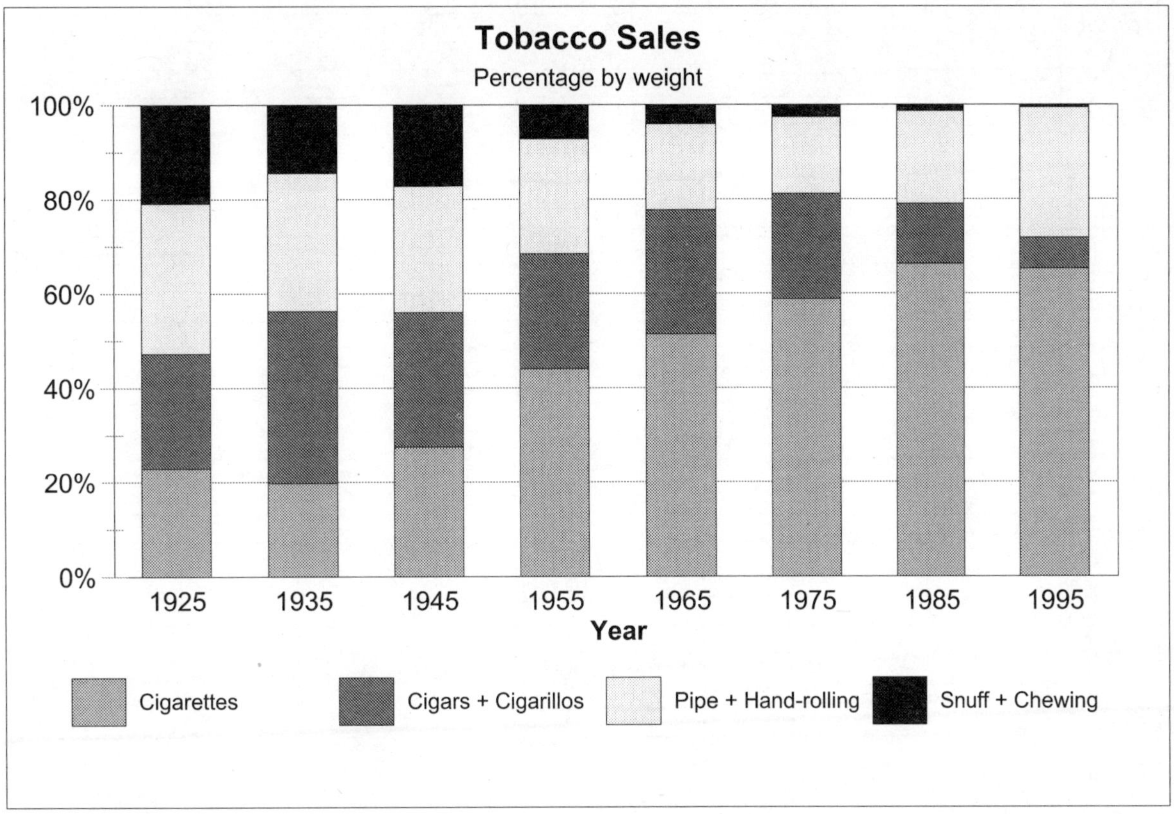

Table 7.4M Prevalence of smoking, males: some selected Danish surveys by age, 1953-1995 *(continues on p.144)*

Frequency Product Source Year	12	13	14	15	16	17	18	19	20-24	25-29	30-34	35-39	40-44	45-49	50-54	55-59	60-64	65-69	70-74	75-79	80+	All ages
53 6 UC U				28					35		32		27		16		6		2			23
53 6 A U				61					83		85		83		79		70		59			78
54 6 UC U				22																		
54 6 A U				78																		
58 2 TC R				46																		
59 2 TC R				43																		
59 9 A A	80	83	90																			
60 1 A U	22								76		82		85		77		70					70
60 2 TC R				44																		
61 1 A U									65													
61 2 TC R				43																		
62 2 TC R				41																		
63 2 TC R				39																		
63 2 A R				71																		
64 2 TC R				38																		
64 8 TC U															⟨43⟩							
64 8 A U															⟨78⟩							
64 14 TC U				44																		
64 14 A U				76																		
65 1 TC U									43													
65 2 TC R				38																		
66 1 TC U									42													
66 2 TC R				38																		
67 1 TC U									40													
67 2 TC R				39																		
67 8 UC R																			⟨20⟩			
67 8 A U																			⟨77⟩			
68 1 A U									72													
68 2 TC R				40																		
69 1 TC U									46													
69 1 A U									72													
69 2 TC R				41																		
69 2 A R				68																		
70 1 A U									69													
70 2 TC R				42					55	56	52		51		37			17				42
70 2 A R				51					65	69	72		77		71			63				68
71 1 TC U									46													
71 1 A U									69													
71 2 TC R				42					55	53	52		48		36			17				41
71 2 A R				48					65	67	71		75		69			60				67
72 1 TC U									47													
72 1 A U									68													
72 2 TC R				39					54	50	47		49		37			18				40
72 2 A R				43					64	64	65		73		68			60				64
72 15 U R				63																		
72 15 U U		16		66																		
73 1 TC U									46													
73 1 A U									66													
73 2 TC R				40					61	51	50		51		37			18				41
73 2 A R				45					68	60	64		71		66			57				63
73 3 UC R				43																		
74 1 A U									64													
74 2 TC R				35					58	52	48		54		41			19				42
74 2 A R				40					65	64	66		72		68			60				64
74 8 TC U																	⟨35⟩					
74 8 A U																	⟨68⟩					
74 12 A U	40								63		65		70		69			61				

Table 7.4F Prevalence of smoking, females: some selected Danish surveys by age, 1953-1995 *(continues on p. 145)*

Frequency / Product / Source / Year	12	13	14	15	16	17	18	19	20-24	25-29	30-34	35-39	40-44	45-49	50-54	55-59	60-64	65-69	70-74	75-79	80+	All ages
53 6 UC U				40					57		47		29		17		6		2			33
53 6 A U				41					59		51		38		31		20		10			40
54 6 UC U				32																		
54 6 A U				39																		
58 2 TC R				38																		
59 2 TC R				36																		
59 9 A A	53	59	75																			
60 1 A U	13								55		56		50		38		23					30
60 2 TC R				34																		
61 1 A U									39													
61 2 TC R				35																		
62 2 TC R				34																		
63 2 TC R				32																		
63 2 A R				41																		
64 2 TC R				32																		
64 8 TC U															⟨41⟩							
64 8 A U															⟨59⟩							
64 14 TC U				40																		
64 14 A U				49																		
65 1 TC U									35													
65 2 TC R				32																		
66 1 TC U									36													
66 2 TC R				33																		
67 1 TC U									34													
67 2 TC R				37																		
67 8 UC R																			⟨12⟩			
67 8 A U																			⟨46⟩			
68 1 A U									46													
68 2 TC R				34																		
69 1 TC U									40													
69 1 A U									50													
69 2 TC R				35																		
69 2 A R				44																		
70 1 A U									47													
70 2 TC R				38					52	52	52		45		31		11					36
70 2 A R				38					53	54	58		55		46		30					47
71 1 TC U									38													
71 1 A U									48													
71 2 TC R				35					51	49	49		45		32		12					36
71 2 A R				38					52	52	55		55		44		28					45
72 1 TC U									40													
72 1 A U									49													
72 2 TC R				42					50	49	48		48		33		11					37
72 2 A R				43					53	51	53		57		44		29					46
72 15 U R				55																		
72 15 U U		34		72																		
73 1 TC U									41													
73 1 A U									50													
73 2 TC R				38					55	49	48		46		35		13					37
73 2 A R				39					57	51	53		55		47		29					45
73 3 UC R				39																		
74 1 A U									48													
74 2 TC R				39					56	44	49		49		33		13					38
74 2 A R				41					57	47	52		56		45		30					46
74 8 TC U																	⟨34⟩					
74 8 A U																	⟨52⟩					
74 12 A U	37								50		50		56		46		30					

Table 7.4M *(continued from p. 142, continued on p. 146)*

Prevalence of smoking, males

Frequency / Product / Source / Year	12	13	14	15	16	17	18	19	20-24	25-29	30-34	35-39	40-44	45-49	50-54	55-59	60-64	65-69	70-74	75-79	80+	All ages
75 2 TC R				37					53	52	48		51		38			16				40
75 2 A R				41					57	63	62		69		65			53				60
75 11 UC U				38					57	54	48		50		38			15				41
75 11 A U				41					62	62	64		70		66			52				61
76 1 MC U									37													
76 1 A A							51				67				63				55			62
76 2 TC R				30					55	53	46		49		42			23				41
76 2 A R				32					61	62	60		68		66			57				61
76 8 A U				〈61〉																		
76 12 A U				35					63		62		69		67			59				
77 1 MC U									36													
77 1 A A							53				65				58				52			59
77 2 TC R				28					52	53	47		50		43			31				40
77 2 A R				30					58	61	60		67		66			60				59
77 8 A U																				〈54〉		
77 16 A U									58	62	63	68	76	77	75	72	70	64	57	53	63	
78 1 MC U									40													
78 1 A A							51				62				60				52			57
78 2 TC R				31					47	50	46		47		42			21				41
78 2 A R				32					53	58	58		66		66			53				57
79 1 TC U									38													
79 2 TC R				30					49	53	48		47		42			21				41
79 2 A R				31					53	60	59		62		65			52				57
79 7 UC R					44																	
79 7 A R					39				62				60						56			59
80 1 MC U																						
80 1 A A							46				59				54				39			53
80 2 TC R				33					46	54	48		46		45			23				42
80 2 A R				33					51	61	61		62		64			53				57
80 13 A R				28																		
80 13 A A	12	19	26	36	52																	
81 1 A A							41				59				60				40			53
81 2 TC R				25					43	53	45		45		48			23				40
81 2 A R				27					46	55	56		61		66			52				54
82 1 A A							43				57				60				40			53
82 2 TC R				29					38	50	47		47		45			24				40
82 2 A R				30					40	55	57		60		61			50				53
83 1 A A							42				53				55				32			48
83 2 TC R				25					45	47	47		42		43			21				39
83 2 A R				28					50	54	59		57		64			49				54
83 4 UC R										55		44		50		39						45
83 4 A A										64		59		65		59						61
83 5 UC U																						
84 1 A A							39				53				54				36			48
84 2 TC R				22					45	47	49		42		42			26				40
84 2 A R				22					46	50	58		55		58			49				51
85 2 TC R				30					42	45	47		43		42			26				40
85 2 A R				30					43	50	55		57		59			49				51
85 17 UC A	4	12	20	32	32																	
85 24 UC *		3		15																		
85 24 UC R		6		19																		
85 24 UC A		8		23																		
86 2 TC R				23					38	53	51		40		43			26				40
86 2 A R				28					39	55	60		58		63			49				53

Table 7.4F *(continued from p. 143, continues on p. 147)*
Prevalence of smoking, females

Frequency / Product / Source / Year	12	13	14	15	16	17	18	19	20-24	25-29	30-34	35-39	40-44	45-49	50-54	55-59	60-64	65-69	70-74	75-79	80+	All ages
75 2 TC R				40					56	49	46		49		33			12				38
75 2 A R				40					57	50	49		56		45			28				46
75 11 UC U				39					56	47	45		48		31			13				37
75 11 A U				40					58	48	49		55		44			29				45
76 1 MC U									36													
76 1 A A							58				53				41				25			46
76 2 TC R				39					59	49	44		50		37			14				39
76 2 A R				39					60	51	49		58		46			30				46
76 8 A U	⟨49⟩																					
76 12 A U				42					57		50		59		48			33				
77 1 MC U									29													
77 1 A A							48				46				37				33			42
77 2 TC R				36					62	54	46		52		38			22				39
77 2 A R				37					63	56	49		59		49			37				47
77 8 A U																					⟨26⟩	
77 16 A U									61	57	64	61	64	66	64	59	53	46	38	34	26	
78 1 MC U									32													
78 1 A A							46				46				40				35			43
78 2 TC R				32					54	55	45		50		38			13				39
78 2 A R				33					54	57	48		56		48			28				46
79 1 TC U									33													
79 2 TC R				34					55	53	42		49		38			13				38
79 2 A R				34					56	54	54		45		47			27				45
79 7 UC R					38																	
79 7 A R					43				52				45						28			46
80 1 MC U									30													
80 1 A A							46				45				39				34			42
80 2 TC R				32					50	49	44		46		41			17				38
80 2 A R				33					52	51	48		52		49			29				44
80 13 A R				36																		
80 13 A A	10	21	35	46	48																	
81 1 A A							49				47				38				41			44
81 2 TC R				34					51	53	44		46		39			17				38
81 2 A R				34					54	56	47		51		46			29				44
82 1 A A							46				49				42				39			45
82 2 TC R				28					50	53	48		45		41			17				38
82 2 A R				28					50	54	50		50		48			28				43
83 1 A A							50				48				42				38			46
83 2 TC R				24					51	54	49		42		41			17				38
83 2 A R				24					52	54	51		47		48			28				43
83 4 UC R										56		45		48		36						44
83 4 A A										57		49		54		44						50
83 5 UC U				33					57	60	55	53	49									50
84 1 A A							49				45				45				34			44
84 2 TC R				26					46	50	49		44		43			22				39
84 2 A R				26					47	51	51		46		49			31				43
85 2 TC R				28					44	49	48		45		38			19				37
85 2 A R				28					44	50	50		48		45			30				42
85 17 UC A	5	11	30	41	45																	
85 24 UC *		11		21																		
85 24 UC R		13		27																		
85 24 UC A		17		37																		
86 2 TC R				26					36	52	52		43		46			24				40
86 2 A R				27					37	53	55		46		52			36				45

Table 7.4M (continued from p. 144)
Prevalence of smoking, males

Year Source Product Frequency	12	13	14	15	16	17	18	19	20-24	25-29	30-34	35-39	40-44	45-49	50-54	55-59	60-64	65-69	70-74	75-79	80+	All ages
87 2 TC R				21					42	50	48		45		39			26				39
87 2 A R				22					43	53	54		58		55			48				50
87 18 UC A				24					44		45		41		44		35		19			38
87 18 A R				23					44	44	49		50		57		53		39		36	
87 18 A A				24					48	45	53		53		59		55		42		42	49
88 2 TC R				18					37	44	47		42		43			28				38
88 2 A R				19					37	46	54		52		56			47				47
88 24 UC *		3		14																		
88 24 UC R		6		11																		
88 24 UC A		9		25																		
89 2 TC R				24					43	44	46		41		42			25				38
89 2 A R				25					44	46	51		49		56			44				47
89 19 U R	1		12																			
89 19 U A	4		17																			
89 19 U *	8		24																			
89 20 A R									30	43				48								43
89 20 A A									35	43	49		52		52							47
89 26 UC R		6		17																		
89 26 UC A		15		40																		
90 2 TC R				26					41	47	47		38		39			28				38
90 2 A R				27					41	49	52		47		54			49				47
90 22 U R			8	9																		
90 22 U A	1	8																				
90 23 U R				8																		
90 23 A A				15					⟨48⟩						⟨53⟩		⟨56⟩		⟨49⟩			
91 2 TC R				22					41	46	47		46		39			26				39
91 2 A R				22					42	48	51		55		53			44				47
91 18 UC A				24					39		48		45		37		33		28			39
91 18 A A				24					41		55		58		44		46		44			47
91 21 U R				16																		
91 21 U A				31																		
91 24 UC *		4		16																		
91 24 UC A		17		26																		
92 2 TC R				20					41	46	46		45		39			27				39
92 2 A R				20					41	47	50		55		49			43				46
93 2 TC R				20																		37
93 2 A R				20					41	47	46		50		53			41				45
94 2 TC R				28																		
94 2 A R				43																		
94 18 UC A					33					39				40				26				36
94 18 A R					30					41				50				38				41
94 18 A A					33					44				52				40				44
94 24 UC *		4		11																		
94 24 UC R		5		14																		
94 24 UC A		11		25																		
95 2 TC R				31																		
95 2 A R				43																		
95 25 UC R				16																		
95 25 UC A				24																		

Source: see *Notes on sources of survey data*, p. 161
Product: MC = manufactured cigarettes
TC = total cigarettes (including hand-rolled)
UC = cigarettes (type unspecified)
A = all products

Frequency: A = all smokers (including occasional)
R = regular or daily smokers
All ages: relevant to ages used and as given in original source
U = unspecified
* = refer to *Notes on sources of survey data*, p. 161

Table 7.4F *(continued from p. 145)*
Prevalence of smoking, females

Frequency / Product / Source / Year	12	13	14	15	16	17	18	19	20-24	25-29	30-34	35-39	40-44	45-49	50-54	55-59	60-64	65-69	70-74	75-79	80+	All ages
87 2 TC R				24					42	49	48		40		42			22				38
87 2 A R				25					43	49	49		44		47			32				42
87 18 UC A				35					50		49		46		45		36		16			39
87 18 A R				33					46	46	47		46		48		42		26		17	
87 18 A A				35					51	49	50		48		49		43		31		19	40
88 2 TC R				25					44	46	50		43		45			21				39
88 2 A R				25					44	47	51		45		49			28				42
88 24 UC *		1		16																		
88 24 UC R		6		17																		
88 24 UC A		7		33																		
89 2 TC R				27					41	53	45		40		44			24				38
89 2 A R				27					41	53	46		42		47			31				41
89 19 U R	1		30																			
89 19 U A	6		39																			
89 19 U *	8		50																			
89 20 A R									31	39				31								35
89 20 A A									38	46	41		33		36							39
89 26 UC R		6		23																		
89 26 UC A		16		30																		
90 2 TC R				22					44	45	47		44		42			23				38
90 2 A R				22					44	46	47		45		46			30				40
90 22 U R			5	17																		
90 22 U A	2	10																				
90 23 U R				12																		
90 23 A A				23					⟨49⟩					⟨46⟩		⟨48⟩		⟨39⟩				
91 2 TC R				20					44	45	50		42		41			27				39
91 2 A R				20					44	46	51		43		44			32				41
91 18 UC A				30					44		46		44		46		32		24			39
91 18 A A				30					44		46		44		49		35		27			41
91 21 U R				21																		
91 21 U A				41																		
91 24 UC *		3		20																		
91 24 UC A		16		32																		
92 2 TC R				26					43	43	49		43		41			23				38
92 2 A R				26					43	43	49		44		44			28				40
93 2 TC R				21																		37
93 2 A R				21					42	44	46		43		45			29				39
94 2 TC R				30																		
94 2 A R				39																		
94 18 UC A					32					46				37				22				37
94 18 A R					29					43				40				27				37
94 18 A A					32					46				41				29				39
94 24 UC *		3		17																		
94 24 UC R		8		24																		
94 24 UC A		16		33																		
95 2 TC R				31																		
95 2 A R				36																		
95 25 UC R				18																		
95 25 UC A				32																		

Source: see *Notes on sources of survey data*, p. 161
Product: MC = manufactured cigarettes
TC = total cigarettes (including hand-rolled)
UC = cigarettes (type unspecified)
A = all products

Frequency: A = all smokers (including occasional)
R = regular or daily smokers
All ages: relevant to ages used and as given in original source
U = unspecified
* = refer to *Notes on sources of survey data*, p. 161

Table 7.5M Number of cigarettes smoked per smoker per day, males: some selected Danish surveys by age, 1953-1995

<table>
<tr><th rowspan="2">Product
Source
Year</th><th colspan="21">Age group</th><th rowspan="2">All ages</th></tr>
<tr><th>12</th><th>13</th><th>14</th><th>15</th><th>16</th><th>17</th><th>18</th><th>19</th><th>20-24</th><th>25-29</th><th>30-34</th><th>35-39</th><th>40-44</th><th>45-49</th><th>50-54</th><th>55-59</th><th>60-64</th><th>65-69</th><th>70-74</th><th>75-79</th><th>80+</th></tr>
<tr><td>53 6 UCE</td><td colspan="3"></td><td colspan="5">9.0</td><td colspan="2">13</td><td colspan="2">15</td><td colspan="2">14</td><td colspan="2">14</td><td colspan="2">11</td><td colspan="3">6.2</td><td>13</td></tr>
<tr><td>54 6 UCE</td><td colspan="3"></td><td colspan="18">13</td><td></td></tr>
<tr><td>64 8 AE*</td><td colspan="21">⟨18⟩</td><td></td></tr>
<tr><td>64 14 TCE</td><td colspan="3"></td><td colspan="18">11</td><td></td></tr>
<tr><td>67 8 A *</td><td colspan="21">⟨14⟩</td><td></td></tr>
<tr><td>67 8 A *</td><td colspan="21">⟨17⟩</td><td></td></tr>
<tr><td>69 2 TCE*</td><td colspan="3"></td><td colspan="18">12</td><td></td></tr>
<tr><td>70 2 TCE*</td><td colspan="3"></td><td colspan="5">9.3</td><td>12</td><td>13</td><td colspan="2">13</td><td colspan="2">13</td><td colspan="3">12</td><td colspan="4">11</td><td>12</td></tr>
<tr><td>71 2 TCE*</td><td colspan="3"></td><td colspan="5">8.9</td><td>11</td><td>13</td><td colspan="2">12</td><td colspan="2">13</td><td colspan="3">13</td><td colspan="4">11</td><td>12</td></tr>
<tr><td>72 2 TCE*</td><td colspan="3"></td><td colspan="5">9.3</td><td>12</td><td>14</td><td colspan="2">14</td><td colspan="2">13</td><td colspan="3">13</td><td colspan="4">11</td><td>13</td></tr>
<tr><td>73 2 TCE*</td><td colspan="3"></td><td colspan="5">9.9</td><td>11</td><td>12</td><td colspan="2">12</td><td colspan="2">12</td><td colspan="3">12</td><td colspan="4">11</td><td>12</td></tr>
<tr><td>74 2 TCE*</td><td colspan="3"></td><td colspan="5">9.7</td><td>12</td><td>14</td><td colspan="2">14</td><td colspan="2">14</td><td colspan="3">13</td><td colspan="4">10</td><td>13</td></tr>
<tr><td>74 8 AE*</td><td colspan="21">⟨17⟩</td><td></td></tr>
<tr><td>74 8 AE*</td><td colspan="21">⟨17⟩</td><td></td></tr>
<tr><td>75 2 TCE*</td><td colspan="3"></td><td colspan="5">9.8</td><td>14</td><td>15</td><td colspan="2">15</td><td colspan="2">15</td><td colspan="3">13</td><td colspan="4">11</td><td>14</td></tr>
<tr><td>75 11 UCE</td><td colspan="3"></td><td colspan="18">11</td><td></td></tr>
<tr><td>76 2 TCE*</td><td colspan="3"></td><td colspan="5">10</td><td>14</td><td>14</td><td colspan="2">15</td><td colspan="2">15</td><td colspan="3">14</td><td colspan="4">12</td><td>14</td></tr>
<tr><td>77 2 TCE*</td><td colspan="3"></td><td colspan="5">12</td><td>14</td><td>15</td><td colspan="2">15</td><td colspan="2">15</td><td colspan="3">14</td><td colspan="4">11</td><td>14</td></tr>
<tr><td>77 16 AE</td><td colspan="8"></td><td>14</td><td>17</td><td>18</td><td>20</td><td>19</td><td>20</td><td>19</td><td>18</td><td>18</td><td>16</td><td>15</td><td>14</td><td>12</td><td></td></tr>
<tr><td>78 2 TCE*</td><td colspan="3"></td><td colspan="5">11</td><td>14</td><td>15</td><td colspan="2">16</td><td colspan="2">16</td><td colspan="3">14</td><td colspan="4">12</td><td>14</td></tr>
<tr><td>79 2 TCE*</td><td colspan="3"></td><td colspan="5">12</td><td>15</td><td>15</td><td colspan="2">16</td><td colspan="2">15</td><td colspan="3">14</td><td colspan="4">12</td><td>15</td></tr>
<tr><td>79 7 UCE*</td><td colspan="4"></td><td colspan="17">16</td><td></td></tr>
<tr><td>80 2 TCE*</td><td colspan="3"></td><td colspan="5">12</td><td>14</td><td>14</td><td colspan="2">16</td><td colspan="2">16</td><td colspan="3">14</td><td colspan="4">13</td><td>15</td></tr>
<tr><td>81 2 TCE*</td><td colspan="3"></td><td colspan="5">12</td><td>13</td><td>15</td><td colspan="2">16</td><td colspan="2">16</td><td colspan="3">15</td><td colspan="4">12</td><td>15</td></tr>
<tr><td>82 2 TCE*</td><td colspan="3"></td><td colspan="5">12</td><td>15</td><td>15</td><td colspan="2">16</td><td colspan="2">16</td><td colspan="3">15</td><td colspan="4">13</td><td>15</td></tr>
<tr><td>83 2 TCE*</td><td colspan="3"></td><td colspan="5">11</td><td>15</td><td>17</td><td colspan="2">17</td><td colspan="2">16</td><td colspan="3">16</td><td colspan="4">13</td><td>16</td></tr>
<tr><td>83 4 UC</td><td colspan="11"></td><td colspan="6">16</td><td colspan="4"></td><td></td></tr>
<tr><td>83 5 UCE*</td><td colspan="21"></td><td></td></tr>
<tr><td>84 2 TCE*</td><td colspan="3"></td><td colspan="5">12</td><td>16</td><td>17</td><td colspan="2">17</td><td colspan="2">17</td><td colspan="3">16</td><td colspan="4">13</td><td>16</td></tr>
<tr><td>85 2 TCE*</td><td colspan="3"></td><td colspan="5">13</td><td>16</td><td>17</td><td colspan="2">17</td><td colspan="2">17</td><td colspan="3">16</td><td colspan="4">14</td><td>16</td></tr>
<tr><td>86 2 TCE*</td><td colspan="3"></td><td colspan="5">14</td><td>14</td><td>18</td><td colspan="2">17</td><td colspan="2">17</td><td colspan="3">15</td><td colspan="4">13</td><td>16</td></tr>
<tr><td>87 2 TCE*</td><td colspan="3"></td><td colspan="5">13</td><td>17</td><td>17</td><td colspan="2">18</td><td colspan="2">17</td><td colspan="3">18</td><td colspan="4">14</td><td>17</td></tr>
<tr><td>87 18 UCE*</td><td colspan="3"></td><td colspan="5">15</td><td colspan="2">17</td><td colspan="2">18</td><td colspan="2">19</td><td colspan="2">17</td><td colspan="2">16</td><td colspan="3">12</td><td>17</td></tr>
<tr><td>88 2 TCE*</td><td colspan="3"></td><td colspan="5">13</td><td>16</td><td>17</td><td colspan="2">16</td><td colspan="2">17</td><td colspan="3">16</td><td colspan="4">12</td><td>16</td></tr>
<tr><td>89 2 TCE*</td><td colspan="3"></td><td colspan="5">12</td><td>16</td><td>17</td><td colspan="2">18</td><td colspan="2">17</td><td colspan="3">16</td><td colspan="4">14</td><td>16</td></tr>
<tr><td>89 20 AE*</td><td colspan="8"></td><td>17</td><td>17</td><td colspan="2">16</td><td colspan="2">13</td><td colspan="2">12</td><td colspan="5"></td><td></td></tr>
<tr><td>90 2 TCE*</td><td colspan="3"></td><td colspan="5">12</td><td>15</td><td>18</td><td colspan="2">17</td><td colspan="2">18</td><td colspan="3">17</td><td colspan="4">13</td><td>16</td></tr>
<tr><td>90 23 AE*</td><td colspan="8"></td><td colspan="2">⟨15⟩</td><td colspan="4"></td><td colspan="2">⟨19⟩</td><td colspan="2">⟨18⟩</td><td colspan="3">⟨16⟩</td><td></td></tr>
<tr><td>91 2 TCE*</td><td colspan="3"></td><td colspan="5">12</td><td>16</td><td>18</td><td colspan="2">18</td><td colspan="2">18</td><td colspan="3">18</td><td colspan="4">14</td><td>17</td></tr>
<tr><td>91 18 UCE*</td><td colspan="3"></td><td colspan="5">10</td><td colspan="2">16</td><td colspan="2">18</td><td colspan="2">20</td><td colspan="2">20</td><td colspan="2">14</td><td colspan="3">16</td><td>17</td></tr>
<tr><td>92 2 TCE*</td><td colspan="3"></td><td colspan="5">13</td><td>17</td><td>18</td><td colspan="2">18</td><td colspan="2">18</td><td colspan="3">17</td><td colspan="4">14</td><td>17</td></tr>
<tr><td>93 2 TCE*</td><td colspan="3"></td><td colspan="18">17</td><td></td></tr>
<tr><td>94 2 TCE*</td><td colspan="3"></td><td colspan="18">21</td><td></td></tr>
<tr><td>94 18 UCE</td><td colspan="4"></td><td colspan="5">16</td><td colspan="4">20</td><td colspan="4">19</td><td colspan="4">14</td><td>18</td></tr>
<tr><td>95 2 TCE*</td><td colspan="3"></td><td colspan="18">19</td><td></td></tr>
<tr><td>95 25 UCE</td><td colspan="3"></td><td colspan="2">11</td><td colspan="16"></td><td></td></tr>
</table>

Source: see *Notes on sources of survey data*, p. 161
Product: MC = manufactured cigarettes
TC = total cigarettes (including hand-rolled)
UC = cigarettes (type unspecified)
A = all products
U = unspecified

Product (cont): E indicates mean estimated from percentage distribution (see also *Consumption category estimation*, p. xxxiv, and Appendix III, p. 789)
All ages: relevant to ages used and as given in original source
* = refer to *Notes on sources of survey data*, p. 161

Table 7.5F Number of cigarettes smoked per smoker per day, females: some selected Danish surveys by age, 1953-1995

Product Source Year	Age group 12	13	14	15	16	17	18	19	20-24	25-29	30-34	35-39	40-44	45-49	50-54	55-59	60-64	65-69	70-74	75-79	80+	All ages
53 6 UCE				6.1					7.4		7.7		7.5		6.2		5.2		4.8			7.3
54 6 UCE				7.3																		
64 8 AE*															⟨12⟩							
64 14 TCE				8.2																		
67 8 A *																			⟨10⟩			
67 8 A *																			⟨7⟩			
69 2 TCE*				10																		
70 2 TCE*				8.9					11	11	11		11		11			8.5				10
71 2 TCE*				8.6					10	11	11		11		10			8.7				10
72 2 TCE*				9.1					11	11	11		11		11			9.5				11
73 2 TCE*				9.1					9.6	11	12		10		10			9.0				10
74 2 TCE*				9.2					11	11	12		12		11			9.3				11
74 8 AE*																	⟨12⟩					
74 8 AE*																	⟨11⟩					
75 2 TCE*				9.2					12	12	12		11		11			9.4				11
75 11 UCE				9.9																		
76 2 TCE*				9.4					11	12	12		12		11			9.3				11
77 2 TCE*				11					12	12	13		12		11			9.6				12
77 16 AE									13	14	15	14	15	15	14	13	13	12	13	13	9.9	
78 2 TCE*				9.9					12	13	13		13		11			9.6				12
79 2 TCE*				9.9					12	12	13		13		12			10				12
79 7 UCE*					13																	
80 2 TCE*				9.8					12	13	13		12		12			10				12
81 2 TCE*				9.6					12	13	13		14		12			11				12
82 2 TCE*				11					12	13	14		13		12			10				13
83 2 TCE*				10					13	13	14		14		12			11				13
83 4 UC												13										
83 5 UCE*				15					14	15	17	16	15									
84 2 TCE*				10					13	14	15		15		12			11				13
85 2 TCE*				11					13	13	15		14		13			11				13
86 2 TCE*				9.5					13	14	14		14		12			11				13
87 2 TCE*				11					13	13	15		14		13			12				13
87 18 UCE				12					13		15		15		14		12		9.6			14
88 2 TCE*				11					12	14	14		15		13			10				13
89 2 TCE*				9.9					13	14	14		14		13			11				13
89 20 AE*									13	13	15		12		11							
90 2 TCE*				10					13	14	15		14		14			11				13
90 23 AE*									⟨13⟩						⟨16⟩		⟨13⟩		⟨11⟩			
91 2 TCE*				13					13	13	15		15		14			12				14
91 18 UCE*				9.7					13		14		15		14		10		9.0			13
92 2 TCE*				11					13	14	14		15		14			12				14
93 2 TCE*				14																		
94 2 TCE*				14																		
94 18 UCE*					13					15				16				10				15
95 2 TCE*				15																		
95 25 UCE				9.7																		

Source: see *Notes on sources of survey data*, p. 161

Product: MC = manufactured cigarettes
TC = total cigarettes (including hand-rolled)
UC = cigarettes (type unspecified)
A = all products
U = unspecified

Product (cont): E indicates mean estimated from percentage distribution (see also *Consumption category estimation*, p. xxxiv, and Appendix III, p. 789)

All ages: relevant to ages used and as given in original source

* = refer to *Notes on sources of survey data*, p. 161

Table 7.6M Number of cigarettes smoked per person per day, males: some selected Danish surveys by age, 1953-1995, with percentage total sales

Product Source Year	12	13	14	15	16	17	18	19	20-24	25-29	30-34	35-39	40-44	45-49	50-54	55-59	60-64	65-69	70-74	75-79	80+	All ages	% Total sales
53 6 UC	2.6								4.5		4.7		3.7		2.2		0.6		0.1			3.1	52%T
54 6 UC				2.9																			51%T
64 8 A *															⟨14⟩								**
64 14 TC				4.7																			72%T
67 8 A *																			⟨13⟩				**
69 2 TC *				4.9																			71%T
70 2 TC *				3.9					6.4	7.2	6.8		6.5		4.5			1.9				5.1	78%T
71 2 TC *				3.8					6.1	7.1	6.4		6.2		4.6			1.9				5.0	76%T
72 2 TC *				3.6					6.7	7.0	6.5		6.2		4.8			1.9				5.0	76%T
73 2 TC *				4.0					7.0	6.3	5.9		6.2		4.5			2.0				4.8	72%T
74 2 TC *				3.4					7.0	7.2	6.7		7.4		5.3			2.0				5.4	77%T
74 8 A *																	⟨12⟩						**
75 2 TC *				3.6					7.2	7.5	7.0		7.4		4.9			1.7				5.4	78%T
75 10 MC				5.7																			---M
75 11 UC				4.5																			66%T
76 2 TC *				3.0					7.5	7.6	6.9		7.3		5.7			2.8				5.7	80%T
77 2 TC *				3.4					7.4	8.0	7.1		7.7		6.0			3.4				5.7	87%T
77 16 A									7.7	10	11	14	15	15	14	13	12	10	8.8	7.3	7.8		105%A
78 2 TC *				3.4					6.4	7.5	7.2		7.3		6.0			2.6				5.9	85%T
79 2 TC *				3.5					7.3	8.1	7.5		7.2		5.9			2.6				6.0	86%T
79 7 UC *					9.2																		122%T
80 2 TC *				4.0					6.7	7.8	7.6		7.4		6.2			3.0				6.1	89%T
81 2 TC *				3.2					5.7	7.9	7.2		6.9		7.0			2.8				5.9	86%T
82 2 TC *				3.4					5.6	7.4	7.3		7.5		6.8			3.1				6.1	81%T
83 2 TC *				2.9					6.8	7.8	8.0		6.8		6.7			2.8				6.1	90%T
83 4 UC *												7.1											**
83 5 UC *																							**
84 2 TC *				2.5					7.3	7.8	8.3		7.2		6.6			3.4				6.3	91%T
85 2 TC *				3.9					6.6	7.9	8.0		7.3		6.8			3.5				6.4	89%T
86 2 TC *				3.3					5.4	9.7	8.4		6.7		6.6			3.3				6.3	92%T
87 2 TC *				2.8					7.2	8.2	8.7		7.7		6.9			3.6				6.6	97%T
87 18 UC *				3.5					7.4		8.0		7.8		7.6		5.6		2.3			6.6	100%T
88 2 TC *				2.3					5.8	7.5	7.7		6.9		6.6			3.4				5.9	94%T
89 2 TC *				2.8					6.9	7.3	8.1		7.0		6.8			3.5				6.2	97%T
89 20 A *									5.9	7.2	7.8		6.8		6.1								**
90 2 TC *				3.2					6.0	8.3	8.1		6.8		6.5			3.7				6.2	98%T
90 23 A *									⟨7.9⟩						⟨10⟩		⟨10⟩		⟨7.7⟩				**
91 2 TC *				2.7					6.7	8.0	8.4		8.1		6.9			3.7				6.6	104%T
91 18 UC *				2.4					6.4		8.5		8.9		7.3		4.8		4.5			6.7	102%T
92 2 TC *				2.6					6.8	8.4	8.3		8.3		6.6			3.8				6.6	103%T
93 2 TC *				6.4																			103%T
94 2 TC *				6.0																			93%T
94 18 UC *					5.4					7.6				7.5				3.5				6.6	107%T
95 2 TC *				5.9																			96%T
95 25 UC				1.7																			**

Source: see *Notes on sources of survey data*, p. 161

Product: MC = manufactured cigarettes
TC = total cigarettes (including hand-rolled)
UC = cigarettes (type unspecified)
A = all products
U = unspecified

All ages: relevant to ages used and as given in original source

% Total sales: estimated % of total sales of M = manufactured or T = total cigarette consumption implied by survey, sexes combined
** = cannot be calculated
--- = adjusted by original author
* = refer to *Notes on sources of survey data*, p. 161

Table 7.6F Number of cigarettes smoked per person per day, females: some selected Danish surveys by age, 1953-1995, with percentage total sales

<table>
<tr><th rowspan="2">Product
Source
Year</th><th colspan="21">Age group</th><th rowspan="2">All ages</th><th rowspan="2">% Total sales</th></tr>
<tr><th>12</th><th>13</th><th>14</th><th>15</th><th>16</th><th>17</th><th>18</th><th>19</th><th>20-24</th><th>25-29</th><th>30-34</th><th>35-39</th><th>40-44</th><th>45-49</th><th>50-54</th><th>55-59</th><th>60-64</th><th>65-69</th><th>70-74</th><th>75-79</th><th>80+</th></tr>
<tr><td>53 6 UC</td><td colspan="3"></td><td colspan="5">2.4</td><td colspan="2">4.3</td><td colspan="2">3.6</td><td colspan="2">2.1</td><td colspan="2">1.0</td><td colspan="2">0.3</td><td colspan="3">0.1</td><td>2.4</td><td>52%T</td></tr>
<tr><td>54 6 UC</td><td colspan="3"></td><td colspan="18">2.4</td><td></td><td>51%T</td></tr>
<tr><td>64 8 A *</td><td colspan="21">⟨7.0⟩</td><td></td><td>**</td></tr>
<tr><td>64 14 TC</td><td colspan="3"></td><td colspan="18">3.3</td><td></td><td>72%T</td></tr>
<tr><td>67 8 A *</td><td colspan="21">⟨2.8⟩</td><td></td><td>**</td></tr>
<tr><td>69 2 TC *</td><td colspan="3"></td><td colspan="18">3.5</td><td></td><td>71%T</td></tr>
<tr><td>70 2 TC *</td><td colspan="3"></td><td colspan="5">3.4</td><td>5.6</td><td>5.5</td><td colspan="2">5.5</td><td colspan="2">4.9</td><td colspan="3">3.2</td><td colspan="4">0.9</td><td>3.8</td><td>78%T</td></tr>
<tr><td>71 2 TC *</td><td colspan="3"></td><td colspan="5">3.0</td><td>5.1</td><td>5.5</td><td colspan="2">5.3</td><td colspan="2">5.1</td><td colspan="3">3.3</td><td colspan="4">1.0</td><td>3.7</td><td>76%T</td></tr>
<tr><td>72 2 TC *</td><td colspan="3"></td><td colspan="5">3.8</td><td>5.7</td><td>5.5</td><td colspan="2">5.4</td><td colspan="2">5.2</td><td colspan="3">3.6</td><td colspan="4">1.0</td><td>4.0</td><td>76%T</td></tr>
<tr><td>73 2 TC *</td><td colspan="3"></td><td colspan="5">3.4</td><td>5.3</td><td>5.4</td><td colspan="2">5.5</td><td colspan="2">4.7</td><td colspan="3">3.6</td><td colspan="4">1.2</td><td>3.8</td><td>72%T</td></tr>
<tr><td>74 2 TC *</td><td colspan="3"></td><td colspan="5">3.6</td><td>6.3</td><td>4.9</td><td colspan="2">5.6</td><td colspan="2">5.7</td><td colspan="3">3.7</td><td colspan="4">1.2</td><td>4.2</td><td>77%T</td></tr>
<tr><td>74 8 A *</td><td colspan="21">⟨5.8⟩</td><td></td><td>**</td></tr>
<tr><td>75 2 TC *</td><td colspan="3"></td><td colspan="5">3.7</td><td>6.4</td><td>6.0</td><td colspan="2">5.4</td><td colspan="2">5.6</td><td colspan="3">3.5</td><td colspan="4">1.2</td><td>4.3</td><td>78%T</td></tr>
<tr><td>75 10 MC</td><td colspan="3"></td><td colspan="18">4.7</td><td></td><td>---M</td></tr>
<tr><td>75 11 UC</td><td colspan="3"></td><td colspan="18">3.7</td><td></td><td>66%T</td></tr>
<tr><td>76 2 TC *</td><td colspan="3"></td><td colspan="5">3.7</td><td>6.6</td><td>5.7</td><td colspan="2">5.3</td><td colspan="2">6.1</td><td colspan="3">4.1</td><td colspan="4">1.3</td><td>4.4</td><td>80%T</td></tr>
<tr><td>77 2 TC *</td><td colspan="3"></td><td colspan="5">3.8</td><td>7.6</td><td>6.5</td><td colspan="2">5.9</td><td colspan="2">6.5</td><td colspan="3">4.3</td><td colspan="4">2.1</td><td>4.6</td><td>87%T</td></tr>
<tr><td>77 16 A</td><td colspan="8"></td><td>8.0</td><td>7.8</td><td>9.6</td><td>8.7</td><td>9.5</td><td>9.7</td><td>8.9</td><td>7.8</td><td>6.9</td><td>5.5</td><td>4.9</td><td>4.3</td><td>2.5</td><td></td><td>105%A</td></tr>
<tr><td>78 2 TC *</td><td colspan="3"></td><td colspan="5">3.2</td><td>6.2</td><td>7.0</td><td colspan="2">5.9</td><td colspan="2">6.4</td><td colspan="3">4.2</td><td colspan="4">1.2</td><td>4.6</td><td>85%T</td></tr>
<tr><td>79 2 TC *</td><td colspan="3"></td><td colspan="5">3.4</td><td>6.5</td><td>6.5</td><td colspan="2">5.4</td><td colspan="2">6.2</td><td colspan="3">4.5</td><td colspan="4">1.3</td><td>4.6</td><td>86%T</td></tr>
<tr><td>79 7 UC *</td><td colspan="4"></td><td colspan="17">5.9</td><td></td><td>122%T</td></tr>
<tr><td>80 2 TC *</td><td colspan="3"></td><td colspan="5">3.2</td><td>6.1</td><td>6.4</td><td colspan="2">5.9</td><td colspan="2">5.5</td><td colspan="3">4.7</td><td colspan="4">1.7</td><td>4.6</td><td>89%T</td></tr>
<tr><td>81 2 TC *</td><td colspan="3"></td><td colspan="5">3.2</td><td>5.9</td><td>6.9</td><td colspan="2">5.9</td><td colspan="2">6.2</td><td colspan="3">4.8</td><td colspan="4">1.8</td><td>4.7</td><td>86%T</td></tr>
<tr><td>82 2 TC *</td><td colspan="3"></td><td colspan="5">3.1</td><td>6.1</td><td>7.2</td><td colspan="2">6.7</td><td colspan="2">5.7</td><td colspan="3">5.0</td><td colspan="4">1.7</td><td>4.8</td><td>81%T</td></tr>
<tr><td>83 2 TC *</td><td colspan="3"></td><td colspan="5">2.4</td><td>6.6</td><td>7.0</td><td colspan="2">6.9</td><td colspan="2">5.9</td><td colspan="3">5.1</td><td colspan="4">1.8</td><td>4.9</td><td>90%T</td></tr>
<tr><td>83 4 UC *</td><td colspan="11"></td><td colspan="6">5.7</td><td colspan="4"></td><td></td><td>**</td></tr>
<tr><td>83 5 UC *</td><td colspan="3"></td><td colspan="5">5</td><td>8</td><td>9</td><td>10</td><td>9</td><td>7</td><td colspan="8"></td><td></td><td>**</td></tr>
<tr><td>84 2 TC *</td><td colspan="3"></td><td colspan="5">2.7</td><td>6.1</td><td>7.0</td><td colspan="2">7.1</td><td colspan="2">6.4</td><td colspan="3">5.3</td><td colspan="4">2.4</td><td>5.2</td><td>91%T</td></tr>
<tr><td>85 2 TC *</td><td colspan="3"></td><td colspan="5">3.0</td><td>5.6</td><td>6.5</td><td colspan="2">7.3</td><td colspan="2">6.2</td><td colspan="3">4.8</td><td colspan="4">2.0</td><td>4.9</td><td>89%T</td></tr>
<tr><td>86 2 TC *</td><td colspan="3"></td><td colspan="5">2.5</td><td>4.7</td><td>7.4</td><td colspan="2">7.1</td><td colspan="2">6.0</td><td colspan="3">5.5</td><td colspan="4">2.5</td><td>5.1</td><td>92%T</td></tr>
<tr><td>87 2 TC *</td><td colspan="3"></td><td colspan="5">2.7</td><td>5.3</td><td>6.4</td><td colspan="2">6.9</td><td colspan="2">5.6</td><td colspan="3">5.6</td><td colspan="4">2.6</td><td>5.0</td><td>97%T</td></tr>
<tr><td>87 18 UC *</td><td colspan="3"></td><td colspan="5">4.3</td><td colspan="2">6.7</td><td colspan="2">7.1</td><td colspan="2">7.0</td><td colspan="2">6.3</td><td colspan="2">4.3</td><td colspan="3">1.5</td><td>5.5</td><td>100%T</td></tr>
<tr><td>88 2 TC *</td><td colspan="3"></td><td colspan="5">2.6</td><td>5.2</td><td>6.3</td><td colspan="2">7.0</td><td colspan="2">6.5</td><td colspan="3">5.9</td><td colspan="4">2.2</td><td>5.1</td><td>94%T</td></tr>
<tr><td>89 2 TC *</td><td colspan="3"></td><td colspan="5">2.6</td><td>5.4</td><td>7.3</td><td colspan="2">6.3</td><td colspan="2">5.7</td><td colspan="3">5.8</td><td colspan="4">2.5</td><td>5.0</td><td>97%T</td></tr>
<tr><td>89 20 A *</td><td colspan="8"></td><td>5.0</td><td>5.9</td><td colspan="2">6.0</td><td colspan="2">4.1</td><td colspan="2">3.8</td><td colspan="5"></td><td></td><td>**</td></tr>
<tr><td>90 2 TC *</td><td colspan="3"></td><td colspan="5">2.2</td><td>5.6</td><td>6.1</td><td colspan="2">6.8</td><td colspan="2">6.2</td><td colspan="3">5.9</td><td colspan="4">2.6</td><td>5.1</td><td>98%T</td></tr>
<tr><td>90 23 A *</td><td colspan="8"></td><td>⟨6.3⟩</td><td></td><td></td><td></td><td></td><td></td><td>⟨7.2⟩</td><td></td><td>⟨6.2⟩</td><td></td><td>⟨4.3⟩</td><td></td><td></td><td></td><td>**</td></tr>
<tr><td>91 2 TC *</td><td colspan="3"></td><td colspan="5">2.5</td><td>5.6</td><td>6.1</td><td colspan="2">7.4</td><td colspan="2">6.1</td><td colspan="3">5.6</td><td colspan="4">3.1</td><td>5.3</td><td>104%T</td></tr>
<tr><td>91 18 UC *</td><td colspan="3"></td><td colspan="5">2.9</td><td colspan="2">5.6</td><td colspan="2">6.5</td><td colspan="2">6.6</td><td colspan="2">6.3</td><td colspan="2">3.2</td><td colspan="3">2.2</td><td>5.0</td><td>102%T</td></tr>
<tr><td>92 2 TC *</td><td colspan="3"></td><td colspan="5">2.9</td><td>5.5</td><td>6.3</td><td colspan="2">6.8</td><td colspan="2">6.4</td><td colspan="3">5.7</td><td colspan="4">2.7</td><td>5.2</td><td>103%T</td></tr>
<tr><td>93 2 TC *</td><td colspan="3"></td><td colspan="18">5.1</td><td></td><td>103%T</td></tr>
<tr><td>94 2 TC *</td><td colspan="3"></td><td colspan="18">4.3</td><td></td><td>93%T</td></tr>
<tr><td>94 18 UC *</td><td colspan="4"></td><td colspan="5">4.2</td><td colspan="4">6.7</td><td colspan="4">6.0</td><td colspan="4">2.3</td><td>5.4</td><td>107%T</td></tr>
<tr><td>95 2 TC *</td><td colspan="3"></td><td colspan="18">4.6</td><td></td><td>96%T</td></tr>
<tr><td>95 25 UC</td><td colspan="3"></td><td colspan="2">1.8</td><td colspan="16"></td><td></td><td>**</td></tr>
</table>

Source: see *Notes on sources of survey data*, p. 161
Product: MC = manufactured cigarettes
TC = total cigarettes (including hand-rolled)
UC = cigarettes (type unspecified)
A = all products
U = unspecified

All ages: relevant to ages used and as given in original source
% Total sales: estimated % of total sales of M = manufactured or T = total cigarette consumption implied by survey, sexes combined
** = cannot be calculated
--- = adjusted by original author
* = refer to *Notes on sources of survey data*, p. 161

Table 7.7M Number of cigarettes smoked per person per day, sales-adjusted, males: some selected Danish surveys[1] by age, 1953-1995, with percentage total sales

Product Source Year	12	13	14	15	16	17	18	19	20-24	25-29	30-34	35-39	40-44	45-49	50-54	55-59	60-64	65-69	70-74	75-79	80+	All ages	% Total sales
53 6 UC				5.0					8.6		9.0		7.1		4.2		1.1		0.2			6.0	52%T
54 6 UC				5.6																			51%T
64 14 TC				6.5																			72%T
69 2 TC *				6.9																			71%T
70 2 TC *				5.0					8.2	9.2	8.7		8.3		5.8			2.4				6.5	78%T
71 2 TC *				5.0					8.0	9.3	8.4		8.2		6.1			2.5				6.6	76%T
72 2 TC *				4.7					8.8	9.2	8.6		8.2		6.3			2.5				6.6	76%T
73 2 TC *				5.5					9.7	8.7	8.2		8.6		6.2			2.8				6.6	72%T
74 2 TC *				4.4					9.1	9.3	8.7		9.6		6.9			2.6				7.0	77%T
75 2 TC *				4.6					9.2	9.6	9.0		9.5		6.3			2.2				6.9	78%T
75 10 MC				5.7																			---M
75 11 UC				6.9																			66%T
76 2 TC *				3.7					9.4	9.5	8.6		9.1		7.1			3.5				7.1	80%T
77 2 TC *				3.9					8.5	9.2	8.1		8.8		6.9			3.9				6.5	87%T
77 16 A									7.4	9.8	11	13	14	14	13	12	12	9.7	8.3	6.9	7.5		105%A
78 2 TC *				4.0					7.5	8.8	8.5		8.6		7.1			3.1				6.9	85%T
79 2 TC *				4.0					8.4	9.4	8.7		8.3		6.8			3.0				6.9	86%T
79 7 UC *					7.5																		122%T
80 2 TC *				4.5					7.5	8.8	8.5		8.3		7.0			3.4				6.9	89%T
81 2 TC *				3.7					6.6	9.1	8.3		8.0		8.1			3.2				6.8	86%T
82 2 TC *				4.2					6.9	9.1	9.0		9.2		8.4			3.8				7.5	81%T
83 2 TC *				3.2					7.6	8.7	8.9		7.6		7.4			3.1				6.8	90%T
84 2 TC *				2.7					8.0	8.6	9.1		7.9		7.2			3.7				6.9	91%T
85 2 TC *				4.4					7.4	8.9	9.0		8.2		7.6			3.9				7.2	89%T
86 2 TC *				3.6					5.9	11	9.2		7.3		7.2			3.6				6.9	92%T
87 2 TC *				2.9					7.5	8.5	9.0		8.0		7.1			3.7				6.8	97%T
87 18 UC *				3.5					7.4		8.0		7.8		7.6		5.6		2.3			6.6	100%T
88 2 TC *				2.4					6.2	8.0	8.2		7.3		7.0			3.6				6.3	94%T
89 2 TC *				2.9					7.1	7.6	8.4		7.2		7.0			3.6				6.4	97%T
90 2 TC *				3.3					6.1	8.5	8.3		6.9		6.6			3.8				6.3	98%T
91 2 TC *				2.6					6.4	7.7	8.1		7.8		6.6			3.6				6.3	104%T
91 18 UC *				2.4					6.3		8.3		8.7		7.1		4.7		4.4			6.6	102%T
92 2 TC *				2.5					6.6	8.1	8.1		8.1		6.4			3.7				6.4	103%T
93 2 TC *				6.2																			103%T
94 2 TC *				6.4																			93%T
94 18 UC *					5.1					7.2				7.1				3.2				6.2	107%T
95 2 TC *				6.1																			96%T

1 Based on those surveys in Table 7.6 with data for both sexes and age range at least 21-64 (see *Cigarette consumption per person*, p. xxxv)

Source: See *Notes on sources of survey data*, p. 161

Product:
MC = manufactured cigarettes
TC = total cigarettes (including hand-rolled)
UC = cigarettes (type unspecified)
A = all products
U = unspecified

All ages: relevant to ages used and as given in original source

% Total sales: Adjustment factor used, estimated % of total sales of M = manufactured or T = total cigarette consumption implied by survey, sexes combined

--- = adjusted by original author

* = refer to *Notes on sources of survey data*, p. 161

Table 7.7F Number of cigarettes smoked per person per day, sales-adjusted, females: some selected Danish surveys[1] by age, 1953-1995, with percentage total sales

<table>
<tr><th rowspan="2">Product
Source
Year</th><th colspan="21">Age group</th><th rowspan="2">All ages</th><th rowspan="2">% Total sales</th></tr>
<tr><th>12</th><th>13</th><th>14</th><th>15</th><th>16</th><th>17</th><th>18</th><th>19</th><th>20-24</th><th>25-29</th><th>30-34</th><th>35-39</th><th>40-44</th><th>45-49</th><th>50-54</th><th>55-59</th><th>60-64</th><th>65-69</th><th>70-74</th><th>75-79</th><th>80+</th></tr>
<tr><td>53 6 UC</td><td colspan="3"></td><td colspan="5">4.6</td><td colspan="2">8.2</td><td colspan="2">6.9</td><td colspan="2">4.0</td><td colspan="2">1.9</td><td colspan="2">0.6</td><td colspan="3">0.2</td><td>4.6</td><td>52%T</td></tr>
<tr><td>54 6 UC</td><td colspan="3"></td><td colspan="18">4.6</td><td></td><td>51%T</td></tr>
<tr><td>64 14 TC</td><td colspan="3"></td><td colspan="18">4.5</td><td></td><td>72%T</td></tr>
<tr><td>69 2 TC *</td><td colspan="3"></td><td colspan="18">4.9</td><td></td><td>71%T</td></tr>
<tr><td>70 2 TC *</td><td colspan="3"></td><td colspan="5">4.4</td><td>7.2</td><td>7.1</td><td colspan="2">7.1</td><td colspan="2">6.3</td><td colspan="3">4.1</td><td colspan="4">1.2</td><td>4.9</td><td>78%T</td></tr>
<tr><td>71 2 TC *</td><td colspan="3"></td><td colspan="5">3.9</td><td>6.7</td><td>7.2</td><td colspan="2">7.0</td><td colspan="2">6.7</td><td colspan="3">4.3</td><td colspan="4">1.3</td><td>4.9</td><td>76%T</td></tr>
<tr><td>72 2 TC *</td><td colspan="3"></td><td colspan="5">5.0</td><td>7.5</td><td>7.2</td><td colspan="2">7.1</td><td colspan="2">6.9</td><td colspan="3">4.7</td><td colspan="4">1.3</td><td>5.3</td><td>76%T</td></tr>
<tr><td>73 2 TC *</td><td colspan="3"></td><td colspan="5">4.7</td><td>7.3</td><td>7.5</td><td colspan="2">7.6</td><td colspan="2">6.5</td><td colspan="3">5.0</td><td colspan="4">1.7</td><td>5.3</td><td>72%T</td></tr>
<tr><td>74 2 TC *</td><td colspan="3"></td><td colspan="5">4.7</td><td>8.2</td><td>6.4</td><td colspan="2">7.3</td><td colspan="2">7.4</td><td colspan="3">4.8</td><td colspan="4">1.6</td><td>5.4</td><td>77%T</td></tr>
<tr><td>75 2 TC *</td><td colspan="3"></td><td colspan="5">4.8</td><td>8.2</td><td>7.7</td><td colspan="2">6.9</td><td colspan="2">7.2</td><td colspan="3">4.5</td><td colspan="4">1.5</td><td>5.5</td><td>78%T</td></tr>
<tr><td>75 10 MC</td><td colspan="3"></td><td colspan="18">4.7</td><td></td><td>---M</td></tr>
<tr><td>75 11 UC</td><td colspan="3"></td><td colspan="18">5.6</td><td></td><td>66%T</td></tr>
<tr><td>76 2 TC *</td><td colspan="3"></td><td colspan="5">4.6</td><td>8.2</td><td>7.1</td><td colspan="2">6.6</td><td colspan="2">7.6</td><td colspan="3">5.1</td><td colspan="4">1.6</td><td>5.5</td><td>80%T</td></tr>
<tr><td>77 2 TC *</td><td colspan="3"></td><td colspan="5">4.3</td><td>8.7</td><td>7.4</td><td colspan="2">6.8</td><td colspan="2">7.4</td><td colspan="3">4.9</td><td colspan="4">2.4</td><td>5.3</td><td>87%T</td></tr>
<tr><td>77 16 A</td><td colspan="8"></td><td>7.6</td><td>7.4</td><td>9.2</td><td>8.3</td><td>9.1</td><td>9.3</td><td>8.5</td><td>7.4</td><td>6.6</td><td>5.3</td><td>4.6</td><td>4.1</td><td>2.4</td><td></td><td>105%A</td></tr>
<tr><td>78 2 TC *</td><td colspan="3"></td><td colspan="5">3.8</td><td>7.3</td><td>8.2</td><td colspan="2">6.9</td><td colspan="2">7.5</td><td colspan="3">4.9</td><td colspan="4">1.4</td><td>5.4</td><td>85%T</td></tr>
<tr><td>79 2 TC *</td><td colspan="3"></td><td colspan="5">3.9</td><td>7.5</td><td>7.5</td><td colspan="2">6.2</td><td colspan="2">7.2</td><td colspan="3">5.2</td><td colspan="4">1.5</td><td>5.3</td><td>86%T</td></tr>
<tr><td>79 7 UC *</td><td colspan="4"></td><td colspan="17">4.8</td><td></td><td>122%T</td></tr>
<tr><td>80 2 TC *</td><td colspan="3"></td><td colspan="5">3.6</td><td>6.9</td><td>7.2</td><td colspan="2">6.6</td><td colspan="2">6.2</td><td colspan="3">5.3</td><td colspan="4">1.9</td><td>5.2</td><td>89%T</td></tr>
<tr><td>81 2 TC *</td><td colspan="3"></td><td colspan="5">3.7</td><td>6.8</td><td>8.0</td><td colspan="2">6.8</td><td colspan="2">7.2</td><td colspan="3">5.6</td><td colspan="4">2.1</td><td>5.4</td><td>86%T</td></tr>
<tr><td>82 2 TC *</td><td colspan="3"></td><td colspan="5">3.8</td><td>7.5</td><td>8.8</td><td colspan="2">8.2</td><td colspan="2">7.0</td><td colspan="3">6.1</td><td colspan="4">2.1</td><td>5.9</td><td>81%T</td></tr>
<tr><td>83 2 TC *</td><td colspan="3"></td><td colspan="5">2.7</td><td>7.3</td><td>7.8</td><td colspan="2">7.7</td><td colspan="2">6.6</td><td colspan="3">5.7</td><td colspan="4">2.0</td><td>5.4</td><td>90%T</td></tr>
<tr><td>84 2 TC *</td><td colspan="3"></td><td colspan="5">3.0</td><td>6.7</td><td>7.7</td><td colspan="2">7.8</td><td colspan="2">7.0</td><td colspan="3">5.8</td><td colspan="4">2.6</td><td>5.7</td><td>91%T</td></tr>
<tr><td>85 2 TC *</td><td colspan="3"></td><td colspan="5">3.4</td><td>6.3</td><td>7.3</td><td colspan="2">8.2</td><td colspan="2">7.0</td><td colspan="3">5.4</td><td colspan="4">2.2</td><td>5.5</td><td>89%T</td></tr>
<tr><td>86 2 TC *</td><td colspan="3"></td><td colspan="5">2.7</td><td>5.1</td><td>8.1</td><td colspan="2">7.7</td><td colspan="2">6.5</td><td colspan="3">6.0</td><td colspan="4">2.7</td><td>5.6</td><td>92%T</td></tr>
<tr><td>87 2 TC *</td><td colspan="3"></td><td colspan="5">2.8</td><td>5.5</td><td>6.6</td><td colspan="2">7.1</td><td colspan="2">5.8</td><td colspan="3">5.8</td><td colspan="4">2.7</td><td>5.2</td><td>97%T</td></tr>
<tr><td>87 18 UC *</td><td colspan="3"></td><td colspan="5">4.3</td><td colspan="2">6.7</td><td colspan="2">7.1</td><td colspan="2">7.0</td><td colspan="2">6.3</td><td colspan="2">4.3</td><td colspan="3">1.5</td><td>5.5</td><td>100%T</td></tr>
<tr><td>88 2 TC *</td><td colspan="3"></td><td colspan="5">2.8</td><td>5.5</td><td>6.7</td><td colspan="2">7.4</td><td colspan="2">6.9</td><td colspan="3">6.3</td><td colspan="4">2.3</td><td>5.4</td><td>94%T</td></tr>
<tr><td>89 2 TC *</td><td colspan="3"></td><td colspan="5">2.7</td><td>5.6</td><td>7.6</td><td colspan="2">6.5</td><td colspan="2">5.9</td><td colspan="3">6.0</td><td colspan="4">2.6</td><td>5.2</td><td>97%T</td></tr>
<tr><td>90 2 TC *</td><td colspan="3"></td><td colspan="5">2.2</td><td>5.7</td><td>6.2</td><td colspan="2">6.9</td><td colspan="2">6.3</td><td colspan="3">6.0</td><td colspan="4">2.6</td><td>5.2</td><td>98%T</td></tr>
<tr><td>91 2 TC *</td><td colspan="3"></td><td colspan="5">2.4</td><td>5.4</td><td>5.9</td><td colspan="2">7.1</td><td colspan="2">5.9</td><td colspan="3">5.4</td><td colspan="4">3.0</td><td>5.1</td><td>104%T</td></tr>
<tr><td>91 18 UC *</td><td colspan="3"></td><td colspan="5">2.8</td><td colspan="2">5.5</td><td colspan="2">6.4</td><td colspan="2">6.5</td><td colspan="2">6.2</td><td colspan="2">3.1</td><td colspan="3">2.2</td><td>4.9</td><td>102%T</td></tr>
<tr><td>92 2 TC *</td><td colspan="3"></td><td colspan="5">2.8</td><td>5.3</td><td>6.1</td><td colspan="2">6.6</td><td colspan="2">6.2</td><td colspan="3">5.5</td><td colspan="4">2.6</td><td>5.0</td><td>103%T</td></tr>
<tr><td>93 2 TC *</td><td colspan="3"></td><td colspan="18">4.9</td><td></td><td>103%T</td></tr>
<tr><td>94 2 TC *</td><td colspan="3"></td><td colspan="18">4.6</td><td></td><td>93%T</td></tr>
<tr><td>94 18 UC *</td><td colspan="4"></td><td colspan="5">4.0</td><td colspan="4">6.3</td><td colspan="4">5.6</td><td colspan="4">2.1</td><td>5.1</td><td>107%T</td></tr>
<tr><td>95 2 TC *</td><td colspan="3"></td><td colspan="18">4.8</td><td></td><td>96%T</td></tr>
</table>

1 Based on those surveys in Table 7.6 with data for both sexes and age range at least 21-64 (see *Cigarette consumption per person*, p. xxxv)

Source: See *Notes on sources of survey data*, p. 161
Product: MC = manufactured cigarettes
TC = total cigarettes (including hand-rolled)
UC = cigarettes (type unspecified)
A = all products
U = unspecified

All ages: relevant to ages used and as given in original source
% Total sales: Adjustment factor used, estimated % of total sales of M = manufactured or T = total cigarette consumption implied by survey, sexes combined
--- = adjusted by original author
* = refer to *Notes on sources of survey data*, p. 161

Table 7.8 Estimated[1] prevalence of smoking and estimated[1] number of cigarettes per person per day (unadjusted and sales-adjusted): summary of Tables 7.4, 7.6 and 7.7, 1953-1995. Males and females aged 15 years and over

Year	Source[2]	Product[3]	Prevalence[4]						Number of cigarettes						
									Unadjusted[7]			Sales-adjusted[8]			
			Manufactured cigarettes		Total cigarettes[5]		All products[6]		Number/ person/day		Total sales %	Manufactured cigarettes number/ person/day		Total cigarettes[9] number/ person/day	
			M	F	M	F	M	F	M	F		M	F	M	F
1953	6	*UC+A*			24	32	77	39	3.1	2.3	52			5.9	4.3
1954	6	*UC+A*			22	32	78	39	2.9	2.3	51			5.6	4.6
1958	2	TC			46	38								(6.4	4.2)
1959	2	TC			43	36								(6.5	4.4)
1960	1	*A*					68	38							
	2	TC			44	34								(6.9	4.3)
1961	1	*A*					62	38							
	2	TC			43	35								(6.6	4.3)
1962	2	TC			41	34								(6.6	4.4)
1963	2	TC+A			39	32	71	41						(6.8	4.5)
1964	2	TC			38	32								(6.6	4.5)
	14	*TC+A*			43	40	76	48	4.7	3.3	72			6.5	4.5
1965	1	*TC*			41	33								(6.8	4.4)
	2	TC			38	32								(6.7	4.5)
1966	1	*TC*			40	34								(6.6	4.5)
	2	TC			38	33								(6.6	4.6)
1967	1	*TC*			38	33								(6.7	4.5)
	2	TC			39	37								(6.4	4.8)
1968	1	*A*					69	44							
	2	TC			40	34								(6.7	4.6)
1969	1	*TC+A*			44	38	69	48						(7.0	4.8)
	2	TC+A			41	35	68	44	4.9	3.5	71			6.9	4.9
1970	1	*A*					66	45							
	2	TC+A			43	37	68	47	5.2	3.9	78			6.7	5.0
1971	1	*TC+A*			44	36	66	46						(7.1	4.7)
	2	TC+A			42	37	66	45	5.1	3.8	76			6.7	5.1
1972	1	*TC+A*			45	38	65	47						(7.3	4.9)
	2	TC+A			41	38	64	46	5.2	4.1	76			6.8	5.3
1973	1	*TC+A*			44	39	63	48						(7.3	5.2)
	2	TC+A			43	38	62	46	5.0	3.9	72			7.0	5.5
	3	UC			43	39								(7.2	5.2)
1974	1	*A*					62	46							
	2	TC+A			43	38	63	46	5.6	4.2	77			7.2	5.4
	12	*A*					62	45							
1975	2	TC			41	38	60	45	5.5	4.2	78			7.1	5.4
	10	MC							5.7	4.7	---	5.7	4.7		
	11	*UC+A*			41	37	61	45	4.5	3.7	66			6.9	5.6

Table 7.8 *(continued)*

Year	Source[2]	Product[3]	Prevalence[4]						Number of cigarettes						
									Unadjusted[7]			Sales-adjusted[8]			
			Manufactured cigarettes		Total cigarettes[5]		All products[6]		Number/ person/day		Total sales %	Manufactured cigarettes number/ person/day		Total cigarettes[9] number/ person/day	
			M	F	M	F	M	F	M	F		M	F	M	F
1976	1	*MC*+**A**	36	35			58	46				(6.1	4.7)		
	2	TC+A			42	39	59	46	5.8	4.4	80			7.3	5.5
	12	*A*					61	48							
1977	1	*MC*+**A**	35	28			57	41				(6.4	4.2)		
	2	TC+A			43	42	59	49	6.1	4.9	87			7.0	5.6
	16	*A*					63	53	10.8[10]	7.3[10]	105			10.3[10]	6.9[10]
6.9[10]															
1978	1	*MC*+**A**	38	31			56	42				(6.2	4.0)		
	2	TC+A			40	38	57	45	5.8	4.5	85			6.8	5.3
1979	1	*TC*			37	32								(7.2	5.0)
	2	TC+A			41	38	56	44	6.0	4.5	86			6.9	5.2
	7	UC+A			44	37	58	45	9.0	5.8	122			7.4	4.8
1980	1	*MC*+**A**		29			50	41							
	2	TC+A			42	38	57	44	6.1	4.5	89			6.9	5.1
1981	1	**A**					51	43							
	2	TC+A			41	38	54	43	5.9	4.7	86			6.9	5.4
1982	1	**A**					50	44							
	2	TC+A			40	38	52	43	6.0	4.8	81			7.4	5.9
1983	1	**A**					47	44							
	2	TC+A			39	38	53	43	6.1	4.9	90			6.8	5.4
1984	1	**A**					46	43							
	2	TC+A			39	39	51	43	6.3	5.2	91			6.9	5.7
1985	2	TC+A			40	37	51	42	6.4	4.9	89			7.2	5.5
1986	2	TC+A			40	40	53	44	6.3	5.0	92			6.9	5.5
1987	2	TC+A			39	37	50	41	6.6	5.0	97			6.9	5.2
	18	A					46	41							
	18	**UC+A**			38	40	49	44	6.5	5.5	100			6.5	5.5
1988	2	TC+A			38	38	47	41	6.0	5.1	94			6.3	5.4
1989	2	TC+A			38	38	47	41	6.2	5.0	97			6.5	5.2
	20	A					42	33							
1990	2	TC+A			38	38	47	40	6.2	5.1	98			6.4	5.2
1991	2	TC+A			39	38	47	40	6.6	5.2	104			6.3	5.0
	18	**UC+A**			38	39	46	40	6.6	5.0	102			6.5	4.9
1992	2	TC+A			39	38	46	40	6.7	5.2	103			6.5	5.0
1993	2	TC+A			37	37	45	39	6.4	5.1	103			6.2	4.9
1994	2	TC+A			28	30	43	39	6.0	4.3	93			6.4	4.6
	18	A					41	37							
	18	**UC+A**			36	36	44	39	6.6	5.2	107			6.2	4.9
1995	2	TC+A			31	31	43	36	5.9	4.6	96			6.1	4.8

See next page for footnotes

1 Surveys covering an age range of at least 21-64 are included. Any gaps in the data for ages 15-20 and 65 years and over are filled in by assumed extensions to the age distribution, given in *Notes on sources of survey data*, p. 161. Method: see *Summary of adult smoking*, p. xxxvi
2 See *Notes on sources of survey data*, p. 161
3 Product: MC = manufactured cigarettes, TC = total cigarettes (including hand-rolled), UC = cigarettes (type unspecified), A = all products, U = unspecified. Frequency of smoking is indicated by: regular or daily smokers in normal type, all smokers (including occasional) in bold, unspecified in italics
4 From Table 7.4
5 This column includes prevalence of smoking classified as UC = cigarettes (type unspecified)
6 This column includes prevalence of smoking classified as U = unspecified product
7 From Table 7.6
8 From Table 7.7, except data in parentheses, which are derived from the prevalence of smoking from Table 7.4 as described in *Summary of adult smoking*, p. xxxvi
9 Number of cigarettes classified as UC = cigarettes (type unspecified) has been adjusted to total cigarette sales and included in this column
10 Grams of tobacco/person/day, adjusted to sales of all tobacco products

Figure 7.3 Estimated prevalence of smoking of (i) manufactured cigarettes, (ii) total cigarettes and (iii) all tobacco products: by year of survey, 1953-1995.
Males and females aged 15 years and over. *Source:* see Table 7.8

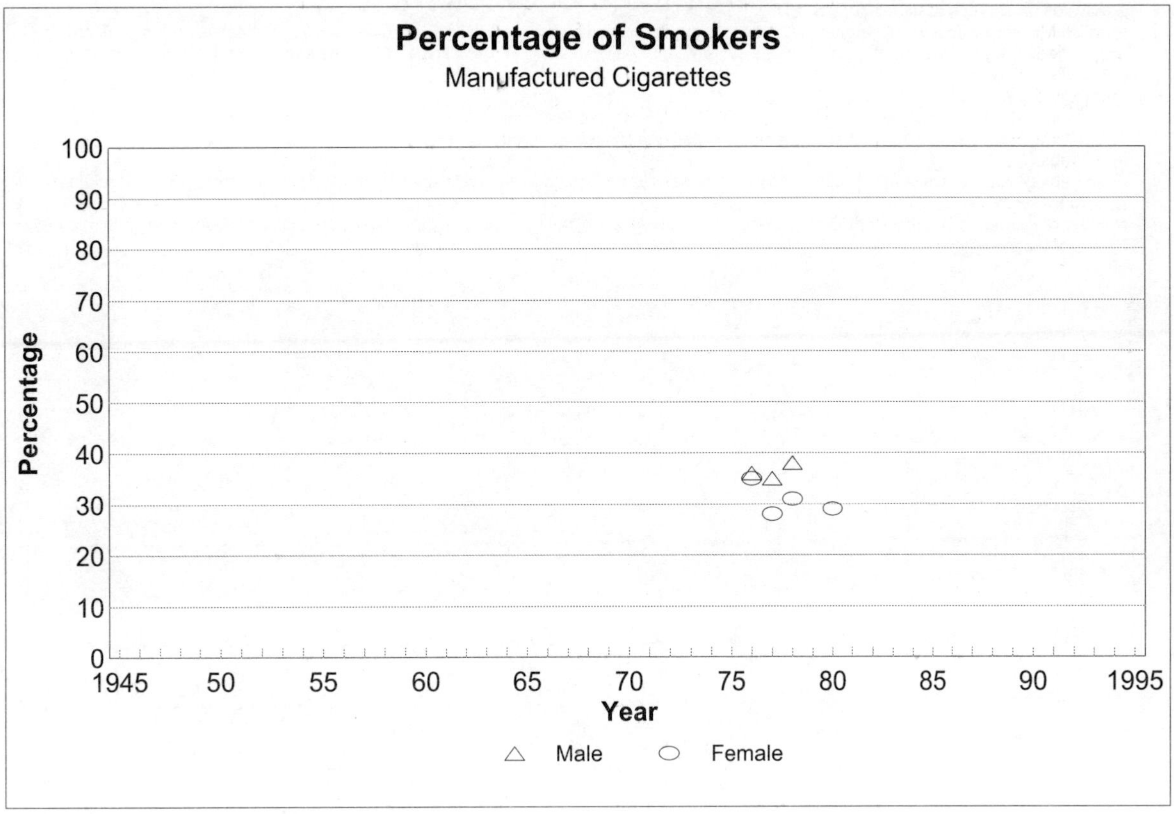

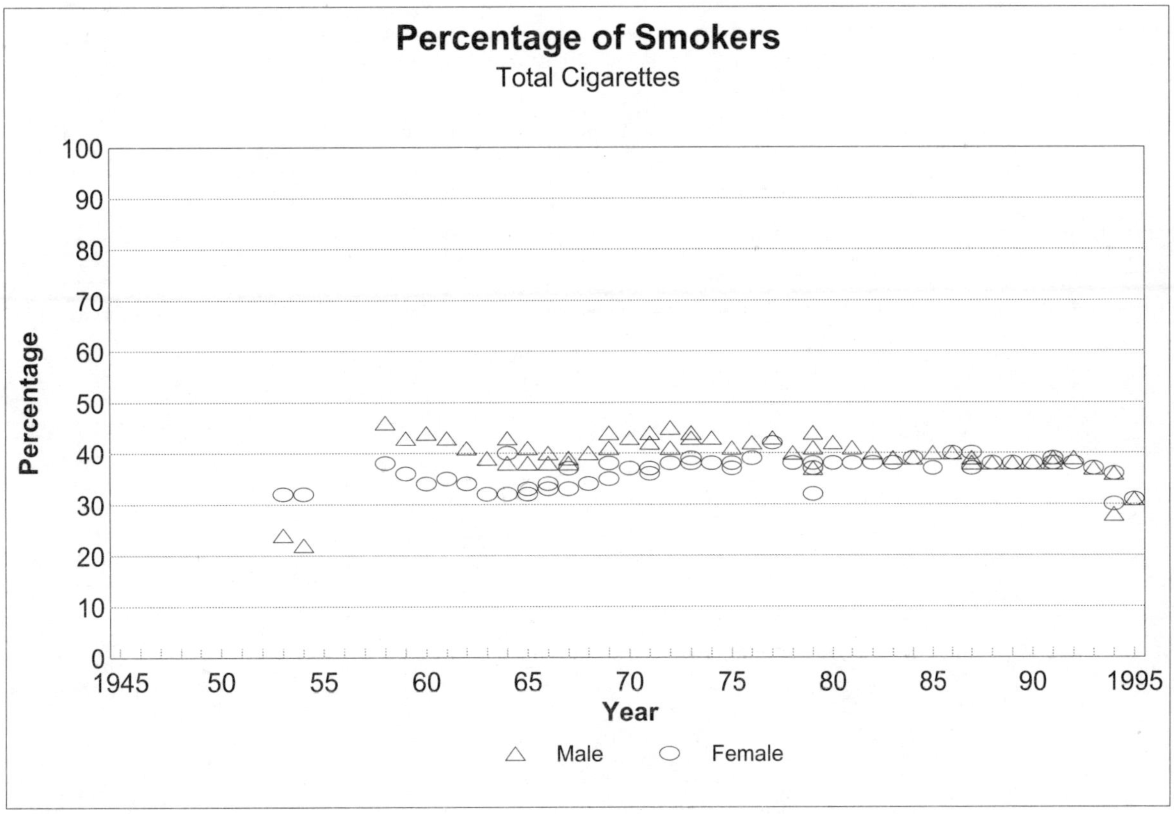

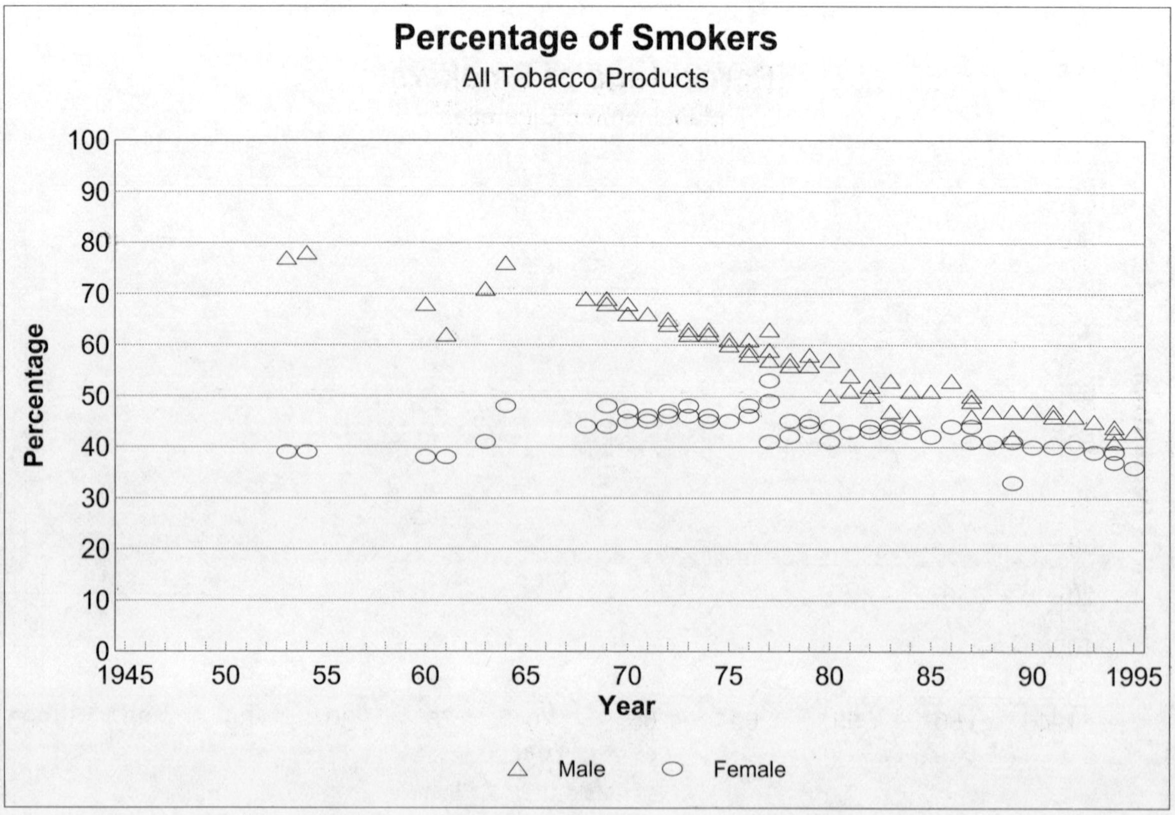
Percentage of Smokers
All Tobacco Products
Percentage
100
90
80
70
60
50
40
30
20
10
0
1945
50
55
60
65
70
75
80
85
90
1995
Year
Male
Female

Figure 7.4 Estimated number of (i) manufactured cigarettes and (ii) total cigarettes smoked per person per day, sales-adjusted, 1953-1995.
Males and females aged 15 years and over. *Source:* see Table 7.8

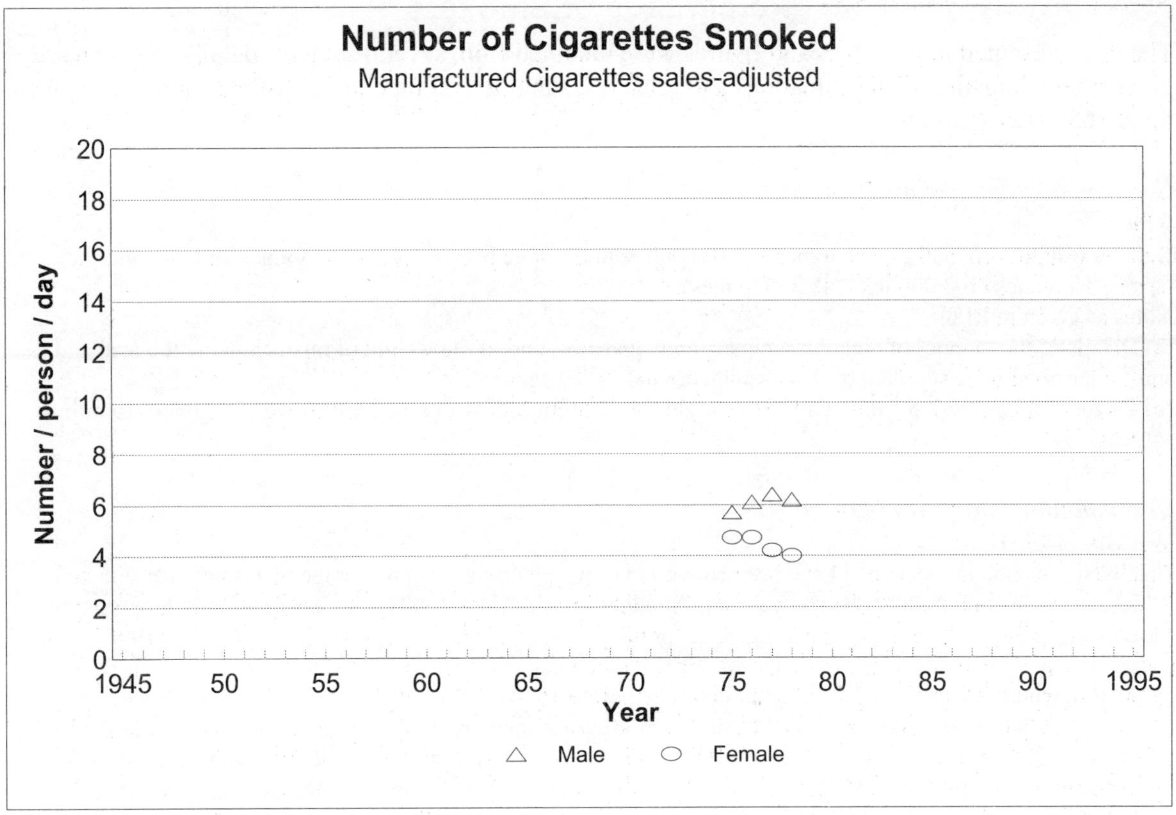

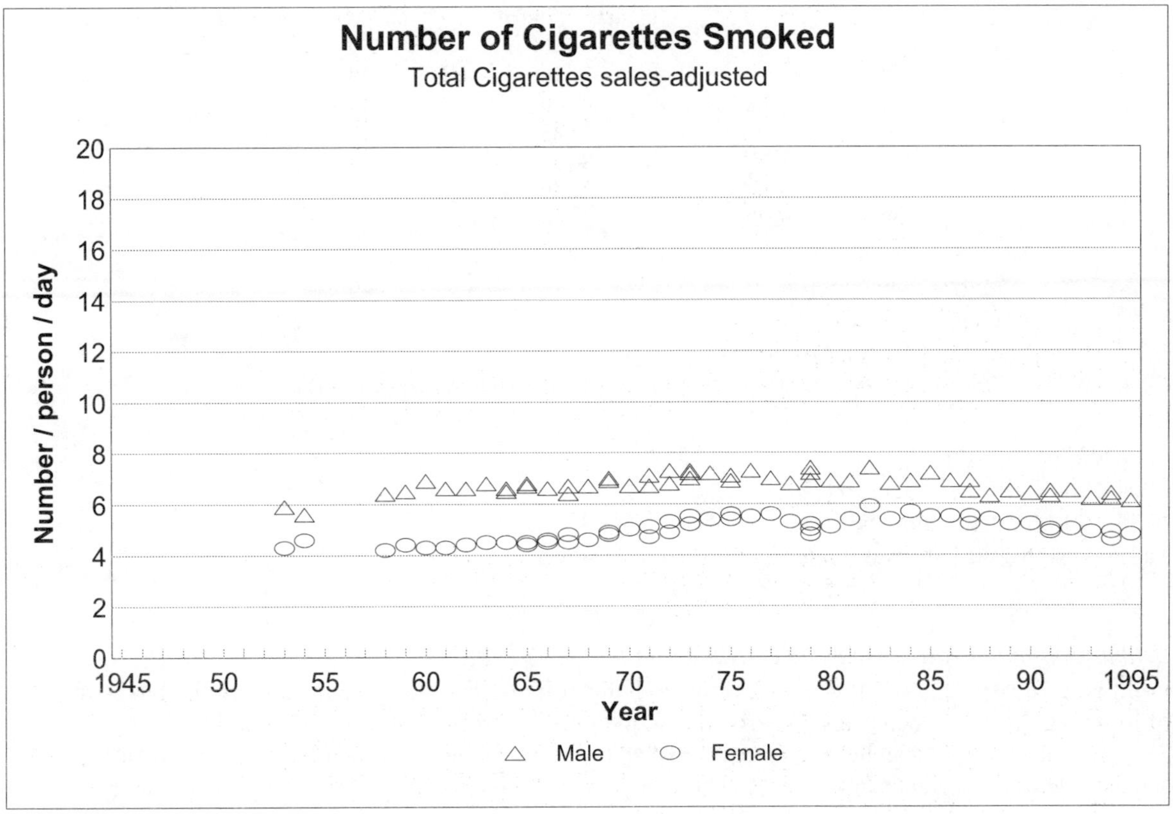

Notes on sources of sales data

The data presented in the tables and figures were obtained from several sources, details of which are given below, together with estimations and related assumptions. Full citations of the sources are given on p. 165 under *References*.

Consumption data before 1974

RP6

Data by weight, originally given to nearest 100 000 pounds, have been converted to tonnes and given to the nearest 10 tonnes (100 000 lbs = 45.359 tonnes).

Notes as given in RP6:

(a) Details of the number of cigarettes, cigars, and cigarillos, and of the weight of pipe, chewing tobacco and snuff consumed were supplied by Tobaksindustrien, Copenhagen.

(b) Factors for conversion from number to weight for cigarettes, cigars and cigarillos were obtained from trade sources.

Consumption data for 1974 onwards

Wicklin (1998)

Data were given in numbers and have been converted to weight assuming an average of 1 g per cigarette and 3.15 g per cigar or cigarillo (based on values in Sundhedsministeriet (1998)). This assumption is supported by Mørck *et al* (1982) which uses 1 g per cigarette for the period 1970-80 but conflicts with Wicklin (1998) which uses 0.65 g per cigarette and 2 g per cigar for all Scandinavian countries (the conventional conversion rates used by WHO), whereas RP6 used 1.2-1.3 g per cigarette before 1974.

The data report taxed sales and exclude cross-border sales. According to Egsmose and Egsmose (1988), a further 10-20% of tobacco is purchased by Danes in tax-free areas. Merzdorf *et al* (1982) and United States Department of Agriculture (USDA) Economic Research Service (1996) provide manufactured cigarette sales data based on production plus imports minus exports. These differ from taxed sales data as follows (selected years):

Year	Taxed sales	Production + imports - exports	Difference (% of taxed sales)
1966	5 566	6 710	20
1970	6 357	7 520	18
1975	7 295	8 640	18
1980	7 151	7 983	12
1985	7 787	8 781	13
1990	6 584	8 049	22
1995	6 429	8 360	30

Plain/Filter cigarette consumption

1960-1981 Maxwell (successive years)

1982-1984 Prener and Jensen (1985)

Cigarette production in Denmark reached 90% filter during the 1990s (USDA (1997)).

Tar yield of cigarettes

1964-1984 Prener and Jensen (1985)

1985-1990 Industry sources

The tar yield per cigarette was limited by EC directive (Directive 90/239/EEC) to 15 mg by the end of 1992, and to 12 mg by the end of 1997 (Harkin *et al* (1997)).

Estimates of hand-rolled cigarette consumption for 1920-1995

Following Merzdorf *et al* (1982) we estimated hand-rolled cigarette consumption on the basis of 80% of loose smoking tobacco sales. We assume an average of 1 g per hand-rolled cigarette.

This gives hand-rolled cigarettes as a proportion of all cigarettes falling from about 30% in 1960 to 16% in 1978 and then increasing again to 26% by 1990. This assumption is supported by USDA Economic Research Service

(1996) which gives separate pipe tobacco and rolling tobacco production figures for 1993-1995, and by WHO (1997) which estimated that roll-your-own cigarettes accounted for 20-25% of total cigarette consumption during the early 1990s. However it conflicts with Mørck *et al* (1982): 'Owing to the tax position, the part played by hand-rolled cigarettes is very small (4-5%). During the last few years, however, this has tended to increase'. It is not clear whether this means that 4-5% of tobacco is used for hand-rolled cigarettes, or that 4-5% of cigarettes are hand-rolled.

Notes on sources of survey data

Each source of survey data—either an individual survey or a series of surveys repeated over a number of years—is cited by a source number. This number is shown in the tables and corresponds to the source numbers given below, where details of the source publication and of the survey methodology are given. Full citations of the sources are given on p. 165 under *References*.

Source number

1 OBSERVA Association and Merzdorf *et al* (1982), quoting OBSERVA

a. Sample size (1976) 1 314, (1980) 1 319, and (1984) 1 252
b. It is unclear whether data relate to age 18+ or age 20+. Figure given in *All ages* column in Table 7.4 for 1960 is for age 20+
c. Assumed extension to age distribution for percentage smokers, age 15-17: males (1976-1978) 25%, (1980-1984) 20%; females 25%. Age 15-19: males (all products to 1974) 40%, (cigarettes) 25%; females (all products to 1979) 20%, (cigarettes to 1979) 20%, (cigarettes 1980) 25%

2 Nielsen *et al* (1978), (1988), Osler (1992a), Nielsen and Sørensen (1995), Joossens *et al* (1994), Wicklin (1998), Statistika Centralbyrån (1995)

a. Annual consumer survey by Gallup Markedsanalyse. Sample size about 20 000
b. Smokers: smoked 'yesterday'
c. Some percentages of cigarette smokers taken from charts
d. Consumption category estimation based on two categories, 1-14 and 15+ cigarettes/smoker/day, and resulting figures should be regarded with caution. There is a discrepancy in the data for 1973, data from Osler (1992a) (used here) give higher estimates than data from Nielsen *et al* (1978) (all ages only)

3 Le Meitour-Kaplan (1977), quoting Nordic Research Association (1973)

a. Survey conducted November-December 1973 in four Nordic countries. Total sample size 6 000. Age group not stated. (See also Norway source 3, Sweden source 4, and Finland source 8)
b. Smokers: smoked 'yesterday'

4 WHO MONICA Project (1988), WHO (1989)

a. Regional survey forming part of WHO MONICA Project:

Region	Population size	Sample size	Participation rate (%)	Sample used*		Date
				Males	Females	
Glostrup	132 000	3 563	79	1 940	1 845	Nov 1982-Feb 1984

* 'Sample used' includes age 25-34; all other figures are for age 35-64 only

b. *All ages* column relates only to age 35-64 and is standardized to world population
c. Regular cigarette smokers: smoked cigarettes daily. All smokers: smoked cigarettes daily or occasionally, or 1 g pipe tobacco or 1 cigar per week. Cigarettes per smoker refers to regular and occasional cigarette smokers
d. Calculation for cigarettes per person based on % regular cigarette smokers and cigarettes per regular or occasional cigarette smoker, so may underestimate

5 Lidegaard (1984)

a. Representative sample of 788 women

b. Data taken from diagram

c. Consumption category estimation based on two categories, 1-10 and 11+ cigarettes/smoker/day, and resulting figures should be regarded with caution

6 Hamtoft and Lindhardt (1955), Osler (1992b)

a. The Danish National Morbidity Survey of 1950, smoking sections conducted August 1952-April 1953 and January-April 1954. Participation rate 83%.

	Sample size	
	Males	Females
1952-1953	11 492	11 800
1954	5 453	5 273

b. Consumption category estimation based on <5 (assume 1-5), 6-15, 16-25, and 26+ cigarettes/smoker/day. Comparable results given directly for the two periods combined were lower (males 11.7, females 5.6)

7 Roed-Petersen (1984)

a. Representative sample in eastern Denmark (Seeland, Lolland-Falster, and Bornholm) in October 1979. Sample size 1 651 (out of intended sample of 2 308, 72%)

b. Smokers: smoked daily during past 3 months

c. Consumption category estimation based on two categories, 1-14 and 15+ cigarettes/smoker/day, and resulting figures should be regarded with caution

d. Assumed extension to age distribution for percentage smokers, age 15: males and females 20%. Number of cigarettes/person/day 1.0

8 Agner and Mørck (date unknown), Hagerup and Larsen (1971), Hagerup *et al* (1981), Schroll (1980)

a. Population studies in Glostrup, studying persons born in specific single years.

Year of examination	Type of examination	Birth year	Number examined	Response rate (%)
1964	Cross-sectional	1914	802	82
1967	Cross-sectional	1897	440	69
1974	Follow-up	1914	666	75
1976	Cross-sectional	1936	1 052	88
1977	Follow-up	1897	246	68

b. Consumption in grams of tobacco (estimated by 1 cigarette = 1 g, 1 cheroot = 3 g, and 1 cigar = 5 g). First results presented in Table 7.5 for 1967 and 1974 are consumption of tobacco per cigarette smoker (including mixed smokers), second results (and results for 1964) are consumption of tobacco per smoker. Only results based on all smokers are included in Table 7.6

c. Consumption category estimation based on 1-14, 15-24, 25+ g/smoker per day

9 Ibsen (1982), Osler (1992a) quoting Lambert *et al* (1961)

a. Nationwide interview survey of 11-14-year-olds. Sample size 3 109

b. Some data taken from graph

10 Todd (1986)

a. Estimated by Todd from available data

11 Nielsen and Krarup (1976)

a. Sample size (males) 5 550, (females) 5 666

b. Consumption category estimation based on 1-7, 8-14, 15-19, and 20+ cigarettes/smoker/day

12 Merzdorf *et al* (1982), quoting tobacco industry

a. Presumably in same series as source 1

13 Ibsen (1982), Holstein *et al* (1990) quoting Ibsen (1981)

a. Stratified sample of 39 schools, representative of all schools in Denmark. Age 9-16. Self-completion questionnaire in class. Sample size 9 158
b. Some data taken from graph
c. 60% of smokers (sexes combined) smoked every day, 95% smoked cigarettes, and 6% smoked more than 10 cigarettes per day

14 Bonnevie (1964)

a. National survey carried out by Elmark & Lorenz Christensen Marketing A/S for *Politiken*. Sample size 1 500
b. Consumption category estimation based on 1-3, 4-8, 9-14, 15-20, 21+ cigarettes/smoker/day

15 Holstein *et al* (1990), Osler (1992a) quoting Vilstrup (1973)

a. Nationwide interview survey of 9-15-year-olds. Sample size 495

16 Appleyard (1987)

a. Baseline of Copenhagen City Heart Study, March 1976-March 1978. Representative sample drawn from 10 administrative wards in Copenhagen. Subjects were invited to health screening and completed a self-administered questionnaire before physical examination. Sample size 14 223, response rate 74%
b. Consumption category estimation based on 1-4, 5-9 10-19 20-29, 30+ grams/smoker/day
c. Assumed extension to age distribution for percentage smokers, age 15-19: males and females 30%. Number of cigarettes/person/day: 3.5

17 Ibsen (1986), Holstein *et al* (1990)

a. Questionnaire survey from a representative sample of Danish schools. Sample size 4 500

18 Osler (1992a, 1992b), Kjøller *et al* (1995) quoting Rasmussen *et al* (1988)

a. Representative nationwide surveys conducted by the Danish Institute for Clinical Epidemiology. Personal interviews at home.

	Date	Sample size		Participation
		Males	Females	rate (%)
1987	Sep 1986-Jun 1987	2 320	2 433	80
1991	Sep 1990-May 1991	1 545	1 659	81
1994	—	2 237	2 431	—

b. Consumption category estimation for 1987 and 1990 based on two categories, 1-14 and 15+ cigarettes/smoker/day, and resulting figures should be regarded with caution. For 1994, based on three categories, 1-4, 5-14 and 15+ cigarettes/smoker/day

19 Hansen and Osler (1990)

a. Survey at 9 elementary schools in the Municipality of Freceriksberg. Approximate ages corresponding to 6th and 8th grades. Sample size (boys grade 6) 162, (boys grade 8) 177, (girls grade 6) 149, (girls grade 8) 186
b. Regular smokers: smoked daily. All smokers: smoked daily or occasionally. Smokers marked as frequency *: smoked daily, occasionally or rarely
c. Assumed extension to age distribution, 1994 only, for percentage smokers, age 15: males and females (cigarettes, and all products regularly) 20%, (all smokers) 25%. Number of cigarettes/person/day 1.0

20 Osler *et al* (1992), (1992a)

a. Questionnaire survey in County Vejle about knowledge and behaviour in relation to cardiovascular risk factors. Sample size (males) 1 330, (females) 1 561
b. There is some discrepancy in the age groups shown by the two sources
c. Consumption category estimation based on two categories, 1-14 and 15+ grams/smoker/day, and resulting figures should be regarded with caution
d. Assumed extension to age distribution ofr percentage smokers, age 15-19: males and females 25%. For age 65+: males 45%, females 30%

21 Due and Holstein (1997) quoting Schmidt (1992), and Osler (1992a) quoting Schmidt

22 van Reek *et al* (1992), van Reek and Adriaanse (1995)

a. A series of surveys of Young Europeans. About 800 children aged 11-15 years interviewed in each EC country except Luxembourg (where only 250 interviewed). Lowest age group 11-12. Interviews conducted at home, with parents absent

b. Regular smokers: smoked daily. All smokers: smoked at least once a week

23 Osler (1992a) quoting Due and Holstein (1991)

a. Danish Longitudinal Health Behaviour Study. Sample size 2 858 at ages 15, 25, 50, 60, 70

b. Regular smokers: smokes daily. All smokers: smokes daily or occasionally

c. Consumption category estimation based on two categories, 1-14 and 15+ grams/smoker/day, and resulting figures should be regarded with caution

24 Ito *et al* (1987), Holstein *et al* (1990), King *et al* (1996), Due and Holstein (1997)

a. Part of the HBSC (Health Behaviour in School-Aged Children) Study, a collaborative cross-national research study sponsored by the WHO. School classes or schools were randomly selected, targeting age groups 11 (not presented here), 13 and 15

Year	Target age 13			Target age 15		
	Sample size		Mean	Sample size		Mean
	Boys	Girls	age	Boys	Girls	age
1985 (Dec 84-Feb 85)	131	114	—	96	99	—
1988	286	288	—	266	301	—
1991	333	310	—	296	333	—
1994	697	717	13.6	696	662	15.6

b. Smokers marked as frequency *: smoked daily. Regular smokers: smoke once a week or more

25 Hibell *et al* (1997)

a. Nationally representative survey forming part of ESPAD (European School Survey Project on Alcohol and Other Drugs). Target was pupils born in 1979, thus age 15-16 at time of survey in March/April 1995. Approximately 95% of this group still in school. Anonymous questionnaire completed and sealed in envelope by pupil, in class. Teachers present, but discouraged from walking round the classroom. Sample size (males) 1 189, (females) 1 250. Response rate (males) 90%, (females) 91%

b. Regular smokers: smoked 1 or more cigarettes per day in last 30 days. All smokers: smoked in last 30 days

c. Consumption category estimation based on 1-5, 6-10, 11-20, 21+ cigarettes/smoker/day

26 Nygaard *et al* (1990)

a. Anonymous questionnaire survey carried out in 1988-1989 in County Roskilde. Approximate ages corresponding to school grades 7 and 9. Sample size 4 044

b. Data taken from diagram

c. Regular smokers: smoked daily. All smokers: smoked daily or only at parties

References

Agner E. and Mørck H. (date unknown). *Smoking and health in old age. Implications for health, evaluated from mortality, incidence of cardiovascular disease and change in pulmonary function in a ten-year follow-up survey*. Glostrup Hospital, University of Copenhagen, Glostrup, Denmark.

Appleyard M. (ed) (1987). The Copenhagen city heart study. A book of tables with data from the first examination (1976-78) and a 5-year follow-up (1981-83). *Scand.J.Soc.Med.,* **(Suppl 41)**, 1-160. Almqvist & Wiksell Periodical Co, Stockholm.

Beese D.H. (ed) (1968). *Tobacco consumption in various countries,* 2nd edition. Tobacco Research Council, London. Research Paper 6.

Beese D.H. (ed) (1972). *Tobacco consumption in various countries,* 3rd edition. Tobacco Research Council, London. Research Paper 6.

Bonnevie P. (1964). Befolkningens rygevaner. (Smoking habits of the Danish population). *Ugeskr Laeger,* **126**, 1433-5.

Due E.P. and Holstein B.E. (1997). Rygevaner blandt 11-15-årige, 1984-1994. (Smoking habits among 11-15-year-old adolescents, 1984-1994). *Ugeskr Laeger,* **159**, 1090-3.

Due P. and Holstein B.E. (1991). *Rygevaner i den danske befolkning—et sundhedssociologisk perspektiv.* Københavns Universitet: Institut for Social Medicin, Copenhagen.§

Egsmose T. and Egsmose L. (1988). Obstacles to a national smoking control programme. In: Aoki M., Hisamichi S. and Tominaga S. (eds) *Smoking and health 1987. Proceedings of the 6th World Conference on Smoking and Health, Tokyo, 9-12 November 1987.* Elsevier Science Publishers B.V. (Biomedical Division), Amsterdam; 417-9. International Congress Series No. 780.

Hagerup L. and Larsen M. (1971). Tobaksrygning og respiratoriske symptomer i en dansk population. (Tobacco smoking and respiratory symptoms in a Danish population). *Ugeskr Laeger,* **133**, 1302-6.

Hagerup L., Eriksen M., Schroll M., Hollnagel H., Agner E. and Larsen S. (eds) (1981). The Glostrup population studies. Collection of epidemiological tables. Reference values for use in cardiovascular population studies. *Scand.J.Soc.Med.,* **(Suppl 20)**, 1-112. Almqvist & Wiksell Periodical Co, Stockholm.

Hamtoft H. and Lindhardt M. (1955). Tobacco consumption in Denmark. I. The Danish national morbidity survey of 1950, communication no. 8. *Dan Med Bull,* **2**, 213-20.

Hansen E.T. and Osler M. (1990). Tobaks- og alkoholvaner blandt skolebørn i Frederiksberg Kommune. (Tobacco and alcohol drinking habits in school pupils in the municipality of Frederiksberg). *Ugeskr Laeger,* **152**, 3531-5.

Harkin A.M., Anderson P. and Goos C. (1997). *Smoking, drinking and drug taking in the European Region.* Alcohol, Drugs and Tobacco Programme, WHO Regional Office for Europe, Copenhagen.

Hibell B., Andersson B., Bjarnason T., Kokkevi A., Morgan M. and Narusk A. (1997). *The 1995 ESPAD report. The European school survey project on alcohol and other drugs. Alcohol and other drug use among students in 26 European countries.* The Swedish Council for Information on Alcohol and Other Drugs. Council of Europe (Pompidou Group).

Holstein B.E., Ito H. and Due P. (1990). Rygevaner blandt 11-15 årige i 1988. (Smoking among children aged 11-15 years in Denmark in 1988). *Ugeskr Laeger,* **152**, 2651-4.

Ibsen K.K. (1981). *Rygning blandt skoleelever—en landsdækkende undersøgelse af 9.000 skolebørns rygevaner.* Københavns Universitet, Institut for Social Medicin, Københavns.§

Ibsen K.K. (1982). Smoking habits in 9000 Danish schoolchildren. *Acta Paediatrica Scandinavica,* **71**, 131-4.

Ibsen K.K. (1986). Rygning og holdning dertil blandt danske skolebørn i 1985 (Smoking and attitudes to smoking among Danish schoolchildren in 1985). *Ugeskr Laeger,* **148**, 2714-5.

Ito H., Holstein B.E. and Ibsen K.K. (1987). Skoleelevers rygevaner og -holdninger i sociologisk belysning. (Schoolchildren's smoking behaviour and attitude. A sociological perspective). *Ugeskr Laeger,* **149**, 396-400.

Joossens L., Naett C., Howie C. and Muldoon A. (1994). *Tobacco and health in the European Union. An overview.* European Bureau for Action on Smoking Prevention (BASP), Brussels.

King A., Wold B., Tudor-Smith C. and Harel Y. (1996). *The health of youth, a cross-national survey.* WHO Regional Publications, Europe, Copenhagen. European Series No. 69.

Kjøller M., Rasmussen N.K., Keiding L., Petersen H.C. and Nielsen G.A. (1995). *Sundhed og sygelighed i Danmark 1994 og udviklingen siden 1987. (Health and disease in Denmark 1994 and changes since 1987).* DIKE, Copenhagen.

Lambert F., Leunbach G. and Knudsen R. (1961). *Skolebørns rygevaner.* Landsforeningen til Kræftens Bekæmpelse, Copenhagen.[§]

Le Meitour-Kaplan A. (1977). Situational Analysis: Profile of women's smoking habits in Continental Western Europe. In: Steinfeld J., Griffiths W., Ball K. and Taylor R.M. (eds) *Health consequences, education, cessation activities, and social action, Volume II. Proceedings of the Third World Conference on Smoking and Health, New York City, June 2-5, 1975.* US Department of Health, Education and Welfare, USA; 309-27. DHEW Publication No (NIH) 77-1413.

Lee P.N. (ed) (1975). *Tobacco consumption in various countries,* 4th edition. Tobacco Research Council, London. Research Paper 6.

Lidegaard O. (1984). Rygevaner blant 15-45 årige kvinder i 1983. (Smoking habits among women aged 15-45 years in 1983). *Ugeskr Laeger,* **146**, 3058-60.

Maxwell J.C.Jr. (successive years). How the brands ranked. Maxwell International Estimates. *World Tobacco.*

Merzdorf J., Reuter U. and Welsch G. (1982). *Daten und Fakten zur Entwicklung des Rauchens in Mitgliedsländern der Europäischen Gemeinschaften (Facts and figures on the development of smoking in the member states of the European Communities).* Kommission der Europäischen Gemeinschaften, Luxemburg. Medizin—EUR 7907 DE.

Mørck H.I., Linde J., Agner E., Hein H.O., Gyntelberg F. and Nielsen P.E. (1982). Tobaksforbrug og rygevaner i Norden 1920-1980. (Tobacco consumption and smoking habits in the Nordic countries). *Nord Med,* **97**, 134-46.

Nielsen P.E. and Krarup N.B. (1976). Tobaksfobruget i Danmark 1920-1975. (Consumption of tobacco in Denmark in the period 1920-1975). *Ugeskr Laeger,* **138**, 2511-6.

Nielsen P.E., Krarup N.B., Astrup J., Gyntelberg F. and Lisse O. (1978). Ændring i danskernes rygevaner 1958-1976. (Alterations in Danish smoking habits 1958-1976). *Ugeskr Laeger,* **140**, 2528-32.

Nielsen P.E. and Sørensen J.F. (1995). Danskernes rygevaner 1988-1993: en opfølgning af tidligere befolkningsundersøgelser (Changes in smoking habits in the Danish population 1988-1993). *Ugeskr Laeger,* **157**, 3451-6.

Nielsen P.E., Zacho J., Olsen J.A. and Olsen C.A. (1988). Ændringer i danskernes rygevaner 1970-1987. (Alteration in the Danes' smoking habits in the period 1970-1987). *Ugeskr Laeger,* **150**, 2229-33.

Nordic Research Association (1973). *1973 Survey. Antalet rökare i fyra nordiska länder i november-december 1973.*

Nygaard B., Barfod A.B.L., Hansen F.H., Jessen T.T., Kryger H. and Meyer L. (1990). Tobak, hash—viden og vaner i skolen. (Tobacco, hash—knowledge and habits in Danish schools). *Ugeskr Laeger,* **152**, 3540-1.

Osler M. (1992a). *Danskernes rygevaner*. Hjerteforeningen, Kræftens Bekæmpelse, Tobaksskaderådet & DIKE, Copenhagen.

Osler M. (1992b). Smoking habits in Denmark from 1953 to 1991: a comparative analysis of results from three nationwide health surveys among adult Danes in 1953-1954, 1986-87 and 1990-1991. *Int J Epidemiol,* **21**, 862-71.

Osler M., Rasmussen N.K. and Lous J. (1992). Voksnes rygevaner—holdning og adfærd i relation til forebyggelse af hjerte-kar-sygdomme. (Smoking habits among adults—attitude and behavior in relation to prevention of cardivascular diseases). *Ugeskr Laeger,* **154**, 543-8.

Prener A. and Jensen O.M. (1985). Lungecancer og cigarettjære i Danmark. (Cancer of the lung and cigarette tar in Denmark). *Ugeskr Laeger,* **147**, 4221-7.

Rasmussen N.K., Groth M., Bredkjær S., Madsen M. and Kamper-Jørgensen F. (1988). *Sundhed og sygelighed i Danmark 1987*. DIKE; 138-42.§

Roed-Petersen B. (1984). Smoking habits in East Denmark at October 1979. *Scand J Soc Med,* **12**, 39-47.

RP6, See Beese (ed) (1968), Beese (ed) (1972), Lee (ed) (1975)

Schmidt D. *Sundhedsstyrelsen. Foreløbig analyse på Sundhedsstyrelsens rusmiddelundersøgelse blandt unge* [Personal communication to Osler M.]§

Schmidt D. (1992). *Unge og rusmidler*. Sundhedsstyrelsen, København.§

Schroll M. (1980). Smoking habits in the Glostrup population of men and women, born in 1914. *Acta Medica Scandinavica,* **208**, 245-56.

Statistika Centralbyrån (1995). *Tobacco consumption 1970-1994 in the member states of the European Union and in Norway and Iceland.* European Commission.

Sundhedsministeriet (1998). *Tobaks- og alkoholforbrug (tobacco and alcohol consumption).* Sundhedsministeriet, Denmark. http://www.sum.dk/cgi-bin/whole doc.cgi/publika/sumital/side37.htm.

Todd G. (1986). *Medicine. Statistics of smoking in the Member States of the European Community*. Commission of the European Communities, Luxembourg.

USDA Economic Research Service (1996). *Tobacco statistics*. Albert R. Mann Library, Cornell University, Ithaca, New York. ERS 94012. (With supplementary material from Tobacco Annual Reports.). http://usda.mannlib.cornell.edu/data-sets/specialty/94012.

USDA (1997). *Tobacco annual report*. USDA/FAS, Washington D.C. AGR Number EZ5016. http://www.fas.usda.gov/scriptsg/gain_display report.exe?Rep_ID=10001496.

van Reek J. and Adriaanse H. (1995). Daily smoking among adolescents in the European Community. *Rev Epidemiol Sante Publique,* **43**, 281-2.

van Reek J., Adriaanse H. and Karaoglou A. (1992). Smoking among children in the European Community. *J Public Health Med,* **14**, 93-4.

Vilstrup K. (1973). Skolebørn og tobak. En undersøgelse af vaner og holdninger blandt 8-16 årige. *Ejnar og Meta Thorsens fond,* 77-83.§

WHO (1989). The WHO MONICA project: a worldwide monitoring system for cardiovascular diseases. In:

World health statistics annual 1989. WHO, Geneva; 25-149.

WHO MONICA Project (1988). Geographical variation in the major risk factors of coronary heart disease in men and women aged 35-64 years. *World Health Stat Q,* **41**, 115-40.

WHO (1997). *Tobacco or health: A global status report*. WHO, Geneva. www.cdc.gov/nccdphp/osh/who/whoampro.htm.

Wicklin B. (ed) (1998). *Tobaksstatistik 1970-1997. Konsumtion av tobaksvaror, priser, inkomster, rökvanor, handel och illegala tillförseln mm i Sverige, Norge, Danmark och Finland (Tobacco statistics 1970-1997. Consumption of tobacco products prices income, smoking habits, trade and attempted smuggling etc. in Sweden, Norway, Denmark and Finland)*. Svenska tobaksbranschföreninger, Örebro, Sweden.

§ Original paper not obtained, but information taken as quoted by another author

Finland 8

Sales data

See Tables 8.1-8.3.

Finland was one of the first countries to adopt manufactured cigarette smoking; production started there in 1859. By the beginning of the 1880s, annual production had reached 100 million cigarettes, and in 1901 this had risen to nearly 500 million cigarettes (Pedersen *et al* (1969) quoting Pernu (1960)). Before the end of the 19th century tobacco was often home grown and smoked in pipes. At the turn of the century hand-rolled cigarettes, snuff, pipes and cigars were all still popular but use of Russian-type manufactured cigarettes, *pilli*, increased rapidly in the 1920s (Karvonen *et al* (1993)). In the 1930s, they accounted for 60% of cigarette consumption (Hutson (1937)). Half the length of this cigarette is filled with tobacco, and the other half is an open mouth-piece made of thin cardboard. On average the *pilli* contains 0.5 g of tobacco and this is usually completely smoked. Until about 1940 a wooden mouth-piece was provided with each pack of manufactured cigarettes of the conventional type (*pölli*) and even this type of cigarette was usually smoked down to a very small butt. By the early 1960s, hand-rolling of cigarettes was very uncommon (Pedersen *et al* (1969)). In the 1950s American-type filter cigarettes became associated with modern life and Russian-type cigarettes gradually lost their popularity (Karvonen *et al* (1993)).

Since 1935, 80-90% of tobacco has been consumed as manufactured cigarettes. Since 1973, pipe and cigarette tobacco accounts for most of the remainder, with consumption of cigars, snuff and chewing tobacco quite low. The same pattern may have been true between 1935 and 1973, although the combinations of categories for which data are available makes this less clear.

From 1920 until 1944 consumption of manufactured cigarettes per adult varied between 3 and 4.5 cigarettes per day. It dipped briefly at the end of the Second World War to 2 cigarettes, after which it increased again to vary between 4.5 and 6 cigarettes from 1950 to 1992. Between 1993 and 1995 it fell below 4 cigarettes per day.

The consumption of all tobacco products combined per adult followed a similar pattern, although the post-war increase was more marked, reaching a peak of about 6.5 g per day in the early 1970s; this was partly due to the increasing average weight of a cigarette. The apparent fall in the estimated consumption in 1974 is an artefact caused by a discrepancy between two sources in the assumed average weight of a cigarette, and estimates before and after this date cannot be compared directly.

Survey data

See Tables 8.4-8.8

Although many early surveys did not specify which tobacco products were covered, the difference between the prevalence of cigarette smoking and tobacco smoking has been small (about 4% in men and 1% in women) because manufactured cigarettes have consistently been the major category. In the early 1960s, the prevalence of regular smoking among those aged 15 years and over was nearly 60% in men and 12-14% in women. The difference in prevalence between men and women has decreased since then. The prevalence among men has decreased steadily, falling below 30% in the mid 1990s, while among women it has remained relatively constant, varying between 15-20%. A further 5-8% of both men and women are occasional smokers.

Some data on adult smoking by age have been available from various non-representative sources since 1962 and from a national source since 1978 (source 6). Among men, the prevalence of smoking has fallen at all ages, while for women, there has been some decrease at age 25-34 in the 1990s but an increase among those aged 35-54. Teenage smoking has been surveyed regularly since 1973 (source 9). Among boys and girls, the prevalence of smoking was similar in 1973, and decreased during the 1970s. Since 1980, the prevalence has changed little, with more boys than girls smoking, notably at age 18.

Comparisons with sales data suggest that surveys of the number of cigarettes smoked under-reported consumption by 20-35% between 1975-1986, but comparisons of surveys of 'daily frequency of smoking' with sales of manufactured cigarettes suggest that under-reporting has decreased since 1985. Between 1967 and 1995, the estimated number of cigarettes smoked per person per day (sales-adjusted) decreased for men from about 9 to 5. For women it remained around 2-3 in the same period.

Table 8.1.1 Total annual sales of tobacco products, 1920-1973

Year	Cigarettes						Cigars and cigarillos[1]		Smoking and chewing tobacco	Snuff	All tobacco products
	Russian style		Other		Total						
	tonnes	millions	tonnes	millions	tonnes	millions	tonnes	millions	tonnes	tonnes	tonnes
1920					1910	2781	90	21	540	50	2590
1921					1450	2132	90	17	320	50	1910
1922					1590	2337	90	18	320	90	2090
1923					1950	2835	140	25	540	90	2720
1924					2040	3002	90	19	640	90	2860
1925					2090	3035	90	19	500	90	2770
1926					2040	3024	90	21	500	90	2720
1927					2310	3423	90	21	450	90	2950
1928					2450	3616	90	21	450	90	3080
1929					2540	3721	90	22	500	90	3220
1930					2680	3913	90	14	500	90	3360
1931					2220	3104	50	8	450	90	2810
1932					2130	2960	50	9	450	50	2680
1933					2270	3037	50	10	410	50	2770
1934					2630	3322	50	11	360	50	3080
1935					2770	3497	50	12	360	50	3220
1936					2810	3616	90	16	410	90	3400
1937					3220	3989	90	19	410	90	3810
1938					3490	4488	90	22	360	90	4040
1939					3310	3963	90	19	450	90	3950
1940					3040	3780	90	15	450	50	3630
1941	950	2080	2680	2393	3630	4473	50	12	450	50	4170
1942	1040	2316	1540	1305	2590	3621	50	7	230	50	2900
1943	1130	2565	1090	1059	2220	3624	50	7	230	50	2540
1944	1090	2414	540	511	1630	2925	50	6	140	50	1860
1945	820	1866	320	274	1130	2140	50	5	180	0	1360
1946	950	2094	950	792	1910	2886	50	5	320	50	2310
1947	1000	2222	1720	1386	2720	3608	50	6	450	50	3270
1948	1000	2220	2490	2038	3490	4258	50	7	590	50	4170
1949	860	1886	2720	2440	3580	4326	50	9	680	50	4350

Table 8.1.1 *(continued)*

Year	Cigarettes						Cigars and cigarillos[1]		Smoking and chewing tobacco tonnes	Snuff tonnes	All tobacco products tonnes
	Russian style		Other		Total						
	tonnes	millions	tonnes	millions	tonnes	millions	tonnes	millions			
1950	950	2104	2680	2476	3630	4580	50	10	820	50	4540
1951	950	2104	2950	2562	3900	4666	50	12	680	50	4670
1952	1040	2331	3310	2856	4350	5187	50	13	590	50	5030
1953	1040	2320	3220	2845	4260	5165	50	12	500	50	4850
1954	1180	2612	3450	2949	4630	5561	50	12	500	50	5220
1955	1180	2668	3490	3036	4670	5704	50	13	410	50	5170
1956	1180	2653	3670	3215	4850	5868	50	9	360	50	5310
1957	950	2135	3950	3410	4900	5545	50	9	590	50	5580
1958	860	1912	3270	3329	4130	5241	50	9	730	0	4900
1959	820	1863	3860	3975	4670	5838	50	10	590	0	5310
1960	770	1723	4220	4564	4990	6287	50	16	500	0	5530
1961	640	1467	4990	5154	5620	6621	50	15	360	0	6030
1962	590	1352	5030	5349	5620	6701	50	18	500	0	6170
1963	590	1393	5810	5838	6400	7231	90	22	640	50	7170
1964	410	950	4580	4596	4990	5546	90	31	950	50	6080
1965	410	920	5580	5597	5990	6517	90	37	820	50	6940
1966	320	750	5620	5633	5940	6383	180	85	820	50	6990
1967	270	629	6030	6055	6300	6684	140	73	950	50	7440
1968	230	482	5850	5866	6080	6348	140	72	1180	50	7440
1969	180	428	6120	6107	6300	6535	180	97	1180	50	7710
1970	140	350	6120	6130	6260	6480	270	190	1000	50	7570
1971	140	300	6670	6700	6800	7000	230	140	1040	0	8070
1972	140	280	7300	7300	7440	7580	230	120	1040	0	8710
1973	140	240	7080	7100	7210	7340	230	140	1000	0	8440

1 Cigarillos included from 1941-1973

Source: see *Notes on sources of sales data*, p. 193

Table 8.1.2 Total annual sales of tobacco products, 1974-1995

Year	Cigarettes		Cigars		Pipe and cigarette tobacco tonnes	Snuff and chewing tobacco tonnes	All tobacco products tonnes
	tonnes	millions	tonnes	millions			
1974	5193	7989	266	133	968	26	6453
1975	5291	8140	286	143	812	27	6416
1976	4190	6446	272	136	1198	28	5688
1977	4317	6642	188	94	1292	28	5825
1978	4354	6698	166	83	1180	31	5731
1979	4555	7007	152	76	1208	31	5946
1980	4627	7119	128	64	905	23	5683
1981	4322	6649	120	60	930	27	5399
1982	4502	6926	108	54	928	27	5565
1983	4641	7140	116	58	906	25	5688
1984	4887	7518	128	64	912	25	5952
1985	4439	6829	132	66	851	27	5449
1986	4697	7226	140	70	784	28	5649
1987	5009	7706	158	79	765	23	5955
1988	4841	7448	152	76	686	116	5795
1989	5022	7726	178	89	684	104	5988
1990	4654	7160	172	86	619	87	5532
1991	4531	6971	152	76	711	92	5486
1992	4485	6900	168	84	889	109	5651
1993	3786	5824	134	67	1072	94	5086
1994	3609	5553	118	59	1062	91	4880
1995	3375	5192	130	65	929	91	4525

Source : see *Notes on sources of sales data*, p. 193

Table 8.1.3 Manufactured cigarettes (i) percentage of total sales as filter cigarettes, 1960-1980, and (ii) sales-weighted average tar yield per cigarette (SWAT), 1970-1992

Year	% Filter	SWAT mg / cig	Year	% Filter	SWAT mg / cig
1960	49.1		1980	96.9	16.9
1961	54.6		1981		15.7
1962	59.9		1982		15.2
1963	62.1		1983		13.3
1964	66.4		1984		13.0
1965	71.3		1985		13.6
1966	74.3		1986		13.0
1967	79.1		1987		12.6
1968	83.3		1988		11.6
1969	85.8		1989		11.4
1970	88.0	25.0	1990		11.5
1971	89.8		1991		10.7
1972	91.2		1992		10.4
1973	93.2				
1974	93.4				
1975	94.2				
1976	95.6	19.1			
1977	95.4	19.1			
1978	95.9	18.3			
1979	96.3	18.4			

Source : see *Notes on sources of sales data,* p. 193

Table 8.2 Consumption of (i) cigarettes and (ii) all tobacco products, 1920-1995 sales-based data, including estimated hand-rolled cigarette consumption. Males and females aged 15 years and over

Year	Manufactured cigarettes		Hand-rolled cigarettes		Total cigarettes		All tobacco products	
	Total annual in millions	Number/ adult/day	Total annual in millions	Number/ adult/day	Total annual in millions	Number/ adult/day	Total annual in tonnes	Grams/ adult/day
1920	2781	3.6					2590	3.4
1921	2132	2.8					1910	2.5
1922	2337	2.9					2090	2.6
1923	2835	3.5					2720	3.4
1924	3002	3.6					2860	3.4
1925	3035	3.6					2770	3.3
1926	3024	3.6					2720	3.2
1927	3423	4.1					2950	3.5
1928	3616	4.1					3080	3.5
1929	3721	4.2					3220	3.7
1930	3913	4.3					3360	3.7
1931	3104	3.4					2810	3.1
1932	2960	3.2					2680	2.9
1933	3037	3.2					2770	2.9
1934	3322	3.5					3080	3.2
1935	3497	3.7					3220	3.4
1936	3616	3.7					3400	3.5
1937	3989	4.0					3810	3.9
1938	4488	4.6					4040	4.1
1939	3963	4.0					3950	4.0

Table 8.2 *(continued)*

Year	Manufactured cigarettes		Hand-rolled cigarettes		Total cigarettes		All tobacco products	
	Total annual in millions	Number/ adult/day	Total annual in millions	Number/ adult/day	Total annual in millions	Number/ adult/day	Total annual in tonnes	Grams/ adult/day
1940	3780	3.8					3630	3.7
1941	4473	4.5					4170	4.2
1942	3621	3.7					2900	2.9
1943	3624	3.7					2540	2.6
1944	2925	3.0					1860	1.9
1945	2140	2.1					1360	1.3
1946	2886	2.8					2310	2.3
1947	3608	3.5					3270	3.2
1948	4258	4.2					4170	4.1
1949	4326	4.2					4350	4.3
1950	4580	4.4					4540	4.4
1951	4666	4.5					4670	4.5
1952	5187	5.0					5030	4.8
1953	5165	4.9					4850	4.6
1954	5561	5.2					5220	4.9
1955	5704	5.3					5170	4.8
1956	5868	5.4					5310	4.9
1957	5545	5.1					5580	5.1
1958	5241	4.8					4900	4.5
1959	5838	5.3					5310	4.8
1960	6287	5.6					5530	4.9
1961	6621	5.8					6030	5.3
1962	6701	5.8					6170	5.3
1963	7231	6.1					7170	6.1
1964	5546	4.6					6080	5.1
1965	6517	5.4					6940	5.7
1966	6383	5.2					6990	5.7
1967	6684	5.4					7440	6.0
1968	6348	5.1					7440	5.9
1969	6535	5.2					7710	6.1
1970	6480	5.1					7570	6.0
1971	7000	5.5					8070	6.3
1972	7580	5.8					8710	6.7
1973	7340	5.6					8440	6.4
1974	7989	6.0					6453	4.9
1975	8140	6.1					6416	4.8
1976	6446	4.8					5688	4.2
1977	6642	4.9					5825	4.3
1978	6698	4.9					5731	4.2
1979	7007	5.1					5946	4.3
1980	7119	5.1					5683	4.1
1981	6649	4.7					5399	3.9
1982	6926	4.9					5565	3.9
1983	7140	5.0					5688	4.0
1984	7518	5.2					5952	4.1
1985	6829	4.7					5449	3.8
1986	7226	5.0					5649	3.9
1987	7706	5.3					5955	4.1
1988	7448	5.1					5795	4.0
1989	7726	5.3					5988	4.1
1990	7160	4.9					5532	3.8
1991	6971	4.7					5486	3.7
1992	6900	4.6					5651	3.8
1993	5824	3.9					5086	3.4
1994	5553	3.7					4880	3.2
1995	5192	3.4					4525	3.0

Source : see *Notes on sources of sales data*, p. 193

Figure 8.1 Daily consumption of (i) manufactured cigarettes, and (ii) all tobacco products, 1920-1995.
Males and females aged 15 years and over. *Source:* see Table 8.2

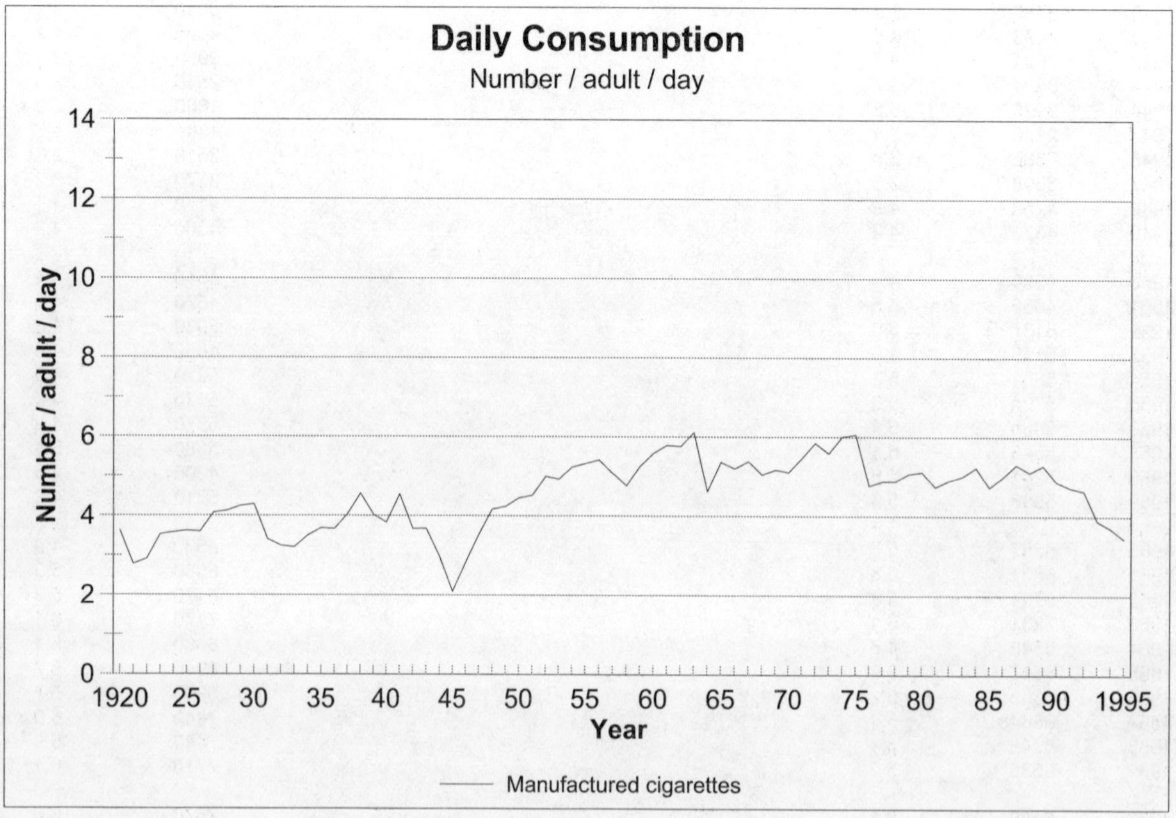

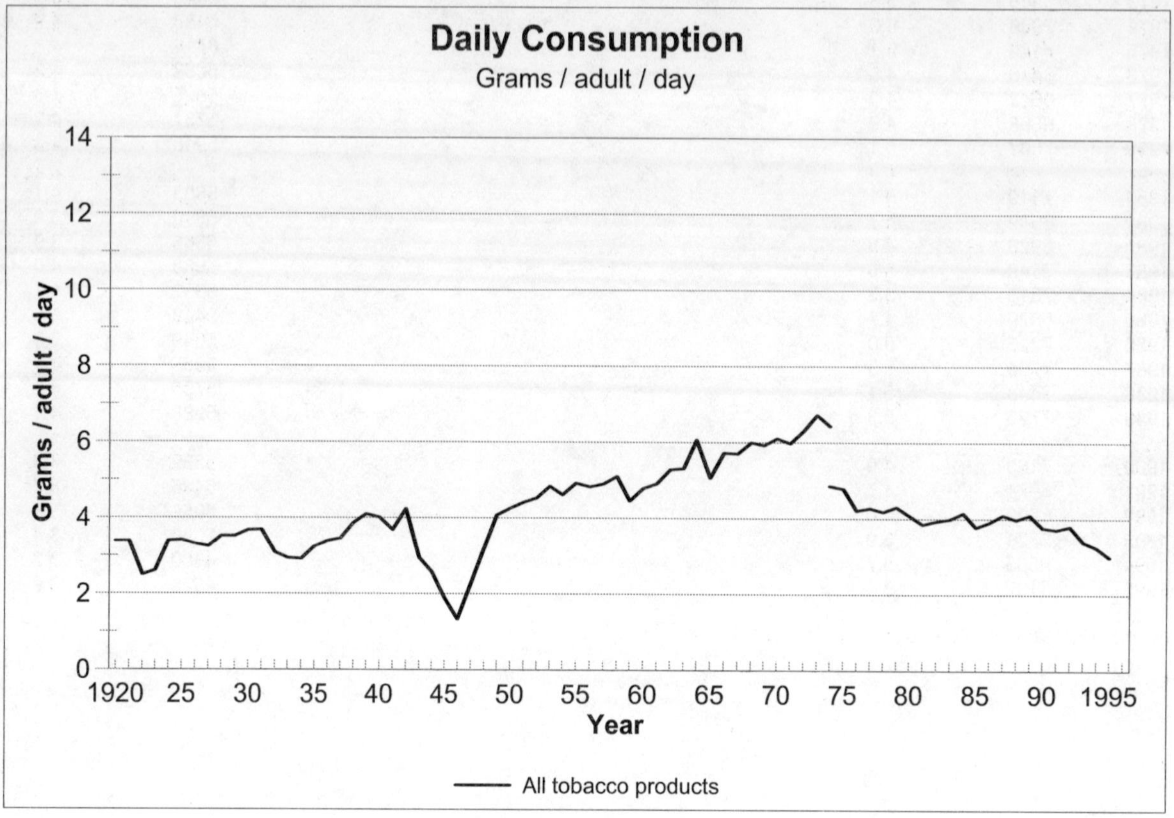

Table 8.3 Percentage sales of tobacco in different forms (by weight), selected years 1925-1995

Year	Cigarettes (%)	Cigars and cigarillos[1] (%)	Other tobacco (%)
1925	75.5	3.2	21.3
1935	86.0	1.6	12.7
1945	83.1	3.7	13.2
1955	90.3	1.0	8.9
1965	86.3	1.3	12.5
1975	82.5	4.5	12.7
1985	81.5	2.4	15.6
1995	74.6	2.9	20.5

1 Cigarillos included 1945-1965

Source : calculated from Tables 8.1.1 & 8.1.2

Figure 8.2 Percentage sales of tobacco in different forms (by weight), selected years 1925-1995
Source: see Table 8.3

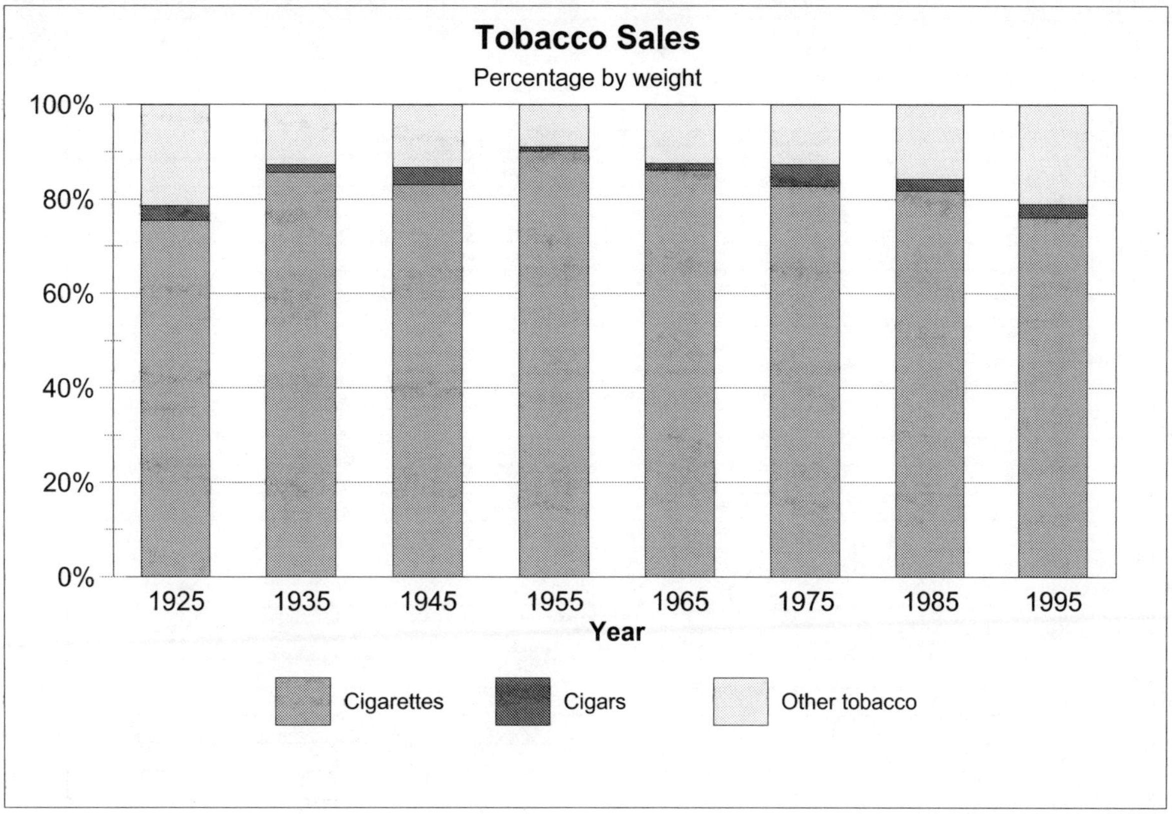

Table 8.4M Prevalence of smoking, males: some selected Finnish surveys by age, 1959-1995 *(continues on p. 178)*

Frequency / Product / Source / Year	12	13	14	15	16	17	18	19	20-24	25-29	30-34	35-39	40-44	45-49	50-54	55-59	60-64	65-69	70-74	75-79	80+	All ages
59 14 UC R													69									
59 15 UC R													57									
60 2 U R				58																		
61 2 U R				57																		
61 22 MC U							47															
61 22 TC U							47															
61 22 A U							53															
61 23 MC U							59															
61 23 TC U							61															
61 23 A U							64															
62 3 TC U													61	59	54	51	44					
62 3 A U													64	62	58	55	48					
63 2 U R				58																		
64 2 U R				56																		
65 2 U R				57																		
66 2 U R				53																		
66 17 A U	8			44					60		58		49									46
67 2 U R				50																		
67 18 UC U				37					55		52		56		50		46		35			
68 2 U R				48																		
69 2 U R				48																		
70 2 U R				44																		
71 2 U R				45																		
71 4 UC U							48		60	50	40	34	54	44	41							
71 17 A U				37					56	56		51		38								46
72 2 U R				46																		
72 11 A R											52		53		52							52
72 12 A R											47		51		51							50
73 1 A A				46																		
73 2 U R				44																		
73 8 UC R				46																		
73 9 TC R			18		39		44															
73 9 TC A			26		48		50															
74 1 A A				42																		
75 1 A A				42																		
75 2 U R				40																		
75 7 UC U							39		49	44	46	43	40	42	42	35	29	27	14			
76 1 A A				40																		
76 2 U R				34																		
76 2 U A				40																		
76 20 U U				38						43		40		41		34		26				38
77 1 A A				40																		
77 2 U R				40																		
77 2 U A				45																		
77 9 TC R			11		30		41															
77 11 A R											45		44		44							44
77 12 A R											46		43		45							44
78 1 A A				37																		
78 5 UC U		13					40		48	33	36	27	28	29	30	26	25	27	3	16		
78 6 MC R				32						39		30		28		26						32
78 6 A R				33						43		34		34		33						36
78 6 A A				42						50		39		39		35						42
79 1 A A				40																		
79 6 MC R				36						37		30		26		22						31
79 6 A R				37						40		36		32		30						36
79 6 A A				46						49		41		35		32						41
79 9 TC R			9		25		34															
79 10 A R				27						37				37								34

Table 8.4F Prevalence of smoking, females: some selected Finnish surveys by age, 1959-1995 *(continues on p 179)*

<table>
<tr><th rowspan="2">Frequency
Product
Source
Year</th><th colspan="21">Age group</th><th rowspan="2">All ages</th></tr>
<tr><th>12</th><th>13</th><th>14</th><th>15</th><th>16</th><th>17</th><th>18</th><th>19</th><th>20-24</th><th>25-29</th><th>30-34</th><th>35-39</th><th>40-44</th><th>45-49</th><th>50-54</th><th>55-59</th><th>60-64</th><th>65-69</th><th>70-74</th><th>75-79</th><th>80+</th></tr>
<tr><td>59 14 UC R</td><td colspan="21"></td><td></td></tr>
<tr><td>59 15 UC R</td><td colspan="21"></td><td></td></tr>
<tr><td>60 2 U R</td><td colspan="3"></td><td colspan="18">14</td><td></td></tr>
<tr><td>61 2 U R</td><td colspan="3"></td><td colspan="18">12</td><td></td></tr>
<tr><td>61 22 MC U</td><td colspan="21"></td><td></td></tr>
<tr><td>61 22 TC U</td><td colspan="21"></td><td></td></tr>
<tr><td>61 22 A U</td><td colspan="21"></td><td></td></tr>
<tr><td>61 23 MC U</td><td colspan="21"></td><td></td></tr>
<tr><td>61 23 TC U</td><td colspan="21"></td><td></td></tr>
<tr><td>61 23 A U</td><td colspan="21"></td><td></td></tr>
<tr><td>62 3 TC U</td><td colspan="21"></td><td></td></tr>
<tr><td>62 3 A U</td><td colspan="21"></td><td></td></tr>
<tr><td>63 2 U R</td><td colspan="3"></td><td colspan="18">13</td><td></td></tr>
<tr><td>64 2 U R</td><td colspan="3"></td><td colspan="18">16</td><td></td></tr>
<tr><td>65 2 U R</td><td colspan="3"></td><td colspan="18">14</td><td></td></tr>
<tr><td>66 2 U R</td><td colspan="3"></td><td colspan="18">15</td><td></td></tr>
<tr><td>66 17 A U</td><td colspan="3">0</td><td colspan="5">8</td><td colspan="2">24</td><td colspan="2">16</td><td colspan="4">12</td><td colspan="5"></td><td>13</td></tr>
<tr><td>67 2 U R</td><td colspan="3"></td><td colspan="18">15</td><td></td></tr>
<tr><td>67 18 UC U</td><td colspan="3"></td><td colspan="5">19</td><td colspan="2">25</td><td colspan="2">16</td><td colspan="2">16</td><td colspan="2">9</td><td colspan="2">4</td><td colspan="3">2</td><td></td></tr>
<tr><td>68 2 U R</td><td colspan="3"></td><td colspan="18">19</td><td></td></tr>
<tr><td>69 2 U R</td><td colspan="3"></td><td colspan="18">17</td><td></td></tr>
<tr><td>70 2 U R</td><td colspan="3"></td><td colspan="18">16</td><td></td></tr>
<tr><td>71 2 U R</td><td colspan="3"></td><td colspan="18">18</td><td></td></tr>
<tr><td>71 4 UC U</td><td colspan="6"></td><td colspan="2">30</td><td>29</td><td>30</td><td>16</td><td>24</td><td>18</td><td>20</td><td>12</td><td colspan="6"></td><td></td></tr>
<tr><td>71 17 A U</td><td colspan="3"></td><td colspan="5">30</td><td>42</td><td colspan="2">29</td><td colspan="2">20</td><td colspan="4">12</td><td colspan="4"></td><td>23</td></tr>
<tr><td>72 2 U R</td><td colspan="3"></td><td colspan="18">19</td><td></td></tr>
<tr><td>72 11 A R</td><td colspan="10"></td><td colspan="2">12</td><td colspan="2">11</td><td colspan="2">7</td><td colspan="5"></td><td>10</td></tr>
<tr><td>72 12 A R</td><td colspan="10"></td><td colspan="2">14</td><td colspan="2">11</td><td colspan="2">9</td><td colspan="5"></td><td>11</td></tr>
<tr><td>73 1 A A</td><td colspan="3"></td><td colspan="18">22</td><td></td></tr>
<tr><td>73 2 U R</td><td colspan="3"></td><td colspan="18">20</td><td></td></tr>
<tr><td>73 8 UC R</td><td colspan="3"></td><td colspan="18">21</td><td></td></tr>
<tr><td>73 9 TC R</td><td colspan="2"></td><td>21</td><td></td><td>32</td><td></td><td>40</td><td colspan="14"></td><td></td></tr>
<tr><td>73 9 TC A</td><td colspan="2"></td><td>33</td><td></td><td>47</td><td></td><td>51</td><td colspan="14"></td><td></td></tr>
<tr><td>74 1 A A</td><td colspan="3"></td><td colspan="18">20</td><td></td></tr>
<tr><td>75 1 A A</td><td colspan="3"></td><td colspan="18">22</td><td></td></tr>
<tr><td>75 2 U R</td><td colspan="3"></td><td colspan="18">17</td><td></td></tr>
<tr><td>75 7 UC U</td><td colspan="6"></td><td colspan="2">38</td><td>36</td><td>30</td><td>24</td><td>19</td><td>14</td><td>12</td><td>14</td><td>9</td><td>7</td><td>5</td><td colspan="3">2</td><td></td></tr>
<tr><td>76 1 A A</td><td colspan="3"></td><td colspan="18">20</td><td></td></tr>
<tr><td>76 2 U R</td><td colspan="3"></td><td colspan="18">17</td><td></td></tr>
<tr><td>76 2 U A</td><td colspan="3"></td><td colspan="18">23</td><td></td></tr>
<tr><td>76 20 U U</td><td colspan="3"></td><td colspan="6">25</td><td colspan="2">28</td><td colspan="2">16</td><td colspan="2">13</td><td colspan="2">9</td><td colspan="4">3</td><td>17</td></tr>
<tr><td>77 1 A A</td><td colspan="3"></td><td colspan="18">19</td><td></td></tr>
<tr><td>77 2 U R</td><td colspan="3"></td><td colspan="18">17</td><td></td></tr>
<tr><td>77 2 U A</td><td colspan="3"></td><td colspan="18">22</td><td></td></tr>
<tr><td>77 9 TC R</td><td colspan="2"></td><td>15</td><td></td><td>27</td><td></td><td>32</td><td colspan="14"></td><td></td></tr>
<tr><td>77 11 A R</td><td colspan="10"></td><td colspan="2">14</td><td colspan="2">9</td><td colspan="2">7</td><td colspan="5"></td><td>10</td></tr>
<tr><td>77 12 A R</td><td colspan="10"></td><td colspan="2">19</td><td colspan="2">9</td><td colspan="2">8</td><td colspan="5"></td><td>12</td></tr>
<tr><td>78 1 A A</td><td colspan="3"></td><td colspan="18">19</td><td></td></tr>
<tr><td>78 5 UC U</td><td></td><td colspan="5">19</td><td colspan="2">32</td><td>28</td><td>23</td><td>14</td><td>18</td><td>14</td><td>14</td><td>11</td><td>5</td><td>7</td><td>4</td><td>3</td><td>0</td><td></td><td></td></tr>
<tr><td>78 6 MC R</td><td colspan="3"></td><td colspan="6">21</td><td colspan="2">23</td><td colspan="2">16</td><td colspan="2">11</td><td colspan="2">7</td><td colspan="4"></td><td>17</td></tr>
<tr><td>78 6 A R</td><td colspan="3"></td><td colspan="6">23</td><td colspan="2">23</td><td colspan="2">16</td><td colspan="2">11</td><td colspan="2">8</td><td colspan="4"></td><td>17</td></tr>
<tr><td>78 6 A A</td><td colspan="3"></td><td colspan="6">37</td><td colspan="2">31</td><td colspan="2">22</td><td colspan="2">14</td><td colspan="2">9</td><td colspan="4"></td><td>24</td></tr>
<tr><td>79 1 A A</td><td colspan="3"></td><td colspan="18">19</td><td></td></tr>
<tr><td>79 6 MC R</td><td colspan="3"></td><td colspan="6">27</td><td colspan="2">24</td><td colspan="2">17</td><td colspan="2">12</td><td colspan="2">7</td><td colspan="4"></td><td>18</td></tr>
<tr><td>79 6 A R</td><td colspan="3"></td><td colspan="6">28</td><td colspan="2">25</td><td colspan="2">18</td><td colspan="2">13</td><td colspan="2">8</td><td colspan="4"></td><td>18</td></tr>
<tr><td>79 6 A A</td><td colspan="3"></td><td colspan="6">39</td><td colspan="2">31</td><td colspan="2">23</td><td colspan="2">15</td><td colspan="2">8</td><td colspan="4"></td><td>23</td></tr>
<tr><td>79 9 TC R</td><td colspan="2"></td><td>9</td><td></td><td>25</td><td></td><td>26</td><td colspan="14"></td><td></td></tr>
<tr><td>79 10 A R</td><td colspan="3"></td><td colspan="6">21</td><td colspan="4">18</td><td colspan="4">10</td><td colspan="4"></td><td>16</td></tr>
</table>

Table 8.4M *(continued from p. 176, continues on p. 180)*
Prevalence of smoking, males

Frequency / Product / Source / Year	12	13	14	15	16	17	18	19	20-24	25-29	30-34	35-39	40-44	45-49	50-54	55-59	60-64	65-69	70-74	75-79	80+	All ages
80 1 A A				39																		
80 6 MC R				28						41		32		26		24						32
80 6 A R				29						44		37		32		28						35
80 6 A A				38						52		41		35		30						41
80 10 A R				31						41				34								37
80 19 U R	1			11			37															
80 19 U A	10			33			58															
81 6 MC R				29						39		36		24		22						31
81 6 A R				30						42		40		32		30						36
81 6 A A				41						48		44		36		33						41
81 9 TC R			15		30		36															
81 10 A R				30						42				35								37
82 6 MC R				25						39		28		26		18						28
82 6 A R				25						41		32		31		24						32
82 6 A A				36						48		38		34		27						38
82 10 A R				26						38				32								33
82 11 UC R										34		29		32		27						29
82 11 A A										47		37		39		34						37
82 11* A R											42		39		34							36
82 12 UC R										38		34		35		29						33
82 12 A A										52		45		43		41						43
82 12* A R											49		43		41							42
82 13 UC R										42		32		27		32						30
82 13 A A										54		44		34		37						39
82 13* A R											39											
83 6 MC R				21						37		28		26		22						28
83 6 A R				22						39		33		32		27						32
83 6 A A				34						48		41		35		28						38
83 9 TC R			15		27		34															
83 10 A R				28						37				29								33
83 21 U R		17		30																		
84 6 MC R				27						38		34		26		24						31
84 6 A R				28						41		37		30		29						34
84 6 A A				36						51		42		34		33						40
84 10 A R				32						36				31								33
85 6 MC R				16					36	36	38	35	28	28	18	25	23					29
85 6 A R				17					36	38	40	39	31	31	24	33	25					32
85 6 A A				30					46	48	49	43	39	37	25	37	28					39
85 9 TC R			13		28		32															
85 10 MC R				30						34				27								
85 10 A R				30						38				34								35
85 10 A A				43						48				37								
86 6 MC R				30						38		34		26		22						31
86 6 A R				30						40		37		28		25						33
86 6 A A				42						49		43		33		28						40
86 21 U *		9		29																		
86 21 U R		13		36																		
86 21 U A		19		42																		
87 6 A R				28						39		39		31		27						33
87 6 A A				42						46		45		33		29						40
87 9 TC R			14		33		37															
87 10 A R				28						38				31								34
87 11 A R											36											
87 12 A R											41											
87 13 A R											38											
88 6 A R				31						37		40		29		27						33
88 6 A A				42						47		46		34		30						40
88 10 A R				30						39				32								35

Table 8.4F *(continued from p. 177, continues on p. 181)*
Prevalence of smoking, females

Frequency / Product / Source / Year	12	13	14	15	16	17	18	19	20-24	25-29	30-34	35-39	40-44	45-49	50-54	55-59	60-64	65-69	70-74	75-79	80+	All ages
80 1 A A				21																		
80 6 MC R				20						25		16		12		7						16
80 6 A R				21						25		16		12		7						17
80 6 A A				34						33		21		13		8						22
80 10 A R				19						17				11								16
80 19 U R	0			10			23															
80 19 U A	4			37			49															
81 6 MC R				21						27		18		14		7						18
81 6 A R				24						28		18		14		8						19
81 6 A A				34						34		23		16		9						23
81 9 TC R			12		25		26															
81 10 A R				20						19				12								17
82 6 MC R				21						20		19		8		8						15
82 6 A R				21						22		20		9		8						16
82 6 A A				30						32		22		11		9						21
82 10 A R				19						21				11								17
82 11 UC R										21		11		8		5						8
82 11 A A										28		20		12		8						14
82 11* A R											26		15		11							15
82 12 UC R										21		12		11		5						10
82 12 A A										34		17		16		8						14
82 12* A R											26		16		12							15
82 13 UC R										26		22		13		12						16
82 13 A A										40		28		17		15						21
82 13* A R											22											
83 6 MC R				21						27		21		10		9						18
83 6 A R				22						28		21		10		9						19
83 6 A A				34						37		25		14		11						25
83 9 TC R			13		23		25															
83 10 A R				18						21				11								17
83 21 U R		11		25																		
84 6 MC R				18						26		20		11		6						17
84 6 A R				18						26		21		12		7						17
84 6 A A				32						33		25		15		8						23
84 10 A R				20						16				10								15
85 6 MC R				11					20	22	19	16	15	8	11	5	8					14
85 6 A R				11					21	22	20	16	15	8	12	5	8					14
85 6 A A				24					32	34	27	19	19	11	16	7	10					21
85 9 TC R			10		25		25															
85 10 MC R				18						21				9								
85 10 A R				19						22				10								17
85 10 A A				29						29				14								
86 6 MC R				25						26		19		12		7						18
86 6 A R				25						26		19		12		8						18
86 6 A A				37						35		23		16		10						25
86 21 U *		6		20																		
86 21 U R		9		27																		
86 21 U A		13		37																		
87 6 A R				23						25		16		16		10						21
87 6 A A				36						35		20		20		12						28
87 9 TC R			10		28		32															
87 10 A R				21						23				12								19
87 11 A R											16											
87 12 A R											15											
87 13 A R											23											
88 6 A R				22						29		23		13		11						20
88 6 A A				36						36		28		16		12						27
88 10 A R				21						25				12								20

Table 8.4M (continued from p. 178)
Prevalence of smoking, males

Year	Source	Product	Frequency	12	13	14	15	16	17	18	19	20-24	25-29	30-34	35-39	40-44	45-49	50-54	55-59	60-64	65-69	70-74	75-79	80+	All ages
89	6	A	R				25						23		20		15		10						19
89	6	A	A				38						33		27		20		12						26
89	9	TC	R			13		29		29															
89	10	A	R				23						24				13								20
90	6	A	R				28						33		38		30		30						32
90	6	A	A				37						42		45		36		31						39
90	10	A	R				38						42				26								36
90	21	UC	R		17		33																		
90	21	UC	A		22		37																		
91	6	A	R				27						39		38		35		25						33
91	6	A	A				39						46		44		39		28						40
91	9	TC	R			14		32		36															
92	6	A	R				30						37		36		35		25						33
92	6	A	A				43						45		42		41		27						40
92	11	A	R											32											
92	12	A	R											37											
92	13	A	R											39											
93	6	A	R				27						32		36		31		22						30
93	6	A	A				34						44		45		36		24						37
93	9	TC	R			15		29		35															
94	6	A	R				26						29		30		26		24						27
94	6	A	A				33						37		39		31		26						34
94	21	UC	R		15		30																		
94	21	UC	*				25																		
95	6	A	R				23						35		36		29		22						29
95	6	A	A				35						43		44		32		26						36
95	9	TC	R			14		30		36															
95	16	UC	R				24																		
95	16	UC	A				36																		

Source: see *Notes on sources of survey data*, p. 193
Product: MC = manufactured cigarettes
TC = total cigarettes (including hand-rolled)
UC = cigarettes (type unspecified)
A = all products

Frequency: A = all smokers (including occasional)
R = regular or daily smokers
All ages: relevant to ages used and as given in original source
U = unspecified
* = refer to *Notes on sources of survey data*, p. 193

Table 8.4F *(continued from p. 179)*
Prevalence of smoking, females

<table>
<tr><th colspan="4">Frequency
Product
Source
Year</th><th colspan="21">Age group</th><th rowspan="2">All ages</th></tr>
<tr><th>Year</th><th>Source</th><th>Product</th><th>Frequency</th><th>12</th><th>13</th><th>14</th><th>15</th><th>16</th><th>17</th><th>18</th><th>19</th><th>20-24</th><th>25-29</th><th>30-34</th><th>35-39</th><th>40-44</th><th>45-49</th><th>50-54</th><th>55-59</th><th>60-64</th><th>65-69</th><th>70-74</th><th>75-79</th><th>80+</th></tr>
<tr><td>89</td><td>6</td><td>A</td><td>R</td><td colspan="3"></td><td colspan="6">25</td><td colspan="2">23</td><td colspan="2">20</td><td colspan="2">15</td><td colspan="2">10</td><td colspan="4"></td><td>19</td></tr>
<tr><td>89</td><td>6</td><td>A</td><td>A</td><td colspan="3"></td><td colspan="6">38</td><td colspan="2">33</td><td colspan="2">27</td><td colspan="2">20</td><td colspan="2">12</td><td colspan="4"></td><td>26</td></tr>
<tr><td>89</td><td>9</td><td>TC</td><td>R</td><td colspan="2"></td><td>13</td><td></td><td>29</td><td></td><td>29</td><td colspan="14"></td><td></td></tr>
<tr><td>89</td><td>10</td><td>A</td><td>R</td><td colspan="3"></td><td colspan="6">23</td><td colspan="4">24</td><td colspan="4">13</td><td colspan="4"></td><td>20</td></tr>
<tr><td>90</td><td>6</td><td>A</td><td>R</td><td colspan="3"></td><td colspan="6">23</td><td colspan="2">23</td><td colspan="2">24</td><td colspan="2">17</td><td colspan="2">11</td><td colspan="4"></td><td>20</td></tr>
<tr><td>90</td><td>6</td><td>A</td><td>A</td><td colspan="3"></td><td colspan="6">36</td><td colspan="2">30</td><td colspan="2">32</td><td colspan="2">21</td><td colspan="2">14</td><td colspan="4"></td><td>27</td></tr>
<tr><td>90</td><td>10</td><td>A</td><td>R</td><td colspan="3"></td><td colspan="6">23</td><td colspan="4">26</td><td colspan="4">14</td><td colspan="4"></td><td>21</td></tr>
<tr><td>90</td><td>21</td><td>UC</td><td>R</td><td></td><td>13</td><td></td><td>32</td><td colspan="17"></td><td></td></tr>
<tr><td>90</td><td>21</td><td>UC</td><td>A</td><td></td><td>21</td><td></td><td>39</td><td colspan="17"></td><td></td></tr>
<tr><td>91</td><td>6</td><td>A</td><td>R</td><td colspan="3"></td><td colspan="6">28</td><td colspan="2">27</td><td colspan="2">24</td><td colspan="2">18</td><td colspan="2">7</td><td colspan="4"></td><td>22</td></tr>
<tr><td>91</td><td>6</td><td>A</td><td>A</td><td colspan="3"></td><td colspan="6">38</td><td colspan="2">32</td><td colspan="2">29</td><td colspan="2">21</td><td colspan="2">9</td><td colspan="4"></td><td>26</td></tr>
<tr><td>91</td><td>9</td><td>TC</td><td>R</td><td colspan="2"></td><td>15</td><td></td><td>27</td><td></td><td>28</td><td colspan="14"></td><td></td></tr>
<tr><td>92</td><td>6</td><td>A</td><td>R</td><td colspan="3"></td><td colspan="6">23</td><td colspan="2">24</td><td colspan="2">25</td><td colspan="2">20</td><td colspan="2">7</td><td colspan="4"></td><td>20</td></tr>
<tr><td>92</td><td>6</td><td>A</td><td>A</td><td colspan="3"></td><td colspan="6">37</td><td colspan="2">34</td><td colspan="2">31</td><td colspan="2">22</td><td colspan="2">8</td><td colspan="4"></td><td>27</td></tr>
<tr><td>92</td><td>11</td><td>A</td><td>R</td><td colspan="10"></td><td colspan="6">17</td><td colspan="5"></td><td></td></tr>
<tr><td>92</td><td>12</td><td>A</td><td>R</td><td colspan="10"></td><td colspan="6">19</td><td colspan="5"></td><td></td></tr>
<tr><td>92</td><td>13</td><td>A</td><td>R</td><td colspan="10"></td><td colspan="6">23</td><td colspan="5"></td><td></td></tr>
<tr><td>93</td><td>6</td><td>A</td><td>R</td><td colspan="3"></td><td colspan="6">22</td><td colspan="2">20</td><td colspan="2">25</td><td colspan="2">15</td><td colspan="2">9</td><td colspan="4"></td><td>19</td></tr>
<tr><td>93</td><td>6</td><td>A</td><td>A</td><td colspan="3"></td><td colspan="6">36</td><td colspan="2">29</td><td colspan="2">33</td><td colspan="2">18</td><td colspan="2">10</td><td colspan="4"></td><td>26</td></tr>
<tr><td>93</td><td>9</td><td>TC</td><td>R</td><td colspan="2"></td><td>13</td><td></td><td>26</td><td></td><td>25</td><td colspan="14"></td><td></td></tr>
<tr><td>94</td><td>6</td><td>A</td><td>R</td><td colspan="3"></td><td colspan="6">22</td><td colspan="2">22</td><td colspan="2">20</td><td colspan="2">19</td><td colspan="2">8</td><td colspan="4"></td><td>19</td></tr>
<tr><td>94</td><td>6</td><td>A</td><td>A</td><td colspan="3"></td><td colspan="6">36</td><td colspan="2">28</td><td colspan="2">25</td><td colspan="2">23</td><td colspan="2">9</td><td colspan="4"></td><td>25</td></tr>
<tr><td>94</td><td>21</td><td>UC</td><td>R</td><td></td><td>11</td><td></td><td>26</td><td colspan="17"></td><td></td></tr>
<tr><td>94</td><td>21</td><td>UC</td><td>*</td><td colspan="3"></td><td>19</td><td colspan="17"></td><td></td></tr>
<tr><td>95</td><td>6</td><td>A</td><td>R</td><td colspan="3"></td><td colspan="6">23</td><td colspan="2">21</td><td colspan="2">24</td><td colspan="2">17</td><td colspan="2">11</td><td colspan="4"></td><td>20</td></tr>
<tr><td>95</td><td>6</td><td>A</td><td>A</td><td colspan="3"></td><td colspan="6">34</td><td colspan="2">29</td><td colspan="2">31</td><td colspan="2">20</td><td colspan="2">12</td><td colspan="4"></td><td>26</td></tr>
<tr><td>95</td><td>9</td><td>TC</td><td>R</td><td colspan="2"></td><td>13</td><td></td><td>26</td><td></td><td>27</td><td colspan="14"></td><td></td></tr>
<tr><td>95</td><td>16</td><td>UC</td><td>R</td><td colspan="3"></td><td colspan="2">24</td><td colspan="16"></td><td></td></tr>
<tr><td>95</td><td>16</td><td>UC</td><td>A</td><td colspan="3"></td><td colspan="2">39</td><td colspan="16"></td><td></td></tr>
</table>

Source: see *Notes on sources of survey data*, p. 193
Product: MC = manufactured cigarettes
TC = total cigarettes (including hand-rolled)
UC = cigarettes (type unspecified)
A = all products

Frequency: A = all smokers (including occasional)
R = regular or daily smokers
All ages: relevant to ages used and as given in original source
U = unspecified
* = refer to *Notes on sources of survey data*, p. 193

Table 8.5M Number of cigarettes smoked per smoker per day, males: some selected Finnish surveys by age, 1959-1995

Product Source Year	12	13	14	15	16	17	18	19	20-24	25-29	30-34	35-39	40-44	45-49	50-54	55-59	60-64	65-69	70-74	75-79	80+	All ages
59 14 UCE*													17									
59 15 UCE*													14									
61 22 TCE							14															
61 23 TCE							17															
62 3 TCE*													<18	17	16	15	14					
71 4 UCE*							18		19	19	21	20	21	20	17							
72 11 A											19											
72 12 A											18											
75 7 UCE							12		15	17	18	17	18	18	17	18	15	14	12			
77 9 MC			7.5		9.9		13															
77 11 A											19											
77 12 A											19											
78 5 UCE*		10					16		20	20	21	22	21	21	22	18	18	17	24	15		
78 6 MCE				16						20		21		20		19						19
79 6 MCE				14						20		21		21		19						19
79 9 MC			7.4		11		13															
80 6 MCE				15						20		21		21		19						19
80 19 UC				7.1			12															
81 6 MCE				15						20		22		21		17						19
81 9 MC			7.6		10		12															
82 6 MCE				15						19		21		21		17						19
82 11 UC												19										
82 11 A											18											
82 12 UC												20										
82 12 A											18											
82 13 UC												22										
83 6 MCE				15						19		22		19		19						19
83 9 MC			7.9		12		13															
84 6 MCE				16						19		23		22		18						20
85 6 MCE				14					16	21	22	22	20	25	23	20	18					20
85 6 AE				15					16	20	21	22	19	25	21	20	19					20
85 9 MC			9.7		12		14															
85 10 MC				14						19				19								18
86 6 MCE				15						19		21		23		20						19
86 6 AE				15						19		21		23		20						19
87 6 AE				15						18		22		21		21						19
88 6 AE				16						21		21		22		19						20
89 6 AE				17						19		22		22		19						20
90 6 AE				16						18		20		24		20						20
91 6 AE				16						19		21		22		19						20
92 6 AE				15						18		21		23		23						20
93 6 AE				15						20		20		21		19						19
94 6 AE				16						19		20		23		20						19
95 6 AE				15						18		20		20		19						19
95 16 UCE				11																		

Source: see *Notes on sources of survey data*, p. 193

Product: MC = manufactured cigarettes
TC = total cigarettes (including hand-rolled)
UC = cigarettes (type unspecified)
A = all products
U = unspecified

Product (cont): E indicates mean estimated from percentage distribution (see also *Consumption category estimation*, p. xxxiv, and Appendix III, p. 789)

All ages: relevant to ages used and as given in original source

* = refer to *Notes on sources of survey data*, p. 193

Table 8.5F Number of cigarettes smoked per smoker per day, females: some selected Finnish surveys by age, 1959-1995

Year Source Product	12	13	14	15	16	17	18	19	20-24	25-29	30-34	35-39	40-44	45-49	50-54	55-59	60-64	65-69	70-74	75-79	80+	All ages
59 14 UCE*																						
59 15 UCE*																						
61 22 TCE																						
61 23 TCE																						
62 3 TCE																						
71 4 UCE*							9.5		10	12	12	11	14	13	11							
72 11 A											11											
72 12 A											11											
75 7 UCE							9.0		10	11	12	11	11	12	11	9.6	9.7	9.8	6.8			
77 9 MC			5.2		7.9		8.9															
77 11 A											11											
77 12 A											11											
78 5 UCE*		10					12			14	19	16	15	12	12	12	18	16	22	7.9	0.0	
78 6 MCE				11						13		15		15		15						13
79 6 MCE				12						13		14		16		12						13
79 9 MC			7.2		8.3		9.2															
80 6 MCE				11						13		16		16		13						13
80 19 UC				6.4			9.0															
81 6 MCE				12						13		16		14		13						14
81 9 MC			6.3		6.8		8.8															
82 6 MCE				12						14		16		14		14						14
82 11 UC												13										
82 11 A											10											
82 12 UC												13										
82 12 A											11											
82 13 UC												16										
83 6 MCE				11						14		15		16		12						14
83 9 MC			6.9		8.9		10															
84 6 MCE				11						15		15		16		17						14
85 6 MCE				11					12	12	13	14	14	16	15	18	11					13
85 6 AE				11					12	12	13	14	14	16	15	18	11					13
85 9 MC			7.6		11		11															
85 10 MC				9.9						13				14								12
86 6 MCE				11						12		15		14		14						13
86 6 AE				11						12		15		13		14						13
87 6 AE				11						13		16		13		13						13
88 6 AE				13						12		14		15		14						14
89 6 AE				13						13		13		16		12						13
90 6 AE				13						15		15		16		14						14
91 6 AE				12						14		15		15		12						14
92 6 AE				11						14		16		17		15						14
93 6 AE				12						12		13		18		14						13
94 6 AE				12						12		14		15		15						13
95 6 AE				12						13		14		16		15						14
95 16 UCE				8.9																		

Source: see *Notes on sources of survey data*, p. 193
Product: MC = manufactured cigarettes
TC = total cigarettes (including hand-rolled)
UC = cigarettes (type unspecified)
A = all products
U = unspecified

Product (cont): E indicates mean estimated from percentage distribution (see also *Consumption category estimation*, p. xxxiv, and Appendix III, p. 789)
All ages: relevant to ages used and as given in original source
* = refer to *Notes on sources of survey data*, p. 193

Table 8.6M Number of cigarettes smoked per person per day, males: some selected Finnish surveys by age, 1959-1995, with percentage total sales

Product Source Year	Age group																					All ages	% Total sales
	12	13	14	15	16	17	18	19	20-24	25-29	30-34	35-39	40-44	45-49	50-54	55-59	60-64	65-69	70-74	75-79	80+		
59 14 UC *														12									**
59 15 UC *														8.1									**
63 3 UC *													⟨11	9.7	8.7	7.6	6.1						**
71 4 UC *								8.6	12	9.5	8.5	6.6	12	8.7	6.7								**
72 11 A													10										**
72 12 A													9										**
75 7 UC								4.7	7.0	7.3	8.2	7.4	7.0	7.4	7.2	6.3	4.4	3.8		1.7			65%m
77 9 MC *			0.8		3.0		5.5																**
77 11 A													9										**
77 12 A													8										**
78 5 UC *				1.4				6.4		9.7	6.5	7.4	6.0	5.7	6.1	6.8	4.6	4.4	4.5	0.7	2.5		84%m
78 6 MC						5.1				8.0		6.5		5.8		5.0						6.3	77%M
79 6 MC						4.9				7.3		6.3		5.4		4.3						5.8	73%M
79 9 MC *			0.7		2.6		4.5																**
80 6 MC						4.1				8.0		6.9		5.7		4.7						6.1	73%M
80 19 UC				0.8			4.5																**
81 6 MC						4.2				7.8		7.7		5.1		3.9						6.0	80%M
81 9 MC *			1.1		3.0		4.5																**
82 6 MC						3.7				7.3		5.9		5.4		3.1						5.4	69%M
82 11 UC *														5.6									**
82 11 A													7										**
82 12 UC *														6.6									**
82 12 A													8										**
82 13 UC *														6.7									**
83 6 MC						3.1				6.9		6.1		4.9		4.0						5.3	69%M
83 9 MC *			1.2		3.2		4.3																**
84 6 MC						4.4				7.3		7.7		5.7		4.4						6.0	73%M
85 6 MC						2.3			5.8	7.5	8.1	7.9	5.6	7.0	4.2	5.2	4.2					5.9	75%M
85 6 A						2.5			5.9	7.7	8.5	8.5	6.1	7.6	5.0	6.7	4.8					6.4	80%m
85 9 MC *			1.3		3.3		4.6																**
85 10 MC						4.2					6.3				5.3								72%M
86 6 MC						4.5				7.3		7.1		5.9		4.3						6.0	75%M
86 6 A						4.6				7.7		7.9		6.3		4.9						6.4	79%m
87 6 A						4.2				7.1		8.4		6.6		5.5						6.4	75%m
88 6 A						4.9				7.6		8.4		6.4		5.1						6.6	82%m
89 6 A						5.2				7.0		8.5		7.0		5.0						6.7	78%m
90 6 A						4.5				6.1		7.5		7.2		5.8						6.3	84%m
91 6 A						4.4				7.5		7.7		7.5		4.6						6.5	89%m
92 6 A						4.6				6.6		7.5		8.0		5.5						6.5	91%m
93 6 A						4.1				6.3		7.3		6.4		4.1						5.7	95%m
94 6 A						4.1				5.4		6.0		5.8		4.7						5.3	94%m
95 6 A						3.5				6.2		7.3		5.7		4.3						5.4	106%m
95 16 UC				2.6																			**

Source: see *Notes on sources of survey data*, p. 193

Product: MC = manufactured cigarettes
TC = total cigarettes (including hand-rolled)
UC = cigarettes (type unspecified)
A = all products
U = unspecified

All ages: relevant to ages used and as given in original source

% Total sales: estimated % of total sales of M = manufactured or T = total cigarette consumption implied by survey, sexes combined
** = cannot be calculated
--- = adjusted by original author
* = refer to *Notes on sources of survey data*, p. 193

Table 8.6F Number of cigarettes smoked per person per day, females: some selected Finnish surveys by age, 1959-1995, with percentage total sales

Product Source Year	Age group 12	13	14	15	16	17	18	19	20-24	25-29	30-34	35-39	40-44	45-49	50-54	55-59	60-64	65-69	70-74	75-79	80+	All ages	% Total sales
59 14 UC *																							**
59 15 UC *																							**
63 3 UC *																							**
71 4 UC *							2.9		3.1	3.5	1.9	1.5	2.5	2.7	1.3								**
72 11 A											1												**
72 12 A											1												**
75 7 UC							3.4		3.6	3.3	2.9	2.1	1.5	1.4	1.4	0.9	0.6	0.5	0.1				65%m
77 9 MC *			0.8		2.1		2.9																**
77 11 A											1												**
77 12 A											1												**
78 5 UC *		2.0					3.7		4.0	4.3	2.3	2.7	1.6	1.7	1.3	0.9	1.0	0.8	0.2	0.0			84%m
78 6 MC				2.4						2.9		2.3		1.7		1.0						2.2	77%M
79 6 MC				3.0						3.2		2.4		1.9		0.9						2.3	73%M
79 9 MC *			0.7		2.1		2.4																**
80 6 MC				2.2						3.3		2.5		2.0		0.8						2.2	73%M
80 19 UC				0.6			2.1																**
81 6 MC				2.5						3.6		2.9		1.9		0.9						2.4	80%M
81 9 MC *			0.8		1.7		2.3																**
82 6 MC				2.5						2.8		3.1		1.2		1.1						2.1	69%M
82 11 UC *												1.1											**
82 11 A											2												**
82 12 UC *												1.2											**
82 12 A											2												**
82 13 UC *												2.6											**
83 6 MC				2.5						3.8		3.0		1.6		1.1						2.5	69%M
83 9 MC *			0.9		2.0		2.5																**
84 6 MC				1.9						4.0		3.1		1.8		1.1						2.4	73%M
85 6 MC				1.2					2.5	2.7	2.5	2.2	2.1	1.3	1.6	0.8	0.9					1.9	75%M
85 6 A				1.2					2.6	2.7	2.5	2.2	2.1	1.3	1.7	0.8	0.9					1.9	80%m
85 9 MC *			0.8		2.7		2.6																**
85 10 MC				1.8						2.6				1.3									72%M
86 6 MC				2.7						3.1		2.9		1.6		1.1						2.3	75%M
86 6 A				2.7						3.2		2.9		1.7		1.1						2.4	79%m
87 6 A				2.5						3.4		2.5		2.1		1.3						2.8	75%m
88 6 A				3.0						3.4		3.3		1.9		1.6						2.7	82%m
89 6 A				3.2						2.9		2.7		2.4		1.2						2.5	78%m
90 6 A				2.9						3.2		3.7		2.7		1.5						2.9	84%m
91 6 A				3.3						3.8		3.6		2.7		0.9						3.0	89%m
92 6 A				2.5						3.3		3.9		3.4		1.0						2.9	91%m
93 6 A				2.6						2.4		3.3		2.5		1.2						2.5	95%m
94 6 A				2.5						2.7		2.8		2.8		1.3						2.5	94%m
95 6 A				2.6						2.7		3.3		2.6		1.7						2.7	106%m
95 16 UC				2.1																			**

Source: see *Notes on sources of survey data*, p. 193
Product: MC = manufactured cigarettes
TC = total cigarettes (including hand-rolled)
UC = cigarettes (type unspecified)
A = all products
U = unspecified

All ages: relevant to ages used and as given in original source
% Total sales: estimated % of total sales of M = manufactured or T = total cigarette consumption implied by survey, sexes combined
** = cannot be calculated
--- = adjusted by original author
* = refer to *Notes on sources of survey data*, p. 193

Table 8.7M Number of cigarettes smoked per person per day, sales-adjusted, males: some selected Finnish surveys[1] by age, 1975-1995, with percentage total sales

Product Source Year	Age group 12	13	14	15	16	17	18	19	20-24	25-29	30-34	35-39	40-44	45-49	50-54	55-59	60-64	65-69	70-74	75-79	80+	All ages	% Total sales
75 7 UC							7.3		11	11	13	11	11	11	11	9.7	6.8	5.9	2.6				65%m
78 5 UC *		1.7					7.7		12	7.8	8.8	7.2	6.8	7.3	8.1	5.5	5.3	5.4	0.8	3.0			84%m
78 6 MC				6.6						10		8.4		7.5		6.4						8.1	77%M
79 6 MC				6.7						10		8.6		7.4		5.8						8.0	73%M
80 6 MC				5.6						11		9.5		7.8		6.4						8.4	73%M
81 6 MC				5.3						9.8		9.6		6.4		4.9						7.6	80%M
82 6 MC				5.3						11		8.5		7.7		4.5						7.8	69%M
83 6 MC				4.5						10		8.9		7.1		5.8						7.7	69%M
84 6 MC				6.0						10		10		7.8		6.0						8.2	73%M
85 6 MC				3.1					7.7	10	11	11	7.5	9.3	5.6	6.9	5.6					7.9	75%M
85 6 A				3.1					7.4	9.7	11	11	7.7	9.6	6.2	8.4	6.0					8.1	80%m
85 10 MC				5.9						8.8				7.4									72%M
86 6 MC				6.0						9.8		9.4		7.8		5.7						7.9	75%M
86 6 A				5.8						9.7		9.9		7.9		6.2						8.1	79%m
87 6 A				5.6						9.4		11		8.8		7.3						8.6	75%m
88 6 A				6.0						9.3		10		7.8		6.2						8.1	82%m
89 6 A				6.7						9.0		11		8.9		6.4						8.6	78%m
90 6 A				5.4						7.3		9.0		8.6		7.0						7.6	84%m
91 6 A				4.9						8.4		8.7		8.4		5.1						7.3	89%m
92 6 A				5.1						7.3		8.3		8.8		6.1						7.2	91%m
93 6 A				4.3						6.7		7.7		6.8		4.3						6.0	95%m
94 6 A				4.4						5.8		6.4		6.2		5.0						5.6	94%m
95 6 A				3.3						5.8		6.9		5.3		4.0						5.1	106%m

1 Based on those surveys in Table 8.6 with data for both sexes and age range at least 21-64 (see *Cigarette consumption per person*, p. xxxv)

Source: See *Notes on sources of survey data*, p. 193

Product:
MC = manufactured cigarettes
TC = total cigarettes (including hand-rolled)
UC = cigarettes (type unspecified)
A = all products
U = unspecified

All ages: relevant to ages used and as given in original source

% Total sales: Adjustment factor used, estimated % of total sales of M = manufactured or T = total cigarette consumption implied by survey, sexes combined

--- = adjusted by original author

* = refer to *Notes on sources of survey data*, p. 193

Table 8.7F Number of cigarettes smoked per person per day, sales-adjusted, females: some selected Finnish surveys[1] by age, 1975-1995, with percentage total sales

Product Source Year	12	13	14	15	16	17	18	19	20-24	25-29	30-34	35-39	40-44	45-49	50-54	55-59	60-64	65-69	70-74	75-79	80+	All ages	% Total sales
75 7 UC							5.2		5.6	5.1	4.5	3.2	2.3	2.2	2.2	1.4	0.9	0.8	0.2				65%m
78 5 UC *		2.4					4.4			4.8	5.1	2.8	3.2	1.9	2.0	1.6	1.1	1.2	1.0	0.2	0.0		84%m
78 6 MC				3.1						3.7		3.0		2.2		1.3						2.8	77%M
79 6 MC				4.2						4.4		3.3		2.6		1.2						3.2	73%M
80 6 MC				3.0						4.5		3.4		2.7		1.2						3.0	73%M
81 6 MC				3.1						4.5		3.6		2.4		1.2						3.0	80%M
82 6 MC				3.6						4.0		4.5		1.7		1.5						3.1	69%M
83 6 MC				3.6						5.5		4.4		2.3		1.5						3.6	69%M
84 6 MC				2.6						5.4		4.2		2.5		1.5						3.3	73%M
85 6 MC				1.7					3.3	3.6	3.3	2.9	2.8	1.7	2.1	1.1	1.2					2.5	75%M
85 6 A				1.6					3.3	3.4	3.2	2.8	2.7	1.6	2.2	1.0	1.1					2.4	80%m
85 10 MC				2.5						3.6				1.8									72%M
86 6 MC				3.6						4.1		3.8		2.2		1.4						3.1	75%M
86 6 A				3.5						4.1		3.6		2.1		1.4						3.0	79%m
87 6 A				3.3						4.5		3.4		2.8		1.8						3.7	75%m
88 6 A				3.6						4.2		4.0		2.4		2.0						3.3	82%m
89 6 A				4.1						3.8		3.4		3.1		1.5						3.2	78%m
90 6 A				3.5						3.8		4.4		3.2		1.8						3.5	84%m
91 6 A				3.7						4.2		4.0		3.0		1.0						3.3	89%m
92 6 A				2.8						3.6		4.3		3.7		1.1						3.2	91%m
93 6 A				2.7						2.5		3.5		2.7		1.3						2.6	95%m
94 6 A				2.7						2.8		3.0		3.0		1.3						2.6	94%m
95 6 A				2.5						2.5		3.2		2.5		1.6						2.5	106%m

1 Based on those surveys in Table 8.6 with data for both sexes and age range at least 21-64 (see *Cigarette consumption per person*, p. xxxv)

Source: See *Notes on sources of survey data*, p. 193
Product: MC = manufactured cigarettes
TC = total cigarettes (including hand-rolled)
UC = cigarettes (type unspecified)
A = all products
U = unspecified

All ages: relevant to ages used and as given in original source
% Total sales: Adjustment factor used, estimated % of total sales of M = manufactured or T = total cigarette consumption implied by survey, sexes combined
--- = adjusted by original author
* = refer to *Notes on sources of survey data*, p. 193

Table 8.8 Estimated[1] prevalence of smoking and estimated[1] number of cigarettes per person per day (unadjusted and sales-adjusted): summary of Tables 8.4, 8.6 and 8.7, 1960-1995. Males and females aged 15 years and over

Year	Source[2]	Product[3]	Prevalence[4]						Number of cigarettes						
									Unadjusted[7]			Sales-adjusted[8]			
			Manufactured cigarettes[5]		Total cigarettes		All products[6]		Number/ person/day		Total sales %	Manufactured cigarettes[9] number/ person/day		Total cigarettes number/ person/day	
			M	F	M	F	M	F	M	F		M	F	M	F
1960	2	U					58	14							
1961	2	U					57	12							
1963	2	U					58	13							
1964	2	U					56	16							
1965	2	U					57	14							
1966	2	U					53	15							
1967	2	U					50	15							
	18	*UC*	50	14								(9.0	2.1)		
1968	2	U					48	19							
1969	2	U					48	17							
1970	2	U					44	16							
1971	2	U					45	18							
	17	*A*					45	20							
1972	2	U					46	19							
1973	1	**A**					46	22							
	2	U					44	20							
	8	UC	46	21								(8.4	3.1)		
1974	1	**A**					42	20							
1975	1	**A**					42	22							
	2	U					40	17							
	7	*UC*	38	18					6.2	1.9	65	9.6	2.9		
1976	1	**A**					40	20							
	2	U					34	17							
	2	**U**					40	23							
	20	*U*					38	17							
1977	1	**A**					40	19							
	2	U					40	17							
	2	**U**					45	22							
1978	1	**A**					37	19							
	5	*UC*	30	16					6.1	2.3	84	7.2	2.7		
	6	MC+A	30	14			34	15	5.9	1.9	77	7.6	2.4		
	6	**A**					40	21							
1979	1	**A**					40	19							
	6	MC+A	30	16			34	17	5.5	2.1	73	7.5	2.8		
	6	**A**					40	21							
	10	A					33	14							

Table 8.8 *(continued)*

Year	Source[2]	Product[3]	Prevalence[4]						Number of cigarettes						
									Unadjusted[7]			Sales-adjusted[8]			
			Manufactured cigarettes[5]		Total cigarettes		All products[6]		Number/ person/day		Total sales %	Manufactured cigarettes[9] number/ person/day		Total cigarettes number/ person/day	
			M	F	M	F	M	F	M	F		M	F	M	F
1980	1	**A**					39	21							
	6	MC+A	30	15			33	15	5.7	1.9	73	7.8	2.7		
	6	**A**					39	20							
	10	A					35	14							
1981	6	MC+A	29	16			34	17	5.6	2.1	80	7.0	2.6		
	6	**A**					40	20							
	10	A					35	15							
1982	6	MC+A	27	14			30	15	5.0	1.9	69	7.3	2.7		
	6	**A**					36	19							
	10	A					32	15							
1983	6	MC+A	26	16			30	15	4.9	2.1	69	7.1	3.1		
	6	**A**					37	22							
	10	A					31	15							
1984	6	MC+A	29	15			32	15	5.7	2.1	73	7.8	2.9		
	6	**A**					39	21							
	10	A					32	13							
1985	6	MC+A	28	12			31	13	6.1	1.6	80	7.7	2.1		
	6	**A**					38	18							
	10	MC+A	29	14			33	15	5.2	1.7	72	7.3	2.4		
	10	**A**					41	20							
1986	6	MC+A	29	16			31	16	6.0	2.1	79	7.6	2.6		
	6	**A**					39	22							
1987	6	A					32	16	6.1	2.1	75	8.1	2.7		
	6	**A**					38	22							
	10	A					32	16							
1988	6	A					32	17	6.3	2.3	82	7.6	2.8		
	6	**A**					39	23							
	10	A					33	17							
1989	6	A					32	16	6.3	2.1	78	8.1	2.7		
	6	**A**					38	22							
	10	A					32	17							
1990	6	A					30	17	5.9	2.4	84	7.1	2.9		
	6	**A**					37	23							
	10	A					34	18							
1991	6	A					31	18	6.1	2.5	89	6.8	2.8		
	6	**A**					38	22							
1992	6	A					31	17	6.1	2.4	91	6.7	2.7		
	6	**A**					38	23							
1993	6	A					29	16	5.5	2.1	95	5.8	2.2		
	6	**A**					36	22							

Table 8.8 *(continued/2)*

Year	Source[2]	Product[3]	Prevalence[4]						Number of cigarettes							
									Unadjusted[7]			Sales-adjusted[8]				
			Manufactured cigarettes[5]		Total cigarettes		All products[6]		Number/ person/day		Total sales %	Manufactured cigarettes[9] number/ person/day		Total cigarettes number/ person/day	
			M	F	M	F	M	F	M	F		M	F	M	F
1994	6	A					26	16	5.0	2.1	94	5.3	2.2		
	6	**A**					32	21							
1995	6	A					28	17	5.2	2.2	106	4.9	2.1		
	6	**A**					35	22							

1 Surveys covering an age range of at least 21-64 are included. Any gaps in the data for ages 15-20 and 65 years and over are filled in by assumed extensions to the age distribution, given in *Notes on sources of survey data*, p. 193. Method: see *Summary of adult smoking*, p. xxxvi

2 See *Notes on sources of survey data*, p. 193

3 Product: MC = manufactured cigarettes, TC = total cigarettes (including hand-rolled), UC = cigarettes (type unspecified), A = all products, U = unspecified. Frequency of smoking is indicated by: regular or daily smokers in normal type, all smokers (including occasional) in bold, unspecified in italics

4 From Table 8.4

5 This column includes prevalence of smoking classified as UC = cigarettes (type unspecified)

6 This column includes prevalence of smoking classified as U = unspecified product

7 From Table 8.6

8 From Table 8.7, except data in parentheses, which are derived from the prevalence of smoking from Table 8.4 as described in *Summary of adult smoking*, p. xxxvi

9 Number of cigarettes classified as UC = cigarettes (type unspecified), and number of times smoked per day classified as A = all products (source 6, from 1985 onwards) have been adjusted to manufactured cigarette sales and included in this column

Figure 8.3 Estimated prevalence of smoking of (i) manufactured cigarettes and (ii) all tobacco products: by year of survey, 1960-1995.
Males and females aged 15 years and over. *Source:* see Table 8.8

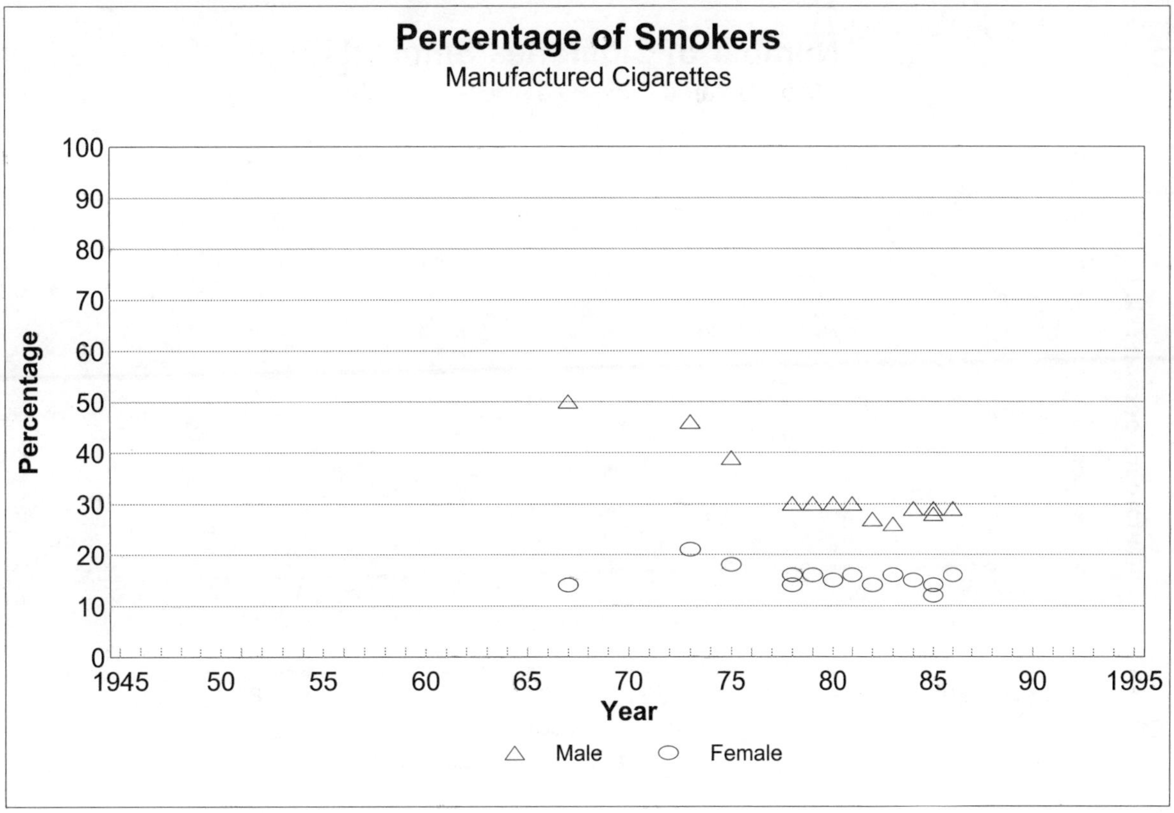

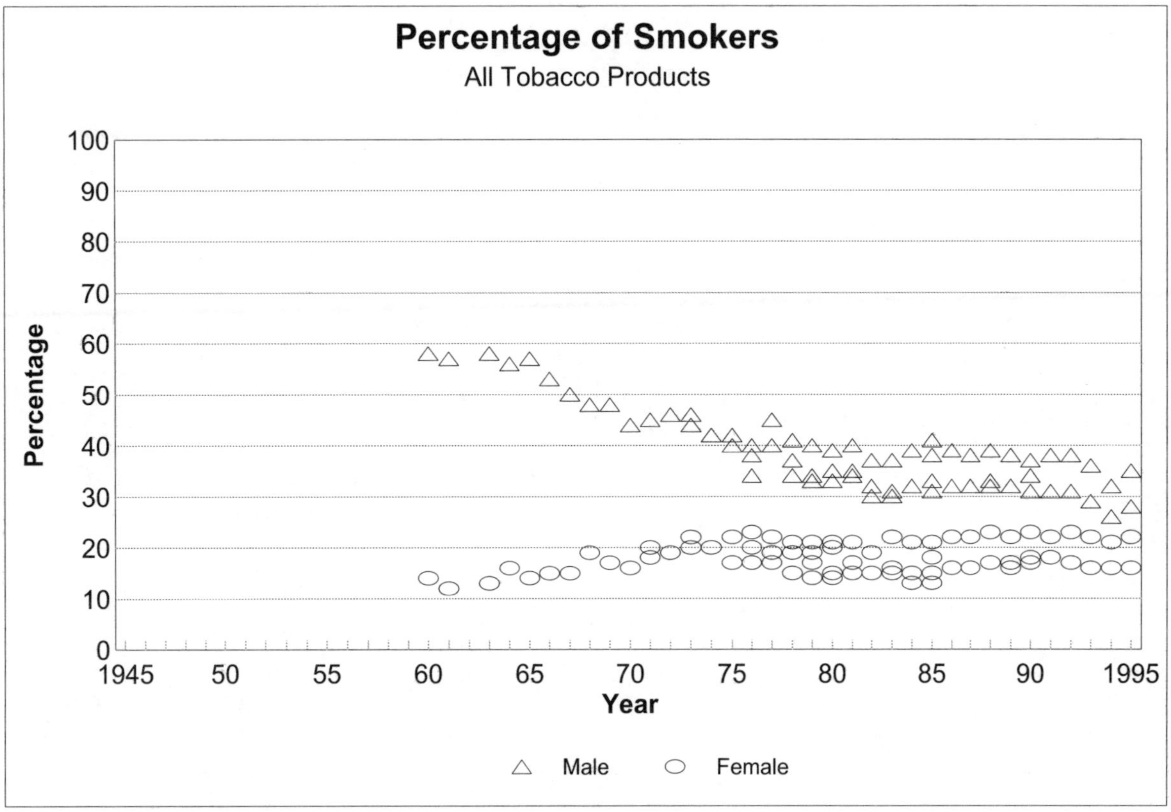

Figure 8.4 Estimated number of cigarettes smoked per person per day, sales-adjusted, 1967-1995.
Males and females aged 15 years and over. *Source:* see Table 8.8

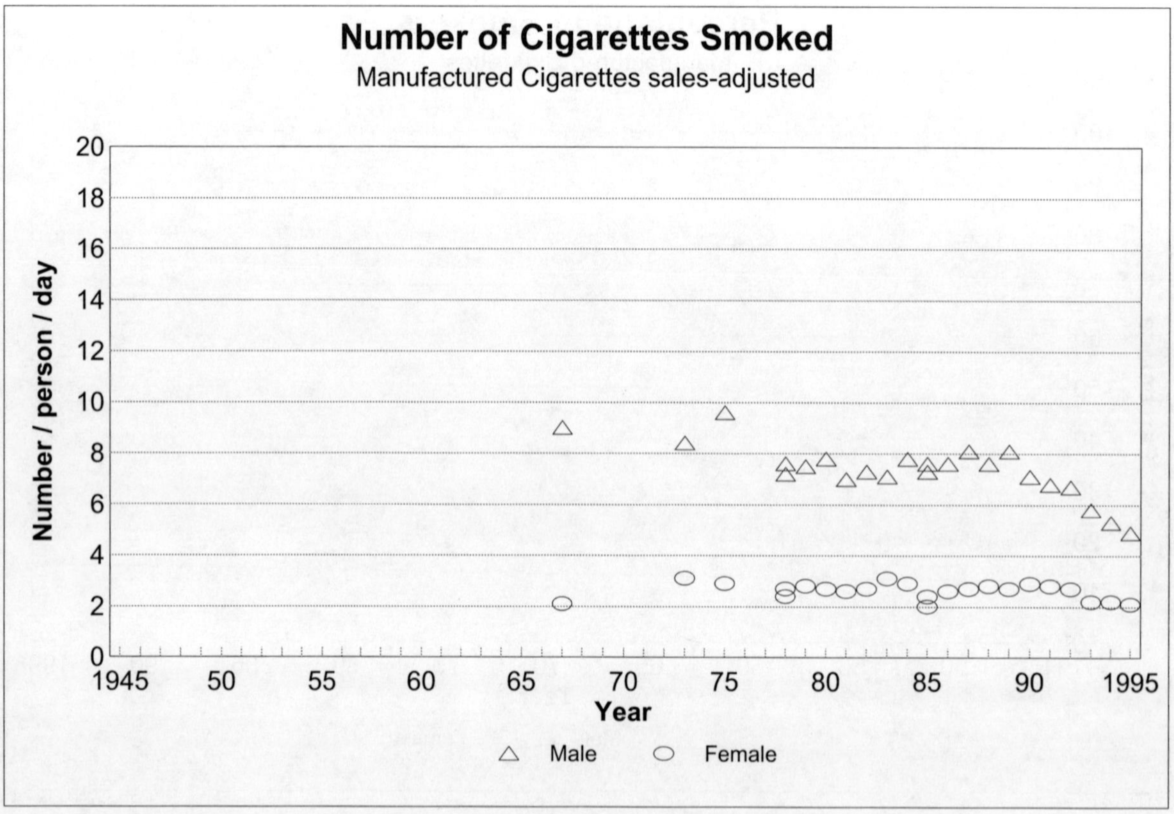

Notes

Notes on sources of sales data

The data presented in the tables and figures were obtained from several sources, details of which are given below, together with estimations and related assumptions. Full citations of the sources are given on p. 197 under *References*.

Consumption data before 1974
RP6
Data by weight, originally given to nearest 100 000 pounds, have been converted to tonnes and given to the nearest 10 tonnes (100 000 lbs = 45.359 tonnes).
Notes as given in RP6:
(a) Details of the number of cigarettes and cigars, and of the weight of pipe and chewing tobacco and snuff consumed were obtained from trade sources.
(b) Factors for conversion from number to weight of cigarettes and cigars were obtained from trade sources.

Consumption data for 1974 onwards
Tilastokeskus (Statistics Finland) (1998)
Consumption figures are wholesale trade purchases from tobacco factories and imports (January-December). Data for the preceding few years (not shown) are slightly different from those shown in Table 8.1.1.

Data were given in numbers and have been converted to weight assuming an average of 0.65 g per cigarette and 2 g per cigar or cigarillo (as given by Tilastokeskus (Statistics Finland) (1998)). These are the conventional conversion rates used by WHO.

Data for snuff and chewing tobacco 1974-1987 excludes imports, 1988-1994 includes imports, 1995 not available (assumed same as 1994 for calculation of total consumption).

Plain/Filter cigarette consumption
Maxwell (successive years)

Tar yield of cigarettes
1970 Mørck *et al* (1982)
1976-1984 National Board of Health (personal communication)
1985-1992 Tilastokeskus (Statistics Finland) (1993)
According to Statistics Finland (personal communication), data on tar content are not available after 1992.

The tar yield per cigarette was limited by EC directive (Directive 90/239/EEC) to 15 mg by the end of 1992, and to 12 mg by the end of 1997; nicotine yield is limited to 1.2 mg (Harkin *et al* (1997)).

Estimates of hand-rolled cigarette consumption for 1920-1995
According to Pedersen *et al* (1969), hand-rolling of cigarettes is very uncommon in Finland and has been assumed to be zero in calculations.

Notes on sources of survey data

Each source of survey data—either an individual survey or a series of surveys repeated over a number of years—is cited by a source number. This number is shown in the tables and corresponds to the source numbers given below, where details of the source publication and of the survey methodology are given. Full citations of the sources are given on p. 197 under *References*.

Source number

1 **Mørck *et al* (1982)**

a. Smokers: presumably included regular and occasional smokers

2 **Valtonen and Rimpelä (1984)**

a. Surveys operated by Finnish Gallup on representative sample of population
b. Smokers: smoked 'yesterday'

3 **Pedersen *et al* (1969), Martelin (1984)**

a. Baseline of a study of male lung cancer in Finland and Norway, May 1962-Feb 1963 (see also Norway source 11). Finnish part of the study was conducted in 3 urban and 3 rural areas. Personal interviews at home or work. Results presented here are weighted by region and urban/rural status. Age groups correspond to men born in 1916-1917, 1911-1915, 1906-1910, 1901-1905 and 1898-1900. Sample size 4 602, response rate 88%
b. The proportion of cigarette smokers (including ex-cigarette smokers) reporting smoking only pilli (Russian style cigarettes) was 20-40%, pölli 40-60% and both types 15-25% in the different areas
c. Consumption category estimation based on two categories, 1-14 and 15+ cigarettes/smoker/day, and resulting figures should be regarded with caution

4 **Martelin (1984), quoting Sievers *et al* (1974)**

a. Consumption category estimation based on two categories, 1-14 and 15+ cigarettes/smoker/day, and resulting figures should be regarded with caution

5 **Martelin (1984), using unpublished data from the Central Statistical Office (ELO survey)**

a. Consumption category estimation based on two categories, 1-14 and 15+ cigarettes/smoker/day, and resulting figures should be regarded with caution
b. Assumed extension to age distribution for percentage smokers, age 83+: males 15% and females 1%

6 **National Public Health Institute/Health Behaviour Research Unit**

a. Annual postal questionnaire sent to a random sample drawn from the National Population Register, two reminders sent to non-respondents. Sample size 3 500-5 000. Response rate 68-85%
b. In Tables 8.5-8, consumption shown as A relates to daily smoking frequency
c. All smokers: has smoked in last month
d. Consumption category estimation based on 1-14, 15-24 and 25+ cigarettes/cigarette smoker/day, or times/smoker/day
e. Assumed extension to age distribution for percentage smokers, age 65+: males (MC/R,-1989) 15%, (MC/R 1990-) 12% (A/R,-1989) 20%, (A/R, 1990-) 17%, (A/A,-1989) 25%, (A/A, 1990-) 20%; females (MC/R and A/R,-1979) 3%, (MC/R and A/R, 1980-) 5%, (A/A,-1979) 4%, (A/A, 1980-) 6%. Number of cigarettes/person/day: males 3.0, females 0.5.

7 **Dr J. Kaprio (personal communication)**

a. Data from Finnish Twin Cohort Study for all twins and 'pseudo-twins' respondents to the questionnaire, treated as individuals
b. Percentages differ from those given by Kaprio *et al* (1978)
c. Consumption category estimation based on 1-9, 10-19, and 20+ cigarettes/smoker/day
d. Assumed extension to age distribution for percentage smokers, age 15-17: males 25% and females 20%. Number of cigarettes/person/day: males 3.0 and females 2.0

8 **Le Meitour-Kaplan (1977), quoting Nordic Research Association (1973)**

a. Survey conducted in four Nordic countries in November-December 1973. Total sample size 6 000. Age group not stated. (See also Denmark source 3, Norway source 3, and Sweden source 4)
b. Smokers: smoked 'yesterday'

9 **M. Rimpela (personal communication) and WHO (1975), Tilastokeskus (Statistics Finland) (1998), Karvonen *et al* (1993)**

a. Juvenile Health Habit Study. National survey conducted alternate years among 14- ,16- and 18-year -olds. Postal questionnaires sent to cross-sectional sample based on consecutive dates of birth. Sample size 300-600 in each sex/age group
b. Regular smokers: smoked 1 or more cigarettes daily. Data for regular smokers differ slightly between sources

c. Calculation of consumption per person based on percentage manufactured and hand-rolled cigarette smokers and number of cigarettes per manufactured cigarette smoker (hand-rolling of cigarettes is rare)

10 Sosiaali- ja terveyshallitus (National Agency for Welfare and Health) (1992)

a. Surveys on health education conducted by Statistics Finland for National Agency for Welfare and Health. Sample size 3 000-4 000 (except 1984: 1 593, and 1990: 1 902)

b. Cigarettes include small cigars

c. Assumed extension to age distribution for percentage smokers, age 65+:males (MC) 15%, (A/R,-1989) 20%, (A/R, 1990) 17%, (A/A) 25%; females (MC) 5%, (A/R, 1979) 3%, (A/R, 1980-) 5%, (A/A) 6%

11-13 WHO MONICA Project (1988), WHO (1989), Vartiainen *et al* (1986, 1994)

a. Surveys in three regions. The 1982 survey formed part of WHO MONICA Project:

	Region	Population size	Sample size	Participation rate (%)	Sample used* Males	Sample used* Females	Date
11	North Karelia	59 800	3 085	80	1 479	1 605	Jan 1982-Apr 1982
12	Kuopio Province	87 900	2 397	85	1 454	1 315	Jan 1982-Apr 1982
13	Turku/Loimaa	74 200	3 019	85	1 580	1 678	Jan 1982-Apr 1982

* 'Sample used' includes age 25-34; all other figures are for age 35-64 only

b. *All ages* column (1982) relates only to age 35-64 and is standardized to world population

c. For earlier years, comparable methods were used, and later surveys followed the WHO MONICA protocol. Results are available only for ages 30-59, so data on the same basis are also presented here for 1982 for comparability.

		1972		1977		1982		1987		1992	
		M	F	M	F	M	F	M	F	M	F
	Sample size										
11	North Karelia	1 959	2 056	2 063	2 020	1 599	1 511	1 521	1 485	759	750
12	Kuopio Province	2 918	2 949	2 933	2 996	1 459	1 143	762	744	768	735
13	Turku/Loimaa					1 506	1 487	756	761	747	720
	Participation rate (%)										
11	North Karelia	94	96	87	91	77	84	79	87	69	82
12	Kuopio Province	91	94	89	92	83	88	82	87	76	85
13	Turku Loimaa					82	87	77	83	75	85

d. Regular cigarette smokers (1982): smoked cigarettes daily. All smokers (1982): smoked cigarettes daily or occasionally, or 1 g pipe tobacco or 1 cigar per week. Regular smokers: had smoked regularly for at least a year and had smoked more than once a day for the last month. Cigarettes per smoker (1982) refers to regular and occasional cigarette smokers. All products per smoker refers to times per day

e. Calculation for cigarettes per person (1982) based on % regular cigarette smokers and cigarettes per regular or occasional cigarette smoker, so may underestimate

14-15 Keys *et al* (1966)

a. Baseline of Seven Countries Study on cardiovascular disease in two rural areas. Interview including smoking questions before medical examinations.

	Location	Description	Sample size	Response rate (%)
14	Karelia, East Finland	Farming and forestry villages	817	99
15	West Finland	Small farming villages	860	97

b. The Russian type of cigarette, with a hollow paper mouthpiece and relatively small amount of tobacco was smoked in East Finland, but rarely in West Finland. There were additionally 'a few' pipe smokers, and cigars are stated to be smoked 'occasionally on festive occasions'

c. Consumption category estimation based on 2 categories, 1-19 and 20+ cigarettes/smoker/day, and resulting figures should be regarded with caution

16 Hibell *et al* (1997)

a. Nationally representative survey forming part of ESPAD (European School Survey Project on Alcohol and Other Drugs). Target was pupils born in 1979, thus age 15-16 at time of survey in March 1995. Approximately 99% of this group still in school. Anonymous questionnaire completed and sealed in envelope by pupil, in class. Teachers present, but discouraged from walking round the classroom. Sample size (males) 1 182, (females) 1 118. Response rate (males) 92%, (females) 91%

b. Regular smokers: smoked 1 or more cigarettes per day in last 30 days. All smokers: smoked in last 30 days

c. Consumption category estimation based on 1-5, 6-10, 11-20, 21+ cigarettes/smoker/day

17 Rimpelä *et al* (1974)

a. Study of asthma in Harjavalta community in 1966. Sample size 1 092 (20% of population), response rate 78%. Mailed follow-up in 1971

b. Assumed extension to age distribution for percentage smokers, age 65+: males 30% and females 3%

18 Heinonen *et al* (1972)

a. Multiphasic screening programme in 13 communities during 1966-1968. Sample size 22 023

b. Smokers: includes those who gave up smoking less than 1 year ago

19 Byckling and Sauri (1985)

a. Cross-sectional study for atherosclerosis precursors. Sample size 1 790

20 Benjamin (1978), quoting Finnish Health and Social Security Department

21 Aarø *et al* (1986), Nutbeam and Aarø (1990), King and Coles (1992), King *et al* (1996), WHO (1997)

a. Part of the HBSC (Health Behaviour in School-Aged Children) Study, a collaborative cross-national research study sponsored by the WHO. School classes or schools were randomly selected, targeting age groups 11 (not presented here), 13 and 15. The target sample size was 1 300 in each age group.

Year	Mean age		Sample size		
	13	15	13	15	Total*
1983-1984	13.6	15.6	—	—	3 618
1986-1987	—	—	—	1 082	—
1990	13.8	15.8	—	—	2,996
1994	13.8	15.8	1 279	1 194	4 187

* Includes age 11

c. Regular smokers: smoke once a week or more. Smokers marked as frequency *: smoked daily

22-23 Hirvonen *et al* (1965)

a. Survey among military conscripts, 1960-1963. Age group not stated.

		Sample size
22	Officer trainees	852
23	Other ranks	1 180

b. Product shown as MC relates to smoking of blended or oriental cigarettes, TC includes paper mouthpiece cigarettes

c. Category consumption estimation based on ≤5, 6-10, 11-15, 16-20, >20 cigarettes/smoker/day

References

Aarø L.E., Wold B., Kannas L. and Rimpelä M. (1986). Health behaviour in school children. A WHO cross-national survey. *Health Promotion,* **1**, 17-33.

Beese D.H. (ed) (1968). *Tobacco consumption in various countries,* 2nd edition. Tobacco Research Council, London. Research Paper 6.

Beese D.H. (ed) (1972). *Tobacco consumption in various countries,* 3rd edition. Tobacco Research Council, London. Research Paper 6.

Benjamin B. (1978). *Tobacco smoking in the world. Report of the WHO Expert Committee on Smoking Control, Geneva 23-28 October 1978*

Byckling T. and Sauri T. (1985). Atherosclerosis precursors in Finnish children and adolescents. XII. Smoking behaviour and its determinants in 12-18-year-old subjects. *Acta Paediatrica Scandinavica,* **Suppl 318**, 195-203.

Harkin A.M., Anderson P. and Goos C. (1997). *Smoking, drinking and drug taking in the European Region.* Alcohol, Drugs and Tobacco Programme, WHO Regional Office for Europe, Copenhagen.

Heinonen O.P., Poppius H., Tamminen M. and Aromaa A. (1972). Tupakointi ja kuolleisuus suomalaisessa väestössä. (Smoking and mortality in a Finnish population). *Duodecim,* **88**, 1239-44.

Hibell B., Andersson B., Bjarnason T., Kokkevi A., Morgan M. and Narusk A. (1997). *The 1995 ESPAD report. The European school survey project on alcohol and other drugs. Alcohol and other drug use among students in 26 European countries.* The Swedish Council for Information on Alcohol and Other Drugs. Council of Europe (Pompidou Group).

Hirvonen L., Lahikainen E.A. and Peltonen T. (1965). Varusmiesten tupakanpoltosta (Smoking habits of Finnish conscripts). *Ann Med milit Fenn,* **40**, 35-56.

Hutson J.B. (1937). *Consumption and production of tobacco in Europe.* USDA, Washington DC. Technical bulletin No. 587.

Kaprio J., Sarna S., Koskenvuo M. and Rantasalo I. (1978). *The Finnish Twin Registry: baseline characteristics. Section II. History of symptoms and illnesses, use of drugs, physical characteristics, smoking, alcohol and physical activity.* Dept of Public Health Science, University of Helsinki, Helsinki.

Karvonen J.S., Rimpelä A.H. and Rimpelä M.K. (1993). Modernization and smoking—regional differences in adolescent smoking in Finland in 1977-1987. *Scand J Soc Med,* **21**, 188-96.

Keys A., Aravanis C., Blackburn H.W., van Buchem F.S.P., *et al* (1966). Epidemiological studies related to coronary heart disease: characteristics of men aged 40-59 in seven countries. *Acta Medica Scandinavica,* **Suppl 460**, 8-392.

King A., Wold B., Tudor-Smith C. and Harel Y. (1996). *The health of youth, a cross-national survey.* WHO Regional Publications, Europe, Copenhagen. European Series No. 69.

King A.J.C. and Coles B. (1992). *The health of Canada's youth. Views and behaviours of 11-, 13- and 15-year-olds from 11 countries.* Health and Welfare Canada, Ottawa.

Le Meitour-Kaplan A. (1977). Situational Analysis: Profile of women's smoking habits in Continental Western Europe. In: Steinfeld J., Griffiths W., Ball K. and Taylor R.M. (eds) *Health consequences, education, cessation activities, and social action, Volume II. Proceedings of the Third World Conference on Smoking and Health, New York City, June 2-5, 1975.* US Department of Health, Education and Welfare, USA; 309-27. DHEW Publication No (NIH) 77-1413.

Lee P.N. (ed) (1975). *Tobacco consumption in various countries,* 4th edition. Tobacco Research Council, London. Research Paper 6.

Martelin T. (1984). *Tupakointitapojen kehitys Suomessa haastattelu—ja kyselytutkimusten valossa. (The development of smoking habits according to survey data in Finland).* National Board of Health, Finland, Helsinki. Health Education, Series Original Reports 1/1984.

Maxwell J.C.Jr. (successive years). How the brands ranked. Maxwell International Estimates. *World Tobacco*

Mørck H.I., Linde J., Agner E., Hein H.O., Gyntelberg F. and Nielsen P.E. (1982). Tobaksforbrug og rygevaner i Norden 1920-1980. (Tobacco consumption and smoking habits in the Nordic countries). *Nord Med,* **97**, 134-46.

Nordic Research Association (1973). *1973 Survey. Antalet rökare i fyra nordiska länder i november-december 1973.* §

Nutbeam D. and Aarø L.E. (1990). Smoking and alienation from school: the implications for health education with young people. Results from the WHO study of health behaviour in schoolchildren. In: Durston B. and Jamrozik K. (eds) *Tobacco & health 1990. The global war. Seventh World Conference on Tobacco and Health, Perth, Western Australia, 1-5 April 1990.* Organising Committee of the Seventh World Conference on Tobacco and Health, 189 Royal Street, East Perth, Western Australia 6004; 539-44.

Pedersen E., Magnus K., Mork T., Hougen A., *et al* (1969). Lung cancer in Finland and Norway, an epidemiological study. *Acta Pathologica et Microbiologica Scandinavica,* **Suppl 199**, 1-74. Munksgaard, Copenhagen.

Pernu J. (1960). An epidemiological study on cancer of the digestive organs and respiratory system: a study based on 7078 cases. *Annales Medicinae Internae Fenniae,* **49 Suppl 3**, 1-117. Duodecim, Helsinki. §

Rimpelä M., Vuori H. and Alanko K. (1974). Changes in smoking habits in Finland, 1966-1971, in the light of a cohort study. *International Journal of Health Education,* **17**, 174-80.

Sievers K., Koskelainen I. and Leppo K. (1974). *Suomalaisten sukupuolielämä. (Sexual life of the Finns).* WSOY, Porvoo.

Sosiaali- ja terveyshallitus (National Agency for Welfare and Health) (1992). *Tupakkatilasto 1991 (Tobacco statistics 1991).* National Agency for Welfare and Health, Helsinki. Health 1992:1.

RP6, See Beese (ed) (1968), Beese (ed) (1972), Lee (ed) (1975)

Tilastokeskus (Statistics Finland) (1993). *Tupakkatilasto (Tobacco statistics) 1992.* Helsinki. Health 1993:2.

Tilastokeskus (Statistics Finland) (1998). *Tupakkatilasto (Tobacco statistics) 1997.* Helsinki. Health 1998:1.

Valtonen H. and Rimpelä M. (1984). *Aikuisväestön tupakointitottumukset 1978-1982. (Smoking habits of the adult Finnish population 1978-1982).* National Board of Health, Finland, Helsinki. Health Education, Series Original Reports 3/1984.

Vartiainen E., Puska P., Jousilahti P., Korhonen H.J., Tuomilehto J. and Nissinen A. (1994). Twenty-year trends in coronary risk factors in North Karelia and in other areas of Finland. *Int J Epidemiol,* **23**, 495-504.

Vartiainen E., Puska P., Koskela K., Nissinen A. and Toumilehto J. (1986). Ten-year results of a community-based anti-smoking program (as part of the North Karelia project in Finland). *Health Education Research Theory and Practice,* **1**, 175-84.

WHO (1989). The WHO MONICA project: a worldwide monitoring system for cardiovascular diseases. In: *World health statistics annual 1989.* WHO, Geneva; 25-149.

WHO MONICA Project (1988). Geographical variation in the major risk factors of coronary heart disease in men and women aged 35-64 years. *World Health Stat Q,* **41**, 115-40.

WHO (1997). *Tobacco or health: A global status report.* WHO, Geneva. www.cdc.gov/nccdphp/osh/who/whoampro.htm.

WHO (1975). Survey on smoking and health in the European Region, 1974-75: preliminary data as at 1 May 1975. *Presented at the Third World Conference on Smoking and Health, New York, 2-5 June 1975.*

§ Original paper not obtained, but information taken as quoted by another author

France 9

Sales data

See Tables 9.1-9.3.

Data on the sales of tobacco in France are available from 1861. The consumption of manufactured cigarettes started around 1880 and reached 0.5 cigarettes per adult per day by 1920. Consumption per adult increased to nearly 6 cigarettes per day between the late 1970s and early 1990s, and then decreased to 5 by 1995. Only during the Second World War was there a dip in the consumption of manufactured cigarettes. Traditionally a high proportion of cigarettes sales in France has been of black tobacco, but in recent years blond cigarettes have overtaken black, the proportion of blond cigarettes rising from 30% in 1980 and 50% in 1985 to 73% by 1995 (Centre de Documentation et d'Information sur le Tabac (CDIT)).

We estimate that consumption of hand-rolled cigarettes per adult declined from about 1.5 to about 0.3 cigarettes per day between 1950 and 1995. Estimates of hand-rolled cigarette consumption are based on sales of 'Scaferlati', which is fine-cut tobacco used for hand-rolling and pipes.

Apart from a fall during the Second World War, the consumption per adult of all tobacco products combined increased from nearly 3 g per day in 1865 to nearly 8 g in the period between the late 1970s and early 1990s. In 1935, 37% of all tobacco consumed was as manufactured cigarettes, increasing to and then remaining at 90% by the early 1980s. Most of the remainder was sold as pipe and hand-rolling tobacco. The percentage of manufactured cigarettes that were filtered increased slowly from 11% in 1960 to 85% in 1995.

Smuggling is not a major feature of the French market. It is estimated at no more than 3% of consumption (Anonymous (2000)).

Survey data

See Tables 9.4-9.8

In 1953, the prevalence of tobacco smoking among those aged 15 years and over was 77% in men and 35% in women. The difference between the percentages of men and women who smoke has decreased since then owing to a steady decrease in the prevalence among men to around 40% in the first half of the 1990s (although one source (source 8) has consistently lower estimates since the 1960s). Estimates for the prevalence among women varied around 15-35%, with no trend evident over time. Several surveys in the 1960s and 1970s showed a high prevalence of occasional smoking: about 10-15% in both sexes.

The percentage of men who smoked other products but not cigarettes dropped from 15% in 1960 to 3-4% since the mid-1970s, with the prevalence somewhat higher for older men. Very few women smoked other tobacco products but not cigarettes. There are few data on prevalence by type of cigarette, but smoking of hand-rolled cigarettes only appears to be 5% among men and negligible among women. Several authors have noted that a higher proportion of men than women prefer black tobacco brands (sources 11 and 12, see *Notes on sources of survey data,* p. 220).

Very few data on adult smoking by age are available before the 1970s. A decrease was seen at all ages in the percentages of men smoking; this appeared greatest among men aged over 65. Among women, there has always been a strong tendency for prevalence to decline with increasing age. Results of surveys of teenage smoking varied considerably, but most showed the prevalence of smoking among girls to be similar to that among boys, particularly when occasional smokers were included.

Comparison of survey and sales data suggests that surveys under-reported consumption by 7-30%. The estimated number of manufactured cigarettes smoked per person per day (sales-adjusted) for men increased from 6 in 1960 to around 7-9 between 1968 and the early 1990s, then decreased again to 6 by 1995, while the number of cigarettes including hand-rolled cigarettes remained around 9 until 1980, after which it decreased to 7. For women the number of cigarettes was 1-2 in the 1960s and 3-4 thereafter.

Table 9.1.1 Total annual sales of tobacco products, 1865-1973

Year	Cigarettes		Cigars		Cigarillos		Smoking tobacco	Chewing tobacco	Snuff	All tobacco products
	tonnes	millions	tonnes	millions	tonnes	millions	tonnes	tonnes	tonnes	tonnes
1865		9		740			18005	1092	7846	
1875		525		837			18607	1029	6859	
1885		886		907			23995	1225	6586	
1895		1309		777			25530	1148	5237	
1905		2258		671			28498	1185	4716	
1913		4048		648			31552	1147	4715	
1924		10029		337			40222	1076	3917	
1932	21860	18186	760	190	160	102	32110	950	2540	58390
1933	21470	17861	700	176	160	103	32020	910	2400	57670
1934	20490	17045	650	163	180	110	31660	910	2310	56200
1935	19790	16464	610	152	190	118	30210	860	2180	53840
1936	20380	16952	630	157	210	130	30570	860	2000	54640
1937	21240	17674	680	169	260	160	29390	820	1860	54250
1938	21940	18253	690	172	260	160	29120	770	1720	54500
1939	23920	19902	610	153	260	160	31660	680	1630	58760
1940	22270	18527	630	157	280	174	29850	540	1410	54970
1941	17940	14924	270	67	180	114	24360	590	1090	44430
1942	13120	10918	240	60	180	114	14920	500	1180	30150
1943	12020	10001	230	58	130	81	11570	450	1180	25580
1944	10670	8878	160	41	140	85	9210	320	820	21310
1945	15910	13233	180	46	140	87	14420	450	860	31970
1946	22160	18433	200	50	140	89	18550	590	860	42500
1947	29180	24274	240	59	150	93	23900	680	910	55050
1948	31360	26089	210	53	120	78	26580	730	860	59860
1949	32950	27415	270	68	160	100	21000	640	770	55790
1950	36560	30418	390	98	240	153	21550	590	770	60110
1951	39510	32873	420	105	250	157	19780	590	730	61280
1952	40660	33824	410	102	300	189	18330	590	680	60960
1953	43770	36415	400	100	360	228	18420	540	640	64130
1954	44240	36801	420	105	380	239	18010	540	590	64180
1955	46060	38315	470	118	440	275	17370	540	590	65470
1956	49350	41059	590	147	470	294	17460	540	540	68960
1957	51590	42919	670	168	530	329	17780	640	500	71700
1958	53400	44422	760	190	570	357	18280	640	450	74100
1959	50830	42284	860	214	520	323	17740	590	410	70930
1960	53980	44904	960	241	520	326	18050	590	410	74510
1961	56060	46638	1060	264	560	351	18140	540	360	76730
1962	57990	48247	1140	285	610	381	18280	540	360	78930
1963	60050	49960	1310	328	600	372	18420	500	320	81190
1964	61020	50767	1510	378	590	371	17280	540	320	81270
1965	65550	54533	1620	406	630	393	16650	500	320	85270
1966	68580	57053	1760	440	670	416	15970	500	270	87740
1967	72570	60377	1800	451	690	434	15510	500	270	91360
1968	76070	63282	1960	491	680	425	15560	500	230	94990
1969	79150	65844	2130	532	660	410	14330	500	230	96990
1970	83720	69650	2180	546	680	426	13340	500	180	100600
1971	86720	72143	2620	656	660	411	12520	500	180	103200
1972	86630	72070	2840	710	640	398	11520	500	140	102260
1973	90610	75379	3180	795	600	378	10700	500	140	105730

Source: see *Notes on sources of sales data*, p. 219

Table 9.1.2 Total annual sales of tobacco products, 1974-1995

Year	Cigarettes tonnes	Cigarettes millions	Cigars and cigarillos tonnes	cigars millions	cigarillos millions	Pipe and hand-rolling tobacco tonnes	Snuff and chewing tobacco tonnes	All tobacco products tonnes
1974	96590	80492	4466	965	379	10263	683	112002
1975	101816	84847	5286	1172	374	9683	685	117470
1976	100646	83872	5973	1358	338	8705	691	116015
1977	103723	86436	7510	1752	314	8260	671	120164
1978	101880	84900	6685	1562	273	7613	655	116833
1979	105491	87909	6683	1568	257	7257	581	120012
1980	105154	87628	6741	1926		7140	516	119551
1981	104518	87098	6155	1865		6972	427	118072
1982	105529	87941	5351	1726		6908	416	118204
1983	107465	89554	4678	1613		6689	416	119248
1984	109384	91153	4188	1551		6469	391	120432
1985	115451	96209	4373	1749		6550	404	126778
1986	113527	94606	3687	1603		5846	372	123432
1987	113069	94224	3217	1532		5529	374	122189
1988	111599	92999	2804	1476		5235	382	120020
1989	113880	94900	2534	83	1376	4988	380	121782
1990	114960	95800	2567	87	1387	4933	397	122857
1991	116520	97100	2568	88	1385	4905	394	124387
1992	115560	96300	2400	82	1295	4969	404	123333
1993	112320	93600	2378	79	1289	5534	391	120623
1994	108120	90100	2438	78	1329	6196	370	117124
1995	105960	88300	2512	74	1385	6444	381	115297

Source : see *Notes on sources of sales data*, p. 219

Table 9.1.3 Manufactured cigarettes (i) percentage of total sales as filter cigarettes, 1958-1995, and (ii) sales-weighted average tar and nicotine yields per cigarette (SWAT and SWAN), 1950-1995 and 1992-1995

Year	% Filter	SWAT mg / cig	SWAN mg / cig
1950		30	
1958	7.5		
1959	8.7		
1960	11.5	28	
1961	14.1		
1962	17.0		
1963	19.0		
1964	21.5		
1965	24.8		
1966	28.7		
1967	31.9		
1968	33.6		
1969	35.6		
1970	38.3		
1971	42.4	24	
1972	44.9		
1973	49.9		
1974	53.8		
1975	56.6		
1976	59.3	18	
1977	59.0		
1978	58.3		
1979	60.5		
1980	61.4		
1981	62.5		
1982	63.8		
1983	65.4		
1984	67.9		
1985	70.2		
1986	71.7	17	
1987	73.3		
1988	74.9		
1989	76.3		
1990	78.5		
1991	80.5		
1992	82.3	13.6	1.03
1993	83.2	13.5	1.04
1994	84.2	13.2	1.01
1995	85.3	12.7	0.97

Source : see *Notes on sources of sales data*, p. 219

Table 9.2 Consumption of (i) cigarettes and (ii) all tobacco products, 1865-1995 sales-based data, including estimated hand-rolled cigarette consumption. Males and females aged 15 years and over

Year	Manufactured cigarettes		Hand-rolled cigarettes		Total cigarettes		All tobacco products	
	Total annual in millions	Number/ adult/day	Total annual in millions	Number/ adult/day	Total annual in millions	Number/ adult/day	Total annual in tonnes	Grams/ adult/day
1865	0	0.0					30000	2.9
1870	0	0.0					30000	3.0
1875	0	0.0					30000	3.0
1880	1000	0.1					33000	3.3
1885	1000	0.1					37000	3.6
1890	1000	0.1					36000	3.5
1895	1000	0.1					36000	3.5
1900	2000	0.2					38000	3.6
1905	2000	0.2					39000	3.7
1910	3000	0.3					42000	4.0
1915	4000	0.4					53000	4.8
1920	5000	0.5					47000	4.3
1925	10000	0.9					51000	4.5
1930	17000	1.5					55000	4.7
1932	18186	1.6					58390	5.0
1933	17861	1.6					57670	5.0
1934	17045	1.5					56200	4.9
1935	16464	1.4					53840	4.7
1936	16952	1.5					54640	4.8
1937	17674	1.5					54250	4.7
1938	18253	1.6					54500	4.8
1939	19902	1.7					58760	5.1
1940	18527	1.7					54970	5.0
1941	14924	1.4					44430	4.1
1942	10918	1.0					30150	2.8
1943	10001	0.9					25580	2.3
1944	8878	0.8					21310	1.9
1945	13233	1.2					31970	2.8
1946	18433	1.6					42500	3.7
1947	24274	2.1					55050	4.7
1948	26089	2.2					59860	5.1
1949	27415	2.3					55790	4.7
1950	30418	2.6	19849	1.7	50267	4.3	60110	5.1
1951	32873	2.8	18218	1.5	51091	4.3	61280	5.2
1952	33824	2.8	16883	1.4	50707	4.3	60960	5.1
1953	36415	3.1	16966	1.4	53381	4.5	64130	5.4
1954	36801	3.1	16588	1.4	53389	4.5	64180	5.4
1955	38315	3.2	15999	1.3	54314	4.5	65470	5.5
1956	41059	3.4	16082	1.3	57141	4.8	68960	5.7
1957	42919	3.6	16376	1.4	59295	4.9	71700	5.9
1958	44422	3.7	16837	1.4	61259	5.0	74100	6.1
1959	42284	3.5	16339	1.3	58623	4.8	70930	5.8
1960	44904	3.7	16625	1.4	61529	5.0	74510	6.1
1961	46638	3.8	16708	1.3	63346	5.1	76730	6.2
1962	48247	3.8	16837	1.3	65084	5.1	78930	6.2
1963	49960	3.9	16966	1.3	66926	5.2	81190	6.3
1964	50767	3.9	15916	1.2	66683	5.1	81270	6.2
1965	54533	4.1	15336	1.2	69869	5.3	85270	6.4
1966	57053	4.3	14709	1.1	71762	5.4	87740	6.6
1967	60377	4.5	14286	1.1	74663	5.5	91360	6.8
1968	63282	4.6	14332	1.1	77614	5.7	94990	7.0
1969	65844	4.7	13199	0.9	79043	5.7	96990	7.0

Table 9.2 *(continued)*

Year	Manufactured cigarettes		Hand-rolled cigarettes		Total cigarettes		All tobacco products	
	Total annual in millions	Number/ adult/day	Total annual in millions	Number/ adult/day	Total annual in millions	Number/ adult/day	Total annual in tonnes	Grams/ adult/day
1970	69650	4.9	12287	0.9	81937	5.8	100600	7.1
1971	72143	5.1	11532	0.8	83675	5.9	103200	7.2
1972	72070	5.0	10611	0.7	82681	5.7	102260	7.1
1973	75379	5.2	9855	0.7	85234	5.9	105730	7.3
1974	80492	5.5	9453	0.6	89945	6.1	112002	7.6
1975	84847	5.7	8919	0.6	93766	6.3	117470	7.9
1976	83872	5.6	8018	0.5	91890	6.2	116015	7.8
1977	86436	5.8	7608	0.5	94044	6.3	120164	8.0
1978	84900	5.6	7012	0.5	91912	6.1	116833	7.7
1979	87909	5.8	6684	0.4	94593	6.2	120012	7.9
1980	87628	5.7	6576	0.4	94204	6.1	119551	7.8
1981	87098	5.6	6422	0.4	93520	6.0	118072	7.6
1982	87941	5.6	6363	0.4	94304	6.0	118204	7.5
1983	89554	5.7	6161	0.4	95715	6.1	119248	7.6
1984	91153	5.7	5958	0.4	97111	6.1	120432	7.6
1985	96209	6.0	6033	0.4	102242	6.4	126778	7.9
1986	94606	5.9	5384	0.3	99990	6.3	123432	7.7
1987	94224	5.8	5093	0.3	99317	6.1	122189	7.5
1988	92999	5.7	4822	0.3	97821	6.0	120020	7.3
1989	94900	5.7	4594	0.3	99494	6.0	121782	7.4
1990	95800	5.7	4544	0.3	100344	6.0	122857	7.4
1991	97100	5.8	4518	0.3	101618	6.1	124387	7.4
1992	96300	5.7	4577	0.3	100877	6.0	123333	7.3
1993	93600	5.5	5097	0.3	98697	5.8	120623	7.1
1994	90100	5.3	5707	0.3	95807	5.6	117124	6.8
1995	88300	5.1	5935	0.3	94235	5.5	115297	6.7

Source : see *Notes on sources of sales data*, p. 219

Figure 9.1 Daily consumption of (i) manufactured and total number of cigarettes, and (ii) all tobacco products, 1920-1995.
Males and females aged 15 years and over. *Source:* see Table 9.2

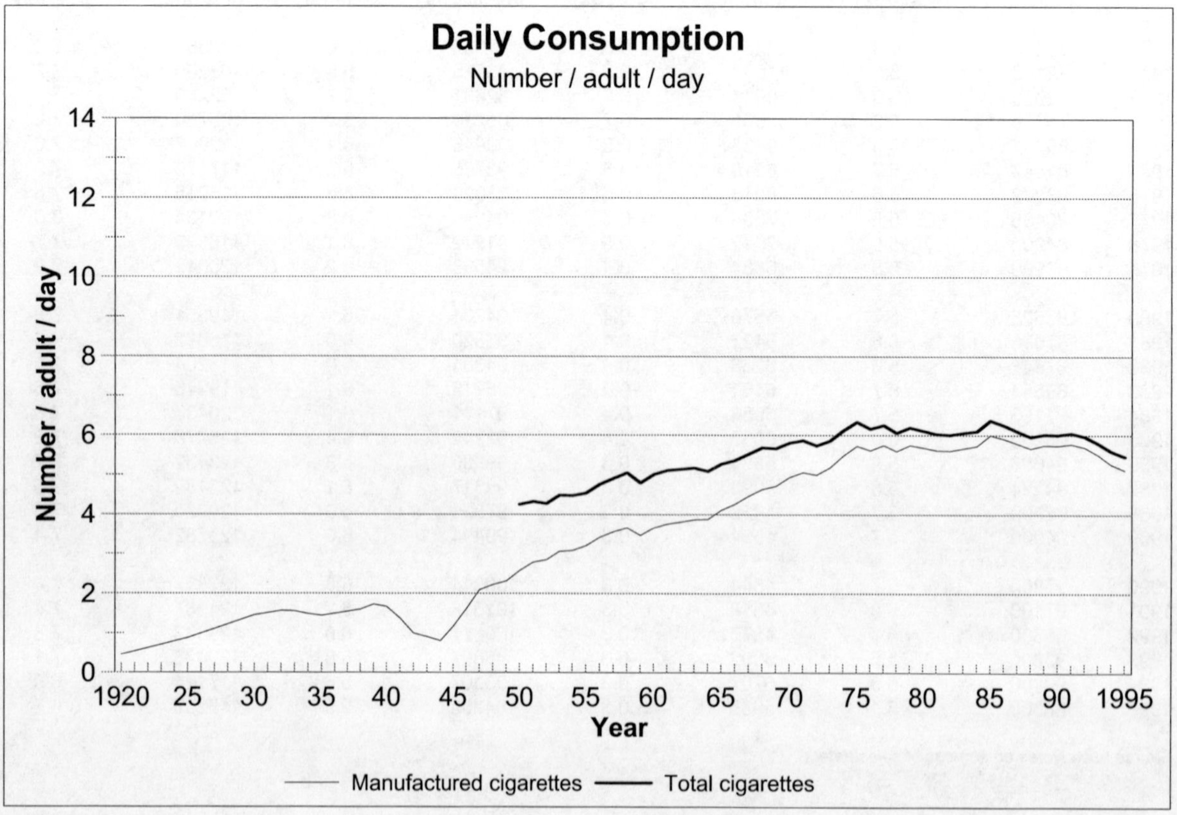

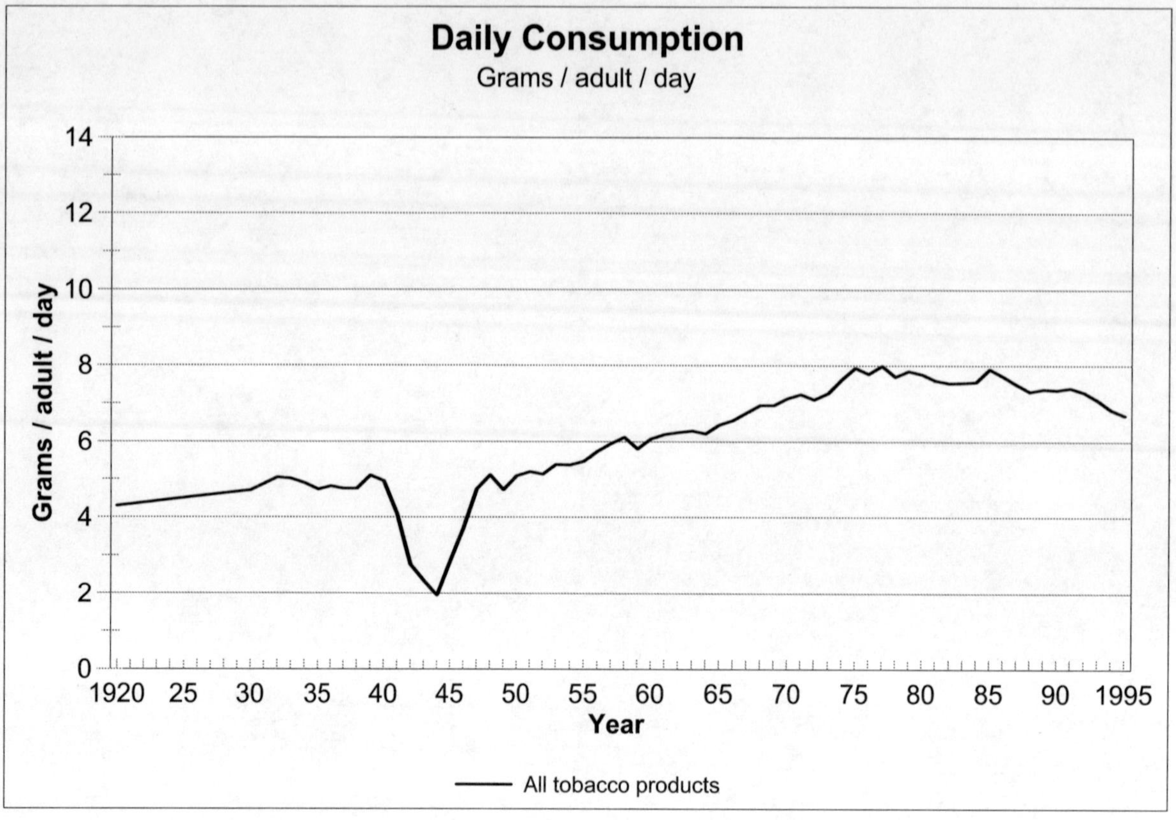

Table 9.3 Percentage sales of tobacco in different forms (by weight), selected years 1935-1995

Year	Cigarettes (%)	Cigars and cigarillos (%)	Pipe and hand-rolling tobacco (%)	Snuff and chewing tobacco(%)
1935	36.8	1.5	56.1	5.6
1945	49.8	1.0	45.1	4.1
1955	70.4	1.4	26.5	1.7
1965	76.9	2.6	19.5	1.0
1975	86.7	4.5	8.2	0.6
1985	91.1	3.4	5.2	0.3
1995	91.9	2.2	5.6	0.3

Source : calculated from Tables 9.1.1 & 9.1.2

Figure 9.2 Percentage sales of tobacco in different forms (by weight), selected years 1935-1995
Source: see Table 9.3

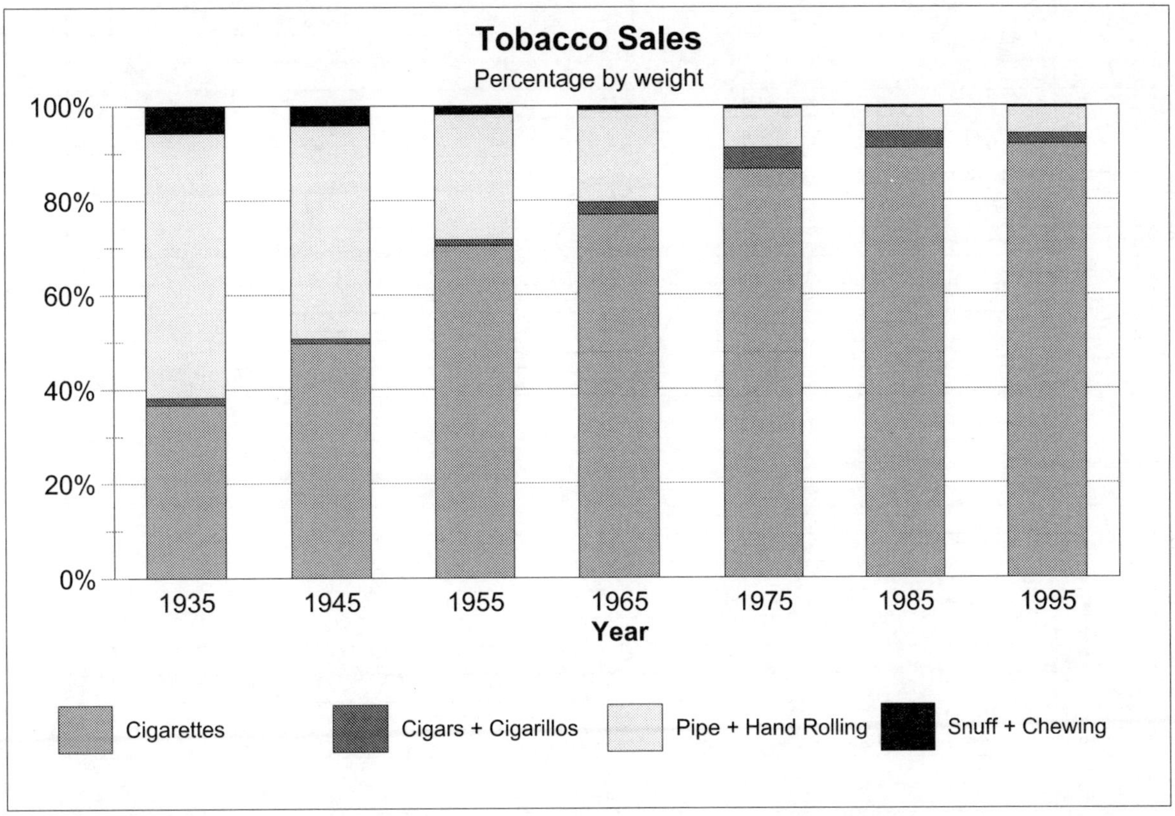

Table 9.4M Prevalence of smoking, males: some selected French surveys by age, 1953-1995 *(continues on p. 208)*

<table>
<tr><th rowspan="2">Frequency
Product
Source
Year</th><th colspan="21">Age group</th><th rowspan="2">All ages</th></tr>
<tr><th>12</th><th>13</th><th>14</th><th>15</th><th>16</th><th>17</th><th>18</th><th>19</th><th>20-24</th><th>25-29</th><th>30-34</th><th>35-39</th><th>40-44</th><th>45-49</th><th>50-54</th><th>55-59</th><th>60-64</th><th>65-69</th><th>70-74</th><th>75-79</th><th>80+</th></tr>
<tr><td>53 1 UC R</td><td colspan="8"></td><td colspan="3">73</td><td colspan="3">73</td><td colspan="3">73</td><td colspan="4">65</td><td>72</td></tr>
<tr><td>53 1 U U</td><td colspan="3"></td><td colspan="18">77</td><td></td></tr>
<tr><td>56 26 UC R</td><td colspan="11"></td><td colspan="3">84</td><td colspan="2">79</td><td colspan="5">69</td><td>77</td></tr>
<tr><td>56 26 A R</td><td colspan="11"></td><td colspan="3">88</td><td colspan="2">82</td><td colspan="5">74</td><td>81</td></tr>
<tr><td>60 1 MC R</td><td colspan="3"></td><td colspan="18">45</td><td></td></tr>
<tr><td>60 1 MC U</td><td colspan="3"></td><td colspan="18">57</td><td></td></tr>
<tr><td>60 1 A U</td><td colspan="3"></td><td colspan="18">73</td><td></td></tr>
<tr><td>60 8 U R</td><td colspan="3"></td><td colspan="18">49</td><td></td></tr>
<tr><td>63 10 UC U</td><td colspan="8"></td><td colspan="13">59</td><td></td></tr>
<tr><td>63 10 A U</td><td colspan="8"></td><td colspan="13">66</td><td></td></tr>
<tr><td>64 13 UC U</td><td colspan="10"></td><td colspan="8">64</td><td colspan="3"></td><td></td></tr>
<tr><td>65 1 U U</td><td colspan="3"></td><td colspan="18">72</td><td></td></tr>
<tr><td>65 8 U R</td><td colspan="3"></td><td colspan="18">50</td><td></td></tr>
<tr><td>68 1 MC R</td><td colspan="3"></td><td colspan="18">45</td><td></td></tr>
<tr><td>68 1 MC A</td><td colspan="3"></td><td colspan="18">62</td><td></td></tr>
<tr><td>68 1 A A</td><td colspan="3"></td><td colspan="18">72</td><td></td></tr>
<tr><td>68 1 U U</td><td colspan="8"></td><td colspan="2">75</td><td colspan="4"></td><td colspan="2">72</td><td colspan="5">65</td><td></td></tr>
<tr><td>70 8 U R</td><td colspan="3"></td><td colspan="18">53</td><td></td></tr>
<tr><td>71 17 U R</td><td colspan="3"></td><td>21</td><td>33</td><td>47</td><td>51</td><td colspan="14"></td><td></td></tr>
<tr><td>71 17 U A</td><td colspan="3"></td><td>60</td><td>64</td><td>69</td><td>70</td><td colspan="14"></td><td></td></tr>
<tr><td>71 19 A U</td><td colspan="6"></td><td>81</td><td>80</td><td>76</td><td colspan="12"></td><td>78</td></tr>
<tr><td>73 1 U U</td><td colspan="21"></td><td></td></tr>
<tr><td>73 1 U U</td><td colspan="3"></td><td colspan="18">64</td><td></td></tr>
<tr><td>74 4 U A</td><td colspan="6"></td><td colspan="15">59</td><td></td></tr>
<tr><td>76 1 MC R</td><td colspan="3"></td><td colspan="18">45</td><td></td></tr>
<tr><td>76 1 MC A</td><td colspan="3"></td><td colspan="18">56</td><td></td></tr>
<tr><td>76 1 A A</td><td colspan="3"></td><td colspan="18">62</td><td></td></tr>
<tr><td>76 4 UC U</td><td colspan="6"></td><td colspan="15">57</td><td></td></tr>
<tr><td>76 4 U A</td><td colspan="6"></td><td colspan="3">74</td><td colspan="2">62</td><td colspan="3">64</td><td colspan="3">51</td><td colspan="4">54</td><td>60</td></tr>
<tr><td>76 5 UC U</td><td colspan="6"></td><td colspan="15">53</td><td></td></tr>
<tr><td>76 5 U U</td><td colspan="6"></td><td colspan="15">57</td><td></td></tr>
<tr><td>76 8 U R</td><td colspan="3"></td><td colspan="18">47</td><td></td></tr>
<tr><td>76 11 UC U</td><td colspan="8"></td><td colspan="12">64</td><td></td><td></td></tr>
<tr><td>76 18 U U</td><td></td><td colspan="2">20</td><td>27</td><td>35</td><td>40</td><td colspan="2">44</td><td colspan="13"></td><td>33</td></tr>
<tr><td>77 3 UC R</td><td colspan="7">30</td><td colspan="14"></td><td></td></tr>
<tr><td>77 3 U A</td><td colspan="7">48</td><td colspan="14"></td><td></td></tr>
<tr><td>77 4 UC R</td><td colspan="6"></td><td colspan="15">41</td><td></td></tr>
<tr><td>77 4 UC A</td><td colspan="6"></td><td colspan="15">47</td><td></td></tr>
<tr><td>77 4 U A</td><td colspan="6"></td><td colspan="15">51</td><td></td></tr>
<tr><td>77 8 U R</td><td colspan="3"></td><td colspan="18">51</td><td></td></tr>
<tr><td>77 25 U R</td><td colspan="6">35</td><td colspan="15"></td><td></td></tr>
<tr><td>77 27 U U</td><td colspan="4">9</td><td colspan="17"></td><td></td></tr>
<tr><td>78 12 MC R</td><td colspan="8"></td><td colspan="13">45</td><td></td></tr>
<tr><td>78 12 TC R</td><td colspan="8"></td><td>61</td><td colspan="2">59</td><td colspan="2">63</td><td colspan="2">52</td><td colspan="2">39</td><td colspan="2">33</td><td colspan="2">28</td><td>50</td></tr>
<tr><td>78 12 A R</td><td colspan="8"></td><td>64</td><td colspan="2">65</td><td colspan="2">67</td><td colspan="2">56</td><td colspan="2">43</td><td colspan="2">40</td><td colspan="2">36</td><td>54</td></tr>
<tr><td>78 17 U R</td><td colspan="3"></td><td>10</td><td>22</td><td>30</td><td>40</td><td colspan="14"></td><td></td></tr>
<tr><td>78 20 UC U</td><td colspan="8"></td><td>55</td><td colspan="12"></td><td></td></tr>
<tr><td>78 20 A U</td><td colspan="8"></td><td>73</td><td colspan="12"></td><td></td></tr>
<tr><td>78 24 UC R</td><td colspan="2">5</td><td colspan="2">20</td><td colspan="2">40</td><td>38</td><td colspan="14"></td><td></td></tr>
<tr><td>79 1 MC R</td><td colspan="3"></td><td colspan="18">37</td><td></td></tr>
<tr><td>79 1 MC A</td><td colspan="3"></td><td colspan="18">42</td><td></td></tr>
<tr><td>79 1 A U</td><td colspan="3"></td><td colspan="18">50</td><td></td></tr>
<tr><td>79 4 U A</td><td colspan="6"></td><td colspan="15">54</td><td></td></tr>
<tr><td>79 4 UC U</td><td colspan="6"></td><td colspan="15">44</td><td></td></tr>
<tr><td>79 4 U A</td><td colspan="6"></td><td colspan="3">52</td><td colspan="2">48</td><td colspan="6">52</td><td colspan="4">38</td><td>48</td></tr>
<tr><td>79 8 U R</td><td colspan="3"></td><td colspan="18">40</td><td></td></tr>
<tr><td>79 21 U U</td><td></td><td colspan="6">26</td><td colspan="14"></td><td></td></tr>
<tr><td>79 28 U U</td><td colspan="5"></td><td colspan="4">64</td><td colspan="12"></td><td></td></tr>
</table>

Table 9.4F Prevalence of smoking, females: some selected French surveys by age, 1953-1995 *(continues on p. 209)*

Frequency / Product / Source / Year	Age group: 12	13	14	15	16	17	18	19	20-24	25-29	30-34	35-39	40-44	45-49	50-54	55-59	60-64	65-69	70-74	75-79	80+	All ages
53 1 UC R									24			20			11			2				17
53 1 U U				35																		
56 26 UC R																						
56 26 A R																						
60 1 MC R				12																		
60 1 MC U				28																		
60 1 A U				28																		
60 8 U R																						
63 10 UC U									15													
63 10 A U									15													
64 13 UC U											15		13		16		6					11
65 1 U U				33																		
65 8 U R																						
68 1 MC R				10																		
68 1 MC A				26																		
68 1 A A				32																		
68 1 U U				66					52								15					
70 8 U R																						
71 17 U R				16	22	28	32															
71 17 U A				67	76	80	76															
71 19 A U																						
73 1 U U				66					50													
73 1 U U				34																		
74 4 U A							28															
76 1 MC R				20																		
76 1 MC A				33																		
76 1 A A				33																		
76 4 UC U							30															
76 4 U A							56			39		26			17			7				31
76 5 UC U							26															
76 5 U U							27															
76 8 U R																						
76 11 UC U									42													
76 18 U U		15		22	31	34	38															28
77 3 UC R	22																					
77 3 U A	43																					
77 4 UC R							18															
77 4 UC A							29															
77 4 U A							29															
77 8 U R				29																		
77 25 U R	24																					
77 27 U U	11																					
78 12 MC R									14													
78 12 TC R									41	21		16		13		7		3		1		14
78 12 A R									41	21		16		13		7		3		1		14
78 17 U R				16	16	28	34															
78 20 UC U																						
78 20 A U																						
78 24 UC R	3		32		46		50															
79 1 MC R				22																		
79 1 MC A				29																		
79 1 A U				30																		
79 4 U A							23															
79 4 UC U							24															
79 4 U A							49			33		18						7				24
79 8 U R																						
79 21 U U			26																			
79 28 U U																						

Table 9.4M *(continued from p.206, continues on p. 210)*
Prevalence of smoking, males

<table>
<tr><th rowspan="2">Frequency / Product / Source / Year</th><th colspan="21">Age group</th><th rowspan="2">All ages</th></tr>
<tr><th>12</th><th>13</th><th>14</th><th>15</th><th>16</th><th>17</th><th>18</th><th>19</th><th>20-24</th><th>25-29</th><th>30-34</th><th>35-39</th><th>40-44</th><th>45-49</th><th>50-54</th><th>55-59</th><th>60-64</th><th>65-69</th><th>70-74</th><th>75-79</th><th>80+</th></tr>
<tr><td>80 3 U A</td><td colspan="2">26</td><td colspan="2">46</td><td colspan="2">63</td><td colspan="15"></td><td>45</td></tr>
<tr><td>80 6 UC R</td><td colspan="3"></td><td colspan="18">41</td><td></td></tr>
<tr><td>80 6 A R</td><td colspan="3"></td><td colspan="5">28</td><td>53</td><td colspan="2">55</td><td colspan="2">50</td><td colspan="2">46</td><td colspan="2">40</td><td colspan="2">34</td><td colspan="2">30</td><td>44</td></tr>
<tr><td>80 7 MC U</td><td colspan="3"></td><td colspan="18">45</td><td></td></tr>
<tr><td>80 7 U U</td><td colspan="3"></td><td colspan="18">52</td><td></td></tr>
<tr><td>80 8 U R</td><td colspan="3"></td><td colspan="18">46</td><td></td></tr>
<tr><td>81 3 U A</td><td colspan="7">43</td><td colspan="14"></td><td></td></tr>
<tr><td>81 5 U A</td><td colspan="6"></td><td colspan="15">50</td><td></td></tr>
<tr><td>81 9 UC U</td><td colspan="4"></td><td colspan="13">49</td><td colspan="4"></td><td></td></tr>
<tr><td>81 9 A U</td><td colspan="4"></td><td colspan="13">54</td><td colspan="4"></td><td></td></tr>
<tr><td>81 22 U U</td><td colspan="2"></td><td colspan="5">36</td><td colspan="14"></td><td></td></tr>
<tr><td>82 5 U A</td><td colspan="6"></td><td colspan="15">49</td><td></td></tr>
<tr><td>82 29 UC R</td><td colspan="3"></td><td colspan="5">24</td><td colspan="13"></td><td></td></tr>
<tr><td>83 3 U A</td><td colspan="2">15</td><td colspan="2">36</td><td colspan="2">45</td><td>57</td><td colspan="14"></td><td>36</td></tr>
<tr><td>83 4 U A</td><td colspan="3"></td><td colspan="6">56</td><td colspan="2">61</td><td colspan="3">54</td><td colspan="3">44</td><td colspan="4">32</td><td>50</td></tr>
<tr><td>83 23 UC R</td><td>2</td><td>9</td><td>20</td><td>34</td><td>45</td><td colspan="16"></td><td>16</td></tr>
<tr><td>84 3 A R</td><td colspan="2">5</td><td colspan="2">20</td><td colspan="2">42</td><td>60</td><td colspan="14"></td><td></td></tr>
<tr><td>84 3 U A</td><td colspan="2">10</td><td colspan="2">34</td><td colspan="2">52</td><td>67</td><td colspan="14"></td><td>37</td></tr>
<tr><td>84 4 U A</td><td colspan="6"></td><td colspan="15">54</td><td></td></tr>
<tr><td>85 5 U U</td><td colspan="3"></td><td colspan="18">50</td><td></td></tr>
<tr><td>85 14 UC R</td><td colspan="9"></td><td colspan="2">51</td><td colspan="2">46</td><td colspan="2">28</td><td colspan="2">27</td><td colspan="4"></td><td>34</td></tr>
<tr><td>85 14 A A</td><td colspan="9"></td><td colspan="2">54</td><td colspan="2">55</td><td colspan="2">33</td><td colspan="2">32</td><td colspan="4"></td><td>41</td></tr>
<tr><td>85 15 UC R</td><td colspan="11"></td><td colspan="2">37</td><td colspan="2">36</td><td colspan="2">36</td><td colspan="4"></td><td>37</td></tr>
<tr><td>85 15 A A</td><td colspan="11"></td><td colspan="2">45</td><td colspan="2">43</td><td colspan="2">40</td><td colspan="4"></td><td>43</td></tr>
<tr><td>85 29 UC R</td><td colspan="3">19</td><td colspan="5">33</td><td colspan="13"></td><td></td></tr>
<tr><td>85 30 U U</td><td colspan="2">13</td><td colspan="2">30</td><td>35</td><td colspan="16"></td><td>23</td></tr>
<tr><td>86 4 U R</td><td colspan="3"></td><td colspan="18">39</td><td></td></tr>
<tr><td>86 4 U A</td><td colspan="3"></td><td colspan="6">59</td><td colspan="2">61</td><td colspan="6">43</td><td colspan="4">28</td><td>46</td></tr>
<tr><td>86 6 UC R</td><td colspan="6"></td><td colspan="3">52</td><td colspan="2">54</td><td colspan="2">48</td><td colspan="2">42</td><td colspan="2">35</td><td colspan="2">27</td><td colspan="2">22</td><td>44</td></tr>
<tr><td>87 8 U R</td><td colspan="3"></td><td colspan="18">43</td><td></td></tr>
<tr><td>87 16 UC R</td><td colspan="9"></td><td colspan="2">45</td><td colspan="2">44</td><td colspan="2">38</td><td colspan="2">32</td><td colspan="4"></td><td>39</td></tr>
<tr><td>87 16 A R</td><td colspan="9"></td><td colspan="2">51</td><td colspan="2">50</td><td colspan="2">46</td><td colspan="2">40</td><td colspan="4"></td><td>46</td></tr>
<tr><td>88 3 U R</td><td colspan="2">1</td><td colspan="2">19</td><td colspan="2">35</td><td>49</td><td colspan="14"></td><td>23</td></tr>
<tr><td>88 3 U A</td><td colspan="2">5</td><td colspan="2">26</td><td colspan="2">51</td><td>61</td><td colspan="14"></td><td>33</td></tr>
<tr><td>88 8 U R</td><td colspan="3"></td><td colspan="18">39</td><td></td></tr>
<tr><td>88 30 U U</td><td colspan="2">5</td><td colspan="2">20</td><td>26</td><td colspan="16"></td><td>14</td></tr>
<tr><td>88 31 UC R</td><td colspan="8">18</td><td colspan="13"></td><td></td></tr>
<tr><td>88 31 UC A</td><td colspan="8">30</td><td colspan="13"></td><td></td></tr>
<tr><td>89 4 U R</td><td colspan="3"></td><td colspan="18">45</td><td></td></tr>
<tr><td>89 4 U A</td><td colspan="3"></td><td colspan="18">48</td><td></td></tr>
<tr><td>90 3 U A</td><td colspan="2">14</td><td colspan="2">34</td><td colspan="2">56</td><td>61</td><td colspan="14"></td><td>39</td></tr>
<tr><td>90 8 U R</td><td colspan="3"></td><td colspan="18">38</td><td></td></tr>
<tr><td>90 23 UC R</td><td>1</td><td>2</td><td>7</td><td>23</td><td>34</td><td colspan="16"></td><td></td></tr>
<tr><td>90 32 U R</td><td colspan="2"></td><td>6</td><td>11</td><td colspan="17"></td><td></td></tr>
<tr><td>90 32 U A</td><td>0</td><td colspan="3">10</td><td colspan="17"></td><td></td></tr>
<tr><td>91 3 U A</td><td colspan="2">9</td><td colspan="2">20</td><td colspan="2">46</td><td>68</td><td colspan="14"></td><td>31</td></tr>
<tr><td>91 4 U R</td><td colspan="6"></td><td colspan="15">38</td><td></td></tr>
<tr><td>91 4 U A</td><td colspan="6"></td><td colspan="3">70</td><td colspan="2">48</td><td colspan="6">46</td><td colspan="4">25</td><td>46</td></tr>
<tr><td>91 6 UC R</td><td colspan="6"></td><td colspan="3">46</td><td colspan="2">51</td><td colspan="2">46</td><td colspan="2">40</td><td colspan="2">30</td><td colspan="2">22</td><td colspan="2">15</td><td>39</td></tr>
<tr><td>91 33 MC U</td><td colspan="6"></td><td colspan="15">39</td><td></td></tr>
<tr><td>91 34 UC R</td><td colspan="9">21</td><td colspan="12"></td><td></td></tr>
<tr><td>91 34 UC A</td><td colspan="9">57</td><td colspan="12"></td><td></td></tr>
<tr><td>92 3 U A</td><td colspan="7">35</td><td colspan="14"></td><td></td></tr>
<tr><td>92 4 UC R</td><td colspan="6"></td><td colspan="15">43</td><td></td></tr>
<tr><td>92 4 A U</td><td colspan="6"></td><td colspan="3">65</td><td colspan="2">60</td><td colspan="2">53</td><td colspan="3">49</td><td colspan="5">25</td><td>48</td></tr>
<tr><td>92 33 MC U</td><td colspan="6"></td><td colspan="3">21</td><td colspan="2">31</td><td colspan="2">26</td><td colspan="8">23</td><td>38</td></tr>
<tr><td>92 35 UC R</td><td colspan="6"></td><td colspan="13">40</td><td colspan="2"></td><td></td></tr>
<tr><td>92 35 U A</td><td colspan="6"></td><td colspan="13">44</td><td colspan="2"></td><td></td></tr>
</table>

Frequency / Product / Source / Year	12	13	14	15	16	17	18	19	20-24	25-29	30-34	35-39	40-44	45-49	50-54	55-59	60-64	65-69	70-74	75-79	80+	All ages
80 3 U A	20		42		61																	42
80 6 UC R				16																		
80 6 A R				20					36	25		17		12		10		4		2		16
80 7 MC U				28																		
80 7 U U				28																		
80 8 U R				16																		
81 3 U A	45																					
81 5 U A							26															
81 9 UC U					40																	
81 9 A U					40																	
81 22 U U			41																			
82 5 U A							26															
82 29 UC R				26																		
83 3 U A	14		25		54		62															36
83 4 U A				54						39		31			17			6				29
83 23 UC R	1	12	16	35	39																	18
84 3 A R	7		23		45		50															
84 3 U A	14		37		60		65															42
84 4 U A							33															
85 5 U U				25																		
85 14 UC R										30		22		11		8						15
85 14 A A										31		28		13		9						18
85 15 UC R												24		16		10						17
85 15 A A												25		17		12						19
85 29 UC R	18			46																		
85 30 U U	12		29		41																	23
86 4 U R				24																		
86 4 U A				55						48		22						9				30
86 6 UC R							42			36		20		13		9		6		2		20
87 8 U R				20																		
87 16 UC R										28		17		10		3						11
87 16 A R										34		22		17		5						16
88 3 U R	3		15		35		40															21
88 3 U A	5		30		48		56															32
88 8 U R				19																		
88 30 U U	5		13		16																	10
88 31 UC R	22																					
88 31 UC A	34																					
89 4 U R				30																		
89 4 U A				33																		
90 3 U A	8		22		52		50															32
90 8 U R				19																		
90 23 UC R	0	3	13	23	38																	
90 32 U R			4	7																		
90 32 U A	2	7																				
91 3 U A	6		22		49		52															29
91 4 U R							26															
91 4 U A							62			52		26						6				35
91 6 UC R							35			36		24		16		9		5		2		20
91 33 MC U							28															
91 34 UC R	26																					
91 34 UC A	47																					
92 3 U A	33																					
92 4 UC R							29															
92 4 A U							62			52		39		20			8					33
92 33 MC U							27			34		25		14								28
92 35 UC R							27															
92 35 U A							29															

Table 9.4M *(continued from p. 208)*
Prevalence of smoking, males

<table>
<tr><th rowspan="2">Frequency
Product
Source
Year</th><th colspan="21">Age group</th><th rowspan="2">All ages</th></tr>
<tr><th>12</th><th>13</th><th>14</th><th>15</th><th>16</th><th>17</th><th>18</th><th>19</th><th>20-24</th><th>25-29</th><th>30-34</th><th>35-39</th><th>40-44</th><th>45-49</th><th>50-54</th><th>55-59</th><th>60-64</th><th>65-69</th><th>70-74</th><th>75-79</th><th>80+</th></tr>
<tr><td>93 4 U R</td><td colspan="6"></td><td colspan="15">36</td><td></td></tr>
<tr><td>93 4 U A</td><td colspan="6"></td><td colspan="3">55</td><td colspan="2">58</td><td colspan="2">42</td><td colspan="2">28</td><td colspan="2">14</td><td colspan="4"></td><td>40</td></tr>
<tr><td>93 33 MC U</td><td colspan="6"></td><td colspan="3">21</td><td colspan="2">31</td><td colspan="2">26</td><td colspan="8">22</td><td>37</td></tr>
<tr><td>93 35 UC R</td><td colspan="6"></td><td colspan="13">36</td><td colspan="2"></td><td></td></tr>
<tr><td>93 35 U A</td><td colspan="6"></td><td colspan="13">40</td><td colspan="2"></td><td></td></tr>
<tr><td>94 3 U A</td><td colspan="8">31</td><td colspan="13"></td><td></td></tr>
<tr><td>94 33 MC U</td><td colspan="6"></td><td colspan="3">21</td><td colspan="2">31</td><td colspan="2">26</td><td colspan="8">22</td><td>36</td></tr>
<tr><td>94 36 UC R</td><td></td><td>11</td><td></td><td>23</td><td colspan="17"></td><td></td></tr>
<tr><td>94 37 U U</td><td colspan="4">6</td><td colspan="2">24</td><td colspan="2">36</td><td colspan="13"></td><td></td></tr>
<tr><td>95 3 U A</td><td colspan="2">5</td><td colspan="2">30</td><td colspan="2">47</td><td>62</td><td colspan="14"></td><td>35</td></tr>
<tr><td>95 4 U U</td><td colspan="6"></td><td colspan="13">41</td><td colspan="2"></td><td></td></tr>
<tr><td>95 33 MC U</td><td colspan="6"></td><td colspan="3">22</td><td colspan="2">31</td><td colspan="2">25</td><td colspan="8">22</td><td>34</td></tr>
<tr><td>95 35 U U</td><td colspan="6"></td><td colspan="13">41</td><td colspan="2"></td><td></td></tr>
</table>

Table 9.5M Number of cigarettes smoked per smoker per day, males:
some selected French surveys by age, 1956-1995

<table>
<tr><th rowspan="2">Product
Source
Year</th><th colspan="21">Age group</th><th rowspan="2">All ages</th></tr>
<tr><th>12</th><th>13</th><th>14</th><th>15</th><th>16</th><th>17</th><th>18</th><th>19</th><th>20-24</th><th>25-29</th><th>30-34</th><th>35-39</th><th>40-44</th><th>45-49</th><th>50-54</th><th>55-59</th><th>60-64</th><th>65-69</th><th>70-74</th><th>75-79</th><th>80+</th></tr>
<tr><td>56 26 A *</td><td colspan="11"></td><td colspan="3">17</td><td colspan="2">15</td><td colspan="5">14</td><td>15</td></tr>
<tr><td>64 13 UCE*</td><td colspan="10"></td><td colspan="8">16</td><td colspan="3"></td><td></td></tr>
<tr><td>71 17 UCE*</td><td colspan="3"></td><td>7</td><td>8</td><td>10</td><td>12</td><td>13</td><td colspan="13"></td><td></td></tr>
<tr><td>71 19 AE</td><td colspan="6"></td><td>15</td><td>16</td><td>18</td><td colspan="12"></td><td>17</td></tr>
<tr><td>76 18 UC</td><td></td><td colspan="7">9.3</td><td colspan="13"></td><td></td></tr>
<tr><td>78 12 TC</td><td colspan="8"></td><td>16</td><td colspan="2">17</td><td colspan="2">16</td><td colspan="2">16</td><td colspan="2">15</td><td colspan="2">15</td><td colspan="2">10</td><td>17</td></tr>
<tr><td>78 20 AE</td><td colspan="8"></td><td>⟨18⟩</td><td colspan="12"></td><td></td></tr>
<tr><td>79 21 UC</td><td colspan="2"></td><td colspan="5">9.6</td><td colspan="14"></td><td></td></tr>
<tr><td>80 6 UC</td><td colspan="3"></td><td colspan="18">16</td><td></td></tr>
<tr><td>81 9 UCE</td><td colspan="4"></td><td colspan="13">17</td><td colspan="4"></td><td></td></tr>
<tr><td>81 22 UC</td><td colspan="2"></td><td colspan="5">9.5</td><td colspan="14"></td><td></td></tr>
<tr><td>83 4 UCE</td><td colspan="3"></td><td colspan="6">14</td><td colspan="2">18</td><td colspan="3">18</td><td colspan="3">17</td><td colspan="4">14</td><td>17</td></tr>
<tr><td>83 4 UC</td><td colspan="3"></td><td colspan="18">15</td><td></td></tr>
<tr><td>85 14 UC</td><td colspan="11"></td><td colspan="6">18</td><td colspan="4"></td><td></td></tr>
<tr><td>85 15 UC</td><td colspan="11"></td><td colspan="6">18</td><td colspan="4"></td><td></td></tr>
<tr><td>85 23 UC</td><td colspan="5">6.1</td><td colspan="16"></td><td></td></tr>
<tr><td>88 31 UCE*</td><td colspan="8">14</td><td colspan="13"></td><td></td></tr>
<tr><td>90 23 UC</td><td colspan="5">5.0</td><td colspan="16"></td><td></td></tr>
<tr><td>91 34 UC</td><td colspan="9">10</td><td colspan="12"></td><td></td></tr>
<tr><td>92 4 UCE</td><td colspan="6"></td><td colspan="15">17</td><td></td></tr>
<tr><td>92 4 UC</td><td colspan="6"></td><td colspan="15">15</td><td></td></tr>
<tr><td>94 37 UC</td><td colspan="4">8.8</td><td colspan="2">8.8</td><td colspan="2">11</td><td colspan="13"></td><td></td></tr>
<tr><td>95 3 UC</td><td colspan="2"></td><td colspan="2">6.0</td><td colspan="2">10</td><td>11</td><td colspan="14"></td><td></td></tr>
<tr><td>95 4 UC</td><td colspan="6"></td><td colspan="13">17</td><td colspan="2"></td><td></td></tr>
<tr><td>95 35 UC</td><td colspan="6"></td><td colspan="13">15</td><td colspan="2"></td><td></td></tr>
</table>

Source: see *Notes on sources of survey data*, p. 220
Frequency: A = all smokers (including occasional)
R = regular or daily smokers
All ages: relevant to ages used and as given in original source
U = unspecified
* = refer to *Notes on sources of survey data*, p. 220

Product: MC = manufactured cigarettes
TC = total cigarettes (including hand-rolled)
UC = cigarettes (type unspecified)
A = all products
E indicates mean estimated from percentage distribution (see also *Consumption category estimation*, p. xxxiv, and Appendix III, p. 789)

Table 9.4F *(continued from p. 209)* Prevalence of smoking, females

<table>
<tr><th rowspan="2">Frequency
Product
Source
Year</th><th colspan="21">Age group</th><th rowspan="2">All ages</th></tr>
<tr><th>12</th><th>13</th><th>14</th><th>15</th><th>16</th><th>17</th><th>18</th><th>19</th><th>20-24</th><th>25-29</th><th>30-34</th><th>35-39</th><th>40-44</th><th>45-49</th><th>50-54</th><th>55-59</th><th>60-64</th><th>65-69</th><th>70-74</th><th>75-79</th><th>80+</th></tr>
<tr><td>93 4 U R</td><td colspan="6"></td><td colspan="15">23</td><td></td></tr>
<tr><td>93 4 U A</td><td colspan="6"></td><td colspan="3">40</td><td colspan="2">44</td><td colspan="2">29</td><td colspan="2">9</td><td colspan="2">5</td><td colspan="4"></td><td>27</td></tr>
<tr><td>93 33 MC U</td><td colspan="6"></td><td colspan="3">25</td><td colspan="2">35</td><td colspan="2">24</td><td colspan="8">16</td><td>28</td></tr>
<tr><td>93 35 UC R</td><td colspan="6"></td><td colspan="13">23</td><td colspan="2"></td><td></td></tr>
<tr><td>93 35 U A</td><td colspan="6"></td><td colspan="13">27</td><td colspan="2"></td><td></td></tr>
<tr><td>94 3 U A</td><td colspan="7">31</td><td colspan="14"></td><td></td></tr>
<tr><td>94 33 MC U</td><td colspan="6"></td><td colspan="3">26</td><td colspan="2">33</td><td colspan="2">25</td><td colspan="8">16</td><td>28</td></tr>
<tr><td>94 36 UC R</td><td></td><td>13</td><td></td><td>25</td><td colspan="17"></td><td></td></tr>
<tr><td>94 37 U U</td><td colspan="4">14</td><td colspan="2">31</td><td colspan="2">47</td><td colspan="13"></td><td></td></tr>
<tr><td>95 3 U A</td><td colspan="2">10</td><td colspan="2">31</td><td colspan="2">57</td><td>55</td><td colspan="14"></td><td>35</td></tr>
<tr><td>95 4 U U</td><td colspan="6"></td><td colspan="13">30</td><td colspan="2"></td><td></td></tr>
<tr><td>95 33 MC U</td><td colspan="6"></td><td colspan="3">25</td><td colspan="2">34</td><td colspan="2">25</td><td colspan="8">16</td><td>28</td></tr>
<tr><td>95 35 U U</td><td colspan="6"></td><td colspan="13">31</td><td colspan="2"></td><td></td></tr>
</table>

Table 9.5F Number of cigarettes smoked per smoker per day, females: some selected French surveys by age, 1956-1995

<table>
<tr><th rowspan="2">Product
Source
Year</th><th colspan="21">Age group</th><th rowspan="2">All ages</th></tr>
<tr><th>12</th><th>13</th><th>14</th><th>15</th><th>16</th><th>17</th><th>18</th><th>19</th><th>20-24</th><th>25-29</th><th>30-34</th><th>35-39</th><th>40-44</th><th>45-49</th><th>50-54</th><th>55-59</th><th>60-64</th><th>65-69</th><th>70-74</th><th>75-79</th><th>80+</th></tr>
<tr><td>56 26 A *</td><td colspan="21"></td><td></td></tr>
<tr><td>64 13 UCE*</td><td colspan="10"></td><td colspan="2">7.9</td><td colspan="2">9.1</td><td colspan="2">9.4</td><td colspan="2">8.6</td><td colspan="3"></td><td>10</td></tr>
<tr><td>71 17 UCE*</td><td colspan="3"></td><td>5</td><td>6</td><td>8</td><td>8</td><td>6</td><td colspan="13"></td><td></td></tr>
<tr><td>71 19 AE</td><td colspan="21"></td><td></td></tr>
<tr><td>76 18 UC</td><td></td><td colspan="7">7.1</td><td colspan="13"></td><td></td></tr>
<tr><td>78 12 TC</td><td colspan="8"></td><td>11</td><td colspan="2">11</td><td colspan="2">12</td><td colspan="2">11</td><td colspan="2">11</td><td colspan="2">8</td><td colspan="2">3</td><td>11</td></tr>
<tr><td>78 20 AE</td><td colspan="21"></td><td></td></tr>
<tr><td>79 21 UC</td><td colspan="2"></td><td colspan="5">7.7</td><td colspan="14"></td><td></td></tr>
<tr><td>80 6 UC</td><td colspan="3"></td><td colspan="18">12</td><td></td></tr>
<tr><td>81 9 UCE</td><td colspan="4"></td><td colspan="13">12</td><td colspan="4"></td><td></td></tr>
<tr><td>81 22 UC</td><td colspan="2"></td><td colspan="5">8.0</td><td colspan="14"></td><td></td></tr>
<tr><td>83 4 UCE</td><td colspan="3"></td><td colspan="6">11</td><td colspan="2">11</td><td colspan="3">14</td><td colspan="3">10</td><td colspan="4">11</td><td>12</td></tr>
<tr><td>83 4 UC</td><td colspan="3"></td><td colspan="18">11</td><td></td></tr>
<tr><td>85 14 UC</td><td colspan="11"></td><td colspan="6">12</td><td colspan="4"></td><td></td></tr>
<tr><td>85 15 UC</td><td colspan="11"></td><td colspan="6">13</td><td colspan="4"></td><td></td></tr>
<tr><td>85 23 UC</td><td colspan="5">7.6</td><td colspan="16"></td><td></td></tr>
<tr><td>88 31 UCE*</td><td colspan="8">11</td><td colspan="13"></td><td></td></tr>
<tr><td>90 23 UC</td><td colspan="5">5.5</td><td colspan="16"></td><td></td></tr>
<tr><td>91 34 UC</td><td colspan="8">9.1</td><td colspan="13"></td><td></td></tr>
<tr><td>92 4 UCE</td><td colspan="6"></td><td colspan="15">15</td><td></td></tr>
<tr><td>92 4 UC</td><td colspan="6"></td><td colspan="15">11</td><td></td></tr>
<tr><td>94 37 UC</td><td colspan="4">6.7</td><td colspan="2">8.6</td><td colspan="2">9.2</td><td colspan="13"></td><td></td></tr>
<tr><td>95 3 UC</td><td colspan="2"></td><td colspan="2">6.2</td><td colspan="2">9.2</td><td>11</td><td colspan="14"></td><td></td></tr>
<tr><td>95 4 UC</td><td colspan="6"></td><td colspan="13">15</td><td colspan="2"></td><td></td></tr>
<tr><td>95 35 UC</td><td colspan="6"></td><td colspan="13">12</td><td colspan="2"></td><td></td></tr>
</table>

Source: see *Notes on sources of survey data*, p. 220
Frequency: A = all smokers (including occasional)
R = regular or daily smokers
All ages: relevant to ages used and as given in original source
U = unspecified
* = refer to *Notes on sources of survey data*, p. 220

Product: MC = manufactured cigarettes
TC = total cigarettes (including hand-rolled)
UC = cigarettes (type unspecified)
A = all products
E indicates mean estimated from percentage distribution (see also *Consumption category estimation*, p. xxxiv, and Appendix III, p. 789)

Table 9.6M Number of cigarettes smoked per person per day, males: some selected French surveys by age, 1956-1995, with percentage total sales

<table>
<tr><th rowspan="2">Product
Source
Year</th><th colspan="21">Age group</th><th rowspan="2">All ages</th><th rowspan="2">% Total sales</th></tr>
<tr><th>12</th><th>13</th><th>14</th><th>15</th><th>16</th><th>17</th><th>18</th><th>19</th><th>20-24</th><th>25-29</th><th>30-34</th><th>35-39</th><th>40-44</th><th>45-49</th><th>50-54</th><th>55-59</th><th>60-64</th><th>65-69</th><th>70-74</th><th>75-79</th><th>80+</th></tr>
<tr><td>56 26 A *</td><td colspan="11"></td><td colspan="3">15</td><td colspan="2">13</td><td colspan="5">10</td><td>12</td><td>**</td></tr>
<tr><td>64 13 UC *</td><td colspan="10"></td><td colspan="8">10</td><td colspan="3"></td><td></td><td>**</td></tr>
<tr><td>71 17 UC *</td><td colspan="3"></td><td>1.4</td><td>2.5</td><td>4.7</td><td>6.0</td><td colspan="14"></td><td></td><td>**</td></tr>
<tr><td>71 19 A</td><td colspan="6"></td><td>12</td><td>13</td><td>14</td><td colspan="12"></td><td>13</td><td>**</td></tr>
<tr><td>76 18 UC</td><td></td><td colspan="7">3.1</td><td colspan="13"></td><td></td><td>**</td></tr>
<tr><td>78 12 TC</td><td colspan="8"></td><td>9.8</td><td colspan="2">10</td><td colspan="2">10</td><td colspan="2">8.4</td><td colspan="2">5.9</td><td colspan="2">5.0</td><td colspan="2">2.8</td><td>8.4</td><td>79%T</td></tr>
<tr><td>78 20 A</td><td colspan="8"></td><td>⟨13⟩</td><td colspan="12"></td><td></td><td>**</td></tr>
<tr><td>79 21 UC</td><td colspan="2"></td><td colspan="5">2.5</td><td colspan="14"></td><td></td><td>**</td></tr>
<tr><td>80 2 MC</td><td colspan="3"></td><td colspan="18">8.6</td><td></td><td>---M</td></tr>
<tr><td>80 6 UC</td><td colspan="3"></td><td colspan="18">6.5</td><td></td><td>68%T</td></tr>
<tr><td>81 9 UC</td><td colspan="4"></td><td colspan="13">8.3</td><td colspan="4"></td><td></td><td>93%T</td></tr>
<tr><td>81 22 UC</td><td colspan="2"></td><td colspan="5">3.4</td><td colspan="14"></td><td></td><td>**</td></tr>
<tr><td>83 4 UC *</td><td colspan="3"></td><td colspan="6">7.8</td><td colspan="2">11</td><td colspan="3">9.7</td><td colspan="3">7.5</td><td colspan="4">4.5</td><td></td><td>95%T</td></tr>
<tr><td>83 4 UC</td><td colspan="3"></td><td colspan="18">7.5</td><td></td><td>87%T</td></tr>
<tr><td>85 14 UC *</td><td colspan="11"></td><td colspan="6">6.2</td><td colspan="4"></td><td></td><td>**</td></tr>
<tr><td>85 15 UC *</td><td colspan="11"></td><td colspan="6">6.6</td><td colspan="4"></td><td></td><td>**</td></tr>
<tr><td>85 23 UC</td><td colspan="5">0.9</td><td colspan="16"></td><td></td><td>**</td></tr>
<tr><td>88 31 UC *</td><td colspan="8">2.5</td><td colspan="13"></td><td></td><td>**</td></tr>
<tr><td>91 34 UC</td><td colspan="9">2.1</td><td colspan="12"></td><td></td><td>**</td></tr>
<tr><td>92 4 UC</td><td colspan="6"></td><td colspan="15">7.1</td><td></td><td>92%T</td></tr>
<tr><td>94 37 UC</td><td colspan="4">0.5</td><td colspan="2">2.1</td><td colspan="2">4.1</td><td colspan="13"></td><td></td><td>**</td></tr>
<tr><td>95 3 UC</td><td colspan="2"></td><td colspan="2">1.8</td><td colspan="2">4.8</td><td>6.9</td><td colspan="14"></td><td></td><td>**</td></tr>
<tr><td>95 4 UC *</td><td colspan="6"></td><td colspan="13">6.7</td><td colspan="2"></td><td></td><td>93%T</td></tr>
<tr><td>95 35 UC *</td><td colspan="6"></td><td colspan="13">6.2</td><td colspan="2"></td><td></td><td>85%T</td></tr>
</table>

Table 9.7M Number of cigarettes smoked per person per day, sales-adjusted, males: some selected French surveys[1] by age, 1978-1995, with percentage total sales

<table>
<tr><th rowspan="2">Product
Source
Year</th><th colspan="21">Age group</th><th rowspan="2">All ages</th><th rowspan="2">% Total sales</th></tr>
<tr><th>12</th><th>13</th><th>14</th><th>15</th><th>16</th><th>17</th><th>18</th><th>19</th><th>20-24</th><th>25-29</th><th>30-34</th><th>35-39</th><th>40-44</th><th>45-49</th><th>50-54</th><th>55-59</th><th>60-64</th><th>65-69</th><th>70-74</th><th>75-79</th><th>80+</th></tr>
<tr><td>78 12 TC</td><td colspan="8"></td><td>12</td><td colspan="2">13</td><td colspan="2">13</td><td colspan="2">11</td><td colspan="2">7.5</td><td colspan="2">6.4</td><td colspan="2">3.6</td><td>11</td><td>79%T</td></tr>
<tr><td>80 2 MC</td><td colspan="3"></td><td colspan="18">8.6</td><td></td><td>---M</td></tr>
<tr><td>80 6 UC</td><td colspan="3"></td><td colspan="18">9.6</td><td></td><td>68%T</td></tr>
<tr><td>81 9 UC</td><td colspan="4"></td><td colspan="13">8.9</td><td colspan="4"></td><td></td><td>93%T</td></tr>
<tr><td>83 4 UC *</td><td colspan="3"></td><td colspan="6">8.2</td><td colspan="2">12</td><td colspan="3">10</td><td colspan="3">7.9</td><td colspan="4">4.7</td><td></td><td>95%T</td></tr>
<tr><td>83 4 UC</td><td colspan="3"></td><td colspan="18">8.6</td><td></td><td>87%T</td></tr>
<tr><td>92 4 UC</td><td colspan="6"></td><td colspan="15">7.7</td><td></td><td>92%T</td></tr>
<tr><td>95 4 UC *</td><td colspan="6"></td><td colspan="13">7.2</td><td colspan="2"></td><td></td><td>93%T</td></tr>
<tr><td>95 35 UC *</td><td colspan="6"></td><td colspan="13">7.4</td><td colspan="2"></td><td></td><td>85%T</td></tr>
</table>

1 Based on those surveys in Table 9.6 with data for both sexes and age range at least 21-64 (see *Cigarette consumption per person*, p. xxxv)

Source: see *Notes on sources of survey data*, p. 220
All ages: relevant to ages used and as given in original source
% Total sales: estimated % of total sales of M = manufactured or T = total cigarette consumption implied by survey, sexes combined, used as adjustment factor in Table 9.7
** = cannot be calculated
--- = adjusted by original author

Product: MC = manufactured cigarettes
TC = total cigarettes (including hand-rolled)
UC = cigarettes (type unspecified)
A = all products
U = unspecified
* = refer to *Notes on sources of survey data*, p. 220

Table 9.6F Number of cigarettes smoked per person per day, females: some selected French surveys by age, 1956-1995, with percentage total sales

Product Source Year	Age group 12	13	14	15	16	17	18	19	20-24	25-29	30-34	35-39	40-44	45-49	50-54	55-59	60-64	65-69	70-74	75-79	80+	All ages	% Total sales
56 26 A *																							**
64 13 UC *											1.2		1.2		1.5		0.5					1.1	**
71 17 UC *				0.8	1.2	2.1	2.5																**
71 19 A																							**
76 18 UC		2.0																					**
78 12 TC									4.5	2.3		1.9		1.4		0.8		0.2		0.0		1.5	79%T
78 20 A																							**
79 21 UC			2.0																				**
80 2 MC				3.1																			---M
80 6 UC				1.9																			68%T
81 9 UC					4.8																		93%T
81 22 UC			3.3																				**
83 4 UC *				5.9						4.3		4.3			1.7			0.7					95%T
83 4 UC				3.2																			87%T
85 14 UC *												1.7											**
85 15 UC *												2.3											**
85 23 UC	1.3																						**
88 31 UC *	2.4																						**
91 34 UC	2.4																						**
92 4 UC							4.2																92%T
94 37 UC	0.9				2.6		4.4																**
95 3 UC			1.9		5.2		6.0																**
95 4 UC *							4.4																93%T
95 35 UC *							3.8																85%T

Table 9.7F Number of cigarettes smoked per person per day, sales-adjusted, females: some selected French surveys[1] by age, 1978-1995, with percentage total sales

Product Source Year	Age group 12	13	14	15	16	17	18	19	20-24	25-29	30-34	35-39	40-44	45-49	50-54	55-59	60-64	65-69	70-74	75-79	80+	All ages	% Total sales
78 12 TC									5.7	2.9		2.4		1.8		1.0		0.3		0.0		1.9	79%T
80 2 MC				3.1																			---M
80 6 UC				2.8																			68%T
81 9 UC					5.2																		93%T
83 4 UC *				6.2						4.5		4.5			1.8			0.7					95%T
83 4 UC				3.7																			87%T
92 4 UC							4.6																92%T
95 4 UC *							4.7																93%T
95 35 UC *							4.5																85%T

1 Based on those surveys in Table 9.6 with data for both sexes and age range at least 21-64 (see *Cigarette consumption per person*, p. xxxv)

Source: see *Notes on sources of survey data*, p. 220
All ages: relevant to ages used and as given in original source
% Total sales: estimated % of total sales of M = manufactured or T = total cigarette consumption implied by survey, sexes combined, used as adjustment factor in Table 9.7
** = cannot be calculated
--- = adjusted by original author

Product: MC = manufactured cigarettes
TC = total cigarettes (including hand-rolled)
UC = cigarettes (type unspecified)
A = all products
U = unspecified
* = refer to *Notes on sources of survey data*, p. 220

Table 9.8 Estimated[1] prevalence of smoking and estimated[1] number of cigarettes per person per day (unadjusted and sales-adjusted): summary of Tables 9.4, 9.6 and 9.7, 1953-1995. Males and females aged 15 years and over

Year	Source[2]	Product[3]	Prevalence[4]						Number of cigarettes						
									Unadjusted[7]			Sales-adjusted[8]			
			Manufactured cigarettes		Total cigarettes[5]		All products[6]		Number/ person/day		Total sales %	Manufactured cigarettes number/ person/day		Total cigarettes[9] number/ person/day	
			M	F	M	F	M	F	M	F		M	F	M	F
1953	1	UC+*U*			69	15	77	35						(7.9	1.4)
1960	1	MC	45	12								(6.2	1.3)		
	1	*MC+A*	57	28			73	28							
	8	U					49								
1963	10	*UC+A*			57	15	64	15						(8.8	1.8)
1965	1	*U*					72	33							
	8	U					50								
1968	1	MC	45	10								(8.1	1.4)		
	1	**MC+A**	62	26			72	32							
1970	8	U					53								
1973	1	*U*					64	34				(7.4	3.1)		
1974	4	**U**					58	28							
1976	1	MC	45	20								(8.4	3.0)		
	1	**MC+A**	56	33			62	33							
	4	*UC*+**U**			56	30	60	28						(8.7	3.8)
	5	*UC+U*			52	27	56	29						(8.9	3.6)
	8	U					47								
	11	*UC*			62	40								(8.2	4.2)
1977	4	UC			41	19								(9.3	3.4)
	4	**UC+U**			47	30	51	30							
	8	U					51	29							
1978	12	MC+A	45	17			56	18				(8.8	2.6)		
	12	TC			52	18			7.9	1.8	79			10.0	2.3
1979	1	MC+*A*	37	22			50	30				(7.9	3.8)		
	1	**MC**	42	29											
	4	**U**					53	24							
	4	*UC*			43	25								(8.6	3.9)
	4	**U**					48	24							
	8	U					40								
1980	2	MC							8.6	3.1	---	8.6	3.1		
	6	UC+A			41	16	45	16	6.5	1.9	68			9.6	2.8
	7	*MC+U*	45	28			52	28				(7.7	3.8)		
	8	U					46	16							
1981	5	**U**					49	27							
	9	*UC+A*			46	33	51	33	7.5	3.8	93			8.1	4.1
1982	5	**U**					48	27							
1983	4	UC+**U**					51	29	7.5	3.2	87			8.6	3.7
1984	4	**U**					53	33						(8.2	4.1)
1985	5	*U*					50	25						(9.3	3.7)

Table 9.8 *(continued)*

Year	Source[2]	Product[3]	Prevalence[4]						Number of cigarettes						
									Unadjusted[7]			Sales-adjusted[8]			
			Manufactured cigarettes		Total cigarettes[5]		All products[6]		Number/ person/day		Total sales %	Manufactured cigarettes number/ person/day		Total cigarettes[9] number/ person/day	
			M	F	M	F	M	F	M	F		M	F	M	F
1986	4	U					39	24							
	4	**U**					48	30							
	6	UC			43	21								(9.2	3.6)
1987	8	U					43	20							
1988	8	U					39	19							
1989	4	U					45	30							
	4	**U**					48	33							
1990	8	U					38	19							
1991	4	U					38	26							
	4	**U**					46	32							
	6	UC			39	21									
	33	*MC*	38	28								(7.4	4.3)		
1992	4	UC+*A*			42	29	48	32	6.8	4.2	92			7.5	4.6
	33	*MC*	24	22								(6.7	4.8)		
	35	UC+**U**			39	25	42	27						(7.9	4.1)
1993	4	U					36	24							
	4	**U**					41	22							
	33	*MC*	24	22								(6.4	4.7)		
	35	UC+**U**			35	21	39	26						(7.9	3.8)
1994	33	*MC*	24	22								(6.2	4.4)		
1995	4	UC+*U*					39	28	6.3	4.0	93			6.8	4.3
	33	*MC*	24	22								(6.0	4.3)		
	35	UC+*U*					40	29	5.9	3.5	85			7.0	4.1

1 Surveys covering an age range of at least 21-64 are included. Any gaps in the data for ages 15-20 and 65 years and over are filled in by assumed extensions to the age distribution, given in *Notes on sources of survey data*, p. 220. Method: see *Summary of adult smoking*, p. xxxvi

2 See *Notes on sources of survey data*, p. 220

3 Product: MC = manufactured cigarettes, TC = total cigarettes (including hand-rolled), UC = cigarettes (type unspecified), A = all products, U = unspecified. Frequency of smoking is indicated by: regular or daily smokers in normal type, all smokers (including occasional) in bold, unspecified in italics

4 From Table 9.4

5 This column includes prevalence of smoking classified as UC = cigarettes (type unspecified)

6 This column includes prevalence of smoking classified as U = unspecified product

7 From Table 9.6

8 From Table 9.7, except data in parentheses, which are derived from the prevalence of smoking from Table 9.4 as described in *Summary of adult smoking*, p. xxxvi

9 Number of cigarettes classified as UC = cigarettes (type unspecified) has been adjusted to total cigarette sales and included in this column

Figure 9.3 Estimated prevalence of smoking of (i) manufactured cigarettes, (ii) total cigarettes and (iii) all tobacco products: by year of survey, 1953-1995.
Males and females aged 15 years and over. *Source:* see Table 9.8

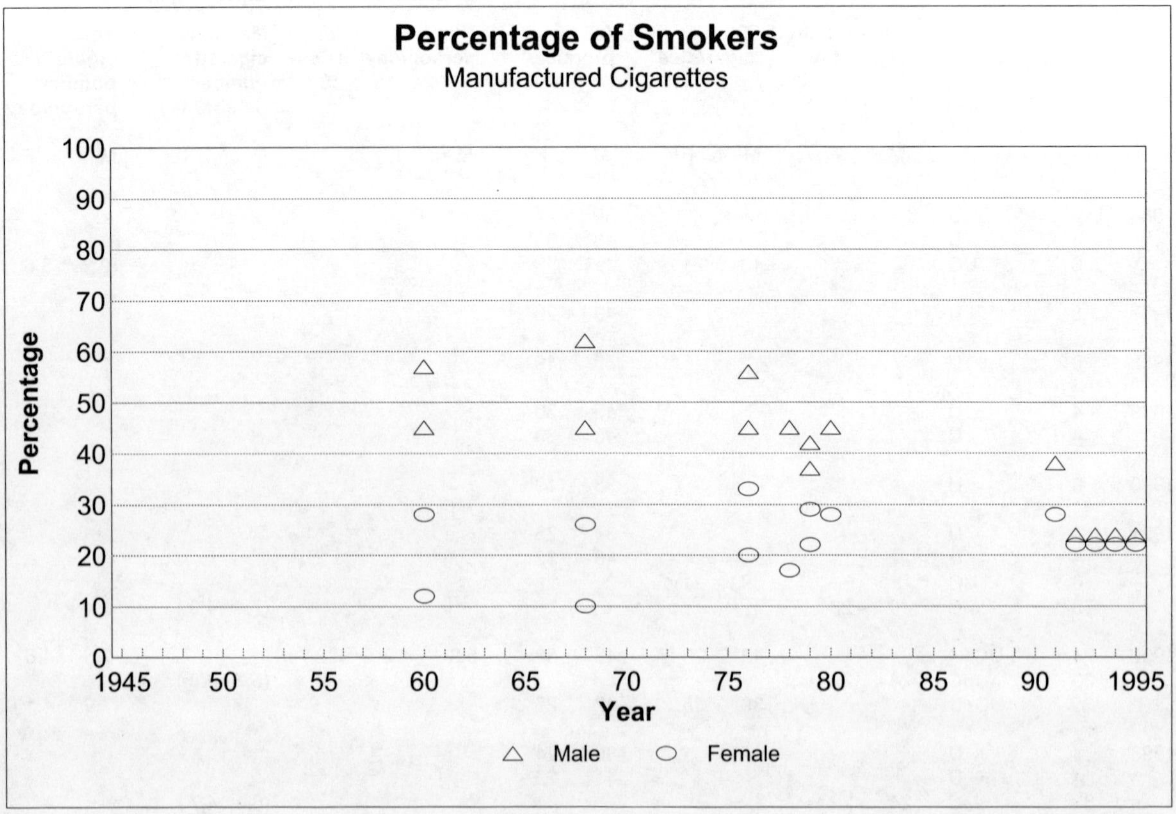

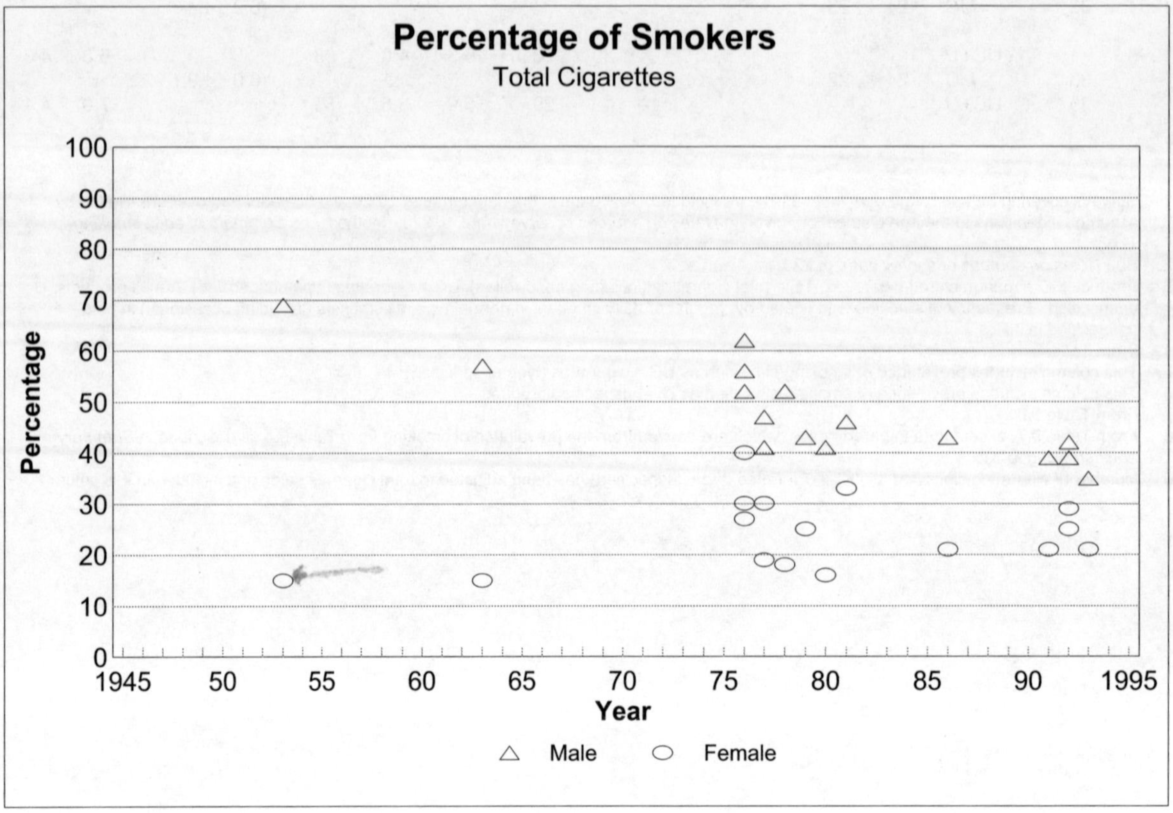

Figure 9.3 *(continued)*

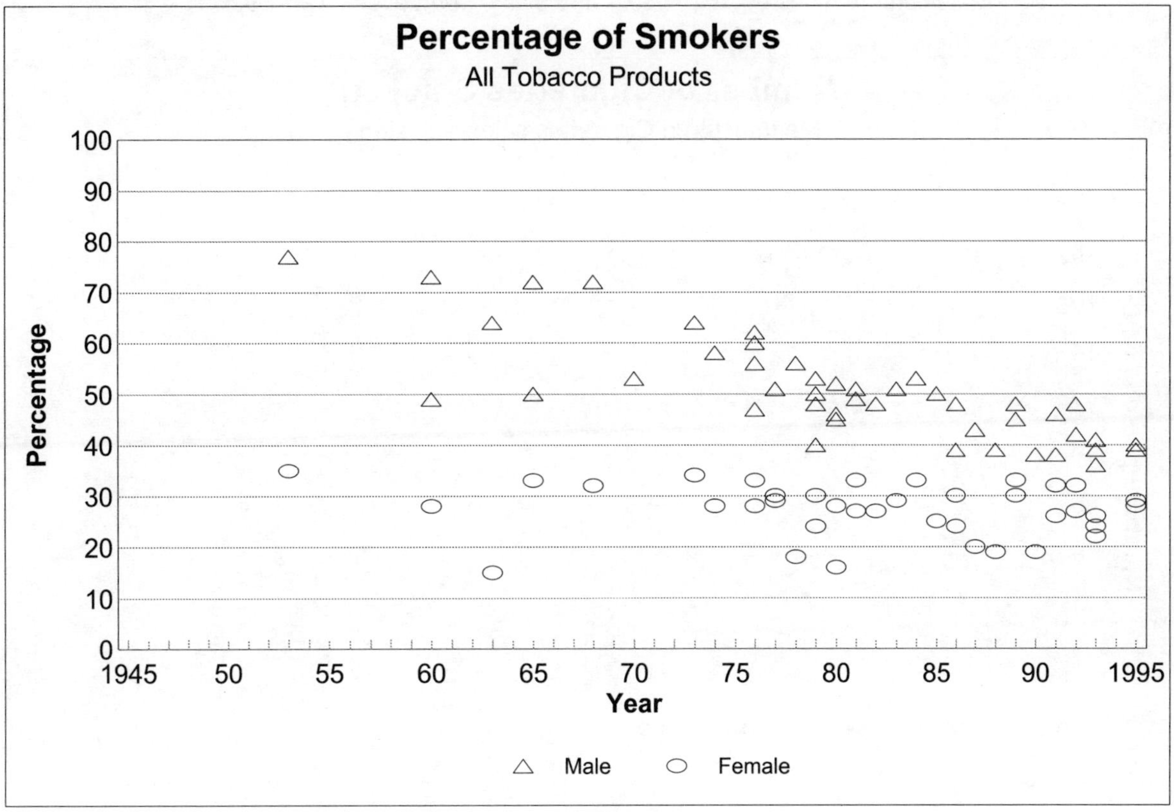

Figure 9.4 Estimated number of (i) manufactured cigarettes and (ii) total cigarettes smoked per person per day, sales-adjusted, 1953-1995.
Males and females aged 15 years and over. *Source:* see Table 9.8

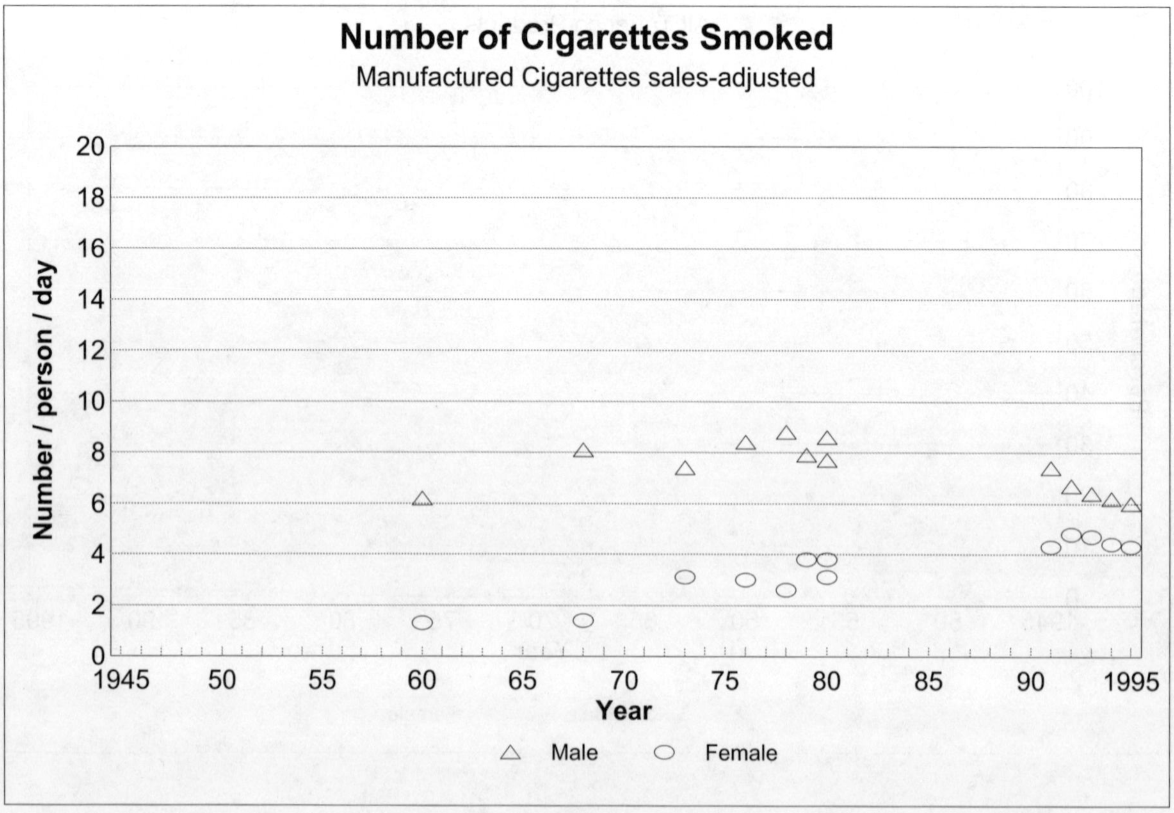

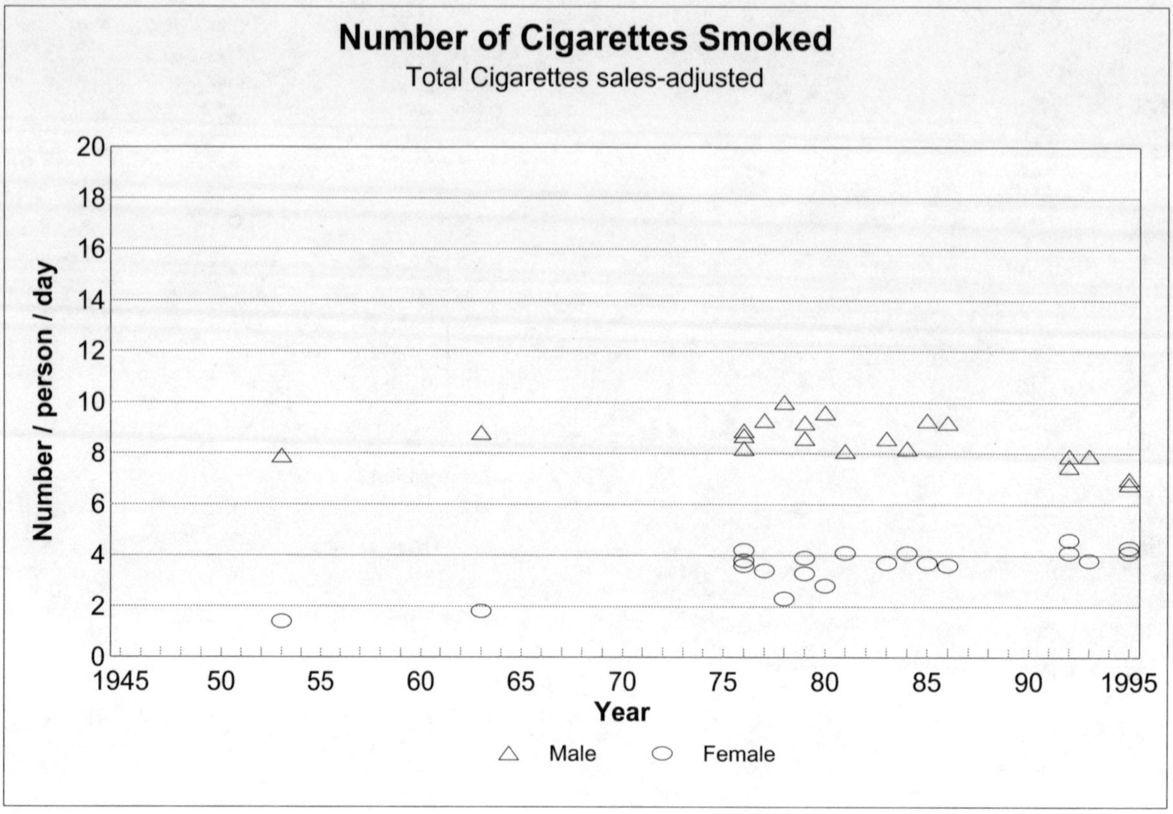

Notes on sources of sales data

The data presented in the tables and figures were obtained from several sources, details of which are given below, together with estimations and related assumptions. Full citations of the sources are given on p. 226 under *References*.

Consumption data before 1932

Hill and Flamant (1985) and Seita (Société Nationale d'Exploitation Industrielle des Tabacs et Allumettes, Paris)

Data shown in Table 9.1.1 are from Seita (selected years shown). Data for individual years are available for 1861-1913 and 1923-1924. Cigarillos are included in the cigarette sales data until 1924.

Estimates shown in Table 9.2 are from Hill and Flammant, and are 5-year averages, based on 1 cigarette = 1 g, 1 cigar = 4 g, and 1 cigarillo = 1 g. Estimates were given to the nearest 1 000 pieces/tonnes.

Consumption data for 1932-1974

RP6

Data by weight, originally given to nearest 100 000 pounds, have been converted to tonnes and given to the nearest 10 tonnes (100 000 lbs = 45.359 tonnes). Where weight conversion factors have been quoted in RP6, the weights have been re-calculated without rounding and then converted to tonnes.

Notes as given in RP6:

Details of the quantities of tobacco products consumed and factors for conversion from number to weight were provided by the French Tobacco Monopoly. These factors were as follows: cigarettes 2.650 lbs per 1 000, cigars 8.820 lbs per 1 000 and cigarillos 3.528 lbs per 1 000.

There are minor discrepancies between the RP6 data and Seita data (not shown) for the same years. These may be due to different treatment of 'restricted sales' (i.e. to certain institutionalized groups) and to minor geographical differences.

Consumption data for 1974 onwards

Seita

Data for cigarettes and cigars were given in numbers and have been converted to weight assuming an average of 1.2 g per cigarette, 4 g per cigar, and 1.6 g per cigarillo (based on values in RP6). In addition, the conversion factor assumed for cigars and cigarillos combined was 3.5 g in 1980 declining by 0.2 g per year to 1.9 g in 1988, reflecting the change in the relative numbers sold during the period when separate data were not available.

Plain/Filter cigarette consumption

1958-1989 Seita yearly bulletins

Data for 1958-1967 were calculated from sales of imports from the common market and other countries and sales of Seita products in France but excluded 'restricted sales' as these were not split by filter and plain cigarette sales. Data for later years were calculated by Seita, apparently on the same basis.

1979-1995 CDIT

For years where data were available from both sources, the values were identical.

Tar and nicotine yield of cigarettes

1950, 1971, 1986 Joossens (1989)

1960, 1976 Todd (1986a)

1992-1995 CDIT

The values for 1992-1995 are based on the top 10 cigarette brands sold in France and, together, make up only around 50% of the market. The tar yield per cigarette was limited by EC directive (Directive 90/239/EEC) to 15 mg by the end of 1992, and to 12 mg by the end of 1997; nicotine yield is limited to 1.2 mg (Harkin *et al* (1997)).

Estimates of hand-rolled cigarette consumption for 1950-1995

For 1950-1985 we have taken as our estimate of hand-rolled cigarette consumption 70% of pipe and hand-rolling tobacco ('Scaferlatis') sales. Following Dymond (1996), we can assume an average weight of 0.76 g per cigarette.

'Scaferlatis' is fine-cut tobacco for hand-rolling and pipes. There is little evidence on which to base estimates of hand-rolled cigarette consumption. CDIT gives the quantities (tonnes) of smoking tobacco and hand-rolling tobacco for 1991 to 1995. This shows the proportion of smoking tobacco used in rolling increasing from 50% to 64% during that period. By contrast Merzdorf *et al* (1982) allocate all 'Scaferlatis' sales to hand-rolled cigarette smoking, ignoring pipes, which (survey source 1) were smoked by 16% of men in 1976.

Our estimate for 1978 give hand-rolled cigarettes as 8% of total cigarette consumption, which can be compared with the smoking prevalences reported by Tuyns and Hu (1982) (survey source 12) in that year. Approximately 9% of cigarette smokers smoked hand-rolled cigarettes only and a further 8% smoked both (sexes combined).

Notes on sources of survey data

Each source of survey data—either an individual survey or a series of surveys repeated over a number of years—is cited by a source number. This number is shown in the tables and corresponds to the source numbers given below, where details of the source publication and of the survey methodology are given. Full citations of the sources are given on p. 226 under *References*.

Source number

1 **Merzdorf *et al* (1982), Hill and Flamant (1985), WHO (1975), Hill (1995, 1998)**

a. Surveys by SOFRES (Institut de Sondage, Études de Marché of Group Metra, Paris) for Seita. Sample size varied between 3 500 (1953) and 24 000
b. Merzdorf *et al* (1982) give 1968 survey as 1967
c. There are some discrepancies in the lower age limit reported by different authors
d. Assumed extension to age distribution for percentage smokers (1953, cigarettes) age 15-19: males 45% and females 15%

2 **Todd (1986a)**

a. Estimated by Todd

3-5 Series of surveys of conducted for CFES (Comité Français d'Éducation pour la Santé, Paris). Results from surveys up to 1991 are largely taken from a summary paper by Sasco *et al* (1995) and are given as source **3** for adolescents and source **4** for adults; surveys attributed by other authors to CFES but not mentioned by Sasco *et al* (1995) are given as source **5**

3,4 **Sasco *et al* (1991, 1994, 1995), Merzdorf *et al* (1982), Todd (1986b), Grizeau *et al* (1997), Guilbert *et al* (1999), Joossens *et al* (1994), CFES (date unknown), WHO (1997), C. Hill (personal communication)**

a. Surveys by CFES. Quota samples representative of the national population. Personal interviews.

	Year	Survey Institute	Sample size
Adults	1974	Sofres	1 000
	1976	Sofres	1 000
	1977	Sofres	1 000
	1979(Jan)	Sofres	1 021
	1979(Dec)	Sofres	1 006
	1983	BVA	2 000
	1984	BVA	2 000
	1986	Omniplus	2 000
	1989	BVA	1 044
	1991	Démoscopie	1 022
	1992	Ipsos	—
	1993	—	—
	1995	Démoscopie	1 000

	Year	Survey Institute	Sample size
Adolescents	1977	Sofres	1 200
	1980	BVA	1 200
	1981	BVA	1 200
	1983	Démoscopie	1 000
	1984	Démoscopie	1 000
	1988	MV2	987
	1990	Ipsos	1 000
	1991	Ipsos	1 000
	1992	—	1 000
	1994	—	1 005
	1995	Ipsos	1 006

There are minor discrepancies in the sample sizes reported by different sources

b. Regular smokers: smoke every day. All smokers: smoke, even if only from time to time. According to Hill, the definition of regular smoking in the 1988 adolescent survey was changed to smoked more than 6 cigarettes per week

c. Most age-specific prevalence data taken from charts. It is not stated to which survey the 1979 adult age-specific prevalence data relate

d. 1983, source 4: age-specific results in Table 9.5 are consumption per regular cigarette smoker, calculated by Todd, using consumption category estimation based on 1-10, 11-20, 21+ cigarettes/smoker/day; calculation of consumption per person based on percentage smokers of any product and number of cigarettes per regular cigarette smoker. They may overestimate for men. The overall age figures in Table 9.5 are from Hill based on consumption per smoker, with derived estimates in Tables 9.6, 9.7, and 9.8

e. 1992: *All ages* column refers to ages 18+. Category consumption estimation based on 1-5, 6-20, >20 cigarettes/smoker/day (Grizeau *et al* (1993)). These estimates have been used for the calculation of cigarettes per person shown in Table 9.6, 9.7 and 9.8, and are somewhat higher than the results for cigarettes per smoker given directly by Hill (1998), also shown in Table 9.5

f. 1995: Calculation of cigarettes per person based on percentage smokers (product unspecified), and number of cigarettes per cigarette smoker, so may overestimate (Guilbert *et al* (1999))

5 Merzdorf *et al* (1982), Hill and Flamant (1985), Hill (1990)

g. Merzdorf *et al* (1982) report a second survey in 1976 (December), sample size 1 052. Hill and Flamant (1985) give slightly different results for December. Hill and Flamant (1985) report surveys in 1981 and 1982, both sample size 1 000

h. Assumed extension to age distribution for percentage smokers (sources 4 and 5), age 15-17: (1974) males 40%, females 30%; (1976-1977) (cigarettes, or regular smokers) males 40%, females 35%, (all or unspecified products, or including occasional smokers) males 45%, females 40%; (1979 on) (cigarettes or regular smokers) males and females 35%, (all or unspecified products, or including occasional smokers) males and females 40%. For age 65+ (1993): males 40%, females 2%. For age 75+ (1995): males 20%, females 2%. Number of cigarettes/person/day (1992-1995), age 15-17: males and females 3.0. For age 75+: males 3.0, females 0.5

6 Service des Statistiques des Etudes et des Systemes d'Information (SESI) (1983), Statistika Centralbyrån (1995), Hill (1990, 1998)

a. Household surveys by INSEE (Institut National de la Statistique et des Études Economiques) for CREDOC, Ministère des Affaires Sociales, Ministère de la Santé, and INSERM (Institut National de la Santé et de la Recherche Médicale). Usually face-to-face interviews with one member of household. Persons living in institutions excluded
1980-1981: 7 323 households, 21 000 individuals, of which 16 200 were age 15+ and included in tobacco questions. Response rate for tobacco questions (males) 43%, (females) 75%
1986-1987: Etude de conditions de vie, 13 154 households from which one person age 18+ selected
1991-1992: L'Enquête Santé, 7 666 interviews representing 21 500 individuals age 14+

b. Percentages of smokers adjusted to exclude non-respondents from base

c. Assumed extension to age distribution for percentage smokers (1986-1987 and 1991-1992, cigarettes), age 15-17: males and females 35%

7 SEITA, IFOP

8 Organisation for Economic Co-operation and Development (1993)

a. No original source

9 Comité National contre le Tabagisme (1982)

a. Survey by IDEM (Institut Développement—Études—Marketing), representative of working population. Sample size 1 001

b. There was one female smoker of only cigars/pipe

c. Consumption category estimation based on ≤5, 5-10 (assumed 6-10), 11-20, and 21+ cigarettes/smoker/day

d. Assumed extension to age distribution for percentage smokers, age 15: males and females 15%. Number of cigarettes/person/day: 1.0. For age 65+: males (cigarettes) 30%, (all products) 40%; females 7%. Number of cigarettes/person/day: males 4.0 and females 0.5

10 Readers Digest (1963)

a. Series of surveys conducted in European countries using identical questionnaires. French survey conducted by SOFRES. Random sample of about 2 000 people

b. It is also reported that 11% of men (12% age <40 and 11% age 40+) smoke a pipe, and that 13% of men (13% age <40 and 12% age 40+) smoke cigars

c. Assumed extension to age distribution for percentage smokers, age 15-20: males (all products) 50%, (cigarettes) 45%; females 15%

11 Wynder *et al* (1981)

a. Subjects randomly selected in 65 départements, as they left factories, stores etc. Sample size (males) 2 163, (females) 1 290. Response rate about 90%, a further 8% excluded owing to history of alcoholism or psychiatric conditions

b. Smokers: includes those who had given up smoking within last year

c. Among cigarette smokers who listed a preferred brand, 86% of men and 49% of women preferred black to blond tobacco

d. Assumed extension to age distribution for percentage smokers, age 15-19: males 50% and females 40%; age 81+: males 40% and females 5%

12 Tuyns and Hu (1982) and Dr A.J. Tuyns (personal communication)

a. Département of Calvados. Tuyns and Hu (1982) stated that 'Calvados can ... be considered as an average French département with regard to tobacco consumption'. Sample size (males) 923, (females 1 053. Response rate (males) 75%, (females) 78%

b. There was only one female smoker of products other than cigarettes

c. Black tobacco brands were the most commonly consumed by 68% of male cigarette (including hand-rolled) smokers and 50% of female smokers

d. Assumed extension to age distribution for percentage smokers, age 15-19:(all products or total cigarettes) males 50% and females 45%; (manufactured cigarettes) males 45% and females 40%. Number of cigarettes/person/day: males 5.0 and females 4.0

13 Fréour *et al* (1969)

a. Study of chronic bronchitis conducted by INSERM in Bordeaux area in 1963-1967. Representative of the regional population. Sample size (males) 1 320, (females) 1 170

b. The all ages data in Tables 9.4-6 are calculated from the prevalence of ever smokers of cigarettes and the proportions of smokers of more than 1 000 cigarettes who had given up smoking, or smoked in specific categories. The age-specific data (females only) are based on the prevalence of ever smokers of cigarettes and the proportion of smokers of more than 1 000 cigarettes who had given up smoking for more than 10 years, and may therefore overestimate as they include some ex-smokers

b. Consumption category estimation based on (males) 0-10, 10-20, 20-30, 30+ and (females) 1-10, 10-20, 20+ cigarettes/smoker/day. This has been interpreted as 1-9, 10-19, 20-29, 30+, but different interpretation would have had considerable impact on the estimates

14-16 WHO (1989), WHO MONICA Project (1988)

a. Three regional surveys forming part of WHO MONICA Project:

	Region	Population size	Sample size	Participation rate (%)	Sample used* Male	Sample used* Female	Date
14	Bas-Rhin	314 200	—	66	731	792	Jan 1985-Sep 1987
15	Haute-Garonne	296 900	2 264	58	678	645	May 1985-Feb 1987
16	Lille	336 000	1 695	69	924	785	Jun 1986-Feb 1989

* Bas-Rhin 'sample used' includes age 25-34; all other figures are for age 35-64 only

b. *All ages* column relates only to age 35-64 and is standardized to world population

c. Regular cigarette smokers: smoked cigarettes daily. All smokers: smoked cigarettes daily or occasionally, or smoked 1 g pipe tobacco or 1 cigar per week. Cigarettes per smoker refers to regular and occasional cigarette smokers

d. Calculation for cigarettes per person based on % regular cigarette smokers and cigarettes per regular or occasional cigarette smoker, so may underestimate

17 Davidson *et al* (1973), Davidson and Choquet (1980)

a. Studies of secondary pupils in Paris and Paris region, Rennes and département (Bretagne), and Marseille and département (Bouches-du-Rhone) during 1971 and 1978-1979. Sample size (1971) 2 339, (1978-1979) 2 088. Studies covered all lycée students, and included some students up to age 20

b. 1971 survey: prevalences averaged over the three regions

c. Regular smokers: smoked daily

d. Consumption category estimation based on <5, 5-9, 10-19, and 20+ cigarettes/smoker/day, excluding about 10% of boys in each age group who smoked pipes, and 10-35% of boys and 35-45% of girls with amount smoked unknown

18 Cooreman *et al* (1978, 1979)

a. Survey in Bas-Rhin in spring 1976, covering all schoolchildren. Sample size 29 138, response rate 93%

19 Lenoir *et al* (1973), Bernard and Boyer (1976)

a. Results combined from a study in 1971 at selection centre (CS) before military service and a study in 1972 at the end of military service (SM)

	Sample size	Average age
CS	47 942	19
SM	27 899	21

In the CS study, 1% smoked only pipe or cigars (no equivalent data for SM study)

b. Numbers of cigarettes include equivalents of 1 pipe or cigarillo = 2 cigarettes and 1 cigar = 5 cigarettes

c. Results presented for individual ages 20-24 have been averaged

d. Consumption category estimation based on <10, 10-20, and 21+ cigarettes/smoker/day

20 Bernard *et al* (1980)

a. Part of a study on anti-smoking campaign during military service

b. Numbers of cigarettes include equivalents of 1 pipe or cigarillo = 2 cigarettes and 1 cigar = 5 cigarettes

c. Consumption category estimation based on <10, 10-20, and 21+ cigarettes/smoker/day

21 Cooreman *et al* (1985), quoting Cooreman *et al* (1982a)

a. Survey in Bas-Rhin. Sample size 7 963. Age group uncertain

22 Cooreman *et al* (1985), quoting Cooreman *et al* (1982b)

a. Survey in Bordeaux. Sample size 15 247. Age group uncertain

23 Oriol *et al* (1988, 1994)

a. Studies conducted in département Yvelines (Ile-de-France). Sample drawn from all types of school (except an international school). Self-completed anonymous questionnaire, distributed by a medical researcher, completed during lesson time generally with a teacher present. Sample size (1983) 2 776, (1990) 1 916. Response rate (1983) 92%

b. Results for 11-year-olds are included in the lowest age group for 1983, and in the all ages results, but are not shown for the age-specific results for 1990

c. Regular smokers: smoked at least 1 cigarette per day on average. Consumption levels based on weekly smoking

24 Neukirch *et al* (1982)

a. Survey of all pupils at a secondary school in Paris. Upper age not stated, results for pupils under age 12 not presented here. Sample size 2 266

b. Smokers: smoked at least 1 cigarette per day

25 Chicou (1978) quoting SOFRES

a. Survey by SOFRES for ONSER and CNCT (Comité National Contre le Tabagisme, Paris). Lower age limit not stated

26 Schwartz *et al* (1961)

a. Patients hospitalized due to work or traffic accident in Paris or large provincial cities (control group in a study of cancer). Study started in 1954, but end year not stated. Age range not stated. Sample size 1 807

b. Smokers: smoked an average of 1 cigarette or 1 g of pipe tobacco a day during the 10 years before interview

c. The amount smoked shown in Tables 9.5-6 relates to all smokers and includes equivalents of 1 g pipe tobacco = 1 cigarette. The amount smoked per smoker was 14.5 cigarettes for cigarette only smokers, 13.6 cigarettes or 21.3 cigarette equivalents for smokers of cigarette *and* pipe, and 16.3 cigarette equivalents for pipe only smokers

27 Poirier *et al* (1979)

a. Anonymous questionnaire survey at 4 schools in Marseilles, November 1976-April 1977, age 11-15. Sample size 1 795, response rate approximately 90%

28 Treguer *et al* (1983)

a. Two studies conducted at the Nancy selection centre before military service, in June and December 1979. Results presented here are average. Age limits are approximate, average age 19.5. Sample size 2 067, response rate 93%

29 Baudier *et al* (1988)

a. Questionnaire survey in schools in Doubs département. Age range not stated, approximate ages shown in Table 9.4 corresponding to school type

Year	School type	Sample size
1982	lyceé	419
1985	lyceé	508
1985	collège	857

b. Regular smokers: smokes daily

30 Sasco *et al* (1991)

a. Study carried out by CIRC (Centre international de la reserche sur le cancer) and ALEC (l'association de lutte étudiante contre le cancer) in 13 representative schools in the Rhône département. Anonymous questionnaire. Results available only for 12-16-year-olds, sample size (1985) 1 867, (1987-1988) 1 909

31 Choquet (1994)

a. Survey of secondary school pupils in Haute-Marne département. Anonymous questionnaires completed in class with teachers absent. Sample size 3 527, response rate 94%. Upper age not stated

b. Regular smokers: smokes daily

c. Consumption category estimation based on 2 categories, 1-9 and 10+ cigarettes/smoker/day, and resulting figures should be regarded with caution

32 **van Reek *et al* (1992), van Reek and Adriaanse (1995)**

a. A series of surveys of Young Europeans. About 800 children aged 11-15 years interviewed in each EC country except Luxembourg (where only 250 interviewed). Lowest age group 11-12. Interviews conducted at home, with parents absent

b. Regular smokers: smoked daily. All smokers: smoked at least once a week

33 **Tobacco industry, CDIT**

a. Assumed extension to age distribution for percentage smokers, age 15-17: males and females 20%

34 **Dautzenberg *et al* (1992, 1995)**

a. Survey representative of Paris secondary school students by Paris Sans Tabac (PST). Anonymous questionnaires completed in class with teachers present. Sample size (1991) 10 043, response rate 93%

b. Dautzenberg *et al* (1995) reported that the study was repeated in 1992 and 1993 and that the prevalence remained stable

c. Regular smokers: smokes daily

35 **Arenes *et al* (1996), Guilbert *et al* (1999)**

a. Baromètre Santé, a random sample phone survey by BVA (Société Brullé-Ville-Associés, Paris) for CFES and INSERM, in cooperation with CNAMTS (la Caisse nationale de l'assurance maladie des travailleurs salarieés), Ministère du travail et des affaires sociales, HCSP (le Haut-Comité de santé publique) and MILDT (la Mission interministérielle à la lutte contre la drogue et la toxicomainie). Same questions as CFES quota samples (source 4). Sample size (1992) 2 099, (1993) 1 950, (1995) 1 993, response rate approximately 75%

b. Calculation of cigarettes per person based on percentage smokers (product unspecified), and number of cigarettes per cigarette smoker, so may overestimate

c. Assumed extension to age distribution for percentage smokers, age 15-17: (manufactured cigarettes) males and females 35%, (unspecified product) males and females 40%. For age 75+: males 20%, females 2%. Number of cigarettes/person/day, age 15-17: males and females 3.0. For age 75+: males 3.0, females 0.5

36 **King and Coles (1992), King *et al* (1996)**

a. Part of the HBSC (Health Behaviour in School-Aged Children) Study, a collaborative cross-national research study sponsored by the WHO. Conducted in Nancy and Toulouse regions. School classes or schools were randomly selected, targeting age groups 11 (not presented here), 13 and 15. The target sample size was 1 300 in each age group.

Target age	Mean age	Sample size
13	13.5	1 283
15	15.5	1 260

b. Regular smokers: smoke once a week or more

37 **Challier *et al* (2000)**

a. Study of all children at 4 schools in the urban area of Nancy, north-eastern France. Questionnaires completed during sports classes with teachers present but discouraged from influencing responses. Full age range 9-25. Sample size 2 396, participation rate 73%

Département = administrative region of France (France consists of 96 départements)

References

Anonymous (2000). *Les consommations de drogues en France. La mesure de l'ampleur des consommations de drogues*. Mission interministerielle de lutte contre la drogue et la toxicomanie. http://www.drogues.gouv.fr/fr/professionnels/etudes_recherches/indicateurs_tendances/57.html.

Arenes J., Grizeau D., Baudier F., Chan-Chee C., *et al* (1996). Evolution des comportements de santé des médecins généralistes en matière de tabagisme de 1992 à 1994. (Changes in smoking habits in doctors 1992-94). *Bulletin epidemiologique hebdomadaire,* **19**, http://www.b3e.jussieu.fr/beh/9619.

Baudier F., Helou J., Bourderont D., Blum D., Thiriet F. and Pinochet C. (1988). Etude de la consommation des drogues licites et illicites chez les jeunes scolarisés du département du Doubs (Consumption of legal and illegal drugs by school students from the region of Doubs). *Archives Francaises de Pediatrie,* **45**, 575-81.

Beese D.H. (ed) (1968). *Tobacco consumption in various countries,* 2nd edition. Tobacco Research Council, London. Research Paper 6.

Beese D.H. (ed) (1972). *Tobacco consumption in various countries,* 3rd edition. Tobacco Research Council, London. Research Paper 6.

Bernard J.-G., Nauroy J., Bizeau J.M. and Bernard J.-J. (1980). Le tabagisme du jeune Français et le service militaire. (Tobacco addiction of the young french male and his military service). *Rev Epidemiol Sante Publique,* **28**, 413-21.

Bernard J.G. and Boyer G. (1976). Etude épidémiologique du tabagisme de l'adulte jeune en France. (Epidemiological study of tobacco smoking among young men in France). *Bull World Health Organ,* **53**, 75-81.

Challier B., Chau N., Prédine R., Choquet M. and Legras B. (2000). Associations of family environment and individual factors with tobacco, alcohol, and illicit drug use in adolescents. *Eur J Epidemiol,* **16**, 33-42.

Chicou F.-J. (1978). La prévention du tabagisme chez les jeunes français. (Prevention of smoking among the young in France). *Revue du Praticien,* **28**, 1423-8.

Choquet M. (1994). La consommation de tabac par les adolescents: évolutions et signication. (Tobacco consumption among adolescents: evolution and significance). *Bull Acad Natl Med,* **178**, 941-54.

Comité Français d'Education pour la Santé (date unknown). *Les femmes de le tabac.* CFES, Paris.

Comité National contre le Tabagisme (1982). La consommation de tabac chez les travailleurs. *Tabac et Sante,* **(45)**, 15.

Cooreman J., Burghard G. and Perdrizet S. (1978). L'adolescent et le tabagisme. Responsabilité des parents et des professeurs. Résultats d'une campagne de sensibilisation (Teenagers and tobacco comsumption. The responsibility of parents and teachers. Results of a sensitizing campaign). *Journal de Medecine de Strasbourg,* **9**, 483-8.

Cooreman J., Neukirch F. and Perdrizet S. (1985). Le tabagisme et les adolescentes scolarisées. *Medecine et Hygiene,* **43**, 3381-4.

Cooreman J., Perdrizet S. and Burghard G. (1982a). La lutte anti-tabagique à l'école primaire. (The results of educational anti-smoking measures at the primary school level). *Archives Francaises de Pediatrie,* **39**, 113-7.

Cooreman J., Perdrizet S., Metz-Marcy G., Welsch M. and Burghard G. (1979). Un auto-questionnaire appliqué à 30 000 adolescents. Evaluation de ce mode de recueil des données. (A self-administered questionnaire applied to 30 000 teen-agers. Assessment of this method of data collection). *Rev Epidemiol Sante Publique,* **27**, 301-5.

Cooreman J., Redon S. and Perdrizet S. (1982b). Etiologie de la toux chronique des lycéens de l'agglomération bordelaise: methodologie de l'enquête et résultats préliminaires. *Bulletin of the International Union Against Tuberculosis,* **57**, 272-9.[§]

Dautzenberg B., Birkui P., Perdrizet S., Paillotet P. and Jouin G. (1992). Tabagisme des élèves des collèges et lycées parisiens. (Smoking among secondary school children in Paris). *Bulletin epidemiologique hebdomadaire,* **34**, 165-6.

Dautzenberg B., Birkui P.J., Perdrizet S., Paillotet P. and Arcival C. (1995). Survey before and after the change of French law of schoolchildren's smoking habits. In: Slama K. (ed) *Tobacco and Health, Ninth World Conference on Tobacco and Health, Paris, Oct 10-14 1994.* Plenum Press, New York and London; 599-601.

Davidson F. and Choquet M. (1980). *Les jeunes et les drogues permises et interdites. Les lycéens, le tabac, l'alcool, les médicaments psychotropes et les drogues illicites. Genèse et évolution de la toxicomaine.* INSERM, Paris.

Davidson F., Choquet M. and Depagne M. (1973). La connaissance et l'usage par les jeunes de produits ayant une affinité psychotrope. Résultats d'une enquête auprès des lycéens. (Results of a survey carried out in secondary schools on the pupils' knowledge and use of psychotropic substances). *Revue d'Epidemiologie, Medecine Sociale et Sante Publique,* **21**, 23-49.

Dymond H.F. (1996). A survey of roll-your-own tobacco use and practice and considerations for the analysis of smoking articles made from it. *Tobacco Science,* **40**, 82-6.

Fréour P., Coudray P. and Fontan M.E.C. (1969). La consommation de tabac. Contribution à son étude en France sur un groupe d'adultes des deux sexes. *Bulletin de l'Institut National de Sante et de la Recherche Medicale,* **24**, 1151-83.

Grizeau D., Baudier F. and Allemand H. (1997). Opinions et comportements des adolescents français face au tabac en 1995. (Opinions and behaviour of French adolescents confronted with tobacco in 1995). *Arch Pediatr,* **4**, 1079-86.

Grizeau D., Baudier F. and Janvrin M.P. (1993). Épidémiologie du tabagisme en France. *Revue du Praticien,* **43**, 1197-202.

Guilbert P., Baudier F. and Arwidson P. (1999). Comparaison de 2 modalités d'enquête sur les comportements et attitudes au sujet de l'alcool, du tabac et des drogues illégales (Comparison of two types of KABP surveys on alcohol, tobacco and illegal drugs). *Rev Epidemiol Sante Publique,* **47**, 129-38.

Harkin A.M., Anderson P. and Goos C. (1997). *Smoking, drinking and drug taking in the European Region.* Alcohol, Drugs and Tobacco Programme, WHO Regional Office for Europe, Copenhagen.

Hill C. (1995). Trends and implications of tobacco use. Lessons from the French experience. In: Slama K. (ed) *Tobacco and health, Ninth World Conference on Tobacco and Health, Oct 10-14 1994, Paris.* Plenum Press, New York and London; 121-7.

Hill C. (1998). Trends in tobacco smoking and consequences on health in France. *Prev Med,* **27**, 514-9.

Hill C. and Flamant R. (1985). Une cause d'épidémie majeure: l'augmentation de la consommation de tabac en France. (A major cause of epidemic: the tobacco consumption increase in France). *Rev Epidemiol Sante Publique,* **33**, 387-95.

Joossens L. (1989). *Documentation Tabac.* CRIOC, Bruxelles. (Hilgers P. (ed) .)

Joossens L., Naett C., Howie C. and Muldoon A. (1994). *Tobacco and health in the European Union. An overview.* European Bureau for Action on Smoking Prevention (BASP), Brussels.

King A., Wold B., Tudor-Smith C. and Harel Y. (1996). *The health of youth, a cross-national survey.* WHO

Regional Publications, Europe, Copenhagen. European Series No. 69.

King A.J.C. and Coles B. (1992). *The health of Canada's youth. Views and behaviours of 11-, 13- and 15-year-olds from 11 countries*. Health and Welfare Canada, Ottawa.

Lee P.N. (ed) (1975). *Tobacco consumption in various countries,* 4th edition. Tobacco Research Council, London. Research Paper 6.

Lenoir P., Bernard J.G. and Boyer G. (1973). Étude épidémiologique du tabagisme de l'adolescent. *Bull Acad Natl Med,* **1572**, 130-6.

Merzdorf J., Reuter U. and Welsch G. (1982). *Daten und Fakten zur Entwicklung des Rauchens in Mitgliedsländern der Europäischen Gemeinschaften (Facts and figures on the development of smoking in the member states of the European Communities)*. Kommission der Europäischen Gemeinschaften, Luxemburg. Medizin—EUR 7907 DE.

Neukirch F., Liard R., Cooreman J. and Perdrizet S. (1982). Prevalence of respiratory symptoms in Parisian teenagers according to smoking habits. *J Epidemiol Community Health,* **36**, 202-4.

Organisation for Economic Co-operation and Development (1993). *OECD health systems. Facts and trends 1960-1991. Health policy studies no 3*. OECD, Paris. (Health policy studies, Volume 1.)

Oriol P., Patois E., Guenin-Tostain F., Benotman H. and Kauffmann F. (1994). Le tabagisme des jeunes de 11-16 ans dans le département des Yvelines en 1990 (Smoking by 11-16-year-olds in the Yvelines department in 1990). *Rev Mal Respir,* **11**, 583-92.

Oriol P., Patois E., Guenin-Tostain F. and Kauffmann F. (1988). Facteurs de risque du tabagisme chez les jeunes de 11 à 16 ans. (Risk factors for smoking in the young age 11 to 16). *Rev Mal Respir,* **5**, 393-400.

Poirier R., Vary M.A., Lanteaume A., Mercier F., Borde G. and Laval P. (1979). Le tabagisme scolaire. Premiers résultats d'une enquête réalisée dans l'agglomération marseillaise (Smoking habit at school. First results of a survey done in Marseille and its suburbs. *Poumon et le Coeur,* **35**, 13-6.

Readers Digest (1963). *Products and people. A digest of the marketing survey of the European Common Market and Britain, 1963* . Reader's Digest Association Limited, London.

RP6, See Beese (ed) (1968), Beese (ed) (1972), Lee (ed) (1975)

Sasco A.J., Grizeau D. and Danzon M. (1995). Is tobacco use finally decreasing in France? *Cancer Detect Prev,* **19**, 210-8.

Sasco A.J., Grizeau D., Pobel D., Chatard O. and Danzon M. (1994). Tabagisme et classe sociale en France de 1974 à 1991 (Smoking and social class in France 1974-1991). *Bull Cancer,* **81**, 355-9.

Sasco A.J., Pobel D., Grizeau D. and Danzon M. (1991). Évolution récente du tabagisme des jeunes en France (Current development of smoking in young people in France). *Pediatrie,* **46**, 555-60.

Schwartz D., Flamant R., Lellouch J. and Denoix P.F. (1961). Results of a French survey on the role of tobacco, particularly inhalation, in different cancer sites. *J Natl Cancer Inst,* **26**, 1085-108.

Service des Statistiques, des Etudes et des Systemes d'Information (SESI) (1983). *Quelques résultats sur les consommateurs de boissons alcoholiques et de tabac en France en 1980. Enquete aupres des menages sur la sante et les soins medicaux—1980-81*. Ministère des Affaires Sociales. Informations Rapides 20.

SOFRES *Les Francais et le tabac. Résultats d'un sondage de la SOFRES effectué entre le 7 et le 10 décembre 1974 auprès d'un échantillon national de 1000 personnes représentatif de la population français âgée de 18 ans et plus.* [§]

Statistika Centralbyrån (1995). *Tobacco consumption 1970-1994 in the member states of the European Union and in Norway and Iceland.* European Commission.

Todd G. (1986a). *Medicine. Statistics of smoking in the Member States of the European Community.* Commission of the European Communities, Luxembourg.

Todd G.F. (1986b). *Cigarette Data Collection : A record of six cigarette smoking parameters in 20 countries.* Unpublished.

Treguer M., D'Houtard A., Deschamps J.P., Martin J., Andre G. and Chau N. (1983). Données épidémiologiques concernant le tabagisme chez les jeunes. *Medecine et Armees,* **11**, 595-600.

Tuyns A.J. and Hu M.X. (1982). Changing smoking patterns in Calvados (France). *British Journal of Addiction,* **77**, 167-83.

van Reek J. and Adriaanse H. (1995). Daily smoking among adolescents in the European Community. *Rev Epidemiol Sante Publique,* **43**, 281-2.

van Reek J., Adriaanse H. and Karaoglou A. (1992). Smoking among children in the European Community. *J Public Health Med,* **14**, 93-4.

WHO (1989). The WHO MONICA project: a worldwide monitoring system for cardiovascular diseases. In: *World health statistics annual 1989.* WHO, Geneva; 25-149.

WHO MONICA Project (1988). Geographical variation in the major risk factors of coronary heart disease in men and women aged 35-64 years. *World Health Stat Q,* **41**, 115-40.

WHO (1997). *Tobacco or health: A global status report.* WHO, Geneva. www.cdc.gov/nccdphp/osh/who/whoampro.htm.

WHO (1975). Survey on smoking and health in the European Region, 1974-75: preliminary data as at 1 May 1975. *Presented at the Third World Conference on Smoking and Health, New York, 2-5 June 1975.* WHO; 1-55.

Wynder E.L., Mushinski M.H., Stellman S.D. and Choay P. (1981). Tobacco usage in France: An epidemiological study. *Prev Med,* **10**, 301-15.

§ Original paper not obtained, but information taken as quoted by another author

Germany 10

Sales data

See Tables 10.1-10.3.

Tobacco processing has a long history in Germany. In 1788 the first tobacco and cigarette factory was founded in Hamburg and in 1882 part-mechanized cigarette production began in Dresden (Kneist (1981)). Attempts to control smoking behaviour also began early. For example, smoking was banned in Bavaria and Kursachsen in the late 1600s and in Berlin in 1723 (Proctor (1997)). A 'Bureau Against the Dangers of Alcohol and Tobacco' was established in 1939 (Davey-Smith *et al* (1994)).

Data are available on consumption of tobacco products from 1906. No data are available for the years of the two world wars, for East Germany, or for 1990, the year of reunification. Data for 1948 suggest that consumption had been very low in the preceding years. Before the First World War consumption per adult was less than 1 manufactured cigarette per day and this increased to around 2 cigarettes between the wars. After the Second World War consumption in West Germany rose steadily until the early 1970s when it reached a peak of 7 manufactured cigarettes per day. It decreased to 6 cigarettes in the 1980s and to about 5.5 cigarettes in unified Germany in the 1990s. We estimate that, at the beginning of the 1950s, consumption of hand-rolled cigarettes per adult was about 1 cigarette per day, but decreased to very low levels by the mid-1960s. In the mid-1970s it started to increase again, returning to 1 cigarette per day in the 1980s.

The consumption of all tobacco products combined per adult was about 6 g per day between the wars. After the Second World War it rose to a peak of nearly 9 g in the early 1970s (West Germany), before falling back below 7 g by 1995. In 1913, 14% of all tobacco was consumed in manufactured cigarettes. From 1925 to 1948 the proportion was around 35%. It increased after the Second World War to about 85% in 1975, but then fell again owing to the increase in consumption of hand-rolled cigarettes. About 70% of manufactured cigarettes were filtered in 1960, rising to over 90% in early 1980s. Consumption of cigars accounted for over 30% of sales until the 1950s. No data are available for smokeless tobacco for recent decades, but in 1913 chewing tobacco and snuff accounted for about 10% of all tobacco consumed, falling to 5% by the mid-1920s (Hutson (1937)).

Survey data

See Tables 10.4-10.8

Representative surveys of smoking have been carried out in West Germany since 1950, but few are available for East Germany. Some series conducted in West Germany, including the mikrocensus (source 67), were continued and reported for both regions after unification. In West Germany in 1950, the prevalence of tobacco smoking among those aged 15 years and over was nearly 90% in men and 20% in women. The difference between the percentages of men and women who smoke has decreased since then, mainly because of a reduction in the prevalence of smoking among men to 32% in 1992. The prevalence among women increased somewhat, with estimates varying around 20-30% in the 1970s and 1980s, and falling below 20% in 1992. A further 4-5% of both men and women smoke occasionally. The prevalence of cigarette smoking among men fell from about 60% in 1950 to about 30% in 1992. Very few women smoked products other than cigarettes.

The prevalence of tobacco smoking, and of cigarette smoking, in East Berlin was similar to that in West Germany when surveyed in 1971 (source 47). In representative surveys conducted shortly before and after reunification, the prevalence in East Germany was a little higher among men and lower among women than in West Germany (sources 64, 67).

Very few data on adult smoking by age in West Germany are available before 1978, while early data for East Germany are mostly on a local basis. More men smoked than women at all ages, except below age 20 where some surveys in the West in the 1980s show that there were more young women who smoked than young men. A lower percentage of smokers in older age groups was more marked in women than in men. There are few data on prevalence by type of cigarette, but one survey in 1984 (source 4) showed that the prevalence of smoking of only hand-rolled cigarettes appeared to be 1% among both men and women, and concentrated among those aged 20-39. In 1992, hand-rolled cigarettes were more popular among young smokers in the West than in the East (source 68, notes).

Comparison of survey and sales data suggests that the mikrocensus under-reported consumption by 40%, both before and after reunification, while other surveys in West Germany under-reported by 10-25%. Between 1950 and the late 1960s, the estimated number of cigarettes smoked per person per day (sales-adjusted) increased for men from about 4 to 10. Although the number of manufactured cigarettes started to fall, the total number of cigarettes (including hand-rolled) remained level through the 1980s, decreasing to about 8 by 1995. For women the increase continued for longer, rising from 1.5 to 5 cigarettes by 1980, and decreasing to 4 by 1995.

Table 10.1.1 Total annual sales of tobacco products, 1906-1973

Year	Cigarettes tonnes	Cigarettes millions	Cigars tonnes	Cigars millions	Fine-cut tobacco tonnes	Pipe tobacco tonnes	All tobacco products tonnes
Germany							
1906		3639			200		
1907		5805			278		
1908		6471			252		
1909		7271			313		
1910		8353			299		
1911		9852			303		
1912		11518			333		
1913		12990			375		
1925	30530	30529	30480	5746	32610		93630
1926	29160	29156	31750	5980	38510		99420
1927	32770	32768	35200	6635	38510		106480
1928	31610	31601	34970	6589	37600		104180
1929	32880	32877	37010	6973	37380		107270
1930	29370	29367	37920	7146	39140		106440
1931	28070	28064	32890	6194	32110		93070
1932	31760	31759	30120	5678	15380	18600	95860
1933	33710	33701	34880	6570	13880	19190	101650
1934	36170	36162	41680	7854	13380	18510	109740
1935	37480	37471	41870	7892	14200	17370	110910
1936	38460	38455	44720	8424	15150	16560	114890
1937	42430	42420	47400	8932	16370	15200	121400
1938	47310	47306	48580	9150	18190	13790	127870
West Germany							
1948	9850	9852	8300	1453	6890	2000	27040
1949	22090	22090	12750	2232	16060	5190	56090
1950	26490	24089	22720	3785	17330	4850	71400
1951	31840	28967	25360	4157	17330	4900	79420
1952	33930	30840	27900	4592	15920	4490	82240
1953	39420	35868	27580	4520	14330	3900	85230
1954	43640	39663	27440	4472	13240	3450	87770
1955	49940	45411	27940	4585	12200	3270	93350
1956	55750	50663	28080	4601	10660	2950	97430
1957	62640	55875	26220	4724	9660	2630	101150
1958	67810	60482	25720	4629	8750	2400	104690
1959	70440	65245	25220	4544	8940	2270	106870
1960	76610	70956	24130	4349	8300	2000	111040
1961	81010	78039	27400	4111	7890	1810	118110
1962	85550	83286	25810	3988	7530	1630	120520
1963	86450	85276	23540	3786	7570	1540	119110
1964	90760	90156	24180	4098	7850	1770	124560
1965	96210	96055	23500	3953	7080	1500	128280
1966	102470	101488	23360	3778	6800	1500	134130
1967	96980	99139	23590	3597	6940	2040	129550
1968	105190	105444	22140	3595	6490	2000	135800
1969	110490	112431	21230	3420	5990	1910	139620
1970	116030	118051	19910	3212	5810	1950	143700
1971	123330	125493	19230	3100	4940	1810	149320
1972	124280	126469	18910	3051	5310	2090	150590
1973	123290	125461	17280	2802	5940	2040	148550

Source: see *Notes on sources of sales data*, p. 263

Table 10.1.2 Total annual sales of tobacco products, 1974-1995

Year	Cigarettes		Cigars & Cigarillos			Fine-cut tobacco	Pipe tobacco	All tobacco products
	tonnes	millions	tonnes	cigars millions	cigarillos millions	tonnes	tonnes	tonnes
West Germany								
1974	125214	127769	16443	2652		5674	1863	149194
1975	122070	124561	15346	2475		5475	1705	144596
1976	126813	129401	15275	2464		6191	1722	150002
1977	113366	115680	15522	2503		10776	1885	141549
1978	120342	122798	14679	2368		10307	1832	147159
1979	122031	124521	13587	2192		10904	1662	148184
1980	125857	128426	12984	974	1120	10658	1732	151230
1981	126534	129117	12426	865	1139	11963	1825	152749
1982	109723	111962	11202	870	937	20719	1919	143563
1983	116159	118530	11023	852	926	17697	1762	146641
1984	116983	119371	10770	795	942	15701	1714	145168
1985	118000	120409	10122	709	923	15398	1611	145131
1986	115153	117503	9490	657	874	15765	1575	141983
1987	115669	118029	8787	575	842	15597	1833	141886
1988	115451	117807	8139	501	812	14804	1331	139725
1989	118128	120539	7570	1221		14269	1256	141223
Unified Germany								
1991	149691	152746	8886	1433		17924	1385	177886
1992	131248	133926	7882	1271		21514	1270	161914
1993	126592	129176	8269	1334		20058	1200	156119
1994	133794	136525	9046	1459		16039	1312	160192
1995	131821	134511	8594	1386		15376	1117	156909

Source : see *Notes on sources of sales data*, p. 263

Table 10.1.3 Manufactured cigarettes (i) percentage of total sales as filter cigarettes, 1960-1983, (ii) sales-weighted average tar yield per cigarette (SWAT), 1961-1985, (iii) sales-weighted average nicotine yield per cigarette (SWAN), 1961-1985, and (iv) total annual sales of cigarette papers 1961-1985

	Year	% Filter	SWAT Moist mg / cig	SWAT Dry mg / cig	SWAN mg / cig	Cigarette papers millions
West Germany						
	1960	67.8				
	1961	72.8	28.3		1.44	4515
	1962	75.9	26.8		1.40	4047
	1963	77.9	25.8		1.35	4345
	1964	80.0	25.5		1.29	4269
	1965	81.6	23.7		1.24	4148
	1966	82.9	22.7	20.7	1.18	3989
	1967	83.3	21.8	19.8	1.14	4518
	1968	82.5	20.9	19.1	1.10	4175
	1969	84.1	20.0	18.4	1.05	4121
	1970	84.2	18.2	17.4	1.00	4056
	1971	84.8	18.5	16.5	0.94	3691
	1972	85.1	17.6	15.5	0.89	3962
	1973	85.2	16.9	15.7	0.91	4868
	1974	84.8	15.9	15.2	0.77	5311
	1975	86.0	15.2	14.1	0.66	5118
	1976	86.4				6167
	1977	86.9				10044
	1978	87.2				9134
	1979	87.5				9711
	1980	88.2				10427
	1981	88.9				12385
	1982	89.0				19086
	1983	92.0				19137
	1984					17116
	1985			12.8	0.78	16765

	Year	% Filter
East Germany		
	1960	<10
	1969	79
	1975	91
	1984	93

Source : see *Notes on sources of sales data*, p. 263

Table 10.2 Consumption of (i) cigarettes and (ii) all tobacco products, 1906-1995 sales-based data, including estimated hand-rolled cigarette consumption. Males and females aged 15 years and over

Year	Manufactured cigarettes		Hand-rolled cigarettes		Total cigarettes		All tobacco products	
	Total annual in millions	Number/ adult/day	Total annual in millions	Number/ adult/day	Total annual in millions	Number/ adult/day	Total annual in tonnes	Grams/ adult/day
Germany								
1906	3639	0.2	140	0.0	3779	0.2		
1907	5805	0.3	194.6	0.0	6000	0.4		
1908	6471	0.4	176.4	0.0	6647	0.4		
1909	7271	0.4	219.1	0.0	7490	0.4		
1910	8353	0.5	209.3	0.0	8562	0.5		
1911	9852	0.6	212.1	0.0	10064	0.6		
1912	11518	0.7	233.1	0.0	11751	0.7		
1913	12990	0.8	262.5	0.0	13252	0.8		
1925	30529	1.8					93630	5.4
1926	29156	1.7					99420	5.7
1927	32768	1.9					106480	6.1
1928	31601	1.8					104180	5.9
1929	32877	1.9					107270	6.1
1930	29367	1.6					106440	6.0
1931	28064	1.6					93070	5.2
1932	31759	1.8	10766	0.6	42525	2.4	95860	5.3
1933	33701	1.9	9716	0.5	43417	2.4	101650	5.6
1934	36162	2.0	9366	0.5	45528	2.5	109740	6.0
1935	37471	2.0	9940	0.5	47411	2.6	110910	6.0
1936	38455	2.1	10605	0.6	49060	2.6	114890	6.2
1937	42420	2.2	11459	0.6	53879	2.9	121400	6.4
1938	47306	2.5	12733	0.7	60039	3.1	127870	6.6
West Germany								
1948	9852	0.7	4823	0.4	14675	1.1	27040	2.0
1949	22090	1.6	11242	0.8	33332	2.5	56090	4.2
1950	24089	1.8	12131	0.9	36220	2.7	71400	5.4
1951	28967	2.2	12131	0.9	41098	3.1	79420	5.9
1952	30840	2.3	11144	0.8	41984	3.1	82240	6.0
1953	35868	2.6	10031	0.7	45899	3.3	85230	6.2
1954	39663	2.8	9268	0.7	48931	3.5	87770	6.2
1955	45411	3.2	8540	0.6	53951	3.8	93350	6.5
1956	50663	3.5	7462	0.5	58125	4.1	97430	6.8
1957	55875	3.9	6762	0.5	62637	4.3	101150	7.0
1958	60482	4.0	6125	0.4	66607	4.4	104690	7.0
1959	65245	4.3	6258	0.4	71503	4.7	106870	7.1
1960	70956	4.7	5810	0.4	76766	5.0	111040	7.3
1961	78039	5.1	4064	0.3	82102	5.4	118110	7.7
1962	83286	5.1	3642	0.2	86928	5.4	120520	7.4
1963	85276	5.2	3910	0.2	89186	5.5	119110	7.3
1964	90156	5.5	3842	0.2	93998	5.7	124560	7.5
1965	96055	5.8	3733	0.2	99788	6.0	128280	7.7
1966	101488	6.0	3590	0.2	105078	6.2	134130	8.0
1967	99139	5.9	4066	0.2	103205	6.1	129550	7.7
1968	105444	6.3	3758	0.2	109202	6.5	135800	8.1
1969	112431	6.6	3709	0.2	116140	6.8	139620	8.2

Table 10.2 *(continued)*

Year	Manufactured cigarettes		Hand-rolled cigarettes		Total cigarettes		All tobacco products	
	Total annual in millions	Number/ adult/day	Total annual in millions	Number/ adult/day	Total annual in millions	Number/ adult/day	Total annual in tonnes	Grams/ adult/day
1970	118051	6.9	3650	0.2	121701	7.2	143700	8.4
1971	125493	7.3	3322	0.2	128815	7.5	149320	8.7
1972	126469	7.3	3566	0.2	130035	7.5	150590	8.7
1973	125461	7.1	4381	0.2	129842	7.4	148550	8.5
1974	127769	7.2	4780	0.3	132549	7.5	149194	8.4
1975	124561	7.0	4606	0.3	129167	7.3	144596	8.2
1976	129401	7.3	5550	0.3	134951	7.6	150002	8.4
1977	115680	6.5	9040	0.5	124719	7.0	141549	7.9
1978	122798	6.8	8221	0.5	131018	7.3	147159	8.2
1979	124521	6.9	8740	0.5	133261	7.3	148184	8.2
1980	128426	7.0	9384	0.5	137810	7.5	151230	8.2
1981	129117	7.0	11146	0.6	140263	7.6	152749	8.2
1982	111962	6.0	17177	0.9	129140	6.9	143563	7.7
1983	118530	6.3	17223	0.9	135753	7.2	146641	7.8
1984	119371	6.3	15404	0.8	134775	7.2	145168	7.7
1985	120409	6.4	15088	0.8	135497	7.2	145131	7.7
1986	117503	6.2	14412	0.8	131914	7.0	141983	7.5
1987	118029	6.2	15209	0.8	133238	7.0	141886	7.5
1988	117807	6.2	14180	0.7	131987	6.9	139725	7.3
1989	120539	6.3	14269	0.7	134808	7.0	141223	7.3
Unified Germany								
1991	152746	6.2	17924	0.7	170671	7.0	177886	7.3
1992	133926	5.4	21514	0.9	155440	6.3	161914	6.6
1993	129176	5.2	20058	0.8	149234	6.0	156119	6.3
1994	136525	5.5	16039	0.6	152564	6.1	160192	6.4
1995	134511	5.4	15376	0.6	149887	6.0	156909	6.3

Source : see *Notes on sources of sales data*, p. 263

Figure 10.1 Daily consumption of (i) manufactured and total number of cigarettes, and (ii) all tobacco products, Germany 1920-1938, West Germany 1948-1989 and Unified Germany 1991-1995.
Males and females aged 15 years and over. *Source:* see Table 10.2

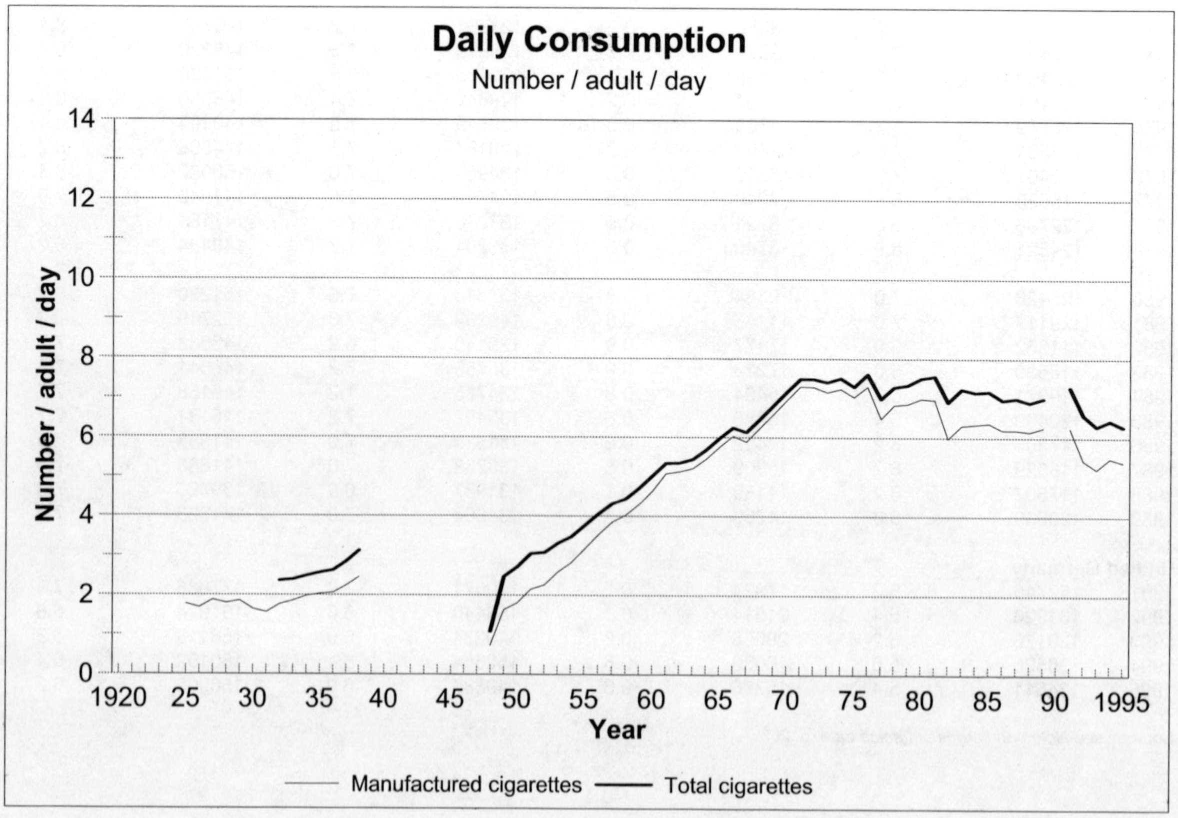

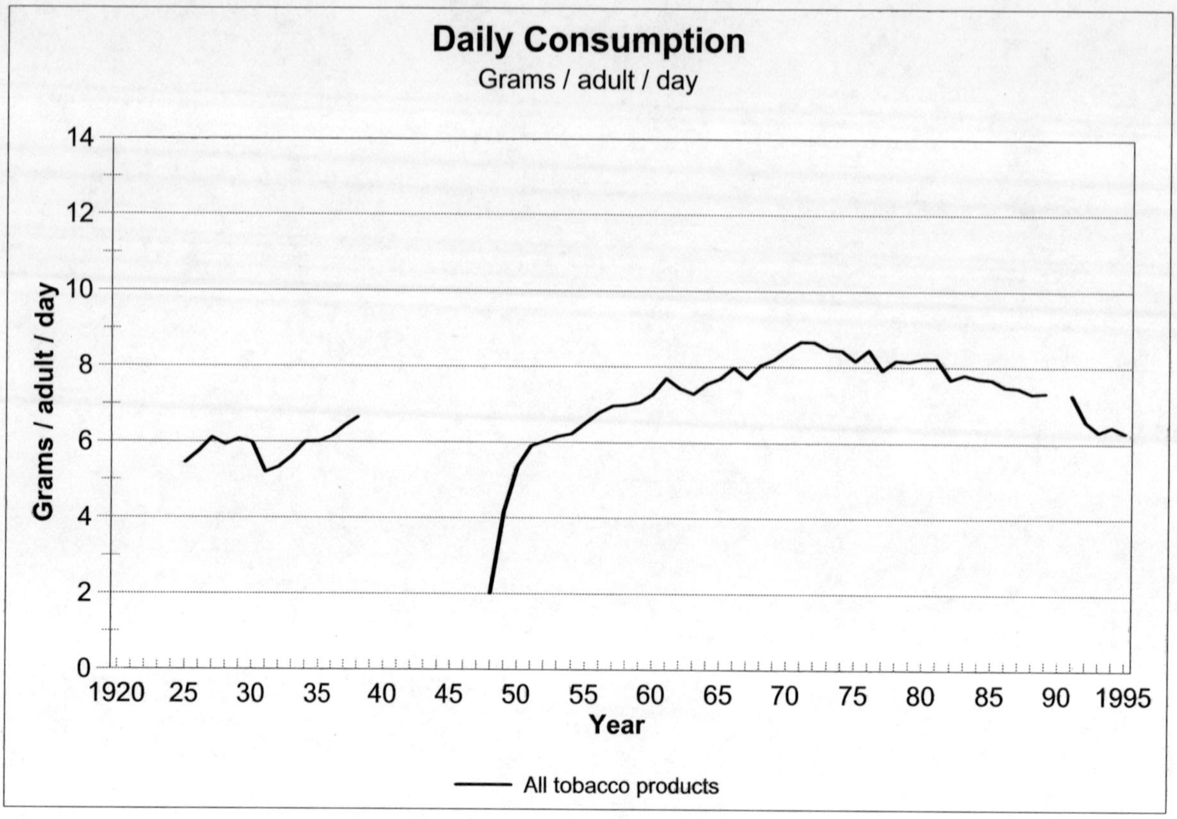

Table 10.3 Percentage sales of tobacco in different forms (by weight), selected years 1925-1995

Year	Cigarettes (%)	Cigars(%)	Loose tobacco	
			Fine-cut (%)	Pipe (%)
1925	32.6	32.6	34.8	
1935	33.8	37.8	12.8	15.7
1948	36.4	30.7	25.5	7.4
1955	72.9	29.9	13.1	3.5
1965	75.0	18.3	5.5	1.2
1975	84.4	10.6	3.8	1.2
1985	81.3	7.0	10.6	1.1
1995	84.0	5.5	9.8	0.7

Note: 1948-1985 relate to West Germany

Source : calculated from Tables 10.1.1 & 10.1.2

Figure 10.2 Percentage sales of tobacco in different forms (by weight), selected years 1925-1995
Source: see Table 10.3

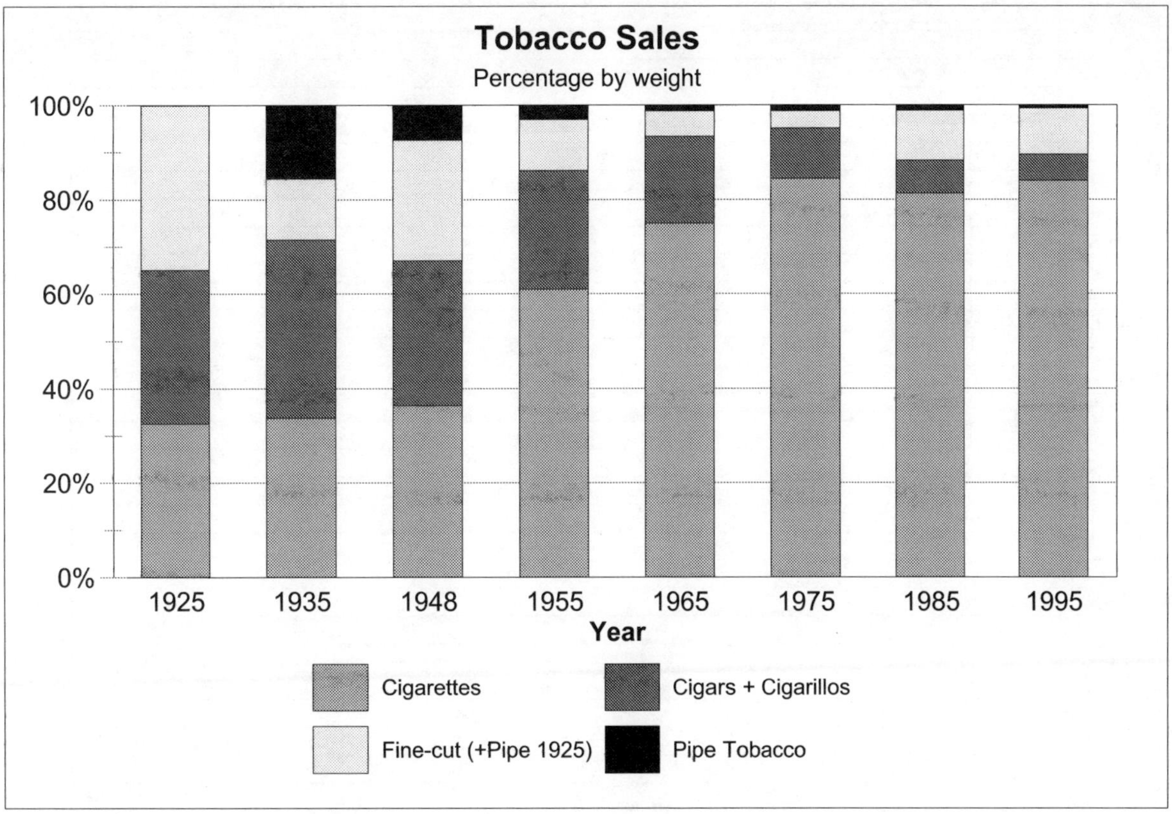

Table 10.4M Prevalence of smoking, males: some selected German surveys by age, 1950-1995 *(continues on p. 242)*

West Germany

<table>
<tr><th rowspan="2">Frequency
Product
Source
Year</th><th colspan="21">Age group</th><th rowspan="2">All ages</th></tr>
<tr><th>12</th><th>13</th><th>14</th><th>15</th><th>16</th><th>17</th><th>18</th><th>19</th><th>20-24</th><th>25-29</th><th>30-34</th><th>35-39</th><th>40-44</th><th>45-49</th><th>50-54</th><th>55-59</th><th>60-64</th><th>65-69</th><th>70-74</th><th>75-79</th><th>80+</th></tr>
<tr><td>50 11 UC U</td><td colspan="2"></td><td colspan="19">60</td><td></td></tr>
<tr><td>50 11 A U</td><td colspan="2"></td><td colspan="19">88</td><td></td></tr>
<tr><td>55 11 UC U</td><td colspan="2"></td><td colspan="19">64</td><td></td></tr>
<tr><td>55 11 A U</td><td colspan="2"></td><td colspan="19">83</td><td></td></tr>
<tr><td>58 12 UC U</td><td colspan="4"></td><td colspan="16">63</td><td></td><td></td></tr>
<tr><td>58 12 A U</td><td colspan="4"></td><td colspan="16">77</td><td></td><td></td></tr>
<tr><td>60 11 UC U</td><td colspan="2"></td><td colspan="19">61</td><td></td></tr>
<tr><td>60 11 A U</td><td colspan="2"></td><td colspan="19">78</td><td></td></tr>
<tr><td>60 13 MC R</td><td colspan="3"></td><td colspan="18">49</td><td></td></tr>
<tr><td>60 13 A U</td><td colspan="3"></td><td colspan="18">77</td><td></td></tr>
<tr><td>63 14 UC U</td><td colspan="8"></td><td colspan="13">56</td><td></td></tr>
<tr><td>63 14 A U</td><td colspan="8"></td><td colspan="13">70</td><td></td></tr>
<tr><td>65 11 UC U</td><td colspan="2"></td><td colspan="19">61</td><td></td></tr>
<tr><td>65 11 A U</td><td colspan="2"></td><td colspan="19">74</td><td></td></tr>
<tr><td>65 12 UC U</td><td colspan="4"></td><td colspan="16">57</td><td></td><td></td></tr>
<tr><td>65 27 U U</td><td colspan="8">42</td><td colspan="13"></td><td></td></tr>
<tr><td>65 28 U U</td><td colspan="2"></td><td colspan="2">41</td><td></td><td colspan="2">59</td><td colspan="14"></td><td></td></tr>
<tr><td>65 29 U U</td><td colspan="2"></td><td colspan="2">45</td><td></td><td colspan="2">62</td><td colspan="14"></td><td></td></tr>
<tr><td>67 5 MC U</td><td colspan="12"></td><td colspan="5">53</td><td colspan="4"></td><td></td></tr>
<tr><td>67 5 A U</td><td colspan="12"></td><td colspan="5">66</td><td colspan="4"></td><td></td></tr>
<tr><td>67 9 U U</td><td></td><td colspan="3">43</td><td colspan="3">61</td><td colspan="14"></td><td></td></tr>
<tr><td>67 15 UC U</td><td colspan="2"></td><td colspan="16">61</td><td colspan="3"></td><td></td></tr>
<tr><td>70 3 A A</td><td colspan="4"></td><td colspan="17">59</td><td></td></tr>
<tr><td>70 8 UC U</td><td colspan="2"></td><td colspan="5">60</td><td colspan="14"></td><td></td></tr>
<tr><td>70 8 A U</td><td colspan="2"></td><td colspan="5">63</td><td colspan="14"></td><td></td></tr>
<tr><td>70 11 UC U</td><td colspan="2"></td><td colspan="19">55</td><td></td></tr>
<tr><td>70 11 A U</td><td colspan="2"></td><td colspan="19">67</td><td></td></tr>
<tr><td>71 13 MC R</td><td colspan="3"></td><td colspan="18">49</td><td></td></tr>
<tr><td>71 16 UC U</td><td colspan="8"></td><td colspan="9">53</td><td colspan="4"></td><td></td></tr>
<tr><td>71 16 A U</td><td colspan="8"></td><td colspan="9">63</td><td colspan="4"></td><td></td></tr>
<tr><td>72 68 U R</td><td colspan="2"></td><td colspan="7">49</td><td colspan="12"></td><td></td></tr>
<tr><td>72 68 U A</td><td colspan="2"></td><td colspan="7">71</td><td colspan="12"></td><td></td></tr>
<tr><td>73 6 U U</td><td colspan="8"></td><td colspan="2">65</td><td colspan="4">64</td><td colspan="3">67</td><td colspan="4"></td><td>60</td></tr>
<tr><td>73 7 * U</td><td colspan="8"></td><td colspan="9">54</td><td colspan="4"></td><td></td></tr>
<tr><td>73 11 UC U</td><td colspan="4"></td><td colspan="17">52</td><td></td></tr>
<tr><td>73 11 A U</td><td colspan="4"></td><td colspan="17">65</td><td></td></tr>
<tr><td>73 31 U A</td><td colspan="9">47</td><td colspan="12"></td><td></td></tr>
<tr><td>74 5 MC U</td><td colspan="12"></td><td colspan="5">42</td><td colspan="4"></td><td></td></tr>
<tr><td>74 5 A U</td><td colspan="12"></td><td colspan="5">49</td><td colspan="4"></td><td></td></tr>
<tr><td>74 11 UC U</td><td colspan="2"></td><td colspan="19">47</td><td></td></tr>
<tr><td>74 11 A U</td><td colspan="2"></td><td colspan="19">55</td><td></td></tr>
<tr><td>74 12 UC U</td><td colspan="4"></td><td colspan="16">46</td><td></td><td></td></tr>
<tr><td>74 22 U A</td><td colspan="7">41</td><td colspan="14"></td><td></td></tr>
<tr><td>74 33 A U</td><td colspan="2"></td><td colspan="7">58</td><td colspan="12"></td><td></td></tr>
<tr><td>75 1 TC A</td><td colspan="2"></td><td colspan="8">50</td><td colspan="2">43</td><td colspan="2">39</td><td colspan="2">43</td><td colspan="5">26</td><td>41</td></tr>
<tr><td>75 1 A A</td><td colspan="2"></td><td colspan="19">48</td><td></td></tr>
<tr><td>75 11 UC U</td><td colspan="2"></td><td colspan="19">50</td><td></td></tr>
<tr><td>75 11 A U</td><td colspan="2"></td><td colspan="19">60</td><td></td></tr>
<tr><td>75 13 MC R</td><td colspan="3"></td><td colspan="18">39</td><td></td></tr>
<tr><td>75 15 UC U</td><td colspan="2"></td><td colspan="16">45</td><td colspan="3"></td><td></td></tr>
<tr><td>75 15 A U</td><td colspan="2"></td><td colspan="19">53</td><td></td></tr>
<tr><td>75 18* U U</td><td colspan="3"></td><td>10</td><td>26</td><td>34</td><td>42</td><td>49</td><td colspan="13"></td><td>47</td></tr>
<tr><td>75 19 U U</td><td colspan="3"></td><td>60</td><td>61</td><td>62</td><td>59</td><td>64</td><td colspan="13"></td><td></td></tr>
</table>

Table 10.4F Prevalence of smoking, females: some selected German surveys by age, 1950-1995 *(continues on p. 243)*

West Germany

Frequency / Product / Source / Year	12	13	14	15	16	17	18	19	20-24	25-29	30-34	35-39	40-44	45-49	50-54	55-59	60-64	65-69	70-74	75-79	80+	All ages
50 11 UC U			21																			
50 11 A U			21																			
55 11 UC U			21																			
55 11 A U			21																			
58 12 UC U																						
58 12 A U																						
60 11 UC U			22																			
60 11 A U			22																			
60 13 MC R				13																		
60 13 A U				23																		
63 14 UC U									16													
63 14 A U									16													
65 11 UC U			24																			
65 11 A U			24																			
65 12 UC U					18																	
65 27 U U	36																					
65 28 U U			33			52																
65 29 U U			12			41																
67 5 MC U													16									
67 5 A U													16									
67 9 U U		23			45																	
67 15 UC U			28																			
70 3 A A					24																	
70 8 UC U																						
70 8 A U																						
70 11 UC U			27																			
70 11 A U			27																			
71 13 MC R				21																		
71 16 UC U																						
71 16 A U																						
72 68 U R			33																			
72 68 U A			64																			
73 6 U U									27													
73 7 * U									26													
73 11 UC U					30																	
73 11 A U					30																	
73 31 U A	39																					
74 5 MC U													19									
74 5 A U													20									
74 11 UC U			29																			
74 11 A U			28																			
74 12 UC U					27																	
74 22 U A	33																					
74 33 A U			44																			
75 1 TC A			40								30		22		17		7					23
75 1 A A			23																			
75 11 UC U			29																			
75 11 A U			29																			
75 13 MC R				20																		
75 15 UC U			23																			
75 15 A U			23																			
75 18* U U				16	28	33	40	36														43
75 19 U U				55	57	62	58	63														

Table 10.4M *(continued from p. 240, continues on p. 244)*
Prevalence of smoking, males

West Germany *(continued)*

<table>
<tr><th rowspan="2">Frequency
Product
Source
Year</th><th colspan="21">Age group</th><th rowspan="2">All ages</th></tr>
<tr><th>12</th><th>13</th><th>14</th><th>15</th><th>16</th><th>17</th><th>18</th><th>19</th><th>20-24</th><th>25-29</th><th>30-34</th><th>35-39</th><th>40-44</th><th>45-49</th><th>50-54</th><th>55-59</th><th>60-64</th><th>65-69</th><th>70-74</th><th>75-79</th><th>80+</th></tr>
<tr><td>76 3 A A</td><td colspan="2"></td><td colspan="19">51</td><td></td></tr>
<tr><td>76 11 UC U</td><td colspan="2"></td><td colspan="19">47</td><td></td></tr>
<tr><td>76 11 A U</td><td colspan="2"></td><td colspan="19">55</td><td></td></tr>
<tr><td>76 13 MC R</td><td colspan="2"></td><td colspan="19">39</td><td></td></tr>
<tr><td>76 31 U A</td><td colspan="9">44</td><td colspan="12"></td><td></td></tr>
<tr><td>76 68 U R</td><td colspan="2"></td><td colspan="7">41</td><td colspan="12"></td><td></td></tr>
<tr><td>76 68 U A</td><td colspan="2"></td><td colspan="7">66</td><td colspan="12"></td><td></td></tr>
<tr><td>77 1 TC A</td><td colspan="2"></td><td colspan="8">52</td><td colspan="2">46</td><td colspan="2">47</td><td colspan="2">38</td><td colspan="5">24</td><td>43</td></tr>
<tr><td>77 1 A A</td><td colspan="2"></td><td colspan="19">48</td><td></td></tr>
<tr><td>77 11 UC U</td><td colspan="2"></td><td colspan="19">45</td><td></td></tr>
<tr><td>77 11 A U</td><td colspan="2"></td><td colspan="19">53</td><td></td></tr>
<tr><td>77 13 MC R</td><td colspan="2"></td><td colspan="19">36</td><td></td></tr>
<tr><td>77 17 UC U</td><td colspan="2"></td><td colspan="15">45</td><td colspan="4"></td><td></td></tr>
<tr><td>77 17 A U</td><td colspan="2"></td><td colspan="15">50</td><td colspan="4"></td><td></td></tr>
<tr><td>78 11 UC U</td><td colspan="2"></td><td colspan="19">47</td><td></td></tr>
<tr><td>78 11 A U</td><td colspan="2"></td><td colspan="19">55</td><td></td></tr>
<tr><td>78 13 MC R</td><td colspan="2"></td><td colspan="19">37</td><td></td></tr>
<tr><td>78 16 UC U</td><td colspan="8"></td><td colspan="9">48</td><td colspan="4"></td><td></td></tr>
<tr><td>78 16 A U</td><td colspan="8"></td><td colspan="9">55</td><td colspan="4"></td><td></td></tr>
<tr><td>78 20 U U</td><td colspan="8">25</td><td colspan="13"></td><td></td></tr>
<tr><td>78 34 UC U</td><td colspan="4"></td><td colspan="14">43</td><td colspan="3"></td><td></td></tr>
<tr><td>78 67 TC R</td><td colspan="2"></td><td colspan="2">4</td><td colspan="2">21</td><td colspan="2">39</td><td>47</td><td>48</td><td colspan="2">44</td><td colspan="2">42</td><td colspan="2">39</td><td>31</td><td colspan="4">27</td><td>34</td></tr>
<tr><td>78 67 A R</td><td colspan="2"></td><td colspan="2">4</td><td colspan="2">22</td><td colspan="2">39</td><td>48</td><td>50</td><td colspan="2">47</td><td colspan="2">45</td><td colspan="2">44</td><td>38</td><td colspan="4">36</td><td>37</td></tr>
<tr><td>78 67 A A</td><td colspan="2"></td><td colspan="2">7</td><td colspan="2">30</td><td colspan="2">49</td><td>56</td><td>57</td><td colspan="2">53</td><td colspan="2">51</td><td colspan="2">49</td><td>45</td><td colspan="4">36</td><td>43</td></tr>
<tr><td>79 1 TC A</td><td colspan="2"></td><td colspan="8">49</td><td colspan="2">43</td><td colspan="2">40</td><td colspan="2">42</td><td colspan="5">28</td><td>41</td></tr>
<tr><td>79 1 A A</td><td colspan="2"></td><td colspan="19">48</td><td></td></tr>
<tr><td>79 2 TC A</td><td colspan="2"></td><td colspan="6">39</td><td colspan="2">56</td><td colspan="2">43</td><td colspan="2">40</td><td colspan="2">42</td><td colspan="5">28</td><td>41</td></tr>
<tr><td>79 2 A A</td><td colspan="2"></td><td colspan="6">39</td><td colspan="2">63</td><td colspan="2">49</td><td colspan="2">43</td><td colspan="2">52</td><td colspan="5">42</td><td>48</td></tr>
<tr><td>79 11 UC U</td><td colspan="2"></td><td colspan="19">44</td><td></td></tr>
<tr><td>79 11 A U</td><td colspan="2"></td><td colspan="19">52</td><td></td></tr>
<tr><td>79 13 MC R</td><td colspan="3"></td><td colspan="18">38</td><td></td></tr>
<tr><td>79 35 U R</td><td>2</td><td>8</td><td>17</td><td>28</td><td>40</td><td colspan="16"></td><td></td></tr>
<tr><td>79 35 U A</td><td>29</td><td>29</td><td>36</td><td>49</td><td>53</td><td colspan="16"></td><td></td></tr>
<tr><td>80 3 A A</td><td colspan="2"></td><td colspan="19">47</td><td></td></tr>
<tr><td>80 11 UC U</td><td colspan="2"></td><td colspan="19">49</td><td></td></tr>
<tr><td>80 11 A U</td><td colspan="2"></td><td colspan="19">53</td><td></td></tr>
<tr><td>80 31 U A</td><td colspan="9">42</td><td colspan="12"></td><td></td></tr>
<tr><td>81 1 TC R</td><td colspan="2"></td><td colspan="6">18</td><td colspan="2">51</td><td colspan="2">37</td><td colspan="2">33</td><td colspan="2">30</td><td colspan="5">18</td><td>31</td></tr>
<tr><td>81 1 TC A</td><td colspan="2"></td><td colspan="6">21</td><td colspan="2">57</td><td colspan="2">42</td><td colspan="2">38</td><td colspan="2">35</td><td colspan="5">23</td><td>36</td></tr>
<tr><td>81 1 A A</td><td colspan="2"></td><td colspan="6">25</td><td colspan="2">68</td><td colspan="2">55</td><td colspan="2">46</td><td colspan="2">45</td><td colspan="5">40</td><td>47</td></tr>
<tr><td>81 3 A A</td><td colspan="2"></td><td colspan="19">46</td><td></td></tr>
<tr><td>81 68 U A</td><td colspan="9">41</td><td colspan="12"></td><td></td></tr>
<tr><td>82 3 A A</td><td colspan="2"></td><td colspan="19">51</td><td></td></tr>
<tr><td>82 21 U A</td><td colspan="2"></td><td colspan="7">35</td><td colspan="2">51</td><td colspan="2">41</td><td colspan="2">44</td><td colspan="2">45</td><td colspan="4"></td><td></td></tr>
<tr><td>83 3 A A</td><td colspan="2"></td><td colspan="19">48</td><td></td></tr>
<tr><td>84 1 A A</td><td colspan="2"></td><td colspan="19">46</td><td></td></tr>
<tr><td>84 3 UC A</td><td colspan="2"></td><td colspan="19">38</td><td></td></tr>
<tr><td>84 3 A A</td><td colspan="2"></td><td colspan="19">49</td><td></td></tr>
<tr><td>84 4 MC A</td><td colspan="2"></td><td colspan="6">22</td><td colspan="2">56</td><td colspan="2">59</td><td colspan="2">47</td><td colspan="2">29</td><td colspan="5">33</td><td>43</td></tr>
<tr><td>84 4 TC A</td><td colspan="2"></td><td colspan="6">24</td><td colspan="2">59</td><td colspan="2">60</td><td colspan="2">47</td><td colspan="2">29</td><td colspan="5">34</td><td>44</td></tr>
<tr><td>84 4 A A</td><td colspan="2"></td><td colspan="6">24</td><td colspan="2">62</td><td colspan="2">66</td><td colspan="2">49</td><td colspan="2">31</td><td colspan="5">40</td><td>47</td></tr>
<tr><td>84 23 UC R</td><td colspan="9"></td><td colspan="2">65</td><td colspan="2">48</td><td colspan="2">43</td><td colspan="2">42</td><td colspan="4"></td><td>45</td></tr>
<tr><td>84 23 A A</td><td colspan="9"></td><td colspan="2">67</td><td colspan="2">53</td><td colspan="2">50</td><td colspan="2">47</td><td colspan="4"></td><td>50</td></tr>
</table>

Table 10.4F (continued from p. 241, continues on p. 245)
Prevalence of smoking, females

West Germany *(continued)*

Frequency / Product / Source / Year	12	13	14	15	16	17	18	19	20-24	25-29	30-34	35-39	40-44	45-49	50-54	55-59	60-64	65-69	70-74	75-79	80+	All ages
76 3 A A			22																			
76 11 UC U			28																			
76 11 A U			28																			
76 13 MC R			21																			
76 31 U A	37																					
76 68 U R			36																			
76 68 U A			61																			
77 1 TC A			45								30		21		23		7					25
77 1 A A	25																					
77 11 UC U	28																					
77 11 A U	29																					
77 13 MC R	28																					
77 17 UC U			26																			
77 17 A U			26																			
78 11 UC U			31																			
78 11 A U			31																			
78 13 MC R			19																			
78 16 UC U									27													
78 16 A U									28													
78 20 U U	21																					
78 34 UC U					28																	
78 67 TC R			2		14		28		36	31	22		16		14		9	4				15
78 67 A R			2		14		28		36	31	22		16		14		9	4				15
78 67 A A			5		22		38		45	39	29		20		18		12	5				19
79 1 TC A			45								41		19		21		12					28
79 1 A A			28																			
79 2 TC A			42						47		41		19		21		18		6			28
79 2 A A			42						47		41		19		21		18		6			28
79 11 UC U			28																			
79 11 A U			28																			
79 13 MC R				22																		
79 35 U R	4	6	29	32	68																	
79 35 U A	21	26	53	52	81																	
80 3 A A			24																			
80 11 UC U			29																			
80 11 A U			29																			
80 31 U A	35																					
81 1 TC R			14						36		31		18		12		10		5			18
81 1 TC A			22						45		36		20		13		11		6			22
81 1 A A			23						47		37		21		13		11		6			23
81 3 A A			25																			
81 68 U A	36																					
82 3 A A			26																			
82 21 U A			36							50		32		22		20						
83 3 A A			28																			
84 1 A A			23																			
84 3 UC A			26																			
84 3 A A			27																			
84 4 MC A			31						46		42		28		21		17		9			28
84 4 TC A			31						49		43		28		23		17		9			29
84 4 A A			31						49		43		28		23		17		9			29
84 23 UC R										50		37		27		21						29
84 23 A A										50		37		27		21						29

Table 10.4M *(continued from p. 242, continues on p. 246)*

Prevalence of smoking, males

West Germany *(continued)*

Frequency / Product / Source / Year	12	13	14	15	16	17	18	19	20-24	25-29	30-34	35-39	40-44	45-49	50-54	55-59	60-64	65-69	70-74	75-79	80+	All ages
85 5 MC U												29										
85 5 A U												36										
85 24 UC R										46		34		34		23						31
85 24 A A										52		41		41		31						37
85 25 UC R										46		41		36		30						36
85 25 A A										53		45		40		34						40
85 26 UC R										42		33		28		28						30
85 26 A A										50		40		36		38						38
85 36 U U										49	51		39		36		31					42
85 37 A R										54		49		39		37						45
88 36 U U										50	54		44		34		35					44
89 67 TC R				16					36	41	42	39	36	32	29	27	24	19	14	10		29
89 67 A R				17					37	43	44	41	39	35	32	31	28	23	18	16		31
89 67 A A				22					44	48	49	47	44	40	37	35	32	27	24	21		36
89 67 A A				43								38						24				
90 36 U U										46	48		40		33		25					39
90 38 U R			5	13																		
90 38 U A	1	12																				
91 39 UC R	14																					
91 39 UC A	23																					
92 40 U R	2																					
92 41 U R	2																					
92 67 TC R				16					34	39	41	41	36	33	28	25	22	18	15	9		28
92 67 A R				16					35	40	43	43	38	36	31	28	25	21	18	13		30
92 67 A A				20					40	45	47	48	43	41	35	31	29	24	22	16		35
92 67 A A				42								36						20				
93 68 A R	29																					
93 68 A A	41																					
94 42 UC R		8		21																		

East Germany

Frequency / Product / Source / Year	12	13	14	15	16	17	18	19	20-24	25-29	30-34	35-39	40-44	45-49	50-54	55-59	60-64	65-69	70-74	75-79	80+	All ages
60 43 UC R										53		49		42		36						46
69 44 UC R	36																					
69 44 UC A	47																					
69 44 A A	48																					
70 45 A R		10																				
70 45 A A		38																				
70 65 U U			15	15	39	26	61	57	54⟩													
71 43 UC R										56		53		51		44						51
71 45 A R			17																			
71 45 A A			40																			
71 46 U U							58															
71 47*UC U							56		58		53		58		52		37					51
71 47 A U							58		63		60		65		68		57					62
71 48*UC U												60	57	55	55	49	43					53
71 48 A U												64	66	63	63	64	61					63
72 45 A R				38																		
72 45 A A				54																		

Table 10.4F *(continued from p. 243, continues on p. 247)*
Prevalence of smoking, females

West Germany *(continued)*

<table>
<tr><td rowspan="2">Frequency
Product
Source
Year</td><td colspan="21">Age group</td><td rowspan="2">All ages</td></tr>
<tr><td>12</td><td>13</td><td>14</td><td>15</td><td>16</td><td>17</td><td>18</td><td>19</td><td>20-24</td><td>25-29</td><td>30-34</td><td>35-39</td><td>40-44</td><td>45-49</td><td>50-54</td><td>55-59</td><td>60-64</td><td>65-69</td><td>70-74</td><td>75-79</td><td>80+</td></tr>
<tr><td>85 5 MC U</td><td colspan="12"></td><td colspan="5">16</td><td colspan="4"></td><td></td></tr>
<tr><td>85 5 A U</td><td colspan="12"></td><td colspan="5">17</td><td colspan="4"></td><td></td></tr>
<tr><td>85 24 UC R</td><td colspan="9"></td><td colspan="2">39</td><td colspan="2">30</td><td colspan="2">17</td><td colspan="2">15</td><td colspan="4"></td><td>21</td></tr>
<tr><td>85 24 A A</td><td colspan="9"></td><td colspan="2">43</td><td colspan="2">35</td><td colspan="2">19</td><td colspan="2">17</td><td colspan="4"></td><td>25</td></tr>
<tr><td>85 25 UC R</td><td colspan="9"></td><td colspan="2">35</td><td colspan="2">24</td><td colspan="2">18</td><td colspan="2">11</td><td colspan="4"></td><td>18</td></tr>
<tr><td>85 25 A A</td><td colspan="9"></td><td colspan="2">42</td><td colspan="2">28</td><td colspan="2">20</td><td colspan="2">14</td><td colspan="4"></td><td>22</td></tr>
<tr><td>85 26 UC R</td><td colspan="9"></td><td colspan="2">25</td><td colspan="2">17</td><td colspan="2">11</td><td colspan="2">7</td><td colspan="4"></td><td>12</td></tr>
<tr><td>85 26 A A</td><td colspan="9"></td><td colspan="2">30</td><td colspan="2">22</td><td colspan="2">13</td><td colspan="2">9</td><td colspan="4"></td><td>15</td></tr>
<tr><td>85 36 U U</td><td colspan="9"></td><td>43</td><td colspan="2">40</td><td colspan="2">24</td><td colspan="2">19</td><td colspan="2">13</td><td colspan="3"></td><td>27</td></tr>
<tr><td>85 37 A R</td><td colspan="9"></td><td colspan="2">43</td><td colspan="2">35</td><td colspan="2">17</td><td colspan="2">11</td><td colspan="4"></td><td>27</td></tr>
<tr><td>88 36 U U</td><td colspan="9"></td><td>47</td><td colspan="2">37</td><td colspan="2">27</td><td colspan="2">19</td><td colspan="2">15</td><td colspan="3"></td><td>27</td></tr>
<tr><td>89 67 TC R</td><td colspan="3"></td><td colspan="5">12</td><td>29</td><td>32</td><td>31</td><td>28</td><td>26</td><td>19</td><td>14</td><td>12</td><td>11</td><td>8</td><td>6</td><td colspan="2">2</td><td>17</td></tr>
<tr><td>89 67 A R</td><td colspan="3"></td><td colspan="5">12</td><td>29</td><td>32</td><td>31</td><td>29</td><td>26</td><td>19</td><td>14</td><td>12</td><td>11</td><td>8</td><td>7</td><td colspan="2">2</td><td>17</td></tr>
<tr><td>89 67 A A</td><td colspan="3"></td><td colspan="5">16</td><td>35</td><td>39</td><td>38</td><td>35</td><td>31</td><td>24</td><td>17</td><td>15</td><td>14</td><td>11</td><td>9</td><td colspan="2">3</td><td>21</td></tr>
<tr><td>89 67 A A</td><td colspan="3"></td><td colspan="9">33</td><td colspan="5">20</td><td colspan="4">7</td><td></td></tr>
<tr><td>90 36 U U</td><td colspan="9"></td><td>41</td><td colspan="2">41</td><td colspan="2">31</td><td colspan="2">19</td><td colspan="2">12</td><td colspan="3"></td><td>28</td></tr>
<tr><td>90 38 U R</td><td colspan="2"></td><td>4</td><td>8</td><td colspan="17"></td><td></td></tr>
<tr><td>90 38 U A</td><td>1</td><td colspan="3">6</td><td colspan="17"></td><td></td></tr>
<tr><td>91 39 UC R</td><td colspan="5">16</td><td colspan="16"></td><td></td></tr>
<tr><td>91 39 UC A</td><td colspan="5">28</td><td colspan="16"></td><td></td></tr>
<tr><td>92 40 U R</td><td>4</td><td colspan="20"></td><td></td></tr>
<tr><td>92 41 U R</td><td>1</td><td colspan="20"></td><td></td></tr>
<tr><td>92 67 TC R</td><td colspan="3"></td><td colspan="5">11</td><td>26</td><td>29</td><td>30</td><td>30</td><td>26</td><td>23</td><td>14</td><td>12</td><td>10</td><td>7</td><td>6</td><td colspan="2">3</td><td>17</td></tr>
<tr><td>92 67 A R</td><td colspan="3"></td><td colspan="5">12</td><td>26</td><td>30</td><td>31</td><td>31</td><td>27</td><td>23</td><td>15</td><td>13</td><td>11</td><td>8</td><td>6</td><td colspan="2">3</td><td>18</td></tr>
<tr><td>92 67 A A</td><td colspan="3"></td><td colspan="5">15</td><td>32</td><td>35</td><td>36</td><td>36</td><td>31</td><td>27</td><td>18</td><td>15</td><td>13</td><td>10</td><td>8</td><td colspan="2">4</td><td>21</td></tr>
<tr><td>92 67 A A</td><td colspan="3"></td><td colspan="9">32</td><td colspan="5">21</td><td colspan="4">7</td><td></td></tr>
<tr><td>93 68 A R</td><td colspan="9">24</td><td colspan="12"></td><td></td></tr>
<tr><td>93 68 A A</td><td colspan="9">35</td><td colspan="12"></td><td></td></tr>
<tr><td>94 42 UC R</td><td></td><td>9</td><td></td><td>29</td><td colspan="17"></td><td></td></tr>
</table>

East Germany

<table>
<tr><td rowspan="2">Frequency
Product
Source
Year</td><td colspan="21">Age group</td><td rowspan="2">All ages</td></tr>
<tr><td>12</td><td>13</td><td>14</td><td>15</td><td>16</td><td>17</td><td>18</td><td>19</td><td>20-24</td><td>25-29</td><td>30-34</td><td>35-39</td><td>40-44</td><td>45-49</td><td>50-54</td><td>55-59</td><td>60-64</td><td>65-69</td><td>70-74</td><td>75-79</td><td>80+</td></tr>
<tr><td>60 43 UC R</td><td colspan="9"></td><td colspan="2">11</td><td colspan="2">11</td><td colspan="2">8</td><td colspan="2">5</td><td colspan="4"></td><td>9</td></tr>
<tr><td>69 44 UC R</td><td colspan="7">3</td><td colspan="14"></td><td></td></tr>
<tr><td>69 44 UC A</td><td colspan="7">7</td><td colspan="14"></td><td></td></tr>
<tr><td>69 44 A A</td><td colspan="7">7</td><td colspan="14"></td><td></td></tr>
<tr><td>70 45 A R</td><td></td><td>3</td><td colspan="19"></td><td></td></tr>
<tr><td>70 45 A A</td><td></td><td>13</td><td colspan="19"></td><td></td></tr>
<tr><td>70 65 U U</td><td colspan="2"></td><td>0</td><td>7</td><td>9</td><td>8</td><td>21</td><td>6</td><td>14〉</td><td colspan="12"></td><td></td></tr>
<tr><td>71 43 UC R</td><td colspan="9"></td><td colspan="2">27</td><td colspan="2">25</td><td colspan="2">23</td><td colspan="2">16</td><td colspan="4"></td><td>23</td></tr>
<tr><td>71 45 A R</td><td colspan="2"></td><td>3</td><td colspan="18"></td><td></td></tr>
<tr><td>71 45 A A</td><td colspan="2"></td><td>17</td><td colspan="18"></td><td></td></tr>
<tr><td>71 46 U U</td><td colspan="6"></td><td colspan="2">32</td><td colspan="13"></td><td></td></tr>
<tr><td>71 47*UC U</td><td colspan="6"></td><td colspan="15">28</td><td></td></tr>
<tr><td>71 47 A U</td><td colspan="6"></td><td colspan="2">32</td><td colspan="2">34</td><td colspan="2">32</td><td colspan="2">35</td><td colspan="2">32</td><td colspan="5">15</td><td>28</td></tr>
<tr><td>71 48 UC U</td><td colspan="21"></td><td></td></tr>
<tr><td>71 48 A U</td><td colspan="21"></td><td></td></tr>
<tr><td>72 45 A R</td><td colspan="3"></td><td>7</td><td colspan="17"></td><td></td></tr>
<tr><td>72 45 A A</td><td colspan="3"></td><td>27</td><td colspan="17"></td><td></td></tr>
</table>

Table 10.4M (continued from p. 244, continues on p. 248)
Prevalence of smoking, males

East Germany *(continued)*

Year	Source	Product	Frequency	12	13	14	15	16	17	18	19	20-24	25-29	30-34	35-39	40-44	45-49	50-54	55-59	60-64	65-69	70-74	75-79	80+	All ages
73	48	UC	U																						
73	48	A	U																						
73	49	UC	U												48										
73	49	A	U												58										
75	45	A	R							56															
75	45	UC	A							62															
75	45	A	A							65															
75	50	U	U						55																
76	51	UC	R	0	2	4	22	30																	
77	43	UC	R										54		47		49		45						49
77	52	U	*	2	2	22	39																		
77	52	U	R	7	11	35	48																		
77	52	U	A	12	22	43	56																		
81	45	A	R		12																				
81	45	A	A		31																				
81	54	UC	R	2																					
81	54	UC	A	15																					
82	45	A	R			25																			
82	45	A	A			47																			
82	55	U	U	18	27	37	51																		
83	45	A	R				40																		
83	45	A	A				53																		
83	46	U	U							55															
83	56	U	*	1	8	19	27																		
83	56	U	R	4	13	26	33																		
83	56	U	A	16	24	37	40																		
83	62	UC	R										52		42		35		30						41
84	43	UC	R										52		42		35		30						40
84	57	UC	R										46		41		28		25						32
84	57	A	A										54		45		34		28						37
84	59	UC	R										59		45		40		29						39
84	59	A	A										64		51		45		38						45
84	60	UC	R										54		37		35		38						37
84	60	A	A										57		41		38		39						40
84	61	UC	R										60		41		38		41						40
84	61	A	A										60		42		40		46						42
85	54	UC	R					41																	
85	54	UC	A					62																	
85	58	UC	R										39		36		27		27						31
85	58	A	A										45		41		37		39						39
86	63	U	R	12	36	44	50																		
86	63	U	A	16	42	50	55																		
88	43	UC	R										52		36		33		29						38
88	62	UC	R										52		36		33		29						38
88	64	U	R				42			60			51		48		36		41		24				
91	43	UC	R										53		45		32		23						39
91	66	U	U										53	52		38		33		22					41
92	62	UC	R										44		42		27		22						35
92	67	TC	R				18					41	47	48	42	38	35	29	27	24	16	16	10		31
92	67	A	R				19					42	48	48	43	39	36	31	29	26	20	19	16		33
92	67	A	A				25					48	54	54	47	43	40	35	33	29	23	22	21		37
92	67	A	A				47									36					22				
93	68	A	R	28																					
93	68	A	A	38																					

Table 10.4F *(continued from p. 245, continues on p. 249)*
Prevalence of smoking, females

East Germany *(continued)*

Frequency Product Source Year	Age group 12	13	14	15	16	17	18	19	20-24	25-29	30-34	35-39	40-44	45-49	50-54	55-59	60-64	65-69	70-74	75-79	80+	All ages
73 48 UC U												22	30	32	24	23	15					24
73 48 A U												22	30	32	24	23	15					24
73 49 UC U												17										
73 49 A U												17										
75 45 A R							31															
75 45 UC A							47															
75 45 A A							47															
75 50 U U						36																
76 51 UC R	0	3	2	11	20																	
77 43 UC R										28		24		22		17						23
77 52 U *	1	2	11	24																		
77 52 U R	3	6	18	30																		
77 52 U A	6	16	31	38																		
81 45 A R		9																				
81 45 A A		26																				
81 54 UC R	1																					
81 54 UC A	6																					
82 45 A R			20																			
82 45 A A			40																			
82 55 U U	7	6	30	33																		
83 45 A R				34																		
83 45 A A				50																		
83 46 U U							39															
83 56 U *	2	6	6	18																		
83 56 U R	4	10	15	31																		
83 56 U A	7	14	28	48																		
83 62 UC R										29		16		16		12						19
84 43 UC R										29		20		15		12						20
84 57 UC R										33		26		20		22						23
84 57 A A										36		27		22		22						24
84 59 UC R										35		16		14		8						13
84 59 A A										40		20		17		10						17
84 60 UC R										20		13		17		12						14
84 60 A A										23		14		19		14						16
84 61 UC R										37		24		27		15						23
84 61 A A										38		24		27		15						23
85 54 UC R					18																	
85 54 UC A					51																	
85 58 UC R										27		13		11		8						11
85 58 A A										34		17		13		9						14
86 63 U R	7	21	42	48																		
86 63 U A	11	28	48	56																		
88 43 UC R										31		21		12		12						19
88 62 UC R										31		21		12		11						20
88 64 U R				20			35			34		23		20		14		9				
91 43 UC R										39		24		12		12						22
91 66 U U										38	34		14		11		10					21
92 62 UC R										32		25		15		8						21
92 67 TC R				10					27	29	29	24	19	12	11	9	9	6	5	2		14
92 67 A R				10					27	29	29	24	20	12	11	9	9	6	5	2		15
92 67 A A				14					34	37	37	30	24	15	13	12	12	9	7	3		19
92 67 A A				31									15					6				
93 68 A R	17																					
93 68 A A	27																					

Table 10.4M *(continued from p. 246)* Prevalence of smoking, males

Unified Germany

Frequency / Product / Source / Year	Age group 12	13	14	15	16	17	18	19	20-24	25-29	30-34	35-39	40-44	45-49	50-54	55-59	60-64	65-69	70-74	75-79	80+	All ages
92 67 TC R				16					35	40	42	41	36	34	28	25	23	17	15	9		29
92 67 A R				17					36	41	44	43	39	36	31	28	25	21	18	13		31
92 67 A A				21					42	47	49	48	43	41	35	32	29	24	22	17		35
92 67 A A				43									36					21				
93 68 A R	29																					
93 68 A A	40																					
95 67 TC R				17					35	39	41	41	37	33	28	24	21	17	13	8		28
95 67 A R				17					36	40	42	43	39	35	31	27	23	19	15	12		29
95 67 A A				22					42	46	48	48	43	40	35	30	26	23	18	14		33
95 67 A A				42									35					19				

Source: see *Notes on sources of survey data*, p. 264
Product: MC = manufactured cigarettes
TC = total cigarettes (including hand-rolled)
UC = cigarettes (type unspecified)
A = all products

Frequency: A = all smokers (including occasional)
R = regular or daily smokers
All ages: relevant to ages used and as given in original source
U = unspecified
* = refer to *Notes on sources of survey data*, p. 264

Prevalence of smoking, females

Unified Germany

Frequency Product Source Year	12	13	14	15	16	17	18	19	20-24	25-29	30-34	35-39	40-44	45-49	50-54	55-59	60-64	65-69	70-74	75-79	80+	All ages
92 67 TC R				11					26	29	30	29	25	21	14	12	10	7	6	3		17
92 67 A R				11					26	30	31	29	25	21	14	12	10	7	6	3		17
92 67 A A				14					32	36	37	35	30	25	17	14	13	10	8	4		21
92 67 A A				32									20					7				
93 68 A R	23																					
93 68 A A	34																					
95 67 TC R				11					25	29	30	30	26	22	16	12	9	8	5	3		17
95 67 A R				11					25	29	31	30	26	23	16	12	9	8	5	3		17
95 67 A A				14					31	35	37	35	31	27	20	14	11	10	7	4		20
95 67 A A				32									21					6				

Source: see *Notes on sources of survey data*, p. 264

Product: MC = manufactured cigarettes
TC = total cigarettes (including hand-rolled)
UC = cigarettes (type unspecified)
A = all products

Frequency: A = all smokers (including occasional)
R = regular or daily smokers

All ages: relevant to ages used and as given in original source

U = unspecified

* = refer to *Notes on sources of survey data*, p. 264

Table 10.5M Number of cigarettes smoked per smoker per day, males: some selected German surveys by age, 1965-1995
(continues on p. 252)

West Germany

<table>
<tr><th rowspan="2">Product
Source
Year</th><th colspan="21">Age group</th><th rowspan="2">All ages</th></tr>
<tr><th>12</th><th>13</th><th>14</th><th>15</th><th>16</th><th>17</th><th>18</th><th>19</th><th>20-24</th><th>25-29</th><th>30-34</th><th>35-39</th><th>40-44</th><th>45-49</th><th>50-54</th><th>55-59</th><th>60-64</th><th>65-69</th><th>70-74</th><th>75-79</th><th>80+</th></tr>
<tr><td>65 28 UCE</td><td></td><td></td><td></td><td></td><td></td><td colspan="2">7</td><td></td><td></td><td></td><td></td><td></td><td></td><td></td><td></td><td></td><td></td><td></td><td></td><td></td><td></td><td></td></tr>
<tr><td>65 29 UCE</td><td></td><td></td><td></td><td></td><td></td><td colspan="2">7</td><td></td><td></td><td></td><td></td><td></td><td></td><td></td><td></td><td></td><td></td><td></td><td></td><td></td><td></td><td></td></tr>
<tr><td>66 30 UCE</td><td colspan="2">3.7</td><td colspan="2">4.8</td><td colspan="2">7.2</td><td colspan="2">8.4</td><td></td><td></td><td></td><td></td><td></td><td></td><td></td><td></td><td></td><td></td><td></td><td></td><td></td><td></td></tr>
<tr><td>67 5 MC</td><td></td><td></td><td></td><td></td><td></td><td></td><td></td><td></td><td></td><td></td><td></td><td></td><td colspan="5">14</td><td></td><td></td><td></td><td></td><td></td></tr>
<tr><td>70 8 UCE*</td><td></td><td></td><td colspan="5">2.1</td><td></td><td></td><td></td><td></td><td></td><td></td><td></td><td></td><td></td><td></td><td></td><td></td><td></td><td></td><td></td></tr>
<tr><td>73 32 UC</td><td colspan="9">12</td><td></td><td></td><td></td><td></td><td></td><td></td><td></td><td></td><td></td><td></td><td></td><td></td><td></td></tr>
<tr><td>74 5 MC</td><td></td><td></td><td></td><td></td><td></td><td></td><td></td><td></td><td></td><td></td><td></td><td></td><td colspan="5">20</td><td></td><td></td><td></td><td></td><td></td></tr>
<tr><td>74 33 A</td><td></td><td></td><td colspan="6">13</td><td></td><td></td><td></td><td></td><td></td><td></td><td></td><td></td><td></td><td></td><td></td><td></td><td></td><td></td></tr>
<tr><td>75 18 UC</td><td></td><td></td><td></td><td colspan="5">12</td><td></td><td></td><td></td><td></td><td></td><td></td><td></td><td></td><td></td><td></td><td></td><td></td><td></td><td></td></tr>
<tr><td>78 34 UC</td><td></td><td></td><td></td><td></td><td colspan="14">20</td><td></td><td></td><td></td><td></td></tr>
<tr><td>78 67 TCE</td><td></td><td></td><td colspan="2">13</td><td colspan="2">14</td><td colspan="2">15</td><td>17</td><td>19</td><td colspan="2">20</td><td colspan="2">20</td><td colspan="2">18</td><td>17</td><td colspan="4">16</td><td>18</td></tr>
<tr><td>79 35 UCE</td><td></td><td>2.5</td><td>2.1</td><td>3.1</td><td></td><td></td><td></td><td></td><td></td><td></td><td></td><td></td><td></td><td></td><td></td><td></td><td></td><td></td><td></td><td></td><td></td><td></td></tr>
<tr><td>81 1 TC</td><td colspan="8">16</td><td colspan="2">19</td><td colspan="2">27</td><td colspan="2">21</td><td colspan="2">17</td><td colspan="5">17</td><td>20</td></tr>
<tr><td>84 4 TCE</td><td></td><td></td><td colspan="19">21</td><td></td></tr>
<tr><td>84 23 UC</td><td></td><td></td><td></td><td></td><td></td><td></td><td></td><td></td><td></td><td></td><td></td><td colspan="6">22</td><td></td><td></td><td></td><td></td><td></td></tr>
<tr><td>85 5 MC</td><td></td><td></td><td></td><td></td><td></td><td></td><td></td><td></td><td></td><td></td><td></td><td></td><td colspan="5">22</td><td></td><td></td><td></td><td></td><td></td></tr>
<tr><td>85 24 UC</td><td></td><td></td><td></td><td></td><td></td><td></td><td></td><td></td><td></td><td></td><td></td><td colspan="6">19</td><td></td><td></td><td></td><td></td><td></td></tr>
<tr><td>85 25 UC</td><td></td><td></td><td></td><td></td><td></td><td></td><td></td><td></td><td></td><td></td><td></td><td colspan="6">20</td><td></td><td></td><td></td><td></td><td></td></tr>
<tr><td>85 26 UC</td><td></td><td></td><td></td><td></td><td></td><td></td><td></td><td></td><td></td><td></td><td></td><td colspan="6">18</td><td></td><td></td><td></td><td></td><td></td></tr>
<tr><td>85 37 UC</td><td></td><td></td><td></td><td></td><td></td><td></td><td></td><td></td><td></td><td colspan="2">18</td><td colspan="2">22</td><td colspan="2">20</td><td colspan="2">17</td><td></td><td></td><td></td><td></td><td>20</td></tr>
<tr><td>88 36 UCE</td><td></td><td></td><td></td><td></td><td></td><td></td><td></td><td></td><td></td><td>19</td><td colspan="2">21</td><td colspan="2">21</td><td colspan="2">19</td><td></td><td></td><td></td><td></td><td></td><td></td></tr>
<tr><td>89 67 TC</td><td></td><td></td><td></td><td colspan="5">14</td><td>15</td><td>17</td><td>18</td><td>19</td><td>19</td><td>19</td><td>18</td><td>18</td><td>16</td><td>15</td><td>15</td><td colspan="2">14</td><td>17</td></tr>
<tr><td>90 36 TC</td><td></td><td></td><td></td><td></td><td></td><td></td><td></td><td></td><td></td><td>19</td><td colspan="2">20</td><td colspan="2">22</td><td colspan="2">19</td><td colspan="2">14</td><td></td><td></td><td></td><td>19</td></tr>
<tr><td>91 39 UCE*</td><td colspan="5">13</td><td></td><td></td><td></td><td></td><td></td><td></td><td></td><td></td><td></td><td></td><td></td><td></td><td></td><td></td><td></td><td></td><td></td></tr>
<tr><td>92 67 TC</td><td></td><td></td><td></td><td colspan="5">14</td><td>15</td><td>16</td><td>18</td><td>19</td><td>19</td><td>19</td><td>19</td><td>18</td><td>16</td><td>15</td><td>15</td><td colspan="2">14</td><td>17</td></tr>
<tr><td>93 68 UC</td><td colspan="9">15</td><td></td><td></td><td></td><td></td><td></td><td></td><td></td><td></td><td></td><td></td><td></td><td></td><td></td></tr>
</table>

East Germany

<table>
<tr><th rowspan="2">Product
Source
Year</th><th colspan="21">Age group</th><th rowspan="2">All ages</th></tr>
<tr><th>12</th><th>13</th><th>14</th><th>15</th><th>16</th><th>17</th><th>18</th><th>19</th><th>20-24</th><th>25-29</th><th>30-34</th><th>35-39</th><th>40-44</th><th>45-49</th><th>50-54</th><th>55-59</th><th>60-64</th><th>65-69</th><th>70-74</th><th>75-79</th><th>80+</th></tr>
<tr><td>69 44 UCE</td><td colspan="7">4.4</td><td></td><td></td><td></td><td></td><td></td><td></td><td></td><td></td><td></td><td></td><td></td><td></td><td></td><td></td><td></td></tr>
<tr><td>71 47 AE</td><td></td><td></td><td></td><td></td><td></td><td></td><td colspan="15">14</td><td></td></tr>
<tr><td>71 48 A</td><td></td><td></td><td></td><td></td><td></td><td></td><td></td><td></td><td></td><td></td><td></td><td colspan="6">15</td><td></td><td></td><td></td><td></td><td></td></tr>
<tr><td>73 48 A</td><td></td><td></td><td></td><td></td><td></td><td></td><td></td><td></td><td></td><td></td><td></td><td></td><td></td><td></td><td></td><td></td><td></td><td></td><td></td><td></td><td></td><td></td></tr>
<tr><td>75 45 UCE*</td><td></td><td></td><td></td><td></td><td></td><td></td><td colspan="2">11</td><td></td><td></td><td></td><td></td><td></td><td></td><td></td><td></td><td></td><td></td><td></td><td></td><td></td><td></td></tr>
<tr><td>78 53 UCE</td><td></td><td></td><td colspan="5">7.8</td><td></td><td></td><td></td><td></td><td></td><td></td><td></td><td></td><td></td><td></td><td></td><td></td><td></td><td></td><td></td></tr>
<tr><td>82 55 UC</td><td>2</td><td>3</td><td>5</td><td>5</td><td></td><td></td><td></td><td></td><td></td><td></td><td></td><td></td><td></td><td></td><td></td><td></td><td></td><td></td><td></td><td></td><td></td><td></td></tr>
<tr><td>84 57 UC</td><td></td><td></td><td></td><td></td><td></td><td></td><td></td><td></td><td></td><td></td><td></td><td colspan="6">16</td><td></td><td></td><td></td><td></td><td></td></tr>
<tr><td>84 59 UC</td><td></td><td></td><td></td><td></td><td></td><td></td><td></td><td></td><td></td><td></td><td></td><td colspan="6">14</td><td></td><td></td><td></td><td></td><td></td></tr>
<tr><td>84 60 UC</td><td></td><td></td><td></td><td></td><td></td><td></td><td></td><td></td><td></td><td></td><td></td><td colspan="6">15</td><td></td><td></td><td></td><td></td><td></td></tr>
<tr><td>84 61 UC</td><td></td><td></td><td></td><td></td><td></td><td></td><td></td><td></td><td></td><td></td><td></td><td colspan="6">16</td><td></td><td></td><td></td><td></td><td></td></tr>
<tr><td>85 54 UCE</td><td></td><td></td><td></td><td></td><td>9.7</td><td></td><td></td><td></td><td></td><td></td><td></td><td></td><td></td><td></td><td></td><td></td><td></td><td></td><td></td><td></td><td></td><td></td></tr>
<tr><td>88 64 UCE</td><td></td><td></td><td></td><td colspan="3">6</td><td colspan="3">14</td><td colspan="2">15</td><td colspan="2">18</td><td colspan="2">15</td><td colspan="2">15</td><td colspan="4">10</td><td></td></tr>
<tr><td>91 66 TC</td><td></td><td></td><td></td><td></td><td></td><td></td><td></td><td></td><td></td><td>14</td><td colspan="2">17</td><td colspan="2">17</td><td colspan="2">15</td><td colspan="2">12</td><td></td><td></td><td></td><td>16</td></tr>
<tr><td>92 67 TC</td><td></td><td></td><td></td><td colspan="5">12</td><td>13</td><td>14</td><td>15</td><td>15</td><td>15</td><td>15</td><td>14</td><td>14</td><td>14</td><td>13</td><td>13</td><td colspan="2">11</td><td>14</td></tr>
<tr><td>93 68 UC</td><td colspan="9">15</td><td></td><td></td><td></td><td></td><td></td><td></td><td></td><td></td><td></td><td></td><td></td><td></td><td></td></tr>
</table>

Table 10.5F Number of cigarettes smoked per smoker per day, females: some selected German surveys by age, 1965-1995
(continues on p. 253)

West Germany

<table>
<tr><th rowspan="2">Product
Source
Year</th><th colspan="21">Age group</th><th rowspan="2">All ages</th></tr>
<tr><th>12</th><th>13</th><th>14</th><th>15</th><th>16</th><th>17</th><th>18</th><th>19</th><th>20-24</th><th>25-29</th><th>30-34</th><th>35-39</th><th>40-44</th><th>45-49</th><th>50-54</th><th>55-59</th><th>60-64</th><th>65-69</th><th>70-74</th><th>75-79</th><th>80+</th></tr>
<tr><td>65 28 UCE</td><td colspan="5"></td><td colspan="2">3</td><td colspan="14"></td><td></td></tr>
<tr><td>65 29 UCE</td><td colspan="5"></td><td colspan="2">2</td><td colspan="14"></td><td></td></tr>
<tr><td>66 30 UCE</td><td colspan="2">3.3</td><td colspan="2">3.8</td><td colspan="2">3.9</td><td colspan="2">3.8</td><td colspan="13"></td><td></td></tr>
<tr><td>67 5 MC</td><td colspan="12"></td><td colspan="5">10</td><td colspan="4"></td><td></td></tr>
<tr><td>70 8 UCE</td><td colspan="21"></td><td></td></tr>
<tr><td>73 32 UC</td><td colspan="9">7</td><td colspan="12"></td><td></td></tr>
<tr><td>74 5 MC</td><td colspan="12"></td><td colspan="5">12</td><td colspan="4"></td><td></td></tr>
<tr><td>74 33 A</td><td colspan="2"></td><td colspan="7">10</td><td colspan="12"></td><td></td></tr>
<tr><td>75 18 UC</td><td colspan="3"></td><td colspan="5">8.6</td><td colspan="13"></td><td></td></tr>
<tr><td>78 34 UC</td><td colspan="4"></td><td colspan="14">16</td><td colspan="3"></td><td></td></tr>
<tr><td>78 67 TCE</td><td colspan="2"></td><td colspan="2">12</td><td colspan="2">13</td><td colspan="2">13</td><td>14</td><td>15</td><td colspan="2">15</td><td colspan="2">15</td><td colspan="2">14</td><td>13</td><td colspan="4">13</td><td>14</td></tr>
<tr><td>79 35 UCE</td><td></td><td>1.6</td><td>2.7</td><td>2.5</td><td colspan="17"></td><td></td></tr>
<tr><td>81 1 TC</td><td colspan="2"></td><td colspan="6">14</td><td colspan="2">15</td><td colspan="2">17</td><td colspan="2">21</td><td colspan="2">19</td><td colspan="2">14</td><td colspan="3">12</td><td>17</td></tr>
<tr><td>84 4 TCE</td><td colspan="2"></td><td colspan="19">11</td><td></td></tr>
<tr><td>84 23 UC</td><td colspan="11"></td><td colspan="6">16</td><td colspan="4"></td><td></td></tr>
<tr><td>85 5 MC</td><td colspan="12"></td><td colspan="5">16</td><td colspan="4"></td><td></td></tr>
<tr><td>85 24 UC</td><td colspan="11"></td><td colspan="6">14</td><td colspan="4"></td><td></td></tr>
<tr><td>85 25 UC</td><td colspan="11"></td><td colspan="6">13</td><td colspan="4"></td><td></td></tr>
<tr><td>85 26 UC</td><td colspan="11"></td><td colspan="6">11</td><td colspan="4"></td><td></td></tr>
<tr><td>85 37 UC</td><td colspan="9"></td><td colspan="2">15</td><td colspan="2">15</td><td colspan="2">13</td><td colspan="2">11</td><td colspan="4"></td><td>14</td></tr>
<tr><td>88 36 UCE</td><td colspan="21"></td><td></td></tr>
<tr><td>89 67 TC</td><td colspan="3"></td><td colspan="5">13</td><td>14</td><td>15</td><td>15</td><td>16</td><td>16</td><td>15</td><td>15</td><td>15</td><td>15</td><td>14</td><td>14</td><td colspan="2">12</td><td>15</td></tr>
<tr><td>90 36 TC</td><td colspan="9"></td><td>16</td><td colspan="2">15</td><td colspan="2">18</td><td colspan="2">15</td><td colspan="2">9.6</td><td colspan="3"></td><td>16</td></tr>
<tr><td>91 39 UCE*</td><td colspan="5">10</td><td colspan="16"></td><td></td></tr>
<tr><td>92 67 TC</td><td colspan="3"></td><td colspan="5">13</td><td>14</td><td>15</td><td>15</td><td>16</td><td>16</td><td>16</td><td>15</td><td>14</td><td>14</td><td>14</td><td>13</td><td colspan="2">12</td><td>15</td></tr>
<tr><td>93 68 UC</td><td colspan="9">14</td><td colspan="12"></td><td></td></tr>
</table>

East Germany

<table>
<tr><th rowspan="2">Product
Source
Year</th><th colspan="21">Age group</th><th rowspan="2">All ages</th></tr>
<tr><th>12</th><th>13</th><th>14</th><th>15</th><th>16</th><th>17</th><th>18</th><th>19</th><th>20-24</th><th>25-29</th><th>30-34</th><th>35-39</th><th>40-44</th><th>45-49</th><th>50-54</th><th>55-59</th><th>60-64</th><th>65-69</th><th>70-74</th><th>75-79</th><th>80+</th></tr>
<tr><td>69 44 UCE</td><td colspan="21"></td><td></td></tr>
<tr><td>71 47 AE</td><td colspan="6"></td><td colspan="15">9.2</td><td></td></tr>
<tr><td>71 48 A</td><td colspan="21"></td><td></td></tr>
<tr><td>73 48 A</td><td colspan="11"></td><td colspan="6">9.0</td><td colspan="4"></td><td></td></tr>
<tr><td>75 45 UCE*</td><td colspan="6"></td><td colspan="2">4</td><td colspan="13"></td><td></td></tr>
<tr><td>78 53 UCE</td><td colspan="2"></td><td colspan="5">4.2</td><td colspan="14"></td><td></td></tr>
<tr><td>82 55 UC</td><td>1</td><td>1</td><td>3</td><td>3</td><td colspan="17"></td><td></td></tr>
<tr><td>84 57 UC</td><td colspan="11"></td><td colspan="6">12</td><td colspan="4"></td><td></td></tr>
<tr><td>84 59 UC</td><td colspan="11"></td><td colspan="6">7</td><td colspan="4"></td><td></td></tr>
<tr><td>84 60 UC</td><td colspan="11"></td><td colspan="6">8</td><td colspan="4"></td><td></td></tr>
<tr><td>84 61 UC</td><td colspan="11"></td><td colspan="6">9</td><td colspan="4"></td><td></td></tr>
<tr><td>85 54 UCE</td><td colspan="4"></td><td>7.3</td><td colspan="16"></td><td></td></tr>
<tr><td>88 64 UCE</td><td colspan="3"></td><td colspan="3">12</td><td colspan="3">11</td><td colspan="2">10</td><td colspan="2">11</td><td colspan="2">10</td><td colspan="2">10</td><td colspan="4">10</td><td></td></tr>
<tr><td>91 66 TC</td><td colspan="9"></td><td>9.5</td><td colspan="2">11</td><td colspan="2">12</td><td colspan="2">11</td><td colspan="2">7.5</td><td colspan="3"></td><td>10</td></tr>
<tr><td>92 67 TC</td><td colspan="3"></td><td colspan="5">11</td><td>12</td><td>12</td><td>13</td><td>12</td><td>13</td><td>12</td><td>12</td><td>12</td><td>12</td><td>11</td><td>9.7</td><td colspan="2">11</td><td>12</td></tr>
<tr><td>93 68 UC</td><td colspan="9">9.4</td><td colspan="12"></td><td></td></tr>
</table>

Table 10.5M *(continued from p. 250)*
Number of cigarettes smoked per smoker per day, males

Unified Germany

<table>
<tr><td rowspan="2">Product
Source
Year</td><td colspan="21">Age group</td><td rowspan="2">All ages</td></tr>
<tr><td>12</td><td>13</td><td>14</td><td>15</td><td>16</td><td>17</td><td>18</td><td>19</td><td>20-24</td><td>25-29</td><td>30-34</td><td>35-39</td><td>40-44</td><td>45-49</td><td>50-54</td><td>55-59</td><td>60-64</td><td>65-69</td><td>70-74</td><td>75-79</td><td>80+</td></tr>
<tr><td>92 67 TC</td><td colspan="3"></td><td colspan="5">13</td><td>15</td><td>16</td><td>17</td><td>18</td><td>18</td><td>19</td><td>18</td><td>17</td><td>16</td><td>15</td><td>15</td><td colspan="2">13</td><td>17</td></tr>
<tr><td>93 68 UC</td><td colspan="9">15</td><td colspan="13"></td></tr>
<tr><td>95 67 TC</td><td colspan="3"></td><td colspan="5">13</td><td>15</td><td>16</td><td>17</td><td>17</td><td>18</td><td>18</td><td>18</td><td>17</td><td>16</td><td>15</td><td>15</td><td colspan="2">13</td><td>16</td></tr>
</table>

Source: see *Notes on sources of survey data*, p. 264

Product:
MC = manufactured cigarettes
TC = total cigarettes (including hand-rolled)
UC = cigarettes (type unspecified)
A = all products
U = unspecified

Product (cont): E indicates mean estimated from percentage distribution (see also *Consumption category estimation*, p. xxxiv, and Appendix III, p. 789)

All ages: relevant to ages used and as given in original source

* = refer to *Notes on sources of survey data*, p. 264

Table 10.5F *(continued from p. 251)* Number of cigarettes smoked per smoker per day, females

Unified Germany

Product Source Year	12	13	14	15	16	17	18	19	20-24	25-29	30-34	35-39	40-44	45-49	50-54	55-59	60-64	65-69	70-74	75-79	80+	All ages
92 67 TC				13					14	14	15	15	15	15	14	14	14	13	13	12		14
93 68 UC	13																					
95 67 TC				12					14	14	14	15	15	15	15	14	14	13	13	12		14

Source: see *Notes on sources of survey data*, p. 264

Product:
- MC = manufactured cigarettes
- TC = total cigarettes (including hand-rolled)
- UC = cigarettes (type unspecified)
- A = all products
- U = unspecified

Product (cont): E indicates mean estimated from percentage distribution (see also *Consumption category estimation*, p. xxxiv, and Appendix III, p. 789)

All ages: relevant to ages used and as given in original source

* = refer to *Notes on sources of survey data*, p. 264

Table 10.6M Number of cigarettes smoked per person per day, males: some selected German surveys by age, 1965-1995, with percentage total sales *(continues on p. 256)*

West Germany

Product Source Year	12	13	14	15	16	17	18	19	20-24	25-29	30-34	35-39	40-44	45-49	50-54	55-59	60-64	65-69	70-74	75-79	80+	All ages	% Total sales
65 28 UC						4																	**
65 29 UC						4																	**
67 5 MC													7.4										**
70 8 UC *			1.3																				**
74 5 MC													8.2										**
74 33 A			7																				**
75 18 UC				5.8																			**
78 34 UC					8.6																		78%T
78 67 TC			0.5		3.0		5.9		7.9	8.8	8.7		8.2		7.2		5.1	4.2				6.2	62%T
79 35 UC		0.2	0.5	1.0																			**
80 10 MC				9.3																			---M
81 1 TC			3.4						11		11		8.0		6.0		3.9					7.2	75%T
82 10 MC				7.7																			---M
84 4 TC *			9.2																				90%T
84 23 UC *												9.9											**
85 5 MC													6.3										**
85 24 UC *												5.9											**
85 25 UC *												7.2											**
85 26 UC *												5.3											**
85 37 UC *										9.8		11		8.0		6.4						8.8	**
88 36 UC *										9.3	11		9.3		6.5								**
89 67 TC				2.2					5.5	6.9	7.4	7.2	6.9	6.3	5.3	4.8	4.0	2.8	2.0	1.4		5.0	58%T
90 36 TC *										8.9	9.5		8.8		6.2		3.5					7.5	**
91 39 UC *	1.8																						**
92 67 TC				2.1					5.2	6.3	7.3	7.5	6.9	6.4	5.4	4.4	3.6	2.7	2.2	1.3		4.9	**
93 68 UC	6.2																						**

East Germany

Product Source Year	12	13	14	15	16	17	18	19	20-24	25-29	30-34	35-39	40-44	45-49	50-54	55-59	60-64	65-69	70-74	75-79	80+	All ages	% Total sales
69 44 UC	1.6																						**
71 47 A							8.6																**
71 48 A *												9.3											**
73 48 A																							**
75 45 UC							6.7																**
82 55 UC	0	1	2	3																			**
84 57 UC *												5.2											**
84 59 UC *												5.5											**
84 60 UC *												5.5											**
84 61 UC *												6.4											**
85 54 UC					4.0																		**
88 64 UC				3			8			7		9		5		6		2					**
91 66 TC *										7.4	8.9		6.3		4.9		2.7					6.4	**
92 67 TC				2.3					5.5	6.6	7.0	6.3	5.7	5.4	4.2	3.8	3.4	2.2	2.1	1.1		4.4	**
93 68 UC	5.7																						**

Table 10.6F Number of cigarettes smoked per person per day, females: some selected German surveys by age, 1965-1995, with percentage total sales *(continues on p. 257)*

West Germany

<table>
<tr><th rowspan="2">Product
Source
Year</th><th colspan="21">Age group</th><th rowspan="2">All ages</th><th rowspan="2">% Total sales</th></tr>
<tr><th>12</th><th>13</th><th>14</th><th>15</th><th>16</th><th>17</th><th>18</th><th>19</th><th>20-24</th><th>25-29</th><th>30-34</th><th>35-39</th><th>40-44</th><th>45-49</th><th>50-54</th><th>55-59</th><th>60-64</th><th>65-69</th><th>70-74</th><th>75-79</th><th>80+</th></tr>
<tr><td>65 28 UC</td><td colspan="5"></td><td colspan="2">1</td><td colspan="14"></td><td></td><td>**</td></tr>
<tr><td>65 29 UC</td><td colspan="5"></td><td colspan="2">1</td><td colspan="14"></td><td></td><td>**</td></tr>
<tr><td>67 5 MC</td><td colspan="12"></td><td colspan="5">1.7</td><td colspan="4"></td><td></td><td>**</td></tr>
<tr><td>70 8 UC</td><td colspan="21"></td><td></td><td>**</td></tr>
<tr><td>74 5 MC</td><td colspan="12"></td><td colspan="5">2.4</td><td colspan="4"></td><td></td><td>**</td></tr>
<tr><td>74 33 A</td><td colspan="2"></td><td colspan="7">4</td><td colspan="12"></td><td></td><td>**</td></tr>
<tr><td>75 18 UC</td><td colspan="3"></td><td colspan="5">3.7</td><td colspan="13"></td><td></td><td>**</td></tr>
<tr><td>78 34 UC</td><td colspan="4"></td><td colspan="14">4.3</td><td colspan="3"></td><td></td><td>78%T</td></tr>
<tr><td>78 67 TC</td><td colspan="2"></td><td colspan="2">0.3</td><td colspan="2">1.8</td><td colspan="2">3.8</td><td>5.0</td><td>4.6</td><td colspan="2">3.3</td><td colspan="2">2.3</td><td colspan="2">1.9</td><td>1.2</td><td colspan="4">0.5</td><td>2.1</td><td>62%T</td></tr>
<tr><td>79 35 UC</td><td></td><td>0.2</td><td>0.9</td><td>0.9</td><td colspan="17"></td><td></td><td>**</td></tr>
<tr><td>80 10 MC</td><td colspan="3"></td><td colspan="18">5.0</td><td></td><td>---M</td></tr>
<tr><td>81 1 TC</td><td colspan="2"></td><td colspan="6">3.1</td><td colspan="2">6.8</td><td colspan="2">6.1</td><td colspan="2">4.2</td><td colspan="2">3.5</td><td colspan="2">1.5</td><td colspan="3">0.7</td><td>3.7</td><td>75%T</td></tr>
<tr><td>82 10 MC</td><td colspan="3"></td><td colspan="18">4.5</td><td></td><td>---M</td></tr>
<tr><td>84 4 TC *</td><td colspan="2"></td><td colspan="19">3.8</td><td></td><td>90%T</td></tr>
<tr><td>84 23 UC *</td><td colspan="11"></td><td colspan="6">4.7</td><td colspan="4"></td><td></td><td>**</td></tr>
<tr><td>85 5 MC</td><td colspan="12"></td><td colspan="5">2.6</td><td colspan="4"></td><td></td><td>**</td></tr>
<tr><td>85 24 UC *</td><td colspan="11"></td><td colspan="6">3.0</td><td colspan="4"></td><td></td><td>**</td></tr>
<tr><td>85 25 UC *</td><td colspan="11"></td><td colspan="6">2.4</td><td colspan="4"></td><td></td><td>**</td></tr>
<tr><td>85 26 UC *</td><td colspan="11"></td><td colspan="6">1.3</td><td colspan="4"></td><td></td><td>**</td></tr>
<tr><td>85 37 UC *</td><td colspan="9"></td><td colspan="2">6.5</td><td colspan="2">5.4</td><td colspan="2">2.2</td><td colspan="2">1.3</td><td colspan="4"></td><td>3.8</td><td>**</td></tr>
<tr><td>88 36 UC</td><td colspan="21"></td><td></td><td>**</td></tr>
<tr><td>89 67 TC</td><td colspan="3"></td><td colspan="5">1.6</td><td>4.0</td><td>4.7</td><td>4.7</td><td>4.5</td><td>4.0</td><td>2.8</td><td>2.1</td><td>1.7</td><td>1.6</td><td>1.1</td><td>0.9</td><td colspan="2">0.3</td><td>2.5</td><td>58%T</td></tr>
<tr><td>90 36 TC *</td><td colspan="9"></td><td>6.8</td><td colspan="2">6.2</td><td colspan="2">5.7</td><td colspan="2">2.8</td><td colspan="2">1.2</td><td colspan="3"></td><td>4.4</td><td>**</td></tr>
<tr><td>91 39 UC *</td><td colspan="5">1.6</td><td colspan="16"></td><td></td><td>**</td></tr>
<tr><td>92 67 TC</td><td colspan="3"></td><td colspan="5">1.4</td><td>3.6</td><td>4.3</td><td>4.6</td><td>4.7</td><td>4.1</td><td>3.5</td><td>2.1</td><td>1.7</td><td>1.4</td><td>1.0</td><td>0.8</td><td colspan="2">0.3</td><td>2.5</td><td>**</td></tr>
<tr><td>93 68 UC</td><td colspan="9">4.8</td><td colspan="12"></td><td></td><td>**</td></tr>
</table>

East Germany

<table>
<tr><th rowspan="2">Product
Source
Year</th><th colspan="21">Age group</th><th rowspan="2">All ages</th><th rowspan="2">% Total sales</th></tr>
<tr><th>12</th><th>13</th><th>14</th><th>15</th><th>16</th><th>17</th><th>18</th><th>19</th><th>20-24</th><th>25-29</th><th>30-34</th><th>35-39</th><th>40-44</th><th>45-49</th><th>50-54</th><th>55-59</th><th>60-64</th><th>65-69</th><th>70-74</th><th>75-79</th><th>80+</th></tr>
<tr><td>69 44 UC</td><td colspan="21"></td><td></td><td>**</td></tr>
<tr><td>71 47 A</td><td colspan="6"></td><td colspan="15">2.6</td><td></td><td>**</td></tr>
<tr><td>71 48 A</td><td colspan="21"></td><td></td><td>**</td></tr>
<tr><td>73 48 A *</td><td colspan="11"></td><td colspan="6">2.2</td><td colspan="4"></td><td></td><td>**</td></tr>
<tr><td>75 45 UC</td><td colspan="6"></td><td colspan="2">1.8</td><td colspan="13"></td><td></td><td>**</td></tr>
<tr><td>82 55 UC</td><td>0</td><td>0</td><td>1</td><td>1</td><td colspan="17"></td><td></td><td>**</td></tr>
<tr><td>84 57 UC *</td><td colspan="11"></td><td colspan="6">2.7</td><td colspan="4"></td><td></td><td>**</td></tr>
<tr><td>84 59 UC *</td><td colspan="11"></td><td colspan="6">0.9</td><td colspan="4"></td><td></td><td>**</td></tr>
<tr><td>84 60 UC *</td><td colspan="11"></td><td colspan="6">1.1</td><td colspan="4"></td><td></td><td>**</td></tr>
<tr><td>84 61 UC *</td><td colspan="11"></td><td colspan="6">2.0</td><td colspan="4"></td><td></td><td>**</td></tr>
<tr><td>85 54 UC</td><td colspan="4"></td><td>1.3</td><td colspan="16"></td><td></td><td>**</td></tr>
<tr><td>88 64 UC</td><td colspan="3"></td><td colspan="3">2</td><td colspan="3">4</td><td colspan="2">3</td><td colspan="2">3</td><td colspan="2">2</td><td colspan="2">1</td><td colspan="4">1</td><td></td><td>**</td></tr>
<tr><td>91 66 TC *</td><td colspan="9"></td><td>3.6</td><td colspan="2">3.6</td><td colspan="2">1.7</td><td colspan="2">1.2</td><td colspan="2">0.7</td><td colspan="3"></td><td>2.1</td><td>**</td></tr>
<tr><td>92 67 TC</td><td colspan="3"></td><td colspan="5">1.0</td><td>3.2</td><td>3.4</td><td>3.6</td><td>3.0</td><td>2.5</td><td>1.5</td><td>1.3</td><td>1.1</td><td>1.1</td><td>0.6</td><td>0.5</td><td colspan="2">0.2</td><td>1.8</td><td>**</td></tr>
<tr><td>93 68 UC</td><td colspan="9">2.4</td><td colspan="12"></td><td></td><td>**</td></tr>
</table>

Table 10.6M (continued from p. 254)
Number of cigarettes smoked per person per day, males

Unified Germany

Product Source Year	12	13	14	15	16	17	18	19	20-24	25-29	30-34	35-39	40-44	45-49	50-54	55-59	60-64	65-69	70-74	75-79	80+	All ages	% Total sales
92 67 TC				2.1					5.2	6.4	7.2	7.2	6.7	6.2	5.1	4.3	3.6	2.6	2.2	1.2		4.9	62%T
93 68 UC	6.0																						**
95 67 TC				2.1					5.1	6.1	6.8	7.0	6.6	6.1	5.1	4.1	3.4	2.5	1.9	1.1		4.6	64%T

Table 10.7M Number of cigarettes smoked per person per day, sales-adjusted, males: some selected German surveys[1] by age, 1978-1995, with percentage total sales

West Germany

Product Source Year	12	13	14	15	16	17	18	19	20-24	25-29	30-34	35-39	40-44	45-49	50-54	55-59	60-64	65-69	70-74	75-79	80+	All ages	% Total sales
78 34 UC					11																		78%T
78 67 TC			0.8		4.9		9.5		13	14	14		13		12		8.3	6.7				10	62%T
80 10 MC				9.3																			---M
81 1 TC			4.6						14		15		11		8.0		5.2					9.6	75%T
82 10 MC				7.7																			---M
84 4 TC *			10																				90%T
89 67 TC				3.8					9.5	12	13	12	12	11	9.1	8.3	6.9	4.8	3.4	2.4		8.6	58%T

Unified Germany

Product Source Year	12	13	14	15	16	17	18	19	20-24	25-29	30-34	35-39	40-44	45-49	50-54	55-59	60-64	65-69	70-74	75-79	80+	All ages	% Total sales
92 67 TC				3.4					8.3	10	12	12	11	10	8.2	6.9	5.8	4.2	3.5	1.9		7.9	62%T
95 67 TC				3.3					8.0	9.6	11	11	10	9.6	8.0	6.5	5.3	3.9	3.0	1.7		7.2	64%T

1 Based on those surveys in Table 10.6 with data for both sexes and age range at least 21-64 (see also *Cigarette consumption per person*, p. xxxv), West Germany and unified Germany only

Source: see *Notes on sources of survey data*, p. 264
All ages: relevant to ages used and as given in original source
% Total sales: estimated % of total sales of M = manufactured or T = total cigarette consumption implied by survey, sexes combined, used as adjustment factor in Table 10.7
** = cannot be calculated
--- = adjusted by original author

Product: MC = manufactured cigarettes
TC = total cigarettes (including hand-rolled)
UC = cigarettes (type unspecified)
A = all products
U = unspecified
* = refer to *Notes on sources of survey data*, p. 264

Table 10.6F *(continued from p. 255)*
Number of cigarettes smoked per person per day, females

Unified Germany

Product Source Year	Age group 12	13	14	15	16	17	18	19	20-24	25-29	30-34	35-39	40-44	45-49	50-54	55-59	60-64	65-69	70-74	75-79	80+	All ages	% Total sales
92 67 TC				1.4					3.5	4.1	4.4	4.3	3.8	3.1	2.0	1.6	1.4	1.0	0.7	0.3		2.4	62%T
93 68 UC	4.4																						**
95 67 TC				1.2					3.4	4.0	4.3	4.4	3.9	3.4	2.3	1.7	1.2	1.0	0.7	0.3		2.4	64%T

Table 10.7F Number of cigarettes smoked per person per day, sales-adjusted, females: some selected German surveys[1] by age, 1978-1995, with percentage total sales

West Germany

Product Source Year	Age group 12	13	14	15	16	17	18	19	20-24	25-29	30-34	35-39	40-44	45-49	50-54	55-59	60-64	65-69	70-74	75-79	80+	All ages	% Total sales
78 34 UC					5.6																		78%T
78 67 TC			0.5		2.9		6.1		8.1	7.4	5.4		3.7		3.1		1.9	0.8				3.4	62%T
80 10 MC				5.0																			---M
81 1 TC			4.2						9.1		8.2		5.6		4.7		2.0		0.9			5.0	75%T
82 10 MC				4.5																			---M
84 4 TC *			4.2																				90%T
89 67 TC				2.8					6.9	8.1	8.1	7.8	6.9	4.8	3.6	2.9	2.8	1.9	1.6	0.5		4.3	58%T

Unified Germany

Product Source Year	Age group 12	13	14	15	16	17	18	19	20-24	25-29	30-34	35-39	40-44	45-49	50-54	55-59	60-64	65-69	70-74	75-79	80+	All ages	% Total sales
92 67 TC				2.2					5.6	6.6	7.1	6.9	6.1	5.0	3.2	2.6	2.2	1.6	1.1	0.5		3.9	62%T
95 67 TC				1.9					5.3	6.3	6.8	6.9	6.1	5.3	3.6	2.7	1.9	1.6	1.1	0.5		3.8	64%T

1 Based on those surveys in Table 10.6 with data for both sexes and age range at least 21-64 (see also *Cigarette consumption per person*, p. xxxv), West Germany and unified Germany only

Source: see *Notes on sources of survey data*, p. 264
All ages: relevant to ages used and as given in original source
% Total sales: estimated % of total sales of M = manufactured or T = total cigarette consumption implied by survey, sexes combined, used as adjustment factor in Table 10.7
** = cannot be calculated
--- = adjusted by original author

Product: MC = manufactured cigarettes
TC = total cigarettes (including hand-rolled)
UC = cigarettes (type unspecified)
A = all products
U = unspecified
* = refer to *Notes on sources of survey data*, p. 264

Table 10.8 Estimated[1] prevalence of smoking and estimated[1] number of cigarettes per person per day (unadjusted and sales-adjusted): summary of Tables 10.4, 10.6 and 10.7, 1950-1995.
Males and females aged 15 years and over

Year	Source[2]	Product[3]	Prevalence[4]						Number of cigarettes						
									Unadjusted[7]			Sales-adjusted[8]			
			Manufactured cigarettes		Total cigarettes[5]		All products[6]		Number/ person/day		Total sales %	Manufactured cigarettes number/ person/day		Total cigarettes[9] number/ person/day	
			M	F	M	F	M	F	M	F		M	F	M	F
West Germany															
1950	11	*UC+A*			60	21	88	21						(4.5	1.3)
1955	11	*UC+A*			64	21	83	21						(6.3	1.6)
1958	12	*UC+A*			62		75								
1960	11	*UC+A*			61	22	78	22						(8.2	2.4)
	13	MC+*A*	49	13			77	23				(8.1	1.7)		
1963	14	*UC+A*			55	16	68	16						(9.3	2.2)
1965	11	*UC+A*			61	24	74	24						(9.5	3.0)
	12	*UC*			56	18								(10.0	2.5)
1967	15	*UC*			60	26								(9.4	3.3)
1970	3	**A**					58	24							
	11	*UC+A*			55	27	67	27						(10.6	4.2)
1971	13	MC	49	21								(11.2	3.8)		
	16	*UC+A*			49		59								
1973	6	*U*					60	24						(11.6	3.7)
	7	*					49	23							
	11	*UC+A*			51	30	64	30						(10.3	4.8)
1974	11	*UC+A*			47	29	55	28						(10.3	5.1)
	12	*UC*			45	26								(10.5	4.8)
1975	1	**TC+A**			41	23	48	23						(10.3	4.6)
	11	*UC+A*			50	29	60	29						(10.2	4.7)
	13	MC	39	20								(10.2	4.2)		
	15	*UC+A*			45	21	53	23						(10.9	4.2)
1976	3	**A**					51	22							
	11	*UC+A*			47	28	55	28						(10.5	5.0)
	13	MC	39	21								(10.5	4.5)		
1977	1	**TC+A**			43	25	48	25						(9.7	4.6)
	11	*UC+A*			45	28	53	29						(9.5	4.7)
	13	MC	36	28								(8.1	5.0)		
	17	*UC+A*			43	22	48	22						(10.2	4.2)
1978	11	*UC+A*			47	31	55	31						(9.7	5.1)
	13	MC	37	19								(9.9	4.1)		
	16	*UC+A*			45	23	51	24						(10.6	4.4)
	34	*UC*			40	24			7.9	3.7	78			10.2	4.7
	67	TC+A			38	16	41	16	7.0	2.3	62			11.3	3.8
	67	**A**					47	21							
1979	1	**TC+A**			41	28	48	28						(9.7	5.2)
	2	**TC+A**			41	27	48	27						(9.8	5.2)
	11	*UC+A*			44	28	52	28						(9.9	5.1)
	13	MC	38	22								(9.6	4.4)		

Table 10.8 *(continued)*

Year	Source[2]	Product[3]	Prevalence[4]						Number of cigarettes						
									Unadjusted[7]			Sales-adjusted[8]			
			Manufactured cigarettes		Total cigarettes[5]		All products[6]		Number/ person/day		Total sales %	Manufactured cigarettes number/ person/day		Total cigarettes[9] number/ person/day	
			M	F	M	F	M	F	M	F		M	F	M	F
West Germany *(continued)*															
1980	3	**A**					47	24							
	10	MC							9.3	5.0	---	9.3	5.0		
	11	*UC+A*			49	29	53	29						(10.4	4.9)
1981	1	TC			32	18			7.6	3.9	75			10.2	5.2
	1	**TC+A**			37	22	48	23						(10.4	5.0)
	3	**A**					46	25							
1982	3	**A**					51	26							
	10	MC							7.7	4.5	---	7.7	4.5		
	21	**U**					41	27						(9.2	4.9)
1983	3	**A**					48	28							
1984	1	**A**					46	23							
	3	**UC+A**			38	26	49	27						(9.4	5.1)
	4	**MC+TC+A**	43	28	44	29	47	29	9.3	3.8	90	(8.5	4.4)	10.4	4.3
1989	67	TC+A			31	18	33	18	5.3	2.7	58			9.1	4.6
	67	**A**					38	22							
1992	67	TC+A			30	18	32	18	5.2	2.7					
	67	**A**					36	22							
East Germany															
1971	47	*A+U*			49	27	59	26	8.2	2.5					
1988	64	UC+U					44	22	6.4	2.3					
1992	67	TC+A			34	15	35	16							
	67	**A**					40	20							
Unified Germany															
1992	67	TC+A			31	18	33	18	5.1	2.5	62			8.2	4.0
	67	**A**					37	22							
1995	67	TC+A			30	18	32	18	5.0	2.5	64			7.8	4.0
	67	**A**					36	22							

1 Surveys covering an age range of at least 21-64 are included. Any gaps in the data for ages 15-20 and 65 years and over are filled in by assumed extensions to the age distribution, given in *Notes on sources of survey data*, p. 264. Method: see *Summary of adult smoking*, p. xxxvi

2 See *Notes on sources of survey data*, p. 264

3 Product: MC = manufactured cigarettes, TC = total cigarettes (including hand-rolled), UC = cigarettes (type unspecified), A = all products, U = unspecified. Frequency of smoking is indicated by: regular or daily smokers in normal type, all smokers (including occasional) in bold, unspecified in italics. * = refer to *Notes on sources of survey data*, p. 264

4 From Table 10.4

5 This column includes prevalence of smoking classified as UC = cigarettes (type unspecified)

6 This column includes prevalence of smoking classified as U = unspecified product

7 From Table 10.6

8 From Table 10.7, except data in parentheses, which are derived from the prevalence of smoking from Table 10.4 as described in *Summary of adult smoking*, p. xxxvi. No sales-adjustment has been carried out for East Germany, nor for West Germany after 1990

9 Number of cigarettes classified as UC = cigarettes (type unspecified) has been adjusted to total cigarette sales and included in this column

Figure 10.3 Estimated prevalence of smoking of (i) manufactured cigarettes, (ii) total cigarettes and (iii) all tobacco products: by year of survey. West Germany 1950-1989, East Germany 1971-1988, and Unified Germany 1992-1995.
Males and females aged 15 years and over. *Source:* see Table 10.8

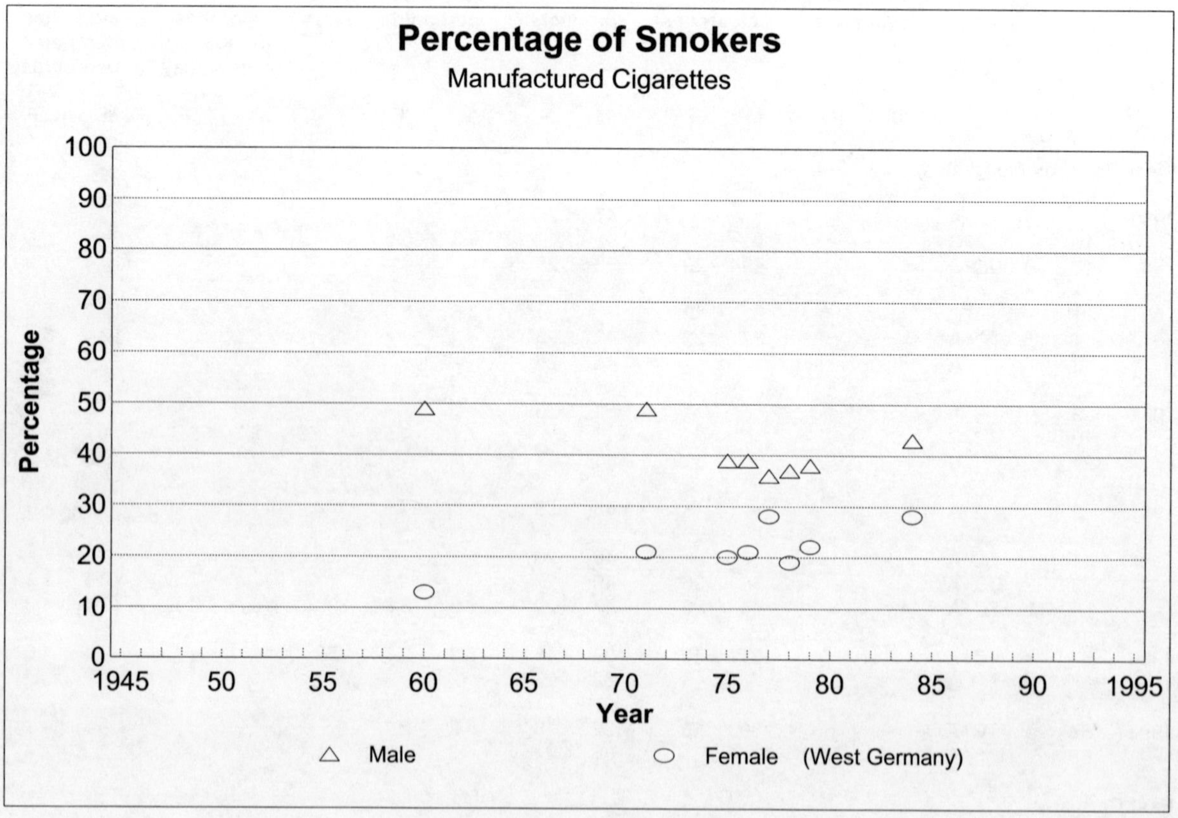

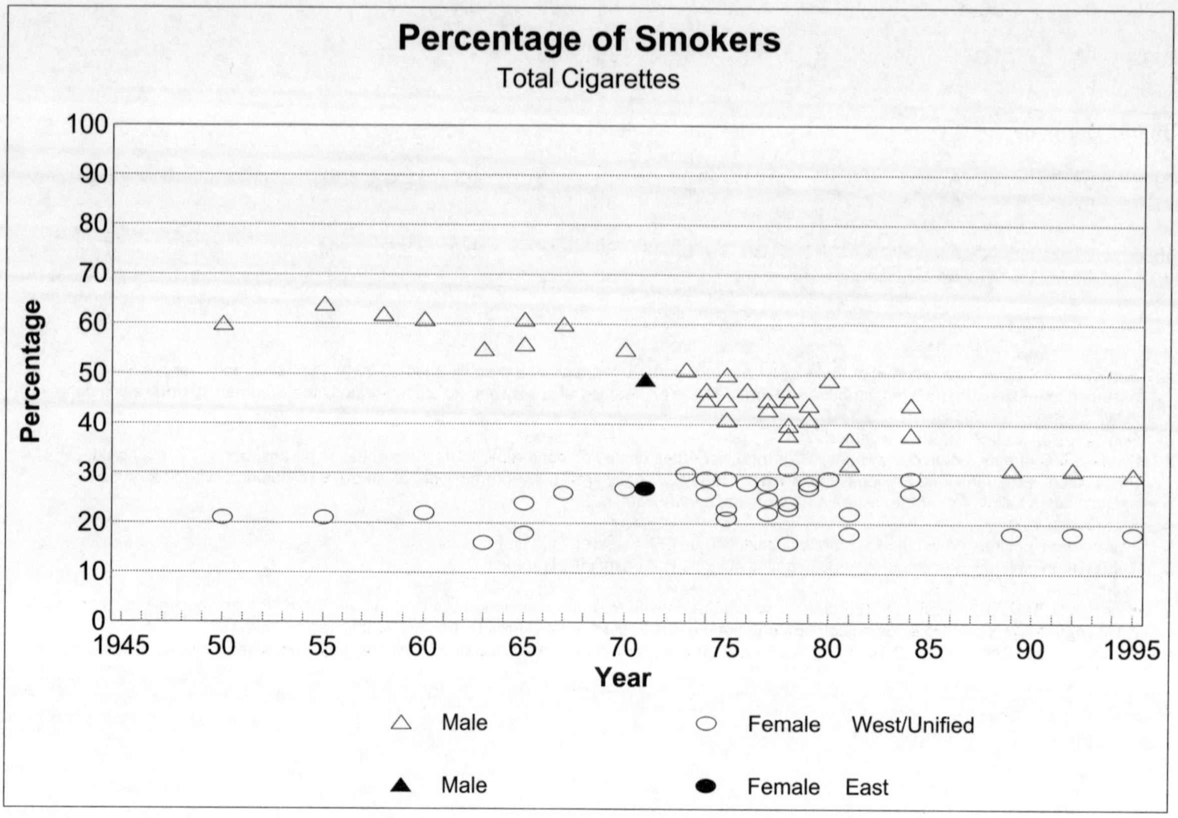

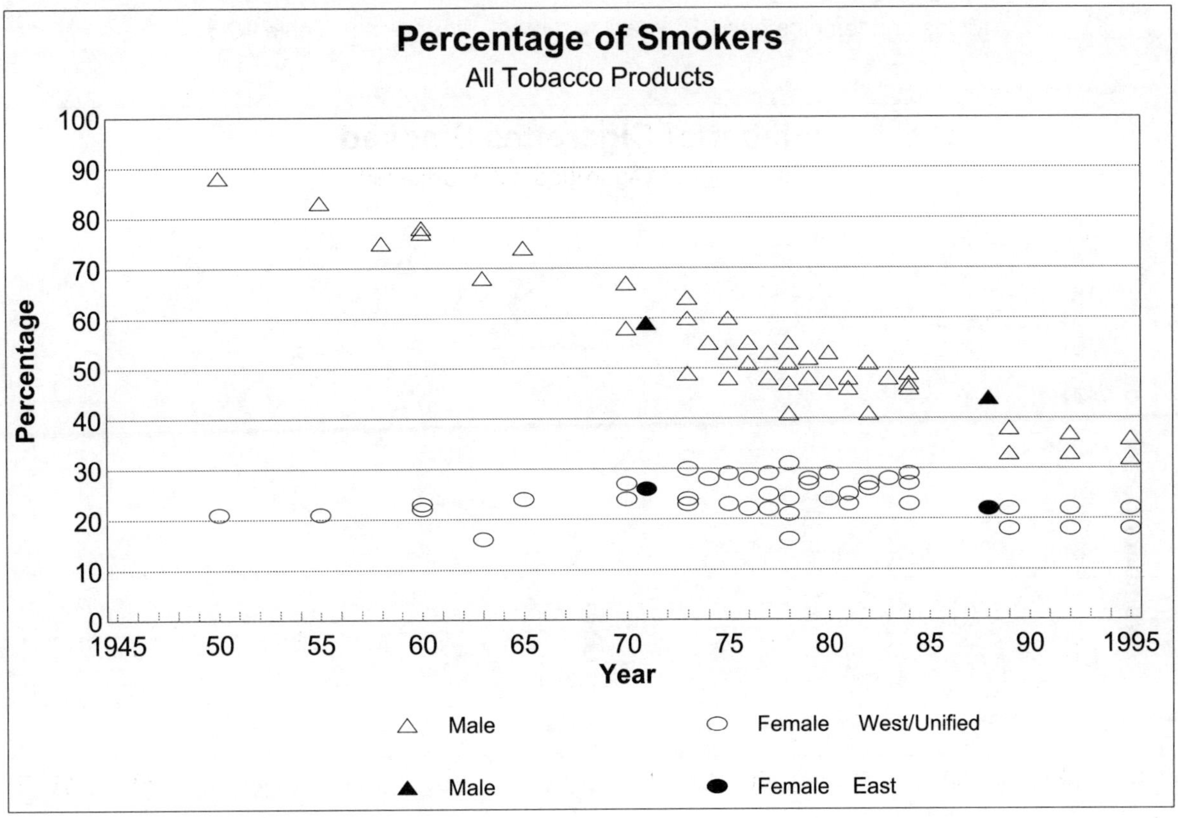
Percentage of Smokers
All Tobacco Products
Percentage
100
90
80
70
60
50
40
30
20
10
0
1945
50
55
60
65
70
75
80
85
90
1995
Year
Male
Female West/Unified
Male
Female East

Figure 10.4 Estimated number of (i) manufactured cigarettes and (ii) total cigarettes smoked per person per day, sales-adjusted. West Germany 1950-1989 and Unified Germany 1992-1995.
Males and females aged 15 years and over. *Source:* see Table 10.8

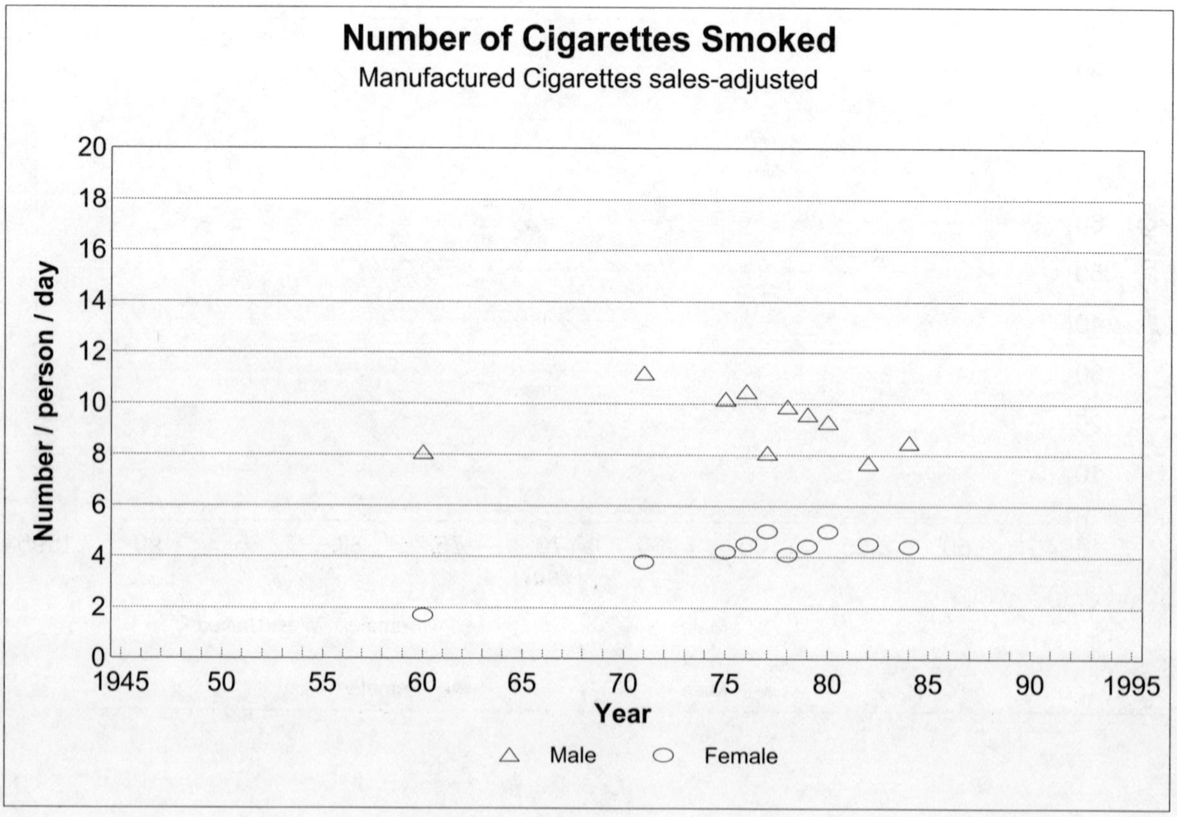

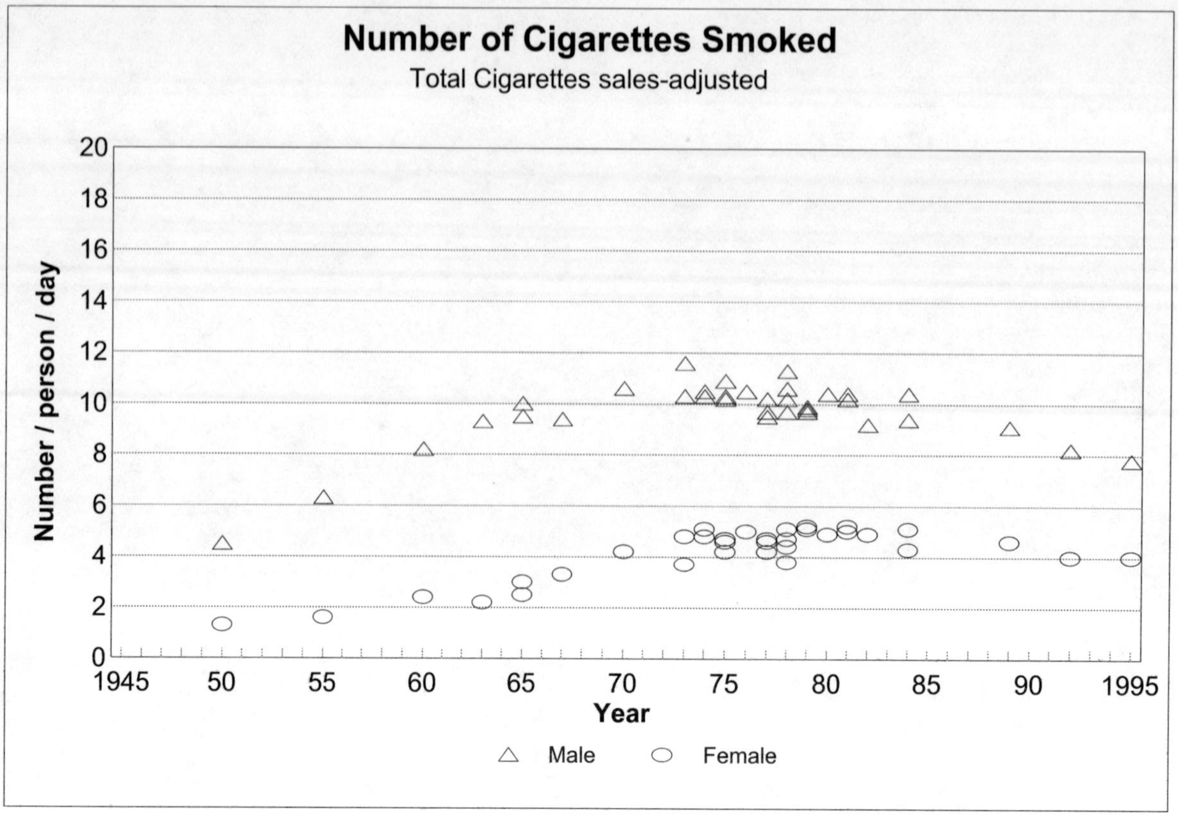

Notes on sources of sales data

The data presented in the tables and figures were obtained from several sources, details of which are given below, together with estimations and related assumptions. Full citations of the sources are given on p. 273 under *References*.

Consumption data for 1906-1913

Statistisches Bundesamt

Data are given on manufactured cigarettes and fine-cut tobacco. Calculation of consumption per adult is based on the population in 1925.

Alternative data presented by Hutson (1937) include consumption of tobacco in various forms for 1913: 12 110 tonnes cigarettes, 39 999 tonnes cigars, 26 374 tonnes smoking mixtures, 5 600 tonnes chewing tobacco and 4 900 tonnes snuff. Data for later years from this source are similar to those given by RP6 (see below).

Consumption data for 1925-1973

RP6

We have followed Statistisches Bundesamt in presenting data starting on 1 April of the named year, and not ending 31 March as in RP6. Data from 1950 are per calendar year. Data for 1948 represent the consumption in West Germany without Baden, Württemberg-Hohenzollern, Saarland, and Berlin; data for 1949 represent West Germany without Saarland and Berlin. Data for 1950-1973 are for West Germany.

Data by weight, originally given to nearest 100 000 pounds, have been converted to tonnes and given to the nearest 10 tonnes (100 000 lbs =45.359 tonnes). Where weight conversion factors have been quoted in RP6, the weights have been re-calculated without rounding and then converted to tonnes.

Notes as given in RP6

(a) Details of the number of cigarettes and cigars and of the weight of fine-cut, pipe and other manufactured tobacco consumed were obtained from the following sources:

1925-49 *Bevölkerung und Wirtschaft*, 1871-1957, published by the Western Germany Federal Statistics Office, Wiesbaden.

1950-63 Estimates from trade sources converted to a calendar year basis.

1964-73 *Finanzen und Steuern—Absatz von Tabakwaren*, published by the Western Germany Federal Statistics Office, Wiesbaden.

(b) Cigarettes consumption in pounds weight was estimated from the number of cigarettes consumed by using a conversion factor of 2.205 lbs per 1 000 up until 1949. From 1950 onwards the conversion factors were provided from trade sources. The conversion factors for cigars were obtained from trade sources for the whole period.

(c) The figures for 1948 onwards include cigarettes which were produced in West Berlin and represent the consumption of tobacco goods in West Germany including West Berlin.

Consumption data for 1974 onwards and sales of cigarette papers 1961-1985

Statistisches Bundesamt (personal communication)

Data for cigarettes, cigars and cigarillos were given as numbers of pieces and have been converted to weights assuming an average of 0.98 g per cigarette and 6.2 g for cigars and cigarillos combined (based on values in RP6).

The data do not make allowance for sales to tourists or for personal imports. Figures for fine-cut include tobacco rolls which became popular during the 1990s; in several European countries tubes with filters for filling with loose tobacco are available but in Germany tobacco rolls which easily fit into the tubes are also available. Originally this had a tax advantage over manufactured cigarettes but an increase in taxation in January 1996 removed much of the advantage of using this product (Anonymous (1996)).

Data are for West Germany only up to 1989 and for Unified Germany from 1991 onwards. No data are available for 1990 itself—reunification took place during that year. No consumption data are available for East Germany, although some indication can be found by comparing the West German data for 1989 with the Unified German data for 1991. Wilde *et al* (1990) gives cigarette consumption per capita in East Germany as follows:

Year	Cigarettes per capita
1960	1 069
1970	1 257
1975	1 451
1980	1 720
1983	1 808
1985	1 833
1986	1 873

Plain/Filter cigarette consumption
West Germany:
1960-1981 Maxwell (successive years)
1982-1983 Todd (1986)
East Germany:
Wilde *et al* (1990)

Tar and nicotine yield of cigarettes
West Germany:
1961-1975 Timm (1976)
Although tar yield is usually expressed as dry yield, this is not available before 1966 and so both dry and moist values are given to show the earlier trend.
1985 Junge *et al* (1989)
East Germany:
No data available.

Anonymous (1996) states that the share of the cigarette market for low tar cigarettes in Germany grew from 19.4% in 1991 to 28.6% in 1995. In former East Germany this grew from 4.6% in 1991 to 18.3% in 1995. Former West Germany's low tar share passed 30% in 1995.

The tar yield per cigarette was limited by EC directive (Directive 90/239/EEC) to 15 mg by the end of 1992, and to 12 mg by the end of 1997 (Harkin *et al* (1997)).

Estimates of hand-rolled cigarette consumption
We have taken as our estimate of hand-rolled cigarette consumption:
before 1961, 70% of fine-cut tobacco sales, at 1 g per cigarette.
1961-1988, 90% of cigarette paper sales
1989 onwards, 80% of fine-cut tobacco sales, at 0.8 g per cigarette
These estimates were based on sometimes conflicting information.

Although fine-cut tobacco (listed separately from pipe tobacco) would be expected to be used predominantly in hand-rolled cigarettes, the data on sales of cigarette papers suggest that consumption of hand-rolled cigarettes was in fact lower, particularly until the mid-1970s.

Estimates for consumption of fine-cut tobacco differ from those given by Merzdorf *et al* (1982) (p. 231) for the period 1974-1979. Merzdorf *et al* (1982) estimated hand-rolled cigarette consumption as 80% of fine-cut tobacco sales, at 1 g per cigarette.

Merzdorf *et al* (1982) (p. 263) estimated that during 1976-1979 consumption of hand-rolled cigarettes amounted to 86% of sales of cigarette papers. However, assuming 1 g of tobacco per cigarette, the estimates of hand-rolled cigarettes based on sales of fine-cut tobacco always exceed sales of cigarette papers.

Dymond (1996) gives mean weights of hand-rolled cigarettes in Germany as 822 mg (1977), 800 mg (1988) and 778 mg (1994).

Estimates for 1985-1988 would have been similar had the later method been used.

Notes on sources of survey data

Each source of survey data—either an individual survey or a series of surveys repeated over a number of years—is cited by a source number. This number is shown in the tables and corresponds to the source numbers given below, where details of the source publication and of the survey methodology are given. Sources 1-42 relate to West Germany, i.e. the former Federal Republic and the equivalent area after unification, sources 43-66 to East Germany, the former Democratic Republic, and sources 67-68 to both areas. Full citations of the sources are given on p. 273 under *References*.

Source number

1 **Baric (1980), Erben (1980), Institut für Markt- und Werbeforshung (IMW) (1981), Junge *et al* (1989)**

a. Representative studies carried out on behalf of BZgA (Bundeszentrale für gesundheitliche Aufklärung, Köln (Federal Centre for Health Education)) by IMW (Institut für Markt- und Werbeforschung, Köln). Sample size 2 000

2 **IMW (1979)**

a. Cigarette smokers: (combination of two categories) smoked cigarettes regularly (5 or more per day) and occasionally (up to 4 per day). Presumably there were no female smokers of products other than cigarettes

3 **Todd (1986), quoting EMNID-Institut**

a. Smokers: includes occasional smokers 'smoking now and then'
b. Assumed extension to age distribution for percentage smokers, age 15: (1970 only) males 20% and females 15%

4 **IMW (1984)**

a. Consumption category estimation by Todd (1986) based on individual number of cigarettes up to 20, then 21-29, 30-39, 40-49, 50+ cigarettes/smoker/day
b. Calculation of consumption per person based on percentage smokers including occasional smokers and number of cigarettes per regular cigarette smokers (1+ cigarettes per day). Therefore they may overestimate

5 **Junge *et al* (1989)**

a. Three nationally representative studies 'Umwelteinwirkungen und Beschwerdehäufigkeiten'

Year		Sample size	
		Males	Females
1967	(May-Sep)	711	964
1974	(Jun-Aug)	733	920
1985	(Aug-Nov)	557	648

First two studies conducted by interviewer—included 32 questions related to smoking. Third study used shortened questionnaire (included five smoking questions) and was sent by post

6 **Le Meitour-Kaplan (1977), quoting Bundesminister für Jugend Familie und Gesundheit (1974), and WHO (1975)**

a. WHO estimates presumably quoting two different surveys (see also source 7)
b. Assumed extension to age distribution for percentage smokers, age 15-19: males 45% and females 27%; age 65+: males 45% and females 10%

7 **WHO (1975)**

a. Cigarette only smokers. Age group unclear
b. Assumed extension to age distribution for percentage smokers, age 15-19: males 40% and females 26%; age 65+: males 30% and females 10%

8 **Koschorreck *et al* (1973)**

a. Representative study in school boys in Bruchsal, North Baden. Anonymous questionnaires completed with teachers absent. Sample size 898, participation rate 98%
b. Results presented here have been adjusted to exclude the 12% of pupils unclassified on smoking
c. Consumption category estimation based on 1-9, 10-29, 30+ cigarettes/smoker/ week

9 Le Meitour-Kaplan (1977)

a. Data taken from 'Official records of the German Federal Centre for Health Education'

10 Todd (1986)

a. Estimated by Todd

11 Merzdorf *et al* (1982), quoting IFD (Institut für Demoskopie, Allensbach) (various years), and Anonymous (1980)

a. Survey details are only available for 1980: Representative cross-section of West Germany, sample size 3 542

a. Assumed extension to age distribution for percentage smokers, age 15: (A and UC) (1973 only) males and females 15%

12 Merzdorf *et al* (1982), quoting DIVO (1958, 1966, 1974)(no details)

a. Assumed extension to age distribution for percentage smokers, age 15:males (1958, A and UC) 20%, (1965, 1974) 15%; females (1965, 1974) 10%. For age 80+:males (1958, A) 10%, (1958, UC) 40%, (1965, 1974) 30%; females (1965, 1974) 5%

13 Merzdorf *et al* (1982), quoting tobacco industry

a. Cigarette smokers: smoked at least one manufactured cigarette per day

14 Readers Digest (1963)

a. Series of surveys conducted in European countries using identical questionnaires. West German survey conducted by IFD. Random sample of about 2 000 people

b. It is also reported that 15% of men (10% age <40 and 19% age 40+) smoke a pipe, and that 27% of men (13% age <40 and 36% age 40+) smoke cigars

c. Assumed extension to age distribution for percentage smokers, age 15-20: males (A) 50%, (UC) 45%; females 16%

15 Merzdorf *et al* (1982), quoting Burda-Verlag (1967, 1976)

a. Assumed extension to age distribution for percentage smokers, age 70+: males 40% and females 10%

16 Merzdorf *et al* (1982), quoting Spiegel-Verlag (1971, 1978)

a. Assumed extension to age distribution for percentage smokers, age 15-19; (A) males (1971) 45%, (1978) 40% and females (1978) 28%; (UC) males (1971, 1978) 40% and females (1978) 27%. For age 65+: (A) males (1971) 45%, (1978) 40% and females (1978) 8%; (UC) males (1971) 35%, (1978) 30% and females (1978) 8%

17 Merzdorf *et al* (1982), quoting Stern (1977)

a. Assumed extension to age distribution for percentage smokers, age 65+:males (A) 40%, (UC) 30%; females 8%

18-19 Laaser *et al* (1977)

a. Study in Cologne schools—23 Gymnasien (Grammar schools) and 17 Berufsschulen (vocational schools). Sample size 6 302

b. Age-specific prevalence shown in Table 10.4 as source **18** based on Gymnasien, **19** on Berufsschulen, taken from graph. All ages-results and other tables based on both school types combined

20 Harreis *et al* (1980)

a. Study in 35 schools, 29 of which were in Baden-Württemberg. Lower age limit 10. Sample size 9 080, response rate 91%

b. Results are also available by school type for age 10-14, showing lower prevalence in Gymnasien than other types

21 Letzel and Johnston (1984)

a. Sample size 1 670, representative sample

b. Assumed extension to age distribution for percentage smokers, age 66+: males 35% and females 8%

22 Aarø *et al* (1981), quoting Tölle (1974)

a. Survey in larger town. Year unknown. Age 10-18

23-26 WHO (1989)

a. Four regional surveys forming part of WHO MONICA Project:

	Region	Population size	Sample size	Participation rate (%)	Sample used* Males	Females	Date
23	Bremen	73 300	1 826	71	809	849	May 1984-Dec 1984
24	Rhein-Neckar Region	235 900	2 865	86	1 492	1 600	Sep 1983-Aug1987
25	Augsburg (urban)	95 300	1 866	75	924	881	Oct 1984-May 1985
26	Augsburg (rural)	109 500	2 118	80	1 098	1 118	Oct 1984-May 1985

* 'Sample used' includes age 25-34; all other figures are for age 35-64 only

b. *All ages* column relates only to age 35-64 and is standardized to world population

c. Regular cigarette smokers: smoked cigarettes daily. All smokers: smoked cigarettes daily or occasionally, or smoked 1 g pipe tobacco or 1 cigar per week. Cigarettes per smoker refers to regular and occasional cigarette smokers

d. Calculation for cigarettes per person based on % regular cigarette smokers and cigarettes per regular or occasional cigarette smoker, so may underestimate

27 Malhotra (1978) quoting Luban-Plozza and Knaak-Sommer (1972)

a. Study in Hamburg schoolchildren, year uncertain. Lower age limit 10

28-29 von Harnack *et al* (1967)

a. Anonymous questionnaire study in 47 schools of all types in Hamburg, urban, shown as source **28**, and Düren, rural, shown as source **29**. Sample size 6 408

b. Consumption category estimation based on 1-7, 8-14, 15-49, 50-99, 100+ cigarettes/smoker/week

30 Bach and Bach (1968)

a. Anonymous questionnaire survey in small town schools in Kirchain/Mittlehessen. Sample size 712, response rate 99%. The proportions attending different school types and their age ranges were:

School type	% of sample	Age range
Gymnasium	50	12-21
Realschule	35	12-18
Volksschule	15	37239

b. The prevalence of smoking was 41% for sexes combined, not reported separately. Among smokers, 72% of boys smoked cigarettes, 19% pipes and 8% cigars, while all girls smoked cigarettes

c. Consumption category estimation based on ≤5, 6-9, 10-20 and 21+ cigarettes/smoker/day

31 Bayerische Staatsministerien des Innern und für Arbeit und Sozialordnung (1982)

a. 'Youth asks youth', series of surveys in Bavaria. Sample size (1973) 2 676, (1976) 2 441, (1980) 2 033

b. Smoker: smokes at least occasionally

32 Malhotra (1978) quoting Benad (1973)

a. Nationwide representative study

b. The prevalence of smoking (sexes combined, age 12-25) was 51%

33 Malhotra (1978) quoting Malhotra (1977)

a. Study in Wuppertal schoolchildren, 1974-1975

34 Mohl (1979)

a. Representative study in West Germany including West Berlin, conducted by GfK (Gesellschaft für Konsum-, Markt-, und Absatzforschung e.V., Nürnberg). Year not stated. Sample size 3 945

b. Assumed extension to age distribution for percentage smokers, age 15: males and females 12%. For age 70+: males 25% and females 6%. Number of cigarettes/smoker/day, age 15: males and females 0.5. For age 70+: males 3.0 and females 0.5

35 Lippert *et al* (1980)

a. Pilot study in schools (Gymnasien and Hauptschüler) before an intervention project in Berlin. School grades 7-9, predominantly aged 13-15. Sample size 818

b. Regular smokers: smoked daily. All smokers: smoked daily or occasionally. Cigarettes per smoker based on smokers of 1+ cigarettes per week

c. Consumption category estimation based on 1-4, 5-9, 10-19 and 20+ cigarettes/smoker/week

36 Hoffmeister *et al* (1994), Rothenbacher *et al* (1996), Junge and Nagel (1999)

a. German Cardiovascular Prevention Study (GCP). Nationally representative samples (West Germany including West Berlin). Subjects invited for physical examination and completed self-administered questionnaire. Results weighted to adjust for non-participation.

Midpoint Year	Dates	Sample size		Participation rate (%)
		Males	Females	
1985	Jun 1984-May 1986	2 417	2 373	67
1988	Sep 1987-Aug 1989	2 649	2 686	71
1990	Apr 1990-Apr 1991	2 623	2 688	69

b. There is a slight discrepancy in the prevalence reported by the different sources

c. Consumption category estimation (1988) based on 1-9, 10-19, 20+ cigarettes/smoker/day. Consumption per smoker (1990) refers to regular and occasional cigarette smokers

d. Calculation of cigarettes per person based on percentage of smokers (unspecified) and cigarettes per cigarette smoker, and should be regarded with caution

37 Scheuermann *et al* (1991)

a. BRUKAMOS study, conducted in Bruchsal, Karlsruhe and Mosbach. Sample size 3 737

b. Smokers: smoked at least 1 cigarette per day, or smoked pipe or cigars

c. Calculation of cigarettes per person based on percentage of smokers of all products, and number of cigarettes per cigarette smoker, so may overestimate

38 van Reek *et al* (1992), van Reek and Adriaanse (1995)

a. A series of surveys of Young Europeans. About 800 children aged 11-15 years interviewed in each EC country except Luxembourg (where only 250 interviewed). Lowest age group 11-12. Interviews conducted at home, with parents absent

b. Regular smokers: smoked daily. All smokers: smoked at least once a week

39 Weiland *et al* (1994)

a. Random sample of schoolchildren in the city of Bochum, school grades 7 and 8. Anonymous questionnaire covering respiratory health and active and passive smoking, completed in class with survey administrators present. Part of a study of asthma. Sample size (males) 978, (females) 1 072

b. Regular smokers: smoke 1+ cigarettes per day. All smokers: smoked in last month

c. Consumption category estimation based on two categories, 1-10 and >10 cigarettes/smoker/day, and resulting figures should be regarded with caution

40-41 Scholz and Kaltenbach (1995)

a. Study in 2 cities, Offenbach (1991-1992) and Hanau (1992). 31 schools of all types. Anonymous questionnaire on smoking, alcohol and drugs. Sample size 2 979

b. Results shown as source **40** relate to inner city, **41** to suburbs

c. Approximate age corresponding to school grade 7

d. Regular smokers: smoked daily

42 King *et al* (1996)

a. Part of the HBSC (Health Behaviour in School-Aged Children) Study, a collaborative cross-national research study sponsored by the WHO. Conducted in the region of Nordrhein-Westfalen. School classes or schools were randomly selected, targeting age groups 11 (not presented here), 13 and 15. The target sample size was 1 300 in each age group.

Target age	Mean age	Sample size
13	13.5	1 121
15	15.5	1 050

c. Regular smokers: smoke once a week or more

43 Heinemann *et al* (1995)

a. Estimates compiled by combining various cross-sectional studies, or baseline of cohort or intervention studies. Results are age-adjusted to 1984 population of Federal Republic of Germany.

Mid-point*	Year	Reference	Area
1960	1960	Werner (1961)	Wurzen, semi-rural
1971	1968	Böthig (1974)	Berlin-Mitte, urban
	1970	Thiele *et al* (1974)	Sternberg, semi-rural
	1970	Wolff (1981)	Gnoien, urban
	1971	Hüttner *et al* (1972a, 1972b)	Berlin-Treptow, Friedrichshain, urban
	1974	Barth *et al* (1978)	Berlin-Lichtenberg, urban
	1974	Faulhaber (unpublished)	Berlin-Pankow
	1974	Knappe (unpublished)	Erfurt (Kaunas-Rotterdam intervention study)
1977	1975/1976	Gräfner (1979)	Schwedt, semi-rural
	1976	Heinemann *et al* (1984), Eckstein *et al* (1983), Eckstein (1986)	2 studies in Schleiz and Dippoldiswalde, rural
	1976	Heinrich (unpublished)	Erfurt (Unformtechnik), urban
	1977	Heinrich (unpublished)	Erfurt (Optima), urban
	1975-1979	Hartung and Hartung (1984)	Chemnitz, urban
1984	1982-1984	Heinemann (unpublished)	Multi-centric CANON-Studie, urban and rural
	1984-1985	Heinemann *et al* (1988), Heinemann (1988)	Multi-centric MONICA I study, urban and rural
1988	1988-1989	MONICA East Germany Team (1993)	Mulit-centric MONICA II study, urban and rural
1991	1991-1992	HIES-Team (1992)	HIES representative survey, urban and rural

*used in Table 10.4

b. Regular smokers: smoked more than 1 cigarette per day, based on different questionnaires in the various studies

c. Some of the studies included here are also presented as separate sources

44 Zuber and Zuber (1973)

a. Anonymous study among pupils at all schools, including vocational school, in Zeulenroda, Ostthüringen. Lower age limit 10. Sample size (males) 710, (females) 663

b. Regular cigarette smokers: smoked daily. All cigarette smokers: smoked weekly. Frequency of pipe and cigar smoking not specified

c. Consumption category estimation based on 1-5, 6-10, >10 cigarettes/smoker/day, males only. All regular female smokers smoked 1-5 cigarettes, except one who smoked 6-10

45 Reissig (1977, 1989)

a. Longitudinal studies conducted by Zentralinstitut für Jugendforschung in Leipzig school pupils. Sample size (first study 1968-1975) 600
b. Approximate ages corresponding to school grades 8-10 (except 1975)
c. Regular smokers: smoked daily. All smokers: smoked daily or occasionally
d. Consumption category estimation (1975 only) based on occasional (assume 0.5), 1-3, 4-10, 11-15, 16-20, 21+ cigarettes/smoker/day

46 Geizerova and Masironi (1988)

a. No original source. Age group not stated for 1971 data, assumed same as for 1983

47 Hüttner *et al* (1972b, 1972a)

a. Representative survey in East Berlin. Sample size 4 983
b. Cigarette smokers: smokers who smoke predominantly cigarettes
c. Consumption category estimation based on 1-4, 5-9, 10-20, 21+ grams/smoker/day
d. Assumed extension to age distribution for percentage smokers, age 15-17: males 30% and females 15%. Number of cigarettes/person/day: males 3.0 and females 1.0

48-49 Herrmann and Liehs (1977)

a. Cross-sectional study comprising interview and medical check.

	Location	Year	Sample size	
			Males	Females
48	4 towns—Halle, Erfurt, Schwerin, Freiberg (males only)	1971 (males), 1973 (females)	8 369	2 505
49	21 towns	1973	13 807	8 324

b. Source 48: Some results were available only for Halle (the age-specific proportion of male smokers who smoke cigarettes or mixed products but not pipe/cigars only), or for Halle, Erfurt and Schwerin (average consumption of tobacco, grams per smoker per day); these have been combined with the prevalence of smoking in the 4 towns to estimate age-specific prevalence of cigarette smoking (Table 10.4) and the consumption per person (Table 10.6)

50 Reissig (1977)

a. Study among young workers in Berlin, Leipzig, Karl-Marx-Stadt and Rostock. Stated to be 'approximately representative of the working youth of the GDR'. Sample size 4 000

51 Wuthe *et al* (1977)

a. Part of a study of lung function in schoolchildren in Berlin-Karow. Confidential interview. Ages 6-16 studied, but only results for age 12-16 presented here. Year not stated. Sample size for age 12-16 (males) 210, (females) 164
b. Regular smokers: smoked 1+ cigarettes per day
c. Most data taken from chart

52 Schlegel and Schulz (1987) quoting Eisenblätter *et al* (1982, 1995)(no details)

a. Study in Berlin-Pankow, 1977-1978
b. Definitions assumed to be the same as for source 56. Smokers marked as frequency *: smoked daily. Regular smokers: smoked >1 cigarette per week. All smokers: smoked >1 cigarette per month

53 Keyl (1979)

a. Interview study in school pupils in a rural district. Approximate ages corresponding to school grades 8-12. Sample size (males) 768, (females) 734
b. The prevalence of smoking was 41% for both sexes; sex-specific results varied between approximately 50-75% for boys and 25-50% for girls for the individual schools, but overall prevalence estimates could not be derived
c. Consumption category estimation based on <3 (assume 1-3), 4-5, 6+ cigarettes/smoker/day, omitting occasional smokers

54 Krecklow (1987)

a. Anonymous questionnaire study in Waren. Sample size (1981, age 12) 1348, (1985, age 16) 613
b. Regular smokers: smoke 1+ cigarettes per day. All smokers: smokes occasionally or 1+ cigarettes per day
c. Consumption category estimation (age 16 only) based on 1-5, 6-10, 11+ cigarettes/smoker/day

55 Piorkowski and Piorkowski (1983)

a. Anonymous questionnaire study in 15 schools in Cottbus county. Questionnaires completed at home after classes on the dangers of smoking. Year not stated. Sample size for grades 5-10 (males) 1 679, (females) 1 541
b. Approximate ages corresponding to school grades 7-10
c. Some data taken from graphs

56 Schlegel and Schulz (1987)

a. Part of an intervention study on cardiovascular risk factors, all schools in Hohenmölsen, a rural district. Self-completion questionniare, not anonymous. Sample size (males) 637, (females) 635
b. Smokers marked as frequency *: smoked daily. Regular smokers: smoked >1 cigarette per week. All smokers: smoked >1 cigarette per month

57-62 WHO (1989), WHO MONICA Project (1988), Heinemann *et al* (1998)

a. Regional surveys forming part of WHO MONICA project:

	Region	Population size	Sample size	Participation rate (%)	Sample used*		Date
					Males	Females	
57	Berlin-Lichtenberg	75 300	1 479	74	598	640	Apr 1984-Jun 1985
58	Cottbus County	307 100	1 330	77	658	739	Oct 1984-Jul 1986
59	Halle County	224 700	2 113	89	1 249	1 311	Nov 1983-Jul 1984
60	Karl-Marx-Stadt County	289 700	2 175	91	1 284	1 394	1982-Dec 1985
61	Rest of DDR	133 700	835	88	528	498	1982-Dec 1985

* 'Sample used' includes age 25-34; all other figures are for age 35-64 only

Results shown as source **62** are for all regions in 1982-1984 and 1987-1989, and for three regions in 1991-1994

b. *All ages* column relates only to age 35-64 and is standardized to world population
c. Regular cigarette smokers: smoked cigarettes daily. All smokers: smoked cigarettes daily or occasionally, or smoked 1 g pipe tobacco or 1 cigar per week. Cigarettes per smoker refers to regular and occasional cigarette smokers
d. Calculation for cigarettes per person based on % regular cigarette smokers and cigarettes per regular or occasional cigarette smoker, so may underestimate

63 Preuss (1991)

a. Anonymous questionnaire study of schoolchildren at all schools in Stendal (county town). Sample size for grades 5-10 (males) 1 401, (females) 1 458
b. Approximate ages corresponding to school grades 7-10

64 Donat (1989)

a. Representative survey by Institüt für Marktforschung Leipzig. Sample size (males) 946, (females) 1 057
b. Regular smokers: smoked at least 1 cigarette per day on average
c. Consumption category estimation based on 1-3, 4-6, 7-10, 11-15, 16-20, >20 cigarettes/smoker/day

65 Theopold (1972) quoting Lickint (no details)

a. Study in schoolchildren in Chemnitz. Year not stated. Last age group relates to age 20

66 Junge and Nagel (1999)

a. Health study in 1991-1992 in East German region, comparable to source 36 in West Germany in 1990-1991

b. Consumption per smoker based on regular and occasional cigarette smokers

c. Calculation of cigarettes per person based on percentage of smokers (unspecified) and cigarettes per cigarette smoker, and should be regarded with caution

67 Statistisches Bundesamt

a. Mikrozensus, sample 0.5% of the population age 10+. Personal interviews

b. Results were originally available by both fine and broad age groups. We have usually presented the finer age groups, but occasionally present both for convenience. We have not presented the results for age 10-14, as they were commonly omitted or marked as unreliable due to small numbers. Results for 1992 reported for both West and East Germany separately and combined

c. Consumption category estimation (1978 only) based on 1-20, 21-40, 41+

68 Der Bundesminister für jugend Familie und Gesundheit (1983), Bundeszentrale für gesundheitliche Aufklärung (BZgA) (1994) and Merzdorf *et al* (1982) quoting BZgA

a. Series of surveys carried out by BZgA on use of alcohol, illegal drugs, medication and tobacco among youth and young adults.
1981: Representative survey in West Germany. Carried out by Infratest Gesundheitsforschung. Sample size 11 711. Age 12-24
1993: Representative multistage survey with results reported for both West and East Germany separately and combined. Carried out by IJF (Institut für Jugendforschung, Institute for Youth Research). Personal interviews. Sample size (West) 2 000, (East) 1 000

b. 1993: Regular smokers: continual smokers. All smokers: continual and occasional smokers. Consumption per smoker is based on all smokers, and the consumption per occasional smoker is said to be about 5 cigarettes per day

c. Among smokers (sexes combined) the percentages smoking different products were:

		Cigarettes			Pipe
		Filter	Plain	Hand-rolled	
1981*	West	76	7	26	1
1993	West	88	1	8	1
1993	East	95	3	2	0

* Multiple response possible

Additional sources (not shown in Tables)

Proctor (1996) quoting Kittel (1944)

a. In a survey of 1 000 servicemen in 1944, 87.3% were smokers, and 0.3% smoked 30+ cigarettes per day. As 101 had started smoking and 7 given up during the war, this implies that 77.9% were smokers in 1939; 4.4% smoked 30+ cigarettes per day

Müller (1939)

a. In a study of lung cancer (years unknown), 84% of a healthy male control group were smokers (sample size 86). The average consumption of cigarette equivalents per smoker per day is estimated as 16, and the consumption per person per day as 14

b. Consumption category estimation based on 1-15, 16-25, 26-35 and >35 cigarette equivalents/smoker/day, where cigarette equivalents are based on 1 cigar = 5 g and 1 cigarette = 0.8 g

References

Aarø L.E., Hauknes A. and Berglund E.-L. (1981). Smoking among Norwegian schoolchildren 1975-1980. I. Extent of smoking in the age group 12-15 years, 1975. *Scand J Psychol,* **22**, 161-9.

Anonymous (1980). German men not smoking as they used to, but women's numbers rise. *Tobacco International,* **182**, 28.

Anonymous (1996). Europe lights up. *Tobacco Europe,* **Jul/Aug**, 17-9.

Bach A. and Bach W. (1968). Schüler und Rauchen. (Schoolchildren and smoking). *Medizinische Welt,* **1**, 83-90.

Baric L. (ed) (1980). *Europäische monographein zur forschung in gesundheitserziehung.* (Volume 2.) Bundeszentrale für Gesundheitliche Aufklärung, Köln.

Barth W., Böthig S., Bährlehner A. *et al* (1978). Interventionsstudie Berlin—Ergebnisse der Screening- und Behandlungsphase. In: *Epidemiologie nichtübertragbarer Krankheiten.* AfAF, Berlin; 186-91. (Series of the Academy for Postgraduate Education, Volume 51.)[§]

Bayerische Staatsministerien des Innern und für Arbeit und Sozialordnung (1982). *Jugend und alkohol, drogen, medikamente, tabak. Jugend fragt jugend. (Youth and alcohol, drugs, medicines, tobacco. Youth asks youth).* Bayerische Staatsministerien des Innern und für Arbeit und Sozialordnung, Munich. RB-Nr. 03A/82/01.

Beese D.H. (ed) (1968). *Tobacco consumption in various countries,* 2nd edition. Tobacco Research Council, London. Research Paper 6.

Beese D.H. (ed) (1972). *Tobacco consumption in various countries,* 3rd edition. Tobacco Research Council, London. Research Paper 6.

Benad A. (1973). Empirische materialien zur situation der 12-bis 25 jährigen in der BRD unter besonderer Berücksichtigung iher Drogenaffinität. *Drogen-Report,* **2**, 2-3.[§]

Böthig S. (1974). *Epidemiologie der Herz-Kreislauf-Krankheiten bei Männern mittleren Alters. Ergebnisse der Erstuntersuchung der Studie Berlin-Mitte* [Thesis]. Humboldt University, Berlin.[§]

Bundesminister für Jugend, Familie und Gesundheit (1974). *Auswirkung des Zigarettenrauchens.* Bonn-Bad Godesberg. Drucksache 7/2070.[§]

Bundeszentrale für gesundheitliche Aufklärung (BZgA) (1994). *Die Drogenaffinität Jugendlicher in der Bundesrepublik Deutschland. Wiederholungsbefragung—1993/1994 (The drug affinity of youths in the Federal Republic of Germany. Repeat survey—1993/1994).* Bundeszentrale für gesundheitliche Aufklärung (BZgA) (December 1994, Referat 2-25), Cologne.

Burda-Verlag (1967). *Verbraucheranalyse.*[§]

Burda-Verlag (1976). Typologie der Wünsche. *Bedürfnisstrukturen von Zielgruppen.*[§]

Davey-Smith G., Ströbele S.A. and Egger M. (1994). Smoking and health promotion in Nazi Germany. *J Epidemiol Community Health,* **48**, 220-3.

Der Bundesminister für jugend Familie und Gesundheit (1983). *Konsum und Mißbrauch von Alkohol, illegalen Drogen, Medikamenten und Tabakwaren durch junge Menschen.* Der Bundesminister für Jugend, Familie und Gesundheit; Bonn.

Donat P. (1989). Schwerpunkte der Verbrauchsentwicklung bei Tabakwaren und alkoholischen Getränken (Important aspects in the development of the consumption of tobacco products and alcoholic beverages). *Z Arztl Fortbild,* **83**, 1071-5.

Dymond H.F. (1996). Making habits of roll-your-own smokers in the Netherlands and tar and nicotine yields from the resultant products. *Tobacco Science,* **40**, 87-91.

Eckstein M. (1986). *Das bevölkerungswirksame Programm zur Bekämpfung von Herz-Kreislauf-Krankheiten und anderen chronischen Krankheiten in Schleiz* [Thesis]. Academy for Postgraduate Education, Berlin.§

Eckstein M., Hellmund W., Winkler M., Heinemann L. and Heine H. (1983). 5-year follow up of the Schleiz project. In: *Hypertension*. Ministry of Public Health and Family, Brussels; 41-56.§

Erben R. (1980). Adult smoking—patterns and trends. In: Ramström L.M. (ed) *The smoking epidemic, a matter of worldwide concern. Proceedings of the fourth world conference on smoking and health, Stockholm, 1979.* Almqvist & Wiskell International, Stockholm; 63-8.

Geizerova H. and Masironi R. (1988). Cigarette smoking in children and adolescents: world review. In: Aoki M., Hisamichi S. and Tominaga S. (eds) *Smoking and health 1987. Proceedings of the 6th World Conference on Smoking and Health, Tokyo, 9-12 November 1987.* Elsevier Science Publishers B.V. (Biomedical Division), Amsterdam; 601-5. International Congress Series No. 780.

Gräfner L. (1979). *Die Häufigkeit von Herz-Kreislauf-Krankheiten bzw. Krankheitsmerkmalen bei 30-59jährigen Schwedter Frauen* [Thesis]. Medical Academy, Erfurt.§

Harkin A.M., Anderson P. and Goos C. (1997). *Smoking, drinking and drug taking in the European Region.* Alcohol, Drugs and Tobacco Programme, WHO Regional Office for Europe, Copenhagen.

Harreis G., Schultze Ch. and Schmidt F. (1980). Das Rauchen von Schülern verlagert sich auf immer jüngere Jahrgänge. (Smoking by pupils shifts to younger and younger generations). *Offentliche Gesundheitswesen,* **42**, 771-8.

Hartung A. and Hartung G. (1984). *Hypertoniescreening in Verbindung mit gynäkologischen Vorsorgeuntersuchungen in einer Industriegroßstadt* [Thesis]. Academy for Postgraduate Education, Berlin.§

Heinemann L. (ed) (1988). *'Mini-DDR-Datenbuch' zu Stand und Trends ausgewählter chronischer Erkrankungen und assoziierter Einflussfaktoren aus Umwelt und Lebensweise. Ansatz einer Gesundheitsberichterstattung.* Academy of Sciences, Berlin.

Heinemann L., Barth W. and Hoffmeister H. (1995). Trend of cardiovascular risk factors in the East German population 1968-1992. *J Clin Epidemiol,* **48**, 787-95.

Heinemann L., Heine H., Assmann A., Schädlich H., *et al* (1988). Risk factors in the population of the GDR-MONICA study (1983/84). *Acta Medica Scandinavica,* **728 (Suppl)**, 144-9.

Heinemann L., Heine H., Hellmund W. and Eckstein M. (1984). Probleme der Durchsetzung gesunder Lebensweise in bevölkerungswirksamen Programmen. *Deutsche Gesundheitswesen,* **39**, 209-12.§

Heinemann L.A.J., Garbe E., Claßen E., Willich S.N., Barth W. and Thiel C. (1998). Trends im kardiovaskulären risikofaktorenprofil in Ostdeutschland. Drei unabhängige Bevölkerungsuntersuchungen im Rahmen des Projekts MONICA Ostdeutschland. (Trends in cardiovascular risk factor profiles in East Germany: three independent population studies as part of the project MONICA East Germany). *Dtsch Med Wochenschr,* **123**, 889-95.§

Herrmann H. and Liehs F. (1977). Die Rauchgewohnheiten und ihr Einfluss auf die Entwicklung chronisch broncho-pulmonaler Erkrankungen—Ergebnisse der epidemiologischen Bronchitisforschung in der DDR. (Smoking habits and their influence on development of chronic bronchopulmonary diseases). *Zeitschrift fur Erkrankungen der Atmungsorgane,* **148**, 5-24.

HIES-Team (1992). *Representative health interview and examination survey: Berlin: New Federal States of Germany, Field report.*§

Hoffmeister H., Mensink G.B.M. and Stolzenberg H. (1994). National trends in risk factors for cardiovascular disease in Germany. *Prev Med,* **23**, 197-205.

Hutson J.B. (1937). *Consumption and production of tobacco in Europe.* USDA, Washington DC. Technical bulletin No. 587.

Hüttner H., Kopske C., Schmidt B. and Wiesner G. (1972a). Rauchgewohnheiten in Berlin (Hauptstadt der DDR) (Smoking habits in Berlin (capital of GDR)). *Deutsche Gesundheitswesen,* **27**, 2094-8.

Hüttner H., Kopske Ch., Schmidt B. and Wiesner G. (1972b). Rauchgewohnheiten in Berlin (Hauptstadt der DDR). 1 (Smoking habits in Berlin (Capital of the GDR). 1). *Deutsche Gesundheitswesen,* **27**, 1999-2003.

Institut für Markt- und Werbeforshung (IMW) (1981). *Effizienzkontrolle 1980 der Bundeszentrale für gesundheitliche Aufklärung, Köln.* IMW, Köln.

Junge B. and Nagel M. (1999). Das Rauchverhalten in Deutschland (Smoking behavior in Germany). *Gesundheitswesen,* **61**, S121-S125.

Junge B., Tiefelsdorf M. and Arab-Kohlmeier L. (1989). Tabakkonsum in der Bundesrepublik Deutschland. Strukturveränderungen in drei Jahrzehnten. *Pravention,* **2**, 35-40.

Keyl K. (1979). Rauchgewohnheiten bei Schülern eines Landkreises. (Smoking habits by pupils in a district of village schools). *Zeitschrift fur Erkrankungen der Atmungsorgane,* **153**, 209-17.

King A., Wold B., Tudor-Smith C. and Harel Y. (1996). *The health of youth, a cross-national survey.* WHO Regional Publications, Europe, Copenhagen. European Series No. 69.

Kittel W. (1944). Hygiene des Rauchens. In: Handloser S. and Hoffmann W. (eds) *Wehrhygiene.* Springer-Verlag, Berlin.[§]

Kneist W. (1981). Rauchen oder Gesundheit. Ein kulturhistorischer Rückblick (Smoking or health. A retrospective view of cultural history). *Zeitschrift fur die Gesamte Hygiene und Ihre Grenzgebiete,* **27**, 477-80.

Koschorreck B., Knopp G. and Blohmke M. (1973). Rauchgewohnheiten bei männlichen Haupt-, Real- und Oberschülern (Smoking habits among male secondary-school students). *Offentliche Gesundheitswesen,* **35**, 1-7.

Krecklow B. (1987). Rauchgewohnheiten von Kindern und Jugendlichen (Smoking habits of children and adolescents). *Z Arztl Fortbild,* **81**, 957-60.

Laaser U., Roegele F., Meurer K.A. and Kaufmann W. (1977). Die Verbreitung des Nikotinabusus bei Schülern; ein Teilergebnis der Kölner Studie zum kardiovaskulären Risikoprofil bei Jugendlichen (The spread of nicotine abuse in students; a partial account of the study in Cologne on the risk profile in adolescents). *Verhandlungen der Deutschen Gesellschaft fur Innere Medizin,* **83**, 1727-9.

Le Meitour-Kaplan A. (1977). Situational Analysis: Profile of women's smoking habits in Continental Western Europe. In: Steinfeld J., Griffiths W., Ball K. and Taylor R.M. (eds) *Health consequences, education, cessation activities, and social action, Volume II. Proceedings of the Third World Conference on Smoking and Health, New York City, June 2-5, 1975.* US Department of Health, Education and Welfare, USA; 309-27. DHEW Publication No (NIH) 77-1413.

Lee P.N. (ed) (1975). *Tobacco consumption in various countries,* 4th edition. Tobacco Research Council, London. Research Paper 6.

Letzel H.W. and Johnston L.C. (1984). The extent of passive smoking in the Federal Republic of Germany. *Prev Med,* **13**, 717-29.

Lippert P.H., Hoffmeister H., Lopez H. and Wünschmann E. (1980). Anmerkungen zu Interventionsprojekten im Jugendalter: das Beispiel Zigarettenrauchen (Problems of intervention projects involving adolescents: cigarette smoking as an example). *Bundesgesundheitsblatt,* **23**, 110-4.

Luban-Plozza B. and Knaak-Sommer L. (1972). *Psychologie des Hasch- und Tabakrauchens.* München.§

Malhotra M. (1977). Tabak bei Schülern. *Suchtgefahren,* **23**, 49-68.§

Malhotra M.K. (1978). Tabakabusus bei Jugendlichen (Tobacco abuse in adolescents). *Fortschr Med,* **96**, 32-4.

Maxwell J.C.Jr. (successive years). How the brands ranked. Maxwell International Estimates. *World Tobacco.*

Merzdorf J., Reuter U. and Welsch G. (1982). *Daten und Fakten zur Entwicklung des Rauchens in Mitgliedsländern der Europäischen Gemeinschaften (Facts and figures on the development of smoking in the member states of the European Communities).* Kommission der Europäischen Gemeinschaften, Luxemburg. Medizin—EUR 7907 DE.

Mohl H. (1979). Raucher-Report '79. Zahlen, Erfahrungen, Meinungen zum Weltgesundheitstag 1980. (Smokers Report '79. Figures, experiences, opinions on World Health Day 1980). *Deutsche Arzteblatt,* **37**, 2348-52.

MONICA East Germany Team (1993). *Das MONICA-Datenbuch Ostdeutschlands. Trends von 1984-1989.* Center for Epidemiology and Health Research, Berlin.§

Müller F.H. (1939). Tabakmißbrauch und Lungencarcinom. *Zeitschrift fur Krebsforschung,* **49**, 57-85.

Piorkowski V.P. and Piorkowski S. (1983). Rauchen in den Schulen des Kreises Cottbus-Land. *Deutsche Gesundheitswesen,* **7**, 267-9.

Preuss K. (1991). Rauchgewohnheiten bei Schülern der 5. bis 10. Klassen in Stendal (Smoking habits in students of the 5th to 10th grades in Stendal). *Z Arztl Fortbild,* **85**, 217-20.

Proctor N.R. (1996). The anti-tobacco campaign of the Nazis: a little known aspect of public health in Germany, 1933-45. *BMJ,* **313**, 1450-3.

Proctor R.N. (1997). The Nazi war on tobacco: ideology, evidence and possible cancer consequences. *Bull Hist Med,* **71**, 435-88.

Readers Digest (1963). *Products and people. A digest of the marketing survey of the European Common Market and Britain, 1963* . Reader's Digest Association Limited, London.

Reissig M. (1977). Zur Verbreitung des Rauchens unter der werktätigen Jugend der DDR und zum Rauchverhalten Leipziger Jugendlicher (Investigations on the extension of smoking among the working youth of the German Democratic Republic and on the smoking habits of Leipzig youth). *Zeitschrift fur Erkrankungen der Atmungsorgane,* **148**, 268-77.

Reissig M. (1989). Die Entwicklung des Rauchverhaltens Jugendlicher (Development of smoking behavior in adolescents). *Arztliche Jugendkunde,* **80**, 220-7.

Rothenbacher D., Brenner H., Arndt V., Fraisse E., Zschenderlein B. and Fliedner T.M. (1996). Smoking patterns and mortality attributable to smoking in a cohort of 3528 construction workers. *Eur J Epidemiol,* **12**, 335-40.

RP6, See Beese (ed) (1968), Beese (ed) (1972), Lee (ed) (1975)

Scheuermann W., Grafnetter D., Östör-Lamm E., Nüssel E. and Ganowa M. (1991). Blood thiocyanate levels and self-reported smoking habits compared in two large cardiovascular population studies. *Cor et Vasa,* **33**, 150-61.

Schlegel V. and Schulz D. (1987). Rauchgewohnheiten 12- bis 16jähriger Schüler im Kreis Hohenmölsen. 1. Mitteilung: Pravalenz an aktuellen Rauchern (Smoking habits of 12-16-year-old students in the district of Hohenmölsen. Part 1. Frequency of actual smokers). *Arztliche Jugendkunde,* **78**, 178-83.

Scholz M. and Kaltenbach M. (1995). Zigaretten-, Alkohol- und Drogenkonsum bei 12- bis 13jährigen Jugendlichen: eine anonyme Befragung bei 2979 Schülern (Cigarette, alcohol and drug use in 12 to 13-year-old adolescents: an anonymous survey of 2 979 students). *Gesundheitswesen,* **57**, 339-44.

Spiegel-Verlag (1971). *Männer und Märkte. Besitz-, Konsum- und informationsverhalten der männlichen Bundesbevölkerung.* Spiegel-Verlag, Hamburg.§

Spiegel-Verlag (1978). *Kauf-, Konsum- und Kommunikationsverhalten der Bundesbevölkerung.* Spiegel-Verlag, Hamburg.§

Statistisches Bundesamt *Befölkerung und Wirtschaft 1872-1972.* Statistisches Bundesamt, Wiesbaden.

Statistisches Bundesamt *Fragen zur Gesundheit (Questions on health).* Metzler Poeschel, Reutlingen. Fachserie 12:Gesundheitswesen. Reihe S.3.

Stern (1977). *Medien-Märkte-Konsumenten.* Markt-profil Genussmittel, Hamburg.§

Theopold W. (1972). Rauchen bei Schülern. *Hess Ärztebl,* **23**, 568-77.

Thiele H.J., Tredt H.J. and Friedemann H. (eds) (1974). *Vielfachreihenuntersuchungen—Erfahrungen und Entwicklungstendenzen* . Volk und Gesundheit, Berlin.§

Timm J. (1976). Trendanalysen zum problem des verbrauches an nikotin und rauchkondensat in der Bundesrepublik Deutschland für die Jahre 1961 bis 1975 (Trend analyses for the problem of nicotine and smoke condensate in FDR for 1961-1975). *Beitrage zur Tabakforschung,* **8**, 404-14.

Todd G. (1986). *Medicine. Statistics of smoking in the Member States of the European Community.* Commission of the European Communities, Luxembourg.

Tölle R. (1974). *Zigarettenrauchen. Zur Psychologie und Psychopathologie des Rauchers.* Springer-Verlag, Berlin.§

van Reek J. and Adriaanse H. (1995). Daily smoking among adolescents in the European Community. *Rev Epidemiol Sante Publique,* **43**, 281-2.

van Reek J., Adriaanse H. and Karaoglou A. (1992). Smoking among children in the European Community. *J Public Health Med,* **14**, 93-4.

von Harnack G.-A., Linn Ch. and Reinecke E. (1967). Über die Verbreitung des Rauchens bei Kindern und Jugendlichen. *Dtsch Med Wochenschr,* **92**, 329-34.

Weiland S.K., Stolpe S. and Keil U. (1994). Die Rauchgewohnheiten von Kindern und Jugendlichen: Eine Herausforderung für die primäre Prävention (Smoking among children and adolescents: a challenge for primary prevention). *Soz Praventivmed,* **39**, 293-8.

Werner E. (1961). Über Rauchgewohnheiten. *Deutsche Gesundheitswesen,* **16**, 2479-83.§

WHO (1989). The WHO MONICA project: a worldwide monitoring system for cardiovascular diseases. In: *World health statistics annual 1989.* WHO, Geneva; 25-149.

WHO (1975). Survey on smoking and health in the European Region, 1974-75: preliminary data as at 1 May 1975. *Presented at the Third World Conference on Smoking and Health, New York, 2-5 June 1975.* WHO; 1-55.

WHO MONICA Project (1988). Geographical variation in the major risk factors of coronary heart disease in men and women aged 35-64 years. *World Health Stat Q,* **41**, 115-40.

Wilde J., Sr., Matthäi C., Mehnert W.H., Staneczek W., Luft D. and Wilde J., Jr. (1990). Lungenkrebs in der DDR unter besonderer Berücksichtigung der histologischen Typen und des Zigarettenkonsums. (Lung cancer in the GDR with special reference to histological types and cigarette consumption). *Archiv fur Geschwulstforschung,* **60**, 25-34.

Wolff E. (1981). *Der Blutdruck in einer ländlichen Bevölkerung: Mehrzeitiges Screening einer ländlichen Population* [Thesis]. University, Greifswald.[§]

Wuthe H., Petro W., Müller E., Pohl S. and Vogel J. (1977). Rauchen im Kindesalter—Ergebnisse einer Schuluntersuchung in Berlin-Karow 1976 (Smoking in the childhood—results of the school study Berlin-Karow 1976). *Zeitschrift fur Erkrankungen der Atmungsorgane,* **148**, 25-34.

Zuber L. and Zuber R. (1973). Rauchgewohnheiten bei Schülern der Klassen 5-12 der erweiterten Oberschule, der polytechnischen Oberschule, der Berufsschule under der Sonderschule der Kreisstadt Zeulenroda (Ostthüringen). *Z Arztl Fortbild,* **67**, 1267-73.

§ Original paper not obtained, but information taken as quoted by another author

Greece 11

Sales data

See Tables 11.1.3-11.2.

From 1920 until the Second World War, the consumption of manufactured cigarettes per adult decreased from 4 cigarettes per day to about 3 cigarettes. During the Second World War there was a dip in the consumption of manufactured cigarettes. Thereafter consumption rose steadily until 1986 when it reached nearly 10 manufactured cigarettes per day. Recent trends are unclear, as imported cigarettes became more popular but were not included in the data until 1994. The consumption of all tobacco products combined followed a similar trend, merely reflecting changes in the estimated average weight of manufactured cigarettes, as the consumption of forms of tobacco other than manufactured cigarettes was negligible. (Tables 11.1.1 and 11.3 on consumption of different tobacco products are not provided.) The proportion of cigarettes that were filtered rose rapidly from zero in 1956 to 90% about 1980.

Survey data

See Tables 11.4-11.8

Very few surveys are available on the smoking situation in Greece, and many of the early sources included here are the control populations of hospital case-control studies; these generally use non-standard definitions of 'a smoker' and the subjects are not representative of the general population. The Eurobarometer survey (source 19) provides data on a consistent basis from 1988.

Estimates of the prevalence of cigarette smoking up to 1985 varied between 40-67% among men aged 15 years and over and between 10-17% among women. Eurobarometer results showed a decrease from over 60% to under 50% for men between 1988 and 1994, while the prevalence among women varied around 24-28%. Few age-specific data are available. At all ages more men than women are reported to smoke, except for a few surveys among teenagers. Most surveys show a lower prevalence of smoking in older age groups, more marked among women than among men. However, this is not seen in two early hospital-based studies for men (sources 6, 7), nor in a recent study (source 29) for women.

Comparison of survey and sales data was only possible in one case, where consumption was under-reported by about 25%. In 1975, the estimated number of cigarettes smoked per person per day (sales-adjusted) was 13 for men and 2 for women. By the mid-1980s, this had increased to 16 and 4 respectively. By 1995 the estimated number had decreased to about 12 for men and increased to about 6 for women, although later estimates may be distorted by problems with the sales data (see above).

Table 11.1.3 Manufactured cigarettes, percentage of total sales as filter cigarettes, 1961-1982

Year	% Filter
1956	0
1961	4.3
1962	5.7
1963	9.4
1964	15.2
1965	17.8
1966	27.6
1967	36.8
1968	51.9
1969	53.7
1970	56.3
1971	70.4
1972	75.2
1973	79.5
1974	82.0
1975	84.5
1976	86.9
1977	88.6
1978	89.5
1979	90.6
1980	91.5
1981	92.0
1982	92.0

Source : see *Notes on sources of sales data*, p. 290

Table 11.2 Consumption of (i) cigarettes and (ii) all tobacco products, 1920-1995 sales-based data, including estimated hand-rolled cigarette consumption. Males and females aged 15 years and over

Year	Manufactured cigarettes		Hand-rolled cigarettes		Total cigarettes		All tobacco products	
	Total annual in millions	Number/ adult/day	Total annual in millions	Number/ adult/day	Total annual in millions	Number/ adult/day	Total annual in tonnes	Grams/ adult/day
1920	3937	3.3					4490	3.7
1921	5203	4.3					5900	4.9
1922	5439	4.4					6170	5.0
1923	4725	3.5					5350	4.0
1924	4663	3.3					5310	3.7
1925	5323	3.6					6030	4.1
1926	4310	3.0					4900	3.4
1927	4221	2.8					4810	3.2
1928	4115	2.7					4670	3.0
1929	4234	2.7					4810	3.1
1930	4123	2.6					4670	3.0
1931	4048	2.6					4580	2.9
1932	3796	2.4					4310	2.7
1933	4049	2.5					4580	2.8
1934	4256	2.6					4850	3.0
1935	4434	2.6					5030	3.0
1936	4625	2.8					5260	3.1
1937	4655	2.7					5310	3.1
1938	5076	3.0					5760	3.4
1939	5179	3.0					5900	3.4
1940	5490	3.1					6260	3.5
1941	4734	2.6					5400	3.0
1942	4964	2.7					5620	3.1
1943	4197	2.3					4760	2.6
1944	2345	1.3					2680	1.5
1945	4248	2.3					4810	2.6
1946	6136	3.3					6990	3.8
1947	7447	3.9					8480	4.5
1948	7841	4.0					8890	4.5
1949	8447	4.4					9620	5.0
1950	8656	4.4					9840	5.0
1951	8607	4.3					9800	4.9
1952	8595	4.2					9750	4.8
1953	8871	4.3					10070	4.8
1954	8964	4.2					10210	4.8
1955	9187	4.3					10430	4.9
1956	9206	4.3					10480	4.8
1957	9578	4.4					10890	5.0
1958	10074	4.6					11430	5.2
1959	10335	4.7					11750	5.3
1960	10563	4.7					12020	5.4
1961	10820	4.8					12290	5.4
1962	11135	4.9					12660	5.5
1963	11719	5.1					13290	5.8
1964	11894	5.1					13520	5.9
1965	12328	5.3					14110	6.1
1966	13073	5.6					14830	6.3
1967	13644	5.7					15470	6.5
1968	14066	5.9					15970	6.6
1969	14432	6.0					16370	6.8

Table 11.2 *(continued)*

Year	Manufactured cigarettes		Hand-rolled cigarettes		Total cigarettes		All tobacco products	
	Total annual in millions	Number/ adult/day	Total annual in millions	Number/ adult/day	Total annual in millions	Number/ adult/day	Total annual in tonnes	Grams/ adult/day
1970	15144	6.3					17190	7.1
1971	15300	6.4					17330	7.2
1972	16250	6.6					18280	7.5
1973	17360	7.0					19550	7.9
1974	18198	7.3					20679	8.3
1975	18889	7.5					21465	8.5
1976	20052	7.9					22786	8.9
1977	20935	8.1					23790	9.2
1978	21949	8.4					24942	9.5
1979	21923	8.3					24912	9.4
1980	21903	8.1					24889	9.2
1981	19673	7.1					22356	8.1
1982	24095	8.6					24095	8.6
1983	25336	9.0					25336	9.0
1984	27019	9.5					27019	9.5
1985	27757	9.7					27757	9.7
1986	28523	9.9					28523	9.9
1987	27825	9.6					27825	9.6
1988	26536	9.1					26536	9.1
1989	25744	8.7					25744	8.7
1990	24856	8.3					24856	8.3
1991	24425	8.0					24425	8.0
1992	21869	7.1					21869	7.1
1993	20807	6.7					20807	6.7
1994	29354	9.3					29354	9.3
1995	28079	8.8					28079	8.8

Source : see *Notes on sources of sales data*, p. 290

Figure 11.1 Daily consumption of (i) manufactured cigarettes, and (ii) all tobacco products, 1920-1995
Males and females aged 15 years and over. *Source:* see Table 11.2

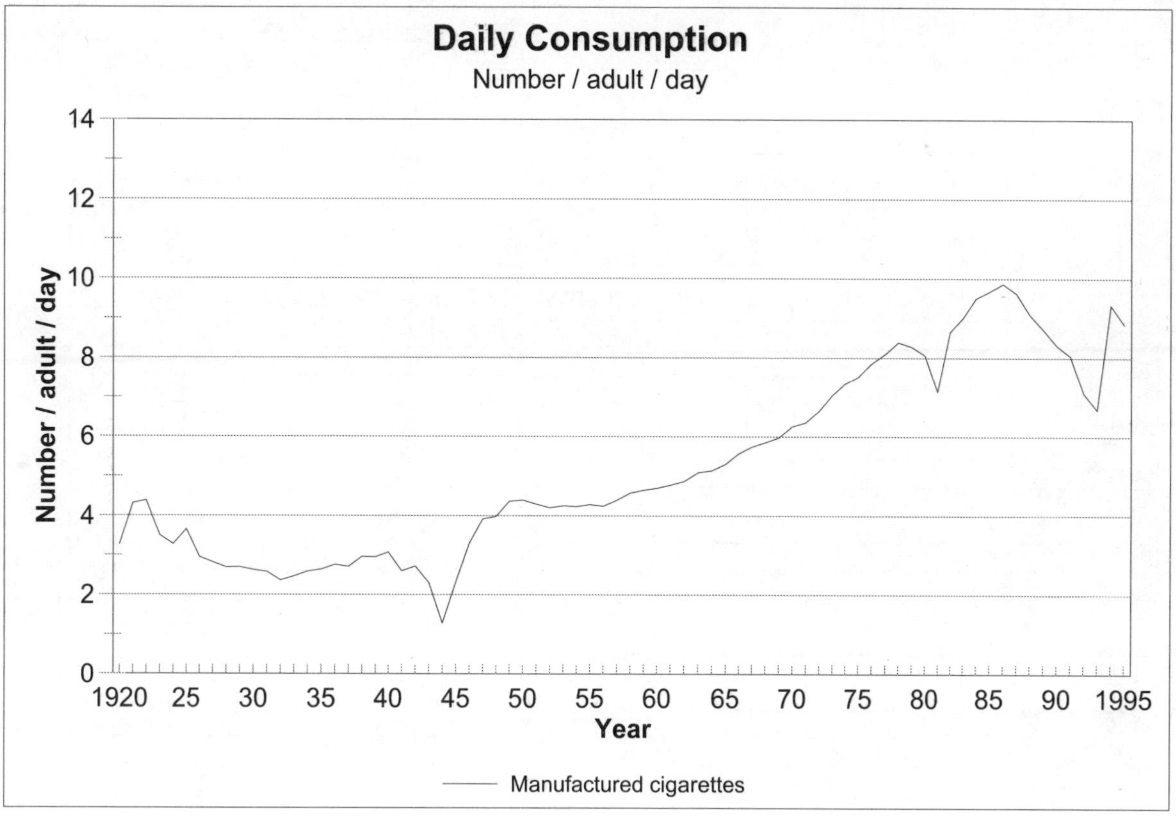

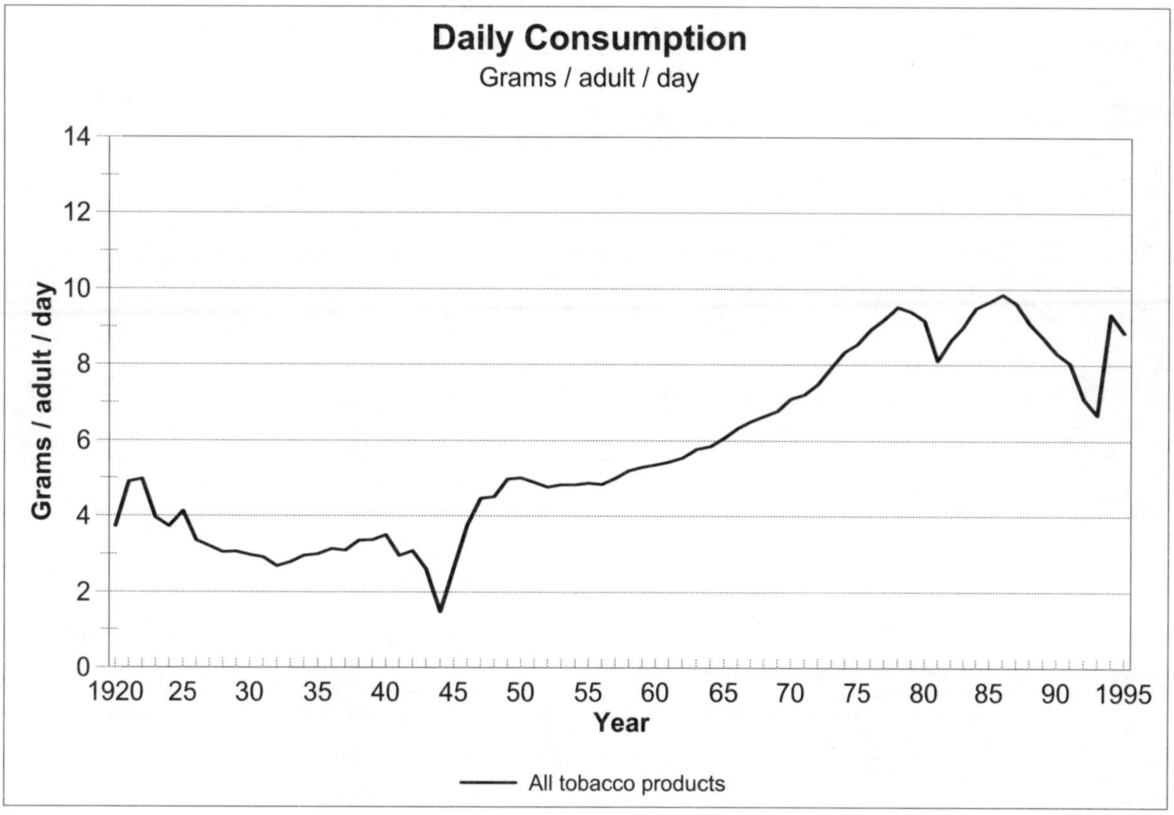

Table 11.4M Prevalence of smoking, males: some selected Greek surveys by age, 1956-1995

<table>
<tr><th rowspan="2">Frequency
Product
Source
Year</th><th colspan="21">Age group</th><th rowspan="2">All ages</th></tr>
<tr><th>12</th><th>13</th><th>14</th><th>15</th><th>16</th><th>17</th><th>18</th><th>19</th><th>20-24</th><th>25-29</th><th>30-34</th><th>35-39</th><th>40-44</th><th>45-49</th><th>50-54</th><th>55-59</th><th>60-64</th><th>65-69</th><th>70-74</th><th>75-79</th><th>80+</th></tr>
<tr><td>56 6*UC R</td><td colspan="8"></td><td colspan="2">61</td><td colspan="2">71</td><td colspan="2">73</td><td colspan="2">75</td><td colspan="2">78</td><td colspan="2">68</td><td>40</td><td></td></tr>
<tr><td>60 9 UC R</td><td colspan="12"></td><td>62</td><td>56</td><td>56</td><td>55</td><td colspan="5"></td><td>57</td></tr>
<tr><td>61 10 UC R</td><td colspan="12"></td><td>66</td><td>60</td><td>66</td><td>61</td><td colspan="5"></td><td>64</td></tr>
<tr><td>68 7 UC *</td><td colspan="10"></td><td colspan="2">70</td><td colspan="2">69</td><td colspan="2">68</td><td colspan="2">58</td><td colspan="2">81</td><td>70</td><td></td></tr>
<tr><td>75 1 MC U</td><td colspan="3"></td><td colspan="18">50</td><td></td></tr>
<tr><td>78 8 U R</td><td colspan="3"></td><td colspan="4">29</td><td colspan="14"></td><td></td></tr>
<tr><td>80 4 A R</td><td colspan="8"></td><td>73</td><td>65</td><td colspan="11"></td><td>71</td></tr>
<tr><td>80 31 U U</td><td colspan="21"></td><td></td></tr>
<tr><td>81 3 A R</td><td colspan="13"></td><td colspan="3">74</td><td colspan="2">61</td><td colspan="3">40</td><td></td></tr>
<tr><td>81 15 UC *</td><td colspan="6"></td><td colspan="2">12</td><td>41</td><td>58</td><td>59</td><td>55</td><td>60</td><td>49</td><td>43</td><td>37</td><td>34</td><td>30</td><td>19</td><td colspan="2">13</td><td>44</td></tr>
<tr><td>82 33 U U</td><td colspan="12"></td><td>75</td><td>74</td><td>73</td><td>74</td><td colspan="5"></td><td>74</td></tr>
<tr><td>83 2 MC U</td><td colspan="3"></td><td colspan="18">67</td><td></td></tr>
<tr><td>84 5 MC *</td><td colspan="3"></td><td>65</td><td colspan="2"></td><td>79</td><td colspan="14"></td><td></td></tr>
<tr><td>84 11 UC R</td><td></td><td colspan="6">26</td><td colspan="14"></td><td></td></tr>
<tr><td>84 12 UC R</td><td></td><td colspan="6">24</td><td colspan="14"></td><td></td></tr>
<tr><td>84 13 U R</td><td colspan="21"></td><td></td></tr>
<tr><td>84 14 U U</td><td colspan="3"></td><td colspan="18">41</td><td></td></tr>
<tr><td>84 30 U R</td><td colspan="6"></td><td colspan="3">52</td><td colspan="2"></td><td colspan="6">56</td><td colspan="4"></td><td>54</td></tr>
<tr><td>85 16 U U</td><td colspan="3"></td><td colspan="18">54</td><td></td></tr>
<tr><td>87 17 U U</td><td colspan="6"></td><td>49</td><td colspan="14"></td><td></td></tr>
<tr><td>87 18 U U</td><td colspan="21"></td><td></td></tr>
<tr><td>87 19 U U</td><td colspan="3"></td><td colspan="18">61</td><td></td></tr>
<tr><td>88 12 UC R</td><td></td><td colspan="6">20</td><td colspan="14"></td><td></td></tr>
<tr><td>88 18 U U</td><td colspan="21"></td><td></td></tr>
<tr><td>88 19 U U</td><td colspan="3"></td><td colspan="18">62</td><td></td></tr>
<tr><td>88 20 UC U</td><td colspan="21"></td><td></td></tr>
<tr><td>88 21 U U</td><td colspan="2"></td><td colspan="3">37</td><td colspan="16"></td><td></td></tr>
<tr><td>88 32 U U</td><td colspan="9"></td><td colspan="8">49</td><td colspan="4"></td><td></td></tr>
<tr><td>89 18 U U</td><td colspan="21"></td><td></td></tr>
<tr><td>89 19 U U</td><td colspan="3"></td><td colspan="18">60</td><td></td></tr>
<tr><td>89 34 UC R</td><td colspan="3"></td><td colspan="10">61</td><td colspan="4">44</td><td colspan="3">13</td><td></td><td></td></tr>
<tr><td>90 18 U U</td><td colspan="21"></td><td></td></tr>
<tr><td>90 19 U U</td><td colspan="3"></td><td colspan="18">54</td><td></td></tr>
<tr><td>90 22 U R</td><td colspan="2"></td><td>3</td><td>6</td><td colspan="17"></td><td></td></tr>
<tr><td>90 22 U A</td><td>0</td><td colspan="3">7</td><td colspan="17"></td><td></td></tr>
<tr><td>90 23 U U</td><td colspan="9"></td><td colspan="3">70</td><td colspan="9"></td><td></td></tr>
<tr><td>91 18 U U</td><td colspan="21"></td><td></td></tr>
<tr><td>91 19 U U</td><td colspan="3"></td><td colspan="18">53</td><td></td></tr>
<tr><td>92 19 U U</td><td colspan="3"></td><td colspan="18">57</td><td></td></tr>
<tr><td>93 23 U U</td><td colspan="21"></td><td></td></tr>
<tr><td>93 24 UC R</td><td colspan="3"></td><td colspan="2">15</td><td colspan="16"></td><td></td></tr>
<tr><td>93 24 UC A</td><td colspan="3"></td><td colspan="2">23</td><td colspan="16"></td><td></td></tr>
<tr><td>94 19 U U</td><td colspan="3"></td><td colspan="18">46</td><td></td></tr>
<tr><td>94 25 U R</td><td colspan="6"></td><td colspan="3">30</td><td colspan="5">50</td><td colspan="7"></td><td></td></tr>
<tr><td>94 25 U A</td><td colspan="6"></td><td colspan="3">44</td><td colspan="5">54</td><td colspan="7"></td><td></td></tr>
<tr><td>94 26 U R</td><td colspan="3"></td><td>49</td><td colspan="17"></td><td></td></tr>
<tr><td>95 27 UC R</td><td colspan="21"></td><td></td></tr>
<tr><td>95 28 U U</td><td colspan="5"></td><td colspan="5">47</td><td colspan="11"></td><td></td></tr>
<tr><td>95 29 U U</td><td colspan="3"></td><td colspan="6">45</td><td colspan="7">50</td><td colspan="5">44</td><td></td></tr>
</table>

Source: see *Notes on sources of survey data*, p. 291
Product: MC = manufactured cigarettes
TC = total cigarettes (including hand-rolled)
UC = cigarettes (type unspecified)
A = all products

Frequency: A = all smokers (including occasional)
R = regular or daily smokers
All ages: relevant to ages used and as given in original source
U = unspecified
* = refer to *Notes on sources of survey data*, p. 291

Table 11.4F Prevalence of smoking, females: some selected Greek surveys by age, 1956-1995

<table>
<tr><th rowspan="2">Frequency
Product
Source
Year</th><th colspan="21">Age group</th><th rowspan="2">All ages</th></tr>
<tr><th>12</th><th>13</th><th>14</th><th>15</th><th>16</th><th>17</th><th>18</th><th>19</th><th>20-24</th><th>25-29</th><th>30-34</th><th>35-39</th><th>40-44</th><th>45-49</th><th>50-54</th><th>55-59</th><th>60-64</th><th>65-69</th><th>70-74</th><th>75-79</th><th>80+</th></tr>
<tr><td>56 6 UC R</td><td colspan="21"></td><td></td></tr>
<tr><td>60 9 UC R</td><td colspan="21"></td><td></td></tr>
<tr><td>61 10 UC R</td><td colspan="21"></td><td></td></tr>
<tr><td>68 7 UC *</td><td colspan="10"></td><td colspan="2">20</td><td colspan="2">10</td><td colspan="2">6</td><td colspan="2">0</td><td colspan="2">0</td><td>0</td><td></td></tr>
<tr><td>75 1 MC U</td><td colspan="3"></td><td colspan="18">10</td><td></td></tr>
<tr><td>78 8 U R</td><td colspan="3"></td><td colspan="4">34</td><td colspan="14"></td><td></td></tr>
<tr><td>80 4 A R</td><td colspan="21"></td><td></td></tr>
<tr><td>80 31 U U</td><td colspan="10"></td><td colspan="11">13</td><td></td></tr>
<tr><td>81 3 A R</td><td colspan="13"></td><td colspan="3">0</td><td colspan="2">5</td><td colspan="3">4</td><td></td></tr>
<tr><td>81 15 UC *</td><td colspan="6"></td><td colspan="2">10</td><td>25</td><td>25</td><td>20</td><td>23</td><td>20</td><td>12</td><td>16</td><td>12</td><td>12</td><td>7</td><td>3</td><td colspan="2">9</td><td>17</td></tr>
<tr><td>82 33 U U</td><td colspan="21"></td><td></td></tr>
<tr><td>83 2 MC U</td><td colspan="3"></td><td colspan="18">28</td><td></td></tr>
<tr><td>84 5 MC *</td><td colspan="3"></td><td>50</td><td colspan="2"></td><td>82</td><td colspan="14"></td><td></td></tr>
<tr><td>84 11 UC R</td><td></td><td colspan="6">19</td><td colspan="14"></td><td></td></tr>
<tr><td>84 12 UC R</td><td></td><td colspan="6">22</td><td colspan="14"></td><td></td></tr>
<tr><td>84 13 U R</td><td colspan="12"></td><td colspan="9">12</td><td></td></tr>
<tr><td>84 14 U U</td><td colspan="3"></td><td colspan="18">12</td><td></td></tr>
<tr><td>84 30 U R</td><td colspan="6"></td><td colspan="3">28</td><td colspan="2"></td><td colspan="6">14</td><td colspan="4"></td><td>20</td></tr>
<tr><td>85 16 U U</td><td colspan="3"></td><td colspan="18">13</td><td></td></tr>
<tr><td>87 17 U U</td><td colspan="6"></td><td>36</td><td colspan="14"></td><td></td></tr>
<tr><td>87 18 U U</td><td colspan="3"></td><td colspan="18">25</td><td></td></tr>
<tr><td>87 19 U U</td><td colspan="3"></td><td colspan="18">25</td><td></td></tr>
<tr><td>88 12 UC R</td><td></td><td colspan="6">21</td><td colspan="14"></td><td></td></tr>
<tr><td>88 18 U U</td><td colspan="3"></td><td colspan="18">26</td><td></td></tr>
<tr><td>88 19 U U</td><td colspan="3"></td><td colspan="18">24</td><td></td></tr>
<tr><td>88 20 UC U</td><td colspan="3"></td><td colspan="18">26</td><td></td></tr>
<tr><td>88 21 U U</td><td colspan="2"></td><td colspan="3">13</td><td colspan="16"></td><td></td></tr>
<tr><td>88 32 U U</td><td colspan="8"></td><td colspan="8">39</td><td colspan="5"></td><td></td></tr>
<tr><td>89 18 U U</td><td colspan="3"></td><td colspan="18">29</td><td></td></tr>
<tr><td>89 19 U U</td><td colspan="3"></td><td colspan="18">27</td><td></td></tr>
<tr><td>89 34 UC R</td><td colspan="3"></td><td colspan="10">28</td><td colspan="4">2</td><td colspan="3">0</td><td></td><td></td></tr>
<tr><td>90 18 U U</td><td colspan="3"></td><td colspan="18">25</td><td></td></tr>
<tr><td>90 19 U U</td><td colspan="3"></td><td colspan="18">26</td><td></td></tr>
<tr><td>90 22 U R</td><td colspan="2"></td><td>1</td><td>2</td><td colspan="17"></td><td></td></tr>
<tr><td>90 22 U A</td><td>0</td><td colspan="3">4</td><td colspan="17"></td><td></td></tr>
<tr><td>90 23 U U</td><td colspan="9"></td><td colspan="3">40</td><td colspan="9"></td><td></td></tr>
<tr><td>91 18 U U</td><td colspan="6"></td><td colspan="15">27</td><td></td></tr>
<tr><td>91 19 U U</td><td colspan="3"></td><td colspan="18">26</td><td></td></tr>
<tr><td>92 19 U U</td><td colspan="3"></td><td colspan="18">24</td><td></td></tr>
<tr><td>93 23 U U</td><td colspan="9"></td><td colspan="7">56</td><td colspan="5"></td><td></td></tr>
<tr><td>93 24 UC R</td><td colspan="3"></td><td colspan="2">14</td><td colspan="16"></td><td></td></tr>
<tr><td>93 24 UC A</td><td colspan="3"></td><td colspan="2">24</td><td colspan="16"></td><td></td></tr>
<tr><td>94 19 U U</td><td colspan="3"></td><td colspan="18">28</td><td></td></tr>
<tr><td>94 25 U R</td><td colspan="6"></td><td colspan="3">19</td><td colspan="5">36</td><td colspan="7"></td><td></td></tr>
<tr><td>94 25 U A</td><td colspan="6"></td><td colspan="3">29</td><td colspan="5">43</td><td colspan="7"></td><td></td></tr>
<tr><td>94 26 U R</td><td colspan="3"></td><td>46</td><td colspan="17"></td><td></td></tr>
<tr><td>95 27 UC R</td><td colspan="4"></td><td>12</td><td>10</td><td>27</td><td colspan="14"></td><td>13</td></tr>
<tr><td>95 28 U U</td><td colspan="21"></td><td></td></tr>
<tr><td>95 29 U U</td><td colspan="3"></td><td colspan="6">28</td><td colspan="7">35</td><td colspan="5">30</td><td></td></tr>
</table>

Source: see *Notes on sources of survey data*, p. 291
Product: MC = manufactured cigarettes
TC = total cigarettes (including hand-rolled)
UC = cigarettes (type unspecified)
A = all products

Frequency: A = all smokers (including occasional)
R = regular or daily smokers
All ages: relevant to ages used and as given in original source
U = unspecified
* = refer to *Notes on sources of survey data*, p. 291

Table 11.5M Number of cigarettes smoked per smoker per day, males: some selected Greek surveys by age, 1956-1993

Product Source Year	12	13	14	15	16	17	18	19	20-24	25-29	30-34	35-39	40-44	45-49	50-54	55-59	60-64	65-69	70-74	75-79	80+	All ages
56 6 UCE*									12		11		13		14		13		13		9.7	
60 9 UCE													19	19	18	18						18
61 10 UCE													15	15	16	17						16
80 4 UCE									21													
80 31 UCE																						
81 3 UCE															20		22			17		
84 30 UCE									22													
88 32 UC													26									
93 24 UCE				14																		

Table 11.6M Number of cigarettes smoked per person per day, males: some selected Greek surveys by age, 1956-1993, with percentage total sales

Product Source Year	12	13	14	15	16	17	18	19	20-24	25-29	30-34	35-39	40-44	45-49	50-54	55-59	60-64	65-69	70-74	75-79	80+	All ages	% Total sales
56 6 UC *									7.4		8.0		9.3		10		9.8		8.5		3.9		**
60 9 UC													12	10	10	9.8						10	**
61 10 UC													10	8.7	11	10						9.9	**
80 4 UC									15														**
80 31 UC																							**
81 3 UC															15		13			6.6			**
84 30 UC									12														74%m
88 32 UC													13										**
93 24 UC				2.0																			**

Table 11.7M Number of cigarettes smoked per person per day, sales-adjusted, males: selected Greek survey[1] by age, 1984, with percentage total sales

Product Source Year	12	13	14	15	16	17	18	19	20-24	25-29	30-34	35-39	40-44	45-49	50-54	55-59	60-64	65-69	70-74	75-79	80+	All ages	% Total sales
84 30 UC									16														74%m

1 Based on those surveys in Table 11.6 with data for both sexes and age range at least 21-64 (see *Cigarette consumption per person*, p. xxxv)

Source: see *Notes on sources of survey data*, p. 291
All ages: relevant to ages used and as given in original source
% Total sales: estimated % of total sales of M = manufactured or T = total cigarette consumption implied by survey, sexes combined, used as adjustment factor in Table 11.7
** = cannot be calculated
--- = adjusted by original author
* = refer to *Notes on sources of survey data*, p. 291

Product: MC = manufactured cigarettes
TC = total cigarettes (including hand-rolled)
UC = cigarettes (type unspecified)
A = all products
U = unspecified
E indicates mean estimated from percentage distribution (see also *Consumption category estimation*, p. xxxiv, and Appendix III, p. 789)

Table 11.5F Number of cigarettes smoked per smoker per day, females: some selected Greek surveys by age, 1956-1993

Product Source Year	Age group																					
	12	13	14	15	16	17	18	19	20-24	25-29	30-34	35-39	40-44	45-49	50-54	55-59	60-64	65-69	70-74	75-79	80+	All ages
56 6 UCE																						
60 9 UCE																						
61 10 UCE																						
80 4 UCE																						
80 31 UCE*											15											
81 3 UCE																						
84 30 UCE	13																					
88 32 UC									13													
93 24 UCE				8.8																		

Table 11.6F Number of cigarettes smoked per person per day, females: some selected Greek surveys by age, 1956-1993, with percentage total sales

Product Source Year	Age group																						
	12	13	14	15	16	17	18	19	20-24	25-29	30-34	35-39	40-44	45-49	50-54	55-59	60-64	65-69	70-74	75-79	80+	All ages	% Total sales
56 6 UC																							**
60 9 UC																							**
61 10 UC																							**
80 4 UC																							**
80 31 UC *											2.0												**
81 3 UC																							**
84 30 UC	2.5																						74%m
88 32 UC									5.1														**
93 24 UC				1.2																			**

Table 11.7F Number of cigarettes smoked per person per day, sales-adjusted, females: selected Greek survey[1] by age, 1984, with percentage total sales

Product Source Year	Age group																						
	12	13	14	15	16	17	18	19	20-24	25-29	30-34	35-39	40-44	45-49	50-54	55-59	60-64	65-69	70-74	75-79	80+	All ages	% Total sales
84 30 UC	3.3																						74%m

1 Based on those surveys in Table 11.6 with data for both sexes and age range at least 21-64 (see *Cigarette consumption per person*, p. xxxv)

Source: see *Notes on sources of survey data*, p. 291
All ages: relevant to ages used and as given in original source
% Total sales: estimated % of total sales of M = manufactured or T = total cigarette consumption implied by survey, sexes combined, used as adjustment factor in Table 11.7
** = cannot be calculated
--- = adjusted by original author
* = refer to *Notes on sources of survey data*, p. 291

Product: MC = manufactured cigarettes
TC = total cigarettes (including hand-rolled)
UC = cigarettes (type unspecified)
A = all products
U = unspecified
E indicates mean estimated from percentage distribution (see also *Consumption category estimation*, p. xxxiv, and Appendix III, p. 789)

Table 11.8 Estimated[1] prevalence of smoking and estimated[1] number of cigarettes per person per day (unadjusted and sales-adjusted): summary of Tables 11.4, 11.6 and 11.7, 1956-1995.
Males and females aged 15 years and over

Year	Source[2]	Product[3]	Prevalence[4]						Number of cigarettes						
									Unadjusted[7]			Sales-adjusted[8]			
			Manufactured cigarettes[5,6]		Total cigarettes		All products		Number/ person/day		Total sales %	Manufactured cigarettes[9] number/ person/day		Total cigarettes number/ person/day	
			M	F	M	F	M	F	M	F		M	F	M	F
1956	6	UC	64						8.1						
1975	1	*MC*	50	10								(13.3	2.1)		
1981	15	UC	40	15											
1983	2	*MC*	67	28								(13.7	4.6)		
1984	14	*U*	41	12								(15.7	3.7)		
	30	UC+U	50	17					12.0	2.3	74	16.2	3.2		
1985	16	*U*	54	13								(16.6	3.2)		
1987	18	*U*		25											
	19	*U*	61	25								(14.7	4.8)		
1988	18	*U*		25											
	19	*U*	62	24								(14.1	4.4)		
	20	*UC*		26											
1989	18	*U*		28											
	19	*U*	60	27								(13.0	4.7)		
	34	UC	48	15											
1990	18	*U*		24											
	19	*U*	54	26								(12.1	4.7)		
1991	18	*U*		27											
	19	*U*	53	26								(11.7	4.6)		
1992	19	*U*	57	24								(10.8	3.6)		
1994	19	*U*	46	28								(12.6	6.2)		
1995	29	*U*	48	32								(11.5	6.3)		

1 Surveys covering an age range of at least 21-64 are included. Any gaps in the data for ages 15-20 and 65 years and over are filled in by assumed extensions to the age distribution, given in *Notes on sources of survey data*, p. 291. Method: see *Summary of adult smoking*, p. xxxvi
2 See *Notes on sources of survey data*, p. 291
3 Product: MC = manufactured cigarettes, TC = total cigarettes (including hand-rolled), UC = cigarettes (type unspecified), A = all products, U = unspecified. Frequency of smoking is indicated by: regular or daily smokers in normal type, all smokers (including occasional) in bold, unspecified in italics
4 From Table 11.4
5 This column includes prevalence of smoking classified as UC = cigarettes (type unspecified)
6 This column includes prevalence of smoking classified as U = unspecified product
7 From Table 11.6
8 From Table 11.7, except data in parentheses, which are derived from the prevalence of smoking from Table 11.4 as described in *Summary of adult smoking*, p. xxxvi
9 Number of cigarettes classified as UC = cigarettes (type unspecified) or U = product unspecified has been adjusted to manufactured cigarette sales and included in this column

Figure 11.3 Estimated prevalence of smoking: by year of survey, 1956-1995.
Males and females aged 15 years and over. *Source:* see Table 11.8

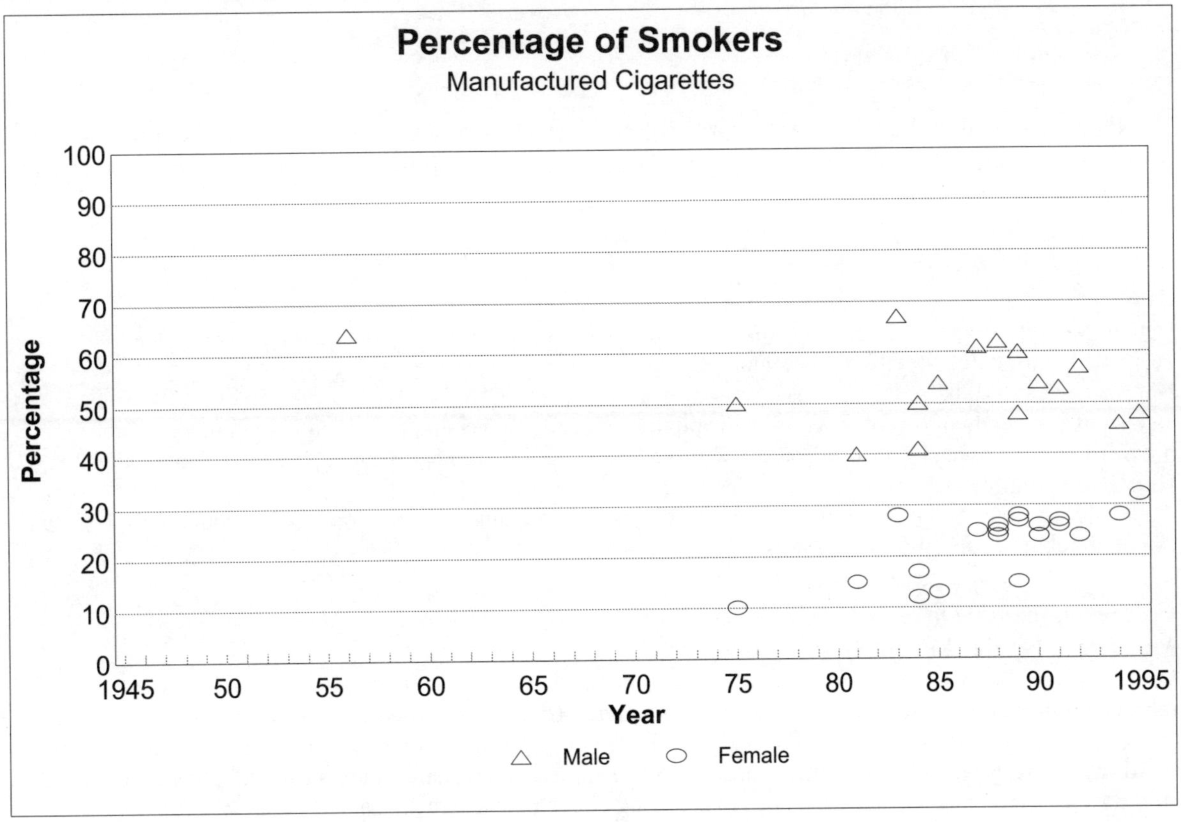

Figure 11.4 Estimated number of cigarettes smoked per person per day, sales-adjusted, 1975-1995.
Males and females aged 15 years and over. *Source:* see Table 11.8

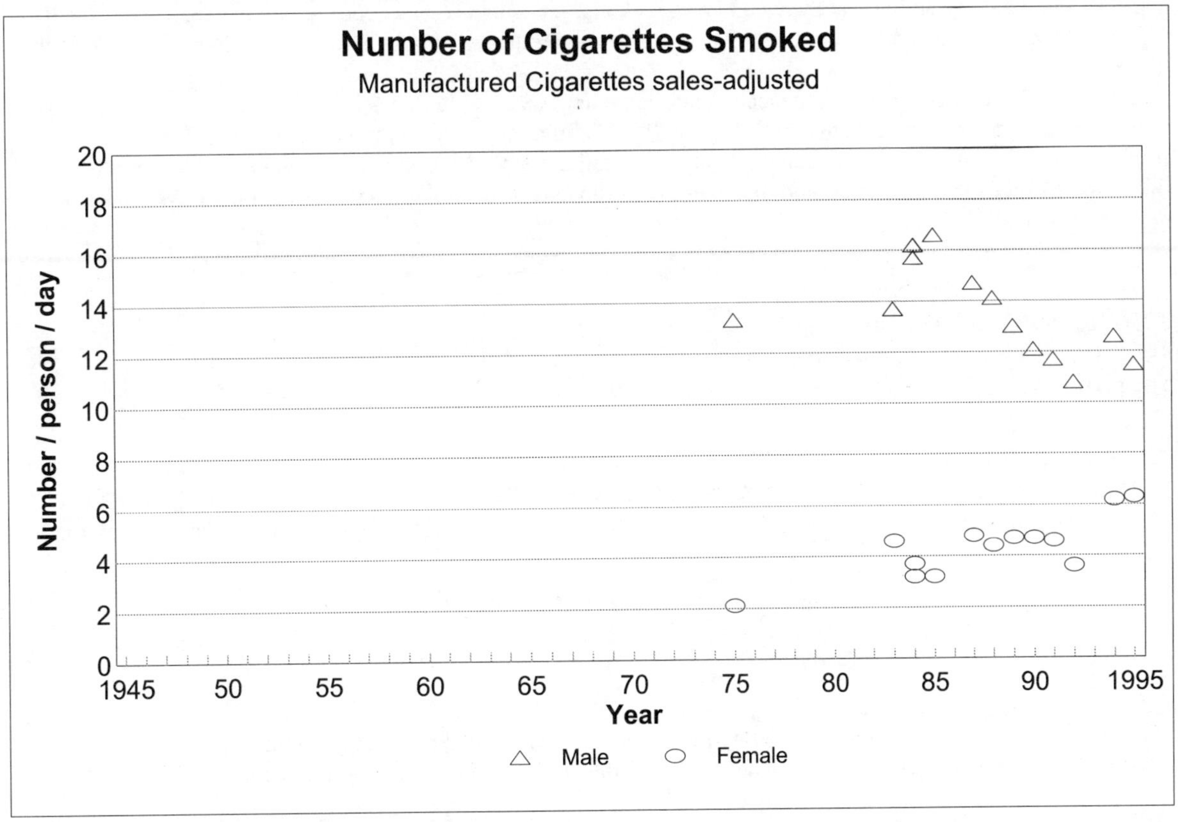

Notes on sources of sales data

The data presented in the tables and figures were obtained from several sources, details of which are given below, together with estimations and related assumptions. Full citations of the sources are given on p. 295 under *References*.

Consumption data before 1974

RP6

Data by weight, originally given to nearest 100 000 pounds, have been converted to tonnes and given to the nearest 10 tonnes (100 000 lbs = 45.359 tonnes).

Notes as given in RP6:

Details of the weight of cigarettes consumed and the factor for conversion from weight to numbers were provided by the National Tobacco Board of Greece. Consumption of other manufactured tobacco goods in Greece is negligible.

Data given by Hutson (1937) show that cigars and smoking mixtures combined accounted for less than 2% of all tobacco consumption in 1926.

Consumption data for 1974 onwards

Ministry of National Economy

Data are given for consumption of manufactured cigarettes only. The weight of cigarettes and the weight of all tobacco products are taken to be the same, as shown under *All tobacco products* in Table 11.2.

Data on imports are included for 1994 and 1995 only (for those years imports were 9 322 million and 9 701 million respectively). The data for previous years represent domestic cigarettes only. Polychronidis (1995) suggests that preference for imported cigarettes among Greek people had arisen in the previous few years only. Thassitis (1983) states that imports of cigarettes were only 1.122 million in 1981 and 1.590 million in 1982.

According to Anonymous (1993), trade sources believed cheap untaxed cigarettes to be coming into Greece from neighbouring Balkan states, in amounts thought to represent between 6% and 7% of the total volume of cigarette sales during 1991-1992.

Data are given for manufactured cigarettes in both weight and numbers, implying a conversion rate of 1.136 g per cigarette until 1981 and 1 g per cigarette thereafter. Thassitis (1983) quotes the Association of Greek Tobacco Industries as saying that the weight of Greek cigarettes had recently reduced by between 20% and 30%. This would suggest a conversion rate of 0.9 or 0.8 g per cigarette, and would give lower estimates of weight than those shown.

Consumption of forms of tobacco other than manufactured cigarettes is negligible. In 1982 cigars and pipe tobacco consumption amounted to 0.1% and 0.2% of cigarette consumption respectively (Thassitis (1983)). Ioannidis and Aravanis (1984) state that a relatively small amount of tobacco is consumed by rural producers in the form of hand rolled cigarettes, and that cigar, cigarillo and pipe smoking represented only 0.28% of total consumption in 1979.

Plain/Filter cigarette consumption

1956 Ioannidis and Aravanis (1984)

1961-1980 Maxwell (successive years)

1981-1982 Thassitis (1983)

Tar yield of cigarettes

Belgian Association for Smoking Prevention (1989) quotes the Drama Tobacco Institute as saying there was a 40% reduction in tar yield in 1983 compared with 1977. They give the share of the market by tar level in 1983 as follows:

Tar range	No of brands	Market share (%)
< 12 mg	7	24
12-15 mg	6	21
> 15 mg	16	55

Greece has been granted a temporary derogation in relation to the EC directive on maximum tar yields. This allows the 12 mg limit on tar yield to be delayed until the end of 2006, with intermediate limits of 20 mg by

December 1992, 18 mg by December 1993 and 15 mg by December 2000 (Joossens *et al* (1994)).

Estimates of hand-rolled cigarette consumption
As consumption of hand-rolled cigarettes is negligible, they have been ignored in all calculations

Notes on sources of survey data

Each source of survey data—either an individual survey or a series of surveys repeated over a number of years—is cited by a source number. This number is shown in the tables and corresponds to the source numbers given below, where details of the source publication and of the survey methodology are given. Full citations of the sources are given on p. 295 under *References*.

Source number

1 **Kalapothaki *et al* (1977)**
   a. Based on data compiled from seven studies covering various segments of Greek population, where the prevalence of smoking was:

	Urban	Semi-urban	Rural
Males	54	48	41
Females	13	8	2

2 **Todd (1986), quoting Mr B. Thassitis (personal communication)**

3 **Rebelakos *et al* (1985)**
   a. Patients hospitalized at major accident hospital in Athens from November 1980 to October 1981 (controls in a study of bladder cancer). Sample size (males) 250, (females) 50
   b. Smokers: includes those who had given up smoking within previous 5 years and excludes smokers who had smoked for less than 1 year; includes a 'few individuals' smoking products other than manufactured cigarettes
   c. Consumption category estimation based on 1-10, 11-20, 21-30, and 31+ cigarettes/smoker/day

4 **Tsakraklides *et al* (1983)**
   a. Study of male soldiers from all over Greece. Over-representative of rural areas and high school education. Anonymous questionnaire completed when soldiers gathered for lecture or medical check. Sample size 6 650
   b. 1% of smokers smoked pipe or cigars
   c. Consumption category estimation based on 1-5, 6-10, 11-20, 21-30, 31-40, and 41+ cigarettes/smoker/day

5 **Keenan (1985)**
   a. Survey in two urban and two rural high schools, grades 9 and 12. Year not stated
   b. Smokers: ever tried smoking

6 **Kanellakis *et al* (1976)**
   a. Study covering 1950-1962. Patients with cancer other than lung cancer (controls in a retrospective study of lung cancer). Sample size 613
   b. Smokers: ever smoked regularly. Although we usually only report on current smoking, this study has been included because it provides very early age-specific data when little else is available
   c. Consumption category estimation based on 1-10, 11-20, 21-35, and 36+ cigarettes/smoker/day
   d. Assumed extension to age distribution for percentage smokers, males only, age 15: 5%. Number of cigarettes/person/day: 5.0

7 Voridis *et al* (1974)

a. Study conducted from 1966 to 1969. Non-coronary hospital patients (controls in a study of myocardial infarction). Sample size (males) 223, (females) 61

b. Heavy smokers: smoked at least 20 cigarettes per day for 10 years (data for age 20-29 are omitted because of this definition)

c. Assumed extension to age distribution for percentage smokers, age 15-19: males 30%. Number of cigarettes/person/day: 5.0

8 Dontas (1980)

a. Combined results from three surveys in Athens, Larissa (industrial town, Central Greece), and Chania (town in agricultural/tourist area, Crete). Year unknown. Sample sizes 6 000 (8% of all schoolchildren), 800 (80% of all schoolchildren), and 700 (85% of all schoolchildren) respectively

b. The paper states that 31.8% of children were regular smokers. Hence, we have interpreted 'Of the boys 45.9% smoked compared with 54.1% of the girls' as meaning 'of the smokers, 45.9% were boys and 54.1% girls'. This implies (assuming equal populations) that 29.2% of boys smoked and 34.4% of girls, but the original percentages have been quoted elsewhere (e.g. Masironi and Roy (1982))

9-10 Keys *et al* (1966)

a. Baseline of Seven Countries Study on cardiovascular disease. Interview including smoking questions before medical examinations.

	Location	Description	Sample size	Response rate (%)
9	Crete	Farming villages	686	98
10	Corfu	Farming villages	529	95

b. Water pipes (hookah) are stated to be smoked occasionally in Crete

c. Consumption category estimation based on 1-9, 10-19, and 20+ cigarettes/smoker/day

11-12 Kokkevi and Stefanis (1991)

a. Results shown as source **11** are from a nationwide study in a representative sample of high schools in 1984. Anonymous questionnaire completed in class, on licit and illicit drug use. Absentee rate 6%, participation rate among those present 100%. Sample size (males) 5 354, (females) 5 359

b. Results from 18 Athens schools (of 38) are shown as source **12**. The study was repeated at these schools in 1988 with a shortened questionnaire. Absentee rate 5%.

	Sample size	
	Males	**Females**
1984	1 065	1 060
1988	1 007	922

c. Smokers: use tobacco regularly now

13 Koumantaki *et al* (1989)

a. Patients hospitalized in Athens with orthopaedic conditions (controls in study of cancer of endometrium). Sample size 164, response rate 95%

b. It was reported that most of the smokers smoked 15-20 cigarettes per day

14 Crofton (1990) quoting Director General of WHO (1988)

a. Adults. Year not stated, probably 1981-1986

15 Moulopoulos *et al* (1987)

a. Study of coronary risk factors in Athens. Random sample of adults invited to medical examination, 1979-1983. Sample size (males) 1 835, (females) 2 244. Response rate 91% during 1979-1981, 87% during 1981-1983

b. Heavy smokers: smokes 20+ cigarettes per day

c. Assumed extension to age distribution for percentage smokers, age 15-17: males and females 5%

16 Masironi and Rothwell (1988)

a. No original source. Age group not stated

17 **Rigatos (1988)**

a. Pupils in Evros, Northern Greece. No original source. Year not stated

b. It is also reported that at age 18, 22.4% of their fathers and 0.5% of their mothers had smoked

18 **Karaoglou and Naett (1991) quoting Europe against Cancer Programme (no details)**

a. Results presented here for 1988-1990 are average of spring and autumn results

b. Assumed extension to age distribution for percentage smokers, females only 1991, age 15-17: 20-%

19 **Joossens *et al* (1994) quoting Commission of the European Communities**

a. Eurobarometer surveys

20 **Chollat-Traquet (1992) quoting Europe Against Cancer (no details)**

a. Age group not specified

21 **Mayer (1989)**

a. No original source. Year not stated. High school students, age not stated

22 **van Reek *et al* (1992), van Reek and Adriaanse (1995)**

a. A series of surveys of Young Europeans. About 800 children aged 11-15 years interviewed in each EC country except Luxembourg (where only 250 interviewed). Lowest age group 11-12. Interviews conducted at home, with parents absent

b. Regular smokers: smoked daily. All smokers: smoked at least once a week

23 **WHO (1997)**

a. No original source

24 **Hibell *et al* (1997)**

a. Part of a nationally representative survey, comparable with ESPAD (European School Survey Project on Alcohol and Other Drugs). Target was pupils born in 1977, thus age 15-16 at time of survey in March-April 1993. Approximately 80% of this group still in school. Anonymous questionnaire completed and sealed in envelope by pupil, in class. Teachers absent. Sample size (males) 1 205, (females) 1 412. Response rate 78%

b. Regular smokers: smoked 1 or more cigarettes per day in last 30 days. All smokers: smoked in last 30 days

c. Consumption category estimation based on 1-5, 6-10, 11-20, 21+ cigarettes/smoker/day

25 **Athanasiou and Macris (1995)**

a. Questionnaire study carried out in a random sample of students and in a group of parents of school- and pre-school children. Student group were described as age 18-25+ and are shown in Table 11.4 as age 18-24. Age of parental group not stated and shown in Table 11.4 as 25-49. Year not stated.

	Sample size	
	Males	**Females**
Students	475	661
Parents	379	391

b. Regular smokers: smokes 5+ cigarettes per week. All smokers: smokes 1+ cigarettes per week

26 **WHO (1997)**

a. WHO study in 1993-1994.

b. Regular smoker: smoked weekly

27 **Elisaf *et al* (1996)**

a. Study of all female students in the final year of high school in Ioannina (city in Northwest Greece). Anonymous questionnaire as part of health check. Year not stated. Sample size 590, predominantly age 17

b. Smokers: smoked daily

28 Psathakis *et al* (1997)

a. Anonymous questionnaire study among male conscripts just after joining Greek army. Mean age 21. Considered representative of young Greek males overall. Sample size 1 200, response rate 88%

29 Tessier *et al* (1999) quoting Prof N. Choulis (personal data)

a. Year not stated

30 Kokkevi *et al* (2000)

a. Nationwide survey of use of addictive substances, carried out by University of Athens. Personal interviews at home. *All ages* results in Table 11.4 are for age 12-64

b. Consumption category estimation based on 1-5, 6-20 and 21+ cigarettes/smoker/day

c. Assumed extension to age distribution for percentage smokers, age 65+: males 30%, females 8%. Number of cigarettes/person/day: males 8.0, females 1.0

31 Tzonou *et al* (1984)

a. Patients hospitalized in Athens 1980-1981, with orthopaedic conditions (controls in study of ovarian cancer). Sample size 250, response rate 100%. Lower age limit not stated (but <34). 60% of the patients were age 55+

b. Category consumption estimation based on two categories, less than half a pack and more than half a pack (assume 1-10, 11+ cigarettes)/smoker/day, and resulting figures should be regarded with caution

32 Kafatos *et al* (1991)

a. Study of all employees of a bank throughout Crete, considered representative of middle-class Cretans. Interview including smoking habits as part of comprehensive medical check. Sample size (males) 247, (females) 129. Participation rate 97%

33 Aravanis *et al* (1988)

a. Study in rural Crete, in the same area and following the same protocol as the Seven Countries study (see source 9). All men in 3 villages, and a random sample in a rural municipality invited to medical examination. Sample size 401, response rate 100%.

b. Results presented exclude 69 men with certain diseases

34 Lindholm *et al* (1992)

a. Study of coronary risk factors in Spili, a village in Crete. All adult residents (age <80) invited to medical examination. Year not stated. Sample size 445, response rate 82%

b. Assumed extension to age distribution for percentage smokers, age 80+: males 10%, females 0%

References

Anonymous (1993). Greek imports of cigarettes rise. *Tobacco Journal International,* **4**, 34-5.

Aravanis C., Mensink R.P., Corcondilas A., Ioanidis P., Feskens E.J.M. and Katan M.B. (1988). Risk factors for coronary heart disease in middle-aged men in Crete in 1982. *Int J Epidemiol,* **17**, 779-83.

Athanasiou K. and Macris G. (1995). Smoking and cancer: exploring the level of knowledge and attitudes of Greek youngsters and parents. In: Slama K. (ed) *Tobacco and Health, 9th World Conference on Tobacco and Health, Paris, 10-14 October 1994*. Plenum Press, New York; 623-5.

Beese D.H. (ed) (1968). *Tobacco consumption in various countries,* 2nd edition. Tobacco Research Council, London. Research Paper 6.

Beese D.H. (ed) (1972). *Tobacco consumption in various countries,* 3rd edition. Tobacco Research Council, London. Research Paper 6.

Belgian Association for Smoking Prevention (1989). *Tobacco, health, economy and the tar-yield of cigarettes.* Belgian Association for Smoking Prevention, Brussels.

Chollat-Traquet C. (1992). *Women and tobacco* . WHO, Geneva.

Crofton J. (1990). Tobacco and the Third World. *Thorax,* **45**, 164-9.

Director General of WHO (1988). *Tobacco or health. Report to the Forty-first World Health Assembly*. WHO, Geneva.[§]

Dontas N.S. (1980). Smoking behavior in Greek schoolchildren. *World Smoking and Health,* **5**, 34-5.

Elisaf M., Papanikolaou N., Letzaris G. and Siamopoulos K.C. (1996). Smoking habit in female students of northwestern Greece: relation to other cardiovascular risk factors. *J R Soc Health,* **116**, 87-90.

Hibell B., Andersson B., Bjarnason T., Kokkevi A., Morgan M. and Narusk A. (1997). *The 1995 ESPAD report. The European school survey project on alcohol and other drugs. Alcohol and other drug use among students in 26 European countries*. The Swedish Council for Information on Alcohol and Other Drugs. Council of Europe (Pompidou Group).

Hutson J.B. (1937). *Consumption and production of tobacco in Europe*. USDA, Washington DC. Technical bulletin No. 587.

Ioannidis P.J. and Aravanis C. (1984). The smoking problem in the South-European countries. Tobacco smoking in Greece. Situational Analysis 1920-1982 (consumption—incidence—economics). In: *Symposium on smoking and health in the South European countries*. Institut d'Estudis de la Salut, Barcelona; 121-2.

Joossens L., Naett C., Howie C. and Muldoon A. (1994). *Tobacco and health in the European Union. An overview*. European Bureau for Action on Smoking Prevention (BASP), Brussels.

Kafatos A., Kouroumalis I., Vlachonikolis I., Theodorou C. and Labadarios D. (1991). Coronary-heart-disease risk-factor status of the Cretan urban population in the 1980s. *Am J Clin Nutr,* **54**, 591-8.

Kalapothaki V., Haniotis D., Xirouchaki E. and Trichopoulos D. (1977). Smoking and mortality in Greece. *Materia Medica Greca,* **5**, 390-6.

Kanellakis A., Trichopoulos D., Michalakopoulos N., Margoudakis S., *et al* (1976). The relationship between smoking of Greek cigarettes and the development of lung cancer. *Materia Medica Greca,* **4**, 351-5.

Karaoglou A. and Naett C. (1991). *Is she still a smoker?* BASP, Brussels. (European Bureau for Action on Smoking Prevention.)

Keenan E. (1985). Smoking and its promotion in Greece. A 20th century Trojan horse. *New York State Journal of Medicine,* 409.

Keys A., Aravanis C., Blackburn H.W., van Buchem F.S.P., *et al* (1966). Epidemiological studies related to coronary heart disease: characteristics of men aged 40-59 in seven countries. *Acta Medica Scandinavica,* **Suppl 460**, 8-392.

Kokkevi A., Loukadakis M., Plagianakou S., Politikou K. and Stefanis C. (2000). Sharp increase in illicit drug use in Greece: trends from a general population survey on licit and illicit drug use. *Eur Addict Res,* **6**, 42-9.

Kokkevi A. and Stefanis C. (1991). The epidemiology of licit and illicit substance use among high school students in Greece. *Am J Public Health,* **81**, 48-52.

Koumantaki Y., Tzonou A., Koumantakis E., Kaklamani E., Aravantinos D. and Trichopoulos D. (1989). A case-control study of cancer of endometrium in Athens. *Int J Cancer,* **43**, 795-9.

Lee P.N. (ed) (1975). *Tobacco consumption in various countries,* 4th edition. Tobacco Research Council, London. Research Paper 6.

Lindholm L.H., Koutis A.D., Lionis C.D., Vlachonikolis I.G., Isacsson Å. and Fioretos M. (1992). Risk factors for ischaemic heart disease in a Greek population. A cross-sectional study of men and women living in the village of Spili in Crete. *Eur Heart J,* **13**, 291-8.

Masironi R. and Rothwell K. (1988). Tendances et effets du tabagisme dans le monde (Smoking trends and effects worldwide). *World Health Stat Q,* **41**, 228-41.

Masironi R. and Roy L. (1982). Cigarettes smoking in young age groups. Geographic prevalence. In: Fontana F. (ed) *Tabacco e giovani (Tobacco and youth), International conference, Venice 9-11 November 1981* . ATTI, Venice; 21-40.

Maxwell J.C.Jr. (successive years). How the brands ranked. Maxwell International Estimates. *World Tobacco.*

Mayer C. (1989). Smoke signals. *Business Traveller* **June**:19-24.

Moulopoulos S.D., Adamopoulos P.N., Diamantopoulos E.I., Nanas S.N., Anthopoulos L.N. and Iliadi-Alexandrou M. (1987). Coronary heart disease risk factors in a random sample of Athenian adults. *Am J Epidemiol,* **126**, 882-92.

Polychronidis C.P. (1995). No future for traditional Greek cigarettes and tobaccos? *Tobacco Journal International,* 48-52.

Psathakis K., Bouros D., Vlasserou F., Tzanakis N. and Slafakas N.M. (1997). Relationship between the age at which smoking begins and frequency of smoking in young males in Greece. *Indoor + Built Environment,* **6**, 362-5.

Rebelakos A., Trichopoulos D., Tzonou A., Zavitsanos X., Velonakis E. and Trichopoulos A. (1985). Tobacco smoking, coffee drinking and occupation as risk factors for bladder cancer in Greece. *J Natl Cancer Inst,* **75**, 455-61.

Rigatos G.A. (1988). The smoking epidemic in Greece. *World Smoking and Health,* **13**, 11.

RP6, See Beese (ed) (1968), Beese (ed) (1972), Lee (ed) (1975)

Tessier J.-F., Nejjari C. and Bennani-Othmani M. (1999). Smoking in Mediterranean countries: Europe, North Africa and the Middle-East. Results from a co-operative study. *International Journal of Tuberculosis and Lung Diseases,* **3**, 927-37.

Thassitis B. (1983). Greek cigarette consumption reaches record levels. *Tobacco Journal International,* **3**, 213-4.

References *(continued)*

Todd G. (1986). *Medicine. Statistics of smoking in the Member States of the European Community*. Commission of the European Communities, Luxembourg.

Tsakraklides V., Mentis A., Efstathiou P. and Trichopoulos D. (1983). Tobacco smoking by young adult males in Greece. *International Journal of Health Education,* **2**, 26-30.

Tzonou A., Day N.E., Trichopoulos D., Walker A., *et al* (1984). Epidemiology of ovarian cancer in Greece: a case-control study. *European Journal of Cancer and Clinical Oncology,* **20**, 1045-52.

van Reek J. and Adriaanse H. (1995). Daily smoking among adolescents in the European Community. *Rev Epidemiol Sante Publique,* **43**, 281-2.

van Reek J., Adriaanse H. and Karaoglou A. (1992). Smoking among children in the European Community. *J Public Health Med,* **14**, 93-4.

Voridis E., Plessas S.T., Trichopoulos T. and Plessas C. (1974). Acute myocardial infarction among smokers of oriental tobacco. *Angiology,* **25**, 309-11.

WHO (1997). *Tobacco or health: A global status report*. WHO, Geneva. www.cdc.gov/nccdphp/osh/who/whoampro.htm.

§ Original paper not obtained, but information taken as quoted by another author

Hungary 12

Sales data

See Tables 12.1-12.2.

In the 1920s and 1930s consumption of manufactured cigarettes per adult was low, below 1 cigarette per day. No estimates of hand-rolled cigarette consumption are available until 1940, at which point about equal numbers of manufactured and hand-rolled cigarettes were smoked. By 1960, consumption had increased to 6 manufactured cigarettes per day, and continued to increase to over 9 in the 1990s, by which time hand-rolled cigarettes had all but disappeared. These figures may be lower than actual consumption, as estimates of smuggling are as high as 25%. The proportion of cigarettes that were filtered rose slowly during the 1960s, then rapidly during the 1970s to about 80% in 1980. The tar yield of cigarettes was high, in the range 18-24 mg per cigarette in 1992.

Data on products other than cigarettes are available only for occasional years. Consumption of all tobacco products per adult rose from 2-5 g per day in 1920 to 5 g in 1940 and 9 g in 1988. Around 20-25% of all tobacco was consumed as manufactured cigarettes before 1940 with the remainder mainly as smoking tobacco; in 1940 this was about equally split between pipe and cigarette tobaccos. By 1988 products other than manufactured cigarettes had virtually disappeared.

Survey data

See Tables 12.4-12.8

Estimates of the prevalence of smoking among men aged 15 years and over have fluctuated, but with some exceptions, have generally decreased from about 50% to about 40% between the mid-1960s and the mid-1990s. Estimates of the prevalence among women in the same period varied, but were mostly around 25%.

There are few age-specific data available on the prevalence of smoking. More men than women smoke at all ages, but the difference between the proportion of boys and girls smoking is small for the two surveys conducted in 1995.

Comparison of survey and sales data was only possible for two surveys. One, a non-representative survey in 1966 (source 2), under-reported consumption by 10%, while a recent study (source 12) under-reported by nearly 50%. Between 1966 and 1995, the estimated number of cigarettes smoked per person per day (sales-adjusted) was about 11-14 for men and about 4-8 for women.

Table 12.1.1 Total annual sales of tobacco products, 1920-1934

Year	Cigarettes		Cigars tonnes	Smoking mixtures tonnes	Cigarette tobacco tonnes	All tobacco products tonnes
	tonnes	millions				
1920	898	898	570	3470	1	4939
1921	1652	1652	719	5898	1	8270
1922	2041	2041	742	7247	1	10031
1923	1299	1299	607	6314	1	8221
1924	1872	1872	591	7194	1	9658
1925	1980	1980	699	8195	1	10875
1926	2113	2113	752	8424	1	11290
1927	2267	2267	950	8872	1	12090
1928	2344	2344	744	9043	1	12132
1929	2199	2199	544	8674	1	11418
1930	2000	2000	409	7910	1	10320
1931	1827	1827	316	7506	1	9650
1932	1793	1793	259	6507	1	8560
1933	1971	1971	237	6588	1	8797
1934	1958	1793	231	6655	1	8845

Source : see *Notes on sources of sales data*, p. 312

Table 12.1.2 Total annual sales of tobacco products, 1940-1995

Year	Cigarettes		Cigars		Pipe tobacco	Cigarette tobacco	All tobacco products
	tonnes	millions	tonnes	millions	tonnes	tonnes	tonnes
1940	3045	3045	345	69	4741	3539	11670
1960	15782	15782					
1961	16793	16793					
1962	16449	16449					
1963	15812	15812					
1964	16393	16393					
1965	18478	18478					
1966	20525	20525					
1967	20936	20936					
1968	21836	21836					
1969	20772	20772					
1970	22502	22502					
1971	24008	24008					
1972	26135	26135					
1973	23603	23603					
1974	23593	23593					
1975	25783	25783					
1976	26250	26250					
1977	25700	25700					
1978	25525	25525					
1979	26050	26050					
1980	28598	28598					
1981	28190	28190					
1982	26435	26435					
1983	24850	24850					
1984	27540	27540					
1985	27280	27280					
1986	27133	27133					
1987	27242	27242					
1988	26628	26628	65	13	50	17	26760
1989	27415	27415					
1990	28849	28849					
1991	26530	26530					
1992	25895	25895					
1993	27769	27769					
1994	28579	28579					
1995	27750	27750					

Source : see *Notes on sources of sales data,* p. 312

Table 12.1.3 Manufactured cigarettes (i) percentage of total sales as filter cigarettes, 1963-1995, and (ii) tar yield per cigarette, 1973 and 1992

Year	% Filter	Tar yield mg / cig
1963	6.4	
1964	10.5	
1965	14.0	
1966	16.5	
1967	19.5	
1968	23.2	
1969	27.3	
1970	37.2	
1971	41.4	
1972	46.8	
1973	52.0	32-34
1974	56.7	
1975	61.0	
1976	67.7	
1977	72.0	
1978	77.3	
1979	78.0	
1980	79.0	
1981	82.2	
1982	84.0	
1988	91.4	
1992		18-24
1993	92.9	
1994	93.2	
1995	93.8	

Source : see *Notes on sources of sales data*, p. 312

Table 12.2 Consumption of (i) cigarettes and (ii) all tobacco products, 1920-1995 sales-based data, including estimated hand-rolled cigarette consumption. Males and females aged 15 years and over

Year	Manufactured cigarettes		Hand-rolled cigarettes		Total cigarettes		All tobacco products	
	Total annual in millions	Number/ adult/day	Total annual in millions	Number/ adult/day	Total annual in millions	Number/ adult/day	Total annual in tonnes	Grams/ adult/day
1920	898	0.4					4939	2.5
1921	1652	0.8					8270	3.9
1922	2041	1.0					10031	4.8
1923	1299	0.6					8221	3.9
1924	1872	0.9					9658	4.6
1925	1980	0.9					10875	5.2
1926	2113	0.9					11290	5.0
1927	2267	1.0					12090	5.4
1928	2344	1.0					12132	5.4
1929	2199	1.0					11418	5.1
1930	2000	0.9					10320	4.6
1931	1827	0.8					9650	4.1
1932	1793	0.8					8560	3.6
1933	1971	0.8					8797	3.7
1934	1958	0.8					8845	3.8
1940	3045	1.2	3539	1.5	6584	2.7	11670	4.8
1960	15782	5.8						
1961	16793	6.1						
1962	16449	6.0						
1963	15812	5.7						
1964	16393	5.8						
1965	18478	6.5						
1966	20525	7.2						
1967	20936	7.2						
1968	21836	7.5						
1969	20772	7.0						
1970	22502	7.5						
1971	24008	8.0						
1972	26135	8.6						
1973	23603	7.7						
1974	23593	7.7						
1975	25783	8.4						
1976	26250	8.6						
1977	25700	8.4						
1978	25525	8.3						
1979	26050	8.5						
1980	28598	9.4						
1981	28190	9.2						
1982	26435	8.7						
1983	24850	8.2						
1984	27540	9.0						
1985	27280	8.9						
1986	27133	8.9						
1987	27242	8.9						
1988	26628	8.7	17	0.0	26645	8.7	26760	8.8
1989	27415	8.9						
1990	28849	9.6						
1991	26530	8.7						
1992	25895	8.5						
1993	27769	9.1						
1994	28579	9.4						
1995	27750	9.1						

Source : see *Notes on sources of sales data*, p. 312

Figure 12.1 Daily consumption of cigarettes, 1920-1995
Males and females aged 15 years and over. *Source:* see Table 12.2

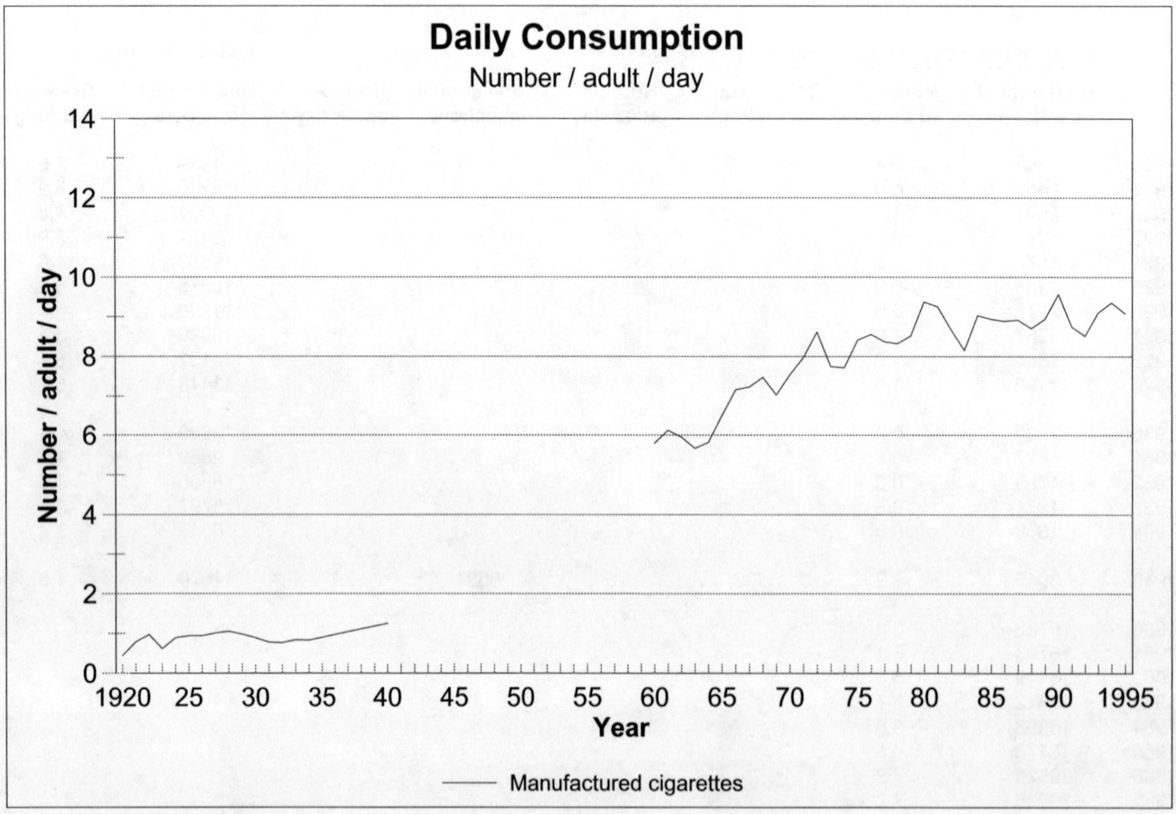

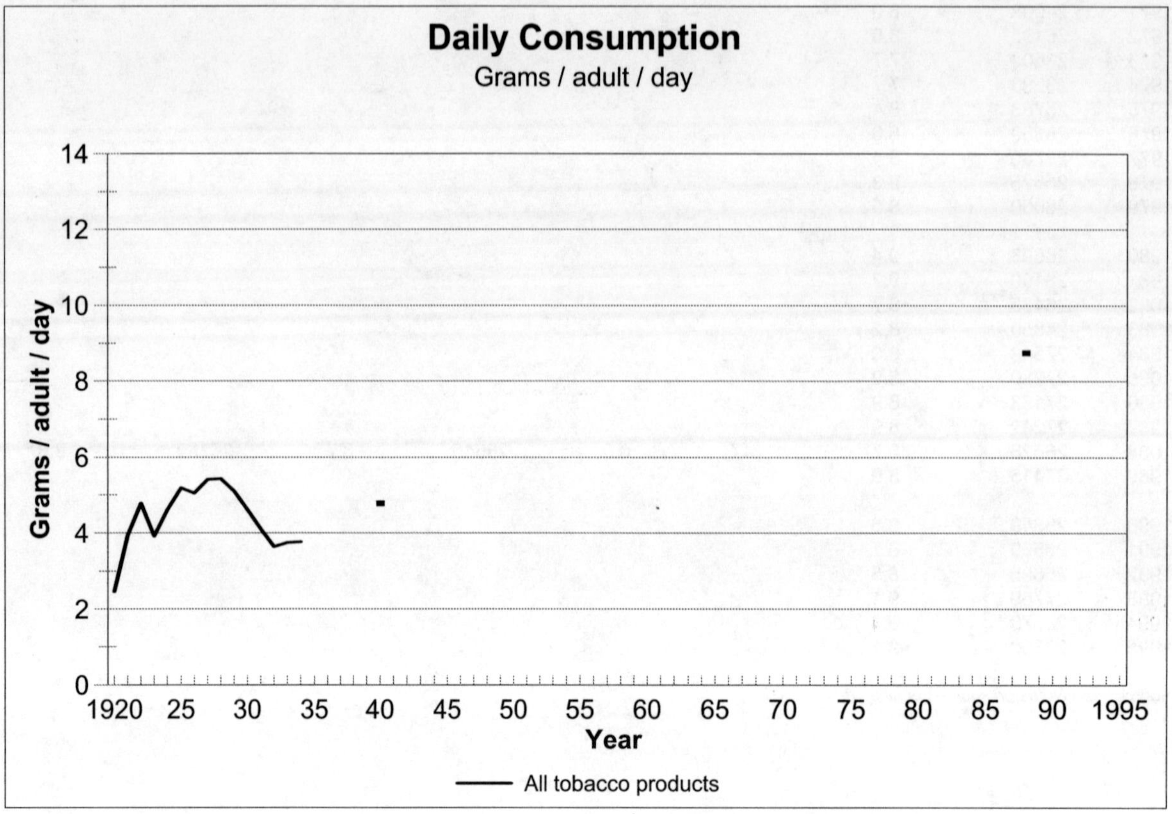

Table 12.3 Percentage sales of tobacco in different forms[1] (by weight), selected years 1925-1988

Year	Cigarettes (%)	Cigars (%)	Smoking mixtures (%)	Pipe tobacco (%)	Cigarette tobacco (%)
1925	18.2	6.4	75.4	–	–
1934	22.1	2.6	75.2	–	–
1940	26.1	3.0	–	40.6	30.3
1988	99.5	0.2	–	0.2	0.1

1 Snuff, not shown, accounts for about 0.1%

Source : calculated from Tables 12.1.1 & 12.1.2

Figure 12.2 Percentage sales of tobacco in different forms (by weight), selected years 1925-1988
Source: see Table 12.3

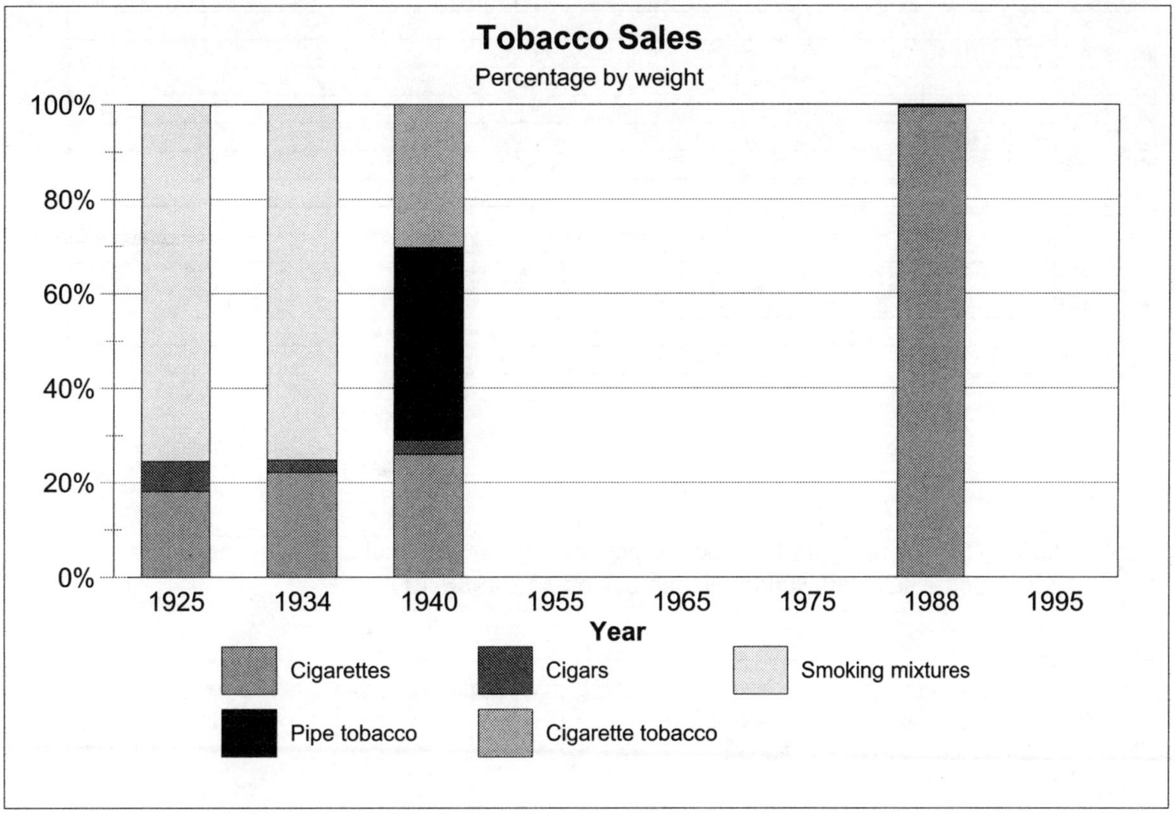

Table 12.4M Prevalence of smoking, males: some selected Hungarian surveys by age, 1965-1995

Year / Source / Product / Frequency	12	13	14	15	16	17	18	19	20-24	25-29	30-34	35-39	40-44	45-49	50-54	55-59	60-64	65-69	70-74	75-79	80+	All ages
65 1 UC U															56							
66 2 U U															57							
75 3 U U													45									
80 4 UC U				31																		
80 5 U U												50										
82 6 UC R										65		47			56		40					49
82 6 A A										66		47			57		41					49
83 7 UC R										63		61			46		47					52
83 7 A A										64		62			47		47					53
84 8 U U												47										
86 5 MC R												61										
86 9 U *		3		21																		
86 9 U R		7		27																		
86 9 U A		15		35																		
89 5 U U												40										
90 9 UC R		11		31																		
90 9 UC A		21		39																		
92 5 U U												63										
92 10 UC R		2			15																	
92 10 UC A		15			44																	
93 5 U U												40										
93 9 UC R		9		25																		
94 11 U U										44												
95 12 UC U						27			33	35		47			39		28			19		34
95 12 A U						29			33	37		48			39		28			20		35
95 13 UC R				32																		
95 13 UC A				36																		
95 14 UC A					36																	

Table 12.5M Number of cigarettes smoked per smoker per day, males: some selected Hungarian surveys by age, 1966-1995

Year / Source / Product	12	13	14	15	16	17	18	19	20-24	25-29	30-34	35-39	40-44	45-49	50-54	55-59	60-64	65-69	70-74	75-79	80+	All ages
66 2 UCE															21							
82 6 UC															21							
83 7 UC															23							
95 12 UC						9.0			15	18		21		20		17			17			18
95 13 UCE				16																		

Source see *Notes on sources of survey data*, p. 312
Frequency: A = all smokers (including occasional)
R = regular or daily smokers
All ages relevant to ages used and as given in original source
U = unspecified
* = refer to *Notes on sources of survey data*, p. 312

Product: MC = manufactured cigarettes
TC = total cigarettes (including hand-rolled)
UC = cigarettes (type unspecified)
A = all products
E indicates mean estimated from percentage distribution (see also *Consumption category estimation*, p. xxxiv, and Appendix III, p. 789)

Table 12.4F Prevalence of smoking, females: some selected Hungarian surveys by age, 1965-1995

Year Source Product Frequency	12	13	14	15	16	17	18	19	20-24	25-29	30-34	35-39	40-44	45-49	50-54	55-59	60-64	65-69	70-74	75-79	80+	All ages
65 1 UC U																						
66 2 U U									18													
75 3 U U					23																	
80 4 UC U				20																		
80 5 U U				25																		
82 6 UC R										49		34		24		10						24
82 6 A A										51		36		25		11						26
83 7 UC R										44		46		31		27						36
83 7 A A										45		47		32		27						37
84 8 U U			27																			
86 5 MC R				23																		
86 9 U *		1		14																		
86 9 U R		2		21																		
86 9 U A		7		29																		
89 5 U U				27																		
90 9 UC R		5		20																		
90 9 UC A		11		29																		
92 5 U U				25																		
92 10 UC R		2			5																	
92 10 UC A		18			30																	
93 5 U U				37																		
93 9 UC R		7		19																		
94 11 U U				27																		
95 12 UC U				23					28	34		37		33		20		13				28
95 12 A U				24					28	35		38		33		20		13				28
95 13 UC R				26																		
95 13 UC A				32																		
95 14 UC A			35																			

Table 12.5F Number of cigarettes smoked per smoker per day, females: some selected Hungarian surveys by age, 1966-1995

Year Source Product	12	13	14	15	16	17	18	19	20-24	25-29	30-34	35-39	40-44	45-49	50-54	55-59	60-64	65-69	70-74	75-79	80+	All ages
66 2 UCE									16													
82 6 UC												17										
83 7 UC												17										
95 12 UC				8.7					11	12		15		14		14		13				13
95 13 UCE				12																		

Source: see *Notes on sources of survey data*, p. 312
Frequency: A = all smokers (including occasional)
R = regular or daily smokers
All ages: relevant to ages used and as given in original source
U = unspecified
* = refer to *Notes on sources of survey data*, p. 312

Product: MC = manufactured cigarettes
TC = total cigarettes (including hand-rolled)
UC = cigarettes (type unspecified)
A = all products
E indicates mean estimated from percentage distribution (see also *Consumption category estimation*, p. xxxiv, and Appendix III, p. 789)

Table 12.6M Number of cigarettes smoked per person per day, males: some selected Hungarian surveys by age, 1966-1995, with percentage total sales

<table>
<tr><th rowspan="2">Product
Source
Year</th><th colspan="21">Age group</th><th rowspan="2">All ages</th><th rowspan="2">% Total sales</th></tr>
<tr><th>12</th><th>13</th><th>14</th><th>15</th><th>16</th><th>17</th><th>18</th><th>19</th><th>20-24</th><th>25-29</th><th>30-34</th><th>35-39</th><th>40-44</th><th>45-49</th><th>50-54</th><th>55-59</th><th>60-64</th><th>65-69</th><th>70-74</th><th>75-79</th><th>80+</th></tr>
<tr><td>66 2 UC</td><td colspan="8"></td><td colspan="13">12</td><td></td><td>91%m</td></tr>
<tr><td>82 6 UC *</td><td colspan="11"></td><td colspan="6">10</td><td colspan="4"></td><td></td><td>**</td></tr>
<tr><td>83 7 UC *</td><td colspan="11"></td><td colspan="6">12</td><td colspan="4"></td><td></td><td>**</td></tr>
<tr><td>95 12 UC</td><td colspan="3"></td><td colspan="5">2.4</td><td>4.9</td><td colspan="2">6.2</td><td colspan="2">9.9</td><td colspan="2">7.9</td><td colspan="2">4.8</td><td colspan="4">3.3</td><td>6.2</td><td>52%m</td></tr>
<tr><td>95 13 UC</td><td colspan="3"></td><td colspan="2">5.2</td><td colspan="17"></td><td>**</td></tr>
</table>

Table 12.7M Number of cigarettes smoked per person per day, sales-adjusted, males: some selected Hungarian surveys[1] by age, 1966-1995, with percentage total sales

<table>
<tr><th rowspan="2">Product
Source
Year</th><th colspan="21">Age group</th><th rowspan="2">All ages</th><th rowspan="2">% Total sales</th></tr>
<tr><th>12</th><th>13</th><th>14</th><th>15</th><th>16</th><th>17</th><th>18</th><th>19</th><th>20-24</th><th>25-29</th><th>30-34</th><th>35-39</th><th>40-44</th><th>45-49</th><th>50-54</th><th>55-59</th><th>60-64</th><th>65-69</th><th>70-74</th><th>75-79</th><th>80+</th></tr>
<tr><td>66 2 UC</td><td colspan="8"></td><td colspan="13">13</td><td></td><td>91%m</td></tr>
<tr><td>95 12 UC</td><td colspan="3"></td><td colspan="5">4.6</td><td>9.4</td><td colspan="2">12</td><td colspan="2">19</td><td colspan="2">15</td><td colspan="2">9.2</td><td colspan="4">6.4</td><td>12</td><td>52%m</td></tr>
</table>

1 Based on those surveys in Table 12.6 with data for both sexes and age range at least 21-64 (see *Cigarette consumption per person*, p. xxxv)

Source: see *Notes on sources of survey data*, p. 312
All ages: relevant to ages used and as given in original source
% Total sales: estimated % of total sales of M = manufactured or T = total cigarette consumption implied by survey, sexes combined, used as adjustment factor in Table 12.7
** = cannot be calculated
--- = adjusted by original author

Product: MC = manufactured cigarettes
TC = total cigarettes (including hand-rolled)
UC = cigarettes (type unspecified)
A = all products
U = unspecified
* = refer to *Notes on sources of survey data*, p. 312

Table 12.6F Number of cigarettes smoked per person per day, females: some selected Hungarian surveys by age, 1966-1995, with percentage total sales

Product Source Year	12	13	14	15	16	17	18	19	20-24	25-29	30-34	35-39	40-44	45-49	50-54	55-59	60-64	65-69	70-74	75-79	80+	All ages	% Total sales
66 2 UC									3.0														91%m
82 6 UC *												4.1											**
83 7 UC *												6.1											**
95 12 UC				2.0					3.2	4.2		5.5		4.6		2.9		1.7				3.7	52%m
95 13 UC				3.2																			**

Table 12.7F Number of cigarettes smoked per person per day, sales-adjusted, females: some selected Hungarian surveys[1] by age, 1966-1995, with percentage total sales

Product Source Year	12	13	14	15	16	17	18	19	20-24	25-29	30-34	35-39	40-44	45-49	50-54	55-59	60-64	65-69	70-74	75-79	80+	All ages	% Total sales
66 2 UC									3.3														91%m
95 12 UC				3.9					6.1	8.1		11		8.9		5.5		3.3				7.1	52%m

1 Based on those surveys in Table 12.6 with data for both sexes and age range at least 21-64 (see *Cigarette consumption per person*, p. xxxv)

Source: see *Notes on sources of survey data*, p. 312
All ages: relevant to ages used and as given in original source
% Total sales: estimated % of total sales of M = manufactured or T = total cigarette consumption implied by survey, sexes combined, used as adjustment factor in Table 12.7
** = cannot be calculated
--- = adjusted by original author

Product: MC = manufactured cigarettes
TC = total cigarettes (including hand-rolled)
UC = cigarettes (type unspecified)
A = all products
U = unspecified
* = refer to *Notes on sources of survey data*, p. 312

Table 12.8 Estimated[1] prevalence of smoking and estimated[1] number of cigarettes per person per day (unadjusted and sales-adjusted): summary of Tables 12.4, 12.6 and 12.7, 1966-1995.
Males and females aged 15 years and over

Year	Source[2]	Product[3]	Prevalence[4]						Number of cigarettes						
									Unadjusted[7]			Sales-adjusted[8]			
			Manufactured cigarettes[5,6]		Total cigarettes		All products		Number/ person/day		Total sales %	Manufactured cigarettes[9] number/ person/day		Total cigarettes number/ person/day	
			M	F	M	F	M	F	M	F		M	F	M	F
1966	2	UC+*U*	53	18					10.6	2.8	91	11.7	3.1		
1975	3	*U*	44	23								(12.1	5.0)		
1980	5	*U*	50	25								(13.7	5.5)		
1984	8	*U*	47	27								(12.7	5.7)		
1986	5	MC	61	23								(14.0	4.2)		
1989	5	*U*	40	27								(11.8	6.4)		
1992	5	*U*	63	25								(13.3	4.2)		
1993	5	*U*	40	37								(10.6	7.8)		
1994	11	*U*	40	24								(13.0	6.1)		
1995	12	*UC+A*	34	27			35	27	6.1	3.5	52	11.7	6.7		

1 Surveys covering an age range of at least 21-64 are included. Any gaps in the data for ages 15-20 and 65 years and over are filled in by assumed extensions to the age distribution, given in *Notes on sources of survey data*, p. 312. Method: see *Summary of adult smoking*, p. xxxvi
2 See *Notes on sources of survey data*, p. 312
3 Product: MC = manufactured cigarettes, TC = total cigarettes (including hand-rolled), UC = cigarettes (type unspecified), A = all products, U = unspecified. Frequency of smoking is indicated by: regular or daily smokers in normal type, all smokers (including occasional) in bold, unspecified in italics
4 From Table 12.4
5 This column includes prevalence of smoking classified as UC = cigarettes (type unspecified)
6 This column includes prevalence of smoking classified as U = unspecified product
7 From Table 12.6
8 From Table 12.7, except data in parentheses, which are derived from the prevalence of smoking from Table 12.4 as described in *Summary of adult smoking*, p. xxxvi
9 Number of cigarettes classified as UC = cigarettes (type unspecified) or U = product unspecified has been adjusted to manufactured cigarette sales and included in this column

Figure 12.3 Estimated prevalence of smoking: by year of survey, 1966-1995. Males and females aged 15 years and over. *Source:* see Table 12.8

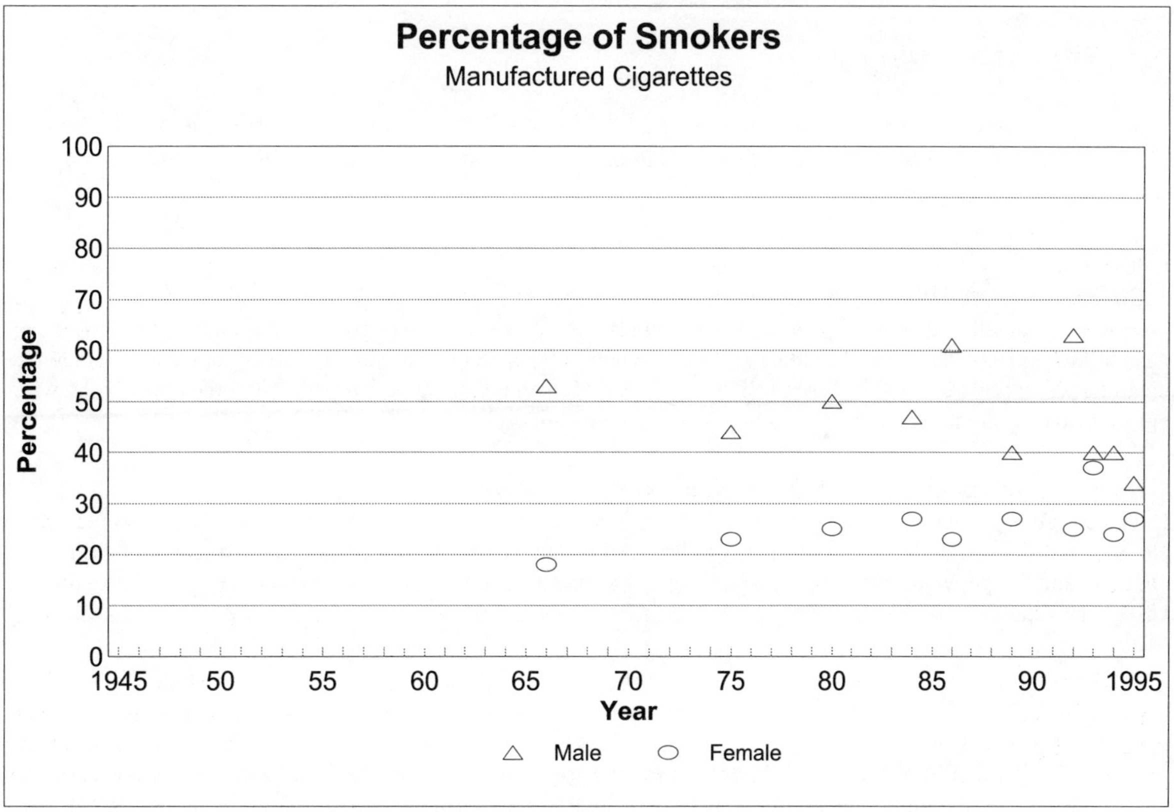

Figure 12.4 Estimated number of cigarettes smoked per person per day, sales-adjusted, 1966-1995. Males and females aged 15 years and over. *Source:* see Table 12.8

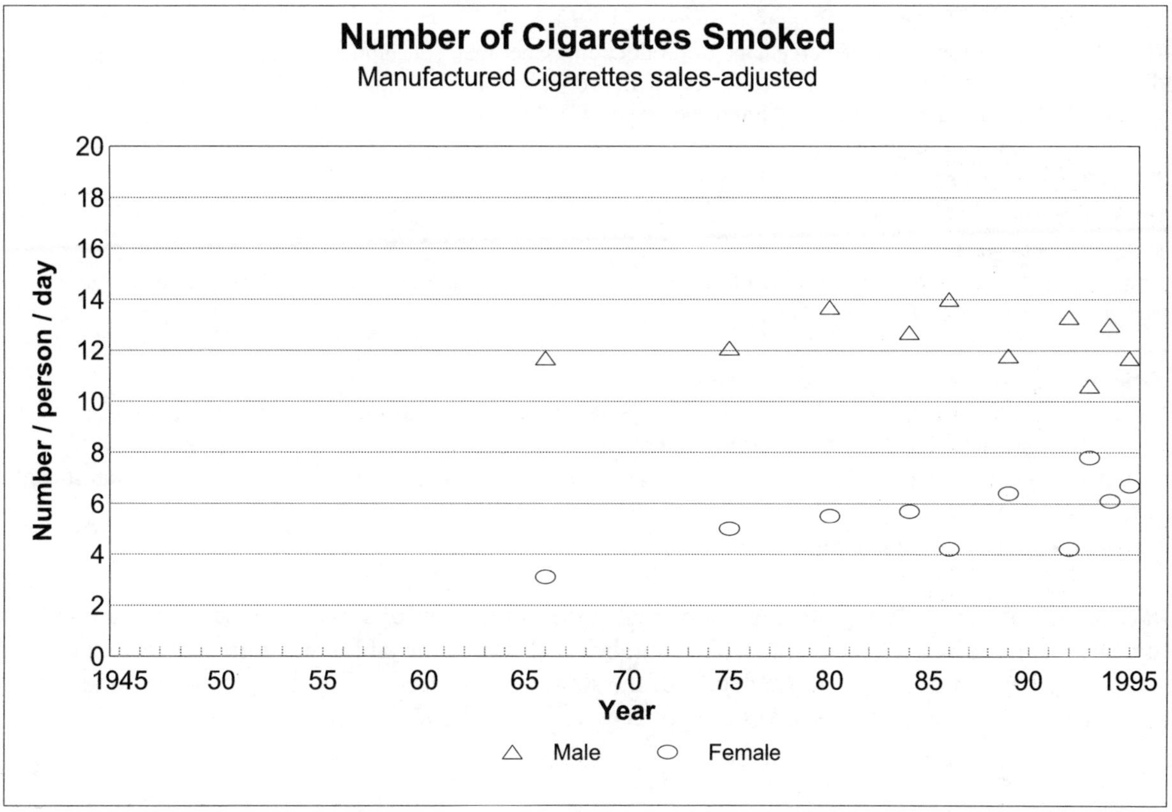

Notes on sources of sales data

The data presented in the tables and figures were obtained from several sources, details of which are given below, together with estimations and related assumptions. Full citations of the sources are given on p. 315 under *References*.

Consumption data

1920-1935 Hutson (1937) quoting Annuaire Statistique Hongrois

Data were originally given to the nearest 1 000 pounds and have been converted to tonnes and given to the nearest tonne (1 000 lbs = 450.359 tonnes). For conversion from weights to numbers we assumed an average cigarette weight of 1 g. 1920 represents 1920-1921, etc. Hutson commented that 'following the close of the war, either the data were incomplete or consumption fluctuated widely'.

1940, and 1988 (products other than cigarettes) Péter (1990)

Data were given as numbers of cigarettes and cigars, and grams of cigarette and pipe tobacco per adult per year. No information is available on the weights of cigarettes or cigars, and we have assumed an average of 1 g per cigarette and 5 g per cigar. Data for cigarettes for 1988 from this source (not shown) were very similar to the USDA data shown.

1960-1995 United States Department of Agriculture (USDA) Economic Research Service (1996)

Data are available only for cigarettes. For conversion from numbers to weights we assumed an average cigarette weight of 1 g. This may be too high a weight, especially for later years when international brands were becoming popular. The share of local brands fell from 80% in the early 1990s to around 60% in 1998 (Anonymous (1998)).

Estimates of smuggling are given, variously, as 10-15% of sales for 1987-1988 (Connolly (1995)), 25% for 1990-1991 (Horne (1992)) and around 15% for 1995-1996 (Anonymous (2000), quoting the Hungarian Tobacco Industry Association). These amounts are additional to the consumption figures given in Table 12.2.

Plain/Filter cigarette consumption

1963-1982 Maxwell (successive years)

1988 Péter (1990)

1993-1995 USDA Economic Research Service (1996)

The USDA figures represent the percentage of production, rather than consumption, that was of filter cigarettes. However, imports and exports are low compared with production. For example, in 1994 imports and exports amounted to 1.3% and 4.6% of production respectively (USDA Economic Research Service (1996)).

Tar yield of cigarettes

1973 Doolittle (1991)

1992 WHO (1997)

Although there is no maximum permitted limit, the tar content of cigarettes is required to be printed on the packet (Harkin *et al* (1997)).

Estimates of hand-rolled cigarette consumption

We estimated hand-rolled cigarette consumption as 100% of cigarette tobacco at 1 g per cigarette. As data are only available for 1940 and 1988, and as consumption of products other than cigarettes was negligible at the later year, we have ignored hand-rolled cigarettes in other calculations such as sales-adjustment.

Notes on sources of survey data

Each source of survey data—either an individual survey or a series of surveys repeated over a number of years—is cited by a source number. This number is shown in the tables and corresponds to the source numbers given below, where details of the source publication and of the survey methodology are given. Full citations of the sources are given on p. 315 under *References*.

Source number

1 **Lamm *et al* (1985)**

a. Study of coronary risk factors, using methods strictly comparable to the Seven Countries Study. All men age 40-59 from 3 small villages in southern Hungary invited for screening. Sample size 1 088, response rate 99%. Analysis was restricted to 1 038 'coronary-free' men

2 **Ormos *et al* (1969)**

a. Systematic questioning of railway passengers (to provide comparison group for a study of lung cancer). Mostly in Csongrád, also Bács-Kiskum, Pest and Szolnok. Sample size (males) 777, (females) 1 044

b. Consumption category estimation based on 1-15, 16-30, >30 cigarettes/smoker/day

c. Assumed extension to age distribution for percentage smokers, age 15-19: males 25% and females 15%. Number of cigarettes/person/day: males 2.0 and females 1.0

3 **Benjamin (1978)**

a. Quoting Statistical Yearbook of Hungarian Central Statistical Office (CSO) 1975

b. Assumed extension to age distribution for percentage smokers, age 15: males 20% and females 15%

4 **Geizerova and Masironi (1988)**

a. No original source

5 **WHO quoted by Chollat-Traquet (1992), Harkin *et al* (1997), Masironi and Rothwell (1988), Piha *et al* (1993), WHO (1996)**

a. Age group not stated

6-7 **WHO (1989), WHO MONICA Project (1988)**

a. Regional surveys forming part of WHO MONICA project:

	Region	Population size	Sample size	Participation rate (%)	Sample used*		Date
					Males	Females	
6	Budapest	94 000	1 472	80	747	692	Apr 1982-Sep 1984
7	Pecs	76 200	—	—	823	846	Jan 1982-Feb 1983

* 'Sample used' includes age 25-34; all other figures are for age 35-64 only

b. *All ages* column relates only to age 35-64 and is standardized to world population

c. Regular cigarette smokers: smoked cigarettes daily. All smokers: smoked cigarettes daily or occasionally, or smoked 1 g pipe tobacco or 1 cigar per week. Cigarettes per smoker refers to regular and occasional cigarette smokers

d. Calculation for cigarettes per person based on % regular cigarette smokers and cigarettes per regular or occasional cigarette smoker, so may underestimate

8 **Kertai (1993)**

a. Microcensus

9 **Nutbeam and Aarø (1990), King and Coles (1992), King *et al* (1996)**

a. Part of the HBSC (Health Behaviour in School-Aged Children) Study, a collaborative cross-national research study sponsored by the WHO. School classes or schools were randomly selected, targeting age groups 11 (not presented here), 13 and 15

Year	Sample size		Mean age	
	Target age 13	Target age 15	Target Age 13	Target age 15
1986-1987	—	1 266	—	—
1990	—	—	14.2	16.2
1993	1 944	1 759	13.8	15.8

Sample size in 1990 was 6 498 (including age 11)

c. Smokers marked as frequency *: smoked daily. Regular smokers: smoke once a week or more

10 Nemeth *et al* (1994)

a. Study conducted at two schools in Györ, an industrial town in north-west Hungary. Anonymous questionnaire on use of legal and illegal substances, completed in class by all pupils who were present on the day. Approximate ages corresponding to school grades 8 and 11. Response rate 100%.

School type	Sample size	
	Males	Females
Elementary	65	55
Gimnázium (selective high school)	34	80

b. Regular smokers: smoked daily. All smokers: smoked at least once in a while

11 Józan (1995)

a. Health Behaviour Survey by Hungarian CSO. Sample size 5 476

b. Assumed extension to age distribution for percentage smokers, age 65+: males 20% and females 13%

12 Scientific Association of Hungarian General Practitioners (1996), and additional unpublished data

a. A health and lifestyle survey, conducted 1995-1996. Representative of the population registered at family practices, thus under-representing younger, male and more highly qualified persons compared with the national population. Sample size (males) 1 109, (females) 1 503

13 Hibell *et al* (1997)

a. Nationally representative survey forming part of ESPAD (European School Survey Project on Alcohol and Other Drugs). Target was pupils born in 1979, thus age 15-16 at time of survey in March 1995. Approximately 95% of this group still in school. Anonymous questionnaire completed and sealed in envelope by pupil, in class. Teachers absent. Sample size (males) 1 199, (females) 1 372. Response rate (males) 88%, (females) 89%

b. Regular smokers: smoked 1 or more cigarettes per day in last 30 days. All smokers: smoked in last 30 days

c. Consumption category estimation based on 1-5, 6-10, 11-20, 21+ cigarettes/smoker/day

14 Anonymous (1997)

a. Study conducted in Budapest by the Field Epidemiology Training Program, Hungarian Ministry of Welfare, at randomly selected schools (20 traditional high schools and 5 vocational/technical schools). All pupils in randomly selected classes completed questionnaire. Sample size (males) 1 470, (females) 1 324

b. Smokers: smoked at least 1 cigarette in last 30 days

References

Anonymous (1997). Prevalence of cigarette smoking among secondary school students—Budapest, Hungary, 1995. *MMWR Morb Mortal Wkly Rep,* **46**, 56-9.

Anonymous (1998). Hungarians flock to light cigarettes. *Tobacco Reporter,* **125**, 6.

Anonymous (2000). Hungary: Hungarian tobacco market stagnates. *Napi Gazdasag* **Jan 28**:3.

Benjamin B. (1978). *Tobacco smoking in the world. Report of the WHO Expert Committee on Smoking Control, Geneva 23-28 October 1978*

Chollat-Traquet C. (1992). *Women and tobacco* . WHO, Geneva.

Connolly G.N. (1995). Tobacco, trade and Eastern Europe. In: Slama K. (ed) *Tobacco and health, Ninth World Conference on Tobacco and Health, Paris, Oct 10-14 1994*. Plenum Press, New York, London; 51-60.

Doolittle D.E. (1991). Beauty and order. *Tobacco Reporter,* **118**, 28-9.

Geizerova H. and Masironi R. (1988). Cigarette smoking in children and adolescents: world review. In: Aoki M., Hisamichi S. and Tominaga S. (eds) *Smoking and health 1987. Proceedings of the 6th World Conference on Smoking and Health, Tokyo, 9-12 November 1987*. Elsevier Science Publishers B.V. (Biomedical Division), Amsterdam; 601-5. International Congress Series No. 780.

Harkin A.M., Anderson P. and Goos C. (1997). *Smoking, drinking and drug taking in the European Region.* Alcohol, Drugs and Tobacco Programme, WHO Regional Office for Europe, Copenhagen.

Hibell B., Andersson B., Bjarnason T., Kokkevi A., Morgan M. and Narusk A. (1997). *The 1995 ESPAD report. The European school survey project on alcohol and other drugs. Alcohol and other drug use among students in 26 European countries*. The Swedish Council for Information on Alcohol and Other Drugs. Council of Europe (Pompidou Group).

Horne B. (1992). New tobacco legislation in Hungary. *Tobacco Journal International,* **4**, 30,32.

Hutson J.B. (1937). *Consumption and production of tobacco in Europe*. USDA, Washington DC. Technical bulletin No. 587.

Józan P. (1995). The main features of tobacco smoking and smoking attributable mortality in Hungary. Some results of the health behaviour survey 1994 [Abstract]. *Tuber Lung Dis,* **76 (Suppl 2)**, 104.

Kertai P. (1993). *Public health priorities in Hungary by the year 2000.* Budapest.

King A., Wold B., Tudor-Smith C. and Harel Y. (1996). *The health of youth, a cross-national survey*. WHO Regional Publications, Europe, Copenhagen. European Series No. 69.

King A.J.C. and Coles B. (1992). *The health of Canada's youth. Views and behaviours of 11-, 13- and 15-year-olds from 11 countries*. Health and Welfare Canada, Ottawa.

Lamm G., Csukás M., Gyárfás J. and Östör E. (1985). Risk factors for coronary heart disease in rural Hungary. *Int J Epidemiol,* **14**, 327-9.

Masironi R. and Rothwell K. (1988). Tendances et effets du tabagisme dans le monde (Smoking trends and effects worldwide). *World Health Stat Q,* **41**, 228-41.

Maxwell J.C.Jr. (successive years). How the brands ranked. Maxwell International Estimates. *World Tobacco.*

Nemeth J., Swaim R.C., Katona E. and Oetting E.R. (1994). Substance use among Hungarian students. *International Journal of the Addictions,* **29**, 1443-67.

Nutbeam D. and Aarø L.E. (1990). Smoking and alienation from school: the implications for health education with young people. Results from the WHO study of health behaviour in schoolchildren. In: Durston B. and Jamrozik K. (eds) *Tobacco & health 1990. The global war. Seventh World Conference on Tobacco and Health, Perth, Western Australia, 1-5 April 1990*. Organising Committee of the Seventh World Conference on Tobacco and Health, 189 Royal Street, East Perth, Western Australia 6004; 539-44.

Ormos J., Karácsonyi G., Biliczki F. and Szőnyi F. (1969). Lung cancer in the Hungarian plain. *Neoplasma,* **16**, 667-75.

Péter Z. (1990). Changes of smoking behavior and tobacco related cancer mortality in Hungary: epidemiological correlation and trends (15th International Cancer Congress, Hamburg) [Abstract]. *J Cancer Res Clin Oncol,* **116(Suppl)**, 969.

Piha T., Besselink E. and Lopez A.D. (1993). Tobacco or health. *World Health Stat Q,* **46**, 188-94.

Scientific Association of Hungarian General Practitioners (1996). *Several relationships between the health status and life-style of the Hungarian population.* Unpublished.

United States Department of Agriculture Economic Research Service (1996). *Tobacco statistics*. Albert R. Mann Library, Cornell University, Ithaca, New York. ERS 94012. (With supplementary material from Tobacco Annual Reports.). http://usda.mannlib.cornell.edu/data-sets/specialty/94012.

WHO (1989). The WHO MONICA project: a worldwide monitoring system for cardiovascular diseases. In: *World health statistics annual 1989*. WHO, Geneva; 25-149.

WHO (1996). *The tobacco epidemic: a global public health emergency,* 118. WHO. (Fact sheet.) http://www.who.int/psa/toh/Alert/apr96/fulltext.html 2.

WHO MONICA Project (1988). Geographical variation in the major risk factors of coronary heart disease in men and women aged 35-64 years. *World Health Stat Q,* **41**, 115-40.

WHO (1997). *Tobacco or health: A global status report*. WHO, Geneva. www.cdc.gov/nccdphp/osh/who/whoampro.htm.

Iceland 13

Sales data

See Tables 13.1-13.3.

The consumption of manufactured cigarettes per adult was about 1 cigarette per day during the 1930s. There was a peak in consumption around the end of the Second World War, then a steady increase until the mid 1980s when it reached 7 cigarettes per day. It decreased to 5 cigarettes per day by 1995. There is no tradition of hand-rolled cigarette consumption in Iceland.

Data on all tobacco products combined are available from 1862. The consumption of all tobacco products per adult (based on estimated adult population) fluctuated around 3-5 g per day before the 1930s. Thereafter it followed a similar pattern to cigarette consumption, rising from about 3 g per day in the 1930s to 8 g per day in the 1970s and 1980s, then decreasing to 6 g per day by 1995. The proportion smoked as manufactured cigarettes was about 40% in the 1930s, with the majority of the remainder being used as snuff. The proportion of cigarettes has since increased to nearly 90% while the proportion used as snuff has decreased, to below 5% since 1974. The proportion smoked as cigars and cigarillos has usually been less than 10% while the proportion smoked in pipes has varied around 5-20%. Very little chewing tobacco is used.

Survey data

See Tables 13.4-13.8

The prevalence of smoking has been reported regularly since 1985, but little information is available for earlier years, or according to the type of tobacco product smoked. In 1985 the prevalence of regular smoking among those aged 15 years and over was 43% in men and 37% in women. It decreased, rapidly over the next 5 years, more for men than for women, so that by 1990 there was little difference between the sexes. The decrease continued slowly, and the prevalence of regular smoking in 1995 was 27% for both men and women. About a further 4% of men and women smoke occasionally. There is no clear pattern in the trends over time by age group, with the prevalence of smoking having decreased in most age groups, but increased in some others. Only one survey (source 4, 1983) reported the prevalence of smoking according to type of tobacco, although this was somewhat obscured by a difference in the definition of frequency of smoking used. This suggests that other products but not cigarettes are smoked by about 40% of male smokers at age 25-34, increasing to about 60% at age 55-64, but by few female smokers.

Nearly all surveys of teenagers showed that more girls than boys smoked. A series of surveys in Reykyavik schools (source 3) showed a substantial decrease in the prevalence of smoking between 1974 and 1986—from 22% to 8% for boys and from 24% to 10% for girls (daily smoking, age 12-16).

It was not possible to estimate the number of cigarettes smoked per person per day by men and women from the survey data available, nor to assess any possible under-statement by comparison of sales and survey data.

Table 13.1.1 Total annual sales of tobacco products, 1862-1973

Year	Cigarettes tonnes	Cigarettes millions	Cigars tonnes	Cigars millions	Smoking tobacco tonnes	Snuff tonnes	All tobacco products tonnes
1862-1865							58
1866-1870							56
1871-1875							63
1876-1880							74
1881-1885							86
1886-1890							82
1891-1895							88
1896-1900							96
1901-1905							100
1906-1910							91
1911-1915							96
1916-1920							112
1921-1925							86
1926-1930							124
1932	37	37	5	1	18	36	100
1933	48	48	5	1	18	36	110
1934	55	55	5	1	18	27	120
1935	39	39	5	1	14	32	100
1936	32	32	5	1	18	32	90
1937	36	36	5	1	18	32	100
1938	38	38	5	1	18	45	120
1939	27	27	5	1	18	32	90
1940	54	54	5	1	32	18	110
1941	66	66	7	1	23	27	130
1942	76	76	9	1	18	32	140
1943	72	72	20	3	5	36	140
1944	77	77	9	1	9	36	130
1945	112	112	5	1	14	32	170
1946	167	167	18	3	18	32	240
1947	157	157	9	1	14	45	230
1948	159	159	5	1	23	36	220
1949	143	143	9	1	14	36	210
1950	148	148	9	1	23	36	220
1951	141	141	5	1	14	36	200
1952	141	141	5	1	23	36	200
1953	162	162	9	1	23	36	230
1954	145	145	14	2	18	36	210
1955	151	151	14	2	18	36	220
1956	173	173	9	1	18	36	240
1957	199	199	14	2	23	41	280
1958	197	197	23	3	18	32	270
1959	194	194	27	4	18	36	280
1960	196	196	23	3	23	32	270
1961	217	217	27	4	27	32	300
1962	229	229	36	5	32	32	330
1963	243	243	45	7	27	32	350
1964	202	202	64	9	45	32	340
1965	232	232	68	10	41	32	370
1966	258	258	75	11	41	32	410
1967	270	270	82	12	41	32	420
1968	250	250	68	10	59	32	410
1969	221	221	68	10	91	27	410
1970	254	254	75	11	82	27	440
1971	254	254	88	13	68	27	440
1972	291	291	109	16	64	27	490
1973	298	298	122	18	59	23	500

Source: see *Notes on sources of sales data*, p. 330

Table 13.1.2 Total annual sales of tobacco products, 1974-1995

Year	Cigarettes		Cigars and cigarillos		Smoking tobacco	Snuff and chewing tobacco	All tobacco products
	tonnes	millions	tonnes	millions	tonnes	tonnes	tonnes
1974	342	342	48	19	57	20	467
1975	335	335	48	19	65	17	465
1976	350	350	50	20	61	17	478
1977	333	333	44	18	51	16	443
1978	349	349	40	16	46	14	450
1979	373	373	38	15	45	14	470
1980	378	378	36	14	45	15	474
1981	407	407	36	14	43	15	501
1982	416	416	35	14	39	15	504
1983	438	438	36	14	37	15	525
1984	447	447	38	15	36	15	536
1985	435	435	36	14	28	13	512
1986	430	430	36	14	23	12	501
1987	441	441	36	14	18	13	508
1988	431	431	34	14	17	12	494
1989	418	418	33	13	16	12	479
1990	413	413	32	13	16	12	472
1991	417	417	32	13	14	13	476
1992	403	403	30	12	14	13	460
1993	384	384	29	12	13	12	439
1994	381	381	29	11	13	13	435
1995	369	369	28	11	12	12	421

Source : see *Notes on sources of sales data,* p. 330

Table 13.1.3 Manufactured cigarettes, percentage of total sales as filter cigarettes, 1975

Year	% Filter
1975	66.2

Source : see *Notes on sources of sales data,* p. 330

Table 13.2 Consumption of (i) cigarettes and (ii) all tobacco products, 1862-1995 sales-based data, including estimated hand-rolled cigarette consumption. Males and females aged 15 years and over

Year	Manufactured cigarettes		Hand-rolled cigarettes		Total cigarettes		All tobacco products	
	Total annual in millions	Number/ adult/day	Total annual in millions	Number/ adult/day	Total annual in millions	Number/ adult/day	Total annual in tonnes	Grams/ adult/day
1862-1865							58	3.4
1866-1870							56	3.2
1871-1875							63	3.5
1876-1880							74	4.1
1881-1885							86	4.7
1886-1890							82	4.7
1891-1895							88	4.7
1896-1900							96	4.8
1901-1905							100	5.0
1906-1910							91	4.2
1911-1915							96	4.4
1916-1920							112	4.8
1921-1925							86	3.5
1926-1930							124	4.7
1932	37	1.3					100	3.4
1933	48	1.6					110	3.8
1934	55	1.9					120	4.1
1935	39	1.3					100	3.4
1936	32	1.1					90	3.1
1937	36	1.2					100	3.4
1938	38	1.3					120	4.1
1939	27	0.9					90	3.1
1940	54	1.6					110	3.3
1941	66	2.0					130	4.0
1942	76	2.3					140	4.3
1943	72	2.2					140	4.3
1944	77	2.3					130	4.0
1945	112	3.4					170	5.2
1946	167	5.1					240	7.3
1947	157	4.8					230	7.0
1948	159	4.4					220	6.0
1949	143	3.9					210	5.8
1950	148	4.1					220	6.1
1951	141	3.8					200	5.4
1952	141	3.8					200	5.4
1953	162	4.3					230	6.1
1954	145	3.8					210	5.5
1955	151	3.9					220	5.7
1956	173	4.4					240	6.1
1957	199	5.0					280	7.1
1958	197	4.9					270	6.7
1959	194	4.8					280	6.9
1960	196	4.7					270	6.5
1961	217	5.1					300	7.0
1962	229	5.3					330	7.6
1963	243	5.5					350	7.9
1964	202	4.5					340	7.5
1965	232	5.1					370	8.1
1966	258	5.5					410	8.7
1967	270	5.6					420	8.8
1968	250	5.1					410	8.4
1969	221	4.5					410	8.3

Table 13.2 *(continued)*

Year	Manufactured cigarettes		Hand-rolled cigarettes		Total cigarettes		All tobacco products	
	Total annual in millions	Number/ adult/day	Total annual in millions	Number/ adult/day	Total annual in millions	Number/ adult/day	Total annual in tonnes	Grams/ adult/day
1970	254	5.1					440	8.8
1971	254	5.0					440	8.6
1972	291	5.6					490	9.4
1973	298	5.6					500	9.4
1974	342	6.3					467	8.6
1975	335	6.0					465	8.4
1976	350	6.2					478	8.4
1977	333	5.8					443	7.7
1978	349	6.0					450	7.7
1979	373	6.3					470	7.9
1980	378	6.3					474	7.8
1981	407	6.6					501	8.2
1982	416	6.7					504	8.1
1983	438	6.9					525	8.3
1984	447	7.0					536	8.3
1985	435	6.7					512	7.9
1986	430	6.6					501	7.6
1987	441	6.6					508	7.6
1988	431	6.3					494	7.2
1989	418	6.0					479	6.9
1990	413	5.9					472	6.8
1991	417	5.9					476	6.7
1992	403	5.6					460	6.4
1993	384	5.3					439	6.1
1994	381	5.2					435	6.0
1995	369	5.0					421	5.7

Source : see *Notes on sources of sales data*, p. 330

Figure 13.1 Daily consumption of (i) manufactured cigarettes, and (ii) all tobacco products, 1920-1995.
Males and females aged 15 years and over. *Source:* see Table 13.2

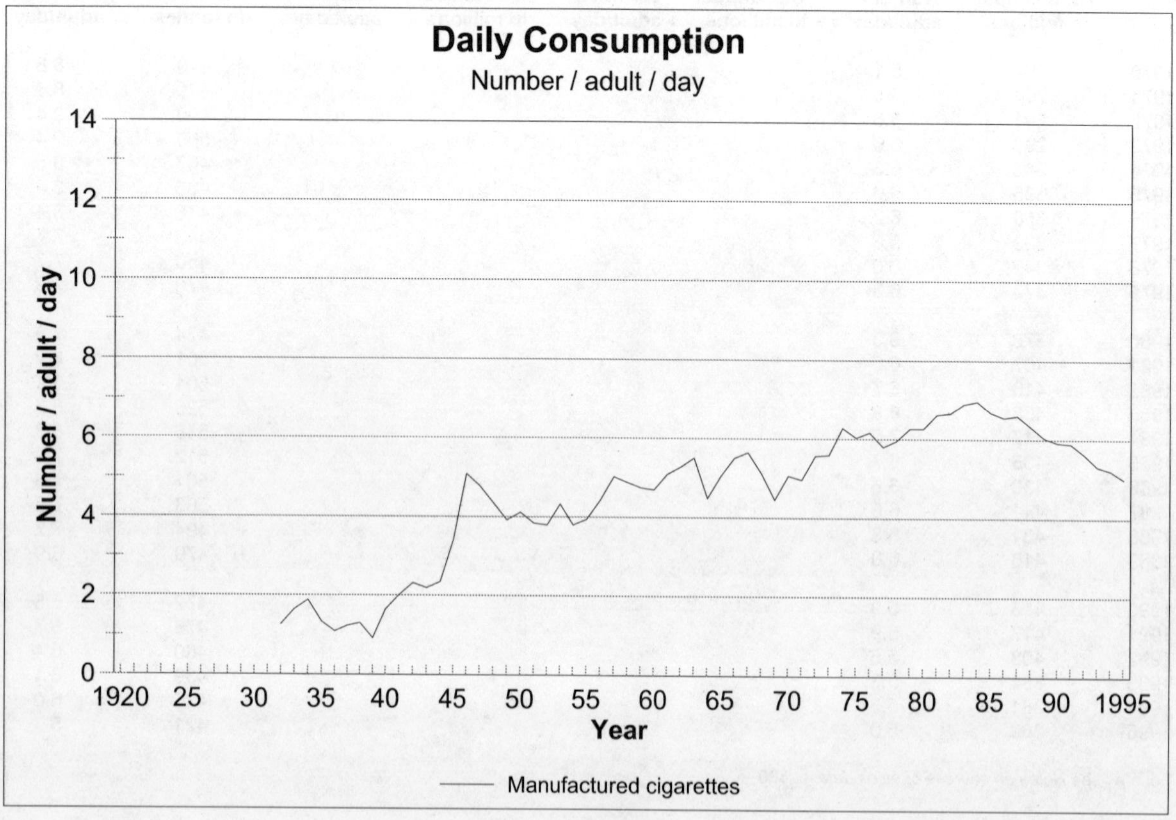

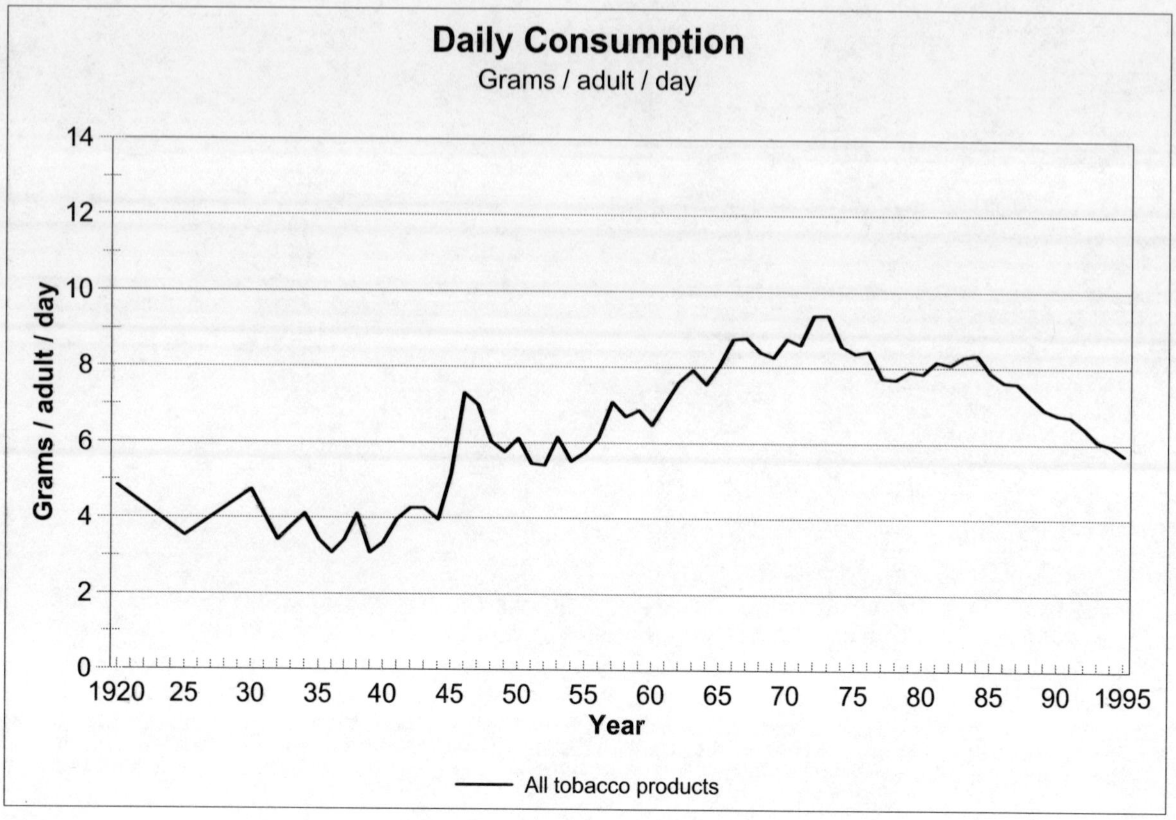

Table 13.3 Percentage sales of tobacco in different forms (by weight), selected years 1935-1995

Year	Cigarettes (%)	Cigars and cigarillos (%)	Smoking tobacco (%)	Snuff and chewing tobacco (%)
1935	39.0	5.0	14.0	32.0
1945	65.9	2.9	8.2	27.1
1955	68.6	6.4	8.2	24.5
1965	62.7	18.4	11.1	19.7
1975	72.0	10.3	13.9	13.9
1985	85.0	7.0	5.6	5.6
1995	87.6	6.6	2.9	2.9

Source : calculated from Tables 13.1.1 & 13.1.2

Figure 13.2 Percentage sales of tobacco in different forms (by weight), selected years 1935-1995
Source: see Table 13.3

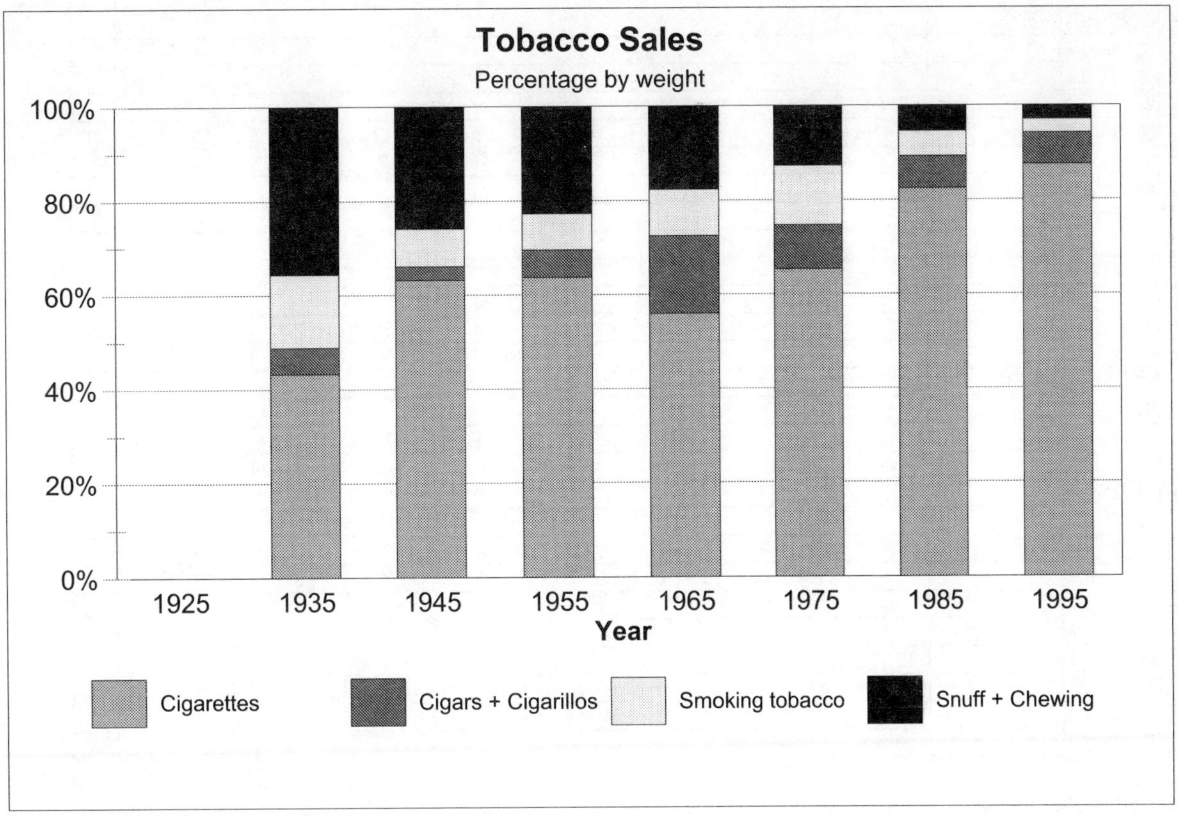

Table 13.4M Prevalence of smoking, males: some selected Icelandic surveys by age, 1968-1995

Year	Source	Product	Frequency	Age group																					
				12	13	14	15	16	17	18	19	20-24	25-29	30-34	35-39	40-44	45-49	50-54	55-59	60-64	65-69	70-74	75-79	80+	All ages
68	2	U	R				55																		
74	3	U	R	22																					
74	3	U	A	31																					
78	2	U	R																						
78	3	U	R	15																					
78	3	U	A	20																					
82	3	U	R	13																					
82	3	U	A	16																					
83	4	UC	R										37		31		26		19						26
83	4	A	A										58		59		47		45						51
85	2	U	R				43																		
86	2	U	R				37																		
86	3	U	R	1	2	8	16	25																	8
86	3	U	A	11																					
87	1	U	R				28						45		42		35		33		29		18		36
87	1	U	A				40																		
87	2	U	R				38																		
88	1	U	R				33																		
88	1	U	A				37																		
88	2	U	R				35																		
89	1	U	R				15					35		36		35		29		32		14			31
89	1	U	A				16					38		40		41		33		37		14			35
89	2	U	R				34																		
90	1	U	R				31																		
90	1	U	A				35																		
90	2	U	R				33																		
90	5	U	R				11	11																	
91	1	U	R				15					33		43		33		35		27		19			31
91	1	U	A				17					37		47		37		36		29		19			34
92	1	U	R				28																		
92	1	U	A				33																		
93	1	U	R				16					28		33		32		24		19		16		17	26
93	1	U	A				19					30		35		36		25		21		17		20	28
93	1*	U	R				26																		
93	1*	U	A				29																		
94	1	U	R				16					32		35		31		31		24		16		3	27
94	1	U	A				19					36		40		35		32		25		17		3	30
94	1*	U	R				28																		
94	1*	U	A				31																		
94	5	U	R				15	26																	
95	1	U	R				17					25		35		30		30		22		20		9	26
95	1	U	A				20					33		41		37		34		27		21		9	32
95	1*	U	R				27																		
95	1*	U	A				32																		
95	6	UC	R				22																		
95	6	UC	A				30																		

Source: see *Notes on sources of survey data*, p. 330

Product: MC = manufactured cigarettes
TC = total cigarettes (including hand-rolled)
UC = cigarettes (type unspecified)
A = all products

Frequency: A = all smokers (including occasional)
R = regular or daily smokers

All ages: relevant to ages used and as given in original source

U = unspecified

* = refer to *Notes on sources of survey data*, p. 330

Table 13.4F Prevalence of smoking, females: some selected Icelandic surveys by age, 1968-1995

Frequency / Product / Source / Year	Age group 12	13	14	15	16	17	18	19	20-24	25-29	30-34	35-39	40-44	45-49	50-54	55-59	60-64	65-69	70-74	75-79	80+	All ages
68 2 U R																						
74 3 U R	24																					
74 3 U A	34																					
78 2 U R				42																		
78 3 U R	19																					
78 3 U A	27																					
82 3 U R	17																					
82 3 U A	22																					
83 4 UC R										46		45		39		34						40
83 4 A A										50		49		44		39						44
85 2 U R				37																		
86 2 U R				35																		
86 3 U R	0	4	11	22	27																	10
86 3 U A	14																					
87 1 U R				28						37		40		31		25		19		15		31
87 1 U A				35																		
87 2 U R				33																		
88 1 U R				32																		
88 1 U A				36																		
88 2 U R				34																		
89 1 U R				16					35		35		41		35		30		21			33
89 1 U A				20					39		41		44		36		32		24			36
89 2 U R				35																		
90 1 U R				30																		
90 1 U A				33																		
90 2 U R				32																		
90 5 U R				13	18																	
91 1 U R				19					34		38		33		30		18		20			30
91 1 U A				23					37		42		35		32		19		20			33
92 1 U R				30																		
92 1 U A				33																		
93 1 U R				19					25		34		33		30		26		13		10	27
93 1 U A				22					29		38		36		31		28		15		12	29
93 1* U R				27																		
93 1* U A				30																		
94 1 U R				14					29		31		32		29		15		21		16	26
94 1 U A				19					34		34		36		30		20		21		18	29
94 1* U R				26																		
94 1* U A				30																		
94 5 U R				20	19																	
95 1 U R				19					28		37		30		24		19		19		20	27
95 1 U A				29					34		42		36		28		24		21		24	32
95 1* U R				27																		
95 1* U A				33																		
95 6 UC R				20																		
95 6 UC A				33																		

Source: see *Notes on sources of survey data*, p. 330
Product: MC = manufactured cigarettes
TC = total cigarettes (including hand-rolled)
UC = cigarettes (type unspecified)
A = all products

Frequency: A = all smokers (including occasional)
R = regular or daily smokers
All ages: relevant to ages used and as given in original source
U = unspecified
* = refer to *Notes on sources of survey data*, p. 330

Table 13.5M Number of cigarettes smoked per smoker per day, males: some selected Icelandic surveys by age, 1983-1995

<table>
<tr><th rowspan="2">Product
Source
Year</th><th colspan="21">Age group</th><th rowspan="2">All ages</th></tr>
<tr><th>12</th><th>13</th><th>14</th><th>15</th><th>16</th><th>17</th><th>18</th><th>19</th><th>20-24</th><th>25-29</th><th>30-34</th><th>35-39</th><th>40-44</th><th>45-49</th><th>50-54</th><th>55-59</th><th>60-64</th><th>65-69</th><th>70-74</th><th>75-79</th><th>80+</th></tr>
<tr><td>83 4 UC</td><td colspan="11"></td><td colspan="6">20</td><td colspan="5"></td><td></td></tr>
<tr><td>95 6 UCE</td><td colspan="3"></td><td colspan="2">12</td><td colspan="16"></td><td></td></tr>
</table>

Table 13.6M Number of cigarettes smoked per person per day, males: some selected Icelandic surveys by age, 1983-1995, with percentage total sales

<table>
<tr><th rowspan="2">Product
Source
Year</th><th colspan="21">Age group</th><th rowspan="2">All ages</th><th rowspan="2">% Total sales</th></tr>
<tr><th>12</th><th>13</th><th>14</th><th>15</th><th>16</th><th>17</th><th>18</th><th>19</th><th>20-24</th><th>25-29</th><th>30-34</th><th>35-39</th><th>40-44</th><th>45-49</th><th>50-54</th><th>55-59</th><th>60-64</th><th>65-69</th><th>70-74</th><th>75-79</th><th>80+</th></tr>
<tr><td>83 4 UC *</td><td colspan="11"></td><td colspan="6">5.3</td><td colspan="5"></td><td></td><td>**</td></tr>
<tr><td>95 6 UC</td><td colspan="3"></td><td colspan="2">2.6</td><td colspan="16"></td><td></td><td>**</td></tr>
</table>

Table 13.7 is omitted because no sales-adjustment was possible

Source: see *Notes on sources of survey data*, p. 330
All ages: relevant to ages used and as given in original source
% Total sales: estimated % of total sales of M = manufactured or T = total cigarette consumption implied by the survey, sexes combined
** = cannot be calculated
--- = adjusted by original author
* = refer to *Notes on sources of survey data*, p. 330

Product:
MC = manufactured cigarettes
TC = total cigarettes (including hand-rolled)
UC = cigarettes (type unspecified)
A = all products
U = unspecified
E indicates mean estimated from percentage distribution (see also *Consumption category estimation*, p. xxxiv, and Appendix III, p. 789)

Table 13.5F Number of cigarettes smoked per smoker per day, females: some selected Icelandic surveys by age, 1983-1995

<table>
<tr><th rowspan="2">Product
Source
Year</th><th colspan="21">Age group</th><th rowspan="2">All ages</th></tr>
<tr><th>12</th><th>13</th><th>14</th><th>15</th><th>16</th><th>17</th><th>18</th><th>19</th><th>20-24</th><th>25-29</th><th>30-34</th><th>35-39</th><th>40-44</th><th>45-49</th><th>50-54</th><th>55-59</th><th>60-64</th><th>65-69</th><th>70-74</th><th>75-79</th><th>80+</th></tr>
<tr><td>83 4 UC</td><td colspan="11"></td><td colspan="6">15</td><td colspan="4"></td><td></td></tr>
<tr><td>95 6 UCE</td><td colspan="3"></td><td colspan="2">10</td><td colspan="16"></td><td></td></tr>
</table>

Table 13.6F Number of cigarettes smoked per person per day, females: some selected Icelandic surveys by age, 1983-1995, with percentage total sales

<table>
<tr><th rowspan="2">Product
Source
Year</th><th colspan="21">Age group</th><th rowspan="2">All ages</th><th rowspan="2">% Total sales</th></tr>
<tr><th>12</th><th>13</th><th>14</th><th>15</th><th>16</th><th>17</th><th>18</th><th>19</th><th>20-24</th><th>25-29</th><th>30-34</th><th>35-39</th><th>40-44</th><th>45-49</th><th>50-54</th><th>55-59</th><th>60-64</th><th>65-69</th><th>70-74</th><th>75-79</th><th>80+</th></tr>
<tr><td>83 4 UC *</td><td colspan="11"></td><td colspan="6">6.0</td><td colspan="4"></td><td></td><td>**</td></tr>
<tr><td>95 6 UC</td><td colspan="3"></td><td colspan="2">2.1</td><td colspan="16"></td><td></td><td>**</td></tr>
</table>

Table 13.7 is omitted because no sales-adjustment was possible

Source: see *Notes on sources of survey data*, p. 330
All ages: relevant to ages used and as given in original source
% Total sales: estimated % of total sales of M = manufactured or T = total cigarette consumption implied by the survey, sexes combined
** = cannot be calculated
--- = adjusted by original author
* = refer to *Notes on sources of survey data*, p. 330

Product: MC = manufactured cigarettes
TC = total cigarettes (including hand-rolled)
UC = cigarettes (type unspecified)
A = all products
U = unspecified
E indicates mean estimated from percentage distribution (see also *Consumption category estimation*, p. xxxiv, and Appendix III, p. 789)

Table 13.8 Estimated[1] prevalence of smoking: summary of Table 13.4, 1985-1995. Males and females aged 15 years and over

Year	Source[2]	Product[3]	Prevalence[4]						Number of cigarettes						
									Unadjusted[7]			Sales-adjusted[8]			
			Manufactured cigarettes		Total cigarettes[5]		All products[6]		Number/ person/day		Total sales %	Manufactured cigarettes number/ person/day		Total cigarettes number/ person/day	
			M	F	M	F	M	F	M	F		M	F	M	F
1985	2	U					43	37							
1986	2	U					37	35							
1987	1	U					35	30							
	1	**U**					39	34							
	2	U					38	33							
1988	1	U					32	31							
	1	**U**					36	34							
	2	U					35	34							
1989	1	U					30	31							
	1	**U**					34	35							
	2	U					33	35							
1990	1	U					30	29							
	1	**U**					35	32							
	2	U					33	32							
1991	1	U					31	29							
	1	**U**					34	32							
1992	1	U					28	29							
	1	**U**					33	32							
1993	1	U					26	27							
	1	**U**					28	29							
1994	1	U					28	26							
	1	**U**					31	29							
1995	1	U					27	27							
	1	**U**					32	32							

1 Surveys covering an age range of at least 21-64 are included. Any gaps in the data for ages 15-20 and 65 years and over are filled in by assumed extensions to the age distribution, given in *Notes on sources of survey data*, p. 330. Method: see *Summary of adult smoking*, p. xxxvi
2 See *Notes on sources of survey data*, p. 330
3 Product: MC = manufactured cigarettes, TC = total cigarettes (including hand-rolled), UC = cigarettes (type unspecified), A = all products, U = unspecified. Frequency of smoking is indicated by: regular or daily smokers in normal type, all smokers (including occasional) in bold, unspecified in italics
4 From Table 13.4
5 This column includes prevalence of smoking classified as UC = cigarettes (type unspecified)
6 This column includes prevalence of smoking classified as U = unspecified product
7,8 No suitable data exist in Tables 13.4 or 13.6 to allow the number of cigarettes per person to be estimated or sales-adjustment to be carried out

Figure 13.3 Estimated prevalence of smoking: by year of survey, 1985-1995. Males and females aged 15 years and over. *Source:* see Table 13.8

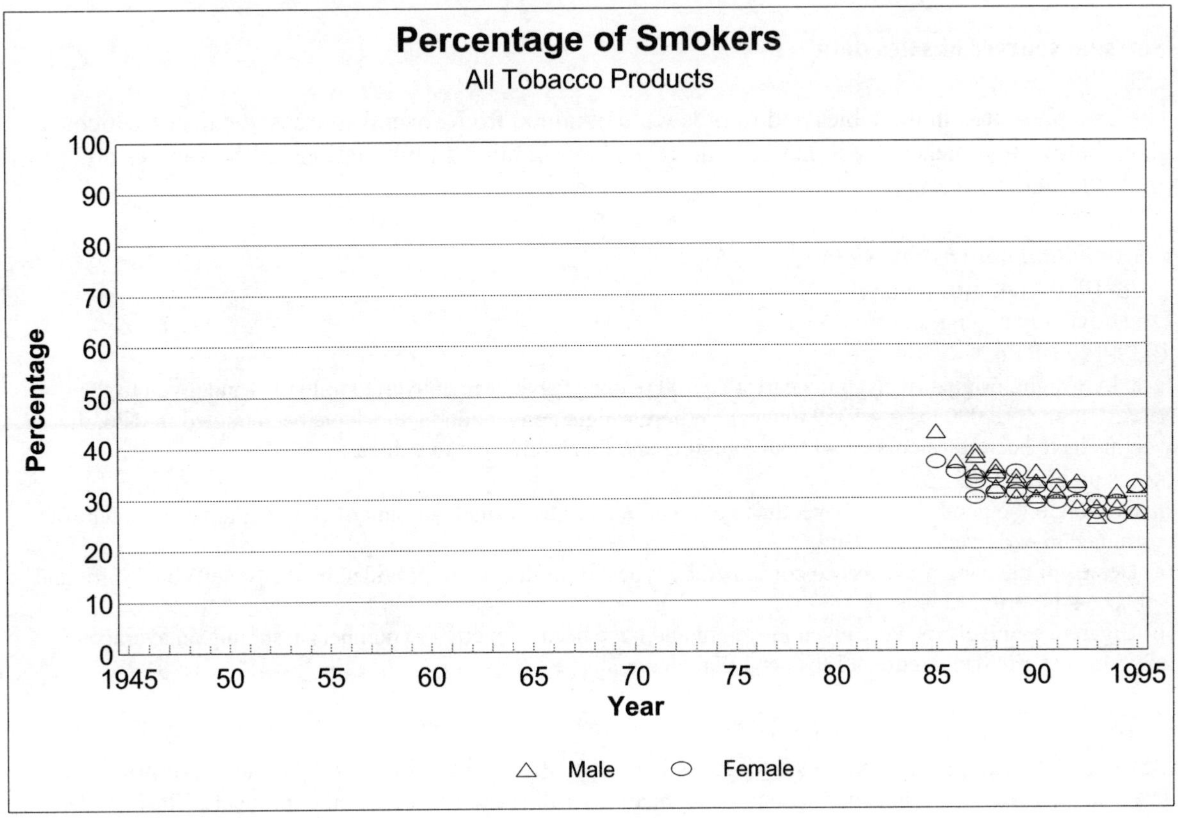

Notes on sources of sales data

The data presented in the tables and figures were obtained from several sources, details of which are given below, together with estimations and related assumptions. Full citations of the sources are given on p. 332 under *References*.

Consumption data before 1974

1825-1930 Statistics Iceland

Data originally in tonnes.

1932-1973 RP6

Data by weight, originally given to nearest 10 000 pounds, have been converted to tonnes and given to the nearest tonne (10 000 lbs = 4.5359 tonnes). Where weight conversion factors have been quoted in RP6, the weights have been re-calculated without rounding and then converted to tonnes.

Notes as given in RP6:

In addition to the goods listed above, the total column includes a small amount of chewing tobacco which was consumed in early years in Iceland.

(a) Details of the weight of tobacco consumed by types of product were provided by the State Wine, Spirit and Tobacco Authority, Reykjavik.

(b) Cigarettes, and cigars were given in weight and have been converted to numbers assuming an average of 2.205 lbs per 1 000 cigarettes, 15 lbs per 1 000 cigars.

Consumption data for 1974 onwards

Statistics Iceland, quoting wholesale figures from the State Wine, Spirit and Tobacco Authority.

The data are given in millions for cigarettes and cigars/cigarillos and tonnes for other products. They are the same as the RP6 data for overlapping years (1960-1973).

For 1965-1994 Statistics Iceland give data for sales of snuff and chewing tobacco separately. The sales of snuff are far greater than sales of chewing tobacco, the latter ranging from 268 kg (1968) to 27 kg (1993). The snuff is said to be mostly of the traditional type. Moist snuff began to attract young people but its import was banned in 1996.

Statistics Iceland suggest conversion factors of 1 g per cigarette and 2 g or 2.5 g per cigar/cigarillo. RP6 uses the equivalent of 1 g per cigarette and 6.8 g per cigar. We use 1 g per cigarette and 2.5 g per cigar/cigarillo for 1974 onwards.

Plain/Filter cigarette consumption

Maxwell (successive years)

Data available only for 1975. The proportion is believed to have increased considerably since then.

Tar yield of cigarettes

The tar yield per cigarette was limited from 1996 to 15 mg (Harkin *et al* (1997)). No other data available.

Estimates of hand-rolled cigarette consumption

There is no tradition for hand rolled cigarettes in Iceland (Statistics Iceland). They have been ignored in all calculations.

Notes on sources of survey data

Each source of survey data—either an individual survey or a series of surveys repeated over a number of years—is cited by a source number. This number is shown in the tables and corresponds to the source numbers given below, where details of the source publication and of the survey methodology are given. Full citations of the sources are given on p. 332 under *References*.

Source number

1 Statistics Iceland (personal communication), Statistika Centralbyrån (1995), quoting the Committee for Tobacco Use Prevention and Statistics Yearbook of Iceland (various years)

a. Three telephone surveys per year by Hagvangur/Price Waterhouse Coopers for the Committee for Tobacco Use Prevention. Response rate (1987) 78%, (1994) 75%.

	Sample size	
	Males	**Females**
1987	1 550	1 673
1988	1 620	1 634
1989	1 579	1 652
1990	1 580	1 681
1991	1 532	1 613
1992	1 569	1 591
1993	1 590	1 637
1994	1 541	1 591
1995	1 513	1 538

b. Age groups sampled were 15-79 in 1987-1992 and 15-89 in 1993-1995. For 1993 onwards, overall prevalence for the 15-79 year age group is shown in Table 13.4, in addition to the breakdown for ages 15-89, for comparison with previous years

c. Assumed extension to age distribution for percentage smokers, age 80+: males and females (1987-1992) 12%. For 1993-1995 the prevalence at age 80-87 has been assumed to apply to age 80+

2 Blöndal *et al* (1991)

a. Sample sizes:

Year	**Sample size**
1968	—
1978	—
1985	2 708
1986	2 288
1987	2 830
1988	2 844
1989	2 841
1990	2 855

3 Magnússon (1988)

a. Series of studies of schoolchildren in Reykjavik by Reykjavik City Medical Office and Reykjavik Cancer Society. All Reykjavik schoolchildren who were not absent for sickness or similar reason were included. Response rate 85-90%

b. Sample size not known but 40% of Icelandic people live in Reykjavik. School is compulsory up to age 15 years

c. Regular smokers: smoke daily

d. Prevalence for males and females calculated from overall prevalence and girl-boy prevalence ratios

4 WHO (1989), WHO MONICA Project (1988)

a. Regional survey forming part of WHO MONICA project:

Region	**Population size**	**Sample size**	**Participation rate (%)**	**Sample used***		**Date**
				Males	**Females**	
Iceland	29 200	1 793	76	828	918	Mar 1983-Nov 1983

* age 25-64; all other figures are for age 35-64 only

b. *All ages* column relates to age 35-64 and is standardized to world population

c. Regular smokers: smoked cigarettes daily. All smokers: smoked cigarettes daily or occasionally, or 1 g pipe tobacco or 1 cigar per week. Cigarettes per smoker refers to regular and occasional cigarette smokers

d. Calculation for cigarettes per person based on % regular cigarette smokers and cigarettes per regular or occasional cigarette smoker, so may underestimate

Notes *(continued)*

5 **WHO (1997)**

a. No original source

6 **Hibell *et al* (1997)**

a. National survey forming part of ESPAD (European School Survey Project on Alcohol and Other Drugs). Target was all pupils born in 1979, thus age 15-16 at time of survey in January 1995. Approximately 98% of this group still in school. Anonymous questionnaire completed and sealed in envelope by pupil, in class. Teachers present in Reykjavik schools, but discouraged from walking round the classroom, and absent elsewhere. Sample size (males) 1 931, (females) 1 878. Response rate (males) 86%, (females) 88%

b. Regular smokers: smoked 1 or more cigarettes per day in last 30 days. All smokers: smoked in last 30 days

c. Consumption category estimation based on 1-5, 6-10, 11-20, 21+ cigarettes/smoker/day

References

Beese D.H. (ed) (1968). *Tobacco consumption in various countries,* 2nd edition. Tobacco Research Council, London. Research Paper 6.

Beese D.H. (ed) (1972). *Tobacco consumption in various countries,* 3rd edition. Tobacco Research Council, London. Research Paper 6.

Blöndal P., Hardarson P., Helgason T. and Ragnarsson J. (1991). Tobaken eller livet? Minskad rökning i Island 1985-1990 (Smoking or living? Reduced smoking in Iceland in 1985-90). *Nord Med,* **106**, 11-2.

Harkin A.M., Anderson P. and Goos C. (1997). *Smoking, drinking and drug taking in the European Region.* Alcohol, Drugs and Tobacco Programme, WHO Regional Office for Europe, Copenhagen.

Hibell B., Andersson B., Bjarnason T., Kokkevi A., Morgan M. and Narusk A. (1997). *The 1995 ESPAD report. The European school survey project on alcohol and other drugs. Alcohol and other drug use among students in 26 European countries.* The Swedish Council for Information on Alcohol and Other Drugs. Council of Europe (Pompidou Group).

Lee P.N. (ed) (1975). *Tobacco consumption in various countries,* 4th edition. Tobacco Research Council, London. Research Paper 6.

Magnússon S. (1988). Smoking habits of school children in Reykjavík, Iceland 1974 to 1986. In: Aoki M., Hisamichi S. and Tominaga S. (eds) *Smoking and health 1987. Proceedings of the 6th World Conference on Smoking and Health, Tokyo, 9-12 November 1987.* Elsevier Science Publishers B.V. (Biomedical Division), Amsterdam; 547-9. International Congress Series No. 780.

Maxwell J.C.Jr. (successive years). How the brands ranked. Maxwell International Estimates. *World Tobacco.*

RP6, See Beese (ed) (1968), Beese (ed) (1972), Lee (ed) (1975)

Statistika Centralbyrån (1995). *Tobacco consumption 1970-1994 in the member states of the European Union and in Norway and Iceland.* European Commission.

WHO (1989). The WHO MONICA project: a worldwide monitoring system for cardiovascular diseases. In: *World health statistics annual 1989.* WHO, Geneva; 25-149.

WHO MONICA Project (1988). Geographical variation in the major risk factors of coronary heart disease in men and women aged 35-64 years. *World Health Stat Q,* **41**, 115-40.

WHO (1997). *Tobacco or health: A global status report.* WHO, Geneva. www.cdc.gov/nccdphp/osh/who/whoampro.htm.

Ireland 14

Sales data

See Tables 14.1-14.3.

From 1920 until 1950 the consumption of manufactured cigarettes per adult increased from 2 to nearly 8 cigarettes per day, apart from a small decline during the Second World War. It varied between 6.5 and 8 cigarettes per day until 1970 when a further increase took it to nearly 10 cigarettes per adult per day in the mid-1970s. It then decreased, and stabilized around 6-7 between 1985 and 1995. Consumption of hand-rolled cigarettes is low in Ireland, only about 0.1 cigarettes per adult per day.

The consumption of all tobacco products combined per adult increased slowly from 5 g to 6 g per day between 1920 and 1940. After a small decline during the war it rose to a maximum of nearly 9 g per day in 1951. Thereafter it remained at about 8 g until the 1970s, when it started to decrease again to 6 g in 1985. In 1925, about 40% of all tobacco was consumed as manufactured cigarettes and nearly 60% was used as loose smoking tobacco. The proportion of manufactured cigarettes increased to 95% in 1995, while smoking tobacco declined to 4% of sales. Although separate data do not exist until recent years, loose tobacco was predominantly used in pipes, but since the late 1970s the proportion used for hand-rolling has increased, and exceeded use in pipes in the early 1990s. The remaining few per cent of consumption comprised snuff in the earlier years, and cigars since the 1960s.

Survey data

See Tables 14.4-14.8

In 1967, the prevalence of tobacco smoking among those aged 15 years and over was about 70% in men and nearly 40% in women. The prevalence of cigarette smoking was 55% in men; very few women smoked products other than cigarettes. By the 1990s the prevalence of smoking among men decreased to about 35% for all smoking and 30% for cigarette smoking, while among women it decreased to 26-28%.

Nationally based data on adult smoking by age are available only for 1977 and 1980. In this 3-year period there was a decrease in smoking prevalence for both sexes at age 15-19, and also among men aged 55 or over.

The prevalence of smoking among teenage girls was much lower than among boys when first surveyed in the late 1950s and early 1960s. By the 1980s, most surveys indicate that it had increased except among older boys (aged 16-18); the prevalence among girls was still generally lower than among boys, but to a lesser extent. By the 1990s most surveys showed that slightly more girls smoked than boys.

Comparison of survey and sales data gave inconsistent results. Some surveys reported consumption similar to sales data but others under-reported consumption by 25%. It has not been possible to make this comparison for any surveys since 1980. Between 1967 and 1980, the estimated number of cigarettes smoked per person per day (sales-adjusted) varied between 10 and 12 for men and increased from 4 to 7 for women. It then decreased to about 7 for men and 5 for women by 1995.

Table 14.1.1 Total annual sales of tobacco products, 1920-1974

Year	Cigarettes tonnes	Cigarettes millions	Cigars tonnes	Cigars millions	Smoking tobacco tonnes	Snuff tonnes	All tobacco products tonnes
1920	1410	1406	0	0	2490	140	4040
1921	1360	1361	0	0	2490	140	3990
1922	1320	1315	0	0	2400	140	3860
1923	1360	1361	0	0	2220	140	3720
1924	1410	1406	0	0	2220	140	3760
1925	1500	1497	0	0	2220	140	3860
1926	1540	1542	0	0	2130	140	3810
1927	1630	1633	0	0	2090	140	3860
1928	1720	1723	0	0	2040	140	3900
1929	1810	1814	0	0	2000	140	3950
1930	1950	1950	0	0	2000	140	4080
1931	2130	2132	0	0	1910	140	4170
1932	2220	2222	0	0	1720	140	4080
1933	2310	2313	0	0	1720	90	4130
1934	2490	2494	0	0	1630	90	4220
1935	2540	2540	0	0	1630	90	4260
1936	2590	2585	0	0	1630	90	4310
1937	2720	2721	0	0	1630	90	4450
1938	2900	2900	0	0	1590	90	4580
1939	3040	3038	0	0	1500	90	4630
1940	3180	3175	0	0	1410	90	4670
1941	2770	2766	0	0	1270	90	4130
1942	2770	2766	0	0	1270	90	4130
1943	3180	3175	0	0	1360	90	4630
1944	3400	3401	0	0	1410	90	4900
1945	3270	3265	0	0	1450	90	4810
1946	4130	4127	0	0	1500	90	5720
1947	4350	4354	0	0	1360	90	5810
1948	4580	4580	0	0	1220	90	5900
1949	4990	4989	0	0	1270	90	6350
1950	5260	5261	0	0	1270	50	6580
1951	5940	5941	0	0	1220	50	7210
1952	5580	5578	0	0	950	50	6580
1953	5350	5400	0	0	1130	50	6530
1954	5220	5220	0	0	950	50	6210
1955	5490	5500	0	0	1000	50	6530
1956	5030	5027	0	0	860	50	5940
1957	4900	4850	0	0	820	50	5760
1958	4810	4765	0	0	820	50	5670
1959	4940	4942	0	0	770	50	5760
1960	5130	5115	0	0	730	50	5900
1961	5310	5325	0	0	730	50	6080
1962	5220	5270	0	0	730	50	5990
1963	5490	5570	0	0	730	50	6260
1964	5260	5360	50	12	770	0	6080
1965	5220	5380	50	12	730	0	5990
1966	5310	5530	50	12	640	0	5990
1967	5260	5603	50	16	640	0	5940
1968	5260	5700	50	16	590	0	5900
1969	5310	5925	50	23	590	0	5940
1970	5260	6070	50	30	540	0	5850
1971	5260	6105	90	40	590	0	5940
1972	5530	6510	90	55	540	0	6170
1973	5850	6975	90	55	540	0	6490
1974	6170	7500	90	60	540	0	6800

Source: see *Notes on sources of sales data*, p. 350

Table 14.1.2 Total annual sales of tobacco products, 1975-1995

<table>
<tr><th>Year</th><th colspan="2">Cigarettes</th><th colspan="2">Cigars</th><th>Pipe tobacco</th><th>Hand-rolling tobacco</th><th>All tobacco products</th></tr>
<tr><th></th><th>tonnes</th><th>millions</th><th>tonnes</th><th>millions</th><th>tonnes</th><th>tonnes</th><th>tonnes</th></tr>
<tr><td>1975</td><td>5990</td><td>7520</td><td>90</td><td>59</td><td colspan="2">500</td><td>6580</td></tr>
<tr><td>1976</td><td>5900</td><td>7490</td><td>90</td><td>65</td><td colspan="2">500</td><td>6490</td></tr>
<tr><td>1977</td><td>5710</td><td>7260</td><td>140</td><td>67</td><td colspan="2">450</td><td>6300</td></tr>
<tr><td>1978</td><td>6168</td><td>7725</td><td>149</td><td></td><td>429</td><td>48</td><td>6794</td></tr>
<tr><td>1979</td><td>6084</td><td>7603</td><td>163</td><td></td><td>386</td><td>50</td><td>6683</td></tr>
<tr><td>1980</td><td>6058</td><td>7518</td><td>161</td><td></td><td>367</td><td>54</td><td>6640</td></tr>
<tr><td>1981</td><td>5910</td><td>7297</td><td>144</td><td></td><td colspan="2">400</td><td>6454</td></tr>
<tr><td>1982</td><td>5560</td><td>6794</td><td>150</td><td></td><td colspan="2">403</td><td>6113</td></tr>
<tr><td>1983</td><td>5387</td><td>6539</td><td>132</td><td></td><td colspan="2">396</td><td>5915</td></tr>
<tr><td>1984</td><td>5267</td><td>6373</td><td>125</td><td></td><td>247</td><td>116</td><td>5755</td></tr>
<tr><td>1985</td><td>5248</td><td>6226</td><td>112</td><td></td><td>231</td><td>121</td><td>5712</td></tr>
<tr><td>1986</td><td>4945</td><td>5887</td><td>109</td><td></td><td>205</td><td>127</td><td>5386</td></tr>
<tr><td>1987</td><td>4728</td><td>5628</td><td>97</td><td></td><td>183</td><td>122</td><td>5130</td></tr>
<tr><td>1988</td><td>4702</td><td>5598</td><td>92</td><td></td><td>164</td><td>118</td><td>5076</td></tr>
<tr><td>1989</td><td>4751</td><td>5656</td><td>87</td><td></td><td>147</td><td>109</td><td>5094</td></tr>
<tr><td>1990</td><td>4872</td><td>5800</td><td>88</td><td></td><td>133</td><td>109</td><td>5202</td></tr>
<tr><td>1991</td><td>5260</td><td>6262</td><td>90</td><td></td><td>135</td><td>122</td><td>5607</td></tr>
<tr><td>1992</td><td>5038</td><td>5998</td><td>84</td><td></td><td>115</td><td>122</td><td>5359</td></tr>
<tr><td>1993</td><td>4820</td><td>5738</td><td>79</td><td></td><td>102</td><td>119</td><td>5120</td></tr>
<tr><td>1994</td><td>5006</td><td>5959</td><td>75</td><td></td><td>90</td><td>120</td><td>5291</td></tr>
<tr><td>1995</td><td>5347</td><td>6365</td><td>79</td><td></td><td>89</td><td>122</td><td>5637</td></tr>
</table>

Source : see *Notes on sources of sales data*, p. 350

Table 14.1.3 Manufactured cigarettes, percentage of total sales as filter cigarettes, 1962-1983

Year	% Filter
1962	10.0
1963	15.0
1964	19.0
1965	35.0
1968	55.0
1969	62.0
1970	66.7
1971	71.0
1972	74.0
1973	78.0
1978	85.0
1980	87.0
1981	87.3
1982	89.0
1983	89.0

Source : see *Notes on sources of sales data*, p. 350

Table 14.2 Consumption of (i) cigarettes and (ii) all tobacco products, 1920-1995 sales-based data, including estimated hand-rolled cigarette consumption. Males and females aged 15 years and over

Year	Manufactured cigarettes		Hand-rolled cigarettes		Total cigarettes		All tobacco products	
	Total annual in millions	Number/ adult/day	Total annual in millions	Number/ adult/day	Total annual in millions	Number/ adult/day	Total annual in tonnes	Grams/ adult/day
1920	1406	1.8					4040	5.0
1921	1361	1.7					3990	5.0
1922	1315	1.6					3860	4.8
1923	1361	1.8					3720	4.9
1924	1406	1.8					3760	4.9
1925	1497	2.0					3860	5.0
1926	1542	2.0					3810	5.0
1927	1633	2.1					3860	5.0
1928	1723	2.2					3900	5.1
1929	1814	2.4					3950	5.2
1930	1950	2.5					4080	5.3
1931	2132	2.8					4170	5.4
1932	2222	2.9					4080	5.3
1933	2313	3.0					4130	5.4
1934	2494	3.3					4220	5.5
1935	2540	3.3					4260	5.6
1936	2585	3.4					4310	5.6
1937	2721	3.5					4450	5.8
1938	2900	3.8					4580	6.0
1939	3038	4.0					4630	6.0
1940	3175	4.0					4670	5.8
1941	2766	3.4					4130	5.1
1942	2766	3.4					4130	5.1
1943	3175	4.1					4630	6.0
1944	3401	4.4					4900	6.4
1945	3265	4.3					4810	6.3
1946	4127	5.4					5720	7.5
1947	4354	5.7					5810	7.6
1948	4580	6.0					5900	7.7
1949	4989	6.5					6350	8.3
1950	5261	6.8	127	0.2	5388	7.0	6580	8.5
1951	5941	7.7	122	0.2	6063	7.9	7210	9.4
1952	5578	7.3	95	0.1	5673	7.4	6580	8.6
1953	5400	7.1	113	0.1	5513	7.2	6530	8.6
1954	5220	6.9	95	0.1	5315	7.0	6210	8.2
1955	5500	7.3	100	0.1	5600	7.5	6530	8.7
1956	5027	6.8	86	0.1	5113	6.9	5940	8.0
1957	4850	6.6	82	0.1	4932	6.7	5760	7.8
1958	4765	6.6	82	0.1	4847	6.7	5670	7.8
1959	4942	6.9	77	0.1	5019	7.0	5760	8.0
1960	5115	7.2	73	0.1	5188	7.3	5900	8.3
1961	5325	7.5	73	0.1	5398	7.6	6080	8.6
1962	5270	7.4	73	0.1	5343	7.5	5990	8.4
1963	5570	7.8	73	0.1	5643	7.9	6260	8.7
1964	5360	7.5	77	0.1	5437	7.6	6080	8.5
1965	5380	7.4	73	0.1	5453	7.6	5990	8.3
1966	5530	7.6	64	0.1	5594	7.7	5990	8.3
1967	5603	7.7	64	0.1	5667	7.8	5940	8.2
1968	5700	7.8	59	0.1	5759	7.9	5900	8.1
1969	5925	8.1	59	0.1	5984	8.2	5940	8.1

Table 14.2 *(continued)*

Year	Manufactured cigarettes		Hand-rolled cigarettes		Total cigarettes		All tobacco products	
	Total annual in millions	Number/ adult/day	Total annual in millions	Number/ adult/day	Total annual in millions	Number/ adult/day	Total annual in tonnes	Grams/ adult/day
1970	6070	8.2	54	0.1	6124	8.3	5850	7.9
1971	6105	8.2	59	0.1	6164	8.2	5940	8.0
1972	6510	8.6	54	0.1	6564	8.7	6170	8.2
1973	6975	9.1	54	0.1	7029	9.2	6490	8.5
1974	7500	9.7	54	0.1	7554	9.8	6800	8.8
1975	7520	9.6	50	0.1	7570	9.7	6580	8.4
1976	7490	9.2	50	0.1	7540	9.3	6490	8.0
1977	7260	8.8	45	0.1	7305	8.8	6300	7.6
1978	7725	9.2	48	0.1	7773	9.3	6794	8.1
1979	7603	8.9	48	0.1	7651	9.0	6683	7.8
1980	7518	8.7	55	0.1	7573	8.8	6640	7.7
1981	7297	8.3	72	0.1	7369	8.4	6454	7.4
1982	6794	7.7	93	0.1	6887	7.8	6113	6.9
1983	6539	7.3	107	0.1	6646	7.4	5915	6.6
1984	6373	7.0	116	0.1	6489	7.1	5755	6.3
1985	6226	6.8	121	0.1	6347	6.9	5712	6.2
1986	5887	6.4	127	0.1	6014	6.5	5386	5.9
1987	5628	6.1	122	0.1	5750	6.2	5130	5.6
1988	5598	6.0	118	0.1	5716	6.2	5076	5.5
1989	5656	6.1	109	0.1	5765	6.2	5094	5.5
1990	5800	6.2	109	0.1	5909	6.4	5202	5.6
1991	6262	6.6	122	0.1	6384	6.8	5607	5.9
1992	5998	6.3	122	0.1	6120	6.4	5359	5.6
1993	5738	5.9	119	0.1	5857	6.0	5120	5.3
1994	5959	6.1	120	0.1	6079	6.2	5291	5.4
1995	6365	6.4	122	0.1	6487	6.5	5637	5.7

Source : see *Notes on sources of sales data,* p. 350

Figure 14.1 Daily consumption of (i) manufactured and total number of cigarettes, and (ii) all tobacco products, 1920-1995.
Males and females aged 15 years and over. *Source:* see Table 14.2

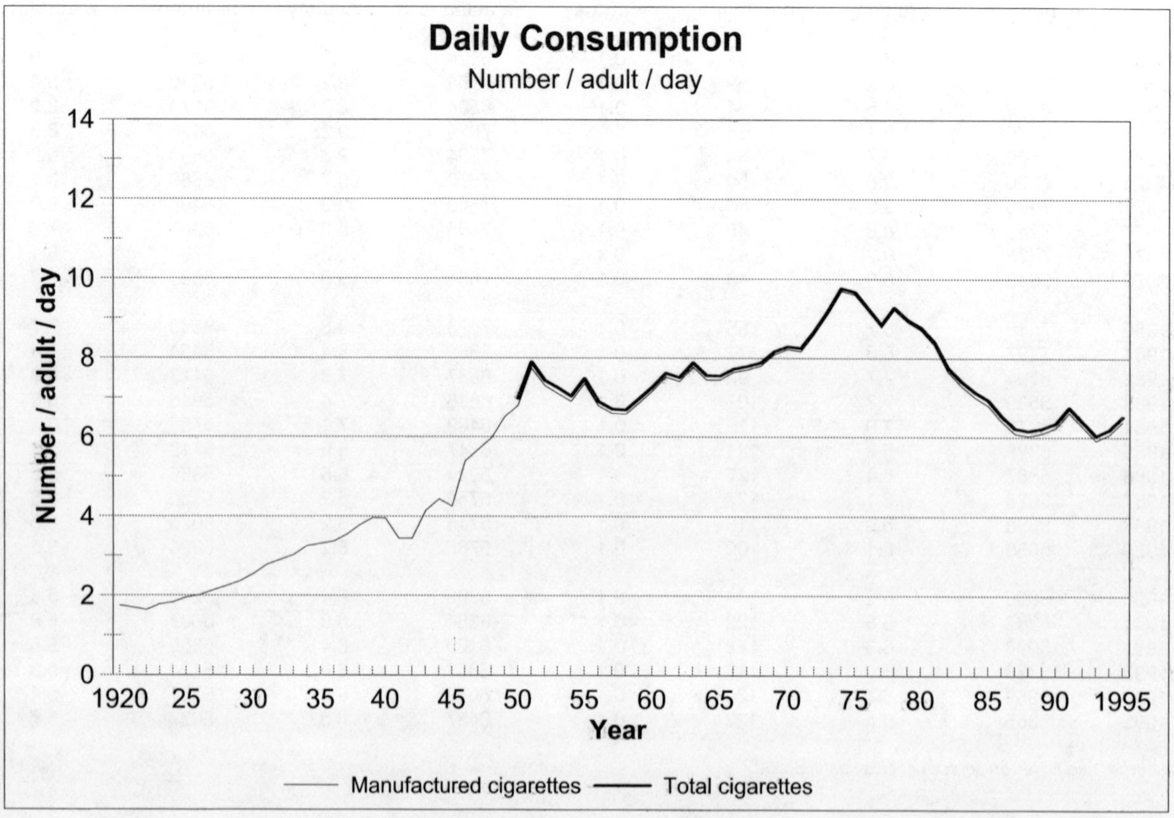

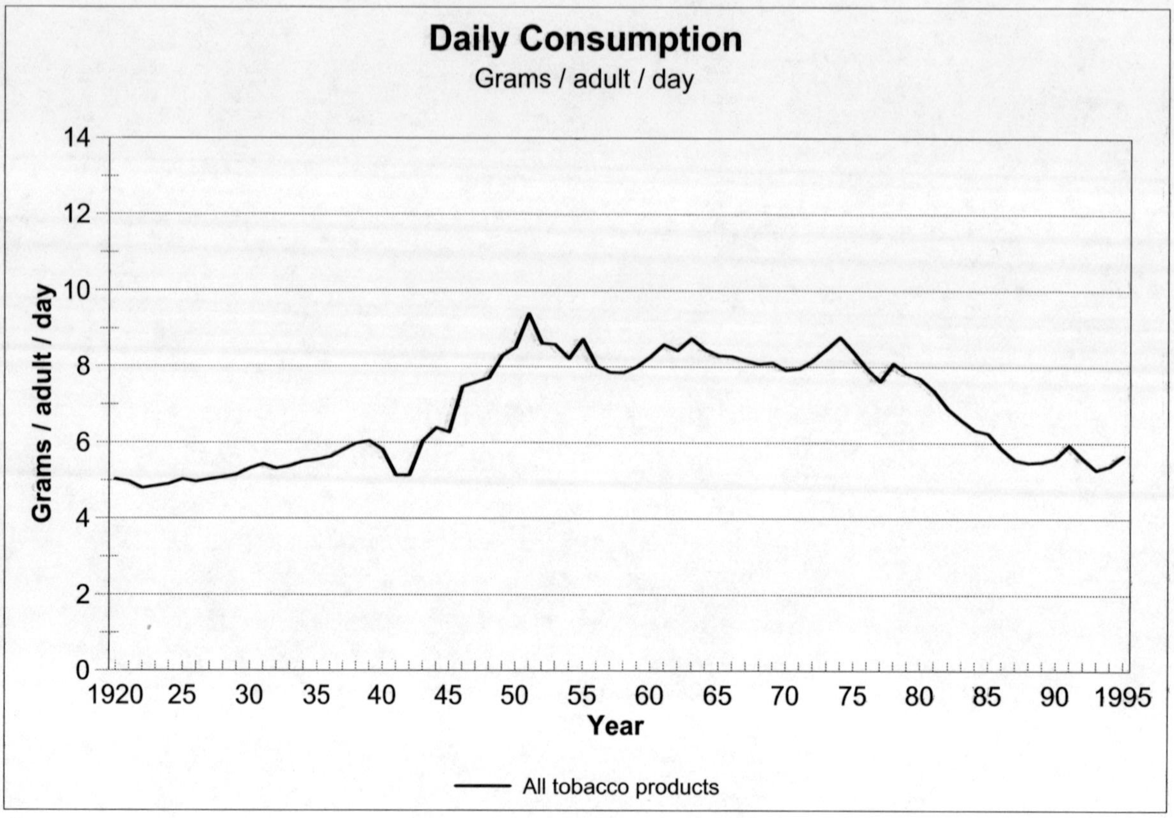

Table 14.3 Percentage sales of tobacco in different forms (by weight), selected years 1925-1995

Year	Cigarettes (%)	Cigars (%)	Other tobacco (%)
1925	38.9	0.0	61.1
1935	59.6	0.0	40.4
1945	68.0	0.0	32.0
1955	84.1	0.0	16.1
1965	87.1	0.8	12.2
1975	91.0	1.4	7.6
1985	91.9	2.0	6.2
1995	94.9	1.4	3.7

Source : calculated from Tables 14.1.1 & 14.1.2

Figure 14.2 Percentage sales of tobacco in different forms (by weight), selected years 1925-1995
Source: see Table 14.3

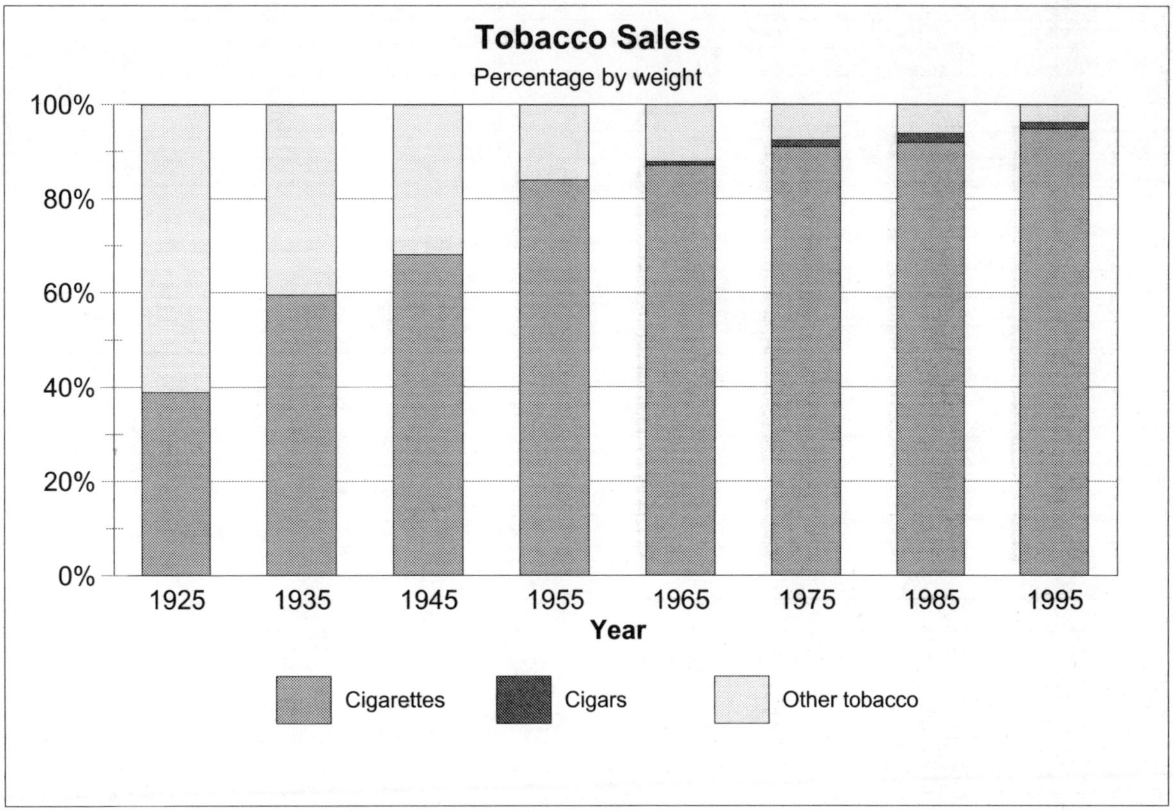

Table 14.4M Prevalence of smoking, males: some selected Irish surveys by age, 1959-1995 *(continues on p. 342)*

<table>
<tr><th rowspan="2">Frequency
Product
Source
Year</th><th colspan="21">Age group</th><th rowspan="2">All ages</th></tr>
<tr><th>12</th><th>13</th><th>14</th><th>15</th><th>16</th><th>17</th><th>18</th><th>19</th><th>20-24</th><th>25-29</th><th>30-34</th><th>35-39</th><th>40-44</th><th>45-49</th><th>50-54</th><th>55-59</th><th>60-64</th><th>65-69</th><th>70-74</th><th>75-79</th><th>80+</th></tr>
<tr><td>59 11 UC R</td><td>22</td><td>19</td><td>27</td><td>29</td><td>43</td><td>45</td><td>52</td><td>42</td><td colspan="13"></td><td>27</td></tr>
<tr><td>59 11 UC A</td><td>38</td><td>32</td><td>46</td><td>47</td><td>64</td><td>62</td><td>67</td><td>83</td><td colspan="13"></td><td>44</td></tr>
<tr><td>61 7 U R</td><td colspan="4"></td><td colspan="17">61</td><td></td></tr>
<tr><td>61 7 U U</td><td colspan="11"></td><td colspan="5">71</td><td colspan="5"></td><td></td></tr>
<tr><td>62 5 UC R</td><td>23</td><td>40</td><td>48</td><td colspan="18"></td><td></td></tr>
<tr><td>67 2 U R</td><td>13</td><td>19</td><td>31</td><td>36</td><td>42</td><td>43</td><td>55</td><td colspan="14"></td><td>32</td></tr>
<tr><td>67 7 MC A</td><td colspan="4"></td><td colspan="17">55</td><td></td></tr>
<tr><td>67 10 U U</td><td colspan="3"></td><td colspan="18">68</td><td></td></tr>
<tr><td>69 12 U U</td><td>8</td><td>8</td><td>17</td><td>20</td><td>36</td><td>35</td><td>28</td><td colspan="14"></td><td>23</td></tr>
<tr><td>70 2 U R</td><td>25</td><td>24</td><td>33</td><td>38</td><td>45</td><td>44</td><td>47</td><td colspan="14"></td><td>35</td></tr>
<tr><td>71 3 U R</td><td>14</td><td>15</td><td>21</td><td>30</td><td>36</td><td>41</td><td>39</td><td colspan="14"></td><td></td></tr>
<tr><td>71 7 MC U</td><td colspan="4"></td><td colspan="17">56</td><td></td></tr>
<tr><td>71 7 A U</td><td colspan="8"></td><td colspan="13">68</td><td></td></tr>
<tr><td>72 8 UC R</td><td colspan="4"></td><td colspan="17">49</td><td></td></tr>
<tr><td>73 8 UC R</td><td colspan="4"></td><td colspan="17">48</td><td></td></tr>
<tr><td>74 8 UC R</td><td colspan="4"></td><td colspan="17">45</td><td></td></tr>
<tr><td>75 7 U R</td><td colspan="4"></td><td colspan="17">51</td><td></td></tr>
<tr><td>75 8 UC R</td><td colspan="4"></td><td colspan="17">45</td><td></td></tr>
<tr><td>76 8 UC R</td><td colspan="4"></td><td colspan="17">43</td><td></td></tr>
<tr><td>77 1 UC U</td><td colspan="3"></td><td colspan="5">35</td><td>47</td><td colspan="2">47</td><td colspan="2">40</td><td colspan="2">47</td><td colspan="2">47</td><td colspan="4">39</td><td>43</td></tr>
<tr><td>77 8 UC R</td><td colspan="4"></td><td colspan="17">44</td><td></td></tr>
<tr><td>78 8 UC R</td><td colspan="4"></td><td colspan="17">40</td><td></td></tr>
<tr><td>79 9 UC U</td><td colspan="3"></td><td colspan="18">37</td><td></td></tr>
<tr><td>80 1 UC U</td><td colspan="3"></td><td colspan="5">26</td><td>42</td><td colspan="2">46</td><td colspan="2">37</td><td colspan="2">45</td><td colspan="2">38</td><td colspan="4">30</td><td>38</td></tr>
<tr><td>80 2 U R</td><td>21</td><td>31</td><td>39</td><td>37</td><td>32</td><td>31</td><td>46</td><td colspan="14"></td><td>34</td></tr>
<tr><td>80 2 U A</td><td>43</td><td>55</td><td>61</td><td>58</td><td>62</td><td>60</td><td>69</td><td colspan="14"></td><td>58</td></tr>
<tr><td>80 8 UC R</td><td colspan="4"></td><td colspan="17">39</td><td></td></tr>
<tr><td>80 13 A U</td><td colspan="3"></td><td colspan="18">49</td><td></td></tr>
<tr><td>81 8 UC R</td><td colspan="4"></td><td colspan="17">39</td><td></td></tr>
<tr><td>82 3 U R</td><td>23</td><td>23</td><td>34</td><td>38</td><td>36</td><td>44</td><td>46</td><td colspan="14"></td><td></td></tr>
<tr><td>82 8 UC R</td><td colspan="4"></td><td colspan="17">34</td><td></td></tr>
<tr><td>83 8 UC R</td><td colspan="4"></td><td colspan="17">34</td><td></td></tr>
<tr><td>83 14 UC R</td><td colspan="2">14</td><td colspan="19"></td><td></td></tr>
<tr><td>83 14 UC A</td><td colspan="2">31</td><td colspan="19"></td><td></td></tr>
<tr><td>84 4 UC R</td><td colspan="2">14</td><td>26</td><td>30</td><td>33</td><td colspan="2">29</td><td colspan="14"></td><td>27</td></tr>
<tr><td>84 4 UC A</td><td colspan="2">28</td><td>36</td><td>40</td><td>43</td><td colspan="2">37</td><td colspan="14"></td><td>38</td></tr>
<tr><td>84 8 UC R</td><td colspan="4"></td><td colspan="17">37</td><td></td></tr>
<tr><td>85 8 UC R</td><td colspan="3"></td><td colspan="18">36</td><td></td></tr>
<tr><td>86 8 UC R</td><td colspan="3"></td><td colspan="18">34</td><td></td></tr>
<tr><td>86 15 * R</td><td colspan="11"></td><td colspan="6">28</td><td colspan="4"></td><td></td></tr>
<tr><td>86 15 UC R</td><td colspan="11"></td><td colspan="6">32</td><td colspan="4"></td><td></td></tr>
<tr><td>86 15 A R</td><td colspan="11"></td><td colspan="2">43</td><td colspan="2">42</td><td colspan="2">32</td><td colspan="4"></td><td>39</td></tr>
<tr><td>87 8 UC R</td><td colspan="3"></td><td colspan="18">30</td><td></td></tr>
<tr><td>87 19 U U</td><td colspan="3"></td><td colspan="18">38</td><td></td></tr>
<tr><td>88 8 UC R</td><td colspan="3"></td><td colspan="18">32</td><td></td></tr>
<tr><td>89 8 UC R</td><td colspan="3"></td><td colspan="18">31</td><td></td></tr>
<tr><td>89 19 U U</td><td colspan="3"></td><td colspan="18">40</td><td></td></tr>
<tr><td>90 8 UC R</td><td colspan="3"></td><td colspan="18">30</td><td></td></tr>
<tr><td>90 16 U R</td><td colspan="2"></td><td>3</td><td>6</td><td colspan="17"></td><td></td></tr>
<tr><td>90 16 U A</td><td>0</td><td colspan="3">5</td><td colspan="17"></td><td></td></tr>
<tr><td>91 8 UC R</td><td colspan="3"></td><td colspan="18">30</td><td></td></tr>
<tr><td>91 15 * R</td><td colspan="11"></td><td colspan="6">25</td><td colspan="4"></td><td></td></tr>
<tr><td>91 15 UC R</td><td colspan="11"></td><td colspan="6">28</td><td colspan="4"></td><td></td></tr>
<tr><td>91 15 A R</td><td colspan="11"></td><td colspan="2">42</td><td colspan="2">31</td><td colspan="2">30</td><td colspan="4"></td><td>36</td></tr>
<tr><td>91 19 U U</td><td colspan="3"></td><td colspan="18">35</td><td></td></tr>
</table>

Table 14.4F Prevalence of smoking, females: some selected Irish surveys by age, 1959-1995 *(continues on p. 343)*

Frequency Product Source Year	12	13	14	15	16	17	18	19	20-24	25-29	30-34	35-39	40-44	45-49	50-54	55-59	60-64	65-69	70-74	75-79	80+	All ages
59 11 UC R	2	4	8	11	12	16	13															8
59 11 UC A	9	14	27	37	29	47	31															25
61 7 U R					38																	
61 7 U U																						
62 5 UC R	4	10	11																			
67 2 U R	1	6	11	13	15	22	20															11
67 7 MC A					38																	
67 10 U U				39																		
69 12 U U	0	2	10	21	34	22	10															10
70 2 U R	3	9	18	25	28	29	28															18
71 3 U R	2	7	11	13	21	19	19															
71 7 MC U					42																	
71 7 A U																						
72 8 UC R					37																	
73 8 UC R					38																	
74 8 UC R					37																	
75 7 U R					42																	
75 8 UC R					34																	
76 8 UC R					34																	
77 1 UC U				30					40	40		34		37		33		20				33
77 8 UC R					34																	
78 8 UC R					31																	
79 9 UC U				33																		
80 1 UC U				23					40	39		32		35		33		22				32
80 2 U R	10	18	29	27	32	34	29															26
80 2 U A	29	40	53	57	63	65	59															52
80 8 UC R					32																	
80 13 A U				36																		
81 8 UC R					32																	
82 3 U R	11	16	26	26	26	34	32															
82 8 UC R					29																	
83 8 UC R					30																	
83 14 UC R	5																					
83 14 UC A	13																					
84 4 UC R	9		18	20	28	32																21
84 4 UC A	24		37	38	42	42																36
84 8 UC R					32																	
85 8 UC R				32																		
86 8 UC R				31																		
86 15 * R												28										
86 15 UC R												28										
86 15 A R												25		26		39						28
87 8 UC R				27																		
87 19 U U				32																		
88 8 UC R				27																		
89 8 UC R				29																		
89 19 U U				31																		
90 8 UC R				27																		
90 16 U R			5	7																		
90 16 U A	1	6																				
91 8 UC R				30																		
91 15 * R												24										
91 15 UC R												24										
91 15 A R												24		25		23						24
91 19 U U				31																		

Table 14.4M (continued from p. 340) Prevalence of smoking, males

Frequency / Product / Source / Year	12	13	14	15	16	17	18	19	20-24	25-29	30-34	35-39	40-44	45-49	50-54	55-59	60-64	65-69	70-74	75-79	80+	All ages
92 8 UC R				31																		
93 8 UC R				29																		
93 17 U R				17																		
94 19 U U				36																		
95 18 UC R				29																		
95 18 UC A				37																		
95 20 U R		17																				

Table 14.5M Number of cigarettes smoked per smoker per day, males: some selected Irish surveys by age, 1959-1995

Product / Source / Year	12	13	14	15	16	17	18	19	20-24	25-29	30-34	35-39	40-44	45-49	50-54	55-59	60-64	65-69	70-74	75-79	80+	All ages
59 11 UCE*	1.2	1.8	3.2	5.1	5.9	7.4	11	9.2														4.2
62 5 UCE*	0.9	1.3	1.1																			
67 2 UC	0.8	1.2	1.9	2.9	5.1	5.6	6.1															3.8
67 7 MC					18																	
70 2 UC	2.6					8.6																5.8
80 1 UC				20																		
80 2 UC	5.6				7.7	8.7	10															
82 3 UC				6.0	7.3	8.7	11															
83 14 UCE	6.5																					
86 15 UC												21										
90 15 UC												23										
95 18 UCE				10																		

Source: see *Notes on sources of survey data*, p. 351
Frequency: A = all smokers (including occasional)
R = regular or daily smokers
All ages: relevant to ages used and as given in original source
U = unspecified
* = refer to *Notes on sources of survey data*, p. 351

Product: MC = manufactured cigarettes
TC = total cigarettes (including hand-rolled)
UC = cigarettes (type unspecified)
A = all products
E indicates mean estimated from percentage distribution (see also *Consumption category estimation*, p. xxxiv, and Appendix III, p. 789)

Table 14.4F *(continued from p. 341)*
Prevalence of smoking, females

Frequency / Product / Source / Year	12	13	14	15	16	17	18	19	20-24	25-29	30-34	35-39	40-44	45-49	50-54	55-59	60-64	65-69	70-74	75-79	80+	All ages
92 8 UC R				26																		
93 8 UC R				28																		
93 17 U R	15																					
94 19 U U				27																		
95 18 UC R				30																		
95 18 UC A				45																		
95 20 U R		23																				

Table 14.5F Number of cigarettes smoked per smoker per day, females: some selected Irish surveys by age, 1959-1995

Product / Source / Year	12	13	14	15	16	17	18	19	20-24	25-29	30-34	35-39	40-44	45-49	50-54	55-59	60-64	65-69	70-74	75-79	80+	All ages
59 11 UCE*	0.7	0.5	0.6	0.8	0.8	0.7	0.4															0.7
62 5 UCE*	0.6	0.7	1.2																			
67 2 UC	1.1	0.4	1.8	1.2	1.7	2.0	3.6															1.4
67 7 MC					13																	
70 2 UC	1.9					4.7																3.4
80 1 UC				17																		
80 2 UC	4.1				5.9	6.0	9.6															
82 3 UC				3.4	5.0	5.9	5.1															
83 14 UCE	2.7																					
86 15 UC												16										
90 15 UC												17										
95 18 UCE				7.9																		

Source: see *Notes on sources of survey data*, p. 351
Frequency: A = all smokers (including occasional)
R = regular or daily smokers
All ages: relevant to ages used and as given in original source
U = unspecified
* = refer to *Notes on sources of survey data*, p. 351

Product: MC = manufactured cigarettes
TC = total cigarettes (including hand-rolled)
UC = cigarettes (type unspecified)
A = all products
E indicates mean estimated from percentage distribution (see also *Consumption category estimation*, p. xxxiv, and Appendix III, p. 789)

Table 14.6M Number of cigarettes smoked per person per day, males: some selected Irish surveys by age, 1959-1995, with percentage total sales

<table>
<tr><th rowspan="2">Product
Source
Year</th><th colspan="21">Age group</th><th rowspan="2">All ages</th><th rowspan="2">% Total sales</th></tr>
<tr><th>12</th><th>13</th><th>14</th><th>15</th><th>16</th><th>17</th><th>18</th><th>19</th><th>20-24</th><th>25-29</th><th>30-34</th><th>35-39</th><th>40-44</th><th>45-49</th><th>50-54</th><th>55-59</th><th>60-64</th><th>65-69</th><th>70-74</th><th>75-79</th><th>80+</th></tr>
<tr><td>59 11 UC *</td><td>0.3</td><td>0.4</td><td>0.9</td><td>1.5</td><td>2.5</td><td>3.3</td><td>5.8</td><td colspan="2">3.9</td><td colspan="12"></td><td>1.1</td><td>**</td></tr>
<tr><td>61 7 MC</td><td colspan="4"></td><td colspan="17">11</td><td></td><td>100%M</td></tr>
<tr><td>62 5 UC *</td><td>0.2</td><td>0.5</td><td>0.6</td><td colspan="18"></td><td></td><td>**</td></tr>
<tr><td>67 2 UC</td><td>0.1</td><td>0.2</td><td>0.6</td><td>1.1</td><td>2.1</td><td>2.4</td><td>3.4</td><td colspan="14"></td><td>1.2</td><td>**</td></tr>
<tr><td>67 7 MC</td><td colspan="4"></td><td colspan="17">10</td><td></td><td>95%M</td></tr>
<tr><td>70 2 UC</td><td>0.7</td><td colspan="6">3.8</td><td colspan="14"></td><td>2.0</td><td>**</td></tr>
<tr><td>71 7 MC</td><td colspan="4"></td><td colspan="17">11</td><td></td><td>102%M</td></tr>
<tr><td>75 6 MC</td><td colspan="3"></td><td colspan="18">12</td><td></td><td>---M</td></tr>
<tr><td>75 7 MC</td><td colspan="4"></td><td colspan="17">11</td><td></td><td>91%M</td></tr>
<tr><td>80 1 UC</td><td colspan="3"></td><td colspan="18">7.6</td><td></td><td>74%T</td></tr>
<tr><td>80 2 UC</td><td colspan="4">1.8</td><td>2.5</td><td>2.7</td><td>4.6</td><td colspan="14"></td><td></td><td>**</td></tr>
<tr><td>80 6 MC</td><td colspan="3"></td><td colspan="18">11</td><td></td><td>---M</td></tr>
<tr><td>82 3 UC</td><td colspan="3"></td><td>2.3</td><td>2.6</td><td>3.8</td><td>5.1</td><td colspan="14"></td><td></td><td>**</td></tr>
<tr><td>83 14 UC</td><td colspan="2">0.9</td><td colspan="19"></td><td></td><td>**</td></tr>
<tr><td>86 15 UC</td><td colspan="11"></td><td colspan="6">6.6</td><td colspan="4"></td><td></td><td>**</td></tr>
<tr><td>90 15 UC</td><td colspan="11"></td><td colspan="6">6.2</td><td colspan="4"></td><td></td><td>**</td></tr>
<tr><td>95 18 UC</td><td colspan="3"></td><td colspan="2">3.0</td><td colspan="16"></td><td></td><td>**</td></tr>
</table>

Table 14.7M Number of cigarettes smoked per person per day, sales-adjusted, males: some selected Irish surveys[1] by age, 1961-1980, with percentage total sales

<table>
<tr><th rowspan="2">Product
Source
Year</th><th colspan="21">Age group</th><th rowspan="2">All ages</th><th rowspan="2">% Total sales</th></tr>
<tr><th>12</th><th>13</th><th>14</th><th>15</th><th>16</th><th>17</th><th>18</th><th>19</th><th>20-24</th><th>25-29</th><th>30-34</th><th>35-39</th><th>40-44</th><th>45-49</th><th>50-54</th><th>55-59</th><th>60-64</th><th>65-69</th><th>70-74</th><th>75-79</th><th>80+</th></tr>
<tr><td>61 7 MC</td><td colspan="4"></td><td colspan="17">11</td><td></td><td>100%M</td></tr>
<tr><td>67 7 MC</td><td colspan="4"></td><td colspan="17">10</td><td></td><td>95%M</td></tr>
<tr><td>71 7 MC</td><td colspan="4"></td><td colspan="17">11</td><td></td><td>102%M</td></tr>
<tr><td>75 6 MC</td><td colspan="3"></td><td colspan="18">12</td><td></td><td>---M</td></tr>
<tr><td>75 7 MC</td><td colspan="4"></td><td colspan="17">12</td><td></td><td>91%M</td></tr>
<tr><td>80 1 UC</td><td colspan="3"></td><td colspan="18">10</td><td></td><td>74%T</td></tr>
<tr><td>80 6 MC</td><td colspan="3"></td><td colspan="18">11</td><td></td><td>---M</td></tr>
</table>

1 Based on those surveys in Table 14.6 with data for both sexes and age range at least 21-64 (see *Cigarette consumption per person*, p. xxxv)

Source: see *Notes on sources of survey data*, p. 351
All ages: relevant to ages used and as given in original source
% Total sales: estimated % of total sales of M = manufactured or T = total cigarette consumption implied by survey, sexes combined, used as adjustment factor in Table 14.7
** = cannot be calculated
--- = adjusted by original author

Product: MC = manufactured cigarettes
TC = total cigarettes (including hand-rolled)
UC = cigarettes (type unspecified)
A = all products
U = unspecified
* = refer to *Notes on sources of survey data*, p. 351

Table 14.6F Number of cigarettes smoked per person per day, females: some selected Irish surveys by age, 1959-1995, with percentage total sales

<table>
<tr><th rowspan="2">Product
Source
Year</th><th colspan="21">Age group</th><th rowspan="2">All ages</th><th rowspan="2">% Total sales</th></tr>
<tr><th>12</th><th>13</th><th>14</th><th>15</th><th>16</th><th>17</th><th>18</th><th>19</th><th>20-24</th><th>25-29</th><th>30-34</th><th>35-39</th><th>40-44</th><th>45-49</th><th>50-54</th><th>55-59</th><th>60-64</th><th>65-69</th><th>70-74</th><th>75-79</th><th>80+</th></tr>
<tr><td>59 11 UC *</td><td>0.0</td><td>0.0</td><td>0.0</td><td>0.1</td><td>0.1</td><td>0.1</td><td>0.0</td><td colspan="14"></td><td>0.1</td><td>**</td></tr>
<tr><td>61 7 MC</td><td colspan="4"></td><td colspan="17">4.2</td><td></td><td>100%M</td></tr>
<tr><td>62 5 UC *</td><td>0.0</td><td>0.1</td><td>0.1</td><td colspan="18"></td><td></td><td>**</td></tr>
<tr><td>67 2 UC</td><td>0.0</td><td>0.0</td><td>0.2</td><td>0.1</td><td>0.2</td><td>0.4</td><td>0.7</td><td colspan="14"></td><td>0.1</td><td>**</td></tr>
<tr><td>67 7 MC</td><td colspan="4"></td><td colspan="17">5</td><td></td><td>95%M</td></tr>
<tr><td>70 2 UC</td><td>0.1</td><td colspan="4"></td><td colspan="2">1.4</td><td colspan="14"></td><td>0.6</td><td>**</td></tr>
<tr><td>71 7 MC</td><td colspan="4"></td><td colspan="17">6</td><td></td><td>102%M</td></tr>
<tr><td>75 6 MC</td><td colspan="3"></td><td colspan="18">7.7</td><td></td><td>---M</td></tr>
<tr><td>75 7 MC</td><td colspan="4"></td><td colspan="17">7.0</td><td></td><td>91%M</td></tr>
<tr><td>80 1 UC</td><td colspan="3"></td><td colspan="18">5.4</td><td></td><td>74%T</td></tr>
<tr><td>80 2 UC</td><td colspan="4">0.9</td><td>1.9</td><td>2.0</td><td>2.8</td><td colspan="14"></td><td></td><td>**</td></tr>
<tr><td>80 6 MC</td><td colspan="3"></td><td colspan="18">6.9</td><td></td><td>---M</td></tr>
<tr><td>82 3 UC</td><td colspan="3"></td><td>0.9</td><td>1.3</td><td>2.0</td><td>1.6</td><td colspan="14"></td><td></td><td>**</td></tr>
<tr><td>83 14 UC</td><td colspan="2">0.1</td><td colspan="19"></td><td></td><td>**</td></tr>
<tr><td>86 15 UC</td><td colspan="11"></td><td colspan="6">4.5</td><td colspan="4"></td><td></td><td>**</td></tr>
<tr><td>90 15 UC</td><td colspan="11"></td><td colspan="6">4.1</td><td colspan="4"></td><td></td><td>**</td></tr>
<tr><td>95 18 UC</td><td colspan="3"></td><td colspan="2">2.4</td><td colspan="16"></td><td></td><td>**</td></tr>
</table>

Table 14.7F Number of cigarettes smoked per person per day, sales-adjusted, females: some selected Irish surveys[1] by age, 1961-1980, with percentage total sales

<table>
<tr><th rowspan="2">Product
Source
Year</th><th colspan="21">Age group</th><th rowspan="2">All ages</th><th rowspan="2">% Total sales</th></tr>
<tr><th>12</th><th>13</th><th>14</th><th>15</th><th>16</th><th>17</th><th>18</th><th>19</th><th>20-24</th><th>25-29</th><th>30-34</th><th>35-39</th><th>40-44</th><th>45-49</th><th>50-54</th><th>55-59</th><th>60-64</th><th>65-69</th><th>70-74</th><th>75-79</th><th>80+</th></tr>
<tr><td>61 7 MC</td><td colspan="4"></td><td colspan="17">4.2</td><td></td><td>100%M</td></tr>
<tr><td>67 7 MC</td><td colspan="4"></td><td colspan="17">5</td><td></td><td>95%M</td></tr>
<tr><td>71 7 MC</td><td colspan="4"></td><td colspan="17">6</td><td></td><td>102%M</td></tr>
<tr><td>75 6 MC</td><td colspan="3"></td><td colspan="18">7.7</td><td></td><td>---M</td></tr>
<tr><td>75 7 MC</td><td colspan="4"></td><td colspan="17">7.7</td><td></td><td>91%M</td></tr>
<tr><td>80 1 UC</td><td colspan="3"></td><td colspan="18">7.3</td><td></td><td>74%T</td></tr>
<tr><td>80 6 MC</td><td colspan="3"></td><td colspan="18">6.9</td><td></td><td>---M</td></tr>
</table>

1 Based on those surveys in Table 14.6 with data for both sexes and age range at least 21-64 (see *Cigarette consumption per person*, p. xxxv)

Source: see *Notes on sources of survey data*, p. 351
All ages: relevant to ages used and as given in original source
% Total sales: estimated % of total sales of M = manufactured or T = total cigarette consumption implied by survey, sexes combined, used as adjustment factor in Table 14.7
** = cannot be calculated
--- = adjusted by original author

Product: MC = manufactured cigarettes
TC = total cigarettes (including hand-rolled)
UC = cigarettes (type unspecified)
A = all products
U = unspecified
* = refer to *Notes on sources of survey data*, p. 351

Table 14.8 Estimated[1] prevalence of smoking and estimated[1] number of cigarettes per person per day (unadjusted and sales-adjusted): summary of Tables 14.4, 14.6 and 14.7, 1961-1994.
Males and females aged 15 years and over

Year	Source[2]	Product[3]	Prevalence[4]						Number of cigarettes						
									Unadjusted[7]			Sales-adjusted[8]			
			Manufactured cigarettes		Total cigarettes[5]		All products[6]		Number/ person/day		Total sales %	Manufactured cigarettes number/ person/day		Total cigarettes[9] number/ person/day	
			M	F	M	F	M	F	M	F		M	F	M	F
1961	7	MC+U					60	37	10.9	4.1	100	10.9	4.1		
1967	7	**MC**	54	38					9.8	4.9	95	10.3	5.1		
	10	*U*					68	39							
1971	7	*MC+A*	55	41			65		10.8	5.9	102	10.6	5.8		
1972	8	UC			48	36								(10.9	6.5)
1973	8	UC			47	37								(11.3	7.1)
1974	8	UC			45	36								(11.8	7.7)
1975	6	MC							11.9	7.7	---	11.9	7.7		
	7	MC+U					50	41	10.7	6.9	91	11.7	7.5		
	8	UC			45	34								(12.1	7.3)
1976	8	UC			43	34								(11.4	7.2)
1977	1	*UC*			43	33								(11.0	6.7)
	8	UC			44	34								(10.9	6.7)
1978	8	UC			40	31								(11.5	7.1)
1979	9	*UC*			37	33						(10.4	7.4)		
1980	1	*UC*			38	31			7.6	5.4	74			10.3	7.3
	6	MC							11.0	6.9	---	11.0	6.9		
	8	UC			39	32								(10.6	6.9)
	13	*A*					49	36							
1981	8	UC			39	32								(10.2	6.7)
1982	8	UC			34	29								(9.3	6.3)
1983	8	UC			34	30								(8.7	6.1)
1984	8	UC			37	32								(8.5	5.8)
1985	8	UC			36	32								(8.1	5.8)
1986	8	UC			34	31								(7.6	5.5)
1987	8	UC			30	27								(7.3	5.2)
	19	*U*					38	32							
1988	8	UC			32	27								(7.4	5.0)
1989	8	UC			31	29								(7.1	5.3)
	19	*U*					40	31							
1990	8	UC			30	27								(7.4	5.3)

Table 14.8 *(continued)*

Year	Source[2]	Product[3]	Prevalence[4]						Number of cigarettes						
									Unadjusted[7]			Sales-adjusted[8]			
			Manufactured cigarettes		Total cigarettes[5]		All products[6]		Number/ person/day		Total sales %	Manufactured cigarettes number/ person/day		Total cigarettes[9] number/ person/day	
			M	F	M	F	M	F	M	F		M	F	M	F
1991	8	UC			30	30								(7.5	6.0)
	19	*U*					35	31							
1992	8	UC			31	26								(7.7	5.2)
1993	8	UC			29	28								(6.8	5.3)
1994	19	*U*					36	27							

1 Surveys covering an age range of at least 21-64 are included. Any gaps in the data for ages 15-20 and 65 years and over are filled in by assumed extensions to the age distribution, given in *Notes on sources of survey data*, p. 351. Method: see *Summary of adult smoking*, p. xxxvi
2 See *Notes on sources of survey data*, p. 351
3 Product: MC = manufactured cigarettes, TC = total cigarettes (including hand-rolled), UC = cigarettes (type unspecified), A = all products, U = unspecified. Frequency of smoking is indicated by: regular or daily smokers in normal type, all smokers (including occasional) in bold, unspecified in italics
4 From Table 14.4
5 This column includes prevalence of smoking classified as UC = cigarettes (type unspecified)
6 This column includes prevalence of smoking classified as U = unspecified product
7 From Table 14.6
8 From Table 14.7, except data in parentheses, which are derived from the prevalence of smoking from Table 14.4 as described in *Summary of adult smoking*, p. xxxvi
9 Number of cigarettes classified as UC = cigarettes (type unspecified) has been adjusted to total cigarette sales and included in this column

Figure 14.3 Estimated prevalence of smoking of (i) cigarettes and (ii) all tobacco products: by year of survey, 1961-1994.
Males and females aged 15 years and over. *Source:* see Table 14.8

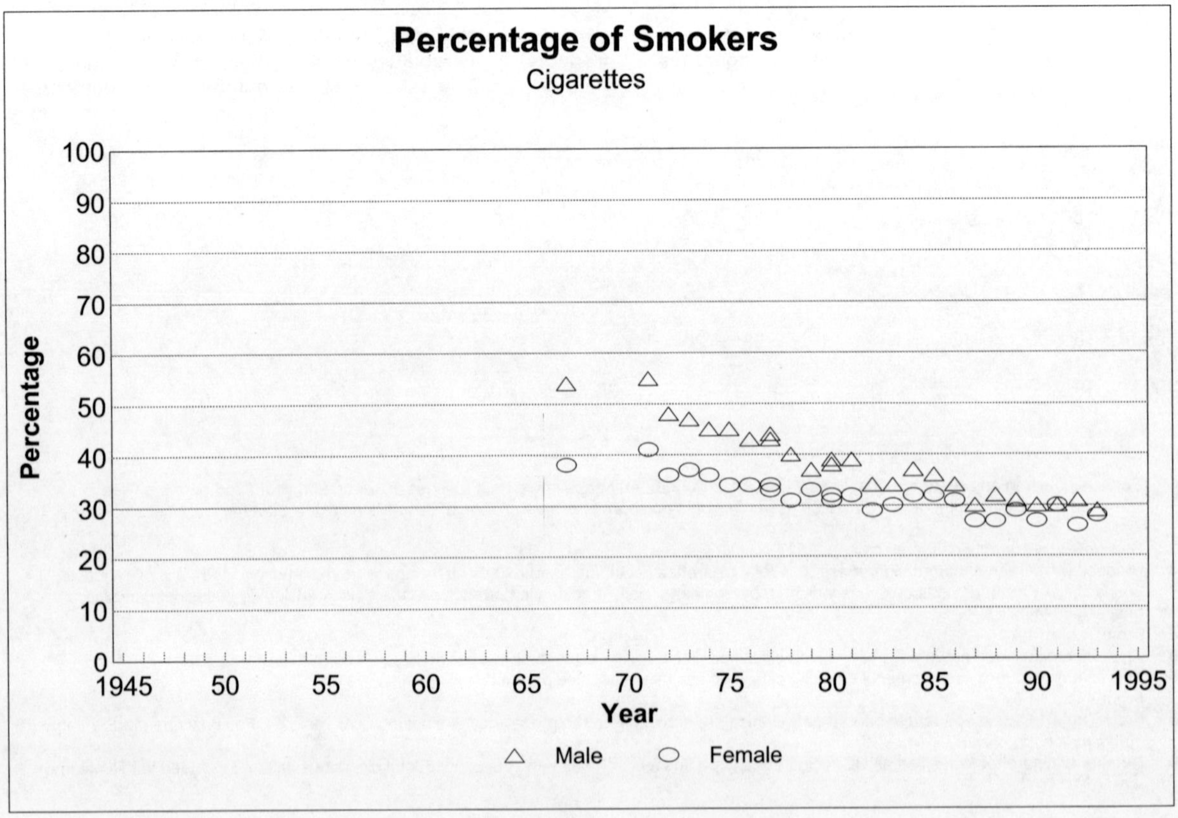

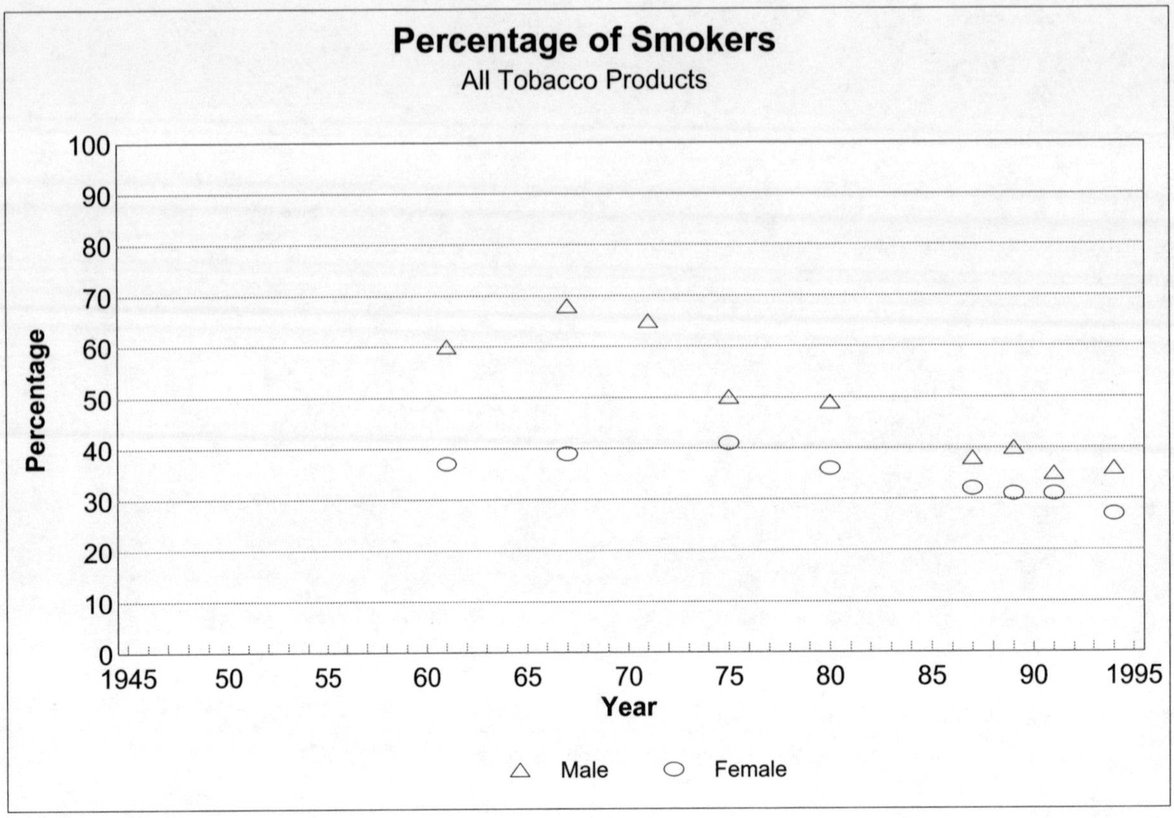

Note: As the smoking of hand-rolled cigarettes is rare, the prevalence of smoking of manufactured cigarettes, and of cigarettes (type unspecified) have been combined here

Figure 14.4 Estimated number of cigarettes smoked per person per day, sales-adjusted, 1961-1993.
Males and females aged 15 years and over. *Source:* see Table 14.8

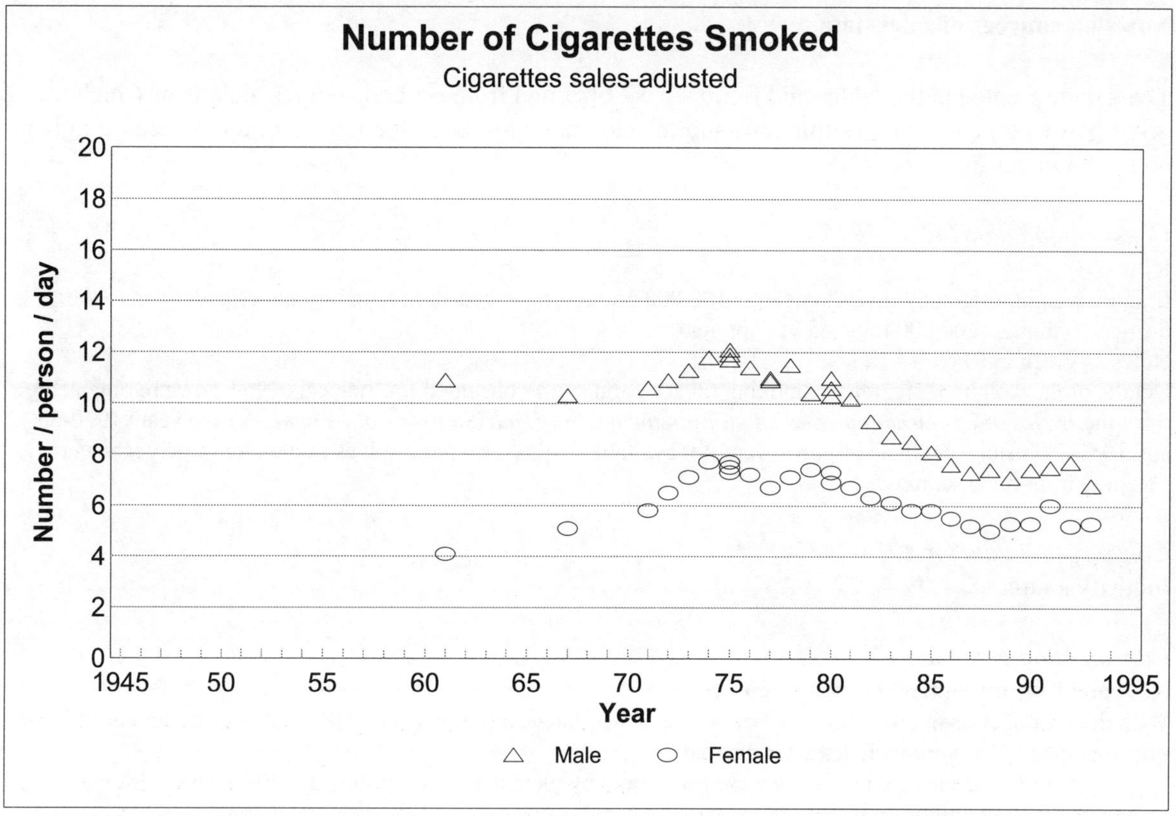

Note : As the smoking of hand-rolled cigarettes is rare, the numbers adjusted to manufactured or total cigarettes have been combined here.

Notes on sources of sales data

The data presented in the tables and figures were obtained from several sources, details of which are given below, together with estimations and related assumptions. Full citations of the sources are given on p. 354 under *References*.

Consumption data before 1975
RP6
Data by weight, originally given to nearest 100 000 pounds, have been converted to tonnes and given to the nearest 10 tonnes (100 000 lbs = 45.359 tonnes).
Notes as given in RP6
Details of the weight of cigarettes, smoking tobacco and snuff consumed for the years 1954-56 were obtained from the *Irish Trade Journal and Statistical Bulletin* and the *Trade Statistics of Ireland.* For the years 1920-53 and 1957-74 official published figures were not available in the form required; estimates for these years were obtained from trade sources.

Consumption data for 1975-1977
Industry sources

Consumption data for 1978-1995
Revenue Commissioners (various years)
With the introduction of an end-product duty on finished tobacco products in 1978, snuff was no longer liable to excise duty, and so is not included after that date.

Up to 1985 data for cigarettes were given both by weight and in millions. For 1986 onwards cigarette data were given in millions only. For conversion to weights, we assumed an average cigarette weight of 0.84 g, based on the average weight of a cigarette in 1985.

Mooney (2000) estimates that official figures for cigarettes consumption (1986-1997) were understated by 5-15% due to smuggling. Tax stamps were introduced in March 1996 to help control smuggling. During the first two weeks of December 1996 a Customs and Gardai special operation seized almost a quarter of a million cigarettes destined for the illicit street trade (Revenue Commissioners (1996)).

Plain/Filter cigarette consumption
1962-1981 Maxwell (successive years)
1982-1983 Todd (1986)

Tar yield of cigarettes
The tar yield per cigarette was limited by EC directive (Directive 90/239/EEC) to 15 mg by the end of 1992, and to 12 mg by the end of 1997 (Harkin *et al* (1997)).

Estimates of hand-rolled cigarette consumption for 1950-1995
We have estimated hand-rolled cigarette consumption as 10% of pipe and hand-rolling ('other') tobacco for 1950-1977, as 100% of hand-rolling tobacco for 1978-1980 and 1984 onwards and as 18%, 23% and 27% of smoking tobacco for 1981-1983 respectively, (based on interpolation). We have assumed 1g per cigarette throughout.

According to Merzdorf *et al* (1982) '... between 5 and 10% of fine-cut pipe tobacco sales are smoked in the form of roll-your-own cigarettes'.

Notes on sources of survey data

Each source of survey data—either an individual survey or a series of surveys repeated over a number of years—is cited by a source number. This number is shown in the tables and corresponds to the source numbers given below, where details of the source publication and of the survey methodology are given. Full citations of the sources are given on p. 354 under *References*.

Source number

1 **Todd (1986) quoting Health Education Bureau**

a. Percentage smokers given from national probability sample. Sample size approximately 5 000 each year. Year commencing July

b. Cigarettes per smoker given from national stratified random sample in summer 1980. Sample size 3 000

2 **O'Rourke *et al* (1968, 1971, 1983a)**

a. Studies of smoking in randomly selected post-primary schools in City and County of Dublin. Anonymous questionnaires completed by all pupils at the schools, with teachers usually absent. Sample size in 1967 (boys) 2 710, (girls) 1 792, in 1970 (boys) 3 015, (girls) 2 468, and in 1980-1981 (boys) 3 068, (girls) 2 085

b. Regular smokers: smoked at least once a week. All smokers (1980 only): smoked regularly, or on holiday, at parties etc

c. Consumption per smoker has been converted from weekly

3 **Todd (1986), quoting O'Rourke *et al* (1983b) and O'Rourke *et al* (in press)**

a. Rural areas.

Year	Sample size	
	Males	Females
1971	2 897	2 853
1982	2 092	2 716

b. Regular smokers: smoked at least 1 cigarette per week every week

4 **Grube and Morgan (1986)**

a. Study conducted in 24 randomly selected post-primary schools (excluding boarding and special schools) in greater Dublin. Years randomly selected within schools. Anonymous questionnaire completed on two occasions a month apart, in class with teachers absent Sample size (males) 1 837, (females) 1 732. Two schools refused to participate

b. Regular smokers: smoke cigarettes daily in last month. All smokers: smoked at least a few cigarettes in last month

5 **Corridan (1963)**

a. Survey in Cork City in April-May 1962, administered by doctor with teachers absent. Sample size (boys) 1 588, (girls) 1 532

b. Regular smokers: smoked 1 or more cigarettes a week

c. Consumption category estimation adult method, which may not be appropriate, based on 1-4, 5-9, 10-19, 20-29, and 30+ cigarettes/smoker/week

6 **Todd (1986)**

a. Estimated by Todd

7 **Herity *et al* (1976), Ward *et al* (1978), Council of Europe (1978), quoting Irish Tobacco Manufacturers' Advisory Committee, and Cleary and Shelley (1983) quoting Research Services (1962)**

a. National quota samples

b. Assumed extension to age distribution for percentage smokers, age 15: males 30%; females (1961) 10%, (1967, 1971) 15%, (1975) 20%. Number of cigarettes/person/day: males: 3.0; females (1961, 1967) 1.0, (1971, 1975) 2.0

8 **Cleary and Shelley (1983) and Department of Health/Health Promotion Unit**

a. Joint National Media Research surveys. 1972 represents July 1972-June 1973 etc. Conducted by (1972-1983) Irish Marketing Surveys Ltd, (1984-1989) Market Research Bureau of Ireland, (1990-1993) Lansdowne market Research. Random samples of around 5 000 each year

b. Regular smokers: smoked at least 1 cigarette on average per day

c. Assumed extension to age distribution for percentage smokers, age 15: males 30%; females (1972-1974) 15%, (1975-1984) 20%

9 **Merzdorf *et al* (1982), quoting Health Education Bureau Research and Information Division (1979)**

10 **Adriaanse *et al* (1986), quoting Cleary and Shelley (1983)**

a. National sample. Age not stated

11 **Flynn (1961)**

a. Survey conducted Sep 1959-Feb 1960 in schools in Co. Westmeath. Included all secondary and vocational schools; also older pupils at all primary schools in larger towns and villages, and some in isolated rural areas. Anonymous questionnaire usually completed in assembly hall, with teachers absent. Sample size (males) 1 389, (females) 1 317. All pupils present on the day participated, but 20 (0.7%) questionnaires rejected

b. Results presented in the *All ages* column of Table 14.4 include a few pupils age 9-11 (117 males and 85 females)

c. Regular smokers: smokes 1+ cigarettes per week. All smokers: smokers regularly or occasionally, including those who smoke only on festive occasions. There were no pipe smokers

d. Consumption category estimation based on 1-4, 5-9, 10-19, 20-29, 30-49, 50-89, 90+ cigarettes/smoker/week. The questionnaire allowed the pupils to give their consumption as daily, weekly or monthly, so the standard method of estimation should be regarded with caution

e. 75% of the pupils' fathers and 43% of their mothers smoke

12 **O'Rourke *et al* (1970)**

a. Study by the Irish Cancer Society of pupils at all vocational schools in Co. Kerry. Sample size (males) 899, (females) 617, comprising over two thirds of vocational school students in the county

13 **International Agency for Research on Cancer (IARC) (1986) quoting Health Education Bureau (1980)**

a. National survey, no further details available. Age not stated

14 **Grube *et al* (1984)**

a. Study of pupils at 27 Catholic primary schools in Dublin. Approximate ages corresponding to 6th class, median age 12.4. Anonymous questionnaires completed in class with student teacher present and regular teacher absent. Sample size (males) 331, (females) 418

b. Regular smokers: smoked daily in last month. All smokers: smoked at least 1 cigarette in last month

c. Consumption category estimation based on 1-2, 3-5, 6-10, 11-15, 16-20, 21+ cigarettes/smoker/day

15 Shelley *et al* (1996)

a. Random sample in county Offaly, reference area for a community prevention and health promotion programme conducted in Kilkenny
b. Smokers of all products: smoked cigarettes daily, 1 g tobacco daily, 1 cigar weekly, or a mixture of tobacco products. Prevalence shown with product * is for cigarette only smokers. It is unclear whether consumption per smoker relates to this group or to all cigarette smokers

16 van Reek *et al* (1992), van Reek and Adriaanse (1995)

a. A series of surveys of Young Europeans. About 800 children aged 11-15 years interviewed in each EC country except Luxembourg (where only 250 interviewed). Lowest age group 11-12. Interviews conducted at home, with parents absent
b. Regular smokers: smoked daily. All smokers: smoked at least once a week

17 WHO (1997)

a. No original source. National survey among 4 000 students
b. Regular smoker: smoked at least one or two cigarettes daily
c. This survey is also reported by Joossens *et al* (1994), except prevalence among girls is given as 13%

18 Hibell *et al* (1997)

a. Nationally representative survey forming part of ESPAD (European School Survey Project on Alcohol and Other Drugs). Target was pupils born in 1979, thus age 15-16 at time of survey in March/April1995. Approximately 80% of this group still in school. Anonymous questionnaire completed and sealed in envelope by pupil, in class. Teachers present, but discouraged from walking round the classroom. Sample size (males) 907, (females) 942. Response rate approximately 96%
b. Regular smokers: smoked 1 or more cigarettes per day in last 30 days. All smokers: smoked in last 30 days
c. Consumption category estimation based on 1-5, 6-10, 11-20, 21+ cigarettes/smoker/day

19 Joossens *et al* (1999) quoting Commission of European Community

a. 1987 represents 1988/1988 etc. Age group not stated

20 Clancy and Manning (1999)

a. Study of 3 418 children randomly selected from 30 schools throughout Republic of Ireland. Self-completion questionnaire on smoking and chest symptoms
b. Regular smokers: no further definition, but it is stated that two thirds of these smokers smoked daily

References

Adriaanse H., van Reek J. and van Zutphen W.M. (1986). Rookgewoonten van atrsen wereldwijd; een overzicht van 100 onderzoekinge naar tabaksgebruik onder artsen in 31 landen in de periode 1951-1985 (Worldwide physicians' smoking habits; a review of 100 surveys into physicians' tobacco consumption in 31 countries in the period 1951-1985. *Ned Tijdschr Geneeskd,* **130**, 2224-9.

Beese D.H. (ed) (1968). *Tobacco consumption in various countries,* 2nd edition. Tobacco Research Council, London. Research Paper 6.

Beese D.H. (ed) (1972). *Tobacco consumption in various countries,* 3rd edition. Tobacco Research Council, London. Research Paper 6.

Clancy L. and Manning P.J. (1999). Smoking prevalence in Irish teenagers [Abstract]. *Nicotine & Tobacco Research,* **1**, 190.

Cleary A. and Shelley E. Bourke G. and Graham I. (eds) (1983). Smoking and health—the facts in Ireland. *Ir.Med.J.,* **76 Suppl**, 1-29. Irish Medical Association, Dublin.

Corridan J.P. (1963). A smoking survey of Cork City children. *Journal of the Irish Medical Association,* **53**, 147-53.

Council of Europe (1978). *Lung cancer in Western Europe,* 3rd edition. Council of Europe, Strasbourg.

Flynn M. (1961). Smoking habits of school children in County Westmeath. *Journal of the Irish Medical Association,* **XLVIII**, 87-97.

Grube J.W., McGree S. and Morgan M. (1984). Smoking behaviours, intentions and beliefs among Dublin primary school children. *Economic and Social Review,* **15**, 265-88.

Grube J.W. and Morgan M. (1986). *Smoking, drinking and other drug use among Dublin post-primary school pupils.* Economic and Social Research Institute, Dublin, Dublin. Paper No. 132.

Harkin A.M., Anderson P. and Goos C. (1997). *Smoking, drinking and drug taking in the European Region.* Alcohol, Drugs and Tobacco Programme, WHO Regional Office for Europe, Copenhagen.

Health Education Bureau (1980). *Tobacco consumption in Ireland: fact sheet 15, Smoking.* Dublin.[§]

Health Education Bureau Research and Information Division (1979). *Smoking Patterns, May 1979. Omnibus Survey.* Dublin.[§]

Herity B.A., Wilson-Davis K. and Bourke G.J. (1976). A study of the smoking habits of medical and non-medical university staff. *Journal of the Irish Medical Association,* **69**, 163-6.

Hibell B., Andersson B., Bjarnason T., Kokkevi A., Morgan M. and Narusk A. (1997). *The 1995 ESPAD report. The European school survey project on alcohol and other drugs. Alcohol and other drug use among students in 26 European countries.* The Swedish Council for Information on Alcohol and Other Drugs. Council of Europe (Pompidou Group).

IARC (1986). *Tobacco smoking.* IARC, Lyon, France. (IARC Monographs on the evaluation of the carcinogenic risk of chemicals to humans, Volume 38.)

Joossens L., Naett C., Howie C. and Muldoon A. (1994). *Tobacco and health in the European Union. An overview.* European Bureau for Action on Smoking Prevention (BASP), Brussels.

Joossens L., Sasco A., Salvador T. and Villalbí J.R. (1999). Las mujeres y el tabaco en la Unión Europea (Women and tobacco in the European Union). *Revista Espanola de Salud Publica,* **73**, 3-11. http://www.msc.es/salud/epidemiologia/resp/199901/colab%5Fmujeres.htm.

Lee P.N. (ed) (1975). *Tobacco consumption in various countries,* 4th edition. Tobacco Research Council,

London. Research Paper 6.

Maxwell J.C.Jr. (successive years). How the brands ranked. Maxwell International Estimates. *World Tobacco.*

Merzdorf J., Reuter U. and Welsch G. (1982). *Daten und Fakten zur Entwicklung des Rauchens in Mitgliedsländern der Europäischen Gemeinschaften (Facts and figures on the development of smoking in the member states of the European Communities)*. Kommission der Europäischen Gemeinschaften, Luxemburg. Medizin—EUR 7907 DE.

Mooney T. (2000). *Towards a tobacco free society: report of the fobacco free policy review group*. Department of Health and Children, Dublin.

O'Rourke A., O'Sullivan N. and Groke M. (1970). A study of children's smoking habits in Kerry. *Irish Nurses' Journal,* **3**, 17-9.

O'Rourke A., O'Sullivan N. and Wilson-Davis K. (1968). A Dublin schools smoking survey. Part I. *Ir J Med Sci,* **7th series, Vol 1**, 123-30.

O'Rourke A., Wilson-Davis K. and Gough C. (1971). Smoking, drugs and alcohol in Dublin secondary schools. *Ir J Med Sci,* **140**, 230-41.

O'Rourke A.H., O'Byrne D.J., Condren L. and Wilson-Davis K. (1983a). Smoking—a study of post-primary schools, 1980-81. *Ir Med J,* **76**, 285-92.

O'Rourke A.H., O'Byrne D.J. and Wilson-Davis K. (1983b). Smoking among schoolchildren. *Journal of the Royal College of General Practitioners,* **33**, 569-72.

Research Services (1962). *Statistics of smoking in the Irish Republic* §

Revenue Commissioners (various years). *Report of the revenue commissioners.*

Revenue Commissioners (1996). *Customs continue operation against illicit tobacco sales (Press release).*

Shelley E., Collins C. and Daly L. (1996). Trends in smoking prevalence: the Kilkenny Health Project population surveys 1985 to 1991. *Ir Med J,* **89**, 182-5.

Todd G. (1986). *Medicine. Statistics of smoking in the Member States of the European Community*. Commission of the European Communities, Luxembourg.

van Reek J. and Adriaanse H. (1995). Daily smoking among adolescents in the European Community. *Rev Epidemiol Sante Publique,* **43**, 281-2.

van Reek J., Adriaanse H. and Karaoglou A. (1992). Smoking among children in the European Community. *J Public Health Med,* **14**, 93-4.

Ward J.B., Healy C. and Dean G. (1978). Urban and Rural Mortality in the Republic of Ireland. *Journal of the Irish Medical Association,* **71**, 73-80.

WHO (1997). *Tobacco or health: A global status report.* WHO, Geneva. www.cdc.gov/nccdphp/osh/who/whoampro.htm.

§ Original paper not obtained, but information taken as quoted by another author

Israel 15

Sales data

See Tables 15.1-15.3.

Comprehensive data on tobacco consumption in Israel are not available. Most data on consumption of cigarettes and other tobacco products are based on Israeli production. Data for cigars and pipe tobacco were not given after 1982 and are therefore not included in the total.

From 1967 until the mid-1980s the consumption of manufactured cigarettes per adult was about 6-7 cigarettes per day. By 1995, it decreased to 4 cigarettes per day. No data on consumption of hand-rolled cigarettes are available in Israel.

The consumption of all tobacco products combined, based on production data and available for certain years only, varied between 5 and 7 g per adult per day from 1970 to 1989. Nearly all tobacco in this period was consumed in manufactured cigarettes. Until 1982 about 1% of all tobacco was used in water-pipes ('Tombac'), and in the 1970s another 1% was used as snuff. In 1982, the last year for which production data were available for cigars and pipe tobacco, consumption of these tobacco products was negligible.

Survey data

See Tables 15.4-15.8

A series of surveys (source 4, see Table 15.4) gives information on smoking almost annually from 1972 to 1983, but relates only to the Jewish population and the data are only available by two broad age groups. A study carried out in 1985-1987 (source 12) presents a more detailed breakdown in age groups. Few data are available for more recent years.

Between 1972 and 1983, the prevalence of tobacco smoking among those aged 15 years and over was around 45% in men and around 30%, perhaps decreasing slightly, in women. Later sources generally gave lower estimates of prevalence, 36-38% in men and 21-25% in women, but one source for 1989 (source 16) gave values similar to the earlier years.

Data on smoking among teenagers is scarce. Surveys in the 1970s showed that more boys smoked than girls, but this difference disappeared after the mid-1980s. At discharge from military service (age 20-22) more young men than young women smoke, but this prevalence has decreased, from about 60% and 40% respectively in the early 1980s, to 40% and 30% in 1995.

Comparison of survey and sales data suggests that surveys reported consumption within plus or minus 15% of manufactured cigarette production data. However, comparisons should be made with caution, since the sales data are incomplete, and the survey-based consumption is calculated from limited data (see notes 4b and 12b). Between 1972 and the mid-1980s, the estimated number of cigarettes smoked per person per day (sales-adjusted) was about 8 to 9 for men and about 4 to 5 for women. By 1995, it decreased to 6 for men and 3 for women.

Table 15.1.1 Total annual production of tobacco products, 1970-1995

Year	Cigarettes tonnes	Cigars tonnes	Pipe tobacco tonnes	Tombac tonnes	Snuff tonnes	All tobacco products tonnes
1970	3868	15	19	60	39	4001
1975	5553	16	17	52	36	5674
1980	5337	9	8	41	27	5422
1982	6043	3	1	35	24	6106
1983	6373			29	23	6425
1984	6714			29	21	6764
1985	6709			29	20	6758
1986	6723			33	21	6777
1987	6888			29	19	6936
1988	5882			27	20	5929
1989	5245			25	18	5288
1990	5440					
1991	5590					
1992	5742					
1993	5525					
1994	5638					
1995	4933					

Source : see *Notes on sources of sales data*, p. 370

Table 15.1.3 Manufactured cigarettes, percentage of total sales as filter cigarettes, 1968-1980

Year	% Filter
1968	77.5
1969	83.0
1970	86.4
1971	93.0
1972	95.0
1973	95.4
1974	96.8
1975	96.9
1976	97.1
1977	97.3
1978	97.6
1979	97.9
1980	98.7

Source : see *Notes on sources of sales data*, p. 370

Table 15.2 Consumption of (i) cigarettes and (ii) all tobacco products, 1967-1995 sales-based data, including estimated hand-rolled cigarette consumption. Males and females aged 15 years and over

Year	Manufactured cigarettes		Hand-rolled cigarettes		Total cigarettes		All tobacco products	
	Total annual in millions	Number/ adult/day	Total annual in millions	Number/ adult/day	Total annual in millions	Number/ adult/day	Total annual in tonnes	Grams/ adult/day
1967	3200	5.4						
1968	3340	5.5						
1969	3682	5.9						
1970	3868	6.0					4001	6.2
1971	4100	6.2						
1972	4400	6.4						
1973	5000	7.1						
1974	5200	7.2						
1975	5553	6.6					5674	6.7
1976	5500	6.4						
1977	5500	6.2						
1978	5800	6.5						
1979	5700	6.2						
1980	5337	5.6					5422	5.7
1981	6000	6.2						
1982	6043	6.2					6106	6.2
1983	6373	6.4					6425	6.5
1984	6714	6.6					6764	6.6
1985	6709	6.4					6758	6.5
1986	6723	6.3					6777	6.4
1987	6888	6.4					6936	6.4
1988	5882	5.3					5929	5.4
1989	5245	4.7					5288	4.7
1990	5440	4.7						
1991	5590	4.5						
1992	5742	4.4						
1993	5525	4.1						
1994	5638	4.1						
1995	4933	3.5						

Source : see *Notes on sources of sales data,* p. 370

Figure 15.1 Daily consumption of (i) manufactured and total number of cigarettes, and (ii) all tobacco products, 1967-1995.
Males and females aged 15 years and over. *Source:* see Table 15.2

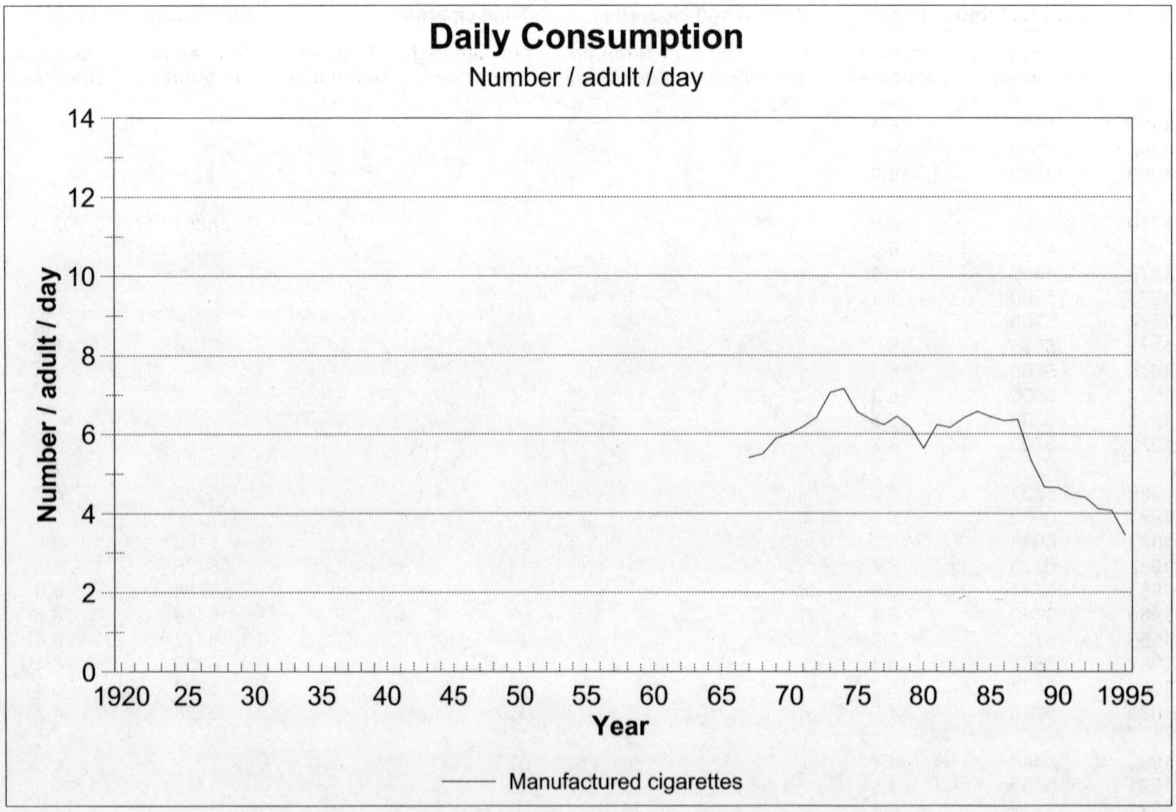

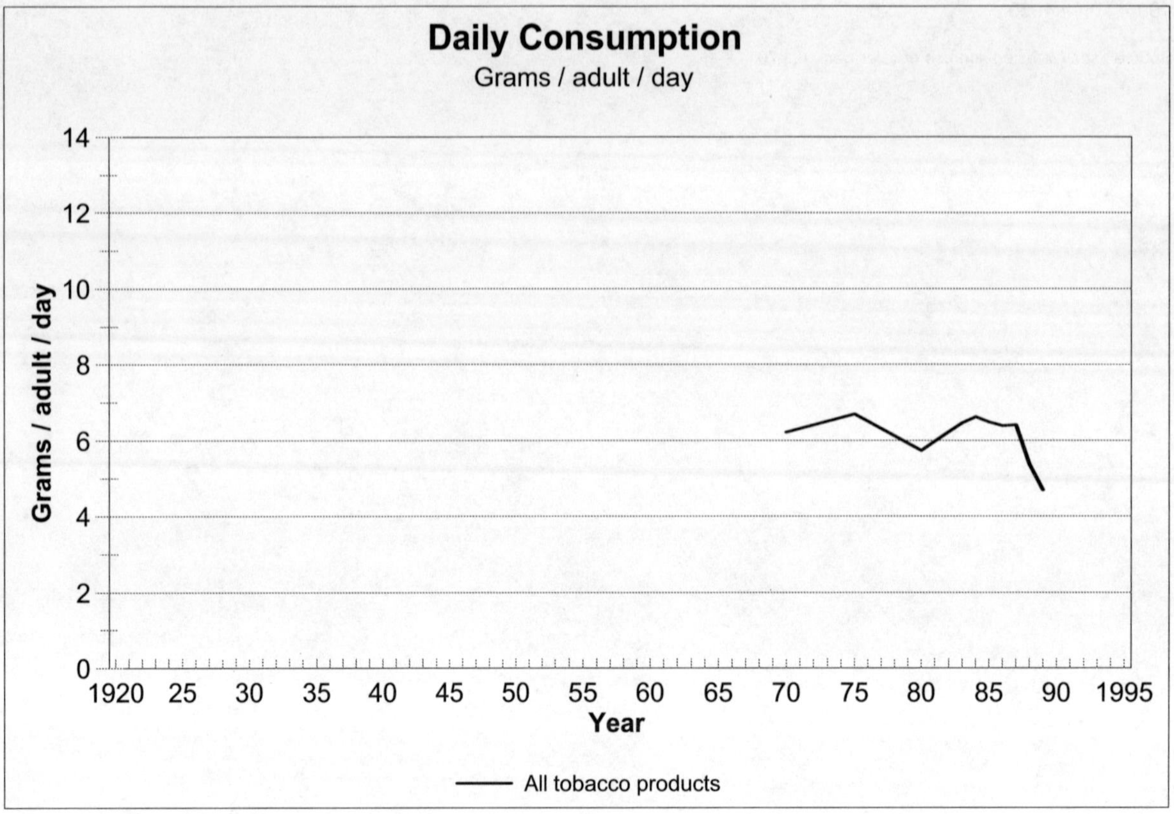

Table 15.3 Percentage sales of tobacco in different forms (by weight), selected years 1975-1985

Year	Cigarettes (%)	Cigars (%)	Pipe tobacco (%)	Tombac (%)	Snuff (%)
1975	97.9	0.3	0.3	0.9	0.6
1985	99.3	0.0	0.0	0.4	0.3

Source : calculated from Table 15.1.2

Figure 15.2 Percentage sales of tobacco in different forms (by weight), selected years 1975-1985
Source: see Table 15.3

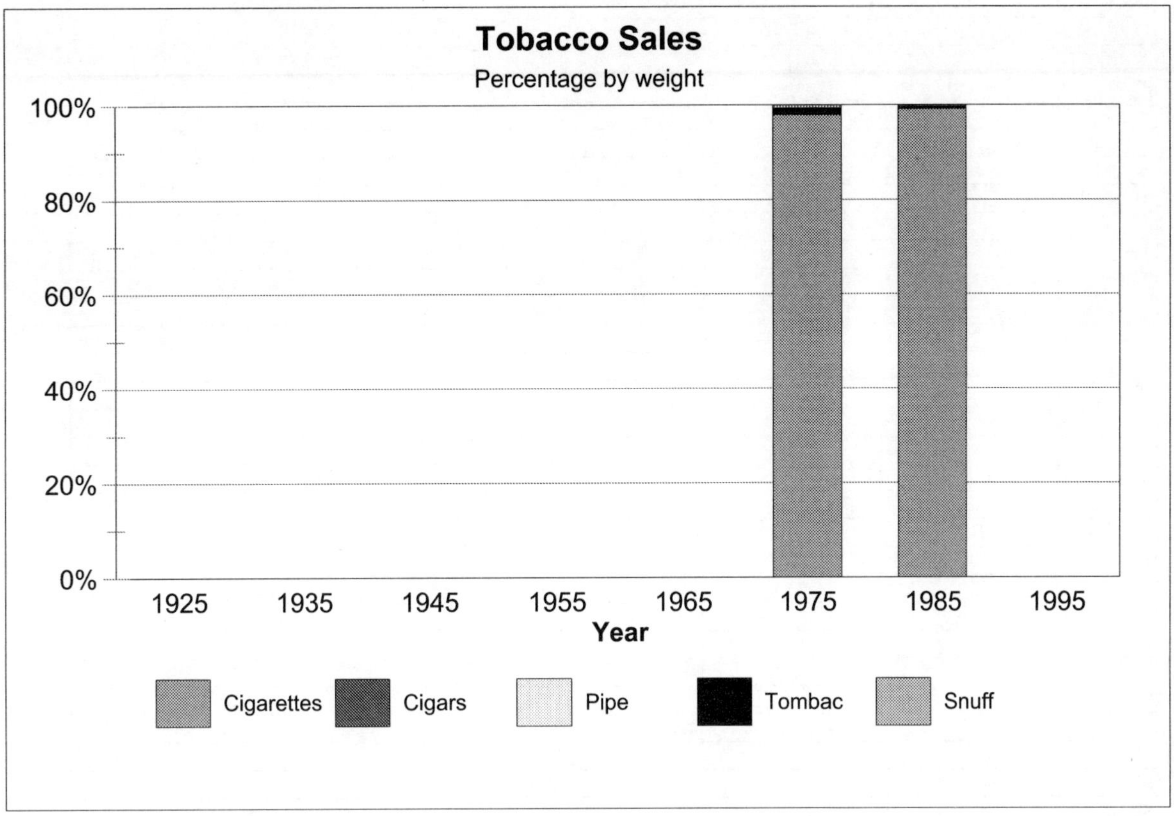

Table 15.4M Prevalence of smoking, males: some selected Israeli surveys by age, 1963-1995

<table>
<tr><th rowspan="2">Frequency
Product
Source
Year</th><th colspan="21">Age group</th><th rowspan="2">All ages</th></tr>
<tr><th>12</th><th>13</th><th>14</th><th>15</th><th>16</th><th>17</th><th>18</th><th>19</th><th>20-24</th><th>25-29</th><th>30-34</th><th>35-39</th><th>40-44</th><th>45-49</th><th>50-54</th><th>55-59</th><th>60-64</th><th>65-69</th><th>70-74</th><th>75-79</th><th>80+</th></tr>
<tr><td>63 1 UC R</td><td colspan="12"></td><td>56</td><td>51</td><td>49</td><td>46</td><td colspan="5">43</td><td></td></tr>
<tr><td>63 1 A U</td><td colspan="12"></td><td>57</td><td>52</td><td>50</td><td>48</td><td colspan="5">45</td><td></td></tr>
<tr><td>70 2 UC U</td><td colspan="3"></td><td colspan="5">31</td><td>61</td><td colspan="2">54</td><td colspan="2">59</td><td colspan="2">52</td><td colspan="2">39</td><td colspan="2">32</td><td colspan="2">34</td><td>50</td></tr>
<tr><td>72 4 U U</td><td colspan="8"></td><td colspan="13">43</td><td></td></tr>
<tr><td>73 4 U U</td><td colspan="8"></td><td colspan="4">55</td><td colspan="9">36</td><td>41</td></tr>
<tr><td>74 4 U U</td><td colspan="8"></td><td colspan="4">56</td><td colspan="9">40</td><td>48</td></tr>
<tr><td>75 4 U U</td><td colspan="8"></td><td colspan="4">63</td><td colspan="9">34</td><td>44</td></tr>
<tr><td>76 4 U U</td><td colspan="8"></td><td colspan="13">45</td><td></td></tr>
<tr><td>78 6 U U</td><td colspan="4"></td><td colspan="3">26</td><td colspan="14"></td><td></td></tr>
<tr><td>79 4 U U</td><td colspan="8"></td><td colspan="4">50</td><td colspan="9">41</td><td>43</td></tr>
<tr><td>79 7 U U</td><td colspan="5"></td><td>31</td><td colspan="15"></td><td></td></tr>
<tr><td>80 3 UC U</td><td colspan="5"></td><td>31</td><td colspan="5"></td><td colspan="2">40</td><td colspan="2">42</td><td colspan="2">34</td><td colspan="4">28</td><td>40</td></tr>
<tr><td>81 4 U U</td><td colspan="8"></td><td colspan="13">47</td><td></td></tr>
<tr><td>81 8 UC A</td><td colspan="2"></td><td>17</td><td>19</td><td>30</td><td colspan="2">23</td><td colspan="14"></td><td>25</td></tr>
<tr><td>81 13 UC U</td><td colspan="8"></td><td>57</td><td colspan="12"></td><td></td></tr>
<tr><td>82 13 UC U</td><td colspan="8"></td><td>60</td><td colspan="12"></td><td></td></tr>
<tr><td>83 4 U U</td><td colspan="8"></td><td colspan="4">50</td><td colspan="9">38</td><td>44</td></tr>
<tr><td>83 9 U U</td><td colspan="2"></td><td colspan="5">17</td><td colspan="14"></td><td></td></tr>
<tr><td>83 13 UC U</td><td colspan="8"></td><td>59</td><td colspan="12"></td><td></td></tr>
<tr><td>84 10 U U</td><td colspan="2"></td><td>34</td><td colspan="18"></td><td></td></tr>
<tr><td>84 13 UC U</td><td colspan="8"></td><td>53</td><td colspan="12"></td><td></td></tr>
<tr><td>85 11 U A</td><td></td><td colspan="5">31</td><td colspan="15"></td><td></td></tr>
<tr><td>85 12 UC R</td><td colspan="8"></td><td>48</td><td colspan="2">49</td><td colspan="2">40</td><td colspan="2">38</td><td colspan="2">27</td><td colspan="4"></td><td>40</td></tr>
<tr><td>85 13 UC U</td><td colspan="8"></td><td>50</td><td colspan="12"></td><td></td></tr>
<tr><td>86 5 U *</td><td></td><td>2</td><td></td><td>6</td><td colspan="17"></td><td></td></tr>
<tr><td>86 5 U R</td><td></td><td>3</td><td></td><td>10</td><td colspan="17"></td><td></td></tr>
<tr><td>86 5 U A</td><td></td><td>4</td><td></td><td>13</td><td colspan="17"></td><td></td></tr>
<tr><td>86 13 UC U</td><td colspan="8"></td><td>50</td><td colspan="12"></td><td></td></tr>
<tr><td>87 13 UC U</td><td colspan="8"></td><td>51</td><td colspan="12"></td><td></td></tr>
<tr><td>87 14 MC R</td><td colspan="3"></td><td colspan="18">38</td><td></td></tr>
<tr><td>88 13 UC U</td><td colspan="8"></td><td>46</td><td colspan="12"></td><td></td></tr>
<tr><td>88 15 UC R</td><td colspan="8"></td><td>46</td><td colspan="12"></td><td></td></tr>
<tr><td>88 15 UC A</td><td colspan="8"></td><td>48</td><td colspan="12"></td><td></td></tr>
<tr><td>89 13 UC U</td><td colspan="8"></td><td>48</td><td colspan="12"></td><td></td></tr>
<tr><td>89 16 U U</td><td colspan="3"></td><td colspan="18">45</td><td></td></tr>
<tr><td>90 13 UC U</td><td colspan="8"></td><td>47</td><td colspan="12"></td><td></td></tr>
<tr><td>91 13 UC U</td><td colspan="8"></td><td>46</td><td colspan="12"></td><td></td></tr>
<tr><td>92 13 UC U</td><td colspan="8"></td><td>40</td><td colspan="12"></td><td></td></tr>
<tr><td>92 17 U U</td><td colspan="6"></td><td colspan="15">38</td><td></td></tr>
<tr><td>92 18 U U</td><td colspan="8"></td><td>48</td><td colspan="2">49</td><td colspan="2"></td><td colspan="8"></td><td></td></tr>
<tr><td>93 13 UC U</td><td colspan="8"></td><td>41</td><td colspan="12"></td><td></td></tr>
<tr><td>94 5 UC R</td><td></td><td>3</td><td></td><td>9</td><td colspan="17"></td><td></td></tr>
<tr><td>94 13 UC U</td><td colspan="8"></td><td>39</td><td colspan="12"></td><td></td></tr>
<tr><td>95 13 UC U</td><td colspan="8"></td><td>41</td><td colspan="12"></td><td></td></tr>
</table>

Source: see *Notes on sources of survey data*, p. 370

Product:
MC = manufactured cigarettes
TC = total cigarettes (including hand-rolled)
UC = cigarettes (type unspecified)
A = all products

Frequency:
A = all smokers (including occasional)
R = regular or daily smokers

All ages: relevant to ages used and as given in original source
U = unspecified
* = refer to *Notes on sources of survey data*, p. 370

Table 15.4F Prevalence of smoking, females: some selected Israeli surveys by age, 1963-1995

Year	Source	Product	Frequency	12	13	14	15	16	17	18	19	20-24	25-29	30-34	35-39	40-44	45-49	50-54	55-59	60-64	65-69	70-74	75-79	80+	All ages
63	1	UC	R																						
63	1	A	U																						
70	2	UC	U				18					31	35		31		27		16		22		7		27
72	4	U	U									30													
73	4	U	U									41			33										36
74	4	U	U									34			28										31
75	4	U	U									40			27										34
76	4	U	U									34													
78	6	U	U					17																	
79	4	U	U									32			27										29
79	7	U	U						19																
80	3	UC	U						19						28		20		16						24
81	4	U	U									29													
81	8	UC	A			4	11	13	33																13
81	13	UC	U									42													
82	13	UC	U									43													
83	4	U	U									35			22										30
83	9	U	U			11																			
83	13	UC	U									42													
84	10	U	U			21																			
84	13	UC	U									40													
85	11	U	A		48																				
85	12	UC	R									24	29		27		18		15						23
85	13	UC	U									39													
86	5	U	*		0		5																		
86	5	U	R		0		8																		
86	5	U	A		1		14																		
86	13	UC	U									39													
87	13	UC	U									38													
87	14	MC	R				25																		
88	13	UC	U									35													
88	15	UC	R									26													
88	15	UC	A									30													
89	13	UC	U									30													
89	16	U	U				30																		
90	13	UC	U									30													
91	13	UC	U									30													
92	13	UC	U									25													
92	17	U	U							25															
92	18	U	U												27										
93	13	UC	U									29													
94	5	UC	R		2		9																		
94	13	UC	U									30													
95	13	UC	U									31													

Source: see *Notes on sources of survey data*, p. 370
Product: MC = manufactured cigarettes
TC = total cigarettes (including hand-rolled)
UC = cigarettes (type unspecified)
A = all products

Frequency: A = all smokers (including occasional)
R = regular or daily smokers
All ages: relevant to ages used and as given in original source
U = unspecified
* = refer to *Notes on sources of survey data*, p. 370

Table 15.5M Number of cigarettes smoked per smoker per day, males: some selected Israeli surveys by age, 1963-1995

Product Source Year	12	13	14	15	16	17	18	19	20-24	25-29	30-34	35-39	40-44	45-49	50-54	55-59	60-64	65-69	70-74	75-79	80+	All ages
63 1 UCE													21	20	19	19	18					20
70 2 UCE*				15					18	19		18		18		15		15		12		18
73 4 UCE*									22				19									
74 4 UCE*									19				20									
75 4 UCE*									21				21									
79 4 UCE*									24				22									
80 3 UCE						13						19										
81 8 UCE			8.3																			
83 4 UCE*									20				19									
85 12 UCE*									21	21		21		20		19						21
88 15 UCE									22													
89 13 UC									22													
90 13 UC									20													
91 13 UC									19													
92 13 UC									18													
93 13 UC									19													
94 13 UC									17													
95 13 UC									17													

Table 15.6M Number of cigarettes smoked per person per day, males: some selected Israeli surveys by age, 1963-1995, with percentage total sales

Product Source Year	12	13	14	15	16	17	18	19	20-24	25-29	30-34	35-39	40-44	45-49	50-54	55-59	60-64	65-69	70-74	75-79	80+	All ages	% Total sales
63 1 UC													12	10	9.5	8.8	7.7					9.9	**
70 2 UC *				4.4					11	10		11		9.5		5.8		4.9		4.1		8.7	96%m
73 4 UC *									12				6.8										100%m
74 4 UC *									11				8.0										92%m
75 4 UC *									13				7.0										110%m
79 4 UC *									12				8.8										113%m
80 3 UC						4.0						7.6											**
81 8 UC			2.1																				**
83 4 UC *									10				7.3										99%m
85 12 UC *									10	10		8.5		7.7		5.2						8.2	85%m
88 15 UC									10														**
89 13 UC									10														**
90 13 UC									⟨9.4⟩														**
91 13 UC									⟨8.7⟩														**
92 13 UC									⟨7.2⟩														**
93 13 UC									⟨7.8⟩														**
94 13 UC									⟨6.6⟩														**
95 13 UC									⟨6.8⟩														**

Source: see *Notes on sources of survey data*, p. 370
All ages: relevant to ages used and as given in original source
% Total sales: estimated % of total sales of M = manufactured or T = total cigarette consumption implied by the survey, sexes combined
** = cannot be calculated
--- = adjusted by original author
* = refer to *Notes on sources of survey data*, p. 370

Product: MC = manufactured cigarettes
TC = total cigarettes (including hand-rolled)
UC = cigarettes (type unspecified)
A = all products
U = unspecified
E indicates mean estimated from percentage distribution (see also *Consumption category estimation*, p. xxxiv, and Appendix III, p. 789)

Table 15.5F Number of cigarettes smoked per smoker per day, females: some selected Israeli surveys by age, 1963-1995

Year	Source	Product	Age group 12	13	14	15	16	17	18	19	20-24	25-29	30-34	35-39	40-44	45-49	50-54	55-59	60-64	65-69	70-74	75-79	80+	All ages
63	1	UCE																						
70	2	UCE*				12					13	13		13		14		12		13		9.7		11
73	4	UCE*									16				15									
74	4	UCE*									16				16									
75	4	UCE*									17				16									
79	4	UCE*									17				15									
80	3	UCE						9.5						13										
81	8	UCE			6.0																			
83	4	UCE*									16				17									
85	12	UCE*									12	15		15		16		16						15
88	15	UCE									16													
89	13	UC									14													
90	13	UC									15													
91	13	UC									13													
92	13	UC									14													
93	13	UC									14													
94	13	UC									12													
95	13	UC									13													

Table 15.6F Number of cigarettes smoked per person per day, females: some selected Israeli surveys by age, 1963-1995, with percentage total sales

Year	Source	Product	Age group 12	13	14	15	16	17	18	19	20-24	25-29	30-34	35-39	40-44	45-49	50-54	55-59	60-64	65-69	70-74	75-79	80+	All ages	% Total sales
63	1	UC																							**
70	2	UC *				2.2					3.9	4.5		4.2		3.7		1.9		2.9		0.6		3.0	96%m
73	4	UC *									6.6				5.1										100%m
74	4	UC *									5.3				4.4										92%m
75	4	UC *									6.6				4.4										110%m
79	4	UC *									5.3				3.9										113%m
80	3	UC						1.8						3.2											**
81	8	UC			0.8																				**
83	4	UC *									5.7				3.6										99%m
85	12	UC *									3.0	4.3		4.2		2.9		2.3						3.5	85%m
88	15	UC									⟨4.3⟩														**
89	13	UC									⟨4.3⟩														**
90	13	UC									⟨4.5⟩														**
91	13	UC									⟨3.9⟩														**
92	13	UC									⟨3.5⟩														**
93	13	UC									⟨4.1⟩														**
94	13	UC									⟨3.6⟩														**
95	13	UC									⟨4.1⟩														**

Source: see *Notes on sources of survey data*, p. 370
All ages: relevant to ages used and as given in original source
% Total sales: estimated % of total sales of M = manufactured or T = total cigarette consumption implied by the survey, sexes combined
** = cannot be calculated
--- = adjusted by original author
* = refer to *Notes on sources of survey data*, p. 370

Product: MC = manufactured cigarettes
TC = total cigarettes (including hand-rolled)
UC = cigarettes (type unspecified)
A = all products
U = unspecified
E indicates mean estimated from percentage distribution (see also *Consumption category estimation*, p. xxxiv, and Appendix III, p. 789)

Table 15.7M Number of cigarettes smoked per person per day, sales-adjusted, males: some selected Israeli surveys[1] by age, 1970-1985, with percentage total sales

Product Source Year	Age group 12	13	14	15	16	17	18	19	20-24	25-29	30-34	35-39	40-44	45-49	50-54	55-59	60-64	65-69	70-74	75-79	80+	All ages	% Total sales
70 2 UC *				4.6					12	10		11		9.9		6.0		5.1		4.3		9.1	96%m
73 4 UC *									12				6.8										100%m
74 4 UC *									11				8.7										92%m
75 4 UC *									12				6.4										110%m
79 4 UC *									11				7.8										113%m
83 4 UC *									10				7.4										99%m
85 12 UC *									12	12		10		9.1		6.1						9.6	85%m

Table 15.7F Number of cigarettes smoked per person per day, sales-adjusted, females: some selected Israeli surveys[1] by age, 1970-1985, with percentage total sales

Product Source Year	Age group 12	13	14	15	16	17	18	19	20-24	25-29	30-34	35-39	40-44	45-49	50-54	55-59	60-64	65-69	70-74	75-79	80+	All ages	% Total sales
70 2 UC *				2.3					4.1	4.7		4.3		3.8		2.0		3.0		0.7		3.1	96%m
73 4 UC *									6.6				5.1										100%m
74 4 UC *									5.8				4.8										92%m
75 4 UC *									6.0				4.0										110%m
79 4 UC *									4.7				3.5										113%m
83 4 UC *									5.8				3.7										99%m
85 12 UC *									3.6	5.1		5.0		3.4		2.7						4.1	85%m

1 Based on those surveys in Table 15.6 with data for both sexes and age range at least 21-64 (see *Cigarette consumption per person*, p. xxxv)

Source: See *Notes on sources of survey data*, p. 370

Product: MC = manufactured cigarettes
TC = total cigarettes (including hand-rolled)
UC = cigarettes (type unspecified)
A = all products
U = unspecified

All ages: relevant to ages used and as given in original source

% Total sales: Adjustment factor used, estimated % of total sales of M = manufactured or T = total cigarette consumption implied by survey, sexes combined

--- = adjusted by original author

* = refer to *Notes on sources of survey data*, p. 370

Table 15.8 Estimated[1] prevalence of smoking and estimated[1] number of cigarettes per person per day (unadjusted and sales-adjusted): summary of Tables 15.4, 15.6 and 15.7, 1970-1992.
Males and females aged 15 years and over

Year	Source[2]	Product[3]	Prevalence[4]						Number of cigarettes						
									Unadjusted[7]			Sales-adjusted[8]			
			Manufactured cigarettes[5]		Total cigarettes		All products[6]		Number/ person/day		Total sales %	Manufactured cigarettes[9] number/ person/day		Total cigarettes number/ person/day	
			M	F	M	F	M	F	M	F		M	F	M	F
1970	2	*UC*	48	26					8.3	3.3	96	8.6	3.5		
1972	9	*U*					41	29				(8.3	4.6)		
1973	4	UC+*U*					43	34	8.7	5.4	100	8.7	5.4		
1974	4	UC+*U*					45	29	8.6	4.6	92	9.4	5.0		
1975	4	UC+*U*					46	32	9.3	5.1	110	8.5	4.7		
1976	4	*U*					43	32				(8.0	4.8)		
1979	4	UC+*U*					43	28	9.7	4.4	113	8.5	3.9		
1981	4	*U*					45	27				(8.4	4.1)		
1983	4	UC+*U*					42	26	8.3	4.4	99	8.4	4.5		
1985	12	UC	38	21					7.7	3.2	85	9.1	3.8		
1987	14	MC	38	25								(8.4	4.4)		
1989	16	*U*					45	30				(6.1	3.3)		
1992	17	*U*					36	24				(5.8	3.1)		

1 Surveys covering an age range of at least 21-64 are included. Any gaps in the data for ages 15-20 and 65 years and over are filled in by assumed extensions to the age distribution, given in *Notes on sources of survey data*, p. 370. Method: see *Summary of adult smoking*, p. xxxvi
2 See *Notes on sources of survey data*, p. 370
3 Product: MC = manufactured cigarettes, TC = total cigarettes (including hand-rolled), UC = cigarettes (type unspecified), A = all products, U = unspecified. Frequency of smoking is indicated by: regular or daily smokers in normal type, all smokers (including occasional) in bold, unspecified in italics
4 From Table 15.4
5 This column includes prevalence of smoking classified as UC = cigarettes (type unspecified)
6 This column includes prevalence of smoking classified as U = unspecified product
7 From Table 15.6
8 From Table 15.7, except data in parentheses, which are derived from the prevalence of smoking from Table 15.4 as described in *Summary of adult smoking*, p. xxxvi
9 Number of cigarettes classified as UC = cigarettes (type unspecified) has been adjusted to manufactured cigarette sales and included in this column

Figure 15.3 Estimated prevalence of smoking of (i) cigarettes and (ii) all tobacco products: by year of survey, 1970-1992.
Males and females aged 15 years and over. *Source:* see Table 15.8

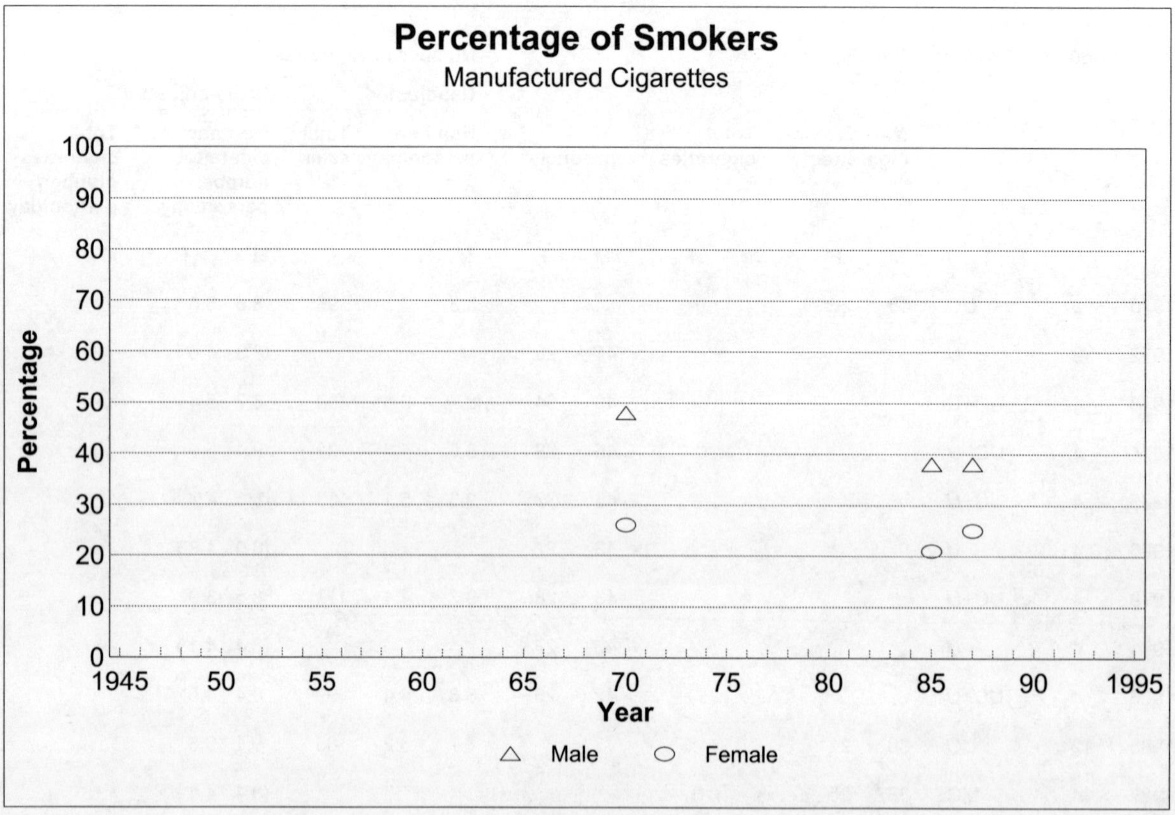

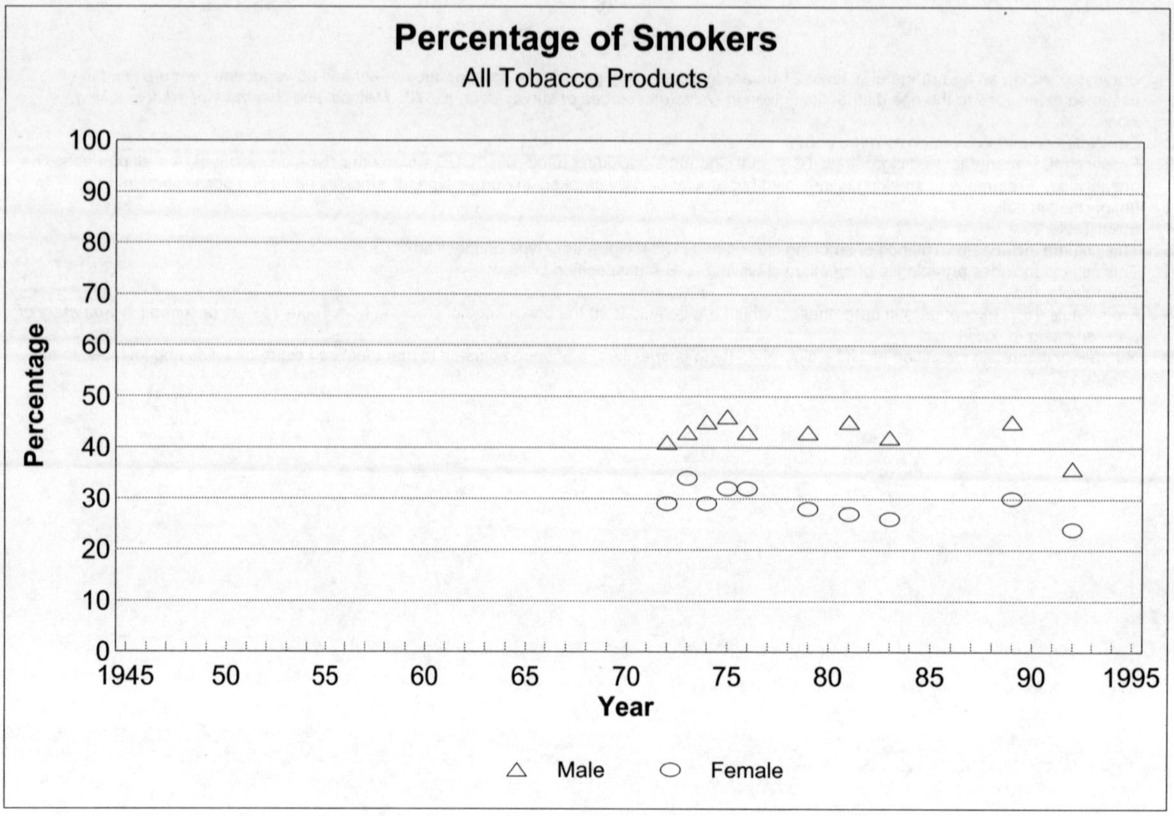

Figure 15.4 Estimated number of cigarettes smoked per smoker per day, sales-adjusted, 1970-1992.
Males and females aged 15 years and over. *Source:* see Table 15.8

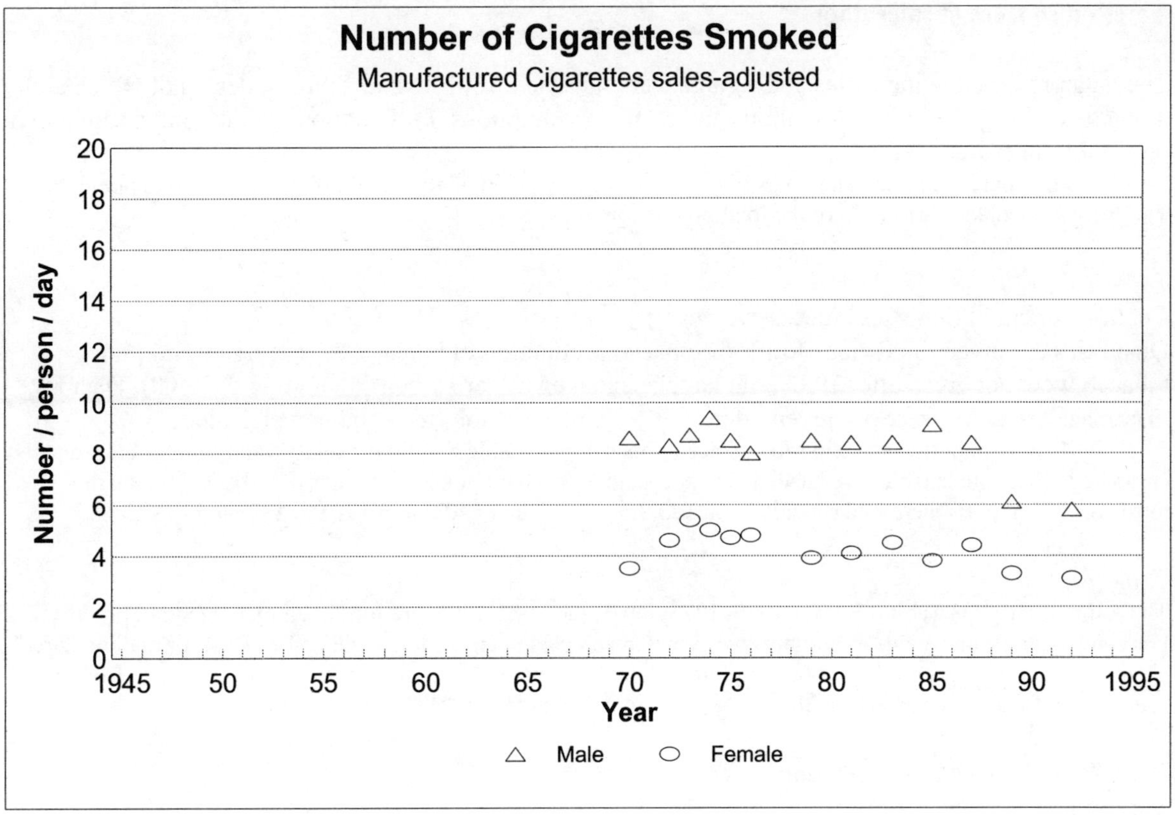

Notes on sources of sales data

The data presented in the tables and figures were obtained from several sources, details of which are given below, together with estimations and related assumptions. Full citations of the sources are given on p. 373 under *References*.

Note that population data up to 1974 are for the Jewish population only, thereafter for total population. The Jewish population was 89% of the total population in 1975.

Table 15.1.1
Central Bureau of Statistics (successive years)
Quantities are given for various forms of tobacco production in Israel. Data for cigars and pipe tobacco were not given after 1982 (and have been taken as zero when calculating the total). Data for 'Tombac' and snuff were not given after 1989. 'Tombac' is tobacco used in water-pipes.

Data on imported and exported tobacco goods are available only in monetary value and for all products combined. (The source tables are headed 'Tobacco and tobacco manufactures' and so probably include raw tobacco.) Net imports increased steadily from $23.8m in 1980 and $40.2m in 1987 to $89.6m in 1995.

Table 15.2
The estimates used in Table 15.2, for 1970, 1975, 1980, and 1982-1995, are for Israeli manufactured products. For conversion from weights to numbers we assumed an average cigarette weight of 1 g. Data for manufactured cigarettes in other years are from Maxwell International Estimates. (In years where data are available from both sources, the figures are very close, the largest difference being 5% in 1980.)

Plain/Filter cigarette consumption
Maxwell (successive years)

Tar yield of cigarettes
No data available.

Estimates of hand-rolled cigarette consumption
No information on smoking of hand-rolled cigarettes is available, and as the production data does not include a category for hand-rolling tobacco, consumption has been assumed to be negligible.

Notes on sources of survey data

Each source of survey data—either an individual survey or a series of surveys repeated over a number of years—is cited by a source number. This number is shown in the tables and corresponds to the source numbers given below, where details of the source publication and of the survey methodology are given. Full citations of the sources are given on p. 373 under *References*.

Source number

1 **Goldbourt and Medalie (1975), Benjamin (1978)**

a. Israel Ischaemic Heart Disease Project. Civil servants. Substantial differences by country of origin and period of immigration. Sample size (males only) 10 000
b. Consumption category estimation based on 1-10, 11-20, and 21+ cigarettes/smoker/day

2 **Kark *et al* (1979), Gofin *et al* (1981)**

a. Health study in Kiryat Hayovel suburb of Jerusalem, 1969-1971. Sample size (males) 2 254, (females) 2 669. Response rate (males, 15-19 years) 50%, (males, 25 years +) 85%, (females) 91%

b. 3% of men were pipe or cigar smokers

c. Low response rate among young men attributed to absence due to army service. Results for this group should be regarded with caution

d. Consumption category estimation based on two categories, 1-19 and 20+ cigarettes/smoker/day, and resulting figures should be regarded with caution

3 **Gofin *et al* (1982)**

a. Jerusalem Lipid Research Clinic Prevalence Study. Sample 17-year-olds and parents of 17-year-olds from Jerusalem. Sample size: (boys) 650, (girls) 557, (men) 1 064, (women) 595. Response rate (boys) 75%, (girls) 76%, (men) 77%, (women) 86%

b. Results shown in *All ages* column relate to age 35+

c. Persons of North African origin had the highest proportion of smokers; those of European origin had the lowest

d. Consumption category estimation based on 1-10, 11-20 and 21+ cigarettes/smoker/day

4 **Epstein and Biger (1987), quoting Ben Sira (1983)**

a. Representative surveys of Jewish population (excluding Kibbutzim) by Israel Institute of Applied Social Research. Study details only available for 1983. At home interviews. Sample size (age 20+) 830, (age 14-18) 282. See source 9 for adolescent part of this study

b. Consumption category estimation based on two categories, percentage smokers and percentage of smokers who smoked 21+ cigarettes/day, and resulting figures should be regarded with caution

c. Assumed extension to age distribution for percentage smokers, age 15-19: males 30% and females (1972-1976, 1979) 20%, (1981, 1983) 15%. Number of cigarettes/person/day: males 5.0 and females 3.0

5 **Nutbeam and Aarø (1990), King *et al* (1996)**

a. Part of the HBSC (Health Behaviour in School-Aged Children) Study, a collaborative cross-national research study sponsored by the WHO. School classes or schools were randomly selected, targeting age groups 11 (not presented here), 13 and 15. The target sample size was 1 300 in each age group.

Year	Location	Mean age		Sample size	
		Target age 13	Target age 15	Target age 13	Target age 15
1985-1986	Jerusalem	—	—	983	980
1994	Nationwide	13.5	15.6	1 646	1 352

c. Regular smokers: smoke once a week or more. Smokers marked as frequency *: smoked daily

6 **Epstein and Biger (1987), quoting Tamir *et al* (1982)**

a. Ort Study, in suburban area near Haifa

7 **Epstein and Biger (1987), quoting Halfon *et al* (1982)**

a. Survey in Jerusalem among 17-year-olds. Smoking most common among those of North African extraction and least common among those of European origin

8 **Zoller and Maymon (1983)**

a. National study of high school adolescents developed by Oranim, the School of Education of the Kibbutz Movement in Israel. Sample size 1 420

b. Smokers: smoke regularly or when given the chance, even if this means just one (or a few) cigarettes per week

c. Consumption category estimation based on 1, 2-5, 5-10 and more than 10 cigarettes/smoker/day (1, 2-4, 5-10 and 11+ assumed)

9 **Epstein and Biger (1987), quoting Ben Sira (1983)**

a. Adolescent part of study described in source 4

b. Assumed extension to age distribution for percentage smokers (1972), age 15-19: males 30% and females 20%

10 Geizerova and Masironi (1988)

a. No original source

11 Isralowitz and Sobel (1988)

a. Year not stated. Anonymous pre-coded questionnaire. Sample size (males) 33, (females) 21; comprising approximately 85% of high-school-age youth in an established kibbutz

12 Green and Harari (1992)

a. The Cordis Study. Employees at 21 factories screened for cardiovascular risk factors, 1985-1987. Personal interviews. Sample size (males) 4 317, (females) 1 698; response rate 60%. Analysis restricted to Jewish subjects only (5 281)

b. Consumption category estimation based on two categories, 1-19 and 20+ cigarettes/smoker/day, and resulting figures should be regarded with caution

c. Assumed extension to age distribution for percentage smokers, age 15-19: males 30% and females 15%; age 65+: males 25% and females 10%. Number of cigarettes/person/day, age 15-19: males 5.0 and females 3.0; age 65+: males 5.0 and females 2.0

13 Ashkenazi and Shemer (1997)

a. Surveys of soldiers on their day of discharge from the Israeli Defence Forces between 1980 and 1995. Total sample size 32 166. See source 15 for comments on representativeness

b. Data taken from charts

14 Mackay (1994)

a. No original source. Age group not stated

15 Kark and Laor (1992)

a. Study of Israeli men and women on release from military service. Age 20-22. Largely representative of all Jewish men and of educated women in Israel. Sample size (males) 1 142, (females) 842

b. Consumption category estimation based on 1-9, 10-19, 20-29 and 30+ cigarettes/smoker/day

16 WHO (1997)

a. No original source. Age group not stated

17 Levy (1993)

a. No original source. Year not stated

b. Assumed extension to age distribution for percentage smokers, age 15-17: males 20% and females 15%

18 WHO(1997)

a. A national survey. Quoted data relate to the age groups with the highest smoking prevalence for each sex

Additional information (not presented in tables)

WHO (1997) gives adult (18+) Jewish smoking prevalence (sexes combined) as 31% in 1993 and 29% in 1994

Meijer *et al* (1996) gives smoking prevalence among students in two high schools in the Jerusalem area (year not specified) as follows:

Grade (age)	n	Current smokers	
		%	male:female ratio
6th (11-12)	155	1	2
7th (12-13)	213	4	1.7
8th (13-14)	132	8	0.9
9th (14-15)	111	21	0.6
10th (15-16)	146	36	1.3
11th (16-17)	90	28	1.2
Total	847	14	1

These smoking rates are considerably higher than those reported by source 5

References

Ashkenazi I. and Shemer J. (1997). Smoking habits of young Israeli soldiers. *Harefuah,* **132**, 502-7.

Ben Sira Z. (1983). *Smoking among adults and youths: trends, predictions and justifications for smoking and its cessation.* Israel Institute for Applied Social Research, Jerusalem.§

Benjamin B. (1978). *Tobacco smoking in the world. Report of the WHO Expert Committee on Smoking Control, Geneva 23-28 October 1978*

Central Bureau of Statistics (successive years). *Statistical abstract of Israel.* Jerusalem, Tel Aviv, Haifa.

Epstein L. and Biger C. (1987). Cigarette smoking in Israel: prevalence and control. *Harefuah,* **112**, 301-6.

Geizerova H. and Masironi R. (1988). Cigarette smoking in children and adolescents: world review. In: Aoki M., Hisamichi S. and Tominaga S. (eds) *Smoking and health 1987. Proceedings of the 6th World Conference on Smoking and Health, Tokyo, 9-12 November 1987.* Elsevier Science Publishers B.V. (Biomedical Division), Amsterdam; 601-5. International Congress Series No. 780.

Gofin J., Kark E., Mainemer N., Kark S.L., *et al* (1981). Prevalence of selected health characteristics of women and comparisons with men: a community health survey in Jerusalem. *Isr J Med Sci,* **17**, 145-59.

Gofin J., Kark J.D., Halfon S.T., Friedlander Y. and Stein Y. (1982). Cigarette smoking and its relation to anthropometric characteristics and biochemical variables in Jerusalem 17-year-olds and adults. *Isr J Med Sci,* **18**, 1233-41.

Goldbourt U. and Medalie J.H. (1975). Characteristics of smokers, nonsmokers and ex-smokers among 10 000 adult males in Israel. 1. Distribution of selected sociodemographic behavioural variables and the prevalence of disease. *Isr J Med Sci,* **11**, 1079-101.

Green M.S. and Harari G. (1992). Past and present smoking behaviour and its association with health-related habits in selected Israeli working populations. The Cordis study. *Int J Epidemiol,* **21**, 494-501.

Halfon S.-T., Kark J.D., Bonar M., Friedlander Y. and Eisenberg S. (1982). Smoking, lipids and lipoproteins in Jerusalem 17-year-olds. *Isr J Med Sci,* **18**, 1150-7.§

Isralowitz R.E. and Sobel R. (1988). Smoking among Kibbutz youth: Patterns, perceptions and determinants. *Journal of Adolescent Health Care,* **9**, 495-7.

Kark J.D. and Laor A. (1992). Cigarette smoking and educational level among young Israelis upon release from military service in 1988—a public health challenge. *Isr J Med Sci,* **28**, 33-7.

Kark S.L., Gofin J., Abramson J., Makler A., *et al* (1979). Prevalence of selected health characteristics of men: a community health survey in Jerusalem. *Isr J Med Sci,* **15**, 732-41.

King A., Wold B., Tudor-Smith C. and Harel Y. (1996). *The health of youth, a cross-national survey.* WHO Regional Publications, Europe, Copenhagen. European Series No. 69.

Levy J. (1993). Israel's roller coaster year. *Tobacco International,* **195**, 30-1.

Mackay J.L. (1994). The fight against tobacco in developing countries. *Tuber Lung Dis,* **75**, 8-24.

Maxwell J.C.Jr. (successive years). How the brands ranked. Maxwell International Estimates. *World Tobacco.*

Meijer B., Branski D., Knol K. and Kerem E. (1996). Cigarette smoking habits among schoolchildren. *Chest,* **110**, 921-6.

Nutbeam D. and Aarø L.E. (1990). Smoking and alienation from school: the implications for health education with young people. Results from the WHO study of health behaviour in schoolchildren. In: Durston B. and Jamrozik K. (eds) *Tobacco & health 1990. The global war. Seventh World Conference on Tobacco and*

Health, Perth, Western Australia, 1-5 April 1990. Organising Committee of the Seventh World Conference on Tobacco and Health, 189 Royal Street, East Perth, Western Australia 6004; 539-44.

Tamir A., Wolff H. and Epstein L.M. (1982). Health-related behaviour in Israel adolescents. *Journal of Adolescent Health Care,* **2**, 261-5.[§]

WHO (1997). *Tobacco or health: A global status report*. WHO, Geneva. www.cdc.gov/nccdphp/osh/who/whoampro.htm.

Zoller U. and Maymon T. (1983). Smoking behaviour of high school students in Israel. *J Sch Health,* **53**, 613-7.

§ Original paper not obtained, but information taken as quoted by another author

Italy 16

Sales data

See Tables 16.1-16.3.

Until 1955, sales data were available only for 5-year periods; they show no evidence of war-time shortages. The data presented are of tobacco sold legally; several authors have reported that smuggled cigarettes may have amounted to a further 10-30% per cent (Merzdorf *et al* (1982), Jones and Mazzi (1996) and others). From 1921 until 1950 the consumption of manufactured cigarettes per adult increased slowly from 1 to 2 per day. Thereafter, consumption continued to rise until the mid-1980s when it reached 6 cigarettes per day, then decreased to 5 per day. Hand-rolled cigarette consumption is estimated to have declined to negligible levels by the mid-1960s.

The consumption of all tobacco products per adult varied between 2 and 3 g per day from 1921 to 1950. After 1950 it started to rise, reaching 6 g by 1985. In 1925, 40% of all tobacco was consumed in manufactured cigarettes. This proportion increased to 98% by 1985. The proportion of manufactured cigarettes that were filtered was already nearly 30% in 1961, and continued to increase, reaching 90% about 1980. The consumption of cigars and cigarillos, and also the use of pipe and hand-rolling tobacco, decreased from about 25% in 1925 to less than 1% in the 1990s. The consumption of smokeless tobacco has been very low since the 1940s.

Survey data

See Tables 16.4-16.8

In 1949, the prevalence of cigarette smoking among those aged 15 years and over was 70% in men and 10% in women. The difference between the percentages of men and women who smoke has decreased since then. The prevalence among men decreased to around 35% by 1995. Estimates of the prevalence among women vary considerably, with some estimates as high as 30% in the 1970s and 1980s, and between 15 and 25% in the 1990s.

Nationally based data on adult smoking by age have been available from 1965. At all ages, the prevalence of smoking has decreased since then among men, and increased among women. However, the prevalence among women aged below about 35 started to decrease in the 1990s. A lower percentage of smokers in older age groups was more marked in women than in men. Around 1% of men smoked other products but not cigarettes, with the prevalence somewhat higher for older men. Only very few women smoke products other than cigarettes.

Most surveys of smoking among teenagers were locally based, making comparisons over time difficult. When first surveyed in 1962, the prevalence of smoking among teenage boys was very high. The prevalence among girls was much lower, although when occasional smokers were included, the difference between the sexes was not great at age 18 years and over. From the late 1970s some surveys show prevalence similar between boys and girls.

Apart from surveys where the original authors made adjustments to include clandestine sales, comparison of survey and sales data suggests that the degree of under-statement increased from 5% in the 1960s to 30% in the 1990s. However, as the extent of the clandestine market is unknown, this result should be regarded with caution. In the period 1949-1995, the estimated number of cigarettes smoked per person per day (sales-adjusted) varied for men between 8 and 10. For women, although estimates varied considerably, it increased from less than 1 to between 2 and 5.

Table 16.1.1 Total annual sales of tobacco products, 1921-1973

Year	Cigarettes		Cigars		Cigarillos		Smoking tobacco	Snuff	All tobacco products
	tonnes	millions	tonnes	millions	tonnes	millions	tonnes	tonnes	tonnes
1921-25	11150	11148	6640	1328	0	0	7760	2090	27630
1926-30	13900	13900	5940	1188	70	29	7760	1720	29400
1931-35	12910	12911	2990	597	920	366	6260	1320	24390
1936-40	17340	17342	2260	451	1720	689	5440	1090	27850
1941-45	20750	20748	2340	468	1320	527	5620	730	30760
1946-50	22350	22347	1960	391	700	278	5220	540	30760
1951-55	33980	33978	2100	420	190	75	5130	540	41940
1956	40400	40398	1700	340	160	62	5260	500	48020
1957	42670	42658	1630	326	140	55	5080	500	50010
1958	44910	44906	1550	309	130	52	5220	500	52300
1959	46590	46584	1490	297	130	51	5260	500	53970
1960	48320	48313	1450	289	130	52	5130	450	55480
1961	51870	51864	1420	284	130	52	4850	450	58730
1962	55840	55826	1390	277	180	71	4540	410	62340
1963	57160	57154	1350	269	160	65	4260	410	63340
1964	58610	58599	1320	263	180	72	4130	360	64590
1965	60630	60621	1140	227	180	72	3810	320	66070
1966	64660	64645	1160	232	180	73	3540	270	69810
1967	66670	66657	1080	216	140	54	3580	270	71740
1968	68470	68454	1100	220	140	56	3400	270	73380
1969	68540	68526	1080	215	120	49	3220	230	73180
1970	69550	69534	940	188	120	46	2900	180	73690
1971	70840	70830	920	183	150	60	2720	180	74810
1972	74180	74165	860	172	130	53	2450	180	77800
1973	80140	80131	790	158	130	50	2310	140	83510

Source: see *Notes on sources of sales data*, p. 394

Table 16.1.2 Total annual sales of tobacco products, 1974-1995

Year	Cigarettes		Cigars and cigarillos[1]		Snuff[1] tonnes	Pipe and hand-rolling[1] tobacco tonnes	All tobacco products tonnes
	tonnes	millions	tonnes	millions			
1974	87500	87500	945	210	140	2000	90585
1975	88800	88800	900	200	130	1800	91630
1976	89700	89700	855	190	120	1700	92375
1977	90300	90300	855	190	110	1500	92765
1978	88800	88800	720	160	100	1400	91020
1979	96800	96800	765	170	100	1300	98965
1980	98700	98700	810	180	90	1200	100800
1981	100900	100900	855	190	80	1200	103035
1982	101600	101600	855	190	80	1000	103535
1983	102300	102300	855	190	70	900	104125
1984	104283	104283				1682	105965
1985	105315	105315				1581	106896
1986	104771	104771				1492	106263
1987	102181	102181				1637	103818
1988	97576	97576				1551	99127
1989	97455	97455				1466	98921
1990	90904	90904				1434	92338
1991	89108	89108				1416	90524
1992	88194	88194				1208	89402
1993	88618	88618	878		36	626	90158
1994	89460	89460				1229	90689
1995	89838	89838				1296	91134

1 Cigars, Cigarillos and Snuff were included with Pipe and hand-rolling tobacco for 1984-1992 and 1994-1995.

Source : see *Notes on sources of sales data,* p. 394

Table 16.1.3 Total annual sales of tobacco products, Italian production and imports, 1982-1995

Year	Italian Production			Imports tonnes	All tobacco products tonnes
	Cigarettes tonnes	Cigars and cigarillos tonnes	Snuff and cut tobacco tonnes		
1982	66811	503	732	35470	103517
1983	68466	500	645	34340	103951
1984	66904	490	554	38012	105960
1985	65594	474	486	40342	106895
1986	64861	465	415	40462	106203
1987	60610	667	374	39169	100819
1988	57086	636	331	41075	99127
1989	54579	606	288	43448	98921
1990	46856	607	260	44612	92335
1991	43218	622	231	46460	90532
1992	42945	534	185	45901	89565
1993	40042	602	213	49354	90210
1994	38929	480	156	51118	90683
1995	37863	187	159	52639	91148

Source : see *Notes on sources of sales data,* p. 394

Table 16.1.4 Manufactured cigarettes (i) percentage of total sales as filter cigarettes, 1961-1983, and (ii) sales-weighted average tar yield per cigarette (SWAT), 1984 and 1993

Year	% Filter	SWAT mg / cig
1961	29.2	
1962	33.6	
1963	38.4	
1964	39.0	
1965	39.6	
1966	43.0	
1967	44.0	
1969	55.7	
1970	60.0	
1971	66.8	
1972	71.8	
1973	77.0	
1974	80.5	
1975	84.3	
1976	85.0	
1977	86.8	
1978	86.7	
1979	84.8	
1980	88.6	
1981	89.3	
1983	93.0	
1984		17.29
1993		10.3

Source : see *Notes on sources of sales data*, p. 394

Table 16.2 Consumption of (i) cigarettes and (ii) all tobacco products, 1921-1995 sales-based data, including estimated hand-rolled cigarette consumption. Males and females aged 15 years and over

Year	Manufactured cigarettes		Hand-rolled cigarettes		Total cigarettes		All tobacco products	
	Total annual in millions	Number/ adult/day	Total annual in millions	Number/ adult/day	Total annual in millions	Number/ adult/day	Total annual in tonnes	Grams/ adult/day
1921-25	11148	1.2					27630	2.9
1926-30	13900	1.4					29400	2.9
1931-35	12911	1.2					24390	2.3
1936-40	17342	1.6					27850	2.5
1941-45	20748	1.8					30760	2.6
1946-50	22347	1.8					30760	2.5
1951-55	33978	2.7	2565	0.2	36543	2.9	41940	3.3
1956	40398	3.0	2367	0.2	42765	3.2	48020	3.6
1957	42658	3.2	2032	0.2	44690	3.3	50010	3.7
1958	44906	3.3	1827	0.1	46733	3.4	52300	3.8
1959	46584	3.4	1578	0.1	48162	3.5	53970	3.9
1960	48313	3.5	1282	0.1	49596	3.6	55480	4.0
1961	51864	3.7	970	0.1	52834	3.8	58730	4.2
1962	55826	4.0	681	0.0	56507	4.0	62340	4.4
1963	57154	4.0	426	0.0	57580	4.1	63340	4.5
1964	58599	4.1	206	0.0	58806	4.1	64590	4.5
1965	60621	4.2	0	0.0	60621	4.2	66070	4.6
1966	64645	4.5	0	0.0	64645	4.5	69810	4.8
1967	66657	4.6	0	0.0	66657	4.6	71740	4.9
1968	68454	4.7	0	0.0	68454	4.7	73380	5.0
1969	68526	4.7	0	0.0	68526	4.7	73180	5.0
1970	69534	4.7	0	0.0	69534	4.7	73690	5.0
1971	70830	4.7	0	0.0	70830	4.7	74810	5.0
1972	74165	4.9	0	0.0	74165	4.9	77800	5.2
1973	80131	5.3	0	0.0	80131	5.3	83510	5.5
1974	87500	5.7	0	0.0	87500	5.7	90585	5.9
1975	88800	5.7	0	0.0	88800	5.7	91630	5.9
1976	89700	5.7	0	0.0	89700	5.7	92375	5.9
1977	90300	5.7	0	0.0	90300	5.7	92765	5.9
1978	88800	5.6	0	0.0	88800	5.6	91020	5.7
1979	96800	6.0	0	0.0	96800	6.0	98965	6.2
1980	98700	6.1	0	0.0	98700	6.1	100800	6.2
1981	100900	6.1	0	0.0	100900	6.1	103035	6.3
1982	101600	6.2	0	0.0	101600	6.2	103535	6.3
1983	102300	6.2	0	0.0	102300	6.2	104125	6.3
1984	104283	6.3	0	0.0	104283	6.3	105965	6.4
1985	105315	6.3	0	0.0	105315	6.3	106896	6.4
1986	104771	6.2	0	0.0	104771	6.2	106263	6.3
1987	102181	6.0	0	0.0	102181	6.0	103818	6.1
1988	97576	5.6	0	0.0	97576	5.6	99127	5.7
1989	97455	5.6	0	0.0	97455	5.6	98921	5.7
1990	90904	5.2	0	0.0	90904	5.2	92338	5.3
1991	89108	5.1	0	0.0	89108	5.1	90524	5.2
1992	88194	5.0	0	0.0	88194	5.0	89402	5.1
1993	88618	5.0	0	0.0	88618	5.0	90158	5.1
1994	89460	5.1	0	0.0	89460	5.1	90689	5.1
1995	89838	5.1	0	0.0	89838	5.1	91134	5.1

Source : see *Notes on sources of sales data*, p. 394

Figure 16.1 Daily consumption of (i) manufactured and total number of cigarettes, and (ii) all tobacco products, 1920-1995.
Males and females aged 15 years and over. *Source:* see Table 16.2

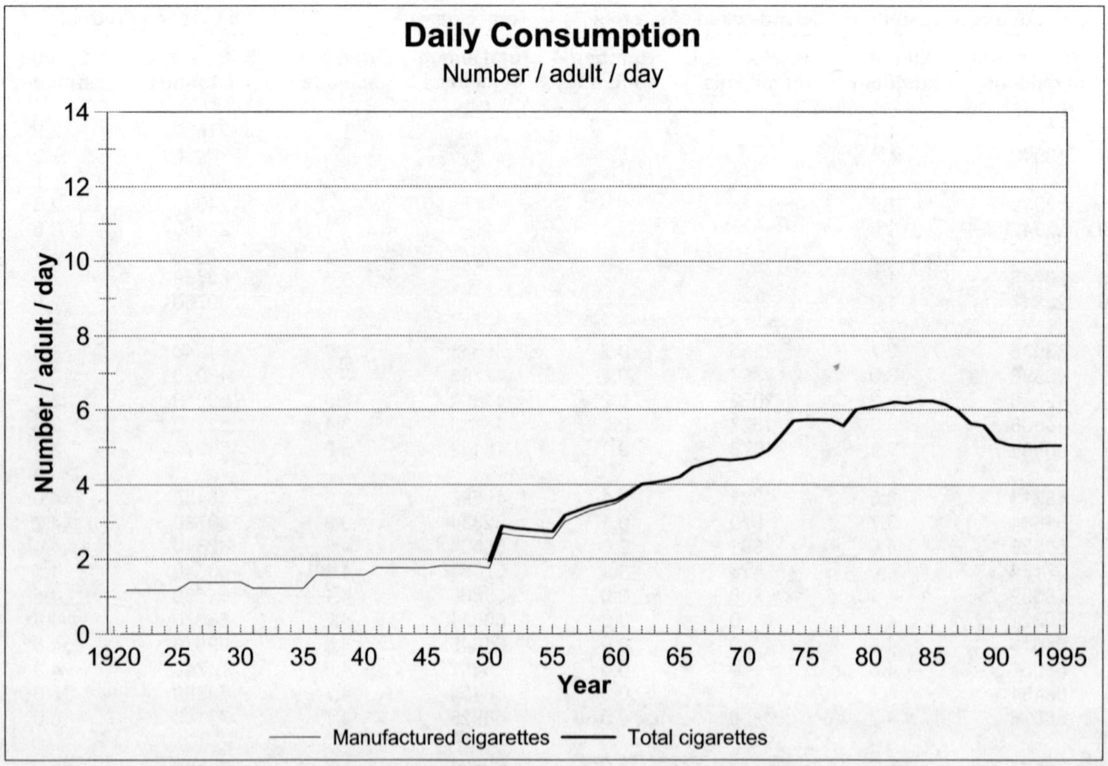

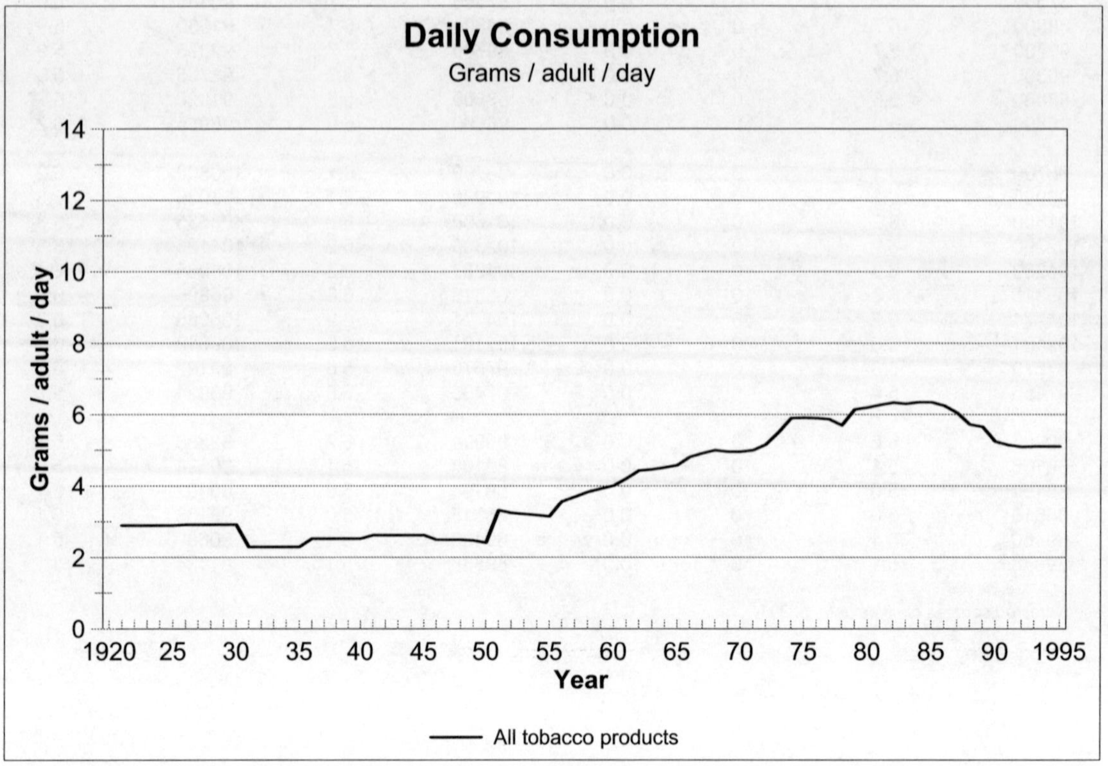

Table 16.3 Percentage sales of tobacco in different forms (by weight), selected years 1925-1993

Year	Cigarettes (%)	Cigars and cigarillos (%)	Pipe and hand-rolling (%)	Snuff (%)
1925	40.4	24.0	28.1	7.6
1935	52.9	16.0	25.7	5.4
1945	67.5	11.9	18.3	2.4
1955	81.0	5.5	12.2	1.3
1965	91.8	2.0	5.8	0.5
1975	96.9	1.0	2.0	0.1
1983	98.2	0.8	0.9	0.1
1993	98.3	1.0	0.7	0.0

Source : calculated from Tables 16.1.1 & 16.1.2

Figure 16.2 Percentage sales of tobacco in different forms (by weight), selected years 1925-1993
Source: see Table 16.3

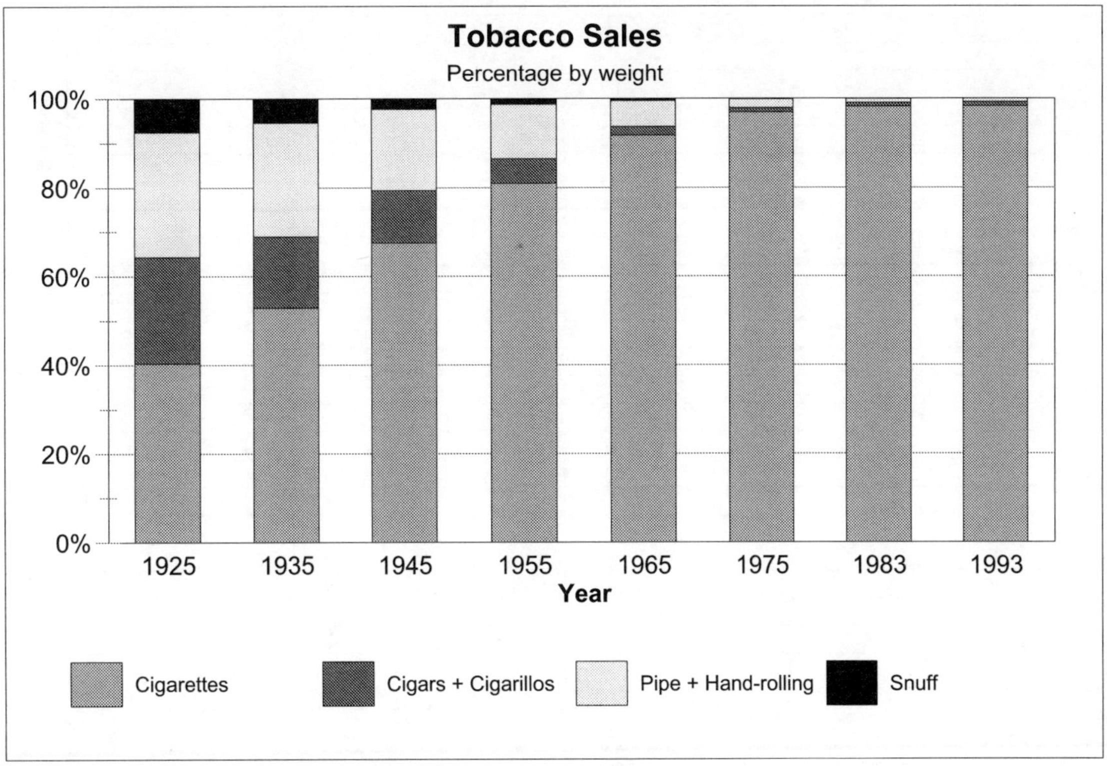

Table 16.4M Prevalence of smoking, males: some selected Italian surveys by age, 1949-1995 *(continues on p. 384)*

Frequency / Product / Source / Year	12	13	14	15	16	17	18	19	20-24	25-29	30-34	35-39	40-44	45-49	50-54	55-59	60-64	65-69	70-74	75-79	80+	All ages
49 14 UC U														71								
57 14 UC U													65									
57 21 UC R														72	66	62						68
60 22 UC R													57	67	63	60						63
60 23 UC R													63	57	61	55						59
62 6 U R				33	43	45	59	73	67〉													
62 6 U A				52	63	61	67	79	75〉													
63 7 UC U															46							
63 7 A U															50							
65 14 UC U							55			61		68			66			53				60
72 6 U R				46	59	69	73	79	82〉													
72 6 U A				64	75	78	85	86	90〉													
73 12 U U			34																			
73 13 U U			39																			
75 14 UC U												53										
76 2 U U									56		57		54		51							55
77 8 UC R					29																	
77 8 UC A					38																	
77 20 U U												62										
79 9 UC A												67										
79 9 A A												68										
79 24 U R		8				25																
80 1*UC U						44					64		61		61		48			31		53
80 1 A U					23				61		65		62		62		52			39		54
80 1 U U			2	6	16	31	43	42														
80 19 U U	1	4	13	19	27	42	48	39														
81 3 U R			13				31															
81 3 U A			24				42															
81 11 MC U																						
82 10 U U										54												
83 1*UC U						33				56		53			52	46		35		25		46
83 16 UC R										60		50			49	46						49
83 16 A A										62		53			52	48						51
85 17 UC R										49		39			36	27						35
85 17 A A										55		42			38	30						38
86 18 UC R										50		49			41	39						44
86 18 A A										56		52			46	41						47
87 1*UC U						31				49		49			44	41		30		19		
87 1 A U						31				50		50			44	41		31		21		41
87 15*UC U						33					47				38				26			38
87 15* A U												40										
87 25 U U												38										
88 3 U R			10				28															
88 3 U A			16				37															
88 25 U U												38										
88 26 UC R			7				24															
88 26 UC A			14				33															
89 18 A A										41		47			39	36						41
89 25 U U												37										
89 27 U U					10																	
89 28 U R			9				20															
89 28 U A			20				31															

Table 16.4F Prevalence of smoking, females: some selected Italian surveys by age, 1949-1995 *(continues on p. 385)*

Frequency / Product / Source / Year	12	13	14	15	16	17	18	19	20-24	25-29	30-34	35-39	40-44	45-49	50-54	55-59	60-64	65-69	70-74	75-79	80+	All ages
49 14 UC U							10															
57 14 UC U					6																	
57 21 UC R																						
60 22 UC R																						
60 23 UC R																						
62 6 U R				6	12	8	23	25	27〉													
62 6 U A				16	29	30	47	60	69〉													
63 7 UC U									27													
63 7 A U									27													
65 14 UC U					9					9		11		8		4						8
72 6 U R				38	53	53	51	57	61〉													
72 6 U A				63	78	78	81	83	81〉													
73 12 U U			24																			
73 13 U U			29																			
75 14 UC U				16																		
76 2 U U									42		29		16		14							26
77 8 UC R			25																			
77 8 UC A			39																			
77 20 U U				32																		
79 9 UC A				18																		
79 9 A A				18																		
79 24 U R	2			24																		
80 1*UC U			10						32		26		18		13		7		3			17
80 1 A U			10						32		26		18		13		7		3			17
80 1 U U			0	2	8	11	16	23														
80 19 U U	0	5	9	23	26	37	39	47														
81 3 U R			12				32															
81 3 U A			25				47															
81 11 MC U				44						49		38		26		20						37
82 10 U U				37																		
83 1*UC U			20							27		24		16		12		6		4		18
83 16 UC R										36		24		11		7						15
83 16 A A										42		30		12		7						17
85 17 UC R										30		30		25		23						26
85 17 A A										33		32		28		25						29
86 18 UC R										33		22		19		13						18
86 18 A A										36		25		21		13						21
87 1*UC U				16						30		25		16		10		7		3		
87 1 A U				16						30		25		16		10		7		2		17
87 15*UC U				31						35				22				10				28
87 15* A U				27																		
87 25 U U				28																		
88 3 U R			7				21															
88 3 U A			12				29															
88 25 U U				27																		
88 26 UC R			5				20															
88 26 UC A			9				27															
89 18 A A										34		30		17		12						23
89 25 U U				28																		
89 27 U U				9																		
89 28 U R			4				9															
89 28 U A			9				17															

Table 16.4M *(continued from p. 382)*
Prevalence of smoking, males

<table>
<tr><th rowspan="2">Frequency / Product / Source / Year</th><th colspan="21">Age group</th><th rowspan="2">All ages</th></tr>
<tr><th>12</th><th>13</th><th>14</th><th>15</th><th>16</th><th>17</th><th>18</th><th>19</th><th>20-24</th><th>25-29</th><th>30-34</th><th>35-39</th><th>40-44</th><th>45-49</th><th>50-54</th><th>55-59</th><th>60-64</th><th>65-69</th><th>70-74</th><th>75-79</th><th>80+</th></tr>
<tr><td>90 15 UC U</td><td colspan="3"></td><td colspan="18">38</td><td></td></tr>
<tr><td>90 25 U U</td><td colspan="3"></td><td colspan="18">38</td><td></td></tr>
<tr><td>90 27 U U</td><td colspan="4"></td><td colspan="3">13</td><td colspan="14"></td><td></td></tr>
<tr><td>90 29 U R</td><td colspan="2"></td><td>2</td><td>6</td><td colspan="17"></td><td></td></tr>
<tr><td>90 29 U A</td><td>0</td><td colspan="3">6</td><td colspan="17"></td><td></td></tr>
<tr><td>90 30 UC R</td><td colspan="2"></td><td colspan="2">8</td><td colspan="4">25</td><td colspan="13"></td><td></td></tr>
<tr><td>90 30 UC A</td><td colspan="2"></td><td colspan="2">16</td><td colspan="4">34</td><td colspan="13"></td><td></td></tr>
<tr><td>91 1*UC U</td><td colspan="3"></td><td colspan="6">29</td><td colspan="2">42</td><td colspan="2">45</td><td colspan="2">42</td><td colspan="2">34</td><td colspan="2">28</td><td colspan="2">17</td><td>37</td></tr>
<tr><td>91 1 A U</td><td colspan="3"></td><td colspan="6">29</td><td colspan="2">43</td><td colspan="2">46</td><td colspan="2">43</td><td colspan="2">35</td><td colspan="2">29</td><td colspan="2">19</td><td>37</td></tr>
<tr><td>91 25 U U</td><td colspan="3"></td><td colspan="18">38</td><td></td></tr>
<tr><td>91 27 U U</td><td colspan="5"></td><td colspan="3">16</td><td colspan="13"></td><td></td></tr>
<tr><td>92 25 U U</td><td colspan="3"></td><td colspan="18">38</td><td></td></tr>
<tr><td>92 27 U U</td><td colspan="6"></td><td colspan="2">24</td><td colspan="13"></td><td></td></tr>
<tr><td>92 31 UC R</td><td colspan="8"></td><td>⟨53⟩</td><td colspan="12"></td><td></td></tr>
<tr><td>93 27 U U</td><td colspan="7"></td><td>23</td><td colspan="13"></td><td></td></tr>
<tr><td>93 32 A U</td><td colspan="3"></td><td colspan="18">38</td><td></td></tr>
<tr><td>93 33 U U</td><td colspan="3">8</td><td colspan="18"></td><td></td></tr>
<tr><td>93 34 U R</td><td colspan="2"></td><td colspan="2">4</td><td colspan="2">10</td><td colspan="2">18</td><td>36⟩</td><td colspan="12"></td><td></td></tr>
<tr><td>93 34 U A</td><td colspan="2"></td><td colspan="2">9</td><td colspan="2">21</td><td colspan="2">28</td><td>47⟩</td><td colspan="12"></td><td></td></tr>
<tr><td>94 1*UC U</td><td colspan="3"></td><td colspan="6">20</td><td colspan="2">42</td><td colspan="2">42</td><td colspan="2">39</td><td colspan="2">31</td><td colspan="2">22</td><td colspan="2">16</td><td>32</td></tr>
<tr><td>94 1 A U</td><td colspan="3"></td><td colspan="6">20</td><td colspan="2">42</td><td colspan="2">42</td><td colspan="2">40</td><td colspan="2">31</td><td colspan="2">22</td><td colspan="2">17</td><td>33</td></tr>
<tr><td>94 25 U U</td><td colspan="3"></td><td colspan="18">38</td><td></td></tr>
<tr><td>94 35 UC *</td><td colspan="4">4</td><td colspan="17"></td><td></td></tr>
<tr><td>94 35 UC R</td><td colspan="4">6</td><td colspan="17"></td><td></td></tr>
<tr><td>94 35 UC A</td><td>4</td><td>7</td><td>25</td><td>34</td><td colspan="17"></td><td>11</td></tr>
<tr><td>95 1 A U</td><td colspan="3"></td><td colspan="6">28</td><td colspan="2">40</td><td colspan="2">44</td><td colspan="2">39</td><td colspan="2">31</td><td colspan="2">24</td><td colspan="2">14</td><td>34</td></tr>
<tr><td>95 32 A U</td><td colspan="3"></td><td colspan="18">35</td><td></td></tr>
<tr><td>95 36 UC R</td><td colspan="3"></td><td colspan="2">22</td><td colspan="16"></td><td></td></tr>
<tr><td>95 36 UC A</td><td colspan="3"></td><td colspan="2">36</td><td colspan="16"></td><td></td></tr>
<tr><td>95 37 U U</td><td colspan="3">14</td><td colspan="6">31</td><td colspan="7">40</td><td colspan="5">20</td><td></td></tr>
</table>

Source: see *Notes on sources of survey data*, p. 395
Product: MC = manufactured cigarettes
TC = total cigarettes (including hand-rolled)
UC = cigarettes (type unspecified)
A = all products

Frequency: A = all smokers (including occasional)
R = regular or daily smokers
All ages: relevant to ages used and as given in original source
U = unspecified
* = refer to *Notes on sources of survey data*, p. 395

Table 16.4F *(continued from p. 383)*
Prevalence of smoking, females

Frequency / Product / Source / Year	Age group 12	13	14	15	16	17	18	19	20-24	25-29	30-34	35-39	40-44	45-49	50-54	55-59	60-64	65-69	70-74	75-79	80+	All ages
90 15 UC U				26																		
90 25 U U				25																		
90 27 U U					10																	
90 29 U R			1	1																		
90 29 U A	2	2																				
90 30 UC R			4				20															
90 30 UC A			8				29															
91 1*UC U				17						26		26		18		12		7		2		17
91 1 A U				17						26		26		18		11		7		2		17
91 25 U U				25																		
91 27 U U						13																
92 25 U U				26																		
92 27 U U							12															
92 31 UC R																						
93 27 U U								27														
93 32 A U				20																		
93 33 U U	3																					
93 34 U R			2		8		9		30〉													
93 34 U A			8		20		17		32〉													
94 1*UC U				10						23		29		20		13		7		2		16
94 1 A U				10						23		29		20		13		7		3		16
94 25 U U				26																		
94 35 UC *	2																					
94 35 UC R	4																					
94 35 UC A	2	5	17	16																		6
95 1 A U				13						24		27		21		13		7		3		17
95 32 A U				23																		
95 36 UC R				22																		
95 36 UC A				37																		
95 37 U U	7			15						23						6						

Source: see *Notes on sources of survey data*, p. 395
Product: MC = manufactured cigarettes
TC = total cigarettes (including hand-rolled)
UC = cigarettes (type unspecified)
A = all products

Frequency: A = all smokers (including occasional)
R = regular or daily smokers
All ages: relevant to ages used and as given in original source
U = unspecified
* = refer to *Notes on sources of survey data*, p. 395

Table 16.5M Number of cigarettes smoked per smoker per day, males: some selected Italian surveys by age, 1949-1995

<table>
<tr><th rowspan="2">Product
Source
Year</th><th colspan="21">Age group</th><th rowspan="2">All ages</th></tr>
<tr><th>12</th><th>13</th><th>14</th><th>15</th><th>16</th><th>17</th><th>18</th><th>19</th><th>20-24</th><th>25-29</th><th>30-34</th><th>35-39</th><th>40-44</th><th>45-49</th><th>50-54</th><th>55-59</th><th>60-64</th><th>65-69</th><th>70-74</th><th>75-79</th><th>80+</th></tr>
<tr><td>49 14 UC</td><td></td><td></td><td></td><td></td><td></td><td></td><td colspan="15">14</td><td></td></tr>
<tr><td>57 14 UC</td><td></td><td></td><td></td><td></td><td colspan="17">13</td><td></td></tr>
<tr><td>57 21 UCE</td><td></td><td></td><td></td><td></td><td></td><td></td><td></td><td></td><td></td><td></td><td></td><td></td><td></td><td>10</td><td>9.8</td><td>9.9</td><td></td><td></td><td></td><td></td><td></td><td>10</td></tr>
<tr><td>60 22 UCE</td><td></td><td></td><td></td><td></td><td></td><td></td><td></td><td></td><td></td><td></td><td></td><td></td><td>17</td><td>14</td><td>13</td><td>13</td><td></td><td></td><td></td><td></td><td></td><td>14</td></tr>
<tr><td>60 23 UCE</td><td></td><td></td><td></td><td></td><td></td><td></td><td></td><td></td><td></td><td></td><td></td><td></td><td>12</td><td>11</td><td>11</td><td>10</td><td></td><td></td><td></td><td></td><td></td><td>11</td></tr>
<tr><td>65 14 UC</td><td></td><td></td><td></td><td></td><td colspan="17">13</td><td></td></tr>
<tr><td>73 12 UCE</td><td></td><td></td><td>1.3</td><td></td><td></td><td></td><td></td><td></td><td></td><td></td><td></td><td></td><td></td><td></td><td></td><td></td><td></td><td></td><td></td><td></td><td></td><td></td></tr>
<tr><td>76 2 UC</td><td></td><td></td><td></td><td></td><td></td><td></td><td></td><td></td><td colspan="2">18</td><td colspan="2">18</td><td colspan="2">19</td><td colspan="2">19</td><td></td><td></td><td></td><td></td><td></td><td>19</td></tr>
<tr><td>77 8 UC</td><td></td><td></td><td colspan="6">6.5</td><td></td><td></td><td></td><td></td><td></td><td></td><td></td><td></td><td></td><td></td><td></td><td></td><td></td><td></td></tr>
<tr><td>79 24 UCE</td><td></td><td></td><td></td><td colspan="5">8.2</td><td></td><td></td><td></td><td></td><td></td><td></td><td></td><td></td><td></td><td></td><td></td><td></td><td></td><td></td></tr>
<tr><td>80 1 UCE</td><td></td><td></td><td colspan="6">11</td><td colspan="2">16</td><td colspan="2">18</td><td colspan="2">19</td><td colspan="2">18</td><td colspan="2">16</td><td colspan="3">14</td><td>17</td></tr>
<tr><td>81 3 UCE</td><td></td><td></td><td colspan="2">7.5</td><td></td><td></td><td colspan="2">11</td><td></td><td></td><td></td><td></td><td></td><td></td><td></td><td></td><td></td><td></td><td></td><td></td><td></td><td></td></tr>
<tr><td>81 11 MCE</td><td></td><td></td><td></td><td></td><td></td><td></td><td></td><td></td><td></td><td></td><td></td><td></td><td></td><td></td><td></td><td></td><td></td><td></td><td></td><td></td><td></td><td></td></tr>
<tr><td>83 1 UCE</td><td></td><td></td><td></td><td colspan="18">18</td><td></td></tr>
<tr><td>85 17 UC</td><td></td><td></td><td></td><td></td><td></td><td></td><td></td><td></td><td></td><td></td><td></td><td colspan="6">17</td><td></td><td></td><td></td><td></td><td></td></tr>
<tr><td>86 18 UC</td><td></td><td></td><td></td><td></td><td></td><td></td><td></td><td></td><td></td><td></td><td></td><td colspan="6">17</td><td></td><td></td><td></td><td></td><td></td></tr>
<tr><td>87 1 UCE</td><td></td><td></td><td></td><td colspan="6">14</td><td colspan="2">18</td><td colspan="2">19</td><td colspan="2">19</td><td colspan="2">17</td><td colspan="2">15</td><td colspan="2">12</td><td>16</td></tr>
<tr><td>87 15 UC</td><td></td><td></td><td></td><td colspan="18">15</td><td></td></tr>
<tr><td>88 3 UCE*</td><td></td><td></td><td colspan="2">9.2</td><td></td><td></td><td colspan="2">12</td><td></td><td></td><td></td><td></td><td></td><td></td><td></td><td></td><td></td><td></td><td></td><td></td><td></td><td></td></tr>
<tr><td>88 26 UCE</td><td></td><td></td><td colspan="2">5.2</td><td></td><td></td><td colspan="2">8.0</td><td></td><td></td><td></td><td></td><td></td><td></td><td></td><td></td><td></td><td></td><td></td><td></td><td></td><td></td></tr>
<tr><td>89 18 UC</td><td></td><td></td><td></td><td></td><td></td><td></td><td></td><td></td><td></td><td colspan="2">15</td><td colspan="2">19</td><td colspan="2">18</td><td colspan="2">16</td><td></td><td></td><td></td><td></td><td>17</td></tr>
<tr><td>89 28 UCE</td><td></td><td></td><td colspan="2">6.6</td><td></td><td></td><td colspan="2">8.9</td><td></td><td></td><td></td><td></td><td></td><td></td><td></td><td></td><td></td><td></td><td></td><td></td><td></td><td></td></tr>
<tr><td>90 15 UC</td><td></td><td></td><td></td><td colspan="18">19</td><td></td></tr>
<tr><td>90 30 UCE</td><td></td><td></td><td colspan="2">10</td><td></td><td></td><td colspan="2">9.7</td><td></td><td></td><td></td><td></td><td></td><td></td><td></td><td></td><td></td><td></td><td></td><td></td><td></td><td></td></tr>
<tr><td>91 1 UCE</td><td></td><td></td><td></td><td colspan="6">17</td><td colspan="2">18</td><td colspan="2">19</td><td colspan="2">20</td><td colspan="2">18</td><td colspan="2">16</td><td colspan="2">13</td><td>18</td></tr>
<tr><td>93 34 UCE</td><td></td><td></td><td colspan="6">9.8</td><td></td><td></td><td></td><td></td><td></td><td></td><td></td><td></td><td></td><td></td><td></td><td></td><td></td><td></td></tr>
<tr><td>94 1 UCE</td><td></td><td></td><td></td><td colspan="6">13</td><td colspan="2">17</td><td colspan="2">19</td><td colspan="2">20</td><td colspan="2">17</td><td colspan="2">16</td><td colspan="2">15</td><td>18</td></tr>
<tr><td>95 1 UCE*</td><td></td><td></td><td></td><td colspan="6">12</td><td colspan="2">15</td><td colspan="2">19</td><td colspan="2">17</td><td colspan="2">16</td><td colspan="2">14</td><td colspan="2">12</td><td>15</td></tr>
<tr><td>95 36 UCE</td><td></td><td></td><td></td><td colspan="2">9.0</td><td></td><td></td><td></td><td></td><td></td><td></td><td></td><td></td><td></td><td></td><td></td><td></td><td></td><td></td><td></td><td></td><td></td></tr>
</table>

Source: see *Notes on sources of survey data*, p. 395
Product: MC = manufactured cigarettes
TC = total cigarettes (including hand-rolled)
UC = cigarettes (type unspecified)
A = all products
U = unspecified

Product (cont): E indicates mean estimated from percentage distribution (see also *Consumption category estimation*, p. xxxiv, and Appendix III, p. 789)
All ages: relevant to ages used and as given in original source
* = refer to *Notes on sources of survey data*, p. 395

Table 16.5F Number of cigarettes smoked per smoker per day, females: some selected Italian surveys by age, 1949-1995

<table>
<tr><th rowspan="2">Product
Source
Year</th><th colspan="21">Age group</th><th rowspan="2">All ages</th></tr>
<tr><th>12</th><th>13</th><th>14</th><th>15</th><th>16</th><th>17</th><th>18</th><th>19</th><th>20-24</th><th>25-29</th><th>30-34</th><th>35-39</th><th>40-44</th><th>45-49</th><th>50-54</th><th>55-59</th><th>60-64</th><th>65-69</th><th>70-74</th><th>75-79</th><th>80+</th></tr>
<tr><td>49 14 UC</td><td colspan="6"></td><td colspan="15">7.9</td><td></td></tr>
<tr><td>57 14 UC</td><td colspan="4"></td><td colspan="17">7.0</td><td></td></tr>
<tr><td>57 21 UCE</td><td colspan="21"></td><td></td></tr>
<tr><td>60 22 UCE</td><td colspan="21"></td><td></td></tr>
<tr><td>60 23 UCE</td><td colspan="21"></td><td></td></tr>
<tr><td>65 14 UC</td><td colspan="4"></td><td colspan="17">5.8</td><td></td></tr>
<tr><td>73 12 UCE</td><td colspan="2"></td><td>0.9</td><td colspan="18"></td><td></td></tr>
<tr><td>76 2 UC</td><td colspan="8"></td><td colspan="2">11</td><td colspan="2">11</td><td colspan="2">11</td><td colspan="2">10</td><td colspan="5"></td><td>11</td></tr>
<tr><td>77 8 UC</td><td colspan="2"></td><td colspan="6">3.5</td><td colspan="13"></td><td></td></tr>
<tr><td>79 24 UCE</td><td colspan="3"></td><td colspan="5">6.7</td><td colspan="13"></td><td></td></tr>
<tr><td>80 1 UCE</td><td colspan="2"></td><td colspan="6">8.9</td><td colspan="2">11</td><td colspan="2">11</td><td colspan="2">11</td><td colspan="2">11</td><td colspan="2">12</td><td colspan="3">8.4</td><td>11</td></tr>
<tr><td>81 3 UCE</td><td colspan="2"></td><td colspan="2">6.6</td><td colspan="2"></td><td colspan="2">7.2</td><td colspan="13"></td><td></td></tr>
<tr><td>81 11 MCE</td><td colspan="3"></td><td colspan="6">10</td><td colspan="2">13</td><td colspan="2">9.6</td><td colspan="2">11</td><td colspan="2">10</td><td colspan="4"></td><td>11</td></tr>
<tr><td>83 1 UCE</td><td colspan="3"></td><td colspan="18">12</td><td></td></tr>
<tr><td>85 17 UC</td><td colspan="11"></td><td colspan="6">10</td><td colspan="4"></td><td></td></tr>
<tr><td>86 18 UC</td><td colspan="11"></td><td colspan="6">11</td><td colspan="4"></td><td></td></tr>
<tr><td>87 1 UCE</td><td colspan="3"></td><td colspan="6">10</td><td colspan="2">12</td><td colspan="2">13</td><td colspan="2">13</td><td colspan="2">12</td><td colspan="2">11</td><td colspan="2">10</td><td>11</td></tr>
<tr><td>87 15 UC</td><td colspan="3"></td><td colspan="18">10</td><td></td></tr>
<tr><td>88 3 UCE*</td><td colspan="2"></td><td colspan="2">7.4</td><td colspan="2"></td><td colspan="2">8.0</td><td colspan="13"></td><td></td></tr>
<tr><td>88 26 UCE</td><td colspan="2"></td><td colspan="2">5.6</td><td colspan="2"></td><td colspan="2">5.7</td><td colspan="13"></td><td></td></tr>
<tr><td>89 18 UC</td><td colspan="9"></td><td colspan="2">11</td><td colspan="2">13</td><td colspan="2">12</td><td colspan="2">9</td><td colspan="4"></td><td>12</td></tr>
<tr><td>89 28 UCE</td><td colspan="2"></td><td colspan="2">8.2</td><td colspan="2"></td><td colspan="2">6.1</td><td colspan="13"></td><td></td></tr>
<tr><td>90 15 UC</td><td colspan="3"></td><td colspan="18">12</td><td></td></tr>
<tr><td>90 30 UCE</td><td colspan="2"></td><td colspan="2">8.8</td><td colspan="2"></td><td colspan="2">8.4</td><td colspan="13"></td><td></td></tr>
<tr><td>91 1 UCE</td><td colspan="3"></td><td colspan="6">16</td><td colspan="2">12</td><td colspan="2">14</td><td colspan="2">13</td><td colspan="2">13</td><td colspan="2">11</td><td colspan="2">11</td><td>14</td></tr>
<tr><td>93 34 UCE</td><td colspan="2"></td><td colspan="6">7.3</td><td colspan="13"></td><td></td></tr>
<tr><td>94 1 UCE</td><td colspan="3"></td><td colspan="6">11</td><td colspan="2">11</td><td colspan="2">13</td><td colspan="2">13</td><td colspan="2">12</td><td colspan="2">11</td><td colspan="2">11</td><td>13</td></tr>
<tr><td>95 1 UCE*</td><td colspan="3"></td><td colspan="6">9.3</td><td colspan="2">10</td><td colspan="2">11</td><td colspan="2">12</td><td colspan="2">11</td><td colspan="2">11</td><td colspan="2">9.6</td><td>11</td></tr>
<tr><td>95 36 UCE</td><td colspan="3"></td><td colspan="2">8.0</td><td colspan="16"></td><td></td></tr>
</table>

Source: see *Notes on sources of survey data*, p. 395
Product: MC = manufactured cigarettes
TC = total cigarettes (including hand-rolled)
UC = cigarettes (type unspecified)
A = all products
U = unspecified

Product (cont): E indicates mean estimated from percentage distribution (see also *Consumption category estimation*, p. xxxiv, and Appendix III, p. 789)
All ages: relevant to ages used and as given in original source
* = refer to *Notes on sources of survey data*, p. 395

Table 16.6M Number of cigarettes smoked per person per day, males: some selected Italian surveys by age, 1949-1995, with percentage total sales

<table>
<tr><th rowspan="2">Product
Source
Year</th><th colspan="21">Age group</th><th rowspan="2">All ages</th><th rowspan="2">% Total sales</th></tr>
<tr><th>12</th><th>13</th><th>14</th><th>15</th><th>16</th><th>17</th><th>18</th><th>19</th><th>20-24</th><th>25-29</th><th>30-34</th><th>35-39</th><th>40-44</th><th>45-49</th><th>50-54</th><th>55-59</th><th>60-64</th><th>65-69</th><th>70-74</th><th>75-79</th><th>80+</th></tr>
<tr><td>49 14 UC *</td><td colspan="6"></td><td colspan="15">9.6</td><td></td><td>---*</td></tr>
<tr><td>57 14 UC *</td><td colspan="4"></td><td colspan="17">8.6</td><td></td><td>---*</td></tr>
<tr><td>57 21 UC</td><td colspan="13"></td><td>7.3</td><td>6.5</td><td>6.1</td><td colspan="5"></td><td>6.8</td><td>**</td></tr>
<tr><td>60 22 UC</td><td colspan="12"></td><td>9.6</td><td>9.5</td><td>8.5</td><td>7.8</td><td colspan="5"></td><td>8.8</td><td>**</td></tr>
<tr><td>60 23 UC</td><td colspan="12"></td><td>7.4</td><td>6.3</td><td>6.9</td><td>5.7</td><td colspan="5"></td><td>6.5</td><td>**</td></tr>
<tr><td>65 14 UC *</td><td colspan="4"></td><td colspan="17">8.0</td><td></td><td>95%T</td></tr>
<tr><td>72 5 UC</td><td colspan="3"></td><td colspan="18">10</td><td></td><td>---*</td></tr>
<tr><td>73 12 UC</td><td colspan="2"></td><td>0.4</td><td colspan="18"></td><td></td><td>**</td></tr>
<tr><td>76 2 UC</td><td colspan="8"></td><td colspan="2">10</td><td colspan="2">10</td><td colspan="2">10</td><td colspan="2">10</td><td colspan="5"></td><td>10</td><td>**</td></tr>
<tr><td>77 8 UC *</td><td colspan="2"></td><td colspan="6">2.5</td><td colspan="13"></td><td></td><td>**</td></tr>
<tr><td>79 24 UC</td><td colspan="3"></td><td colspan="5">2.0</td><td colspan="13"></td><td></td><td>**</td></tr>
<tr><td>80 1 UC</td><td colspan="2"></td><td colspan="8">6.7</td><td colspan="2">12</td><td colspan="2">12</td><td colspan="2">11</td><td colspan="2">7.9</td><td colspan="3">4.3</td><td>9.0</td><td>88%T</td></tr>
<tr><td>80 4 MC</td><td colspan="3"></td><td colspan="18">10</td><td></td><td>---M</td></tr>
<tr><td>81 3 UC</td><td colspan="2"></td><td colspan="2">0.9</td><td colspan="2"></td><td colspan="2">3.3</td><td colspan="13"></td><td></td><td>**</td></tr>
<tr><td>81 11 MC</td><td colspan="21"></td><td></td><td>**</td></tr>
<tr><td>83 1 UC</td><td colspan="3"></td><td colspan="18">8.0</td><td></td><td>79%T</td></tr>
<tr><td>85 17 UC *</td><td colspan="11"></td><td colspan="6">5.9</td><td colspan="4"></td><td></td><td>**</td></tr>
<tr><td>86 18 UC *</td><td colspan="11"></td><td colspan="6">7.4</td><td colspan="4"></td><td></td><td>**</td></tr>
<tr><td>87 1 UC</td><td colspan="3"></td><td colspan="6">4.2</td><td colspan="2">8.7</td><td colspan="2">9.5</td><td colspan="2">8.3</td><td colspan="2">7.0</td><td colspan="2">4.5</td><td colspan="2">2.4</td><td></td><td>73%T</td></tr>
<tr><td>87 15 UC</td><td colspan="3"></td><td colspan="18">5.8</td><td></td><td>71%T</td></tr>
<tr><td>88 3 UC *</td><td colspan="2"></td><td colspan="2">0.9</td><td colspan="2"></td><td colspan="2">3.3</td><td colspan="13"></td><td></td><td>**</td></tr>
<tr><td>88 26 UC</td><td colspan="2"></td><td colspan="2">0.4</td><td colspan="2"></td><td colspan="2">1.9</td><td colspan="13"></td><td></td><td>**</td></tr>
<tr><td>89 28 UC</td><td colspan="2"></td><td colspan="2">0.6</td><td colspan="2"></td><td colspan="2">1.8</td><td colspan="13"></td><td></td><td>**</td></tr>
<tr><td>90 15 UC</td><td colspan="3"></td><td colspan="18">7.1</td><td></td><td>98%T</td></tr>
<tr><td>90 30 UC</td><td colspan="2"></td><td colspan="2">0.9</td><td colspan="2"></td><td colspan="2">2.4</td><td colspan="13"></td><td></td><td>**</td></tr>
<tr><td>91 1 UC</td><td colspan="3"></td><td colspan="6">4.9</td><td colspan="2">7.5</td><td colspan="2">8.6</td><td colspan="2">8.2</td><td colspan="2">6.2</td><td colspan="2">4.5</td><td colspan="2">2.2</td><td>6.6</td><td>85%T</td></tr>
<tr><td>94 1 UC</td><td colspan="3"></td><td colspan="6">2.6</td><td colspan="2">7.3</td><td colspan="2">8.0</td><td colspan="2">8.0</td><td colspan="2">5.3</td><td colspan="2">3.5</td><td colspan="2">2.3</td><td>5.9</td><td>75%T</td></tr>
<tr><td>95 1 UC *</td><td colspan="3"></td><td colspan="6">3.3</td><td colspan="2">6.1</td><td colspan="2">8.5</td><td colspan="2">6.6</td><td colspan="2">4.9</td><td colspan="2">3.4</td><td colspan="2">1.6</td><td>5.3</td><td>70%T</td></tr>
<tr><td>95 36 UC</td><td colspan="3"></td><td colspan="2">2.0</td><td colspan="16"></td><td></td><td>**</td></tr>
</table>

Table 16.7M Number of cigarettes smoked per person per day, sales-adjusted, males: some selected Italian surveys[1] by age, 1949-1995, with percentage total sales

<table>
<tr><th rowspan="2">Product
Source
Year</th><th colspan="21">Age group</th><th rowspan="2">All ages</th><th rowspan="2">% Total sales</th></tr>
<tr><th>12</th><th>13</th><th>14</th><th>15</th><th>16</th><th>17</th><th>18</th><th>19</th><th>20-24</th><th>25-29</th><th>30-34</th><th>35-39</th><th>40-44</th><th>45-49</th><th>50-54</th><th>55-59</th><th>60-64</th><th>65-69</th><th>70-74</th><th>75-79</th><th>80+</th></tr>
<tr><td>49 14 UC *</td><td colspan="6"></td><td colspan="15">9.6</td><td></td><td>---*</td></tr>
<tr><td>57 14 UC *</td><td colspan="4"></td><td colspan="17">8.6</td><td></td><td>---*</td></tr>
<tr><td>65 14 UC *</td><td colspan="4"></td><td colspan="17">8.4</td><td></td><td>95%T</td></tr>
<tr><td>72 5 UC</td><td colspan="3"></td><td colspan="18">10</td><td></td><td>---*</td></tr>
<tr><td>80 1 UC</td><td colspan="2"></td><td colspan="8">7.6</td><td colspan="2">13</td><td colspan="2">13</td><td colspan="2">12</td><td colspan="2">9.0</td><td colspan="3">4.9</td><td>10</td><td>88%T</td></tr>
<tr><td>80 4 MC</td><td colspan="3"></td><td colspan="18">10</td><td></td><td>---M</td></tr>
<tr><td>83 1 UC</td><td colspan="3"></td><td colspan="18">10</td><td></td><td>79%T</td></tr>
<tr><td>87 1 UC</td><td colspan="3"></td><td colspan="6">5.7</td><td colspan="2">12</td><td colspan="2">13</td><td colspan="2">11</td><td colspan="2">9.6</td><td colspan="2">6.1</td><td colspan="2">3.3</td><td></td><td>73%T</td></tr>
<tr><td>87 15 UC</td><td colspan="3"></td><td colspan="18">8.1</td><td></td><td>71%T</td></tr>
<tr><td>90 15 UC</td><td colspan="3"></td><td colspan="18">7.3</td><td></td><td>98%T</td></tr>
<tr><td>91 1 UC</td><td colspan="3"></td><td colspan="6">5.8</td><td colspan="2">8.9</td><td colspan="2">10</td><td colspan="2">9.7</td><td colspan="2">7.3</td><td colspan="2">5.3</td><td colspan="2">2.6</td><td>7.8</td><td>85%T</td></tr>
<tr><td>94 1 UC</td><td colspan="3"></td><td colspan="6">3.5</td><td colspan="2">9.8</td><td colspan="2">11</td><td colspan="2">11</td><td colspan="2">7.1</td><td colspan="2">4.7</td><td colspan="2">3.1</td><td>7.9</td><td>75%T</td></tr>
<tr><td>95 1 UC *</td><td colspan="3"></td><td colspan="6">4.7</td><td colspan="2">8.8</td><td colspan="2">12</td><td colspan="2">9.5</td><td colspan="2">7.0</td><td colspan="2">4.9</td><td colspan="2">2.3</td><td>7.6</td><td>70%T</td></tr>
</table>

1 Based on those surveys in Table 16.6 with data for both sexes and age range at least 21-64 (see *Cigarette consumption per person*, p. xxxv)

Source: see *Notes on sources of survey data*, p. 395
All ages: relevant to ages used and as given in original source
% Total sales: estimated % of total sales of M = manufactured or T = total cigarette consumption implied by survey, sexes combined, used as adjustment factor in Table 16.7
** = cannot be calculated
--- = adjusted by original author

Product: MC = manufactured cigarettes
TC = total cigarettes (including hand-rolled)
UC = cigarettes (type unspecified)
A = all products
U = unspecified
* = refer to *Notes on sources of survey data*, p. 395

Table 16.6F Number of cigarettes smoked per person per day, females: some selected Italian surveys by age, 1949-1995, with percentage total sales

<table>
<tr><th rowspan="2">Product
Source
Year</th><th colspan="21">Age group</th><th rowspan="2">All ages</th><th rowspan="2">% Total sales</th></tr>
<tr><th>12</th><th>13</th><th>14</th><th>15</th><th>16</th><th>17</th><th>18</th><th>19</th><th>20-24</th><th>25-29</th><th>30-34</th><th>35-39</th><th>40-44</th><th>45-49</th><th>50-54</th><th>55-59</th><th>60-64</th><th>65-69</th><th>70-74</th><th>75-79</th><th>80+</th></tr>
<tr><td>49 14 UC *</td><td colspan="6"></td><td colspan="15">0.8</td><td></td><td>---*</td></tr>
<tr><td>57 14 UC *</td><td colspan="4"></td><td colspan="17">0.4</td><td></td><td>---*</td></tr>
<tr><td>57 21 UC</td><td colspan="21"></td><td></td><td>**</td></tr>
<tr><td>60 22 UC</td><td colspan="21"></td><td></td><td>**</td></tr>
<tr><td>60 23 UC</td><td colspan="21"></td><td></td><td>**</td></tr>
<tr><td>65 14 UC *</td><td colspan="4"></td><td colspan="17">0.4</td><td></td><td>95%T</td></tr>
<tr><td>72 5 UC</td><td colspan="3"></td><td colspan="18">5.1</td><td></td><td>---*</td></tr>
<tr><td>73 12 UC</td><td colspan="2"></td><td>0.2</td><td colspan="18"></td><td></td><td>**</td></tr>
<tr><td>76 2 UC</td><td colspan="8"></td><td colspan="2">4</td><td colspan="2">4</td><td colspan="2">2</td><td colspan="2">1</td><td colspan="5"></td><td>3</td><td>**</td></tr>
<tr><td>77 8 UC *</td><td colspan="2"></td><td colspan="6">1.4</td><td colspan="13"></td><td></td><td>**</td></tr>
<tr><td>79 24 UC</td><td colspan="3"></td><td colspan="5">1.6</td><td colspan="13"></td><td></td><td>**</td></tr>
<tr><td>80 1 UC</td><td colspan="2"></td><td colspan="8">2.3</td><td colspan="2">3.0</td><td colspan="2">1.9</td><td colspan="2">1.5</td><td colspan="2">0.8</td><td colspan="3">0.2</td><td>1.8</td><td>88%T</td></tr>
<tr><td>80 4 MC</td><td colspan="3"></td><td colspan="18">2.0</td><td></td><td>---M</td></tr>
<tr><td>81 3 UC</td><td colspan="2"></td><td colspan="2">0.8</td><td colspan="2"></td><td colspan="2">2.3</td><td colspan="13"></td><td></td><td>**</td></tr>
<tr><td>81 11 MC</td><td colspan="3"></td><td colspan="6">4.4</td><td colspan="2">6.5</td><td colspan="2">3.7</td><td colspan="2">2.9</td><td colspan="2">2.0</td><td colspan="4"></td><td>4.0</td><td>**</td></tr>
<tr><td>83 1 UC</td><td colspan="3"></td><td colspan="18">2.1</td><td></td><td>79%T</td></tr>
<tr><td>85 17 UC *</td><td colspan="11"></td><td colspan="6">2.6</td><td colspan="4"></td><td></td><td>**</td></tr>
<tr><td>86 18 UC *</td><td colspan="11"></td><td colspan="6">2.0</td><td colspan="4"></td><td></td><td>**</td></tr>
<tr><td>87 1 UC</td><td colspan="3"></td><td colspan="6">1.7</td><td colspan="2">3.6</td><td colspan="2">3.2</td><td colspan="2">2.1</td><td colspan="2">1.3</td><td colspan="2">0.7</td><td colspan="2">0.3</td><td></td><td>73%T</td></tr>
<tr><td>87 15 UC</td><td colspan="3"></td><td colspan="18">2.9</td><td></td><td>71%T</td></tr>
<tr><td>88 3 UC *</td><td colspan="2"></td><td colspan="2">0.5</td><td colspan="2"></td><td colspan="2">1.7</td><td colspan="13"></td><td></td><td>**</td></tr>
<tr><td>88 26 UC</td><td colspan="2"></td><td colspan="2">0.3</td><td colspan="2"></td><td colspan="2">1.2</td><td colspan="13"></td><td></td><td>**</td></tr>
<tr><td>89 28 UC</td><td colspan="2"></td><td colspan="2">0.3</td><td colspan="2"></td><td colspan="2">0.5</td><td colspan="13"></td><td></td><td>**</td></tr>
<tr><td>90 15 UC</td><td colspan="3"></td><td colspan="18">3.1</td><td></td><td>98%T</td></tr>
<tr><td>90 30 UC</td><td colspan="2"></td><td colspan="2">0.3</td><td colspan="2"></td><td colspan="2">1.7</td><td colspan="13"></td><td></td><td>**</td></tr>
<tr><td>91 1 UC</td><td colspan="3"></td><td colspan="6">2.7</td><td colspan="2">3.2</td><td colspan="2">3.6</td><td colspan="2">2.3</td><td colspan="2">1.5</td><td colspan="2">0.8</td><td colspan="2">0.3</td><td>2.4</td><td>85%T</td></tr>
<tr><td>94 1 UC</td><td colspan="3"></td><td colspan="6">1.1</td><td colspan="2">2.6</td><td colspan="2">3.9</td><td colspan="2">2.6</td><td colspan="2">1.5</td><td colspan="2">0.8</td><td colspan="2">0.3</td><td>2.2</td><td>75%T</td></tr>
<tr><td>95 1 UC *</td><td colspan="3"></td><td colspan="6">1.2</td><td colspan="2">2.5</td><td colspan="2">3.1</td><td colspan="2">2.5</td><td colspan="2">1.4</td><td colspan="2">0.7</td><td colspan="2">0.3</td><td>1.9</td><td>70%T</td></tr>
<tr><td>95 36 UC</td><td colspan="3"></td><td colspan="2">1.8</td><td colspan="16"></td><td></td><td>**</td></tr>
</table>

Table 16.7F Number of cigarettes smoked per person per day, sales-adjusted, females: some selected Italian surveys[1] by age, 1949-1995, with percentage total sales

<table>
<tr><th rowspan="2">Product
Source
Year</th><th colspan="21">Age group</th><th rowspan="2">All ages</th><th rowspan="2">% Total sales</th></tr>
<tr><th>12</th><th>13</th><th>14</th><th>15</th><th>16</th><th>17</th><th>18</th><th>19</th><th>20-24</th><th>25-29</th><th>30-34</th><th>35-39</th><th>40-44</th><th>45-49</th><th>50-54</th><th>55-59</th><th>60-64</th><th>65-69</th><th>70-74</th><th>75-79</th><th>80+</th></tr>
<tr><td>49 14 UC *</td><td colspan="6"></td><td colspan="15">0.8</td><td></td><td>---*</td></tr>
<tr><td>57 14 UC *</td><td colspan="4"></td><td colspan="17">0.4</td><td></td><td>---*</td></tr>
<tr><td>65 14 UC *</td><td colspan="4"></td><td colspan="17">0.4</td><td></td><td>95%T</td></tr>
<tr><td>72 5 UC</td><td colspan="3"></td><td colspan="18">5.1</td><td></td><td>---*</td></tr>
<tr><td>80 1 UC</td><td colspan="2"></td><td colspan="8">2.6</td><td colspan="2">3.4</td><td colspan="2">2.2</td><td colspan="2">1.7</td><td colspan="2">0.9</td><td colspan="3">0.2</td><td>2.0</td><td>88%T</td></tr>
<tr><td>80 4 MC</td><td colspan="3"></td><td colspan="18">2.0</td><td></td><td>---M</td></tr>
<tr><td>83 1 UC</td><td colspan="3"></td><td colspan="18">2.7</td><td></td><td>79%T</td></tr>
<tr><td>87 1 UC</td><td colspan="3"></td><td colspan="6">2.3</td><td colspan="2">5.0</td><td colspan="2">4.4</td><td colspan="2">2.8</td><td colspan="2">1.8</td><td colspan="2">1.0</td><td colspan="2">0.4</td><td></td><td>73%T</td></tr>
<tr><td>87 15 UC</td><td colspan="3"></td><td colspan="18">4.0</td><td></td><td>71%T</td></tr>
<tr><td>90 15 UC</td><td colspan="3"></td><td colspan="18">3.2</td><td></td><td>98%T</td></tr>
<tr><td>91 1 UC</td><td colspan="3"></td><td colspan="6">3.2</td><td colspan="2">3.8</td><td colspan="2">4.2</td><td colspan="2">2.7</td><td colspan="2">1.8</td><td colspan="2">0.9</td><td colspan="2">0.4</td><td>2.8</td><td>85%T</td></tr>
<tr><td>94 1 UC</td><td colspan="3"></td><td colspan="6">1.5</td><td colspan="2">3.5</td><td colspan="2">5.2</td><td colspan="2">3.5</td><td colspan="2">2.0</td><td colspan="2">1.1</td><td colspan="2">0.4</td><td>3.0</td><td>75%T</td></tr>
<tr><td>95 1 UC *</td><td colspan="3"></td><td colspan="6">1.7</td><td colspan="2">3.6</td><td colspan="2">4.5</td><td colspan="2">3.6</td><td colspan="2">2.0</td><td colspan="2">1.0</td><td colspan="2">0.4</td><td>2.7</td><td>70%T</td></tr>
</table>

1 Based on those surveys in Table 16.6 with data for both sexes and age range at least 21-64 (see *Cigarette consumption per person*, p. xxxv)

Source: see *Notes on sources of survey data*, p. 395

All ages: relevant to ages used and as given in original source

% Total sales: estimated % of total sales of M = manufactured or T = total cigarette consumption implied by survey, sexes combined, used as adjustment factor in Table 16.7

** = cannot be calculated

--- = adjusted by original author

Product: MC = manufactured cigarettes

TC = total cigarettes (including hand-rolled)

UC = cigarettes (type unspecified)

A = all products

U = unspecified

* = refer to *Notes on sources of survey data*, p. 395

Table 16.8 Estimated[1] prevalence of smoking and estimated[1] number of cigarettes per person per day (unadjusted and sales-adjusted): summary of Tables 16.4, 16.6 and 16.7, 1949-1995.
Males and females aged 15 years and over

Year	Source[2]	Product[3]	Prevalence[4]						Number of cigarettes						
									Unadjusted[7]			Sales-adjusted[8]			
			Manufactured cigarettes		Total cigarettes[5]		All products[6]		Number/ person/day		Total sales %	Manufactured cigarettes number/ person/day		Total cigarettes[9] number/ person/day	
			M	F	M	F	M	F	M	F		M	F	M	F
1949	14	*UC*			70	10			9.5	0.8	10	9.5	0.8		
1957	14	*UC*			64	6			8.5	0.4	10	8.5	0.4		
1963	7	*UC+A*			46	27	50	27						(5.6	2.6)
1965	14	*UC*			59	8			7.9	0.4	95			8.3	0.4
1972	5	UC							10.3	5.1	10	10.3	5.1		
1975	14	*UC*			53	16								(9.4	2.3)
1977	20	*U*					62	32							
1979	9	**UC+A**			67	18	68	18						(10.2	2.2)
1980	1	UC+*A*			52	17	54	17	9.2	1.8	88			10.4	2.1
	4	MC							10.0	2.0	---	10.0	2.0		
1981	11	*MC*		30						3.3					
1982	10	*U*					52	31							
1983	1	UC			45	17			8.0	2.1	79			10.1	2.7
1987	1	UC+*A*			40	17	41	17	6.8	2.0	73			9.4	2.8
	15	UC+A			38	25	40	27	5.7	2.9	71			8.1	4.0
	25	*U*					38	28							
1988	25	*U*					38	27							
1989	25	*U*					37	28							
1990	15	*UC*			38	26			7.1	3.1	98			7.3	3.2
	25	*U*					38	25							
1991	1	UC+*A*			36	17	37	17	6.5	2.3	85			7.7	2.7
	25	*U*					38	25							
1992	25	*U*					38	26							
1993	32	*A*					38	20							
1994	1	UC+*A*			32	16	33	16	5.7	2.0	75			7.7	2.6
	25	*U*					38	26							
1995	1	UC+*A*					34	16	5.4	1.8	70			7.7	2.6
	32	*A*					35	23							
	37	*U*					33	16							

See footnotes on next page

Table 16.8 *(continued)*

1 Surveys covering an age range of at least 21-64 are included. Any gaps in the data for ages 15-20 and 65 years and over are filled in by assumed extensions to the age distribution, given in *Notes on sources of survey data*, p. 395. Method: see *Summary of adult smoking*, p. xxxvi
2 See *Notes on sources of survey data*, p. 395
3 Product: MC = manufactured cigarettes, TC = total cigarettes (including hand-rolled), UC = cigarettes (type unspecified), A = all products, U = unspecified. Frequency of smoking is indicated by: regular or daily smokers in normal type, all smokers (including occasional) in bold, unspecified in italics
4 From Table 16.4
5 This column includes prevalence of smoking classified as UC = cigarettes (type unspecified)
6 This column includes prevalence of smoking classified as U = unspecified product
7 From Table 16.6
8 From Table 16.7, except data in parentheses, which are derived from the prevalence of smoking from Table 16.4 as described in *Summary of adult smoking*, p. xxxvi
9 Number of cigarettes classified as UC = cigarettes (type unspecified) has been adjusted to total cigarette sales and included in this column
10 Assumed to have been estimated to include clandestine sales, so not sales-adjusted

Figure 16.3 Estimated prevalence of smoking of (i) cigarettes and (ii) all tobacco products: by year of survey, 1949-1995.
Males and females aged 15 years and over. *Source:* see Table 16.8

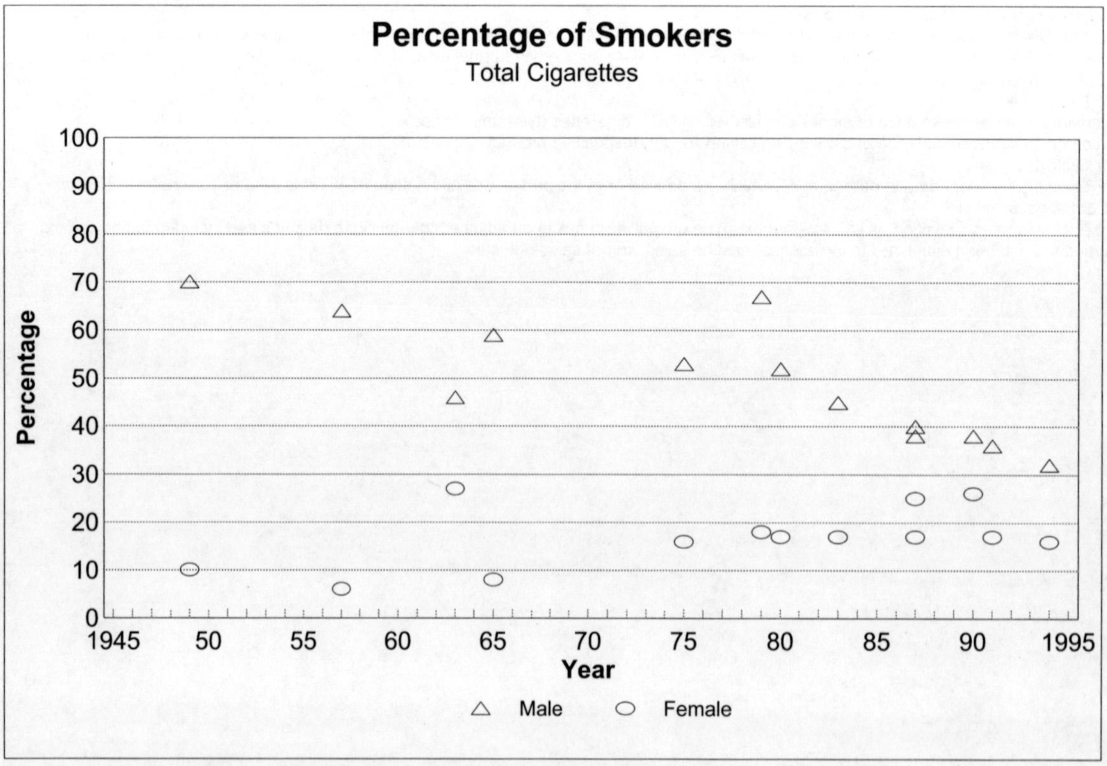

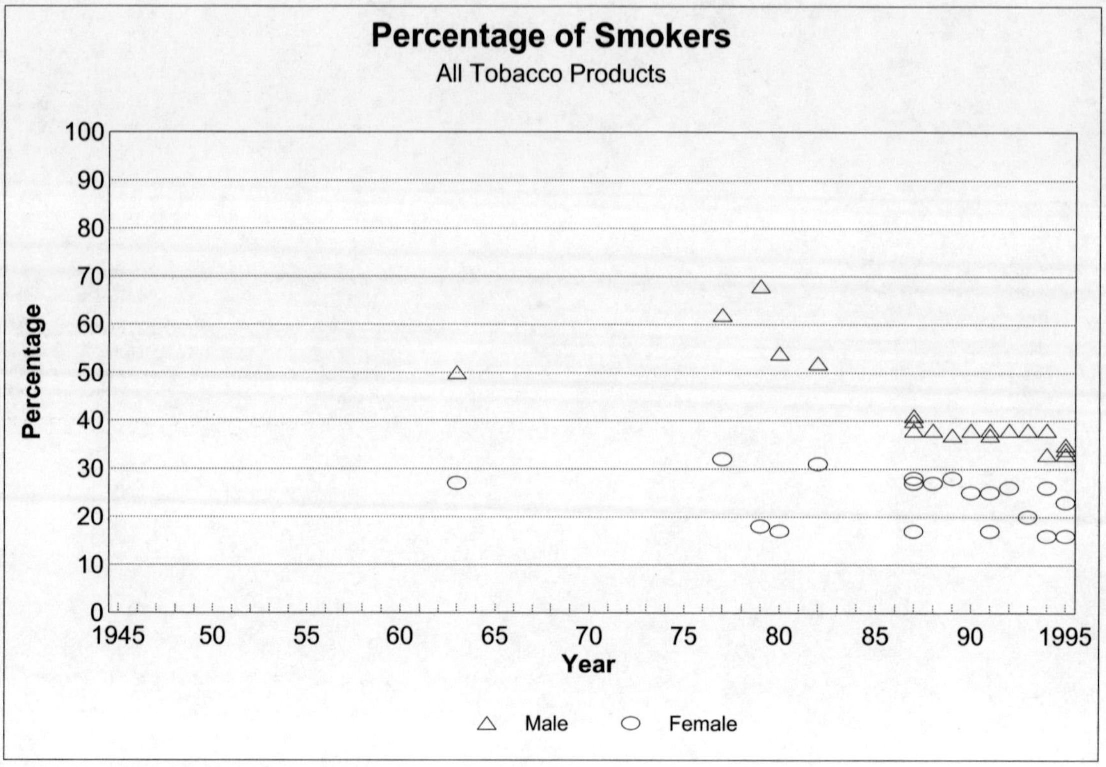

Figure 16.4 Estimated number of cigarettes smoked per person per day, sales-adjusted, 1949-1995.
Males and females aged 15 years and over. *Source:* see Table 16.8

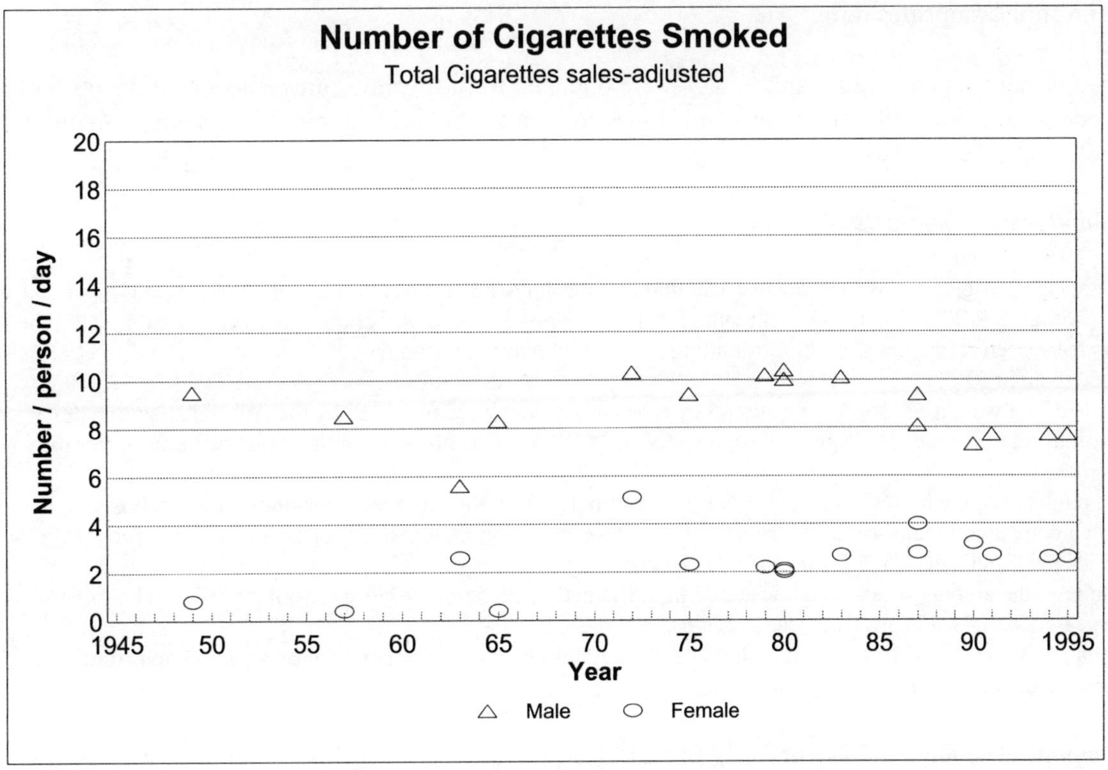

Note: As the sales of hand-rolled cigarettes have been estimated to be negligible from the 1960s onwards, manufactured and total cigarette data have been combined here.

Notes on sources of sales data

The data presented in the tables and figures were obtained from several sources, details of which are given below, together with estimations and related assumptions. Full citations of the sources are given on p. 400 under *References*.

Consumption data before 1974

RP6

Data by weight, originally given to nearest 100 000 pounds, have been converted to tonnes and given to the nearest 10 tonnes (100 000 lbs = 45.359 tonnes). Where weight conversion factors have been quoted in RP6, the weights have been recalculated without rounding and then converted to tonnes.

Notes as given in RP6:

a) Details of the weight of tobacco consumed by types of product were provided by the Amministrazione dei Monopoli di Stato, Rome. The figures for the years up to 1960 were published in the *Industrial Balance of the Administration*.

(b) The numbers of cigarettes consumed have been estimates from the cigarette consumption in pounds weight by using a conversion factor of 2.205 lbs per 1 000. The conversion factors used for cigars and cigarillos were 11.025 lbs per 1 000 and 5.513 lbs per 1 000 respectively.

(c) Details of the amount of tobacco consumed in individual years before 1956 were not provided. The figures for the years 1921 to 1955 are five-year averages.

(d) A change in the accounting period took place during 1964 when the financial year was converted from a year ended 30th June to a calendar year basis.

Consumption data for 1974-1995 (Table 16.1.2)

1974-1983 AMS (Amministrazione dei Monopoli di Stato, Roma). Responsabile per la Direzione Centralerelazioni con la Stampa

Data were given in numbers and have been converted to weight assuming an average of 1 g per cigarette and 4.5 g per cigar or cigarillo (based on a weighted average of the values in RP6). Totals derived using these conversion factors match the totals given by ISTAT (Table 16.1.3) very well.

1984-1995 Federazione Italiana Tabaccai (1999), Joossens *et al* (1994)

Data were given in tonnes. For conversion to numbers, we assumed an average cigarette weight of 1 g. For 1993 the breakdown of 'cigars and cigarillos' was 651 tonnes cigars and 227 tonnes cigarillos (Joossens *et al* (1994)).

Consumption data for 1982-1995 (Table 16.1.3)

Intituto Centrale di Statistica (ISTAT) (various years)

Sales by type of product are only available for home-produced tobacco, and imported tobacco is only given for combined products. Data in this format are also shown for 1982 and 1983, for comparison with Table 12.1.2, suggesting that about 1.5% of imported tobacco comprises products other than cigarettes.

Plain/Filter cigarette consumption

1961-1981 Maxwell (successive years)

1983 Todd (1986)

Tar yield of cigarettes

1984 La Vecchia (1985)

1993 Joossens *et al* (1994)

The value shown for 1984 is derived from tar yields of 18 brands of cigarettes bought in 1983 and 1984 combined using market share information for the years 1977-1979. The value shown for 1993 is derived from a table of tar/cigarette ranges and associated market shares.

The tar yield per cigarette was limited by EC directive (Directive 90/239/EEC) to 15 mg by the end of 1992, and to 12 mg by the end of 1997 (Harkin *et al* (1997)).

Estimates of hand-rolled cigarette consumption for 1951-1995
We have taken as our estimate of hand-rolled cigarette consumption 50% of pipe and hand-rolling tobacco sales up to 1955, decreasing by 5% per year until 1965, and none thereafter, at 1 g per cigarette.
There is little evidence on which to base estimates of hand-rolled cigarette consumption. Mastrandrea *et al* (1984) state that 'although reliable data are lacking, it seems that hand-rolling of cigarettes was a well-established habit in Italy, as in other countries, especially up to about 1950'. Merzdorf *et al* (1982) based estimates on the assumption that all pipe and hand-rolling tobacco was used in hand-rolled cigarettes. However, La Vecchia (personal communication) considered that 'hand-rolled cigarettes practically disappeared in Italy between the mid-1950s and the mid-1960s, and almost the totality of pipe and hand-rolling tobacco has been used in pipes over the last two or three decades'.

Notes on sources of survey data

Each source of survey data—either an individual survey or a series of surveys repeated over a number of years—is cited by a source number. This number is shown in the tables and corresponds to the source numbers given below, where details of the source publication and of the survey methodology are given. Full citations of the sources are given on p. 400 under *References*.

Source number

1 **Istituto Centrale de Statistica (1982), Bolzan *et al* (1982), La Vecchia (1986), Ferraroni *et al* (1989), La Vecchia *et al* (1990, 1994), Pagano *et al* (1996)**

a. National Health Surveys (1980-1994) and National Multipurpose Survey (1995) conducted by the ISTAT. Representative of civilian non-institutionalized population. Interviews (1980-1994) or self-completion questionnaires (1995) at home, with all household members, but proxy interviews permitted for members not present.

Year	Dates	Sample size				Participation rate (%)	Proxies (%)
		Households	Individuals	Adults (15+)			
				Males	Females		
1980	Nov 1980	25 018	75 397			94	—
1983	Nov-Dec 1983	31 025	89 765	34 787	37 497	94	8
1987	Nov 1986-Apr 1987	25 427	77 151	30 096	32 176	>90	—
1991	Dec 1990-May 1991	25 878	67 400	27 135	28 854	89	8
1994	Jan-Mar 1994	5 700	15 513	6 307	6 741	>90	28
1995	Nov 1995	21 629	60 933	24 497	26 088	>90	25

b. Cigarette smokers: smokers who smoked mainly cigarettes

c. Approximately 1% of subjects aged 10-14 described themselves as smokers in both 1986-1987 and 1990-1991

d. Consumption category estimation (except *All ages* data) based on (1980) 1-5, 6-10, 11-20, 21-30, and 31+ cigarettes/smoker/day, (1987-1994) <15 (assume 1-14), 15-24, 25+ cigarettes/smoker/day, (1995) <15 cigarettes or pipes/cigars (assume 1-14) and 15+ cigarettes/smoker/day. 1995 estimates should be regarded with caution. Comparison was possible for *All ages* data between category estimates (not shown) and direct means (as shown in Table 16.5) for 1991 when results were very similar, and for 1994 when category estimates were lower by about 0.8 cigarettes for both males and females

e. Assumed extension to age distribution for age 70+, number of cigarettes/person/day: males 3.0 and females 0.1

2 **The Research Group ATS-RF2 of the Italian National Research Council (1981)**

a. Subjects invited for medical examination as part of project screening for atherosclerosis risk factors. Pooled results from nine population samples in eight regions throughout Italy (Veneto, Pavia, Bologna, Siena, Rome, Naples, Cagliari, Palermo). Sample size (males) 3 189, (females) 3 510. Participation rate 62%

3 Monarca *et al* (1987), Donato *et al* (1994)

a. Study of high school pupils in 10 towns (North: Pavia, Genova. Central: Perugia, Urbino, Latina, S Benedetto del Tronto. South and Islands: Brindisi, Cagliari, Sassari). Questionnaires completed anonymously in class with teachers present. Approximate ages corresponding to 9th and 13th grades.

Year	Sample size			
	Males		Females	
	9th	13th	9th	13th
1981	2 051	2 168	1 983	2 074
1988	2 596	1 937	2 625	2 217

b. Regular smokers: smoked at least one cigarette every day. All smokers: smoked at least one cigarette a month

c. Consumption category estimation based on (1981) 1-4, 5-9, 10-19, >20 (assume 20+) cigarettes/smoker/day; (1988) on two categories 1-9 and 10+ cigarettes/smoker/day and resulting figures should be regarded with caution

4 Todd (1986)

a. Cigarettes sold legally; figures estimated by Todd

5 WHO (1975), probably quoting figures from ISTAT

a. WHO estimates of average national consumption (Table 16.6). They represent 154% of cigarettes sold legally. As they have presumably been estimated to include clandestine sales, no adjustment has been made

6 Modolo (1977)

a. Surveys of senior high school students in Perugia (central Italy). Upper age limit not stated. Sample size in 1962 (boys) 1 250, (girls) 609 and in 1972 (boys) 1 915, (girls) 1 655

b. Regular smokers: smoked 1 or more cigarettes per day

7 Readers Digest (1963)

a. Series of surveys conducted in European countries using identical questionnaires. Italian survey conducted by Misura S.p.A. Random sample of about 2 000 people

b. It is also reported that 4% of men (5% age <40 and 5% age 40+ (*sic*)) smoke a pipe, and that 4% of men (3% age <40 and 7% age 40+) smoke cigars

c. Merzdorf *et al* (1982) commented that '... the strikingly high proportion of female smokers ... is all the more surprising in view of the fact that in other countries the proportion of women who smoke was consistently underestimated in this study'

d. Assumed extension to age distribution for percentages smokers, age 15-20: (A) males 50% and females 27%; (UC) males 46% and females 27%

8 Bartolini *et al* (1977)

a. Interview study of young people in Perugia, considered representative of those not attending high school. Sample size 931

b. Calculation of consumption per person assumed that consumption per smoker related to 'all' smokers

9 Merzdorf *et al* (1982), quoting industry research

10 Analisi e Strategie de Mercato (ASM) (personal communication)

a. Representative sample. Sample size (males) 547, (females) 576

b. Assumed extension to age distribution for percentage smokers, age 65+: males 40% and females 5%

11 ASM (1981)

a. Quota sample, representative of the Italian adult female population. Sample size 1 096

b. Consumption category estimation based on packs per week <2, 2-4, 5-6, 7, 8-10, 11-13, 14, and 15+ cigarettes/smoker (equivalents assumed 1-5, 6-14, 15-19, 20, 21-29, 30-39, 40, and 41+ cigarettes/smoker/day)

c. Assumed extension to age distribution (females only) for percentage smokers, age 65+: females 5%. Number of cigarettes/person/day: 0.5

12 Tonelli *et al* (1980)

a. Survey of 3rd grade pupils in junior high schools throughout Bologna. Sample size (males) 907, (females) 1 017

b. Consumption category estimation based on weekly consumption of <6, 6-10, and 11+ cigarettes/smoker

13 Modolo *et al* (1980)

a. Survey of schoolchildren in Rome

14 La Vecchia (1986), quoting Doxa (1950,1958,1966,1978)

a. Surveys by DOXA Marketing Research Institute on behalf of Italian State Monopoly (and in 1957 of the U.S. Department of Agriculture). Sample size 4 000-6 000. 1949 survey used non-random sampling

c. In 1949, over 5% of smokers used hand-rolled cigarettes only and over 25% used both manufactured and hand-rolled cigarettes

d. Figures for 1949 and 1957 represent 277% and 136% respectively of cigarettes sold legally and have not been adjusted (1949 calculation based on 1946-1950 consumption and 1950 population)

e. Assumed extension to age distribution for percentage smokers, age 15-17: (1949) males 50% and females 8%. Number of cigarettes/person/day: males 5.0 and females 1.0. For age 15: (1957, 1965) males 40% and females (1957) 5%, (1965) 8%. Number of cigarettes/person/day: males 3.0 and females 1.0

15 La Vecchia and Scarpino (1993)

a. Nationally representative surveys conducted by DOXA for the European Economic Community. Personal interviews at home. Sample size (1987) 1 054, (1990) 1 033

b. Age-specific cigarette smoking prevalence and all product prevalence shown in Table 16.4 as 1987 are based on the two surveys combined

16-18 WHO (1989), WHO MONICA Project (1988), Cesana *et al* (1995)

a. Three regional surveys forming part of WHO MONICA project:

	Region	Population size	Sample size	Participation rate (%)	Sample used* Male	Sample used* Female	Date
16	Area Latina	260 000	1 834	76	893	893	May 1982-Mar 1985
17	Friuli	394 100	1 795	81	935	923	Dec 1985-Sep 1987
18	Brianza	333 200	1 773	71	819	839	Apr 1986-Mar 1987

* 'Sample used' includes age 25-34; all other figures are for age 35-64 only

b. *All ages* column relates only to age 35-64 and is standardized to world population

c. A second study was carried out in Brianza in 1989-1990. Participation rate 70%, sample used 1 605. All results for that study reported by Cesana *et al* (1995) relate to age 25-64. For comparison, the prevalence of smoking (all products) in the first study for age 25-64 was (males) 48%, (females) 24%, and the average cigarettes per smoker was (males) 18, (females) 12. There were minor discrepancies in the age-specific results reported by the different sources for the first study

d. Regular cigarette smokers: smoked cigarettes daily. All smokers: smoked cigarettes daily or occasionally, or smoked 1 g pipe tobacco or 1 cigar per week. Cigarettes per smoker refers to regular and occasional cigarette smokers

e. Calculation for cigarettes per person based on % regular cigarette smokers and cigarettes per regular or occasional cigarette smoker, so may underestimate

19 Pastega (1982)

a. Survey in 4 junior and 5 senior high schools in Venice. Questionnaires completed anonymously in class with teachers absent. Year unknown. Sample size 2 196

20 Modolo *et al* (1980)

a. Overall results from survey covering north, central, and southern regions. Age group unknown (adults)

21-23 Keys *et al* (1966)

a. Baseline of Seven Countries Study on cardiovascular disease, in three rural villages. Interview including smoking questions before medical examinations.

	Location	Sample size	Response rate (%)
21	Nicotera, far south	607	97
22	Crevalcore, Po valley	994	99
23	Montegiorgio, Province of Marche (east coast)	719	99

b. Results for additional occupational groups (railwaymen in Rome) are not presented here
c. Pipe and cigar consumption is stated to be negligible in Italy, especially in rural areas
d. Consumption category estimation based on 1-9, 10-19, 20+ cigarettes/smoker/day

24 Casson *et al* (1982)

a. Survey of school pupils in Chioggia. Approximate ages corresponding to junior and senior high schools. Sample size 2 616, response rate 56%
b. Regular smokers: smoked daily
c. Consumption category estimation (upper school) based on 1-5, 6-10, 11-15, 16-20, >20 cigarettes/smoker/day, taken from chart. Approximately 90% of lower school smokers smoked <5 cigarettes per day

25 Joossens *et al* (1994) quoting Commission of the European Communities

a. Eurobarometer surveys

26 Casadidio *et al* (1993)

a. Anonymous survey of high school pupils in two Local Health Units of Marche region (central Italy). Questionnaires completed in class without intervention from teachers present. Approximate ages corresponding to 9th and 13th grades. Sample size (males) 368, (females) 559
b. Regular smokers: smokes daily. All smokers: smokes daily or occasionally
c. Consumption category estimation based on 1-4, 5-9, 10-19, 20+ cigarettes/smoker/day

27 Arciti *et al* (1995)

a. Follow-up study in Liguria of 1 894 pupils who had not participated in any smoking control programme. Pupils were enrolled in first year of senior high, vocational or teacher training school

28 Donato *et al* (1991)

a. Survey of high school pupils in Brescia (northern Italy), using same methodology as source 3. Participation rate 90%.

Year	Sample size			
	Males		Females	
	9th	13th	9th	13th
1989	287	318	366	393

b. Regular smokers: smoked at least one cigarette every day. All smokers: smoked at least one cigarette a week
c. Consumption category estimation based on 1-4, 5-9, 10-19, 20+ cigarettes/smoker/day

29 van Reek *et al* (1992), van Reek and Adriaanse (1995)

a. A series of surveys of Young Europeans. About 800 children aged 11-15 years interviewed in each EC country except Luxembourg (where only 250 interviewed). Lowest age group 11-12. Interviews conducted at home, with parents absent
b. Regular smokers: smoked daily. All smokers: smoked at least once a week

30 Pasquale *et al* (1992)

a. Survey of high school pupils in Valle Camonica, a mountain community in Brescia (northern Italy). Questionnaires completed anonymously in class. Approximate ages corresponding to 9th and 13th grades. Sample size 1 391, participation rate 78%

b. Regular smokers: smoked at least one cigarette every day. All smokers: smoked at least one cigarette a week

c. Consumption category estimation based on 1-4, 5-9, 10-19, 20+ cigarettes/smoker/day

31 Ferrante *et al* (1993)

a. Survey of young men from all Italian regions, at a military training centre. Age 20. Year not stated. Sample size 1 153

32 Centro di Documentazione e Informazione sul Tabacco (1996)

a. Surveys conducted by Abacus (1993) and ISPO (1995). Age not stated

33 Maglione *et al* (1994)

a. Survey of 8th grade pupils at 13 high schools in Benevento (Campania Region). Year not stated

34 Marin *et al* (1999)

a. Anonymous questionnaire survey of 9th, 11th and 13th grade high school pupils at 14 high schools in Belluno and Bassano del Grappa. Conducted in 1993-1994. Upper age limit not stated. Sample size (males) 1 756, (females) 2 329

b. Regular smokers: smokes every day. All smokers: smokers every day or occasionally

c. Consumption category estimation based on <6, 6-10, 11-15, 16-20 and >20 cigarettes/smoker/day

35 Gruppo Collaborativo SIDRIA (1998)

a. S.I.D.R.I.A.(Studi Italiani sui Disturbi Respiratori nell'Infanzia e l'Ambiento, Italian Studies on Respiratory Disorders in Childhood and the Environment). A collaborative study of 8th grade pupils and their families in 10 regions of northern and central Italy. Oct 1994-Mar 1995. Sample size (males) 11 360, (females) 10 486. Participation rate 96%

b. Smokers were defined as those who smoked regularly apart from trying a few cigarettes, and then allocated as regulars smokers: smoked at least 1 cigarette per week, or frequency *: smoked daily

36 Hibell *et al* (1997)

a. Nationally representative survey forming part of ESPAD (European School Survey Project on Alcohol and Other Drugs). Target was pupils born in 1979, thus age 15-16 at time of survey in April-June 1995. Approximately 60% of this group still in school. Anonymous questionnaire completed and sealed in envelope by pupil, in class. Teachers present, but discouraged from walking round the classroom. Sample size (males) 943, (females) 582. Response rate (males) 92%, (females) 94%

b. Results for Italy should be treated with caution compared to other participating countries, due to a high level of inconsistency, and smaller sample size

c. Regular smokers: smoked 1 or more cigarettes per day in last 30 days. All smokers: smoked in last 30 days

d. Consumption category estimation based on 1-5, 6-10, 11-20, 21+ cigarettes/smoker/day

37 Tessier *et al* (1999) quoting Prof A. Quaranta

a. Based on national statistics, but no details. Lower age limit and year not stated

Analisi e Strategie di Mercato (1981). *Smoking habits of Italian women*. ASM srl, Rome.

Arciti C., Pistone M., Persici P., Barbieri A. and Santi L. (1995). Methodologies and results of an antismoking program addressed to schoolchildren and teachers. In: Slama K. (ed) *Tobacco and Health, Ninth World Conference on Tobacco and Health, Paris, Oct 10-14 1994*. Plenum Press, New York and London; 681-4.

Bartolini E., Minelli L. and Cicchitelli G. (1977). *Indagine sull'abitudine di fumare tra i giovani non studenti.*

Beese D.H. (ed) (1968). *Tobacco consumption in various countries,* 2nd edition. Tobacco Research Council, London. Research Paper 6.

Beese D.H. (ed) (1972). *Tobacco consumption in various countries,* 3rd edition. Tobacco Research Council, London. Research Paper 6.

Bolzan M., Fabbris L., Fontana F., Porzia E. and Zanella F. (1982). Frequenza e intensità del fumo tra i giovani in Italia (Frequency and intensity of smoking among youth in Italy). In: Fontana F. (ed) *Tabacco e giovani (Tobacco and youth), International conference, Venice 9-11 November 1981*. ATTI, Venice; 199-210.

Casadidio A., Monarca S., Donato F., Bruni A., *et al* (1993). Indagine sul tabagismo tra studenti di Scuola Media Superiore della U.S.L. No 9 e 19 della Regione Marche (Tobacco smoking among high-school students of Local Health Units No. 9 and 19 in the Le Marche region). *Ann Ig,* **5**, 397-408.

Casson F., Boscolo P., Mantovan C., Boscolo A.B., *et al* (1982). Indagine sul fumo di sigaretta negli studenti di Chioggia (Italia). In: Fontana F. (ed) *Tabacco e giovani (Tobacco and youth), International conference, Venice 9-11 November 1981*. ATTI, Venice; 245-53.

Centro di Documentazione e Informazione sul Tabacco (1996). *I dati e i numeri*. CDIT, Milan.

Cesana G.C., de Vito G., Ferrario M., Sega R. and Mocarelli P. (1995). Trends of smoking habits in northern Italy (1986-1990). The WHO MONICA project in Area Brianza, Italy. *Eur J Epidemiol,* **11**, 251-8.

Donato F., Chiesa R., Monarca S. and Duca P. (1991). Il fumo di tabacco tra gli studenti di scuola media superiore di Brescia: analisi delle relazioni tra abitudine fumatoria e conoscenze, atteggiamenti, fattori socio-ambientali e comportamentali (Cigarette smoking among high school students in Brescia: analysis of relations between smoking habit and knowledge, attitudes socioeconomic and behavioral factors). *Epidemiol Prev,* **13**, 43-9.

Donato F., Monarca S., Chiesa R., Feretti D. and Nardi G. (1994). Smoking among high school students in 10 Italian towns: patterns and covariates. *International Journal of the Addictions,* **29**, 1537-57.

Doxa (1950). *Inchiesta Sulle Abitudini e Preferenze dei Fumatori Italiani.* Sondaggi Doxa No. 2.[§]

Doxa (1958). *Nuovi Studi Sulle Abitudini e Preferenze dei Fumatori Italiani.* Sondaggi Doxa No. 5.[§]

Doxa (1966). Una nuova indagine sui fumatori. *Boll Doxa,* **20**, 20-1.[§]

Doxa (1978). *Quanti fumano (e chi fuma) regolarmente o saltuariamente, sigarette sigari e la pipa.* Unpublished.[§]

Federazione Italiana Tabaccai (1999). http://www.tabaccai.it/home.htm and subsequent pages.

Ferrante E., Muzzolon R., Fuso L., Pistelli R., Corbo G.M. and Ciappi G. (1993). The relationship between sporting activity and smoking habits in young adults. *Mil Med,* **158**, 696-7.

Ferraroni M., La Vecchia C., Pagano R., Negri E. and Decarli A. (1989). Smoking in Italy, 1986-1987. *Tumori,* **75**, 521-6.

Gruppo Collaborativo SIDRIA (1998). Abitudine al fumo di sigarette tra gli studenti di III media in diverse aree italiane. (Cigarette smoking habit among eighth graders in different Italian areas). *Epidemiol Prev,* **22**, 155-64.

Harkin A.M., Anderson P. and Goos C. (1997). *Smoking, drinking and drug taking in the European Region.* Alcohol, Drugs and Tobacco Programme, WHO Regional Office for Europe, Copenhagen.

Hibell B., Andersson B., Bjarnason T., Kokkevi A., Morgan M. and Narusk A. (1997). *The 1995 ESPAD report. The European school survey project on alcohol and other drugs. Alcohol and other drug use among students in 26 European countries*. The Swedish Council for Information on Alcohol and Other Drugs. Council of Europe (Pompidou Group).

Intituto Centrale di Statistica (ISTAT) (various years). *Annuario statistico Italiano*. ISTAT, Italy.

Istituto Centrale de Statistica (1982). *Indagine statistica sulle condizioni di salute della popolazione e sul ricorso al servizi sanitari, November 1980*. Istituto Centrale di Statistica. Supplement 12 Bollettino Mensile di Statistica.

Jones A. and Mazzi M.G. (1996). Tobacco consumption and taxation in Italy: an application of the QUAIDS model. *Applied Economics,* **28**, 595-603.

Joossens L., Naett C., Howie C. and Muldoon A. (1994). *Tobacco and health in the European Union. An overview*. European Bureau for Action on Smoking Prevention (BASP), Brussels.

Keys A., Aravanis C., Blackburn H.W., van Buchem F.S.P., *et al* (1966). Epidemiological studies related to coronary heart disease: characteristics of men aged 40-59 in seven countries. *Acta Medica Scandinavica,* **Suppl 460**, 8-392.

La Vecchia C. (1985). Patterns of cigarette smoking and trends in lung cancer mortality in Italy. *J Epidemiol Community Health,* **39**, 157-64.

La Vecchia C. (1986). Smoking in Italy, 1949-1983. *Prev Med,* **15**, 274-81.

La Vecchia C., Negri E. and Pagano R. (1990). Recent decline of smoking in younger Italian women [Letter]. *Int J Epidemiol,* **19**, 221.

La Vecchia C., Pagano R., Decarli A. and Ferraroni M. (1994). Smoking in Italy, 1990-1991. *Tumori,* **80**, 175-80.

La Vecchia C. and Scarpino V. (1993). Smoking in Italy, 1987-90. *Tob Control,* **2**, 231-5.

Lee P.N. (ed) (1975). *Tobacco consumption in various countries,* 4th edition. Tobacco Research Council, London. Research Paper 6.

Maglione T., De Maria C., Assante M. and Pennino G. (1994). Prevalenza dell'abitudine al fumo tra gli studenti di 3° media di Benevento (Cigarette smoking among secondary school students in Benevento, Italy). *Epidemiol Prev,* **18**, 237-40.

Marin V., Franchin D., Ghio L., Ravazzolo E. and Moretti G. (1999). Abitudini ed opinioni sul fumo di un campione di studenti di scuola media superiore (Smoking habits and opinions of a sample of high school students). *Ann Ig,* **11**, 219-26.

Mastrandrea V., La Rosa F. and Cresci A. (1984). Trends of lung cancer mortality in Italy in relation to consumption of tobacco products. *Am J Epidemiol,* **120**, 257-64.

Maxwell J.C.Jr. (successive years). How the brands ranked. Maxwell International Estimates. *World Tobacco.*

Merzdorf J., Reuter U. and Welsch G. (1982). *Daten und Fakten zur Entwicklung des Rauchens in Mitgliedsländern der Europäischen Gemeinschaften (Facts and figures on the development of smoking in the member states of the European Communities)*. Kommission der Europäischen Gemeinschaften, Luxemburg. Medizin—EUR 7907 DE.

Modolo M.A. (1977). Survey on legislative action in Italy: The advertising ban. In: *Smoking and Health II. Health consequences, education, cessation activities, and governmental action.* USDHEW; 861-5. DHEW

Publication No. (NIH) 77-1413.

Modolo M.A., Minelli L. and Cicchitelli G. (1980). Smoking habits in Italy. *World Smoking and Health,* **5**, 34-6.

Monarca S., Modolo M.A., Stopponi V., Catanelli M., Romizi R. and Santi L. (1987). Alcohol, tobacco and psychoactive medicine consumption among high school students of 10 Italian towns. *International Journal of the Addictions,* **22**, 1243-54.

Pagano R., La Vecchia C. and Decarli A. (1996). Smoking in Italy, 1994. *Tumori,* **82**, 309-13.

Pasquale L., Donato F., Oneda M.L., Tiberti R., Bonomelli D. and Peretti P. (1992). Diffusione del tabagismo tra i giovani di una comunità montana dell'Italia settentrionale (Smoking habits among high school students in a mountain community in North Italy). *Igiene Moderna,* **97**, 314-31.

Pastega G. (1982). Indagini sul fumo di sigarette in alcune scuole del comune di Venezia. In: Fontana F. (ed) *Tabacco e giovani (Tobacco and youth), International conference, Venice 9-11 November 1981*. ATTI, Venice; 179-97.

Readers Digest (1963). *Products and people. A digest of the marketing survey of the European Common Market and Britain, 1963* . Reader's Digest Association Limited, London.

RP6, See Beese (ed) (1968), Beese (ed) (1972), Lee (ed) (1975)

Tessier J.-F., Nejjari C. and Bennani-Othmani M. (1999). Smoking in Mediterranean countries: Europe, North Africa and the Middle-East. Results from a co-operative study. *International Journal of Tuberculosis and Lung Diseases,* **3**, 927-37.

The Research Group ATS-RF2 of the Italian National Research Council (1981). Distribution of some risk factors for atherosclerosis in nine Italian population samples. *Am J Epidemiol,* **113**, 338-46.

Todd G. (1986). *Medicine. Statistics of smoking in the Member States of the European Community.* Commission of the European Communities, Luxembourg.

Tonelli E., Faggioli A., Stampi S., Gatto M.R. and Costa V. (1980). Indagine epidemiologica sulle abitudini al fumo tra i ragazzi di Bologna. (Epidemiological survey of smoking habits among Bologna schoolchildren). *Igiene Moderna,* **74**, 187-211.

van Reek J. and Adriaanse H. (1995). Daily smoking among adolescents in the European Community. *Rev Epidemiol Sante Publique,* **43**, 281-2.

van Reek J., Adriaanse H. and Karaoglou A. (1992). Smoking among children in the European Community. *J Public Health Med,* **14**, 93-4.

WHO (1989). The WHO MONICA project: a worldwide monitoring system for cardiovascular diseases. In: *World health statistics annual 1989.* WHO, Geneva; 25-149.

WHO MONICA Project (1988). Geographical variation in the major risk factors of coronary heart disease in men and women aged 35-64 years. *World Health Stat Q,* **41**, 115-40.

WHO (1975). Survey on smoking and health in the European Region, 1974-75: preliminary data as at 1 May 1975. *Presented at the Third World Conference on Smoking and Health, New York, 2-5 June 1975.* WHO; 1-55.

§ Original paper not obtained, but information taken as quoted by another author

Japan 17

Sales data

See Tables 17.1-17.3.

From 1920 until about 1943 the consumption of manufactured cigarettes per adult increased slowly from 2 to 3 cigarettes per day. Towards the end of the Second World War there was a sharp drop in consumption, but thereafter consumption continued to increase until the late 1970s when it reached a peak of nearly 10 manufactured cigarettes per day. It had decreased to 9 cigarettes per day by the 1990s. We estimate that, apart from an increase just after the Second World War, consumption of hand-rolled cigarettes has declined steadily since 1920. In the early 1920s (and also just after the war), more hand-rolled cigarettes were consumed than manufactured cigarettes. As more manufactured cigarettes were smoked, smoking of hand-rolled cigarettes virtually disappeared during the 1960s.

The consumption of all tobacco products per adult was about 4 g per day from 1920 to 1944; it dropped to 2 g per day in 1945. After the war it increased to nearly 10 g per day by the late 1970s. It decreased to 9 g per adult per day by 1984, after which estimates cannot be made. Almost all tobacco has been consumed in cigarettes since 1920; the consumption of other products was negligible. In 1925, 54% of tobacco was consumed in manufactured cigarettes and 46% was used for hand-rolling. Virtually all tobacco was consumed as filtered manufactured cigarettes after the 1970s.

Survey data

See Tables 17.4-17.8

Information on smoking for those aged 20 years and over has been available annually since 1958 from industry sources. As no data are available on smoking among teenagers until the 1980s, it has been particularly difficult to estimate the overall adult (aged 15 years and over) prevalence of smoking in Japan as shown in Table 17.8. The assumed extensions to the age distribution for ages 15-19 are of a more speculative nature than in other countries. However, we hope any error will be relatively unimportant as the assumed extensions apply only to a small proportion of the adult population and are consistent over the years.

From 1958 until the mid-1970s, the estimated prevalence of cigarette smoking among those aged 15 years and over was about 70-75% in men. It had declined to below 60% by the 1990s. Among women it remained at about 10-15%. From 1968 to 1975, when separate data on occasional smoking were available, the prevalence of regular smoking was 2-4% lower in both sexes.

Data on adult smoking by age have been available since 1965. The prevalence of smoking decreased somewhat among men at all ages, more so over age 40. The prevalence has increased among younger women and decreased among older women, so that the pattern of prevalence with age, increasing in the 1960s, levelled out by 1980 and reversed thereafter.

According to Shimao (1988), an Act prohibiting minors from smoking came into force in 1900, as the Government was worried about the ill-effects of smoking on soldiers. The law was well observed until the 1950s, but smoking in junior and senior high schools has since become a problem. The existence of the Act meant that this was regarded as a problem of juvenile delinquency rather than of health. Surveys on teenage smoking, locally based in the 1980s, and nationally based from 1990 (source 18), show the prevalence of smoking to be much lower among girls than among boys.

Comparison of survey and sales data suggests that there has been a gradual shift from overstatement of about 10% in the 1960s to understatement by 10% in the 1990s. Between

1958 and the mid-1970s, the estimated number of cigarettes smoked per person per day (sales-adjusted) increased for men from about 8 to 17.5, and declined to 15 in 1995. For women it increased from 1 in 1958 to nearly 3 in 1995.

Table 17.1.1 Total annual sales of tobacco products, 1920-1973

Year	Cigarettes		Cigars		Fine-cut tobacco	Pipe tobacco	All tobacco products
	tonnes	millions	tonnes	millions	tonnes	tonnes	tonnes
1920	20960	20954	20	3	26220	0	47200
1921	22740	22732	20	3	26130	0	48880
1922	24030	24031	20	3	25170	0	49230
1923	27220	27220	30	5	24630	0	51890
1924	28950	28943	20	3	23770	0	52740
1925	27280	27273	30	4	23630	0	50940
1926	27210	27205	20	3	23810	0	51040
1927	29180	29178	20	3	23900	0	53110
1928	30960	30954	20	3	22950	0	53930
1929	31670	31664	20	3	23590	0	55280
1930	30210	30201	10	1	23540	0	53750
1931	29370	29368	10	1	22860	0	52240
1932	31840	31831	10	1	23180	0	55020
1933	33540	33536	20	3	22720	0	56290
1934	36630	36625	20	3	22230	50	58920
1935	37910	37907	20	3	21590	0	59520
1936	38480	38477	10	2	20910	0	59410
1937	40650	40641	10	1	21590	0	62250
1938	40980	40974	10	1	20180	0	61170
1939	48130	48125	10	1	18600	0	66740
1940	51390	51381	10	2	19600	0	71000
1941	52440	52428	10	1	18730	0	71180
1942	53840	53830	10	1	19280	0	73120
1943	54270	54258	0	0	18910	0	73180
1944	45780	45770	10	1	18510	0	64290
1945	14690	14691	0	0	16330	0	31020
1946	15720	15715	0	0	31660	0	47380
1947	17850	17843	0	0	29350	0	47190
1948	34270	34263	20	3	22630	230	57150
1949	52750	52744	30	5	13110	50	65940
1950	65310	65298	10	2	9840	50	75210
1951	74010	73995	10	1	8980	50	83040
1952	80190	80177	0	0	8030	50	88260
1953	89530	89516	0	0	7300	50	96880
1954	95630	95614	0	0	7210	50	102890
1955	97660	97646	0	0	6490	50	104190
1956	97250	97212	10	1	5810	50	103110
1957	101420	101403	10	1	5220	50	106690
1958	107410	107415	10	1	4850	50	112320
1959	113170	113196	10	1	4260	50	117490
1960	122740	122760	10	1	3720	50	126510
1961	134400	134431	10	1	3040	50	137490
1962	142020	142013	10	2	2490	50	144570
1963	150950	151111	10	1	2040	50	153050
1964	160660	160807	10	1	1770	50	162480
1965	171280	171449	10	1	1500	50	172820
1966	181300	181488	10	2	1410	50	182770
1967	193910	193932	20	3	1040	90	195060
1968	196720	196709	10	2	950	90	197780
1969	211330	211316	10	2	860	50	212250
1970	222120	222132	10	2	640	50	222820
1971	235500	235449	10	2	410	50	235970
1972	252690	252665	10	2	410	90	253210
1973	266760	266692	10	2	410	90	267270

Source: see *Notes on sources of sales data,* p. 425

Table 17.1.2 Total annual sales of tobacco products, 1970-1995

Year	Cigarettes tonnes	Cigarettes millions	Cigars tonnes	Cigars millions	Fine-cut tobacco tonnes	Pipe tobacco tonnes	All tobacco products tonnes
1970	222880	222880	129	19	614	113	223736
1971	236324	236324	129	19	405	131	236989
1972	253984	253984	204	30	408	184	254780
1973	268727	268727	272	40	376	224	269599
1974	287118	287118	286	42	359	286	288049
1975	293112	293112	190	28	360	338	294000
1976	291448	291448	238	35	327	286	292299
1977	303845	303845	959	141	294	223	305321
1978	304719	304719	925	136	292	183	306119
1979	310774	310774	476	70	94	163	311507
1980	307665	307665	252	37	13	153	308083
1981	312054	312054	197	29	18	152	312421
1982	315073	315073	177	26	10	144	315404
1983	311731	311731	170	25	9	136	312046
1984	312597	312597	156	23	8	119	312880
1985	310726	310726	68	10			
1986	308438	308438	54	8			
1987	308286	308286	54	8			
1988	306415	306415	54	8			
1989	313800	313800					
1990	322000	322000					
1991	328300	328300					
1992	328900	328900					
1993	332600	332600					
1994	334400	334400					
1995	334700	334700					

Source : see *Notes on sources of sales data*, p. 425

Table 17.1.3 Total annual sales of various types of cigarettes, 1970-1988

Year	Filter cigarettes millions	Non-filter cigarettes millions	Cigarettes with mouthpiece millions	Imperial Household millions	Imported cigarettes millions
1970	200588	21062	482	3	745
1971	218404	16652	393	3	872
1972	238335	14005	326	3	1315
1973	254488	11952	252	3	2032
1974	273438	10507	210	3	2960
1975	280124	9551	167	3	3267
1976	280127	8458	145	3	2715
1977	292916	7901	0	3	3025
1978	293860	7264	0	3	3592
1979	300185	6599	0	0	3990
1980	298109	5852	0	0	3704
1981	302192	5354	0	0	4508
1982	305406	4850	0	0	4817
1983	301657	4387	0	0	5687
1984	302046	4004	0	0	6547
1985	299517	3709			7500
1986	293288	3250			11900
1987	275054	2932			30300
1988	266593	2622			37200

Source : see *Notes on sources of sales data*, p. 425

Table 17.1.4 Manufactured cigarettes (i) percentage of total sales as filter cigarettes, 1960-1995, (ii) sales-weighted average tar yield per cigarette (SWAT), 1969-1995 and (iii) sales-weighted average nicotine (SWAN), 1969-1995

Year	% Filter	SWAT mg / cig	SWAN mg / cig
1960	7.9		
1961	12.0		
1962	11.2		
1963	17.4		
1964	24.8		
1965	42.5		
1966	58.0		
1967	76.0		
1968	82.0		
1969	87.0	20.7	1.64
1970	89.7	20.3	1.62
1971	92.5	19.9	1.57
1972	94.2	19.3	1.50
1973	95.1	18.7	1.43
1974	96.1	18.0	1.31
1975	96.5	17.6	1.28
1976	97.1	17.4	1.22
1977	97.0	17.2	1.20
1978	97.6	16.5	1.10
1979	98.0	16.1	1.06
1980	97.8	15.9	1.04
1981	98.1	15.5	1.02
1982	98.4	15.5	1.01
1983	98.6	15.1	1.00
1984	98.7	14.6	0.98
1985	98.8	14.2	0.97
1986	98.9	13.8	0.96
1987	98.9	13.7	1.00
1988	99.0	13.3	1.00
1989		12.7	1.06
1990		12.4	1.04
1991		11.7	1.00
1992		11.0	0.94
1993	99.5	10.0	0.83
1994	99.4	9.5	0.78
1995	99.5	9.0	0.74

Source : see *Notes on sources of sales data,* p. 425

Table 17.2 Consumption of (i) cigarettes and (ii) all tobacco products, 1920-1995 sales-based data, including estimated hand-rolled cigarette consumption. Males and females aged 15 years and over

Year	Manufactured cigarettes		Hand-rolled cigarettes		Total cigarettes		All tobacco products	
	Total annual in millions	Number/ adult/day	Total annual in millions	Number/ adult/day	Total annual in millions	Number/ adult/day	Total annual in tonnes	Grams/ adult/day
1920	20954	1.6	26220	2.0	47174	3.7	47200	3.7
1921	22732	1.7	26130	2.0	48862	3.8	48880	3.8
1922	24031	1.8	25170	1.9	49201	3.7	49230	3.7
1923	27220	2.0	24630	1.8	51850	3.9	51890	3.9
1924	28943	2.1	23770	1.8	52713	3.9	52740	3.9
1925	27273	2.0	23630	1.7	50903	3.7	50940	3.7
1926	27205	2.0	23810	1.7	51015	3.7	51040	3.7
1927	29178	2.1	23900	1.7	53078	3.8	53110	3.8
1928	30954	2.2	22950	1.6	53904	3.8	53930	3.8
1929	31664	2.2	23590	1.6	55254	3.8	55280	3.8
1930	30201	2.0	23540	1.6	53741	3.6	53750	3.6
1931	29368	2.0	22860	1.5	52228	3.5	52240	3.5
1932	31831	2.1	23180	1.5	55011	3.6	55020	3.6
1933	33536	2.2	22720	1.5	56256	3.7	56290	3.7
1934	36625	2.3	22230	1.4	58855	3.8	58920	3.8
1935	37907	2.4	21590	1.4	59497	3.8	59520	3.8
1936	38477	2.4	20910	1.3	59387	3.7	59410	3.7
1937	40641	2.5	21590	1.3	62231	3.8	62250	3.8
1938	40974	2.5	20180	1.2	61154	3.7	61170	3.7
1939	48125	2.9	18600	1.1	66725	4.0	66740	4.0
1940	51381	3.1	19600	1.2	70981	4.3	71000	4.3
1941	52428	3.1	18730	1.1	71158	4.2	71180	4.2
1942	53830	3.2	19280	1.1	73110	4.3	73120	4.3
1943	54258	3.1	18910	1.1	73168	4.2	73180	4.2
1944	45770	2.6	18510	1.1	64280	3.7	64290	3.7
1945	14691	0.9	16330	0.9	31021	1.8	31020	1.8
1946	15715	0.8	31660	1.7	47375	2.5	47380	2.5
1947	17843	1.0	29350	1.6	47193	2.6	47190	2.6
1948	34263	1.8	22630	1.2	56893	3.0	57150	3.0
1949	52744	2.7	13110	0.7	65854	3.4	65940	3.4
1950	65298	3.3	9840	0.5	75138	3.8	75210	3.8
1951	73995	3.7	8980	0.4	82975	4.1	83040	4.1
1952	80177	3.9	8030	0.4	88207	4.3	88260	4.3
1953	89516	4.3	7300	0.3	96816	4.6	96880	4.6
1954	95614	4.5	7210	0.3	102824	4.8	102890	4.8
1955	97646	4.5	6490	0.3	104136	4.8	104190	4.8
1956	97212	4.4	5810	0.3	103022	4.6	103110	4.6
1957	101403	4.5	5220	0.2	106623	4.7	106690	4.7
1958	107415	4.6	4850	0.2	112265	4.8	112320	4.8
1959	113196	4.8	4260	0.2	117456	5.0	117490	5.0
1960	122760	5.1	3720	0.2	126480	5.3	126510	5.3
1961	134431	5.6	3040	0.1	137471	5.7	137490	5.7
1962	142013	5.7	2490	0.1	144503	5.8	144570	5.8
1963	151111	5.9	2040	0.1	153151	6.0	153050	6.0
1964	160807	6.2	1770	0.1	162577	6.2	162480	6.2
1965	171449	6.4	1500	0.1	172949	6.5	172820	6.5
1966	181488	6.7	1410	0.1	182898	6.7	182770	6.7
1967	193932	7.0	1040	0.0	194972	7.1	195060	7.1
1968	196709	7.0	950	0.0	197659	7.1	197780	7.1
1969	211316	7.5	860	0.0	212176	7.5	212250	7.5

Table 17.2 *(continued)*

Year	Manufactured cigarettes		Hand-rolled cigarettes		Total cigarettes		All tobacco products	
	Total annual in millions	Number/ adult/day	Total annual in millions	Number/ adult/day	Total annual in millions	Number/ adult/day	Total annual in tonnes	Grams/ adult/day
1970	222880	7.8	641	0.0	223521	7.8	223736	7.8
1971	236324	8.2	405	0.0	236729	8.2	236989	8.2
1972	253984	8.6	408	0.0	254392	8.6	254780	8.6
1973	268727	8.9	376	0.0	269103	9.0	269599	9.0
1974	287118	9.5	359	0.0	287477	9.5	288049	9.5
1975	293112	9.5	360	0.0	293472	9.5	294000	9.6
1976	291448	9.4	327	0.0	291775	9.4	292299	9.4
1977	303845	9.7	294	0.0	304139	9.7	305321	9.7
1978	304719	9.6	292	0.0	305011	9.6	306119	9.6
1979	310774	9.6	94	0.0	310868	9.6	311507	9.6
1980	307665	9.4	13	0.0	307678	9.4	308083	9.4
1981	312054	9.5	18	0.0	312072	9.5	312421	9.5
1982	315073	9.4	10	0.0	315083	9.4	315404	9.5
1983	311731	9.3	9	0.0	311740	9.3	312046	9.3
1984	312597	9.2	8	0.0	312605	9.2	312880	9.2
1985	310726	9.0						
1986	308438	8.8						
1987	308286	8.7						
1988	306415	8.6						
1989	313800	8.6						
1990	322000	8.8						
1991	328300	8.9						
1992	328900	8.8						
1993	332600	8.8						
1994	334400	8.8						
1995	334700	8.8						

Source : see *Notes on sources of sales data*, p. 425

Figure 17.1 Daily consumption of (i) manufactured and total number of cigarettes, and (ii) all tobacco products, 1920-1995.
Males and females aged 15 years and over. *Source:* see Table 17.2

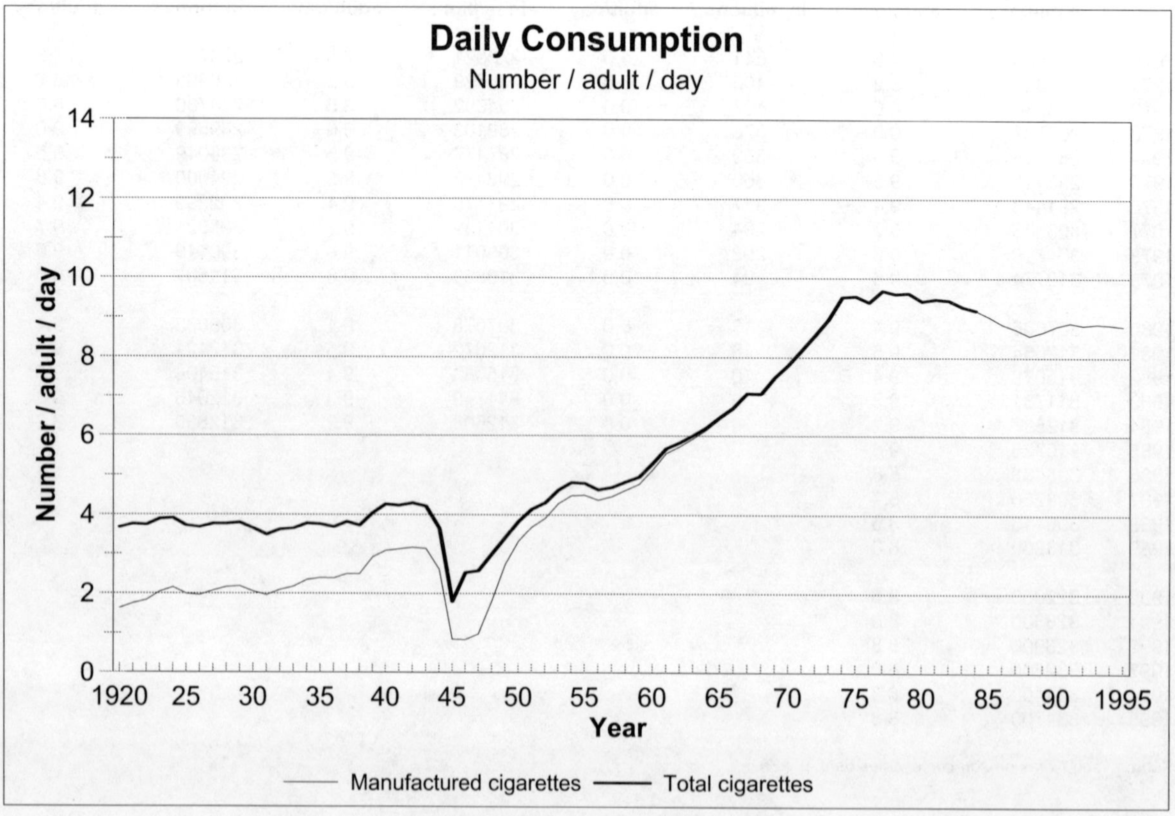

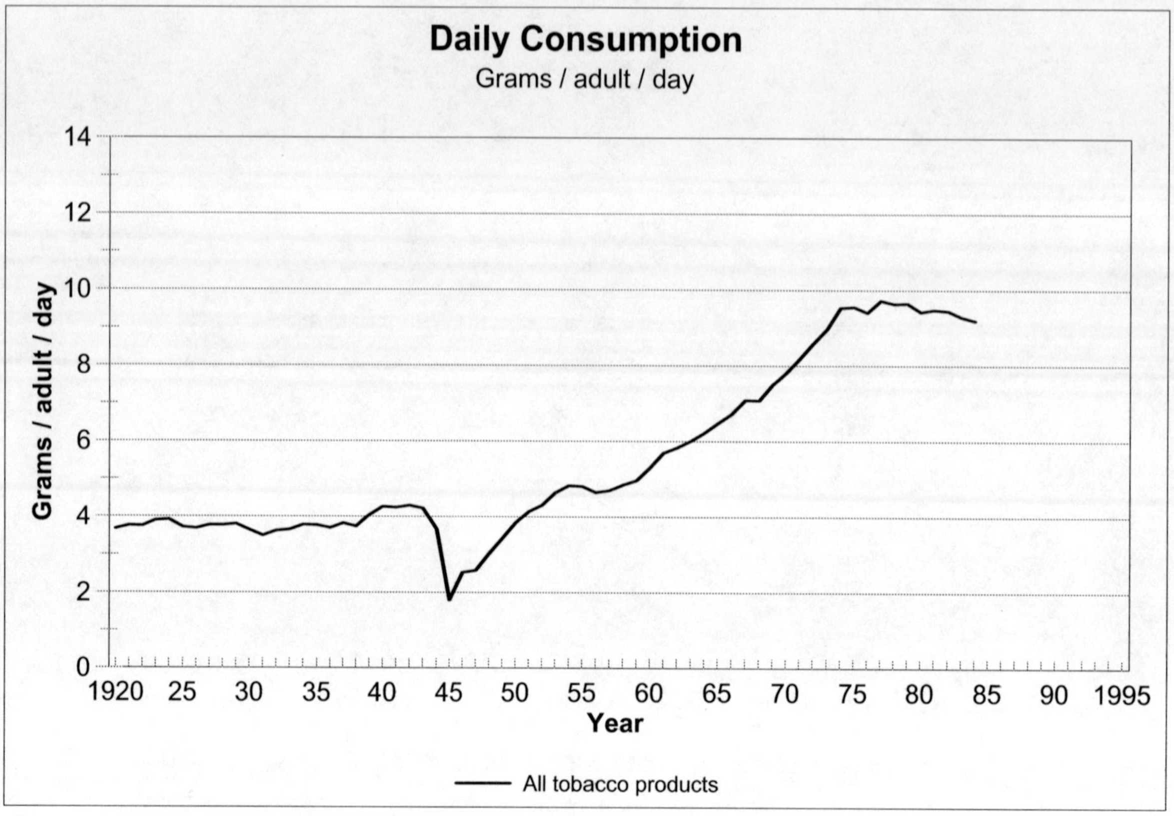

Table 17.3 Percentage sales of tobacco in different forms (by weight), selected years 1925-1984

Year	Cigarettes (%)	Cigars (%)	Fine-cut tobacco (%)	Pipe tobacco (%)
1925	53.6	0.1	46.4	0.0
1935	63.7	0.0	36.3	0.0
1945	47.4	0.0	52.6	0.0
1955	93.7	0.0	6.2	0.0
1965	99.1	0.0	0.9	0.0
1975	99.7	0.1	0.1	0.1
1984	99.9	0.0	0.0	0.0

Source : calculated from Tables 17.1.1 & 17.1.2

Figure 17.2 Percentage sales of tobacco in different forms (by weight), selected years 1925-1984
Source: see Table 17.3

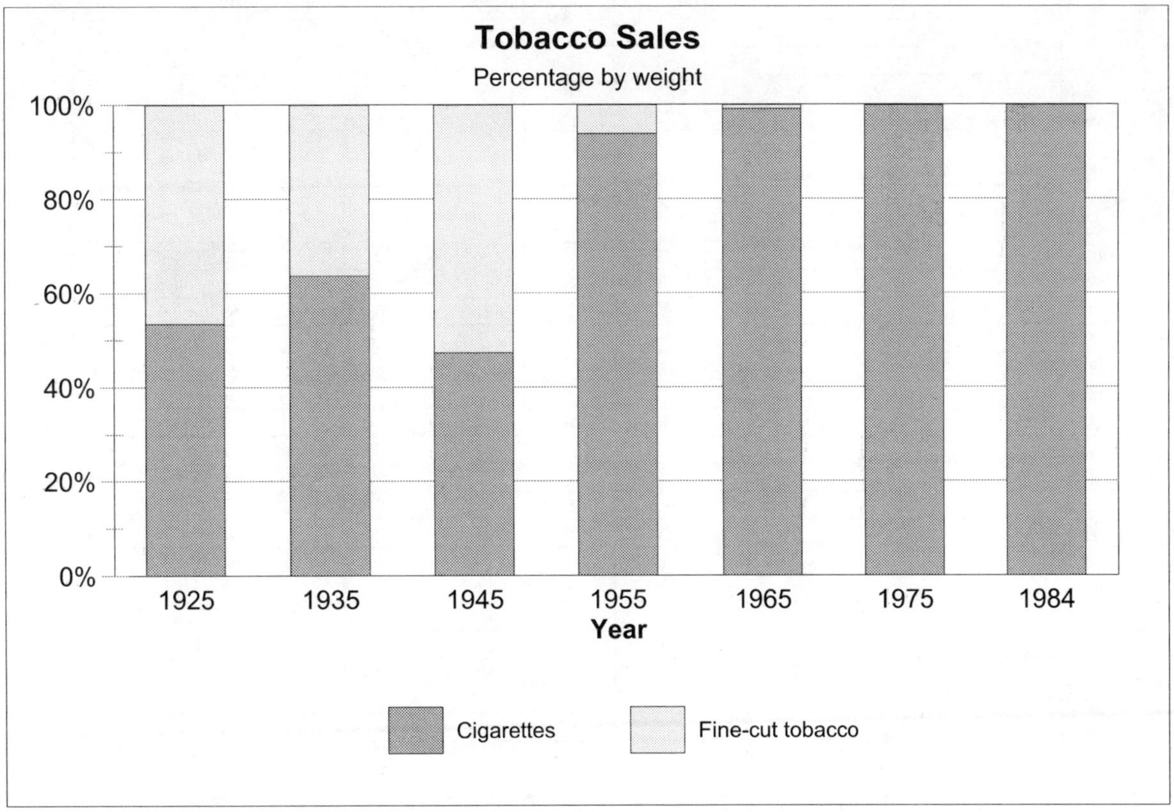

Table 17.4M Prevalence of smoking, males: some selected Japanese surveys by age, 1950-1995 *(continues on p. 414)*

Frequency Product Source Year	Age group																					
	12	13	14	15	16	17	18	19	20-24	25-29	30-34	35-39	40-44	45-49	50-54	55-59	60-64	65-69	70-74	75-79	80+	All ages
50 2 U U															82							
58 1 UC A															76							
58 3 UC R													72	73	72	66						71
59 1 UC A															83							
60 1 UC A															81							
60 4 UC R													75	84	78	73						78
61 1 UC A															82							
61 5 UC U																	76					
62 1 UC A															79							
63 1 UC A															77							
64 1 UC A															76							
65 1 UC A									81		85		87		81				75			82
65 6 U R													80		76		70			63		
65 6 U A													82		78		71			65		
66 1 UC A									84		85		87		83				78			84
67 1 UC A									83		84		86		82				73			82
68 1 UC R															75							
68 1 UC A									78		79		83		81				71			79
69 1 UC R															75							
69 1 UC A									79		81		84		80				71			79
70 1 UC R															73							
70 1 UC A									80		78		81		78				68			78
71 1 UC R															73							
71 1 UC A									79		77		80		79				70			77
72 1 UC R															74							
72 1 UC A									80		77		81		80				69			78
73 1 UC R															75							
73 1 UC A									80		79		82		78				70			78
74 1 UC R									79		76		78		77				68			76
74 1 UC A									83		80		81		78				70			79
75 1 UC R															73							
75 1 UC A									82		77		76		79				66			76
76 1 UC A									81		75		75		78				64			75
77 1 UC A									80		76		75		76				67			75
78 1 UC A									78		76		75		76				66			75
79 1 UC A									80		76		71		75				62			73
80 1 UC A									77		73		69		70				60			70
81 1 UC A									76		76		69		70				61			71
82 1 UC A									76		75		68		72				59			70
82 7 U R		1	3	7																		
82 7 U A		3	4	11																		
82 8 U R					6	13	17															12
82 9 U R					35	46	48															43
82 10 U A					26	42	51															
83 1 UC A									71		71		65		66				57			66
83 11 U U		3	6	12																		7
83 12 U U		7	4	20	7	18																
84 1 UC A									71		71		64		67				53			66
85 1 UC A									72		70		63		63				55			65
85 13 U U						50																
86 1 UC A									71		70		61		60				52			63
87 1 UC A									71		69		61		59				50			62
87 14 U U							41															
88 1 UC A									66		67		63		60				50			61
88 15 U U		1	2	3	20	38	50															

Table 17.4F Prevalence of smoking, females: some selected Japanese surveys by age, 1950-1995 *(continues on p. 415)*

<table>
<tr><th rowspan="2">Frequency
Product
Source
Year</th><th colspan="21">Age group</th><th rowspan="2">All ages</th></tr>
<tr><th>12</th><th>13</th><th>14</th><th>15</th><th>16</th><th>17</th><th>18</th><th>19</th><th>20-24</th><th>25-29</th><th>30-34</th><th>35-39</th><th>40-44</th><th>45-49</th><th>50-54</th><th>55-59</th><th>60-64</th><th>65-69</th><th>70-74</th><th>75-79</th><th>80+</th></tr>
<tr><td>50 2 U U</td><td colspan="8"></td><td colspan="13">13</td><td></td></tr>
<tr><td>58 1 UC A</td><td colspan="8"></td><td colspan="13">12</td><td></td></tr>
<tr><td>58 3 UC R</td><td colspan="8"></td><td colspan="13"></td><td></td></tr>
<tr><td>59 1 UC A</td><td colspan="8"></td><td colspan="13">15</td><td></td></tr>
<tr><td>60 1 UC A</td><td colspan="8"></td><td colspan="13">13</td><td></td></tr>
<tr><td>60 4 UC R</td><td colspan="8"></td><td colspan="13"></td><td></td></tr>
<tr><td>61 1 UC A</td><td colspan="8"></td><td colspan="13">14</td><td></td></tr>
<tr><td>61 5 UC U</td><td colspan="8"></td><td colspan="4"></td><td colspan="9">17</td><td></td></tr>
<tr><td>62 1 UC A</td><td colspan="8"></td><td colspan="13">13</td><td></td></tr>
<tr><td>63 1 UC A</td><td colspan="8"></td><td colspan="13">12</td><td></td></tr>
<tr><td>64 1 UC A</td><td colspan="8"></td><td colspan="13">11</td><td></td></tr>
<tr><td>65 1 UC A</td><td colspan="8"></td><td colspan="2">7</td><td colspan="2">14</td><td colspan="2">19</td><td colspan="2">23</td><td colspan="5">23</td><td>16</td></tr>
<tr><td>65 6 U R</td><td colspan="8"></td><td colspan="4"></td><td colspan="2">9</td><td colspan="2">12</td><td colspan="2">14</td><td colspan="3">16</td><td></td></tr>
<tr><td>65 6 U A</td><td colspan="8"></td><td colspan="4"></td><td colspan="2">9</td><td colspan="2">13</td><td colspan="2">15</td><td colspan="3">17</td><td></td></tr>
<tr><td>66 1 UC A</td><td colspan="8"></td><td colspan="2">11</td><td colspan="2">14</td><td colspan="2">22</td><td colspan="2">24</td><td colspan="5">24</td><td>18</td></tr>
<tr><td>67 1 UC A</td><td colspan="8"></td><td colspan="2">11</td><td colspan="2">16</td><td colspan="2">21</td><td colspan="2">23</td><td colspan="5">20</td><td>18</td></tr>
<tr><td>68 1 UC R</td><td colspan="8"></td><td colspan="13">12</td><td></td></tr>
<tr><td>68 1 UC A</td><td colspan="8"></td><td colspan="2">8</td><td colspan="2">14</td><td colspan="2">18</td><td colspan="2">21</td><td colspan="5">20</td><td>15</td></tr>
<tr><td>69 1 UC R</td><td colspan="8"></td><td colspan="13">12</td><td></td></tr>
<tr><td>69 1 UC A</td><td colspan="8"></td><td colspan="2">10</td><td colspan="2">13</td><td colspan="2">17</td><td colspan="2">21</td><td colspan="5">20</td><td>15</td></tr>
<tr><td>70 1 UC R</td><td colspan="8"></td><td colspan="13">12</td><td></td></tr>
<tr><td>70 1 UC A</td><td colspan="8"></td><td colspan="2">10</td><td colspan="2">13</td><td colspan="2">16</td><td colspan="2">23</td><td colspan="5">20</td><td>16</td></tr>
<tr><td>71 1 UC R</td><td colspan="8"></td><td colspan="13">11</td><td></td></tr>
<tr><td>71 1 UC A</td><td colspan="8"></td><td colspan="2">10</td><td colspan="2">14</td><td colspan="2">16</td><td colspan="2">18</td><td colspan="5">19</td><td>15</td></tr>
<tr><td>72 1 UC R</td><td colspan="8"></td><td colspan="13">11</td><td></td></tr>
<tr><td>72 1 UC A</td><td colspan="8"></td><td colspan="2">13</td><td colspan="2">13</td><td colspan="2">15</td><td colspan="2">21</td><td colspan="5">19</td><td>16</td></tr>
<tr><td>73 1 UC R</td><td colspan="8"></td><td colspan="13">12</td><td></td></tr>
<tr><td>73 1 UC A</td><td colspan="8"></td><td colspan="2">11</td><td colspan="2">12</td><td colspan="2">16</td><td colspan="2">18</td><td colspan="5">21</td><td>15</td></tr>
<tr><td>74 1 UC R</td><td colspan="8"></td><td colspan="2">9</td><td colspan="2">10</td><td colspan="2">14</td><td colspan="2">17</td><td colspan="5">19</td><td>13</td></tr>
<tr><td>74 1 UC A</td><td colspan="8"></td><td colspan="2">13</td><td colspan="2">14</td><td colspan="2">18</td><td colspan="2">21</td><td colspan="5">21</td><td>17</td></tr>
<tr><td>75 1 UC R</td><td colspan="8"></td><td colspan="13">12</td><td></td></tr>
<tr><td>75 1 UC A</td><td colspan="8"></td><td colspan="2">13</td><td colspan="2">14</td><td colspan="2">16</td><td colspan="2">18</td><td colspan="5">17</td><td>15</td></tr>
<tr><td>76 1 UC A</td><td colspan="8"></td><td colspan="2">14</td><td colspan="2">14</td><td colspan="2">15</td><td colspan="2">17</td><td colspan="5">18</td><td>15</td></tr>
<tr><td>77 1 UC A</td><td colspan="8"></td><td colspan="2">16</td><td colspan="2">13</td><td colspan="2">15</td><td colspan="2">16</td><td colspan="5">17</td><td>15</td></tr>
<tr><td>78 1 UC A</td><td colspan="8"></td><td colspan="2">15</td><td colspan="2">16</td><td colspan="2">17</td><td colspan="2">17</td><td colspan="5">17</td><td>16</td></tr>
<tr><td>79 1 UC A</td><td colspan="8"></td><td colspan="2">16</td><td colspan="2">14</td><td colspan="2">16</td><td colspan="2">16</td><td colspan="5">15</td><td>15</td></tr>
<tr><td>80 1 UC A</td><td colspan="8"></td><td colspan="2">16</td><td colspan="2">14</td><td colspan="2">14</td><td colspan="2">13</td><td colspan="5">15</td><td>14</td></tr>
<tr><td>81 1 UC A</td><td colspan="8"></td><td colspan="2">17</td><td colspan="2">15</td><td colspan="2">17</td><td colspan="2">14</td><td colspan="5">14</td><td>15</td></tr>
<tr><td>82 1 UC A</td><td colspan="8"></td><td colspan="2">17</td><td colspan="2">16</td><td colspan="2">16</td><td colspan="2">14</td><td colspan="5">13</td><td>15</td></tr>
<tr><td>82 7 U R</td><td></td><td>0</td><td>0</td><td>1</td><td colspan="4"></td><td colspan="13"></td><td></td></tr>
<tr><td>82 7 U A</td><td></td><td>1</td><td>2</td><td>3</td><td colspan="4"></td><td colspan="13"></td><td></td></tr>
<tr><td>82 8 U R</td><td colspan="4"></td><td>3</td><td>4</td><td>4</td><td></td><td colspan="13"></td><td>3</td></tr>
<tr><td>82 9 U R</td><td colspan="8"></td><td colspan="13"></td><td></td></tr>
<tr><td>82 10 U A</td><td colspan="4"></td><td>3</td><td>4</td><td>14</td><td></td><td colspan="13"></td><td></td></tr>
<tr><td>83 1 UC A</td><td colspan="8"></td><td colspan="2">15</td><td colspan="2">15</td><td colspan="2">13</td><td colspan="2">12</td><td colspan="5">12</td><td>14</td></tr>
<tr><td>83 11 U U</td><td></td><td>2</td><td>3</td><td>2</td><td colspan="4"></td><td colspan="13"></td><td>2</td></tr>
<tr><td>83 12 U U</td><td></td><td>0</td><td>5</td><td>10</td><td>2</td><td>6</td><td colspan="2"></td><td colspan="13"></td><td></td></tr>
<tr><td>84 1 UC A</td><td colspan="8"></td><td colspan="2">17</td><td colspan="2">15</td><td colspan="2">13</td><td colspan="2">11</td><td colspan="5">13</td><td>14</td></tr>
<tr><td>85 1 UC A</td><td colspan="8"></td><td colspan="2">17</td><td colspan="2">14</td><td colspan="2">13</td><td colspan="2">13</td><td colspan="5">12</td><td>14</td></tr>
<tr><td>85 13 U U</td><td colspan="4"></td><td colspan="3">10</td><td></td><td colspan="13"></td><td></td></tr>
<tr><td>86 1 UC A</td><td colspan="8"></td><td colspan="2">16</td><td colspan="2">13</td><td colspan="2">12</td><td colspan="2">11</td><td colspan="5">11</td><td>13</td></tr>
<tr><td>87 1 UC A</td><td colspan="8"></td><td colspan="2">16</td><td colspan="2">15</td><td colspan="2">13</td><td colspan="2">12</td><td colspan="5">11</td><td>13</td></tr>
<tr><td>87 14 U U</td><td colspan="6"></td><td>7</td><td></td><td colspan="13"></td><td></td></tr>
<tr><td>88 1 UC A</td><td colspan="8"></td><td colspan="2">15</td><td colspan="2">15</td><td colspan="2">13</td><td colspan="2">12</td><td colspan="5">11</td><td>13</td></tr>
<tr><td>88 15 U U</td><td></td><td>0</td><td>0</td><td>0</td><td>4</td><td>22</td><td>25</td><td></td><td colspan="13"></td><td></td></tr>
</table>

Table 17.4M *(continued from p. 412)*
Prevalence of smoking, males

Year / Source / Product / Frequency	12	13	14	15	16	17	18	19	20-24	25-29	30-34	35-39	40-44	45-49	50-54	55-59	60-64	65-69	70-74	75-79	80+	All ages
89 1 UC A									68		69		65		57		50					61
89 16 UC A	1	3	9	8	19	31	37															
89 17 UC A	2	3	8	10	21	26	40															
90 1 UC A									66		69		63		57		49					61
90 18 U R		1	2	5	8	15	20															8
90 18 U A		4	6	10	14	20	26															13
90 19 U R		1	4	6																		4
90 19 U A		2	7	10																		7
91 1 UC A									69		68		64		57		51					61
92 1 UC A									66		67		65		53		49					60
92 20 UC R	2	4	2	16	38	44	38															
93 1 UC A									65		66		66		54		47					60
94 1 UC A									63		69		62		56		46					59
95 1 UC A									65		66		62		58		45					59
95 21 U R							25															
95 21 U A							37															

Source: see *Notes on sources of survey data*, p. 426
Product: MC = manufactured cigarettes
TC = total cigarettes (including hand-rolled)
UC = cigarettes (type unspecified)
A = all products

Frequency: A = all smokers (including occasional)
R = regular or daily smokers
All ages: relevant to ages used and as given in original source
U = unspecified
* = refer to *Notes on sources of survey data*, p. 426

Table 17.4F *(continued from p. 413)*
Prevalence of smoking, females

Frequency / Product / Source / Year	12	13	14	15	16	17	18	19	20 - 24	25 - 29	30 - 34	35 - 39	40 - 44	45 - 49	50 - 54	55 - 59	60 - 64	65 - 69	70 - 74	75 - 79	80+	All ages
89 1 UC A									16		15		14		10		9					13
89 16 UC A	1	1	2	3	8	14	15															
89 17 UC A	0	1	3	4	6	13	15															
90 1 UC A									20		17		14		12		9					14
90 18 U R		1	1	2	1	3	3															2
90 18 U A		2	2	4	3	5	5															3
90 19 U R		1	1	1																		1
90 19 U A		2	3	4																		3
91 1 UC A									18		18		14		12		10					14
92 1 UC A									17		18		13		12		8					13
92 20 UC R	0	2	2	5	17	29	23															
93 1 UC A									21		18		13		11		8					13
94 1 UC A									20		19		15		12		8					15
95 1 UC A									23		19		14		13		8					15
95 21 U R							7															
95 21 U A							16															

Source: see *Notes on sources of survey data*, p. 426
Product: MC = manufactured cigarettes
TC = total cigarettes (including hand-rolled)
UC = cigarettes (type unspecified)
A = all products

Frequency: A = all smokers (including occasional)
R = regular or daily smokers
All ages: relevant to ages used and as given in original source
U = unspecified
* = refer to *Notes on sources of survey data*, p. 426

Table 17.5M Number of cigarettes smoked per smoker per day, males: some selected Japanese surveys by age, 1958-1995

Year	Source	Product	12	13	14	15	16	17	18	19	20-24	25-29	30-34	35-39	40-44	45-49	50-54	55-59	60-64	65-69	70-74	75-79	80+	All ages
58	3	UCE*													19	21	20	20						20
60	4	UCE*													19	19	17	17						18
61	5	UCE*													16									
66	1	UC									19													
67	1	UC									20													
68	1	UC									20													
69	1	UC									21													
70	1	UC									20		22		22		21		18					21
71	1	UC									21		22		22		22		19					21
72	1	UC									21		23		23		23		20					22
73	1	UC									22		23		23		23		20					22
74	1	UC									22		24		23		23		20					23
75	1	UC									24													
76	1	UC									24													
77	1	UC									24													
78	1	UC									24													
79	1	UC									24													
80	1	UC									25													
81	1	UC									25													
82	1	UC									25													
83	1	UC									25													
83	11	UCE		14	11	12																		12
84	1	UC									22		27		27		25		21					25
85	1	UC									25													
86	1	UC									25													
87	1	UC									25													
88	1	UC									25													
88	15	UCE					10																	
89	1	UC									25													
90	1	UC									25													
90	18	UCE*		6.7	6.5	8.6	9.4	10	11															
91	1	UC									25													
92	1	UC									24													
93	1	UC									25													
94	1	UC									25													
95	1	UC									25													

Source: see *Notes on sources of survey data*, p. 426

Product:
- MC = manufactured cigarettes
- TC = total cigarettes (including hand-rolled)
- UC = cigarettes (type unspecified)
- A = all products
- U = unspecified

Product (cont): E indicates mean estimated from percentage distribution (see also *Consumption category estimation*, p. xxxiv, and Appendix III, p. 789)

All ages: relevant to ages used and as given in original source

* = refer to *Notes on sources of survey data*, p. 426

Table 17.5F Number of cigarettes smoked per smoker per day, females: some selected Japanese surveys by age, 1958-1995

Product Source Year	Age group 12	13	14	15	16	17	18	19	20-24	25-29	30-34	35-39	40-44	45-49	50-54	55-59	60-64	65-69	70-74	75-79	80+	All ages
58 3 UCE*																						
60 4 UCE*																						
61 5 UCE*													9.8									
66 1 UC									11													
67 1 UC									14													
68 1 UC									14													
69 1 UC									14													
70 1 UC									14		14		16		15		13					14
71 1 UC									16		15		15		13		14					15
72 1 UC									13		15		16		14		13					14
73 1 UC									13		16		17		16		14					15
74 1 UC									14		15		17		16		14					16
75 1 UC									17													
76 1 UC									16													
77 1 UC									16													
78 1 UC									16													
79 1 UC									16													
80 1 UC									16													
81 1 UC									16													
82 1 UC									17													
83 1 UC									16													
83 11 UCE		10	8.6	10																		9.4
84 1 UC									15		17		20		18		15					17
85 1 UC									17													
86 1 UC									16													
87 1 UC									17													
88 1 UC									16													
88 15 UCE					9																	
89 1 UC									17													
90 1 UC									18													
90 18 UCE*		6.6	5.4	8.4	7.3	8.4	7.5															
91 1 UC									18													
92 1 UC									17													
93 1 UC									17													
94 1 UC									17													
95 1 UC									17													

Source: see *Notes on sources of survey data*, p. 426

Product:
MC = manufactured cigarettes
TC = total cigarettes (including hand-rolled)
UC = cigarettes (type unspecified)
A = all products
U = unspecified

Product (cont): E indicates mean estimated from percentage distribution (see also *Consumption category estimation*, p. xxxiv, and Appendix III, p. 789)

All ages: relevant to ages used and as given in original source

* = refer to *Notes on sources of survey data*, p. 426

Table 17.6M Number of cigarettes smoked per person per day, males: some selected Japanese surveys by age, 1958-1995, with percentage total sales

<table>
<tr><th rowspan="2">Product
Source
Year</th><th colspan="21">Age group</th><th rowspan="2">All ages</th><th rowspan="2">% Total sales</th></tr>
<tr><th>12</th><th>13</th><th>14</th><th>15</th><th>16</th><th>17</th><th>18</th><th>19</th><th>20-24</th><th>25-29</th><th>30-34</th><th>35-39</th><th>40-44</th><th>45-49</th><th>50-54</th><th>55-59</th><th>60-64</th><th>65-69</th><th>70-74</th><th>75-79</th><th>80+</th></tr>
<tr><td>58 3 UC *</td><td colspan="12"></td><td>14</td><td>15</td><td>14</td><td>13</td><td colspan="5"></td><td>14</td><td>**</td></tr>
<tr><td>60 4 UC *</td><td colspan="12"></td><td>14</td><td>16</td><td>14</td><td>12</td><td colspan="5"></td><td>14</td><td>**</td></tr>
<tr><td>61 5 UC *</td><td colspan="12"></td><td colspan="9">12</td><td></td><td>**</td></tr>
<tr><td>66 1 UC *</td><td colspan="8"></td><td colspan="13">16</td><td></td><td>113%M</td></tr>
<tr><td>67 1 UC *</td><td colspan="8"></td><td colspan="13">16</td><td></td><td>116%M</td></tr>
<tr><td>68 1 UC</td><td colspan="8"></td><td colspan="13">15</td><td></td><td>104%M</td></tr>
<tr><td>69 1 UC</td><td colspan="8"></td><td colspan="13">15</td><td></td><td>98%M</td></tr>
<tr><td>70 1 UC</td><td colspan="8"></td><td colspan="13">15</td><td></td><td>97%M</td></tr>
<tr><td>70 1 UC *</td><td colspan="8"></td><td colspan="2">16</td><td colspan="2">17</td><td colspan="2">18</td><td colspan="2">17</td><td colspan="5">12</td><td>16</td><td>105%M</td></tr>
<tr><td>71 1 UC</td><td colspan="8"></td><td colspan="13">16</td><td></td><td>94%M</td></tr>
<tr><td>71 1 UC *</td><td colspan="8"></td><td colspan="2">17</td><td colspan="2">17</td><td colspan="2">17</td><td colspan="2">17</td><td colspan="5">13</td><td>17</td><td>102%M</td></tr>
<tr><td>72 1 UC</td><td colspan="8"></td><td colspan="13">16</td><td></td><td>93%M</td></tr>
<tr><td>72 1 UC *</td><td colspan="8"></td><td colspan="2">17</td><td colspan="2">18</td><td colspan="2">18</td><td colspan="2">18</td><td colspan="5">13</td><td>17</td><td>100%M</td></tr>
<tr><td>73 1 UC</td><td colspan="8"></td><td colspan="13">17</td><td></td><td>93%M</td></tr>
<tr><td>73 1 UC *</td><td colspan="8"></td><td colspan="2">18</td><td colspan="2">18</td><td colspan="2">19</td><td colspan="2">18</td><td colspan="5">14</td><td>18</td><td>99%M</td></tr>
<tr><td>74 1 UC</td><td colspan="8"></td><td colspan="2">18</td><td colspan="2">18</td><td colspan="2">18</td><td colspan="2">18</td><td colspan="5">14</td><td>17</td><td>91%M</td></tr>
<tr><td>75 1 UC</td><td colspan="8"></td><td colspan="13">17</td><td></td><td>92%M</td></tr>
<tr><td>76 1 UC *</td><td colspan="8"></td><td colspan="13">18</td><td></td><td>100%M</td></tr>
<tr><td>77 1 UC *</td><td colspan="8"></td><td colspan="13">18</td><td></td><td>96%M</td></tr>
<tr><td>78 1 UC *</td><td colspan="8"></td><td colspan="13">18</td><td></td><td>98%M</td></tr>
<tr><td>79 1 UC *</td><td colspan="8"></td><td colspan="13">18</td><td></td><td>95%M</td></tr>
<tr><td>80 1 UC *</td><td colspan="8"></td><td colspan="13">17</td><td></td><td>94%M</td></tr>
<tr><td>81 1 UC *</td><td colspan="8"></td><td colspan="13">18</td><td></td><td>96%M</td></tr>
<tr><td>82 1 UC *</td><td colspan="8"></td><td colspan="13">18</td><td></td><td>97%M</td></tr>
<tr><td>83 1 UC *</td><td colspan="8"></td><td colspan="13">17</td><td></td><td>92%M</td></tr>
<tr><td>83 11 UC</td><td></td><td>0.4</td><td>0.7</td><td>1.4</td><td colspan="17"></td><td>0.8</td><td>**</td></tr>
<tr><td>84 1 UC *</td><td colspan="8"></td><td colspan="2">16</td><td colspan="2">19</td><td colspan="2">17</td><td colspan="2">17</td><td colspan="5">11</td><td>16</td><td>92%M</td></tr>
<tr><td>85 1 UC *</td><td colspan="8"></td><td colspan="13">16</td><td></td><td>92%M</td></tr>
<tr><td>86 1 UC *</td><td colspan="8"></td><td colspan="13">16</td><td></td><td>90%M</td></tr>
<tr><td>87 1 UC *</td><td colspan="8"></td><td colspan="13">15</td><td></td><td>92%M</td></tr>
<tr><td>88 1 UC *</td><td colspan="8"></td><td colspan="13">15</td><td></td><td>91%M</td></tr>
<tr><td>89 1 UC *</td><td colspan="8"></td><td colspan="13">15</td><td></td><td>92%M</td></tr>
<tr><td>90 1 UC *</td><td colspan="8"></td><td colspan="13">15</td><td></td><td>91%M</td></tr>
<tr><td>91 1 UC *</td><td colspan="8"></td><td colspan="13">15</td><td></td><td>91%M</td></tr>
<tr><td>92 1 UC *</td><td colspan="8"></td><td colspan="13">15</td><td></td><td>88%M</td></tr>
<tr><td>93 1 UC *</td><td colspan="8"></td><td colspan="13">15</td><td></td><td>89%M</td></tr>
<tr><td>94 1 UC *</td><td colspan="8"></td><td colspan="13">15</td><td></td><td>89%M</td></tr>
<tr><td>95 1 UC *</td><td colspan="8"></td><td colspan="13">15</td><td></td><td>91%M</td></tr>
</table>

Source: see *Notes on sources of survey data*, p. 426
Product: MC = manufactured cigarettes
TC = total cigarettes (including hand-rolled)
UC = cigarettes (type unspecified)
A = all products
U = unspecified

All ages: relevant to ages used and as given in original source
% Total sales: estimated % of total sales of M = manufactured or T = total cigarette consumption implied by survey, sexes combined
** = cannot be calculated
--- = adjusted by original author
* = refer to *Notes on sources of survey data*, p. 426

Table 17.6F Number of cigarettes smoked per person per day, females: some selected Japanese surveys by age, 1958-1995, with percentage total sales

Product Source Year	12	13	14	15	16	17	18	19	20-24	25-29	30-34	35-39	40-44	45-49	50-54	55-59	60-64	65-69	70-74	75-79	80+	All ages	% Total sales
58 3 UC *																							**
60 4 UC *																							**
61 5 UC *													1.6										**
66 1 UC *									1.9														113%M
67 1 UC *									2.5														116%M
68 1 UC									1.7														104%M
69 1 UC									1.6														98%M
70 1 UC									1.7														97%M
70 1 UC *									1.4		1.8		2.5		3.4		2.5					2.2	105%M
71 1 UC									1.6														94%M
71 1 UC *									1.6		2.0		2.5		2.4		2.8					2.1	102%M
72 1 UC									1.6														93%M
72 1 UC *									1.7		1.9		2.4		3.0		2.4					2.2	100%M
73 1 UC									1.8														93%M
73 1 UC *									1.4		2.0		2.6		2.8		3.0					2.3	99%M
74 1 UC									1.2		1.4		2.4		2.7		2.6					2.0	91%M
75 1 UC									2.0														92%M
76 1 UC *									2.5														100%M
77 1 UC *									2.4														96%M
78 1 UC *									2.6														98%M
79 1 UC *									2.5														95%M
80 1 UC *									2.3														94%M
81 1 UC *									2.4														96%M
82 1 UC *									2.6														97%M
83 1 UC *									2.2														92%M
83 11 UC		0.2	0.3	0.2																		0.2	**
84 1 UC *									2.5		2.6		2.6		2.0		2.0					2.3	92%M
85 1 UC *									2.3														92%M
86 1 UC *									2.1														90%M
87 1 UC *									2.3														92%M
88 1 UC *									2.1														91%M
89 1 UC *									2.2														92%M
90 1 UC *									2.6														91%M
91 1 UC *									2.5														91%M
92 1 UC *									2.3														88%M
93 1 UC *									2.4														89%M
94 1 UC *									2.5														89%M
95 1 UC *									2.6														91%M

Source: see *Notes on sources of survey data*, p. 426

Product: MC = manufactured cigarettes
TC = total cigarettes (including hand-rolled)
UC = cigarettes (type unspecified)
A = all products
U = unspecified

All ages: relevant to ages used and as given in original source

% Total sales: estimated % of total sales of M = manufactured or T = total cigarette consumption implied by survey, sexes combined
** = cannot be calculated
--- = adjusted by original author

* = refer to *Notes on sources of survey data*, p. 426

Table 17.7M Number of cigarettes smoked per person per day, sales-adjusted, males: some selected Japanese surveys[1] by age, 1966-1995, with percentage total sales

Product Source Year	Age group 12	13	14	15	16	17	18	19	20-24	25-29	30-34	35-39	40-44	45-49	50-54	55-59	60-64	65-69	70-74	75-79	80+	All ages	% Total sales
66 1 UC *									14														113%M
67 1 UC *									14														116%M
68 1 UC									14														104%M
69 1 UC									15														98%M
70 1 UC									16														97%M
70 1 UC *									15		16		17		16		12					15	105%M
71 1 UC									17														94%M
71 1 UC *									16		17		17		17		13					16	102%M
72 1 UC									17														93%M
72 1 UC *									17		18		18		18		13					17	100%M
73 1 UC									18														93%M
73 1 UC *									18		18		19		18		14					18	99%M
74 1 UC									19		20		20		20		15					19	91%M
75 1 UC									19														92%M
76 1 UC *									18														100%M
77 1 UC *									19														96%M
78 1 UC *									19														98%M
79 1 UC *									19														95%M
80 1 UC *									18														94%M
81 1 UC *									18														96%M
82 1 UC *									18														97%M
83 1 UC *									18														92%M
84 1 UC *									17		21		19		18		12					18	92%M
85 1 UC *									17														92%M
86 1 UC *									17														90%M
87 1 UC *									17														92%M
88 1 UC *									17														91%M
89 1 UC *									17														92%M
90 1 UC *									17														91%M
91 1 UC *									17														91%M
92 1 UC *									17														88%M
93 1 UC *									17														89%M
94 1 UC *									16														89%M
95 1 UC *									16														91%M

1 Based on those surveys in Table 17.6 with data for both sexes and age range at least 21-64 (see *Cigarette consumption per person*, p. xxxv)

Source: See *Notes on sources of survey data*, p. 426
Product: MC = manufactured cigarettes
TC = total cigarettes (including hand-rolled)
UC = cigarettes (type unspecified)
A = all products
U = unspecified

All ages: relevant to ages used and as given in original source
% Total sales: Adjustment factor used, estimated % of total sales of M = manufactured or T = total cigarette consumption implied by survey, sexes combined
--- = adjusted by original author
* = refer to *Notes on sources of survey data*, p. 426

Table 17.7F Number of cigarettes smoked per person per day, sales-adjusted, females: some selected Japanese surveys[1] by age, 1966-1995, with percentage total sales

Product	Age group																						
Source Year	12	13	14	15	16	17	18	19	20-24	25-29	30-34	35-39	40-44	45-49	50-54	55-59	60-64	65-69	70-74	75-79	80+	All ages	% Total sales
66 1 UC *									1.7														113%M
67 1 UC *									2.2														116%M
68 1 UC									1.6														104%M
69 1 UC									1.6														98%M
70 1 UC									1.8														97%M
70 1 UC *									1.3		1.7		2.4		3.3		2.4					2.1	105%M
71 1 UC									1.7														94%M
71 1 UC *									1.6		1.9		2.4		2.3		2.7					2.1	102%M
72 1 UC									1.7														93%M
72 1 UC *									1.7		1.9		2.4		3.0		2.4					2.2	100%M
73 1 UC									1.9														93%M
73 1 UC *									1.4		2.0		2.6		2.9		3.1					2.3	99%M
74 1 UC									1.3		1.5		2.6		3.0		2.9					2.2	91%M
75 1 UC									2.2														92%M
76 1 UC *									2.5														100%M
77 1 UC *									2.5														96%M
78 1 UC *									2.6														98%M
79 1 UC *									2.6														95%M
80 1 UC *									2.4														94%M
81 1 UC *									2.5														96%M
82 1 UC *									2.7														97%M
83 1 UC *									2.4														92%M
84 1 UC *									2.7		2.8		2.8		2.2		2.2					2.5	92%M
85 1 UC *									2.5														92%M
86 1 UC *									2.3														90%M
87 1 UC *									2.5														92%M
88 1 UC *									2.3														91%M
89 1 UC *									2.4														92%M
90 1 UC *									2.9														91%M
91 1 UC *									2.7														91%M
92 1 UC *									2.6														88%M
93 1 UC *									2.7														89%M
94 1 UC *									2.8														89%M
95 1 UC *									2.9														91%M

1 Based on those surveys in Table 17.6 with data for both sexes and age range at least 21-64 (see *Cigarette consumption per person*, p. xxxv)

Source: See *Notes on sources of survey data*, p. 426
Product: MC = manufactured cigarettes
TC = total cigarettes (including hand-rolled)
UC = cigarettes (type unspecified)
A = all products
U = unspecified

All ages: relevant to ages used and as given in original source
% Total sales: Adjustment factor used, estimated % of total sales of M = manufactured or T = total cigarette consumption implied by survey, sexes combined
--- = adjusted by original author
* = refer to *Notes on sources of survey data*, p. 426

Table 17.8 Estimated[1] prevalence of smoking and estimated[1] number of cigarettes per person per day (unadjusted and sales-adjusted): summary of Tables 17.4, 17.6 and 17.7, 1950-1995.
Males and females aged 15 years and over

Year	Source[2]	Product[3]	Prevalence[4]						Number of cigarettes						
									Unadjusted[7]			Sales-adjusted[8]			
			Manufactured cigarettes		Total cigarettes[5]		All products[6]		Number/ person/day		Total sales %	Manufactured cigarettes[9] number/ person/day		Total cigarettes number/ person/day	
			M	F	M	F	M	F	M	F		M	F	M	F
1950	2	*U*					75	12				(6.1	0.8)		
1958	1	**UC**			70	11						(8.4	1.1)		
1959	1	**UC**			76	13						(8.6	1.2)		
1960	1	**UC**			75	12						(9.4	1.2)		
1961	1	**UC**			76	13						(10.1	1.3)		
1962	1	**UC**			73	12						(10.4	1.3)		
1963	1	**UC**			71	11						(10.8	1.4)		
1964	1	**UC**			71	10						(11.3	1.3)		
1965	1	**UC**			75	14						(11.4	1.7)		
1966	1	**UC**			77	16			13.7	1.7	113	12.2	1.5		
1967	1	**UC**			76	16			14.5	2.2	116	12.5	1.9		
1968	1	UC			70	11			13.4	1.5	104	12.9	1.5		
	1	**UC**			73	14									
1969	1	UC			70	11			13.6	1.5	98	13.8	1.5		
	1	**UC**			74	14									
1970	1	UC			69	11			14.7	2.0	105	14.1	1.9		
	1	**UC**			73	14									
1971	1	UC			69	10			15.1	2.0	102	14.8	1.9		
	1	**UC**			73	14									
1972	1	UC			70	11			15.6	2.0	100	15.5	2.0		
	1	**UC**			74	14									
1973	1	UC			72	11			16.1	2.1	99	16.3	2.1		
	1	**UC**			74	14									
1974	1	UC			72	12			15.9	1.8	91	17.5	2.0		
	1	**UC**			75	16									
1975	1	UC			70	12			16.1	1.9	92	17.5	2.0		
	1	**UC**			73	14									
1976	1	**UC**			72	15			16.8	2.4	100	16.8	2.4		
1977	1	**UC**			72	14			16.6	2.3	96	17.4	2.4		
1978	1	**UC**			71	15			16.8	2.5	98	17.1	2.5		
1979	1	**UC**			70	15			16.4	2.4	95	17.2	2.5		
1980	1	**UC**			68	14			16.0	2.2	94	17.0	2.3		

Table 17.8 *(continued)*

Year	Source[2]	Product[3]	Prevalence[4]						Number of cigarettes						
									Unadjusted[7]			Sales-adjusted[8]			
			Manufactured cigarettes		Total cigarettes[5]		All products[6]		Number/ person/day		Total sales %	Manufactured cigarettes[9] number/ person/day		Total cigarettes number/ person/day	
			M	F	M	F	M	F	M	F		M	F	M	F
1981	1	**UC**			68	15			16.4	2.3	96	17.0	2.4		
1982	1	**UC**			67	15			16.3	2.5	97	16.8	2.5		
1983	1	**UC**			64	13			15.3	2.1	92	16.7	2.3		
1984	1	**UC**			63	14			15.1	2.2	92	16.4	2.4		
1985	1	**UC**			63	13			14.7	2.2	92	16.1	2.4		
1986	1	**UC**			61	12			14.4	2.0	90	15.9	2.2		
1987	1	**UC**			60	13			14.2	2.2	92	15.4	2.4		
1988	1	**UC**			59	13			13.9	2.0	91	15.3	2.2		
1989	1	**UC**			59	12			14.1	2.1	92	15.4	2.3		
1990	1	**UC**			59	14			13.8	2.4	91	15.2	2.7		
1991	1	**UC**			60	14			14.2	2.4	91	15.5	2.6		
1992	1	**UC**			58	13			13.7	2.2	88	15.5	2.5		
1993	1	**UC**			57	14			13.8	2.3	89	15.5	2.5		
1994	1	**UC**			57	14			13.7	2.4	89	15.3	2.7		
1995	1	**UC**			57	15			13.7	2.5	91	15.2	2.7		

1 Surveys covering an age range of at least 21-64 are included. Any gaps in the data for ages 15-20 and 65 years and over are filled in by assumed extensions to the age distribution, given in *Notes on sources of survey data*, p. 426. Method: see *Summary of adult smoking*, p. xxxvi
2 See *Notes on sources of survey data*, p. 426
3 Product: MC = manufactured cigarettes, TC = total cigarettes (including hand-rolled), UC = cigarettes (type unspecified), A = all products, U = unspecified. Frequency of smoking is indicated by: regular or daily smokers in normal type, all smokers (including occasional) in bold, unspecified in italics
4 From Table 17.4
5 This column includes prevalence of smoking classified as UC = cigarettes (type unspecified)
6 This column includes prevalence of smoking classified as U = unspecified product
7 From Table 17.6
8 From Table 17.7, except data in parentheses, which are derived from the prevalence of smoking from Table 17.4 as described in *Summary of adult smoking*, p. xxxvi
9 Number of cigarettes classified as UC = cigarettes (type unspecified) has been adjusted to manufactured cigarette sales and included in this column

Figure 17.3 Estimated prevalence of cigarette smoking: by year of survey, 1958-1995. Males and females aged 15 years and over. *Source:* see Table 17.8

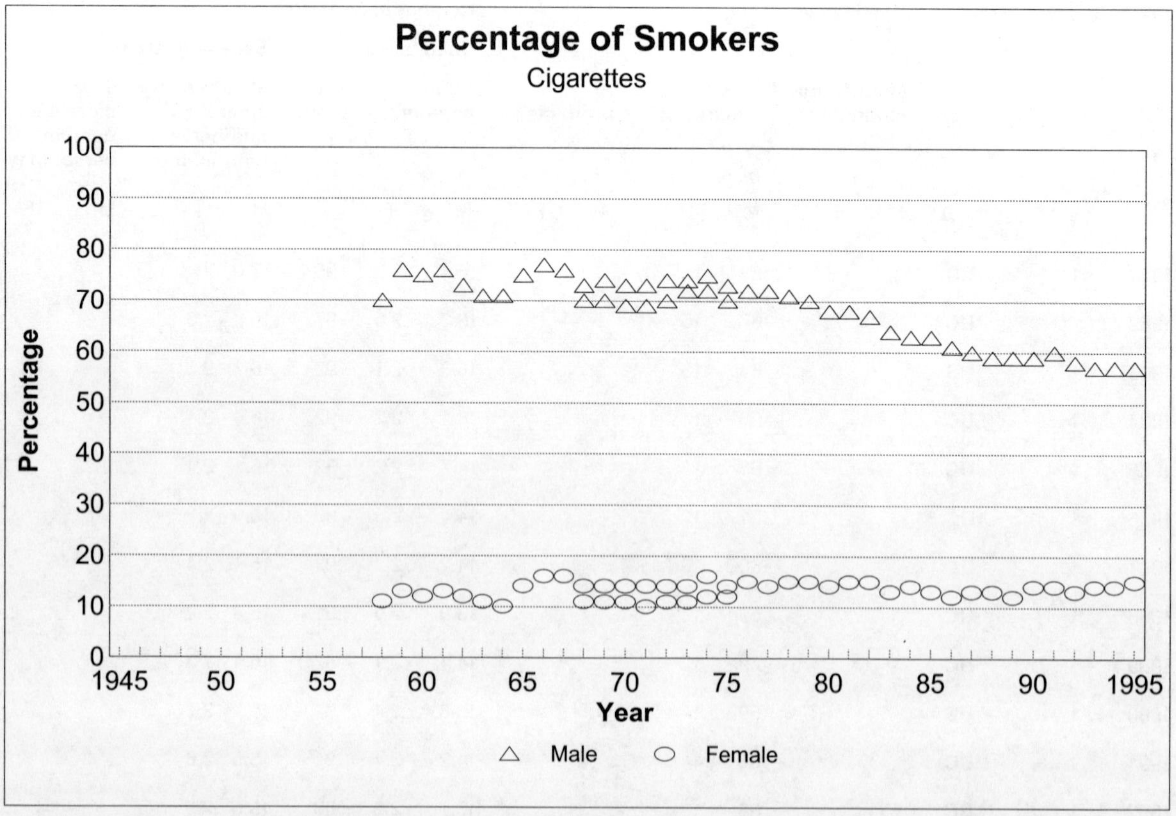

Figure 17.4 Estimated number of manufactured cigarettes smoked per day, sales-adjusted, 1950-1995.
Males and females aged 15 years and over. *Source:* see Table 17.8

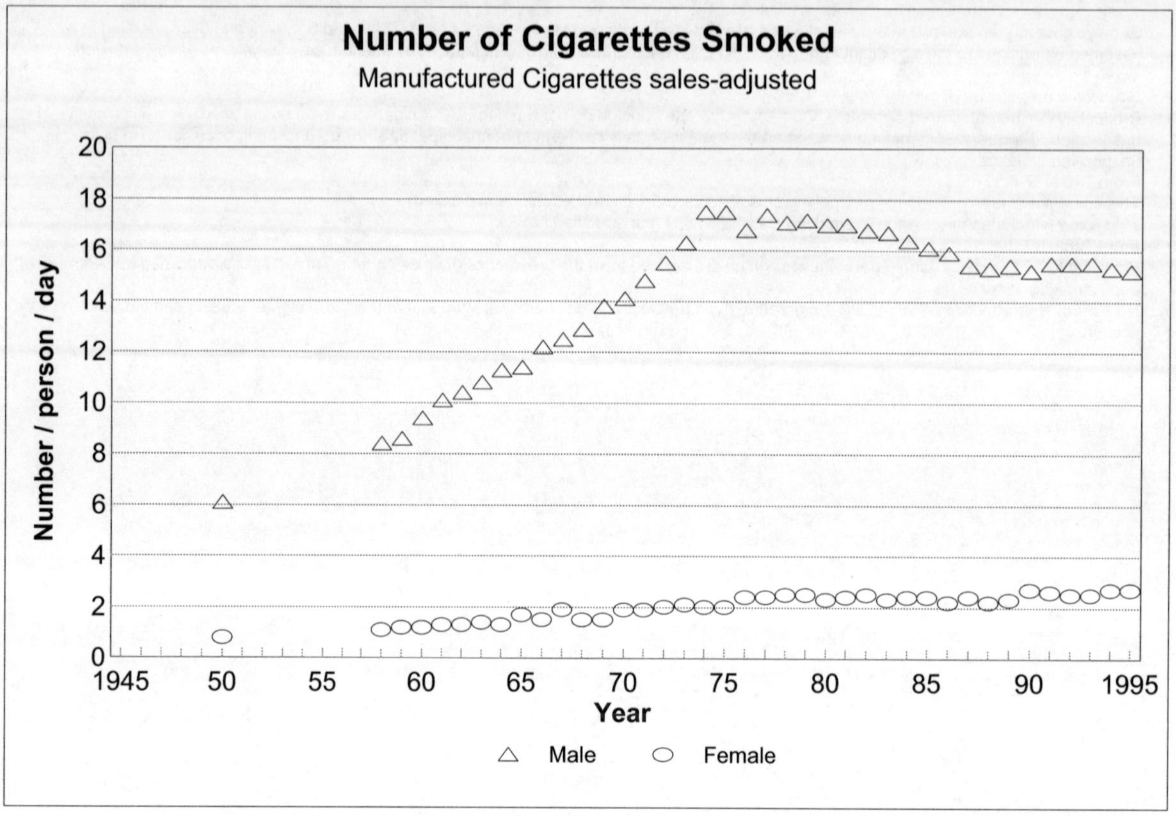

Notes on sources of sales data

The data presented in the tables and figures were obtained from several sources, details of which are given below, together with estimations and related assumptions. Full citations of the sources are given on p. 429 under *References*.

Consumption data before 1974

RP6

Data by weight, originally given to nearest 100 000 pounds, have been converted to tonnes and given to the nearest 10 tonnes (100 000 lbs = 45.359 tonnes). Where weight conversion factors have been quoted in RP6, the weights have been re-calculated without rounding and then converted to tonnes.

Notes as given in RP6:

a) Details of the number of cigarettes and cigars, and of the weight of fine-cut and pipe tobacco consumed were obtained from Sales of Manufactured Tobacco Classified by Brands, 1904-1955, published by the Japan Monopoly Corporation. The figures for 1956-1973 were provided by the Japan Monopoly Corporation.

(b) Cigarettes were given in numbers and have been converted to weight assuming an average of 2.205 lbs per 1 000 cigarettes up to 1955. From 1956 onwards details of the number and weight of cigarettes consumed were provided by the Japan Monopoly Corporation. The conversion factor used for cigars was 15 lbs per 1 000 cigars.

Consumption data for 1974-1995 and additional data for 1970-1973

Japan Tobacco Inc.

Data are for fiscal years beginning with April

Tables 17.1.2 and 17.1.3 show various categories which were excluded from RP6, but are presented here for completeness. The data for 1970-1988 include imports which were excluded from RP6 (eg. 0.3% of cigarettes, 49% of pipe tobacco, and 56% of cigars in 1970). Sales to Imperial Household Agency (assumed to be cigarettes) have also been included (available for 1970-1984). Data from RP6 do not include cigarillos; these are included with cigars from 1974-1988. Data for domestic and imported pipe tobacco are shown combined. Data for fine-cut tobacco are not comparable over time, being variously grouped under domestic cigarettes (1970-1981), imports (1982-1984), and domestic cigars/pipe tobacco/fine-cut tobacco (1985-1988) (not shown).

The tobacco products market opened up to competition in 1985 and data are not available from that year for imports of products other than cigarettes. In 1984 imports accounted for 2% cigarettes, 70% pipe tobacco, and 52% cigars. From 1989 onwards only cigarette data are available.

Data for cigarettes and cigars were given in numbers and have been converted to weight assuming an average of 1 g per cigarette, 6.8 g per cigar or cigarillo (based on values in RP6). Fukumoto *et al* (1997) gives the weight of tobacco in cigarettes as 1 g for plain cigarettes and an average of 0.67 g for filter cigarettes, so our estimates of weight may be too high for later years.

Plain/Filter cigarette consumption

1960-1981 Maxwell (successive years)

1982-1988 Statistics Bureau Management and Co-ordination Agency (personal communication)

1993-1995 United States Department of Agriculture (USDA) Economic Research Service (1996)

For 1982 onwards the data based on production rather than of sales. In 1988 imports represented 12% of sales.

Tar and Nicotine yield of cigarettes

Sato and Araki (2000)

Consumption of hand-rolled cigarettes for 1920-1988

We have taken as our estimate of hand-rolled cigarette consumption 100% of fine-cut tobacco sales, at 1 g per cigarette

Notes on sources of survey data

Each source of survey data—either an individual survey or a series of surveys repeated over a number of years—is cited by a source number. This number is shown in the tables and corresponds to the source numbers given below, where details of the source publication and of the survey methodology are given. Full citations of the sources are given on p. 429 under *References*.

Source number

1 Onodera (1988), Sato and Araki (2000), Health-net (2000), and Japan Tobacco Incorporated

a. Annual nationwide market survey by Japan Tobacco Inc (formerly Japan Public Monopoly Corporation). Sample size 6 000-16 000

b. Consumption per smoker is per regular smoker. For calculation of cigarette consumption per person, percentage regular smokers was used if available; * indicates that the percentage including occasional smokers was used, and therefore cigarette consumption per person is likely to be too high

c. Assumed extension to age distribution for percentage smokers, age 15-19: males 40%; females (before 1980) 5%, (1980-1985) 8%, (1986-1989) 12%, (1990 onwards) 15%. Number of cigarettes/person/day: males 4.0, females (before 1976) 0.5, (1976 onwards) 1.0

2 Sato and Araki (2000) quoting Ministry of Health and Welfare (1993)

a. Assumed extension to age distribution for percentage smokers, age 15-19: males 40%; females 5%

3-4 Keys *et al* (1966)

a. Baseline of Seven Countries Study on cardiovascular disease. Interview including smoking questions before medical examinations.

	Location	Description	Sample size	Response rate (%)
3	Tanushimaru, Kyushu	Farming village	509	100
4	Ushibuka, Kyushu	Fishing village on offshore island	504	99.6

b. Consumption category estimation based on two categories, 1-19 and 20+ cigarettes/smoker/day, and resulting figures should be regarded with caution

5 Kiyohara *et al* (1990)

a. Baseline of a prospective study in Hisayama, a rural community near Fukuoka city. Medical examination, with personal interview covering smoking. 90% of the population age 40+ were examined, analysis restricted to those without history of stroke or infarction. Sample size (males) 699, (females) 904

b. Smokers: includes those who gave up in last year

c. Consumption category estimation for males based on 1-9, 10-19, 20+ cigarette/smoker/day. For females, based on two categories, 1-9 and 10+ cigarettes/smoker/day and resulting figures should be regarded with caution

6 Hirayama (1967)

a. Prospective study in 29 selected districts, including over 90% of the adult population. Sample size 265 118

b. Results presented have been adjusted to exclude 'unknown' and 'no answer' categories

7 Ogawa *et al* (1988)

a. Survey covering entire student population of 3 junior high schools in Nagoya City. Questionnaire completed anonymously in class. Approximate ages corresponding to school grades 1-3. Sample size 3 090

8-9 Shibata *et al* (1990)

a. Survey at 19 senior high schools in Kyushu. Result shown as source **8** were from 15 ordinary co-educational schools, source **9** from 4 male vocational schools. All pupils in selected classes completed anonymous questionnaire in class with teachers present. Approximate ages corresponding to school grades 1-3. Sample size (males) 3 088, (females) 1 601. Response rate 96% for both sexes

10 Kawabata *et al* (1991a) quoting Nozu (no details)

a. Akita prefecture

b. Smokers: smoke 'just about every day' or 'once in a while but not every day'

11 Shiramizu and Shibata (1985)

a. Survey at 11 junior high schools. Approximate ages corresponding to school grades 1-3. Sample size (boys) 4 303, (girls) 4 172

b. Consumption category estimation based on <5, 6-10, and 11+ cigarettes/smoker/day

12 Kawabata *et al* (1991a) quoting Kawabata *et al* (no details)

a. 5 prefectures

13 Shimao (1988)

a. Estimates based on reports by several research workers, which showed marked variation. Age corresponds to senior high school. Year not stated

14 Geizerova *et al* (1990)

a. No original source. Schoolchildren in Nagoya City

15 Matsuzaki (1990)

a. Study at 3 junior high and 5 senior high schools in central Hokkaido, an area with a high adult smoking prevalence. Self-administered questionnaire after anti-smoking lecture. Sample size (males) 870, (females) 762. Response rate 95%

b. Consumption category estimation based on 0-5 (assume 1-5), 6-10, 11-20, 21-30, 31+ cigarettes/smoker/day

16 Kawabata *et al* (1991a)

a. 'Japan Know Your Body' study, conducted in 9 prefectures. 49 schools participated, including elementary, junior and senior high schools. Total sample size 12 892 at ages 6-18. Results reported here are for approximate ages corresponding to elementary grade 6 to senior high grade 3, sample size (males) 3 400, (females) 3 418

b. Smokers: smoked in last month

17 Kawabata *et al* (1991a, 1991b)

a. Japan Adolescent Smoking Survey (JASS) study conducted in 9 prefectures. 51 schools participated, including elementary, junior and senior high schools. Total sample size 9 921 at ages 9-18

b. Smokers: smoked in last month

18 Osaki and Minowa (1993, 1996)

a. Nationwide survey at randomly selected high schools in 1990-1991. Teachers distributed and collected questionnaires but left the classroom while students completed anonymous questionnaire. Participating schools were 33 senior and 70 junior high schools, response rate 66% and 70% respectively; pupils (males) 29 568 and (females) 27 621, response rate (junior high) 97%, (senior high) 91%

b. Results in Table 17.4-5 are for approximate ages corresponding to school grades, Table 17.6 for actual age

c. Regular smokers: smoked almost every day (3 or more times each week). All smokers: smoked in last month
d. Prevalence estimates calculated excluding *unspecified* from base. Consumption category estimation based on 1-4, 5-9, 10-14, 15-19, 20+ cigarettes/smoker/day. This applied to all smokers. 9% were unable to estimate and 12% did not answer, so that the number replying positively was greater than the number smoking regularly. Estimates by Osaki *et al* (1999) on a similar basis and a fitted model were lower

19 Wada and Fukui (1994)

a. Survey at 12 junior high schools in Chiba, selected to represent different regional characteristics. All pupils of all classes, or selected classes of all grades participated except one school where only 3rd grade classes participated. Anonymous questionnaires, sealed in envelope by pupil. Sample size (males) 2 702, (females) 2 530
b. Regular smokers: smokes almost every day. All smokers: smokes now and then, or almost every day

20 Minagawa (1995)

a. Northern Japan. All pupils in the schools participated at the same time. Anonymous questionnaires completed in class and sealed in envelope by pupils, under examination conditions with teachers present. Total sample size at age 9-18, 4 100
b. Regular smokers: smoked 1+ cigarettes per week

21 Honjo and Kawachi (2000) quoting Minowa *et al* (2000)

a. Approximate age corresponding to 12th grade
b. All smokers: smoked in last month

References

Beese D.H. (ed) (1968). *Tobacco consumption in various countries,* 2nd edition. Tobacco Research Council, London. Research Paper 6.

Beese D.H. (ed) (1972). *Tobacco consumption in various countries,* 3rd edition. Tobacco Research Council, London. Research Paper 6.

Fukumoto M., Kubo H. and Ogamo A. (1997). Determination of nicotine content of popular cigarettes. *Vet Hum Toxicol,* **39**, 225-7.

Geizerova H., Masironi R. and Fergusson J. (1990). Smoking among children and adolescents. In: Durstan B. and Jamrozik K. (eds) *Tobacco and health 1990. The global war. Proceedings of the Seventh World Conference on Tobacco and Health; Perth, Western Australia; 1-5 April 1990.* Organising Committee of the Seventh World Conference on Tobacco and Health, 189 Royal Street, East Perth, Western Australia 6004; 303-5.

Health-net (2000). http://www.health-net.or.jp/kenkonet/tobacco/product.

Hirayama T. (1967). *Smoking in relation to death rates of 265,118 men and women in Japan.* National Cancer Center Reaseach Institute, Tokyo.

Honjo K. and Kawachi I. (2000). Effects of market liberalisation on smoking in Japan. *Tob Control,* **9**, 193-200.

Kawabata T., Maruya N., Nakamura M., Hiyama T., *et al* (1991a). Smoking and alcohol drinking behavior among Japanese adolescents—results from 'Japan Know Your Body Study'. *Nippon Koshu Eisei Zasshi,* **38**, 885-99.

Kawabata T., Minagawa K., Nishioka N., Nakamura M., *et al* (1991b). Standardization of definitions concerning smoking behavior among Japanese adolescents—results from the Japan Adolescent Smoking Survey. *Nippon Koshu Eisei Zasshi,* **38**, 859-67.

Keys A., Aravanis C., Blackburn H.W., van Buchem F.S.P., *et al* (1966). Epidemiological studies related to coronary heart disease: characteristics of men aged 40-59 in seven countries. *Acta Medica Scandinavica,* **Suppl 460**, 8-392.

Kiyohara Y., Ueda K. and Fujishima M. (1990). Smoking and cardiovascular disease in the general population in Japan. *J Hypertens,* **8(suppl)**, S9-S15.

Lee P.N. (ed) (1975). *Tobacco consumption in various countries,* 4th edition. Tobacco Research Council, London. Research Paper 6.

Matsuzaki M. (1990). Smoking habits of school children in the northern part of Japan. In: Durston B. and Jamrozik K. (eds) *Tobacco & health 1990. The global war. Seventh World Conference on Tobacco and Health, Perth, Western Australia, 1-5 April 1990.* Organising Committee of the Seventh World Conference on Tobacco and Health, 189 Royal Street, East Perth, Western Australia 6004; 287-9.

Maxwell J.C.Jr. (successive years). How the brands ranked. Maxwell International Estimates. *World Tobacco.*

Minagawa K. (1995). Comparison of smoking prevalence among adolescents between England and Japan, 1992. In: Slama K. (ed) *Tobacco and Health, Ninth World Conference on Tobacco and Health, Paris, Oct 10-14 1994.* Plenum Press, New York and London; 585-8.

Ministry of Health and Welfare (1993). *Smoking and health,* 2nd edition. Health Promotion and Fitness Foundation, Tokyo.[§]

Minowa M., Suzuki K., Wada K. and Osaki Y. (2000). *Miseinen no kitsuen-kodo ni kansuru zenkoku cyousa hokokush. (Report of nationwide survey of smoking prevalence among minors),* March 1998.[§]

Ogawa H., Tominaga S., Gellert G. and Aoki K. (1988). Smoking among Junior High School students in Nagoya, Japan. *Int J Epidemiol,* **17**, 814-20.

Onodera N. (1988). Non-smokers' right and public health. In: Aoki M., Hisamichi S. and Tominaga S. (eds) *Smoking and health 1987. Proceedings of the 6th World Conference on Smoking and Health, Tokyo, 9-12 November 1987.* Elsevier Science Publishers B.V. (Biomedical Division), Amsterdam; 307-10. International Congress Series No. 780.

Osaki Y., Kawaminami K. and Minowa M. (1999). Estimating adolescent cigarette consumption in Japan. *J Epidemiol,* **9**, 56-60.

Osaki Y. and Minowa M. (1993). Nationwide survey of smoking prevalence among school students in Japan. *Nippon Koshu Eisei Zasshi,* **40**, 39-47.

Osaki Y. and Minowa M. (1996). Cigarette smoking among junior and senior high school students in Japan. *J Adolesc Health,* **18**, 59-65.

RP6, See Beese (ed) (1968), Beese (ed) (1972), Lee (ed) (1975)

Sato H. and Araki S. (2000). Yields and daily consumption of cigarettes in Japan in 1969-1996. *J Epidemiol,* **10**, 7-15.

Shibata A., Fukuda K. and Hirohata T. (1990). Smoking habits among senior high school students and related factors. *Kurume Med J,* **37**, 129-40.

Shimao T. (1988). Smoking and its control in Japan. In: Aoki M., Hisamichi S. and Tominaga S. (eds) *Smoking and health 1987. Proceedings of the 6th World Conference on Smoking and Health, Tokyo, 9-12 November 1987.* Elsevier Science Publishers B.V. (Biomedical Division), Amsterdam; 53-60. International Congress Series No. 780.

Shiramizu M. and Shibata A. (1985). A study on factors concerned with smoking behaviors among pupils of junior high school. Part 2. Knowledge of disease caused by smoking and living environment associated with smoking behavior. *Nippon Eiseigaku Zasshi,* **40**, 651-8.

USDA Economic Research Service (1996). *Tobacco statistics.* Albert R. Mann Library, Cornell University, Ithaca, New York. ERS 94012. (With supplementary material from Tobacco Annual Reports.). http://usda.mannlib.cornell.edu/data-sets/specialty/94012.

Wada K. and Fukui S. (1994). Prevalence of tobacco smoking among junior high school students in Japan and background life style of smokers. *Addiction,* **89**, 331-43.

§ Original paper not obtained, but information taken as quoted by another author

Netherlands 18

Sales data

See Tables 18.1-18.3.

Except for the years of the Second World War, data on the consumption of tobacco products have been available since 1923. Before the war, consumption of manufactured cigarettes per adult increased from 1 to 2 cigarettes per day between 1923 and 1939. After the war, consumption continued to increase, with some fluctuations, reaching a peak of 7 cigarettes per day towards the end of the 1970s. It had fallen to 4 cigarettes per day by 1985 and remained at that level until 1995. Although estimates of hand-rolled cigarette consumption vary, one source gives the consumption of hand-rolled cigarettes per adult as being between 2 and 3 cigarettes per day in the 1920s and 1930s (see *Notes on sources of sales data*, p. 451), and about 2 cigarettes during the 1950s. From 1960 onwards, consumption of hand-rolled cigarettes per adult increased slowly from about 2.5 cigarettes per day to 4 in the mid 1980s, then decreased to 3 by 1995. Consumption of hand-rolled cigarettes was higher than that of manufactured cigarettes before the Second World War and again after 1984.

Before the Second World War, tobacco products could be bought very cheaply (Hutson (1937)) and the consumption of tobacco products per adult was high, about 11 g per day. During the war consumption dropped considerably, but reached its pre-war level again in the 1960s and 1970s. It decreased to nearly 7 g per adult per day in 1995. In 1925, 10% of all tobacco was consumed as manufactured cigarettes, increasing to over 50% between about 1970 and 1983. For a few years manufactured cigarette consumption was overtaken by cut tobacco, mostly used for hand-rolling, but reached 50% again by 1995. Cut tobacco consumption had declined from 60% of total tobacco consumption in the 1920s to 30% in the 1960s and 1970s, but rose again to nearly 50% in the mid-1980s. Consumption of cigars and cigarillos accounted for over 30% of all tobacco consumption until the 1940s, but declined to below 10% by the mid 1980s.

Survey data

See Tables 18.4-18.8

In 1958, the prevalence of tobacco smoking among those aged 15 years and over was 85% in men and around 35% in women. The prevalence of cigarette smoking (including hand-rolled cigarettes) was 70% in men; very few women smoked products other than cigarettes. Trends in the prevalence of smoking are complex owing to the need to study three categories: all products, all cigarettes, and manufactured cigarettes. Estimates for all three are available between 1967 and 1979. For men, the prevalence in each category fell over this period, from about 80%, 65%, and 50% to 55%, 45%, and 25% respectively; the steepest fall was for manufactured cigarettes. For women, the prevalence of both all cigarette smoking and manufactured cigarette smoking was about 42% in 1967. A gap then opened up between these two categories. The prevalence of cigarette smoking fell only slightly to 37% in 1979 while the prevalence of manufactured cigarette smoking fell to 33%. The steep fall in prevalence of manufactured cigarette smoking among men was such that it fell below the level for women, and this trend continued into the early 1980s. More recent data are available only for all or unspecified products. Most sources show the prevalence continuing to fall, to about 40% among men and 30% among women by 1995, although some recent industry estimates (source 27) are higher—about 50% among men and 40% among women.

Data on adult smoking by age are available since 1958, but mostly for the all products category. The decrease in the prevalence of smoking was seen at all ages in men, but occurred only among younger age groups in women. The prevalence of smoking was about equal in all age groups for men, but the prevalence in women and of cigarette smoking in men decreased with age.

A series of surveys at the beginning of the 20th century (source 16) showed that smoking was very common among boys. It was then assumed that few girls smoked. The prevalence decreased among teenage boys and increased among girls until, by the mid-1970s, most surveys reported that more girls smoked than boys. Prevalence has since dropped for both boys and girls, and has been about equal since the mid-1980s.

Comparison of survey and sales data suggests that most surveys under-reported consumption by 20-30%. Between 1958 and about 1980, the estimated number of cigarettes smoked per person per day (sales-adjusted) remained about 10-12 for men and increased for women from 3 to 8. It then decreased to 8 for men and 6 for women by 1995. The estimated number of manufactured cigarettes smoked per person per day by men and women was about equal in the late 1970s and early 1980s, falling from 7 in 1979 to 5 in 1982.

Table 18.1.1 Total annual sales of tobacco products, 1923-1973

Year	Cigarettes		Cigars		Cigarillos		Cut tobacco	All tobacco products
	tonnes	millions	tonnes	millions	tonnes	millions	tonnes	tonnes
1923	1960	1958	5960	1043			12700	20620
1924	2510	2507	5930	1037			14610	23040
1925	1980	1982	6080	1063			10610	18670
1926	2370	2369	6540	1145			12560	21480
1927	2590	2591	6850	1198			11840	21280
1928	2790	2791	7240	1267			11750	21780
1929	3180	3180	7690	1346			11290	22170
1930	3590	3590	7830	1370			11570	22990
1931	3550	3554	7820	1369			12290	23670
1932	3660	3655	7740	1355			12930	24330
1933	3910	3914	8050	1409			12750	24710
1934	3930	3926	6910	1015	940	414	10520	22290
1935	4010	4009	7130	1048	860	380	10570	22570
1936	3970	3969	7590	1116	800	353	10980	23340
1937	4350	4349	8060	1185	710	314	10800	23920
1938	4770	4766	8420	1238	710	311	10070	23960
1939	5230	5234	9100	1338	770	340	11390	26490
1946	3330	3332	3570	525	600	264	4720	12220
1947	5360	5362	4260	626	630	278	8030	18280
1948	5330	5334	4580	673	480	211	8940	19330
1949	6090	6092	5070	745	410	181	11250	22820

Table 18.1.1 *(continued)*

Year	Cigarettes		Cigars		Cigarillos		Cut tobacco	All tobacco products
	tonnes	millions	tonnes	millions	tonnes	millions	tonnes	tonnes
1950	8050	8048	4460	655	300	134	11700	24510
1951	8440	8442	4040	594	280	123	10610	23380
1952	9470	9472	4690	690	270	121	10430	24880
1953	10140	10134	5330	783	250	112	10020	25740
1954	11300	11296	5780	850	330	145	9890	27300
1955	11740	11734	6160	906	340	150	8300	26540
1956	13150	13149	6410	942	340	151	8210	28110
1957	13460	13457	6580	967	440	195	8120	28600
1958	13050	13043	6590	968	460	202	8890	28980
1959	13450	13452	6910	1016	550	244	9390	30310
1960	13760	13753	7310	1074	680	299	9530	31270
1961	14640	14635	7810	1148	680	299	9660	32790
1962	15190	15190	7530	1107	720	319	9210	32660
1963	16300	16297	8320	1223	880	389	9480	34980
1964	14080	14073	7770	1142	1090	479	9890	32820
1965	17950	17950	7660	1126	930	409	11200	37750
1966	14200	14201	7480	1100	910	401	10480	33070
1967	16650	16647	7270	1068	820	363	11340	36080
1968	18500	18497	7460	1096	910	403	11880	38760
1969	16250	16251	6500	955	780	342	11700	35230
1970	18680	18675	7200	1058	800	354	11790	38470
1971	19560	19559	6380	937	840	371	11750	38530
1972	21660	21660	6140	903	770	338	12610	41180
1973	23430	23423	6330	930	760	334	13430	43940

Source: see *Notes on sources of sales data,* p. 451

Table 18.1.2 Total annual sales of tobacco products, 1974-1995

Year	Cigarettes		Cigars and cigarillos				Other tobacco	All tobacco products
	tonnes	millions	tonnes	total millions	≥ 3g millions	< 3g millions	tonnes	tonnes
1974	23428	23428	6703	1197	896	301	14446	44577
1975	23892	23892	6726	1201	900	301	14223	44841
1976	22523	22523	6619	1182	874	308	14900	44042
1977	26875	26875	6070	1084	812	272	15801	48746
1978	23463	23463	5891	1052	784	268	14811	44165
1979	26784	26784	5191	927	677	250	15301	47276
1980	22975	22975	5051	902	648	254	14669	42695
1981	21189	21189	4592	820			15509	41290
1982	22127	22127	4211	752			15737	42075
1983	23113	23113	4049	723			18073	45235
1984	16032	16032	3870	691			18336	38238
1985	16289	16289	3791	677			18407	38487
1986	16528	16528	3545	633			18309	38382
1987	16185	16185	3315	592			17560	37060
1988	16263	16263	2957	528			17230	36450
1989	16345	16345	2906	519			16996	36247
1990	17300	17300	2727	487			16587	36614
1991	18398	18398	2710	484			17408	38516
1992	17590	17590	2671	477			15588	35849
1993	16116	16116	2610	466			14096	32822
1994	16530	16530	2638	471			14754	33922
1995	17150	17150	2548	455			14424	34122

Source : see *Notes on sources of sales data,* p. 451

Table 18.1.3 Manufactured cigarettes, percentage of total sales as filter cigarettes, 1960-1993

Year	% Filter	Year	% Filter
1960	12.1	1975	50.9
1961	12.9	1976	54.0
1962	14.4	1977	55.7
1963	15.7	1978	57.9
1964	17.6	1979	60.5
1965	19.5		
1966	21.0	1980	65.0
1967	23.0		
1968	27.2	1982	69.0
1969	32.1	1983	71.0
1970	37.0	1993	85.0
1971	40.3		
1972	43.7		
1973	46.8		
1974	49.0		

Source : see *Notes on sources of sales data*, p. 451

Table 18.2 Consumption of (i) cigarettes and (ii) all tobacco products, 1923-1995 sales-based data, including estimated hand-rolled cigarette consumption. Males and females aged 15 years and over

Year	Manufactured cigarettes		Hand-rolled cigarettes		Total cigarettes		All tobacco products	
	Total annual in millions	Number/ adult/day	Total annual in millions	Number/ adult/day	Total annual in millions	Number/ adult/day	Total annual in tonnes	Grams/ adult/day
1923	1958	1.1					20620	11.8
1924	2507	1.4					23040	12.9
1925	1982	1.1					18670	10.2
1926	2369	1.3					21480	11.5
1927	2591	1.4					21280	11.2
1928	2791	1.4					21780	11.3
1929	3180	1.6					22170	11.2
1930	3590	1.8					22990	11.5
1931	3554	1.7					23670	11.6
1932	3655	1.8					24330	11.7
1933	3914	1.8					24710	11.7
1934	3926	1.8					22290	10.4
1935	4009	1.9					22570	10.5
1936	3969	1.8					23340	10.7
1937	4349	2.0					23920	10.7
1938	4766	2.1					23960	10.6
1939	5234	2.3					26490	11.5
1946	3332	1.3					12220	4.9
1947	5362	2.1					18280	7.3
1948	5334	2.1					19330	7.6
1949	6092	2.4					22820	8.8

Table 18.2 *(continued)*

Year	Manufactured cigarettes		Hand-rolled cigarettes		Total cigarettes		All tobacco products	
	Total annual in millions	Number/ adult/day	Total annual in millions	Number/ adult/day	Total annual in millions	Number/ adult/day	Total annual in tonnes	Grams/ adult/day
1950	8048	3.1					24510	9.4
1951	8442	3.2					23380	8.8
1952	9472	3.6					24880	9.3
1953	10134	3.8					25740	9.6
1954	11296	4.2					27300	10.0
1955	11734	4.3					26540	9.6
1956	13149	4.7					28110	10.1
1957	13457	4.8					28600	10.2
1958	13043	4.6					28980	10.1
1959	13452	4.6					30310	10.5
1960	13753	4.7	7560	2.6	21313	7.3	31270	10.7
1961	14635	4.9	7660	2.6	22295	7.5	32790	11.0
1962	15190	5.0	7310	2.4	22500	7.4	32660	10.7
1963	16297	5.2	7520	2.4	23817	7.7	34980	11.2
1964	14073	4.4	7850	2.5	21923	6.9	32820	10.4
1965	17950	5.6	8890	2.8	26840	8.3	37750	11.7
1966	14201	4.3	8320	2.5	22521	6.9	33070	10.1
1967	16647	5.0	9056	2.7	25703	7.7	36080	10.9
1968	18497	5.5	9757	2.9	28254	8.4	38760	11.5
1969	16251	4.8	9719	2.9	25970	7.6	35230	10.3
1970	18675	5.4	9914	2.9	28589	8.3	38470	11.1
1971	19559	5.6	9999	2.8	29558	8.4	38530	11.0
1972	21660	6.1	10953	3.1	32613	9.2	41180	11.6
1973	23423	6.5	11669	3.2	35092	9.7	43940	12.2
1974	23428	6.4	13001	3.5	36429	9.9	44577	12.2
1975	23892	6.4	13085	3.5	36977	9.9	44841	12.0
1976	22523	6.0	13708	3.6	36231	9.6	44042	11.6
1977	26875	7.0	14695	3.8	41570	10.8	48746	12.7
1978	23463	6.0	14239	3.7	37702	9.7	44165	11.4
1979	26784	6.8	14383	3.6	41167	10.4	47276	12.0
1980	22975	5.7	13935	3.5	36910	9.2	42695	10.6
1981	21189	5.2	14733	3.6	35922	8.8	41290	10.2
1982	22127	5.4	15107	3.7	37234	9.0	42075	10.2
1983	23113	5.6	17350	4.2	40463	9.7	45235	10.9
1984	16032	3.8	17785	4.2	33817	8.0	38238	9.1
1985	16289	3.8	17855	4.2	34144	8.0	38487	9.0
1986	16528	3.8	18309	4.2	34837	8.1	38382	8.9
1987	16185	3.7	17560	4.0	33745	7.7	37060	8.5
1988	16263	3.7	17230	3.9	33493	7.6	36450	8.3
1989	16345	3.7	16996	3.8	33341	7.5	36247	8.2
1990	17300	3.9	16587	3.7	33887	7.6	36614	8.2
1991	18398	4.1	17408	3.9	35806	8.0	38516	8.6
1992	17590	3.9	15588	3.4	33178	7.3	35849	7.9
1993	16116	3.5	14096	3.1	30212	6.6	32822	7.2
1994	16530	3.6	14754	3.2	31284	6.8	33922	7.4
1995	17150	3.7	14424	3.1	31574	6.9	34122	7.4

Source : see *Notes on sources of sales data,* p. 451

Figure 18.1 Daily consumption of (i) manufactured and total number of cigarettes, and (ii) all tobacco products, 1923-1995.
Males and females aged 15 years and over. *Source:* see Table 18.2

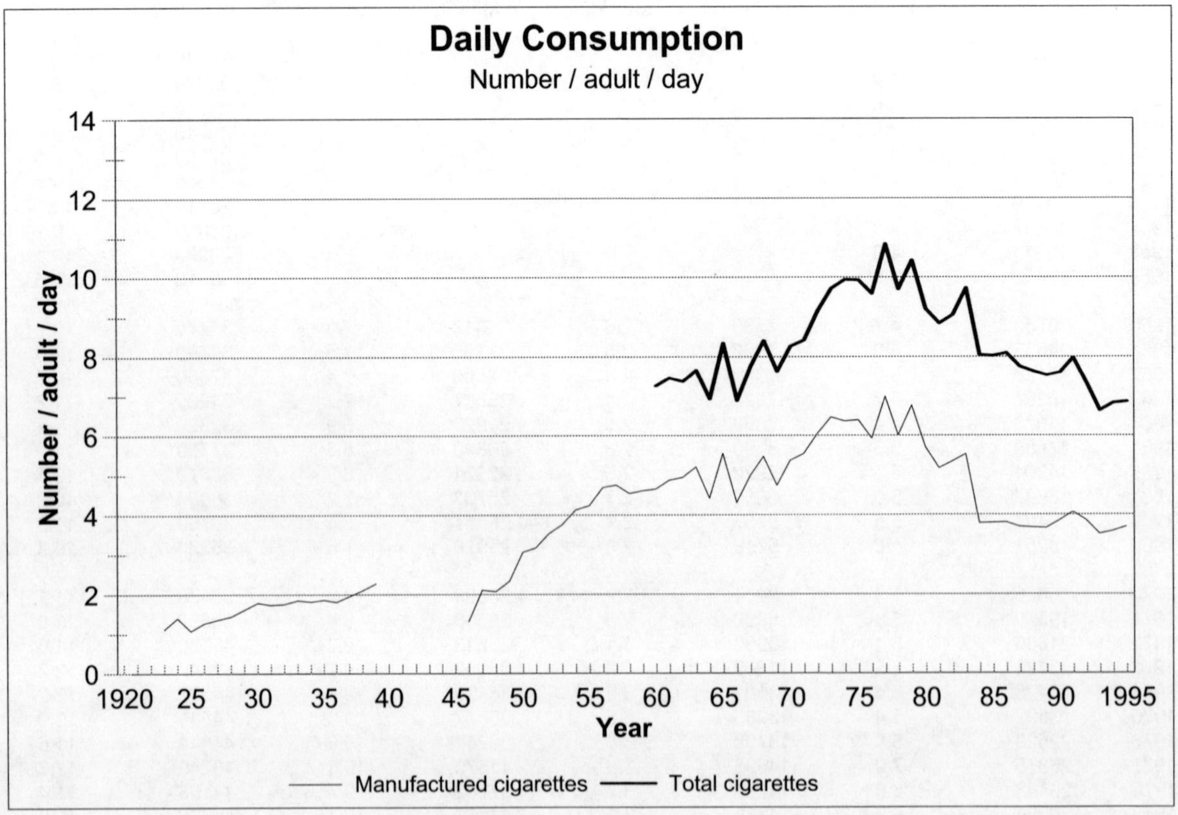

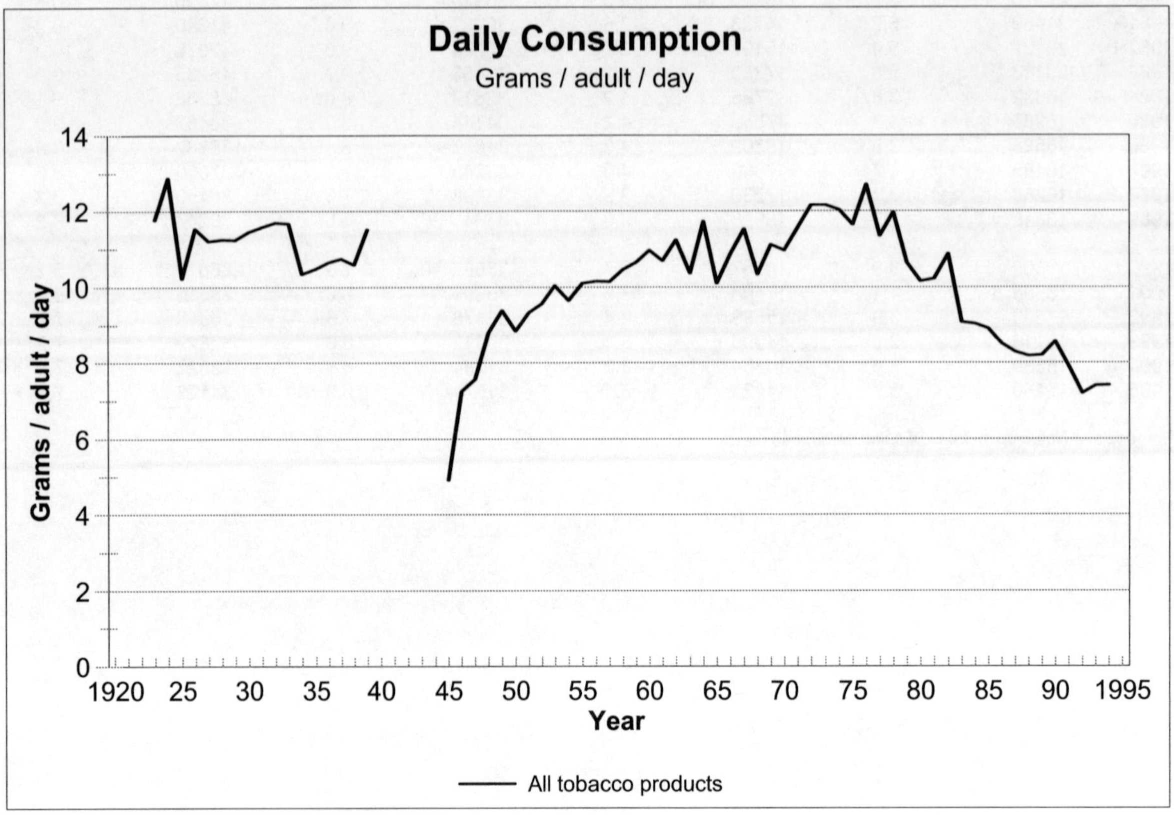

Table 18.3	Percentage sales of tobacco in different forms (by weight), selected years 1925-1995

Year	Cigarettes (%)	Cigars and cigarillos (%)	Cut tobacco (%)
1925	10.6	32.6	56.8
1935	17.8	35.4	46.8
1946	27.3	34.1	38.6
1955	44.2	24.5	31.3
1965	47.5	22.8	29.7
1975	53.3	15.0	31.7
1985	42.3	9.9	47.8
1995	50.3	7.5	42.3

Source : calculated from Tables 18.1.1 & 18.1.2

Figure 18.2 Percentage sales of tobacco in different forms (by weight), selected years 1925-1995
Source: see Table 18.3

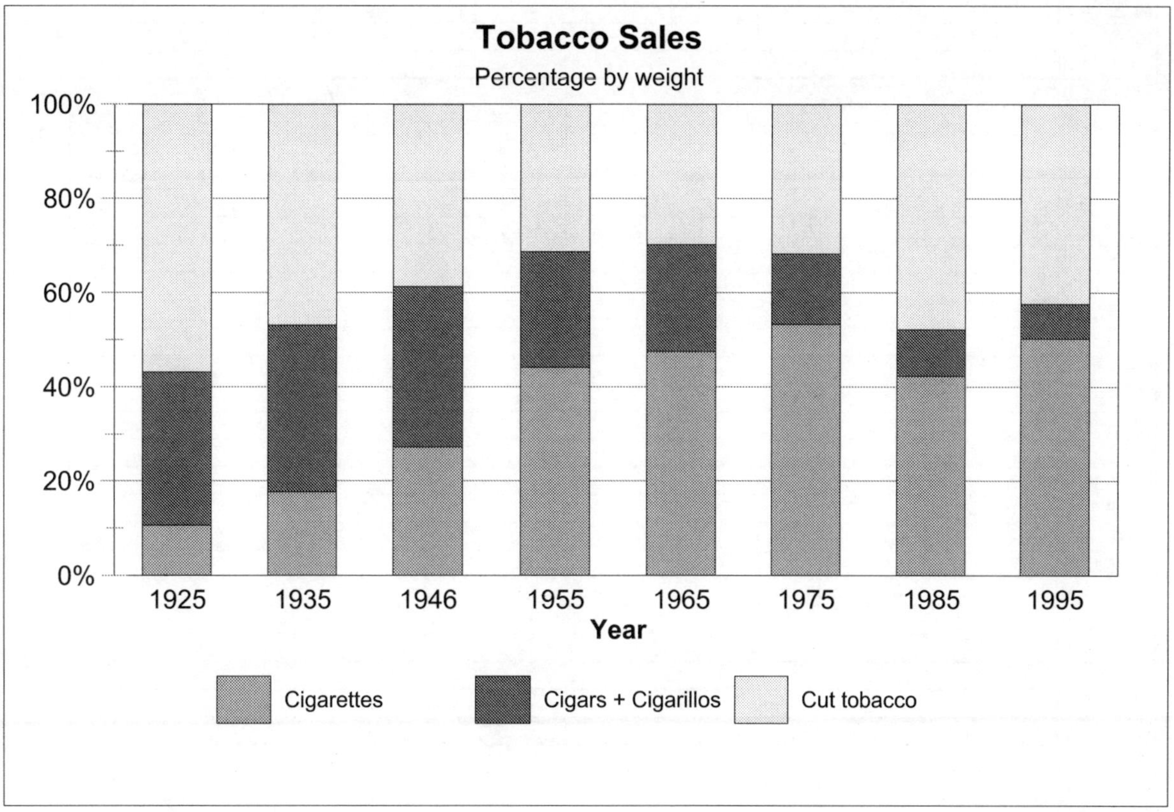

Table 18.4M Prevalence of smoking, males: some selected Dutch surveys by age, 1910-1995 *(continues on p. 440)*

Frequency / Product / Source / Year	Age group																					All ages
	12	13	14	15	16	17	18	19	20-24	25-29	30-34	35-39	40-44	45-49	50-54	55-59	60-64	65-69	70-74	75-79	80+	
10 16 U U	76																					
47 18 U U																81						
57 17 U *	47																					
58 1 A U											91			91			89			89		90
58 2 UC U															74							
58 2 A U															89							
60 19 UC R													83	82	69	66						75
60 20 UC A															64							
60 20 A A															84							
63 3 UC U															63							
63 3 A U															82							
63 4 A R										78			85			81				76		82
63 21 U U												87										
65 14 UC R	26	30	41	50	59	52	56	61														
65 14 UC A	31	34	44	50	61	52	57	63														
65 20 A A																66						
66 5 TC U												67										
66 5 A U												81										
67 7 MC U							59										47					52
67 7 TC U						65				74			70			62				38		64
67 7 A U						58				79			80			82				83		78
70 7 MC U							53										42					47
70 7 TC U				41				70		71			69			58				30		59
70 7 A U						55				77			77			78				74		75
70 8 A U											72											
70 11 UC U													61									
70 11 A U															75							
70 20 A A																	56					
71 5 TC U												58										
71 5 A U												69										
72 5 UC U												59										
72 5 A U												70										
72 8 MC U							48										41					44
72 8 TC U											57											
72 8 A U							66										72					68
73 5 UC U												55										
73 5 A U												66										
74 5 UC U												53										
74 5 A U												62										
75 8 MC U							36										36					36
75 8 TC U											53											
75 8 A U						46				68			69			68				66		66
76 5 UC U												48										
76 5 A U												57										
77 20 A A																		40				
78 5 UC U											49											
78 5 A U											58											
78 5 UC U												48										
78 5 A U						36				57			63			59				53		56
78 6 U U						40			53	61												
78 13 U *	21	37																				

Table 18.4F Prevalence of smoking, females: some selected Dutch surveys by age, 1910-1995 *(continues on p. 441)*

Frequency / Product / Source / Year	Age group 12	13	14	15	16	17	18	19	20-24	25-29	30-34	35-39	40-44	45-49	50-54	55-59	60-64	65-69	70-74	75-79	80+	All ages
10 16 U U																						
47 18 U U																						
57 17 U *	11																					
58 1 A U									46				32		18				5			29
58 2 UC U									37													
58 2 A U									38													
60 19 UC R																						
60 20 UC A																						
60 20 A A																						
63 3 UC U									32													
63 3 A U									32													
63 4 A R									45			38			20			3				32
63 21 U U				30																		
65 14 UC R																						
65 14 UC A																						
65 20 A A																						
66 5 TC U				40																		
66 5 A U				40																		
67 7 MC U				56								30										41
67 7 TC U				59						56		46			26			12				42
67 7 A U				57					58			46			26			13				42
70 7 MC U				55								30										40
70 7 TC U		44						62		56		48			26			11				42
70 7 A U				57					57			48			27			13				42
70 8 A U		41																				
70 11 UC U					47																	
70 11 A U									37													
70 20 A A																						
71 5 TC U				40																		
71 5 A U				40																		
72 5 UC U				44																		
72 5 A U				44																		
72 8 MC U				57								30										40
72 8 TC U		41																				
72 8 A U				57								30										40
73 5 UC U				42																		
73 5 A U				42																		
74 5 UC U				42																		
74 5 A U				42																		
75 8 MC U				48								27										36
75 8 TC U		40																				
75 8 A U				48					58			47			29			12				40
76 5 UC U				37																		
76 5 A U				37																		
77 20 A A																						
78 5 UC U		36																				
78 5 A U		38																				
78 5 UC U				39																		
78 5 A U				42					49			44			31			15				39
78 6 U U				46					56	47												
78 13 U *	10	42																				

Table 18.4M *(continued from p. 438, continues on p. 442)*
Prevalence of smoking, males

<table>
<tr><th rowspan="2">Frequency
Product
Source
Year</th><th colspan="21">Age group</th><th rowspan="2">All ages</th></tr>
<tr><th>12</th><th>13</th><th>14</th><th>15</th><th>16</th><th>17</th><th>18</th><th>19</th><th>20 - 24</th><th>25 - 29</th><th>30 - 34</th><th>35 - 39</th><th>40 - 44</th><th>45 - 49</th><th>50 - 54</th><th>55 - 59</th><th>60 - 64</th><th>65 - 69</th><th>70 - 74</th><th>75 - 79</th><th>80+</th></tr>
<tr><td>79 5 MC U</td><td colspan="3"></td><td colspan="6">20</td><td colspan="5">30</td><td colspan="3">31</td><td colspan="4">18</td><td>26</td></tr>
<tr><td>79 5 TC U</td><td colspan="3"></td><td colspan="5">28</td><td>45</td><td colspan="2">55</td><td colspan="3">52</td><td colspan="3">49</td><td colspan="4">29</td><td>45</td></tr>
<tr><td>79 5 A U</td><td colspan="3"></td><td colspan="5">29</td><td>47</td><td colspan="2">61</td><td colspan="3">58</td><td colspan="3">59</td><td colspan="4">47</td><td>52</td></tr>
<tr><td>79 6 U U</td><td colspan="3"></td><td colspan="5">33</td><td>51</td><td colspan="2">61</td><td colspan="10"></td><td></td></tr>
<tr><td>79 8 MC U</td><td colspan="3"></td><td colspan="8">29</td><td colspan="10">23</td><td>26</td></tr>
<tr><td>79 8 A U</td><td colspan="3"></td><td colspan="5">29</td><td colspan="3">56</td><td colspan="3">58</td><td colspan="3">61</td><td colspan="4">57</td><td>52</td></tr>
<tr><td>79 12 UC U</td><td>3</td><td colspan="2">15</td><td colspan="2">27</td><td colspan="3">54</td><td colspan="13"></td><td>24</td></tr>
<tr><td>79 13 U *</td><td>17</td><td colspan="2">30</td><td colspan="18"></td><td></td></tr>
<tr><td>80 5 A U</td><td colspan="3"></td><td colspan="5">30</td><td colspan="3">56</td><td colspan="3">54</td><td colspan="3">56</td><td colspan="4">52</td><td>52</td></tr>
<tr><td>81 5 A U</td><td colspan="3"></td><td colspan="5">27</td><td colspan="3">49</td><td colspan="3">50</td><td colspan="3">51</td><td colspan="4">51</td><td>47</td></tr>
<tr><td>81 6 U U</td><td colspan="3"></td><td colspan="5">31</td><td>47</td><td colspan="2">52</td><td colspan="10"></td><td></td></tr>
<tr><td>81 13 U *</td><td>16</td><td colspan="2">23</td><td colspan="18"></td><td></td></tr>
<tr><td>82 5 MC U</td><td colspan="3"></td><td colspan="8">19</td><td colspan="10">22</td><td>21</td></tr>
<tr><td>82 5 A U</td><td colspan="3"></td><td colspan="5">18</td><td colspan="3">45</td><td colspan="3">44</td><td colspan="3">45</td><td colspan="4">43</td><td>41</td></tr>
<tr><td>82 13 U A</td><td>6</td><td colspan="2">22</td><td colspan="18"></td><td></td></tr>
<tr><td>83 5 A U</td><td colspan="3"></td><td colspan="5">23</td><td colspan="3">46</td><td colspan="3">50</td><td colspan="3">47</td><td colspan="4">41</td><td>44</td></tr>
<tr><td>83 9 TC R</td><td colspan="3"></td><td colspan="2">17</td><td colspan="2">30</td><td>39</td><td>42</td><td colspan="12"></td><td>32</td></tr>
<tr><td>83 9 TC A</td><td colspan="3"></td><td colspan="2">21</td><td colspan="2">38</td><td>46</td><td>44</td><td colspan="12"></td><td>37</td></tr>
<tr><td>83 13 U A</td><td>5</td><td colspan="2">17</td><td colspan="18"></td><td></td></tr>
<tr><td>83 15 A A</td><td>12</td><td>16</td><td>22</td><td>27</td><td>29</td><td>26</td><td>33</td><td colspan="14"></td><td></td></tr>
<tr><td>84 5 A U</td><td colspan="3"></td><td colspan="5">17</td><td colspan="3">48</td><td colspan="3">48</td><td colspan="3">49</td><td colspan="4">43</td><td>44</td></tr>
<tr><td>84 13 U A</td><td>4</td><td colspan="2">19</td><td colspan="18"></td><td></td></tr>
<tr><td>85 5 A U</td><td colspan="3"></td><td colspan="5">22</td><td colspan="3">46</td><td colspan="3">48</td><td colspan="3">47</td><td colspan="4">42</td><td>43</td></tr>
<tr><td>85 13 U A</td><td>7</td><td colspan="2">22</td><td colspan="18"></td><td></td></tr>
<tr><td>85 20 UC A</td><td colspan="17"></td><td colspan="4">34</td><td></td></tr>
<tr><td>85 20 A A</td><td colspan="17"></td><td colspan="4">42</td><td></td></tr>
<tr><td>86 5 A U</td><td colspan="3"></td><td colspan="5">22</td><td colspan="3">46</td><td colspan="3">46</td><td colspan="3">45</td><td colspan="4">41</td><td>42</td></tr>
<tr><td>86 13 U A</td><td>2</td><td colspan="2">19</td><td colspan="18"></td><td></td></tr>
<tr><td>86 22 U *</td><td></td><td>4</td><td></td><td>21</td><td colspan="17"></td><td></td></tr>
<tr><td>87 5 A U</td><td colspan="3"></td><td colspan="5">21</td><td colspan="3">41</td><td colspan="3">47</td><td colspan="3">44</td><td colspan="4">39</td><td>41</td></tr>
<tr><td>87 13 U A</td><td>3</td><td colspan="2">18</td><td colspan="18"></td><td></td></tr>
<tr><td>87 23 U U</td><td colspan="3"></td><td colspan="18">49</td><td></td></tr>
<tr><td>88 5 A U</td><td colspan="3"></td><td colspan="5">19</td><td colspan="3">39</td><td colspan="3">41</td><td colspan="3">39</td><td colspan="4">35</td><td>37</td></tr>
<tr><td>89 5 A U</td><td colspan="3"></td><td colspan="5">17</td><td colspan="3">37</td><td colspan="3">42</td><td colspan="3">37</td><td colspan="4">34</td><td>36</td></tr>
<tr><td>89 23 U U</td><td colspan="3"></td><td colspan="18">45</td><td></td></tr>
<tr><td>89 24 U *</td><td colspan="2">4</td><td colspan="19"></td><td></td></tr>
<tr><td>89 24 U R</td><td colspan="2">6</td><td colspan="19"></td><td></td></tr>
<tr><td>89 24 U A</td><td colspan="2">13</td><td colspan="19"></td><td></td></tr>
<tr><td>89 25 A U</td><td colspan="4"></td><td colspan="17">44</td><td></td></tr>
<tr><td>90 5 A U</td><td colspan="3"></td><td colspan="5">21</td><td colspan="3">41</td><td colspan="3">43</td><td colspan="3">41</td><td colspan="4">34</td><td>39</td></tr>
<tr><td>90 13 U A</td><td>2</td><td colspan="2">15</td><td colspan="18"></td><td></td></tr>
<tr><td>90 25 A U</td><td colspan="4"></td><td colspan="17">43</td><td></td></tr>
<tr><td>90 26 U R</td><td colspan="2"></td><td>3</td><td>9</td><td colspan="17"></td><td></td></tr>
<tr><td>90 26 U A</td><td>1</td><td colspan="3">9</td><td colspan="17"></td><td></td></tr>
<tr><td>91 5 A U</td><td colspan="3"></td><td colspan="5">22</td><td colspan="3">39</td><td colspan="3">43</td><td colspan="3">40</td><td colspan="4">33</td><td>38</td></tr>
<tr><td>91 23 U U</td><td colspan="3"></td><td colspan="18">46</td><td></td></tr>
<tr><td>91 24 U *</td><td colspan="2"></td><td colspan="2">10</td><td colspan="17"></td><td></td></tr>
<tr><td>91 24 U R</td><td colspan="2"></td><td colspan="2">14</td><td colspan="17"></td><td></td></tr>
<tr><td>91 24 U A</td><td colspan="2"></td><td colspan="2">18</td><td colspan="17"></td><td></td></tr>
<tr><td>91 25 A U</td><td colspan="4"></td><td colspan="17">44</td><td></td></tr>
<tr><td>92 5 A U</td><td colspan="3"></td><td colspan="5">23</td><td colspan="3">38</td><td colspan="3">43</td><td colspan="3">40</td><td colspan="4">32</td><td>38</td></tr>
<tr><td>92 13 U A</td><td>3</td><td colspan="2">22</td><td colspan="2">40</td><td colspan="3">52</td><td colspan="13"></td><td></td></tr>
<tr><td>92 25 A U</td><td colspan="4"></td><td colspan="5">39</td><td colspan="4">46</td><td colspan="4">43</td><td colspan="4">36</td><td>43</td></tr>
<tr><td>93 5 A U</td><td colspan="3"></td><td colspan="5">24</td><td colspan="3">40</td><td colspan="3">40</td><td colspan="3">38</td><td colspan="4">30</td><td>37</td></tr>
<tr><td>93 25 A U</td><td colspan="4"></td><td colspan="17">42</td><td></td></tr>
<tr><td>93 27 A U</td><td colspan="6"></td><td colspan="11">54</td><td colspan="4"></td><td></td></tr>
</table>

Table 18.4F *(continued from p. 439, continues on p. 443)*
Prevalence of smoking, females

Frequency Product Source Year	Age group 12	13	14	15	16	17	18	19	20-24	25-29	30-34	35-39	40-44	45-49	50-54	55-59	60-64	65-69	70-74	75-79	80+	All ages
79 5 MC U				39						41					28			12				33
79 5 TC U				39					55	51		40			30			13				38
79 5 A U				39					55	51		40			30			13				38
79 6 U U				44					59	51												
79 8 MC U				41								27										33
79 8 A U				39					52			40			30			13				38
79 12 UC U	2	17		38		51																26
79 13 U *	8	35																				
80 5 A U				31					44			38			28			11				34
81 5 A U				30					48			39			28			13				36
81 6 U U				34					55	46												
81 13 U *	10	27																				
82 5 MC U				31								23										27
82 5 A U				27					45			36			27			13				33
82 13 U A	4	21																				
83 5 A U				28					48			39			25			12				35
83 9 TC R				28		26		48	48													37
83 9 TC A				33		33		50	53													42
83 13 U A	3	22																				
83 15 A A	10	17	27	32	32	31	37															
84 5 A U				24					44			36			29			12				33
84 13 U A	4	23																				
85 5 A U				23					44			39			29			13				34
85 13 U A	3	24																				
85 20 UC A																						
85 20 A A																						
86 5 A U				22					45			37			29			12				34
86 13 U A	4	22																				
86 22 U *		5		20																		
87 5 A U				22					42			37			31			12				33
87 13 U A	2	19																				
87 23 U U				39																		
88 5 A U				19					38			34			25			11				29
89 5 A U				20					35			35			26			13				29
89 23 U U				34																		
89 24 U *	2																					
89 24 U R	7																					
89 24 U A	13																					
89 25 A U					31																	
90 5 A U				21					38			36			29			12				31
90 13 U A	2	12																				
90 25 A U					32																	
90 26 U R			3	9																		
90 26 U A	1	8																				
91 5 A U				19					37			37			28			13				30
91 23 U U				33																		
91 24 U *			11																			
91 24 U R			17																			
91 24 U A			24																			
91 25 A U					33																	
92 5 A U				21					37			38			28			14				31
92 13 U A	2	17		46		42																
92 25 A U					36					40				28				12				31
93 5 A U				20					35			35			27			13				30
93 25 A U					31																	
93 27 A U							46															

Table 18.4M *(continued from p. 440)*
Prevalence of smoking, males

Year	Source	Frequency	Product	12	13	14	15	16	17	18	19	20-24	25-29	30-34	35-39	40-44	45-49	50-54	55-59	60-64	65-69	70-74	75-79	80+	All ages
94	5	A	U				24					37			40			36			29				36
94	23	U	U				45																		
94	25	A	U					43																	
94	27	A	U							53															
95	5	A	U				25					42			43			38			32				39
95	13	U	A	4	23		43		48																
95	25	A	U					41																	
95	27	A	U							54															

Table 18.5M Number of cigarettes smoked per smoker per day, males: some selected Dutch surveys by age, 1958-1995

Year	Source	Product	12	13	14	15	16	17	18	19	20-24	25-29	30-34	35-39	40-44	45-49	50-54	55-59	60-64	65-69	70-74	75-79	80+	All ages
58	1	TC									18													
60	19	UCE													13	12	11	11						11
65	14	UCE	1	1	2	3	3	5	5	5														
72	8	TC *				20																		
79	5	TC				11					14	16		17			16			14				15
81	5	TC *				23																		
81	6	UC *				15					19	22												
81	13	UC	2	5																				
83	9	TCE				9.1		11		15	18													
83	15	UCE	4.2			7.2		9.3																
89	25	TC					19																	
90	25	TC					17																	
91	25	TC					17																	
92	25	TC					17																	
93	25	TC					17																	
94	25	TC					17																	
95	25	TC					17																	

Source: see *Notes on sources of survey data*, p. 452
Frequency: A = all smokers (including occasional)
R = regular or daily smokers
All ages: relevant to ages used and as given in original source
U = unspecified
* = refer to *Notes on sources of survey data*, p. 452

Product: MC = manufactured cigarettes
TC = total cigarettes (including hand-rolled)
UC = cigarettes (type unspecified)
A = all products
E indicates mean estimated from percentage distribution (see also *Consumption category estimation*, p. xxxiv, and Appendix III, p. 789)

Table 18.4F *(continued from p. 441)* Prevalence of smoking, females

Frequency / Product / Source / Year	12	13	14	15	16	17	18	19	20-24	25-29	30-34	35-39	40-44	45-49	50-54	55-59	60-64	65-69	70-74	75-79	80+	All ages
94 5 A U				22					33			35			27			13				29
94 23 U U				36																		
94 25 A U					32																	
94 27 A U							47															
95 5 A U				21					36			38			27			14				31
95 13 U A	5	26		45		48																
95 25 A U					31																	
95 27 A U							47															

Table 18.5F Number of cigarettes smoked per smoker per day, females: some selected Dutch surveys by age, 1958-1995

Product / Source / Year	12	13	14	15	16	17	18	19	20-24	25-29	30-34	35-39	40-44	45-49	50-54	55-59	60-64	65-69	70-74	75-79	80+	All ages
58 1 TC									8													
60 19 UCE																						
65 14 UCE																						
72 8 TC *				12																		
79 5 TC				10					13	13		13			12			9				13
81 5 TC *				19																		
81 6 UC *				14					20	18												
81 13 UC	1	6																				
83 9 TCE				8.5		11		13	14													
83 15 UCE	4.7			7.2		7.3																
89 25 TC					17																	
90 25 TC					16																	
91 25 TC					15																	
92 25 TC					16																	
93 25 TC					17																	
94 25 TC					16																	
95 25 TC					15																	

Source: see *Notes on sources of survey data*, p. 452
Frequency: A = all smokers (including occasional)
R = regular or daily smokers
All ages: relevant to ages used and as given in original source
U = unspecified
* = refer to *Notes on sources of survey data*, p. 452

Product: MC = manufactured cigarettes
TC = total cigarettes (including hand-rolled)
UC = cigarettes (type unspecified)
A = all products
E indicates mean estimated from percentage distribution (see also *Consumption category estimation*, p. xxxiv, and Appendix III, p. 789)

Table 18.6M Number of cigarettes smoked per person per day, males: some selected Dutch surveys by age, 1958-1995, with percentage total sales

<table>
<tr><th rowspan="2">Product
Source
Year</th><th colspan="21">Age group</th><th rowspan="2">All ages</th><th rowspan="2">% Total sales</th></tr>
<tr><th>12</th><th>13</th><th>14</th><th>15</th><th>16</th><th>17</th><th>18</th><th>19</th><th>20-24</th><th>25-29</th><th>30-34</th><th>35-39</th><th>40-44</th><th>45-49</th><th>50-54</th><th>55-59</th><th>60-64</th><th>65-69</th><th>70-74</th><th>75-79</th><th>80+</th></tr>
<tr><td>58 1 TC</td><td colspan="8"></td><td colspan="13">13</td><td></td><td>101%T</td></tr>
<tr><td>60 19 UC</td><td colspan="12"></td><td>10</td><td>9.6</td><td>7.3</td><td>7.1</td><td colspan="5"></td><td>8.5</td><td>**</td></tr>
<tr><td>65 14 UC</td><td>0</td><td>0</td><td>1</td><td>1</td><td>2</td><td>2</td><td>3</td><td>3</td><td colspan="13"></td><td></td><td>**</td></tr>
<tr><td>72 8 TC</td><td colspan="3"></td><td colspan="18">11</td><td></td><td>---T</td></tr>
<tr><td>79 5 TC</td><td colspan="3"></td><td colspan="5">3.1</td><td>6.3</td><td colspan="2">8.8</td><td colspan="3">8.8</td><td colspan="3">7.8</td><td colspan="4">4.1</td><td>6.8</td><td>56%T</td></tr>
<tr><td>79 10 MC</td><td colspan="3"></td><td colspan="18">6.5</td><td></td><td>---M</td></tr>
<tr><td>81 5 TC *</td><td colspan="3"></td><td colspan="18">11</td><td></td><td>---T</td></tr>
<tr><td>81 6 UC *</td><td colspan="3"></td><td colspan="5">5</td><td>9</td><td colspan="2">11</td><td colspan="10"></td><td></td><td>---T</td></tr>
<tr><td>81 13 UC</td><td>0</td><td colspan="2">1</td><td colspan="18"></td><td></td><td>**</td></tr>
<tr><td>83 9 TC</td><td colspan="3"></td><td colspan="2">1.9</td><td colspan="2">4.2</td><td>6.8</td><td>8.0</td><td colspan="12"></td><td></td><td>**</td></tr>
<tr><td>83 15 UC</td><td colspan="3">0.7</td><td colspan="2">2.0</td><td colspan="2">2.6</td><td colspan="14"></td><td></td><td>**</td></tr>
<tr><td>89 25 TC</td><td colspan="4"></td><td colspan="17">7.3</td><td></td><td>81%T</td></tr>
<tr><td>90 25 TC</td><td colspan="4"></td><td colspan="17">6.4</td><td></td><td>72%T</td></tr>
<tr><td>91 25 TC</td><td colspan="4"></td><td colspan="17">6.5</td><td></td><td>69%T</td></tr>
<tr><td>92 25 TC</td><td colspan="4"></td><td colspan="17">6.1</td><td></td><td>71%T</td></tr>
<tr><td>93 25 TC</td><td colspan="4"></td><td colspan="17">6.2</td><td></td><td>82%T</td></tr>
<tr><td>94 25 TC</td><td colspan="4"></td><td colspan="17">6.0</td><td></td><td>79%T</td></tr>
<tr><td>95 25 TC</td><td colspan="4"></td><td colspan="17">6.1</td><td></td><td>76%T</td></tr>
</table>

Table 18.7M Number of cigarettes smoked per person per day, sales-adjusted, males: some selected Dutch surveys[1] by age, 1958-1995, with percentage total sales

<table>
<tr><th rowspan="2">Product
Source
Year</th><th colspan="21">Age group</th><th rowspan="2">All ages</th><th rowspan="2">% Total sales</th></tr>
<tr><th>12</th><th>13</th><th>14</th><th>15</th><th>16</th><th>17</th><th>18</th><th>19</th><th>20-24</th><th>25-29</th><th>30-34</th><th>35-39</th><th>40-44</th><th>45-49</th><th>50-54</th><th>55-59</th><th>60-64</th><th>65-69</th><th>70-74</th><th>75-79</th><th>80+</th></tr>
<tr><td>58 1 TC</td><td colspan="8"></td><td colspan="13">13</td><td></td><td>101%T</td></tr>
<tr><td>72 8 TC</td><td colspan="3"></td><td colspan="18">11</td><td></td><td>---T</td></tr>
<tr><td>79 5 TC</td><td colspan="3"></td><td colspan="5">5.5</td><td>11</td><td colspan="2">16</td><td colspan="3">16</td><td colspan="3">14</td><td colspan="4">7.4</td><td>12</td><td>56%T</td></tr>
<tr><td>79 10 MC</td><td colspan="3"></td><td colspan="18">6.5</td><td></td><td>---M</td></tr>
<tr><td>81 5 TC *</td><td colspan="3"></td><td colspan="18">11</td><td></td><td>---T</td></tr>
<tr><td>81 6 UC *</td><td colspan="3"></td><td colspan="5">5</td><td>9</td><td colspan="2">11</td><td colspan="10"></td><td></td><td>---T</td></tr>
<tr><td>89 25 TC</td><td colspan="4"></td><td colspan="17">9.0</td><td></td><td>81%T</td></tr>
<tr><td>90 25 TC</td><td colspan="4"></td><td colspan="17">8.8</td><td></td><td>72%T</td></tr>
<tr><td>91 25 TC</td><td colspan="4"></td><td colspan="17">9.4</td><td></td><td>69%T</td></tr>
<tr><td>92 25 TC</td><td colspan="4"></td><td colspan="17">8.6</td><td></td><td>71%T</td></tr>
<tr><td>93 25 TC</td><td colspan="4"></td><td colspan="17">7.6</td><td></td><td>82%T</td></tr>
<tr><td>94 25 TC</td><td colspan="4"></td><td colspan="17">7.6</td><td></td><td>79%T</td></tr>
<tr><td>95 25 TC</td><td colspan="4"></td><td colspan="17">8.0</td><td></td><td>76%T</td></tr>
</table>

1 Based on those surveys in Table 18.6 with data for both sexes and age range at least 21-64 (see *Cigarette consumption per person*, p. xxxv)

Source: see *Notes on sources of survey data*, p. 452
All ages: relevant to ages used and as given in original source
% Total sales: estimated % of total sales of M = manufactured or T = total cigarette consumption implied by survey, sexes combined, used as adjustment factor in Table 18.7
** = cannot be calculated
--- = adjusted by original author

Product: MC = manufactured cigarettes
TC = total cigarettes (including hand-rolled)
UC = cigarettes (type unspecified)
A = all products
U = unspecified
* = refer to *Notes on sources of survey data*, p. 452

Table 18.6F Number of cigarettes smoked per person per day, females: some selected Dutch surveys by age, 1958-1995, with percentage total sales

<table>
<tr><th rowspan="2">Product
Source
Year</th><th colspan="21">Age group</th><th rowspan="2">All ages</th><th rowspan="2">% Total sales</th></tr>
<tr><th>12</th><th>13</th><th>14</th><th>15</th><th>16</th><th>17</th><th>18</th><th>19</th><th>20-24</th><th>25-29</th><th>30-34</th><th>35-39</th><th>40-44</th><th>45-49</th><th>50-54</th><th>55-59</th><th>60-64</th><th>65-69</th><th>70-74</th><th>75-79</th><th>80+</th></tr>
<tr><td>58 1 TC</td><td colspan="8"></td><td colspan="13">3.0</td><td></td><td>101%T</td></tr>
<tr><td>60 19 UC</td><td colspan="21"></td><td></td><td>**</td></tr>
<tr><td>65 14 UC</td><td colspan="21"></td><td></td><td>**</td></tr>
<tr><td>72 8 TC</td><td colspan="3"></td><td colspan="18">4.9</td><td></td><td>---T</td></tr>
<tr><td>79 5 TC</td><td colspan="3"></td><td colspan="5">3.9</td><td>7.2</td><td colspan="2">6.6</td><td colspan="3">5.2</td><td colspan="3">3.6</td><td colspan="4">1.2</td><td>4.9</td><td>56%T</td></tr>
<tr><td>79 10 MC</td><td colspan="3"></td><td colspan="18">7.1</td><td></td><td>---M</td></tr>
<tr><td>81 5 TC *</td><td colspan="3"></td><td colspan="18">6.8</td><td></td><td>---T</td></tr>
<tr><td>81 6 UC *</td><td colspan="3"></td><td colspan="5">5</td><td>11</td><td colspan="2">8</td><td colspan="10"></td><td></td><td>---T</td></tr>
<tr><td>81 13 UC</td><td>0</td><td colspan="2">2</td><td colspan="18"></td><td></td><td>**</td></tr>
<tr><td>83 9 TC</td><td colspan="3"></td><td colspan="2">2.8</td><td colspan="2">3.8</td><td>6.3</td><td>7.7</td><td colspan="12"></td><td></td><td>**</td></tr>
<tr><td>83 15 UC</td><td colspan="3">0.9</td><td colspan="2">2.3</td><td colspan="2">2.4</td><td colspan="14"></td><td></td><td>**</td></tr>
<tr><td>89 25 TC</td><td colspan="4"></td><td colspan="17">5.1</td><td></td><td>81%T</td></tr>
<tr><td>90 25 TC</td><td colspan="4"></td><td colspan="17">4.8</td><td></td><td>72%T</td></tr>
<tr><td>91 25 TC</td><td colspan="4"></td><td colspan="17">4.7</td><td></td><td>69%T</td></tr>
<tr><td>92 25 TC</td><td colspan="4"></td><td colspan="17">4.5</td><td></td><td>71%T</td></tr>
<tr><td>93 25 TC</td><td colspan="4"></td><td colspan="17">4.8</td><td></td><td>82%T</td></tr>
<tr><td>94 25 TC</td><td colspan="4"></td><td colspan="17">4.9</td><td></td><td>79%T</td></tr>
<tr><td>95 25 TC</td><td colspan="4"></td><td colspan="17">4.5</td><td></td><td>76%T</td></tr>
</table>

Table 18.7F Number of cigarettes smoked per person per day, sales-adjusted, females: some selected Dutch surveys[1] by age, 1958-1995, with percentage total sales

<table>
<tr><th rowspan="2">Product
Source
Year</th><th colspan="21">Age group</th><th rowspan="2">All ages</th><th rowspan="2">% Total sales</th></tr>
<tr><th>12</th><th>13</th><th>14</th><th>15</th><th>16</th><th>17</th><th>18</th><th>19</th><th>20-24</th><th>25-29</th><th>30-34</th><th>35-39</th><th>40-44</th><th>45-49</th><th>50-54</th><th>55-59</th><th>60-64</th><th>65-69</th><th>70-74</th><th>75-79</th><th>80+</th></tr>
<tr><td>58 1 TC</td><td colspan="8"></td><td colspan="13">2.9</td><td></td><td>101%T</td></tr>
<tr><td>72 8 TC</td><td colspan="3"></td><td colspan="18">4.9</td><td></td><td>---T</td></tr>
<tr><td>79 5 TC</td><td colspan="3"></td><td colspan="5">7.0</td><td>13</td><td colspan="2">12</td><td colspan="3">9.3</td><td colspan="3">6.5</td><td colspan="4">2.2</td><td>8.8</td><td>56%T</td></tr>
<tr><td>79 10 MC</td><td colspan="3"></td><td colspan="18">7.1</td><td></td><td>---M</td></tr>
<tr><td>81 5 TC *</td><td colspan="3"></td><td colspan="18">6.8</td><td></td><td>---T</td></tr>
<tr><td>81 6 UC *</td><td colspan="3"></td><td colspan="5">5</td><td>11</td><td colspan="2">8</td><td colspan="10"></td><td></td><td>---T</td></tr>
<tr><td>89 25 TC</td><td colspan="4"></td><td colspan="17">6.3</td><td></td><td>81%T</td></tr>
<tr><td>90 25 TC</td><td colspan="4"></td><td colspan="17">6.6</td><td></td><td>72%T</td></tr>
<tr><td>91 25 TC</td><td colspan="4"></td><td colspan="17">6.8</td><td></td><td>69%T</td></tr>
<tr><td>92 25 TC</td><td colspan="4"></td><td colspan="17">6.3</td><td></td><td>71%T</td></tr>
<tr><td>93 25 TC</td><td colspan="4"></td><td colspan="17">5.9</td><td></td><td>82%T</td></tr>
<tr><td>94 25 TC</td><td colspan="4"></td><td colspan="17">6.2</td><td></td><td>79%T</td></tr>
<tr><td>95 25 TC</td><td colspan="4"></td><td colspan="17">5.9</td><td></td><td>76%T</td></tr>
</table>

1 Based on those surveys in Table 18.6 with data for both sexes and age range at least 21-64 (see *Cigarette consumption per person*, p. xxxv)

Source: see *Notes on sources of survey data*, p. 452
All ages: relevant to ages used and as given in original source
% Total sales: estimated % of total sales of M = manufactured or T = total cigarette consumption implied by survey, sexes combined, used as adjustment factor in Table 18.7
** = cannot be calculated
--- = adjusted by original author

Product: MC = manufactured cigarettes
TC = total cigarettes (including hand-rolled)
UC = cigarettes (type unspecified)
A = all products
U = unspecified
* = refer to *Notes on sources of survey data*, p. 452

Table 18.8 Estimated[1] prevalence of smoking and estimated[1] number of cigarettes per person per day (unadjusted and sales-adjusted): summary of Tables 18.4, 18.6 and 18.7, 1945-1995.
Males and females aged 15 years and over

Year	Source[2]	Product[3]	Prevalence[4]						Number of cigarettes						
									Unadjusted[7]			Sales-adjusted[8]			
			Manufactured cigarettes		Total cigarettes[5]		All products[6]		Number/ person/day		Total sales %	Manufactured cigarettes number/ person/day		Total cigarettes[9] number/ person/day	
			M	F	M	F	M	F	M	F		M	F	M	F
1958	1	TC+*A*					86	33	11.9	2.8	101			11.8	2.8
	2	*UC+A*			71	37	85	38						(10.2	4.3)
1963	3	*UC+A*			61	33	78	33						(10.7	4.7)
	4	A					78	31							
	21	*U*					87	30							
1966	5	*TC+A*			67	40	81	40						(9.4	4.5)
1967	7	*MC+TC+A*	52	40	64	42	78	42				(6.2	3.9)	(10.2	5.3)
1970	7	*MC+TC+A*	47	40	59	41	74	42				(6.4	4.4)	(10.7	5.9)
	8	*A*					72	41							
	11	*UC+A*			60	46	73	37						(10.2	6.3)
1971	5	*TC+A*			58	40	69	40						(10.9	6.0)
1972	5	*UC+A*			59	44	70	44						(11.5	6.9)
	8	*MC+TC+A*	44	41	57	41	69	44	11.4	4.9	---			11.4	4.9
1973	5	*UC+A*			55	42	66	42						(12.1	7.4)
1974	5	*UC+A*			53	42	62	42						(12.2	7.7)
1975	8	*MC+TC+A*	36	36	53	40	65	41				(7.2	5.7)	(12.4	7.5)
1976	5	*UC+A*			48	37	57	37						(11.9	7.3)
1978	5	*UC+A*			49	36	58	38						(12.3	7.2)
	5	*UC+A*			48	39	56	38						(11.8	7.7)
1979	5	*MC+TC+A*	26	33	46	37	53	37	7.1	4.6	56			12.7	8.2
	8	*MC+A*	26	33			54	37				(6.7	6.9)		
	10	MC							6.5	7.1	---	6.5	7.1		
1980	5	*A*					52	33							
1981	5	TC+*A*					47	34	10.8	6.8	---			10.8	6.8
1982	5	*MC+A*	21	26			41	32				(5.3	5.4)		
1983	5	*A*					44	33							
1984	5	*A*					44	32							
1985	5	*A*					44	32							
1986	5	*A*					43	32							
1987	5	*A*					41	31							
	23	*U*					49	39							
1988	5	*A*					37	28							

Table 18.8 *(continued)*

Year	Source[2]	Product[3]	Prevalence[4]						Number of cigarettes						
									Unadjusted[7]			Sales-adjusted[8]			
			Manufactured cigarettes		Total cigarettes[5]		All products[6]		Number/ person/day		Total sales %	Manufactured cigarettes number/ person/day		Total cigarettes[9] number/ person/day	
			M	F	M	F	M	F	M	F		M	F	M	F
1989	5	*A*					36	28							
	23	*U*					45	34							
	25	TC+*A*					43	31	7.2	5.0	81			8.9	6.2
1990	5	*A*					39	30							
	25	TC+*A*					42	31	6.3	4.7	72			8.7	6.5
1991	5	*A*					38	29							
	23	*U*					46	33							
	25	TC+*A*					44	32	6.4	4.6	69			9.3	6.7
1992	5	*A*					38	30							
	25	TC+*A*					42	31	6.0	4.4	71			8.5	6.2
1993	5	*A*					37	28							
	25	TC+*A*					42	31	6.1	4.7	82			7.5	5.8
	27	*A*					49	39							
1994	5	*A*					36	28							
	23	*U*					45	36							
	25	TC+*A*					43	32	5.9	4.8	79			7.5	6.2
	27	*A*					49	40							
1995	5	*A*					39	30							
	25	TC+*A*					40	31	6.0	4.5	76			7.9	5.8
	27	*A*					49	39							

1 Surveys covering an age range of at least 21-64 are included. Any gaps in the data for ages 15-20 and 65 years and over are filled in by assumed extensions to the age distribution, given in *Notes on sources of survey data*, p. 452. Method: see *Summary of adult smoking*, p. xxxvi

2 See *Notes on sources of survey data*, p. 452

3 Product: MC = manufactured cigarettes, TC = total cigarettes (including hand-rolled), UC = cigarettes (type unspecified), A = all products, U = unspecified. Frequency of smoking is indicated by: regular or daily smokers in normal type, all smokers (including occasional) in bold, unspecified in italics

4 From Table 18.4

5 This column includes prevalence of smoking classified as UC = cigarettes (type unspecified)

6 This column includes prevalence of smoking classified as U = unspecified product

7 From Table 18.6

8 From Table 18.7, except data in parentheses, which are derived from the prevalence of smoking from Table 18.4 as described in *Summary of adult smoking*, p. xxxvi

9 Number of cigarettes classified as UC = cigarettes (type unspecified) has been adjusted to total cigarette sales and included in this column. For 1958, adjustment to sales of total cigarettes uses hand-rolled estimate for 1960

Figure 18.3 Estimated prevalence of smoking of (i) manufactured cigarettes, (ii) total cigarettes and (iii) all tobacco products: by year of survey, 1958-1995.
Males and females aged 15 years and over. *Source:* see Table 18.8

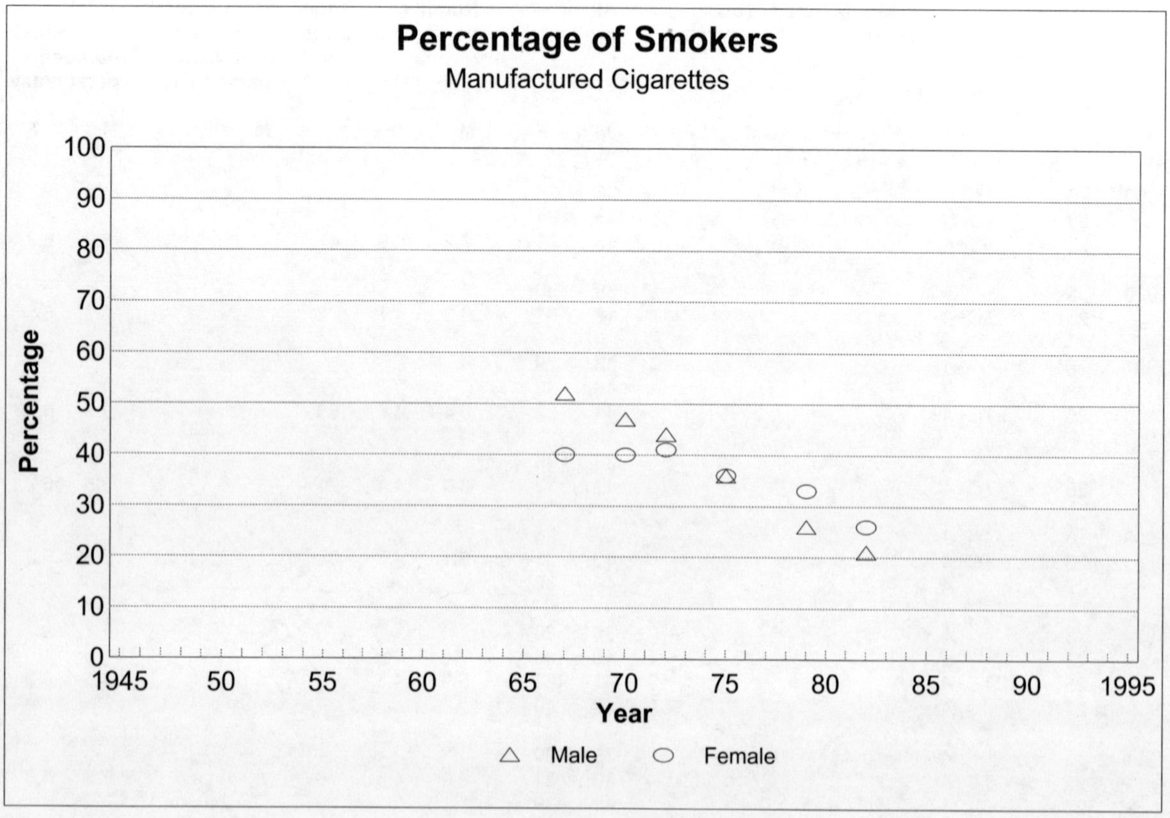

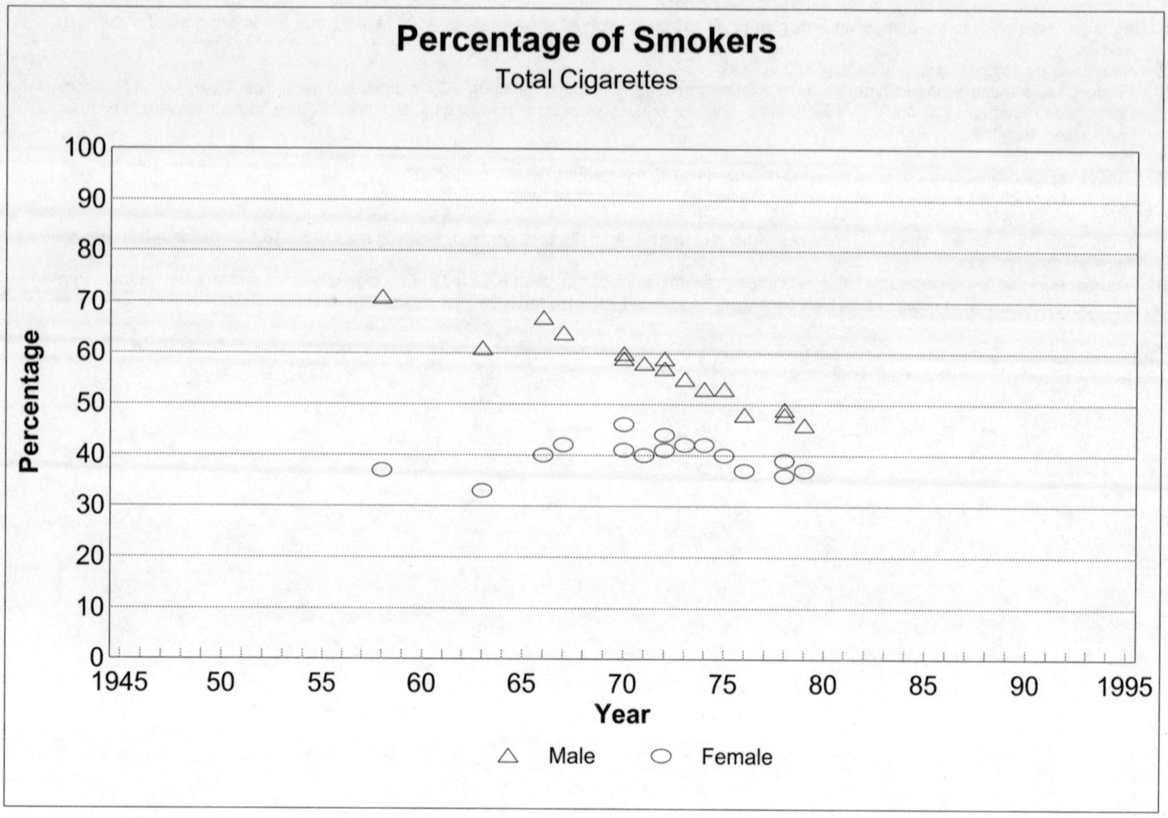

Figure 18.3 *(continued)*

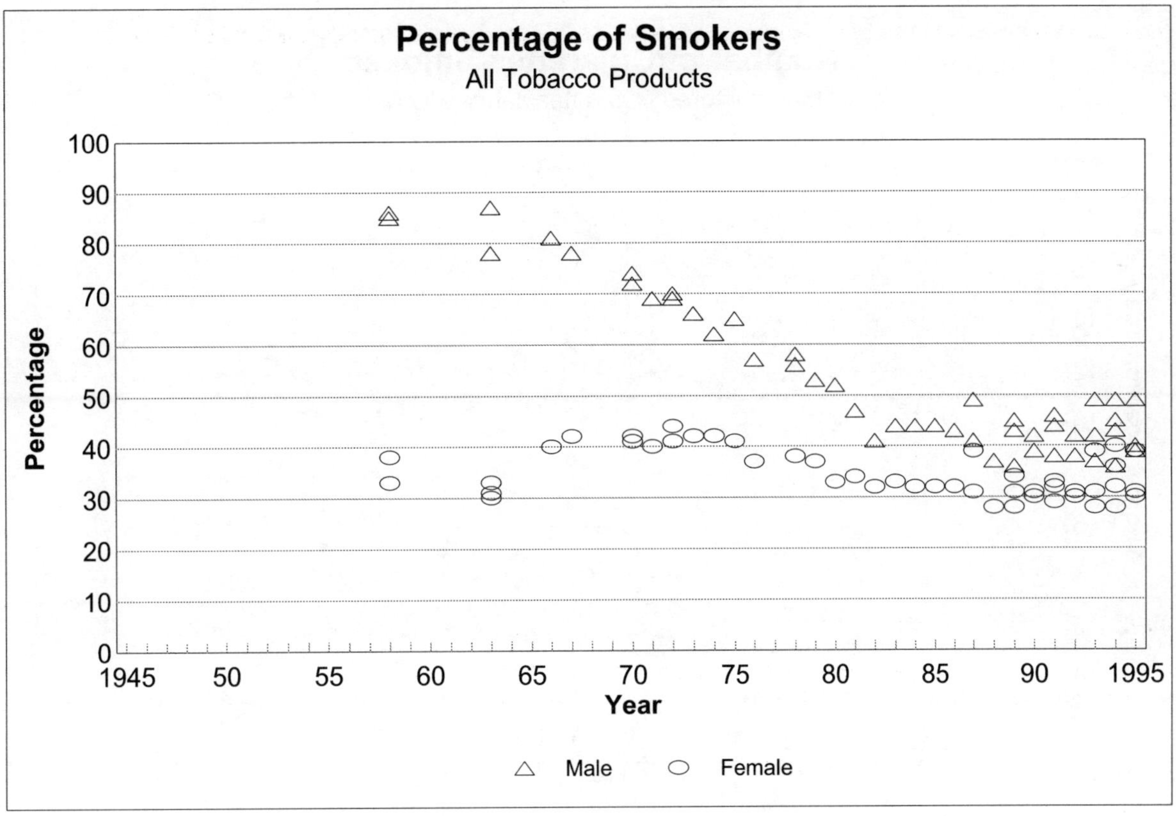

Figure 18.4 Estimated number of (i) manufactured and (ii) total cigarettes smoked per person per day, sales-adjusted, 1958-1995.
Males and females aged 15 years and over. *Source:* see Table 18.8

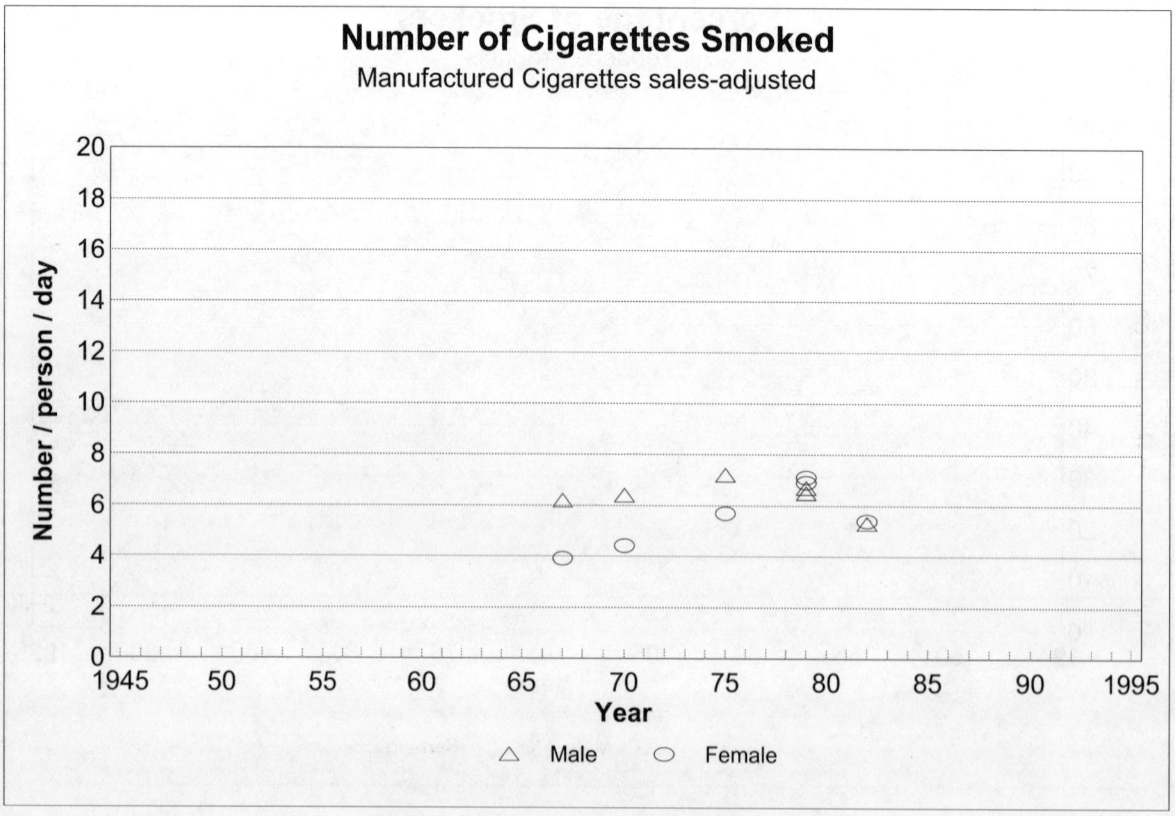

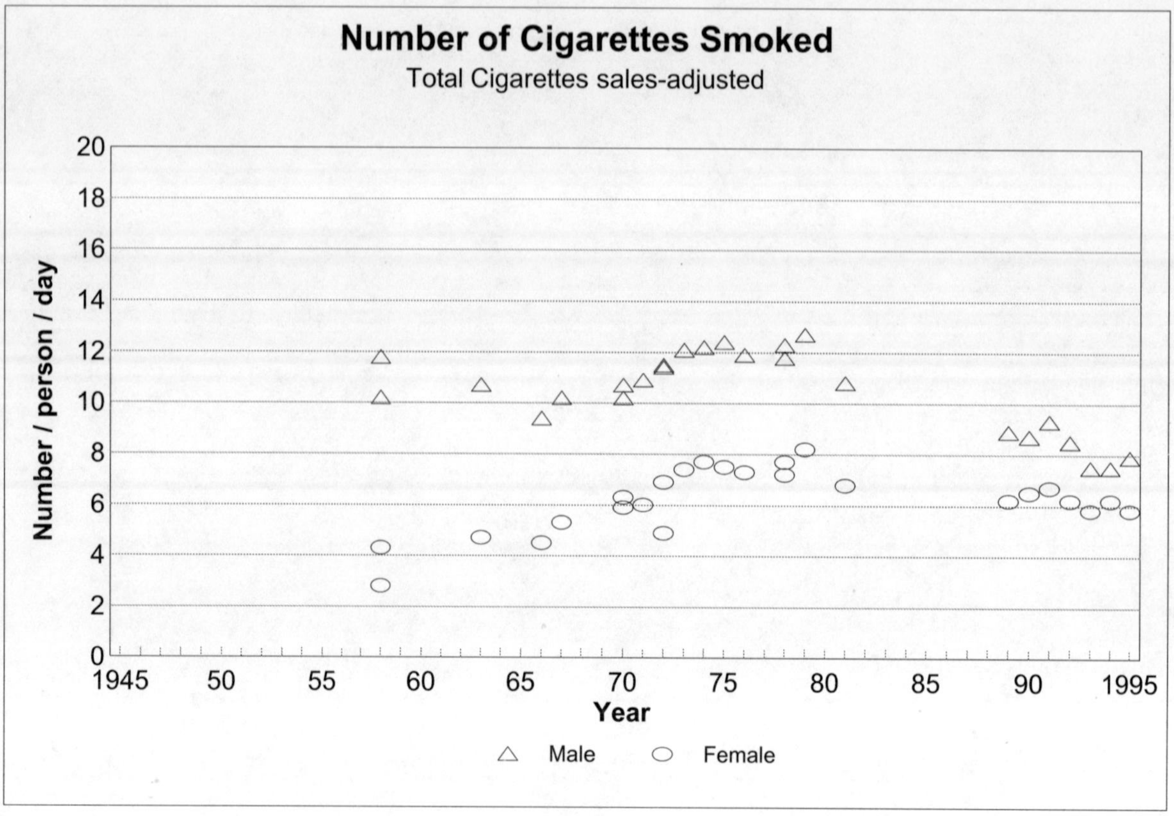

Notes on sources of sales data

The data presented in the tables and figures were obtained from several sources, details of which are given below, together with estimations and related assumptions. Full citations of the sources are given on p. 456 under *References*.

Consumption data before 1974
RP6
Data by weight, originally given to nearest 100 000 pounds, have been converted to tonnes and given to the nearest 10 tonnes (100 000 lbs = 45.359 tonnes). Where weight conversion factors have been quoted in RP6, the weights have been re-calculated without rounding and then converted to tonnes.
Notes as given in RP6:
(a) Details of the number of cigarettes, cigars and cigarillos and of the weight of cut tobacco consumed were obtained from *Produktiestatistieken Tabakverwerkende Industrie*, 1956, published by the Netherlands Central Bureau of Statistics and *Statistics of Banderoles Issued*, published by the Stichting Tabakverwerkende Industrie.
(b) Cigarette consumption in pounds weight has been estimated from the number of cigarettes consumed by using a conversion factor of 2.205 lbs per 1 000. The conversion factors used for cigars and cigarillos were 15 lbs per 1 000 and 5 lbs per 1 000 respectively.
(c) The source of the figures of tobacco consumption given above also provides information for the years 1940-45. These years have been omitted as, according to the Central Bureau of Statistics, the figures are quite unreliable.

Consumption data for 1974 onwards
Centraal Bureau voor de Statistiek
Stichting Volksgezondheid en Roken (Foundation for Smoking and Health) (1998)
Dutch Association of Cigar Manufacturers
Data are based on delivery of fiscal bands. Data were given in numbers and have been converted to weight assuming an average of 1 g per cigarette and 5.6 g per cigar or cigarillo (based on a weighted average of the values in RP6). Due to growing popularity of cigarillos relative to cigars in recent years (United States Department of Agriculture (USDA) Economic Research Service (1996)), the conversion factor for cigars and cigarillos combined may overestimate.

Plain/Filter cigarette consumption
1960-1980 Maxwell (successive years)
1982-1983 Todd (1986)
1993 Joossens *et al* (1994)

Tar yield of cigarettes
The Netherlands conforms to EU regulations on tar and nicotine yields of cigarettes although the implementation of the 15 mg limit was delayed until July 1994 (Joossens *et al* (1994)). No other data available.

Estimates of hand-rolled cigarette consumption
1960-1966 Merzdorf *et al* (1982), quoting Stichting Sigarettenindustrie (1980)
Hand-rolled cigarette consumption was estimated as 80% of fine-cut tobacco sales, at 1 g per cigarette.
1967-1985 Stichting Volksgezondheid en Roken (Foundation for Smoking and Health) (successive years)
Hand-rolled cigarette consumption was estimated as 80% of shag sales in 1967, increasing to 97% in 1985, at 1 g per cigarette.
1986-1989 we estimate 100% of cut tobacco at 1 g per cigarette.
1990-1995 Stichting Volksgezondheid en Roken (Foundation for Smoking and Health) (1998)
The source data are presented as millions of hand-rolled cigarettes at 1 g per cigarette.

For comparison, alternative estimates by de Haas (1973) up to 1972, and by de Haas and de Haas-Posthuma (1980) for 1970-1979 are shown here.

Year	Total annual in millions	Number/ adult/day	As percentage of estimate in Table 18.2
1925-1929	4 621	2.4	
1930-1934	5 751	2.8	
1935-1939	5 117	2.3	
1946-1949	3 494	1.4	
1950-1954	5 512	2.0	
1955-1959	5 505	1.9	
1960-1964	6 093	2.0	81
1965-1969	7 535	2.2	77
1970-1972	8 200	2.3	75
1970-1974	11 196	3.1	102
1975-1979	13 441	3.5	91

These data were originally given on a per capita basis, and have been converted using the mid-point population. de Haas (1973) used estimates of numbers of hand-rolled cigarettes based on 1.25 g per cigarette, which can largely explain the difference between these estimates and those of other authors, who used a basis of 1 g per cigarette.

Dymond (1996) reports the following average weights of hand-rolled cigarettes:

Year	Mean weight of fine-cut tobacco/hand-rolled cigarette (mg)
1978	869
1987	782
1994	771

Notes on sources of survey data

Each source of survey data—either an individual survey or a series of surveys repeated over a number of years—is cited by a source number. This number is shown in the tables and corresponds to the source numbers given below, where details of the source publication and of the survey methodology are given. Full citations of the sources are given on p. 456 under *References*.

Source number

1-2 These two sources relate to the same survey
1 van Reek (1983) and personal communication
2 Merzdorf *et al* (1982), quoting Gadourek and Nass (1963)

a. Based on research project 'Risky habits'. Sample size 1 297, regional based. Percentage female smokers given by van Reek included those who smoked 1 or more cigarettes per week
b. Smokers: defined themselves as such
c. Consumption per smoker is consumption of cigarettes in grams
d. Assumed extension to age distribution for percentage smokers, age 15-20: (A) males 60% and females 40%; (UC) males 50% and females 40%

3-4 These two sources relate to the same survey
3 Merzdorf *et al* (1982), quoting Readers Digest (1963)
4 van Reek (1983) and personal communication

a. Series of surveys conducted in European countries using identical questionnaires. Dutch survey conducted by Nederlandse Stichting voor Statistiek, 'Products and people' study. Random sample of about 2 000 people

b. It is also reported that 17% of men (14% age <40 and 20% age 40+) smoke a pipe, and that 46% of men (32% age <40 and 56% age 40+) smoke cigars

c. Assumed extension to age distribution for percentage smokers, age 15-20 (21) : (A) males 60% and females 40%; (UC) males 50% and females 40%

5-6 NIPO (Nederlands Instituut voor de Publieke Opinie en het Marktonderzoek) surveys for Stichting Volksgezondheid en Roken
1966, 1971, and 1979: de Haas and de Haas-Posthuma (1980)
1972-1978: Merzdorf *et al* (1982), quoting personal communication and Baan (1984)
1980-1985: Stichting Volksgezondheid en Roken (Foundation for Smoking and Health) (successive years) (successive years)
1981: van Reek (1983)
1982: van Reek (1983, 1984)

a. Interviews were conducted at home with all members of household. Proxy interviews were conducted if the subject was not at home when the interviewer called, for example in 1979, this applied to 53% of males and 18% of females (among 15-19-year-olds: 63% males, 53% females). As this procedure was found to have produced systematic bias in 15-24-year-olds, the results shown as source **6** in Table 18.4 were adjusted by van Reek (1982) by increasing the prevalence estimates by 4 percentage points. Results shown as source **6** in Table 18.5 were additionally adjusted to match taxable sales

b. There were two surveys in 1973 and 1976 (averages shown). For 1978 data given by Merzdorf *et al* (1982) are shown for age groups 13+ and 15+.

Year	**Sample size**
1971-1976	13 000-15 000
1978	15 466
1979	21 058
1980	16 977
1981	15 070
1982	13 841
1983	16 133
1984	17 384
1985	22 479

Additional notes related to 1981

c. Consumption per smoker is consumption of cigarettes in grams, adjusted (by van Reek) for 32% under-reporting. (This agrees exactly with our method of calculation on consumption per person.)

d. van Reek (1984) gives the same table of consumption per smoker, but relating to 1982

e. Consumption per person based on percentage smokers (all products) and number of cigarettes per cigarette smoker, so may overestimate

7 TON (Tijdschriften Onderzoek Nederland) surveys
1967: de Haas (1973), de Haas and de Haas-Posthuma (1980), van Reek (1983, 1984)
1970: de Haas (1973), van Reek (1983, 1984)

a. Sample size: (1967) 9 200 from 8 000 households, (1970) 12 648 from 10 000 households. Household response rate (1967) 83%, (1970) 84%

8 NOP (Nationaal Onderzoek Persmedia) surveys
1970: Merzdorf *et al* (1982)
1972: Merzdorf *et al* (1982) quoting Ministerie van Volksgezondheid en Milieu Hygiene (1975), van Reek (1984)
1975: Merzdorf *et al* (1982)
1979: van Reek (1983,1984)

a. Sample size:(1972) 30 746, (1975) 10 215, (1979) 9 930

Additional notes related to 1970

b. Relates to same survey as source 7 (before 1972, NOP surveys were called TON surveys)

Additional notes related to 1972

c. Consumption per smoker is consumption of cigarettes in grams, adjusted (by van Reek) for 23% under-reporting (by our method of calculation on consumption per person, the survey represents 89% of total cigarette consumption).

9 Sijlbing (1984)

a. Report for SWOAD (Stichting voor Wetenschappelijk Onderzoek van Alkohol- en Druggebruik, Amsterdam). Sample size 1 306, representative national sample. Interviews in September 1983
b. Regular cigarette smokers: defined themselves as such. Calculations of consumption based on all smokers (including occasional)
c. Consumption category estimation based on <3, 3-5, 6-10, 11-15, 16-20, 21-25, and 26+ cigarettes/smoker/day

10 Todd (1986)

a. Estimated by Todd

11 Merzdorf *et al* (1982), quoting Ministerie van Volksgezondheid en Milieu Hygiene (1975)

a. Assumed extension to age distribution for percentage smokers, age 15-19: (A) males 60% and females 40%. For age 15: (UC) males 30% and females 20%

12 Merzdorf *et al* (1982), quoting Nederlandse Stichting voor Statistiek

a. First age group 10-12

13 Stichting Volksgezondheid en Roken (Foundation for Smoking and Health) (successive years) and personal communication

a. Representative surveys conducted by NIPO. Children were interviewed outside the parental home. Lowest age group 10-12. Sample size: (1978) 712, (1979) 2 474, (1981) 2 592, (1982) 2 435, (1983) 2 457, (1984) 2 390, (1985) 2 434, (1992) 5 000
b. Smokers: (1978-1981) ever smoked; (1982 onwards) smoked in last 4 weeks

14 Wafelbakker (1968)

a. Study among pupils and ex-pupils of a technical school in Leiden, 1965-66. Sample size 1 310
b. Regular smokers: smoked pipes, or 1+ cigarettes per week. All smokers: additionally includes occasional smokers
c. Category consumption estimation based on 1-9, 10-39 and 40+ cigarettes/smoker/week, with pipe smokers included in the first category

15 van der Wal (1985)

a. Nationwide survey on smoking, alcohol and cannabis, conducted by school medical services in 300 schools. Sample size 24 989
b. Survey covered age 10+, but only results for age 12+ are presented here
c. Consumption category estimation based on 1, 2, 3-4, 5-6, 7-9, 10-14, 15-19, 20-24, and 25+ cigarettes/smoker/day

16 van Reek *et al* (1985), quoting van Proosdij (1957)

a. 17 local surveys by de Bond van Nederlandse Onderwijzers (Association of Dutch Teachers) in period 1907-1916. Total sample size 68 296 boys, aged 6-12. Results presented here for age group 10-12. It is also reported that 26% of boys smoked at age 6-7, and that it was assumed that few girls smoked

17 van Proosdij *et al* (1958)

a. Anonymous questionnaire survey, carried out with the assistance of NOV (Nederlandse Onderwijzers Vereniging, National Association of Teachers) at 24 primary schools in Amsterdam. Total sample size for school grades 4-6, 2 443. Results presented here are for approximate age corresponding to grade 6, sample size (males) 431, (females) 307
b. Smokers: has smoked more than once

18 Council of Europe (1978) quoting Warsink (1948) (no details of reference)

a. Controls in a study of lung cancer, sample size 100. No other details available, assumed to be males only. Age group and year unknown

19-20 Keys *et al* (1966), Djordjević *et al* (1970), van Reek *et al* (1991a)

a. Source **19**: Baseline of Seven Countries Study on cardiovascular disease. Interview including smoking questions before medical examinations. Study conducted in Zutphen, a small commercial town in eastern Netherlands. The target was to interview 43% of the population in the relevant age group. Sample size 917, response rate 84%

b. Source **20**: Follow-up study. Analysis is restricted to 358 subjects who were followed until 1985 (excluding 430 who died by 1985 and 90 who refused to participate after 1960)

c. Results taken from Keys *et al* (1966) are based on smokers of 1+ cigarettes per day, and pipe and cigar smoking are stated to be common. However, according to van Reek *et al* (1991a), frequency of smoking was undefined and would probably have been interpreted as 1+ cigarette, pipe or cigar per week

d. Consumption category estimation based on 1-9, 10-19, and 20+ cigarettes/smoker/day

21 Organisation for Economic Co-operation and Development (1993)

a. No original source

22 van Reek *et al* (1990), King and Coles (1992), King *et al* (1996)

a. Part of the HBSC (Health Behaviour in School-Aged Children) Study, a collaborative cross-national research study sponsored by the WHO. School classes or schools were randomly selected, targeting age groups 11 (not presented here), 13 and 15. The target sample size was 1 300 in each age group

b. Smokers marked as frequency *: smoked daily. Regular smokers: smoke once a week or more

23 Joossens *et al* (1999) quoting Commission of European Community

a. 1987 represents 1987/1988 etc. Age group not stated

24 van Reek *et al* (1991b, 1993)

a. Dutch Cohort Study. Baseline survey in 1989 at 36 randomly selected secondary schools. Questionnaires completed in class with teachers present. Sample size 1 454. Followup survey in 1991, postal questionnaire to home address achieved 76% response, increased to 82% by telephone interviews. Sample size 1 192

b. Approximate age corresponding to school grade

c. Smokers marked as frequency *: regular daily smoker. Regular smoker: smoked last week. All smokers: smoked last month

25 van Baal (1997), Statistika Centralbyrån (1995)

a. Netherlands Health Interview Survey. Representative of the non-institutionalized adult population. Sample size 6 000-7 000 per year

b. Data for cigarettes per person shown in Table 18.6 were given by Van Baal (1997)

c. Assumed extension to age distribution for percentage smokers, age 15: males and females 15%. Number of cigarettes/person/day: males and females 1.0

26 van Reek *et al* (1992), van Reek and Adriaanse (1995)

a. A series of surveys of Young Europeans. About 800 children aged 11-15 years interviewed in each EC country except Luxembourg (where only 250 interviewed). Lowest age group 11-12. Interviews conducted at home, with parents absent

b. Regular smokers: smoked daily. All smokers: smoked at least once a week

27 USDA (1996) quoting Dutch Cigarette Manufacturers Association

a. It is also reported that in 1995, among smokers of both sexes combined, 35% smoked cigarettes only, 24% smoked roll-your-own, 34% smoked cigarettes and roll-your own, and 7% smoked other products

b. Assumed extension to age distribution for percentage smokers age 15-17: males 20% and females 18%. For age 66+: males 30%, females 14%

Additional information (not presented in tables)

de Haas (1974) quoting Wiberdink and van Blaaderen-Stok (1957) reported that: 'In the fifties 5-10% of 15-year-old boys were regular smokers'

References

Baan B. (1984). De rol van de huisarts in de bestrijding en preventie van de rookgewoonte. *Practitioner,* 759-7.

Beese D.H. (ed) (1968). *Tobacco consumption in various countries,* 2nd edition. Tobacco Research Council, London. Research Paper 6.

Beese D.H. (ed) (1972). *Tobacco consumption in various countries,* 3rd edition. Tobacco Research Council, London. Research Paper 6.

Council of Europe (1978). *Lung cancer in Western Europe,* 3rd edition. Council of Europe, Strasbourg.

de Haas J.H. (1973). Rookpatroon in Nederland. Gaan mannen minder roken? *Hart Bulletin,* **4**, 77-86.

de Haas J.H. (1974). *Smoking trends in the Netherlands.* WHO, Geneva.

de Haas J.H. and de Haas-Posthuma J.H. (1980). *Zo rookt Nederland. Evolutie van het landelijk rookpatroon in Nederland naar sexe en leeftijd, in samenhang met welstand. (Smoking habits in the Netherlands. Evolution of the national smoking pattern in the Netherlands according to sex and age, in conjunction with level of prosperity).* Stichting Volksgezondheid en Roken, 's-Gravenhage.

Djordjević B.S., Balog B., Božinović Lj., Josipović V., *et al* (1970). Three cohorts of men followed five years in Serbia. *Circulation,* **XLI and XLII (Suppl I)**, 123-37.

Dymond H.F. (1996). Making habits of roll-your-own smokers in the Netherlands and tar and nicotine yields from the resultant products. *Tobacco Science,* **40**, 87-91.

Gadourek I. and Nass A.G. (1963). *Riskante gewoonten en zorg voor eigen welzijn.* Groningen.[§]

Hutson J.B. (1937). *Consumption and production of tobacco in Europe.* USDA, Washington DC. Technical bulletin No. 587.

Joossens L., Sasco A., Salvador T. and Villalbí J.R. (1999). Las mujeres y el tabaco en la Unión Europea (Women and tobacco in the European Union). *Revista Espanola de Salud Publica,* **73**, 3-11. http://www.msc.es/salud/epidemiologia/resp/199901/colab%5Fmujeres.htm.

Joossens L., Naett C., Howie C. and Muldoon A. (1994). *Tobacco and health in the European Union. An overview.* European Bureau for Action on Smoking Prevention (BASP), Brussels.

Keys A., Aravanis C., Blackburn H.W., van Buchem F.S.P., *et al* (1966). Epidemiological studies related to coronary heart disease: characteristics of men aged 40-59 in seven countries. *Acta Medica Scandinavica,* **Suppl 460**, 8-392.

King A., Wold B., Tudor-Smith C. and Harel Y. (1996). *The health of youth, a cross-national survey.* WHO Regional Publications, Europe, Copenhagen. European Series No. 69.

King A.J.C. and Coles B. (1992). *The health of Canada's youth. Views and behaviours of 11-, 13- and 15-year-olds from 11 countries.* Health and Welfare Canada, Ottawa.

Lee P.N. (ed) (1975). *Tobacco consumption in various countries,* 4th edition. Tobacco Research Council, London. Research Paper 6.

Maxwell J.C.Jr. (successive years). How the brands ranked. Maxwell International Estimates. *World Tobacco.*

Merzdorf J., Reuter U. and Welsch G. (1982). *Daten und Fakten zur Entwicklung des Rauchens in Mitgliedsländern der Europäischen Gemeinschaften (Facts and figures on the development of smoking in the member states of the European Communities).* Kommission der Europäischen Gemeinschaften, Luxemburg. Medizin—EUR 7907 DE.

Ministerie van Volksgezondheid en Milieu Hygiene (1975). *Maatregeln tot beperking van het roken. Advies van de Gezondheidsraad.* Nr 23 der Schriftenreihe Verslagen, Adviezen, Rapporten.§

Organisation for Economic Co-operation and Development (1993). *OECD health systems. Facts and trends 1960-1991. Health policy studies no 3.* OECD, Paris. (Health policy studies, Volume 1.)

Readers Digest (1963). *Products and people. A digest of the marketing survey of the European Common Market and Britain, 1963* . Reader's Digest Association Limited, London.

RP6, See Beese (ed) (1968), Beese (ed) (1972), Lee (ed) (1975)

Sijlbing G. (1984). *Het gebruik van drugs, alcohol en tabak.* SWOAD, Amsterdam.

Statistika Centralbyrån (1995). *Tobacco consumption 1970-1994 in the member states of the European Union and in Norway and Iceland.* European Commission.

Stichting Sigarettenindustrie (1980). *De sigaret—feiten en ontwikkeling* Den Haag.§

Stichting Volksgezondheid en Roken (Foundation for Smoking and Health) (successive years). *Jaarverslag (Annual report).* Stichting Volksgezondheid en Roken, 's-Gravenhage.

Stichting Volksgezondheid en Roken (Foundation for Smoking and Health) (1998). *Jaarverslag (Annual report) '97.* Stichting Volksgezondheid en Roken (Stivoro). http://www.stivoro.nl/actueel/jaarvers/jaarv97/index.htm.

Todd G. (1986). *Medicine. Statistics of smoking in the Member States of the European Community.* Commission of the European Communities, Luxembourg.

USDA (1996). *Tobacco Annual 1996.* AGR Number NL6080. http://www.fas.usda.gov.

USDA Economic Research Service (1996). *Tobacco statistics.* Albert R. Mann Library, Cornell University, Ithaca, New York. ERS 94012. (With supplementary material from Tobacco Annual Reports.). http://usda.mannlib.cornell.edu/data-sets/specialty/94012.

van Baal M. (1997). *Trendcijfers gezondheidsenquête; Aspecten van (on)gezond gedrag, 1989-1996 (Trend figures Netherlands Health Interview Survey; aspects of (un)healthy behaviour, 1989-1996).* Centraal Bureau voor de Statistiek, Voorburg/Heerlen. (Maandbericht gezondheidsstatistiek, Volume 16.)

van der Wal H.J. (1985). *Roken, drinken, cannabisgebruik. (The use of tobacco, alcohol and cannabis).* SWOAD, Amsterdam.

van Proosdij C. (1957). *Roken (Smoking)* [Thesis]. Geemente Universiteit, Amsterdam.§

van Proosdij C., de Jong Z. and van Proosdij-Hartzema E.G. (1958). Een onderzoek naar de rookgewonten op 24 lagere scholen te Amsterdam. (An inquiry into smoking habits in 24 primary schools of Amsterdam). *Ned Tijdschr Geneeskd,* **102**, 902-5.

van Reek J. (1982). Changes in the prevalence of smoking among teen-agers and young adults in the Netherlands during the twentieth century. In: Fontana F. (ed) *Tabacco e giovani (Tobacco and youth), International conference, Venice 9-11 November 1981.* ATTI, Venice; 337-41.

van Reek J. (1983). Rookgedrag in Nederland van 1958-1982. (Smoking behaviour in The Netherlands from 1958 to 1982). *Tijdschrift voor Alcohol en Drugs,* **9**, 99-103.

van Reek J. (1984). Smoking behaviour in the Netherlands and the United Kingdom. *Rev Epidemiol Sante Publique,* **32**, 383-90.

van Reek J. and Adriaanse H. (1995). Daily smoking among adolescents in the European Community. *Rev*

Epidemiol Sante Publique, **43**, 281-2.

van Reek J., Adriaanse H. and Aarø L.E. (1990). Smoking by schoolchildren in eleven European countries. In: Durston B. and Jamrozik K. (eds) *Tobacco & health 1990. The global war. Seventh world conference on tobacco and health, 1st-5th April 1990, Perth, Western Australia.* Organising committee of the Seventh World Conference on Tobacco and Health, 189 Royal Street, East Perth, Western Australia 6004; 301-2.

van Reek J., Adriaanse H. and Karaoglou A. (1992). Smoking among children in the European Community. *J Public Health Med,* **14**, 93-4.

van Reek J., Adriaanse H., Ramstrøm L. and Kromhout D. (1991a). Smoking recidivism among an age cohort of men in Zutphen (The Netherlands): 1960-1985. *Rev Epidemiol Sante Publique,* **39**, 297-300.

van Reek J., Drop M.J. and Joosten J. (1985). Het rookgedrag van Nederlandse schoolkinderen en de invloed van leeftijdgenoten en ouders. (The influence of peer pressure and parental smoking behaviour upon smoking among Dutch schoolchildren). *Tijdschrift voor Alcohol en Drugs,* **11**, 74-9.

van Reek J., Knibbe R. and van Iwaarden T. (1991b). Policy relevance of a survey on smoking and drinking behaviour among Dutch school children. *Health Policy,* **18**, 261-8.

van Reek J., Knibbe R. and van Iwaarden T. (1993). Policy elements as predictors of smoking and drinking behaviour: the Dutch Cohort Study of secondary schoolchildren. *Health Policy,* **26**, 5-18.

Wafelbakker F. (1968). Rookgewoonten bij manlijke adolescenten 1. (Smoking habits in male adolescents). *Ned Tijdschr Geneeskd,* **46**, 518-25.

Wiberdink J. and van Blaaderen-Stok C.L. (1957). Bestrijding van longkanker door beperking van tabaksgebruik. (Fight against lung cancer by restriction of tobacco consumption). *Ned Tijdschr Geneeskd,* **101**, 1695-700.[§]

§ Original paper not obtained, but information taken as quoted by another author

New Zealand 19

Sales data

See Tables 19.1-19.3.

From 1920 until the late 1970s the consumption of manufactured cigarettes per adult increased, with some fluctuations, from 1 to 8 cigarettes per day. It decreased to 3.5 cigarettes per day in 1995. Evidence on consumption of hand-rolled cigarettes is conflicting; we estimate that consumption per adult decreased from 3.5 cigarettes per day in 1950 to 0.5 by 1980, and remained about that level until 1995.

Consumption of all tobacco products per adult fluctuated between 5 and 7 g per day from 1920 to 1945; after rising in the late 1940s, it remained at about 9-10 g from 1950 to 1980 and fell to about 4.5 g by 1995. In the 1920s and 1930s, 25-35% of all tobacco was consumed as manufactured cigarettes, increasing to over 90% between 1975 and 1988, but then decreasing again to 82% in 1995. The remainder was pipe and hand-rolling tobacco, which was predominantly used in hand-rolled cigarettes. Consumption of cigars was negligible.

Survey data

See Tables 19.4-19.8

In 1964, the prevalence of smoking in a sample of Europeans was over 50% among men and 30% among women. The prevalence among Maori women was double that of European women. Census results in 1976 and 1981 provide a detailed age breakdown. In 1976, the prevalence of cigarette smoking among those aged 15 years and over was 40% in men and 32% in women. In 1981, the prevalence declined to about 35% in men and 30% in women. Annual surveys have since shown that the prevalence of smoking continued to fall among both men and women until about 1990, since when it has remained about 27% for both sexes. There are no data on prevalence by type of cigarette.

The prevalence of smoking decreased among men at all ages, notably among those aged over 55; among women, decreases were greatest for those between 25 and 64 years of age. More men than women smoked in the older age groups, but in the younger age groups there is equality or the reverse, and the age at which this switch occurs is gradually increasing—from 15-19 in 1976, 20-24 in 1981, and 25-34 in the mid-1980s.

The prevalence of smoking among girls was lower than among boys when first surveyed in 1960. Although comparisons are difficult owing to different or unknown definitions of 'a smoker' and absence of repeat surveys, the prevalence between about 1970 and 1985 seems to have increased among girls but decreased among boys; most surveys indicate that the prevalence among girls has been higher than among boys since the mid-1970s. A series of surveys among pupils in Wellington in the 1990s shows an increase in prevalence for both boys and girls.

Comparison of survey and sales data suggests that the censuses under-reported consumption by about 30-35%. Between 1976 and 1995, the estimated number of cigarettes smoked per person per day (sales-adjusted) decreased from about 10 to 4 for men, and from 6 to 3 for women.

Table 19.1.1 Total annual sales of (i) tobacco products, 1920-1973, and (ii) cigarette papers, 1935-1973

Year	Cigarettes tonnes	Cigarettes millions	Pipe and hand-rolling tobacco tonnes	All tobacco products tonnes	Cigarette papers millions
1920	580	511	1410	1990	
1921	440	392	1220	1670	
1922	500	443	1180	1680	
1923	560	495	1180	1740	
1924	610	542	1180	1790	
1925	690	606	1360	2050	
1926	730	645	1320	2050	
1927	780	686	1410	2180	
1928	770	683	1360	2140	
1929	820	719	1450	2270	
1930	710	626	1500	2210	
1931	560	498	1540	2110	
1932	460	406	1540	2000	
1933	480	426	1540	2030	
1934	530	463	1590	2110	
1935	660	584	1540	2200	1350
1936	810	712	1680	2490	1589
1937	940	828	1720	2660	1517
1938	1040	916	1770	2810	1980
1939	1070	943	1910	2970	1476
1940	970	852	1910	2870	1808
1941	1020	900	1950	2970	1843
1942	1130	1000	1720	2860	1670
1943	1150	1018	1540	2700	1899
1944	1290	1134	1450	2740	1656
1945	1340	1180	1630	2970	1597
1946	1790	1582	1860	3650	1455
1947	2320	2044	1860	4180	3281
1948	1910	1682	2000	3900	2155
1949	1940	1714	2000	3940	1875
1950	2250	1984	2310	4560	2383
1951	2440	2152	2360	4800	2218
1952	2360	2080	2360	4720	2782
1953	2370	2091	2490	4870	2340
1954	2610	2306	2450	5060	2282
1955	2910	2567	2360	5270	2253
1956	2980	2629	2040	5020	2823
1957	3170	2792	2220	5390	2203
1958	2960	2606	2130	5090	2287
1959	2850	2509	2130	4980	2542
1960	3490	3082	2180	5670	2377
1961	3580	3160	2180	5760	2228
1962	3810	3360	2040	5850	2070
1963	4200	3703	2000	6190	1971
1964	4300	3796	1770	6070	1680
1965	4650	4102	1540	6190	1487
1966	5170	4557	1450	6620	1324
1967	5150	4542	1270	6420	1178
1968	5270	4649	1180	6450	1125
1969	5460	4818	1090	6550	985
1970	5620	4952	1070	6690	911
1971	5800	5118	950	6760	810
1972	6130	5405	950	7080	1000
1973	6270	5525	860	7130	857

Source: see *Notes on sources of sales data*, p. 473

Table 19.1.2 Total annual sales of tobacco products, 1974-1995

Year	Cigarettes		Loose tobacco tonnes	All tobacco products tonnes
	tonnes	millions		
1974	6519	5769	782	7301
1975	7039	6229	749	7788
1976	7040	6230	702	7742
1977	7171	6346	666	7837
1978	7083	6268	610	7693
1979	6927	6130	575	7502
1980	6770	5991	548	7318
1981	6970	6168	553	7523
1982	6907	6112	539	7446
1983	6881	6089	546	7427
1984	7047	6236	534	7581
1985	6389	5654	493	6882
1986	5902	5223	501	6403
1987	6058	5361	511	6569
1988	6051	5355	552	6603
1989	4825	4270	554	5379
1990	5073	4489	602	5675
1991	4536	4014	652	5188
1992	3917	3466	768	4685
1993	3821	3381	810	4631
1994	3837	3396	694	4531
1995	3598	3184	771	4369

Source : see *Notes on sources of sales data,* p. 473

Table 19.1.3 Manufactured cigarettes (i) percentage of total sales as filter cigarettes, 1961-1978, (ii) sales-weighted average tar yield per cigarette (SWAT), 1990 and 1995, and (iii) sales-weighted nicotine yield per cigarette (SWAN), 1994-1995

Year	% Filter	SWAT mg/cig	SWAN mg/cig
1961	42.7		
1962	48.0		
1963	52.7		
1964	55.0		
1965	60.0		
1973	90.7		
1974	92.4		
1975	93.0		
1976	94.0		
1977	94.6		
1978	95.4		
1990		13.2	
1994			1.19
1995		13.7	1.18

Source : see *Notes on sources of sales data,* p. 473

Table 19.2 Consumption of (i) cigarettes and (ii) all tobacco products, 1920-1995 sales-based data, including estimated hand-rolled cigarette consumption. Males and females aged 15 years and over

Year	Manufactured cigarettes		Hand-rolled cigarettes		Total cigarettes		All tobacco products	
	Total annual in millions	Number/ adult/day	Total annual in millions	Number/ adult/day	Total annual in millions	Number/ adult/day	Total annual in tonnes	Grams/ adult/day
1920	511	1.8					1990	6.8
1921	392	1.2					1670	5.1
1922	443	1.3					1680	5.1
1923	495	1.5					1740	5.3
1924	542	1.6					1790	5.4
1925	606	1.7					2050	5.6
1926	645	1.8					2050	5.6
1927	686	1.9					2180	6.0
1928	683	1.9					2140	5.9
1929	719	2.0					2270	6.2
1930	626	1.6					2210	5.5
1931	498	1.2					2110	5.3
1932	406	1.0					2000	5.0
1933	426	1.1					2030	5.1
1934	463	1.2					2110	5.3
1935	584	1.5					2200	5.5
1936	712	1.6					2490	5.7
1937	828	1.9					2660	6.1
1938	916	2.1					2810	6.4
1939	943	2.2					2970	6.8
1940	852	1.9					2870	6.6
1941	900	2.1					2970	6.8
1942	1000	2.3					2860	6.5
1943	1018	2.3					2700	6.2
1944	1134	2.6					2740	6.3
1945	1180	2.7					2970	6.8
1946	1582	3.3					3650	7.7
1947	2044	4.3					4180	8.8
1948	1682	3.5					3900	8.2
1949	1714	3.6					3940	8.3
1950	1984	4.0	1802	3.6	3786	7.6	4560	9.2
1951	2152	4.3	1841	3.7	3993	8.0	4800	9.6
1952	2080	4.1	1841	3.6	3921	7.7	4720	9.3
1953	2091	4.0	1942	3.7	4033	7.8	4870	9.4
1954	2306	4.4	1911	3.6	4217	8.0	5060	9.6
1955	2567	4.8	1841	3.4	4408	8.2	5270	9.8
1956	2629	4.8	1591	2.9	4220	7.7	5020	9.2
1957	2792	5.0	1732	3.1	4524	8.1	5390	9.7
1958	2606	4.6	1661	2.9	4267	7.5	5090	9.0
1959	2509	4.4	1661	2.9	4170	7.3	4980	8.7
1960	3082	5.3	1700	2.9	4782	8.2	5670	9.7
1961	3160	5.3	1700	2.9	4860	8.2	5760	9.7
1962	3360	5.5	1591	2.6	4951	8.1	5850	9.6
1963	3703	5.9	1560	2.5	5263	8.5	6190	9.9
1964	3796	6.0	1381	2.2	5177	8.1	6070	9.5
1965	4102	6.3	1201	1.8	5303	8.2	6190	9.5
1966	4557	6.9	1131	1.7	5688	8.6	6620	10.0
1967	4542	6.8	991	1.5	5533	8.2	6420	9.6
1968	4649	6.8	920	1.4	5569	8.2	6450	9.5
1969	4818	7.0	850	1.2	5668	8.2	6550	9.5

Table 19.2 *(continued)*

Year	Manufactured cigarettes		Hand-rolled cigarettes		Total cigarettes		All tobacco products	
	Total annual in millions	Number/ adult/day	Total annual in millions	Number/ adult/day	Total annual in millions	Number/ adult/day	Total annual in tonnes	Grams/ adult/day
1970	4952	7.1	835	1.2	5787	8.3	6690	9.5
1971	5118	7.2	741	1.0	5859	8.2	6760	9.5
1972	5405	7.3	741	1.0	6146	8.3	7080	9.5
1973	5525	7.4	671	0.9	6196	8.3	7130	9.5
1974	5769	7.5	610	0.8	6379	8.3	7301	9.5
1975	6229	7.9	584	0.7	6813	8.6	7788	9.9
1976	6230	7.7	548	0.7	6778	8.4	7742	9.6
1977	6346	7.9	519	0.6	6865	8.5	7837	9.8
1978	6268	7.7	476	0.6	6744	8.2	7693	9.4
1979	6130	7.4	448	0.5	6578	8.0	7502	9.1
1980	5991	7.2	427	0.5	6418	7.7	7318	8.8
1981	6168	7.3	431	0.5	6599	7.8	7523	8.9
1982	6112	7.1	420	0.5	6532	7.6	7446	8.7
1983	6089	7.0	426	0.5	6515	7.4	7427	8.5
1984	6236	7.0	417	0.5	6653	7.5	7581	8.5
1985	5654	6.3	385	0.4	6039	6.7	6882	7.6
1986	5223	5.8	391	0.4	5614	6.2	6403	7.1
1987	5361	5.8	399	0.4	5760	6.3	6569	7.1
1988	5355	5.8	431	0.5	5786	6.2	6603	7.1
1989	4270	4.6	432	0.5	4702	5.0	5379	5.7
1990	4489	4.7	470	0.5	4959	5.2	5675	6.0
1991	4014	4.2	509	0.5	4523	4.8	5188	5.5
1992	3466	3.6	599	0.6	4065	4.2	4685	4.9
1993	3381	3.5	632	0.7	4013	4.1	4631	4.8
1994	3396	3.5	541	0.6	3937	4.0	4531	4.6
1995	3184	3.2	601	0.6	3785	3.8	4369	4.4

Source : see *Notes on sources of sales data,* p. 473

Figure 19.1 Daily consumption of (i) manufactured and total number of cigarettes, and (ii) all tobacco products, 1920-1995.
Males and females aged 15 years and over. *Source:* see Table 19.2

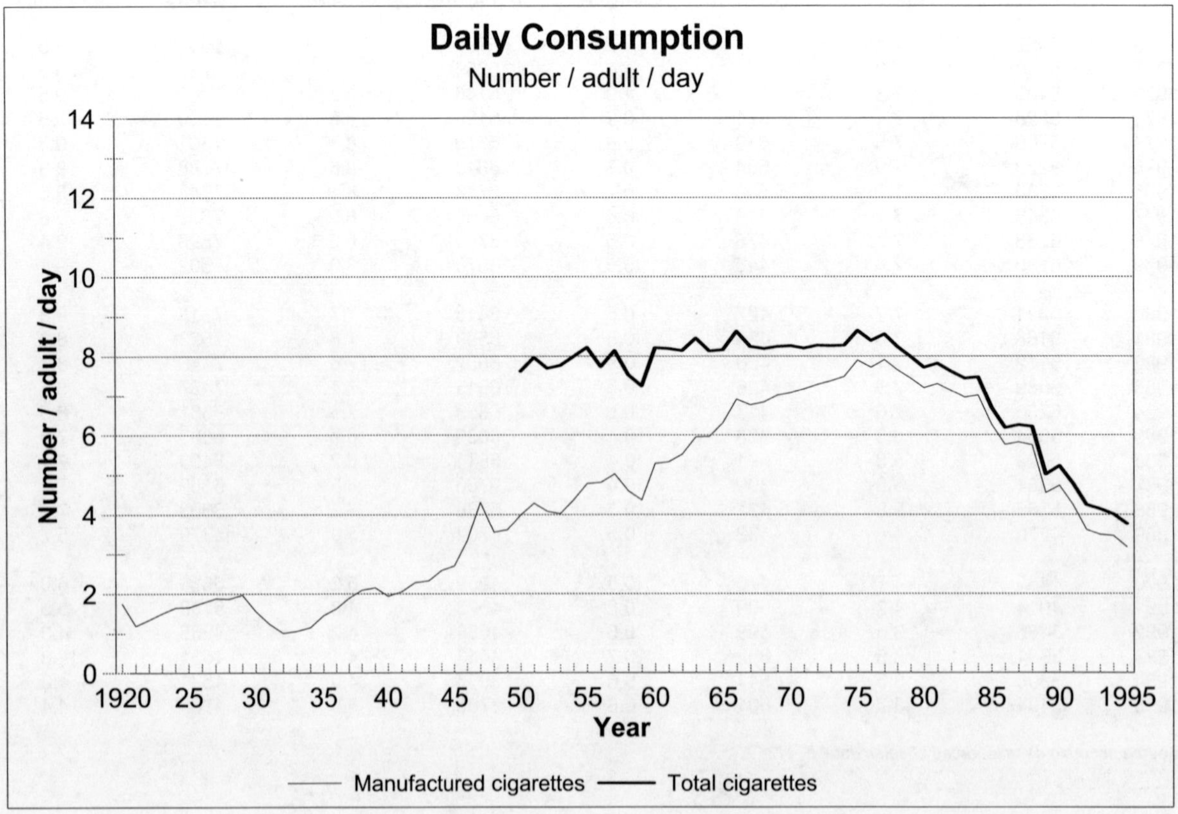

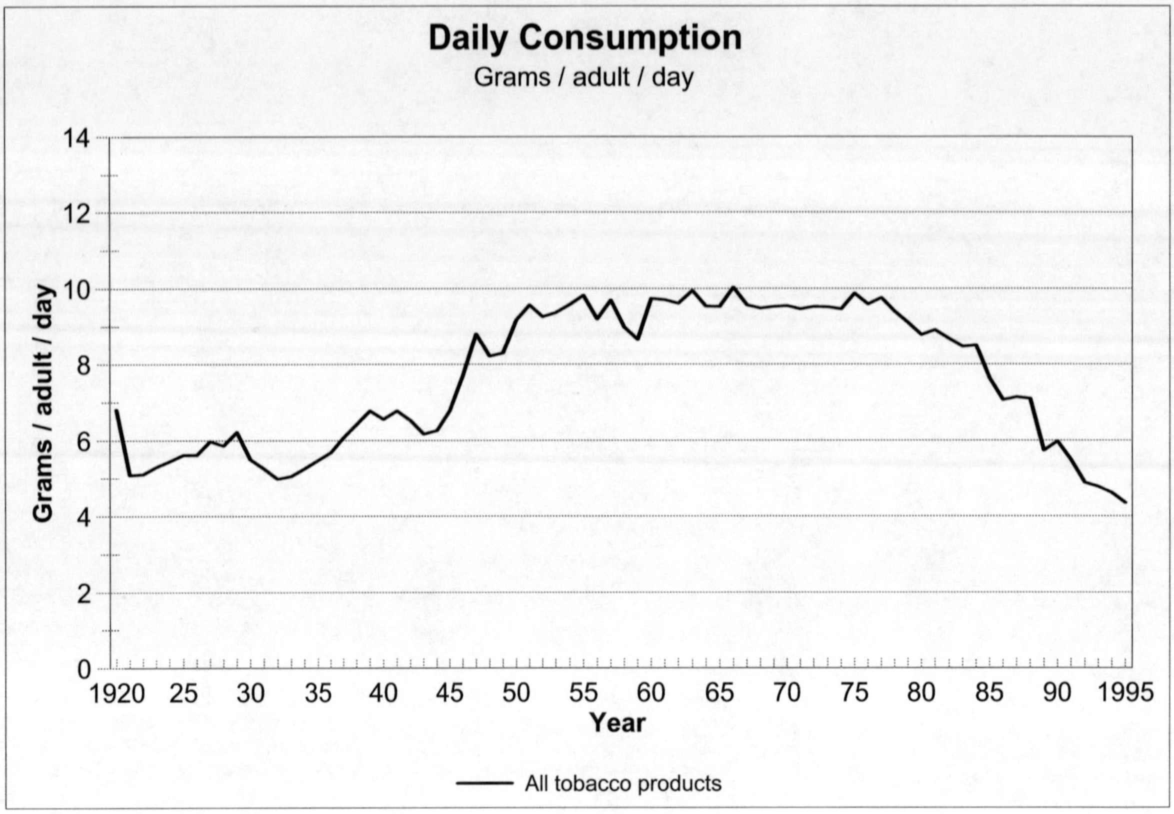

Table 19.3 Percentage sales of tobacco in different forms (by weight), selected years 1925-1995

Year	Cigarettes (%)	Other tobacco (%)
1925	33.7	66.3
1935	30.0	70.0
1945	45.1	54.9
1955	55.2	44.8
1965	75.1	24.9
1975	90.4	9.6
1985	92.8	7.2
1995	82.4	17.6

Source : calculated from Tables 19.1.1 & 19.1.2

Figure 19.2 Percentage sales of tobacco in different forms (by weight), selected years 1925-1995
Source: see Table 19.3

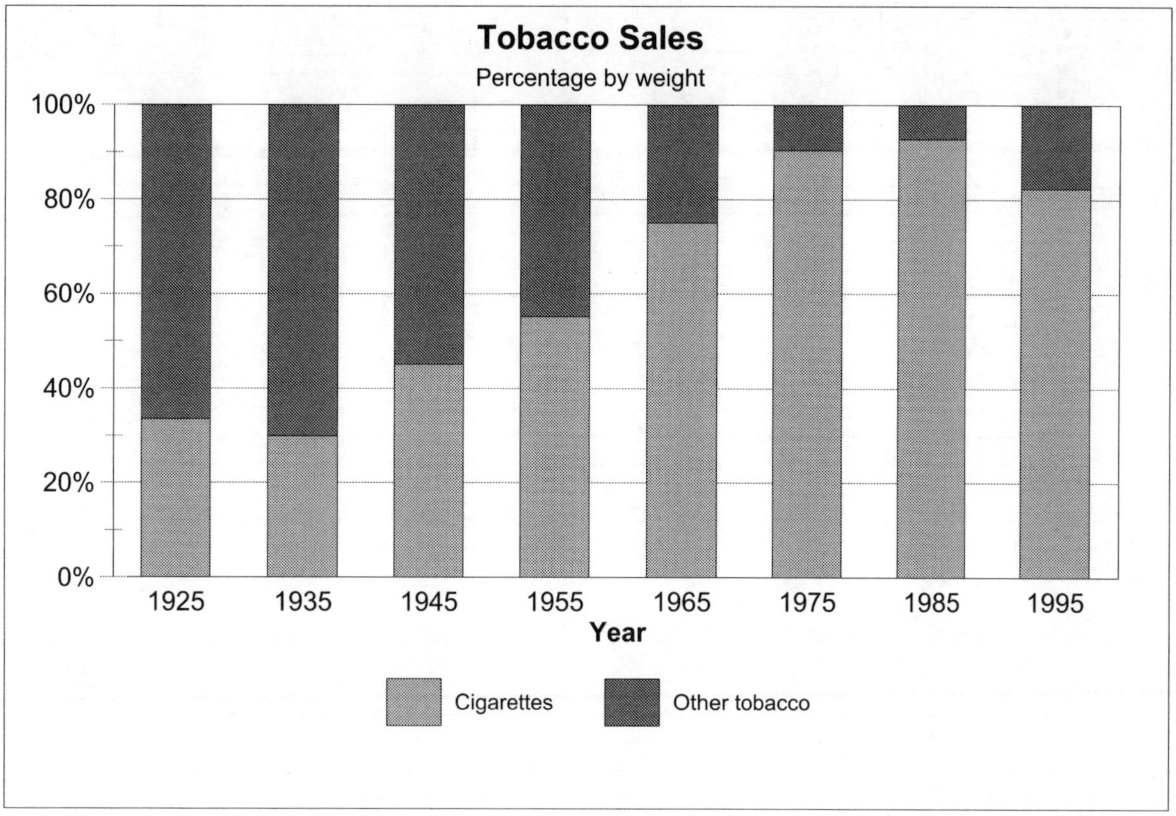

Table 19.4M Prevalence of smoking, males: some selected New Zealand surveys by age, 1960-1995

Frequency / Product / Source / Year	Age group																					All ages
	12	13	14	15	16	17	18	19	20-24	25-29	30-34	35-39	40-44	45-49	50-54	55-59	60-64	65-69	70-74	75-79	80+	
60 7 UC *	24																					
60 7 UC R	35																					
60 7 UC A	40		53	54	41	37																47
64 11 UC R																						
64 12 A R									55													
68 4 U R	15																					
68 4 U A	32																					
69 6 UC R		2	9	13	1																	
69 6 UC A		21	38	38	30																	
72 8 U U		30																				
74 3 UC R																						
75 2 UC U				41																		
75 13 U A	35		46	48	56																	45
76 1 UC R	30								42	43	44	43	44	45	44	57	38	35	31	27	20	40
76 5 UC *	11		18																			
76 5 UC U	30		29																			
77 14 U A			35		50																	
81 1 UC R	27								40	38	37	38	38	38	38	36	32	29	25	20		35
81 4 U R	13																					
81 4 U A	24																					
82 10 UC R												31		27		28						29
82 10 A A												37		33		33						34
83 15 TC R				34						38		37				29						35
83 16 UC R			15																			
83 16 UC A			23																			
84 15 TC R				35						39		35				27						34
85 9 U R		16		14																		
85 15 TC R				31						35		31				24						30
85 17 UC R		1																				
85 17 U A		11																				
86 15 TC R				31						32		29				24						29
87 15 TC R				32						34		34				22						31
87 17 UC R				11																		
87 17 U A				21																		
88 15 TC R				27						38		31				20						29
89 13 U A	26																					
89 15 TC R				28						30		28				20						27
90 15 TC R				30						32		30				18						28
90 19 UC R							28															
90 19 U A							37															
91 15 TC R				28						35		27				18						27
91 18 U R			8																			
91 18 U A			12																			
92 15 TC R				25						34		29				18						27
92 19 UC R			11																			
92 19 UC A			22																			
93 15 TC R				28						35		30				19						28
93 18 U R			8																			
93 18 U A			15																			
94 15 TC R				28						36		30				17						28
95 15 TC R				25						35		29				19						27
95 18 U R			12																			
95 18 U A			18																			

Source: see *Notes on sources of survey data*, p. 474

Product: MC = manufactured cigarettes
TC = total cigarettes (including hand-rolled)
UC = cigarettes (type unspecified)
A = all products

Frequency: A = all smokers (including occasional)
R = regular or daily smokers

All ages: relevant to ages used and as given in original source

U = unspecified

* = refer to *Notes on sources of survey data*, p. 474

Table 19.4F Prevalence of smoking, females: some selected New Zealand surveys by age, 1960-1995

<table>
<tr><td rowspan="2">Frequency
Product
Source
Year</td><td colspan="21">Age group</td><td rowspan="2">All ages</td></tr>
<tr><td>12</td><td>13</td><td>14</td><td>15</td><td>16</td><td>17</td><td>18</td><td>19</td><td>20-24</td><td>25-29</td><td>30-34</td><td>35-39</td><td>40-44</td><td>45-49</td><td>50-54</td><td>55-59</td><td>60-64</td><td>65-69</td><td>70-74</td><td>75-79</td><td>80+</td></tr>
<tr><td>60 7 UC *</td><td colspan="8">6</td><td colspan="13"></td><td></td></tr>
<tr><td>60 7 UC R</td><td colspan="8">13</td><td colspan="13"></td><td></td></tr>
<tr><td>60 7 UC A</td><td colspan="2">17</td><td>28</td><td>29</td><td>25</td><td colspan="3">20</td><td colspan="13"></td><td>25</td></tr>
<tr><td>64 11 UC R</td><td colspan="3"></td><td colspan="18">61</td><td></td></tr>
<tr><td>64 12 A R</td><td colspan="8"></td><td colspan="10">35</td><td colspan="3">0</td><td>31</td></tr>
<tr><td>68 4 U R</td><td colspan="3"></td><td colspan="2">7</td><td colspan="16"></td><td></td></tr>
<tr><td>68 4 U A</td><td colspan="3"></td><td colspan="2">25</td><td colspan="16"></td><td></td></tr>
<tr><td>69 6 UC R</td><td></td><td>3</td><td>10</td><td>6</td><td colspan="2">9</td><td colspan="15"></td><td></td></tr>
<tr><td>69 6 UC A</td><td></td><td>21</td><td>37</td><td>32</td><td colspan="2">25</td><td colspan="15"></td><td></td></tr>
<tr><td>72 8 U U</td><td></td><td colspan="4">31</td><td colspan="16"></td><td></td></tr>
<tr><td>74 3 UC R</td><td colspan="3"></td><td colspan="6">33</td><td colspan="2">37</td><td colspan="2">36</td><td colspan="2">40</td><td colspan="6">19</td><td>31</td></tr>
<tr><td>75 2 UC U</td><td colspan="21"></td><td></td></tr>
<tr><td>75 13 U A</td><td colspan="2">38</td><td>43</td><td>51</td><td colspan="3">63</td><td colspan="14"></td><td>46</td></tr>
<tr><td>76 1 UC R</td><td colspan="3"></td><td colspan="5">30</td><td>39</td><td>38</td><td>38</td><td>35</td><td>35</td><td>36</td><td>34</td><td>31</td><td>26</td><td>20</td><td>15</td><td>11</td><td>6</td><td>32</td></tr>
<tr><td>76 5 UC *</td><td colspan="2">6</td><td colspan="2">27</td><td colspan="17"></td><td></td></tr>
<tr><td>76 5 UC U</td><td colspan="2">29</td><td colspan="2">43</td><td colspan="17"></td><td></td></tr>
<tr><td>77 14 U A</td><td colspan="2"></td><td colspan="2">35</td><td>40</td><td colspan="16"></td><td></td></tr>
<tr><td>81 1 UC R</td><td colspan="3"></td><td colspan="5">30</td><td>40</td><td>35</td><td>33</td><td>33</td><td>31</td><td>31</td><td>31</td><td>28</td><td>25</td><td>20</td><td>15</td><td colspan="2">8</td><td>30</td></tr>
<tr><td>81 4 U R</td><td colspan="3"></td><td colspan="2">33</td><td colspan="16"></td><td></td></tr>
<tr><td>81 4 U A</td><td colspan="3"></td><td colspan="2">47</td><td colspan="16"></td><td></td></tr>
<tr><td>82 10 UC R</td><td colspan="11"></td><td colspan="2">26</td><td colspan="2">26</td><td colspan="2">22</td><td colspan="4"></td><td>25</td></tr>
<tr><td>82 10 A A</td><td colspan="11"></td><td colspan="2">30</td><td colspan="2">27</td><td colspan="2">23</td><td colspan="4"></td><td>27</td></tr>
<tr><td>83 15 TC R</td><td colspan="3"></td><td colspan="6">40</td><td colspan="2">35</td><td colspan="4">31</td><td colspan="6">21</td><td>31</td></tr>
<tr><td>83 16 UC R</td><td colspan="2"></td><td colspan="2">24</td><td colspan="17"></td><td></td></tr>
<tr><td>83 16 UC A</td><td colspan="2"></td><td colspan="2">38</td><td colspan="17"></td><td></td></tr>
<tr><td>84 15 TC R</td><td colspan="3"></td><td colspan="6">40</td><td colspan="2">34</td><td colspan="4">29</td><td colspan="6">22</td><td>31</td></tr>
<tr><td>85 9 U R</td><td></td><td colspan="2">26</td><td colspan="3">18</td><td colspan="15"></td><td></td></tr>
<tr><td>85 15 TC R</td><td colspan="3"></td><td colspan="6">40</td><td colspan="2">34</td><td colspan="4">29</td><td colspan="6">19</td><td>30</td></tr>
<tr><td>85 17 UC R</td><td></td><td>1</td><td colspan="19"></td><td></td></tr>
<tr><td>85 17 U A</td><td></td><td>9</td><td colspan="19"></td><td></td></tr>
<tr><td>86 15 TC R</td><td colspan="3"></td><td colspan="6">37</td><td colspan="2">34</td><td colspan="4">32</td><td colspan="6">21</td><td>31</td></tr>
<tr><td>87 15 TC R</td><td colspan="3"></td><td colspan="6">36</td><td colspan="2">35</td><td colspan="4">26</td><td colspan="6">19</td><td>28</td></tr>
<tr><td>87 17 UC R</td><td colspan="3"></td><td>19</td><td colspan="17"></td><td></td></tr>
<tr><td>87 17 U A</td><td colspan="3"></td><td>33</td><td colspan="17"></td><td></td></tr>
<tr><td>88 15 TC R</td><td colspan="3"></td><td colspan="6">39</td><td colspan="2">35</td><td colspan="4">28</td><td colspan="6">16</td><td>29</td></tr>
<tr><td>89 13 U A</td><td colspan="7">43</td><td colspan="14"></td><td></td></tr>
<tr><td>89 15 TC R</td><td colspan="3"></td><td colspan="6">37</td><td colspan="2">33</td><td colspan="4">25</td><td colspan="6">16</td><td>27</td></tr>
<tr><td>90 15 TC R</td><td colspan="3"></td><td colspan="6">34</td><td colspan="2">32</td><td colspan="4">28</td><td colspan="6">16</td><td>27</td></tr>
<tr><td>90 19 UC R</td><td colspan="6"></td><td>35</td><td colspan="14"></td><td></td></tr>
<tr><td>90 19 U A</td><td colspan="6"></td><td>50</td><td colspan="14"></td><td></td></tr>
<tr><td>91 15 TC R</td><td colspan="3"></td><td colspan="6">33</td><td colspan="2">30</td><td colspan="4">24</td><td colspan="6">16</td><td>26</td></tr>
<tr><td>91 18 U R</td><td colspan="2"></td><td colspan="2">12</td><td colspan="17"></td><td></td></tr>
<tr><td>91 18 U A</td><td colspan="2"></td><td colspan="2">22</td><td colspan="17"></td><td></td></tr>
<tr><td>92 15 TC R</td><td colspan="3"></td><td colspan="6">33</td><td colspan="2">36</td><td colspan="4">27</td><td colspan="6">14</td><td>27</td></tr>
<tr><td>92 19 UC R</td><td colspan="2"></td><td colspan="2">12</td><td colspan="17"></td><td></td></tr>
<tr><td>92 19 UC A</td><td colspan="2"></td><td colspan="2">26</td><td colspan="17"></td><td></td></tr>
<tr><td>93 15 TC R</td><td colspan="3"></td><td colspan="6">30</td><td colspan="2">34</td><td colspan="4">26</td><td colspan="6">16</td><td>26</td></tr>
<tr><td>93 18 U R</td><td colspan="2"></td><td colspan="2">11</td><td colspan="17"></td><td></td></tr>
<tr><td>93 18 U A</td><td colspan="2"></td><td colspan="2">25</td><td colspan="17"></td><td></td></tr>
<tr><td>94 15 TC R</td><td colspan="3"></td><td colspan="6">34</td><td colspan="2">33</td><td colspan="4">25</td><td colspan="6">16</td><td>26</td></tr>
<tr><td>95 15 TC R</td><td colspan="3"></td><td colspan="6">33</td><td colspan="2">36</td><td colspan="4">25</td><td colspan="6">14</td><td>26</td></tr>
<tr><td>95 18 U R</td><td colspan="2"></td><td colspan="2">14</td><td colspan="17"></td><td></td></tr>
<tr><td>95 18 U A</td><td colspan="2"></td><td colspan="2">29</td><td colspan="17"></td><td></td></tr>
</table>

Source: see *Notes on sources of survey data*, p. 474

Product: MC = manufactured cigarettes
TC = total cigarettes (including hand-rolled)
UC = cigarettes (type unspecified)
A = all products

Frequency: A = all smokers (including occasional)
R = regular or daily smokers

All ages: relevant to ages used and as given in original source

U = unspecified

* = refer to *Notes on sources of survey data*, p. 474

Table 19.5M Number of cigarettes smoked per smoker per day, males: some selected New Zealand surveys by age, 1960-1990

	Age group																					
Product Source Year	12	13	14	15	16	17	18	19	20-24	25-29	30-34	35-39	40-44	45-49	50-54	55-59	60-64	65-69	70-74	75-79	80+	All ages
60 7 UCE	2.1																					
64 11 UCE																						
64 12 AE									23													
69 6 UCE*		1.9	2.6	3.0	1.9																	
74 3 UCE																						
75 13 UCE	2.8																					
76 1 UCE				14					17	18	19	20	20	21	20	19	17	16	14	12		20
81 1 UCE				14					17	18	19	19	20	20	20	19	18	16	14	12		18
82 10 UC												21										
87 17 UCE				11																		
89 13 UCE	3.9																					
90 19 UCE							17															

Table 19.6M Number of cigarettes smoked per person per day, males: some selected New Zealand surveys by age, 1960-1990, with percentage total sales

	Age group																						
Product Source Year	12	13	14	15	16	17	18	19	20-24	25-29	30-34	35-39	40-44	45-49	50-54	55-59	60-64	65-69	70-74	75-79	80+	All ages	% Total sales
60 7 UC	0.7																						**
64 11 UC																							**
64 12 A									13														**
69 6 UC *		0.4	1.0	1.1	0.6																		**
74 3 UC																							**
75 13 UC	1.3																						**
76 1 UC				4.2					7.2	7.8	8.5	8.6	8.8	9.2	8.8	11	6.6	5.4	4.3	2.9		7.9	71%T
81 1 UC				3.6					6.6	6.7	6.9	7.4	7.4	7.5	7.5	6.9	5.7	4.5	3.6	2.4		6.1	66%T
82 10 UC *												6.0											**
87 17 UC				1.2																			**
89 13 UC	1.0																						**
90 19 UC							4.7																**

Table 19.7M Number of cigarettes smoked per person per day, sales-adjusted, males: some selected New Zealand surveys[1] by age, 1976-1981, with percentage total sales

	Age group																						
Product Source Year	12	13	14	15	16	17	18	19	20-24	25-29	30-34	35-39	40-44	45-49	50-54	55-59	60-64	65-69	70-74	75-79	80+	All ages	% Total sales
76 1 UC				5.9					10	11	12	12	12	13	12	15	9.3	7.6	6.1	4.1		11	71%T
81 1 UC				5.4					10	10	10	11	11	11	11	10	8.6	6.8	5.4	3.6		9.2	66%T

1 Based on those surveys in Table 19.6 with data for both sexes and age range at least 21-64 (see *Cigarette consumption per person*, p. xxxv)

Source: see *Notes on sources of survey data*, p. 474
All ages: relevant to ages used and as given in original source
% Total sales: estimated % of total sales of M = manufactured or T = total cigarette consumption implied by survey, sexes combined, used as adjustment factor in Table 19.7
** = cannot be calculated
--- = adjusted by original author
* = refer to *Notes on sources of survey data*, p. 474

Product: MC = manufactured cigarettes
TC = total cigarettes (including hand-rolled)
UC = cigarettes (type unspecified)
A = all products
U = unspecified
E indicates mean estimated from percentage distribution (see also *Consumption category estimation*, p. xxxiv, and Appendix III, p. 789)

Table 19.5F Number of cigarettes smoked per smoker per day, females: some selected New Zealand surveys by age, 1960-1990

Product Source Year	12	13	14	15	16	17	18	19	20-24	25-29	30-34	35-39	40-44	45-49	50-54	55-59	60-64	65-69	70-74	75-79	80+	All ages
60 7 UCE	1.3																					
64 11 UCE				13																		
64 12 AE									17													
69 6 UCE*		2.1	2.9	1.9	2.6																	
74 3 UCE				12																		
75 13 UCE	1.6																					
76 1 UCE				13					15	15	15	16	16	16	15	14	13	12	11	9.8		16
81 1 UCE				12					15	15	16	16	16	16	15	14	14	12	11	10		14
82 10 UC												15										
87 17 UCE				10																		
89 13 UCE	1.5																					
90 19 UCE							12															

Table 19.6F Number of cigarettes smoked per person per day, females: some selected New Zealand surveys by age, 1960-1990, with percentage total sales

Product Source Year	12	13	14	15	16	17	18	19	20-24	25-29	30-34	35-39	40-44	45-49	50-54	55-59	60-64	65-69	70-74	75-79	80+	All ages	% Total sales
60 7 UC	0.2																						**
64 11 UC				8																			**
64 12 A									5.8											0.0		5.2	**
69 6 UC *		0.5	1.1	0.6	0.6																		**
74 3 UC				3.7																			**
75 13 UC	0.7																						**
76 1 UC				3.8					5.7	5.7	5.8	5.5	5.6	5.6	5.0	4.2	3.4	2.4	1.6	0.8		5.1	71%T
81 1 UC				3.6					5.9	5.3	5.1	5.3	5.0	4.9	4.7	4.0	3.3	2.5	1.7	0.8		4.2	66%T
82 10 UC *												3.7											**
87 17 UC				1.9																			**
89 13 UC	0.6																						**
90 19 UC							4.2																**

Table 19.7F Number of cigarettes smoked per person per day, sales-adjusted, females: some selected New Zealand surveys[1] by age, 1976-1981, with percentage total sales

Product Source Year	12	13	14	15	16	17	18	19	20-24	25-29	30-34	35-39	40-44	45-49	50-54	55-59	60-64	65-69	70-74	75-79	80+	All ages	% Total sales
76 1 UC				5.4					8.1	8.1	8.2	7.8	7.9	7.9	7.1	5.9	4.8	3.4	2.3	1.1		7.2	71%T
81 1 UC				5.4					8.9	8.0	7.7	8.0	7.5	7.4	7.1	6.0	5.0	3.8	2.6	1.2		6.3	66%T

1 Based on those surveys in Table 19.6 with data for both sexes and age range at least 21-64 (see *Cigarette consumption per person*, p. xxxv)

Source: see *Notes on sources of survey data*, p. 474
All ages: relevant to ages used and as given in original source
% Total sales: estimated % of total sales of M = manufactured or T = total cigarette consumption implied by survey, sexes combined, used as adjustment factor in Table 19.7
** = cannot be calculated
--- = adjusted by original author
* = refer to *Notes on sources of survey data*, p. 474

Product: MC = manufactured cigarettes
TC = total cigarettes (including hand-rolled)
UC = cigarettes (type unspecified)
A = all products
U = unspecified
E indicates mean estimated from percentage distribution (see also *Consumption category estimation*, p. xxxiv, and Appendix III, p. 789)

Table 19.8 Estimated[1] prevalence of smoking and estimated[1] number of cigarettes per person per day (unadjusted and sales-adjusted): summary of Tables 19.4, 19.6 and 19.7, 1964-1995.
Males and females aged 15 years and over

Year	Source[2]	Product[3]	Prevalence[4]						Number of cigarettes						
									Unadjusted[7]			Sales-adjusted[8]			
			Manufactured cigarettes		Total cigarettes[5]		All products[6]		Number/ person/day		Total sales %	Manufactured cigarettes number/ person/day		Total cigarettes[9] number/ person/day	
			M	F	M	F	M	F	M	F		M	F	M	F
1964	11	UC				61				7.6					
	12	A					52	31	11.4	4.9					
1974	3	UC				31				3.7					
1975	2	*UC*			41										
1976	1	UC			40	32			7.3	4.6	71			10.4	6.4
1981	1	UC			35	29			6.1	4.3	66			9.2	6.5
1983	15	TC			35	31								(8.7	6.3)
1984	15	TC			34	31								(8.7	6.3)
1985	15	TC			30	30								(7.5	5.9)
1986	15	TC			29	31								(6.7	5.7)
1987	15	TC			31	28								(7.2	5.3)
1988	15	TC			29	29								(7.0	5.5)
1989	15	TC			27	27								(5.6	4.5)
1990	15	TC			28	27								(5.9	4.6)
1991	15	TC			27	25								(5.5	4.1)
1992	15	TC			26	27								(4.7	3.8)
1993	15	TC			28	26								(4.8	3.5)
1994	15	TC			28	26								(4.6	3.5)
1995	15	TC			27	26								(4.3	3.3)

1 Surveys covering an age range of at least 21-64 are included. Any gaps in the data for ages 15-20 and 65 years and over are filled in by assumed extensions to the age distribution, given in *Notes on sources of survey data*, p. 474. Method: see *Summary of adult smoking*, p. xxxvi
2 See *Notes on sources of survey data*, p. 474
3 Product: MC = manufactured cigarettes, TC = total cigarettes (including hand-rolled), UC = cigarettes (type unspecified), A = all products, U = unspecified. Frequency of smoking is indicated by: regular or daily smokers in normal type, all smokers (including occasional) in bold, unspecified in italics
4 From Table 19.4
5 This column includes prevalence of smoking classified as UC = cigarettes (type unspecified)
6 This column includes prevalence of smoking classified as U = unspecified product
7 From Table 19.6
8 From Table 19.7, except data in parentheses, which are derived from the prevalence of smoking from Table 19.4 as described in *Summary of adult smoking*, p. xxxvi
9 Number of cigarettes classified as UC = cigarettes (type unspecified) has been adjusted to total cigarette sales and included in this column

Figure 19.3 Estimated prevalence of cigarette smoking by year of survey, 1964-1995. Males and females aged 15 years and over. *Source:* see Table 19.8

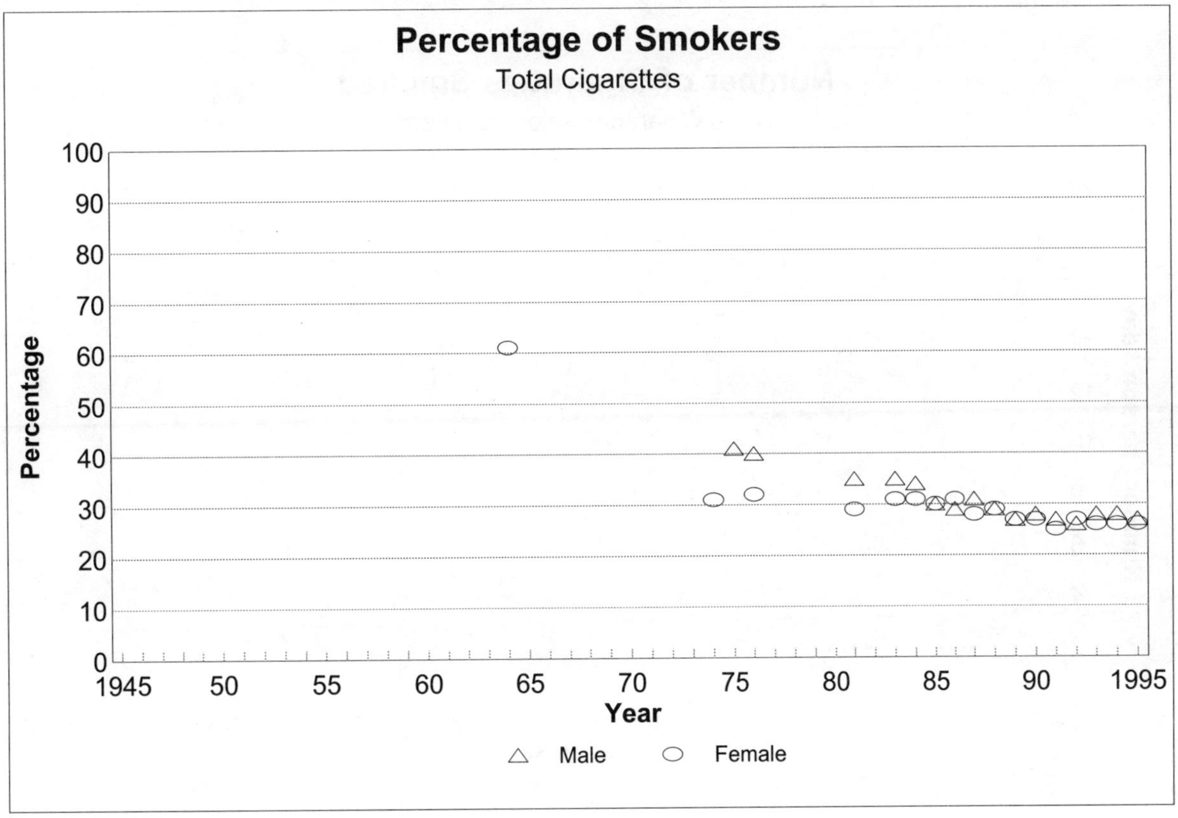

Figure 19.4 Estimated number of cigarettes smoked per person per day, sales-adjusted, 1976-1995.
Males and females aged 15 years and over. *Source:* see Table 19.8

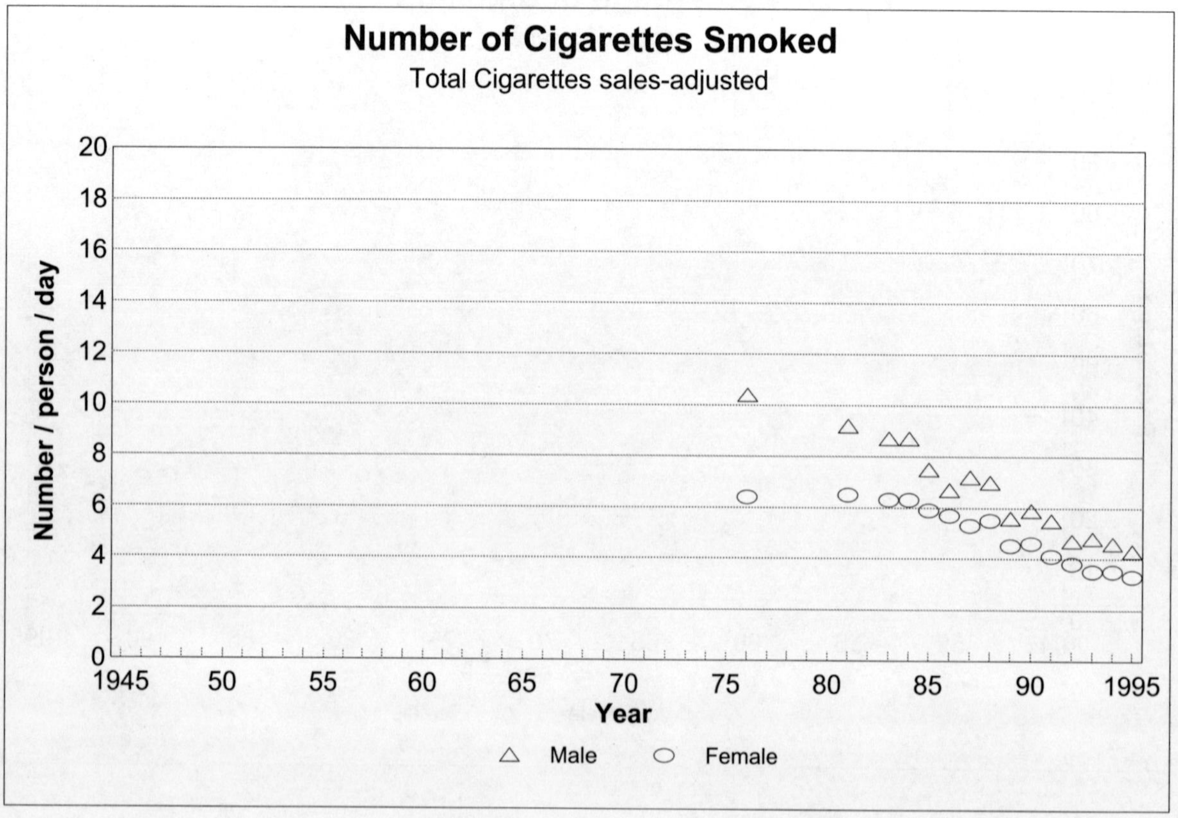

Notes on sources of sales data

The data presented in the tables and figures were obtained from several sources, details of which are given below, together with estimations and related assumptions. Full citations of the sources are given on p. 477 under *References*.

Consumption data before 1974

RP6

Data by weight, originally given to nearest 100 000 pounds, have been converted to tonnes and given to the nearest 10 tonnes (100 000 lbs = 45.359 tonnes). When weight conversion factors have been quoted in RP6, the weights have been re-calculated without rounding and then converted to tonnes.

Notes as given in RP6:

(a) Details of the weight of cigarettes and tobacco consumed were provided by the New Zealand Department of Statistics, Wellington.

(b) A factor of 2.5 lbs per 1 000 cigarettes, provided by the New Zealand Department of Statistics, was used for converting the weight of cigarettes consumed to numbers.

(c) The figures on sales of cigarette papers (produced in New Zealand and imported) show releases from bond of cigarette papers and tubes subject to Customs and Excise duties. These figures exclude cigarette papers for use in factory manufacture. This data provides an indication of the extent of the hand-rolling of cigarettes in New Zealand, but the retail sales do not, of course, take account of subsequent wastage.

Consumption data for 1974 onwards

Ministry of Health New Zealand (1999)

Data are given for tobacco products released for sale. Data for cigars were not available and have not been included in calculation of the total. However, as Laugesen (1996) gives the quantity of cigars released for sale 1990-1995 as between 3 and 11 tonnes this will have little effect.

Data for cigarettes were given in numbers. For conversion to weight, we assume an average cigarette weight of 0.9 g for 1974-1984 and 0.8 g thereafter based on the following data from Laugesen (1996).

Year	Tobacco/cigarette, g
1960	1.1
1965	1.0
1977-1978	0.9
1990	0.8
1991	0.8
1992	0.8
1993	0.8
1994	0.8
1995	0.8
1996	0.8

Plain/Filter cigarette consumption

Maxwell (successive years)

Tar yield of cigarettes

Laugesen (1996)

Estimates of hand-rolled cigarette consumption for 1950-1995

We have taken as our estimate of hand-rolled cigarette consumption 78% of pipe and hand-rolling tobacco/'other' tobacco sales, at 1 g per cigarette.

Estimation of hand-rolled cigarette consumption is difficult owing to the varying data sources available at different times. Data on cigarette papers, available from 1935-1973 (see Table 19.1.1), provide an indication of the extent of hand-rolling of cigarettes, but the retail sales do not, of course, take account of subsequent wastage. However, the relationship between cigarette papers and tobacco consumption, assuming 1 g per cigarette, does not suggest any steady trend, fluctuating between 85% and 120% (occasionally even higher).

Estimates of hand-rolled cigarette consumption in the latest available year were also given in the introductions to successive editions of RP6.

Year	Annual (millions)	Number/adult/day	Percentage of cigarette papers	Percentage of tobacco used in hand-rolled cigarettes (assuming 1 g per cigarette)
1966	1 200	1.8	83	91
1970	660	0.9	63	72
1973	548	0.7	64	64

In the period 1970-1979 production figures were available separately for pipe and hand-rolling tobacco (in the Monthly Abstract of Statistics). Hand-rolling tobacco as a percentage of the total remained steady throughout this period, with a mean of 78%.

Jackson and Beaglehole (1985) uses the assumption that 50% of packet tobacco was used for hand-rolling. Ministry of Health New Zealand (1999) states that loose tobacco is mainly cigarette tobacco but includes a small amount of pipe tobacco. Both these sources use a conversion rate of 1 g per cigarette. Laugesen (1996) suggest that between 1991 and 1995 some smokers changed from smoking manufactured cigarettes to using cheaper hand-rolled cigarettes, enabling them to use less tobacco for the same number of cigarettes.

Notes on sources of survey data

Each source of survey data—either an individual survey or a series of surveys repeated over a number of years—is cited by a source number. This number is shown in the tables and corresponds to the source numbers given below, where details of the source publication and of the survey methodology are given. Full citations of the sources are given on p. 477 under *References*.

Due to constraints of space, we have usually only given results for all ethnic groups combined, although many of the sources cited also give results for ethnic groups separately. Smoking prevalence is generally higher among Maori, especially women, than among Europeans.

Source number

1 **Department of Statistics (1979, 1983), Hay and Foster (1984)**

a. Census results. Completion of the census schedule is required by law. In 1976, visitors to New Zealand were included, but in 1981 only those usually resident were included. Response rate to smoking questions (1976) 97%, (1981) 99%

b. Census returns were overseen by the head of household, which may have led to understatement of smoking by teenagers

c. Number of cigarettes smoked refers to number smoked 'yesterday'

d. Consumption category estimation (not *All ages* results) based on 0-4, 5-9, 10-14, 15-19, ..., 45-49, and 50+ cigarettes/smoker/day. Estimated consumption for *All ages* (not shown) was lower than the direct means (shown in Table 19.5) by 1-2 cigarettes per smoker for 1976, but the same for 1981

2 **Hay (1976)**

a. No original reference. Age group not stated

3 **Hay and Christmas (1976), quoting National Research Bureau (1975)**

a. Surveys carried out in 1974 and 1975 for Cancer Society of New Zealand. Subjects randomly selected from 19 areas. Personal interviews at home. Only results for females available. Sample size (males) 1 200, (females) 1 200

b. Smokers: smoked yesterday

c. Consumption category estimation based on <10, 10-19, 20-29, 30-39, and 40+ cigarettes/smoker/day

4 **Mitchell (1983)**

a. Surveys in three Gisborne city high schools. Approximate ages corresponding to 5th form. Sample size (1968) 514, (1981) 583

b. Results presented here have been combined over Maori and Europeans. Between the two surveys, there was an increase in the proportion of students who were Maori from 24% to 39%

c. Regular smokers: smokes often (at least a packet a week). All smokers: smokes often or 'occasionally (once a week)', but not 'rarely (a puff or two during the year)'

5 Beaglehole *et al* (1978)

a. Confidential interviews, baseline study for intervention programme at 2 high schools. Approximate ages corresponding to 3rd and 4th forms. Sample size (males) 552, (females) 436

b. Smokers marked as frequency *: smokes more than 2 cigarettes per day

c. The median number of cigarettes per week was 5 and 20 for 3rd and 4th form boys respectively, and 3 for 4th form girls (not stated for 3rd form girls)

6 Newman *et al* (1970)

a. Study of high school students, representing urban and rural areas, all socio-economic levels and both North and South Islands. Confidential questionnaires. Approximate ages corresponding to 3rd-6th forms. Year not stated. Sample size (males) 975, (females) 1 049

b. Smokers: smoked in last month

c. Consumption category estimation based on <1, 1, 2, 3+ packs/smoker/week (assumed means 10, 20, 40, 60 cigarettes). As these categories are not contiguous and as the lowest category includes occasional smokers, these estimates should be regarded with caution

7 Gardiner *et al* (1961)

a. Survey at 9 secondary schools, selected to give variety of racial, social, urban/rural and regional coverage. Anonymous questionnaires completed by all pupils in class with teachers usually absent. Year not stated. Sample size (males) 2 407, (females) 1 867

b. All smokers: has smoked in last 4 weeks. Regular smokers: has smoked in last 4 weeks and usually smokes 1+ cigarettes per week. Smokers marked as frequency *: has smoked in last 4 weeks and usually smokes 5+ cigarettes per week

c. Consumption category estimation based on 1-4, 5-9, 10-19, 20-39, 40+ cigarettes/smoker/week

8 Stanhope and Prior (1975)

a. Study of cardiorespiratory risk factors at a high school in Rotorua. Questionnaire completed with parental help before medical examination, but smoking information obtained by confidential interview. Sample size 294

9 Ree (1986)

a. Confidential questionnaire completed by all pupils at a high school in northern King Country, small town/rural area. Sample size (males) 145, (females) 182. Response rate 84%

b. Smokers: smoked at least 1 cigarette on most days of week

10 WHO (1989), WHO MONICA Project (1988)

a. Regional survey forming part of WHO MONICA project:

Region	Population size	Sample size	Participation rate (%)	Sample used		Date
				Males	Females	
Auckland	256 700	1 950	81	1 018	567	Jan 1982-July 1982

All figures are for age 35-64 only

b. *All ages* column is standardized to world population

c. Regular cigarette smokers: smoked cigarettes daily. All smokers: smoked cigarettes daily or occasionally, or smoked 1 g pipe tobacco or 1 cigar per week. Cigarettes per smoker refers to regular and occasional cigarette smokers

d. Calculation for cigarettes per person based on % regular cigarette smokers and cigarettes per regular or occasional cigarette smoker, so may underestimate

11 Doll (1972) quoting Dr Ian Prior

a. Maori women. Age group not stated. Sample size 384

b. Consumption category estimation based on 1-10 (assume 1-9), 10-19, 20+ cigarettes/smoker/day

c. Assumed extension to age distribution for percentage smokers, age 15-19: males 35%, females 30%. Number of cigarettes/person/day: males and females 3.0

12 Prior *et al* (1968), Evans *et al* (1969), Doll (1972)

a. Random sample of Europeans in Carterton, a country town. Interview before medical examination. Sample size (males) 210, (females (228). Response rate 92%

b. Consumption category estimation based on 1-9, 10-20, 21+ cigarettes or <1, 1-3, >3 oz tobacco /smoker/day

13 Stanhope (1978), Shaw *et al* (1991)

a. Survey of rheumatic fever and coronary risk factors in 1975 at a secondary school in Wairoa, a rural area with largely Maori population. Medical examination and confidential interview of 3rd-5th form pupils. The tobacco related part of the survey was repeated in 1989.

Year	Sample size		Response
	Males	Females	rate (%)
1975	364	351	96
1989	237	198	87

b. Smokers: smoked in last month

c. Consumption category estimation based on <20, 20-39, 40+ cigarettes/smoker/week. For 1975, these estimates can be compared with the weekly consumption medians (males 15.2, females 13.9) and geometric means (males 10.7, females 11.4) presented by Stanhope (1978)

14 Nye *et al* (1980)

a. Study of pupils at a Dunedin high school. Approximate ages corresponding to 4th and 6th forms. Sample size 4th form (males) 53, (females) 49; 6th form (males) 34, (females) 55

15 Ministry of Health New Zealand (1999)

a. OTR Spectrum Research. Face-to-face interviews with about 10 000 people each year. Part of AGB McNair Omnibus survey

b. Although there are some smokers who smoke manufactured cigarettes, or hand-rolled cigarettes, less than daily, when the two types of cigarettes are considered together there are no occasional smokers of cigarettes

16 Flight *et al* (1984)

a. Study of pupils at 9 randomly selected schools in Northland. At each school, a 1 in 4 sample of 4th form pupils were interviewed and medically examined. Approximate age corresponding to school form. Year not stated. Sample size (males) 152, (females) 200. Response rate 96%

b. Regular smokers: smoked 7+ cigarettes per week

17 Stanton *et al* (1989, 1996)

a. Dunedin Multidisciplinary Health and Development Study, a longitudinal study of children born at Dunedin's only obstetric hospital April 1972-March 1973. Over-representative of higher socio-economic levels and Europeans. Questions about smoking were included in confidential interviews from age 9. Sample size 1 139. Follow-up rate (age 13) 82%, (age 15) 95%, (age 18) 97%

b. Regular smokers: usually smoked at least one cigarette per day. All smokers: smoked in last month

c. Consumption category estimation based on 1-4, 5-9, 10+ cigarettes/smoker/day. (Categories for age 18 are labelled 1-5, 6-10, 10+ but have been assumed the same as for age 15)

18 Reeder *et al* (1999)

a. Series of surveys of 4th form pupils at Wellington schools. All 35 secondary schools were invited and 15 participated (one school was missing from the 1993 survey and another withdrew after 1993). The participating schools represented higher socio-economic areas than the non-participating schools, and included the two schools with the highest number of Maori pupils. Anonymous questionnaires completed during school hours. Approximate ages corresponding to 4th form. Sample size (males) 2 944, (females) 2 890. Response rate approximately 70%

b. Regular smokers: smoked daily. All smokers: smoked in the last month

19 Ford *et al* (1995), Laugesen and Scragg (1999)

a. Nationally representative sample of 4th form school pupils. 99 schools participated (response rate 79%) representing all school types with at least 100 pupils. All pupils completed the anonymous questionnaire but only pupils age 14-15 were included in analysis. Student response rate 73%, sample size analysed 14 097

b. Regular smokers: smoked daily, reported only for the 85 schools which also participated in a similar survey in 1997. All smokers: smoked at least one cigarette a month

References

Beaglehole R., Eyles E. and Harding W. (1978). Cigarette smoking habits, attitudes and associated social factors in adolescents. *N Z Med J,* **87**, 239-42.

Beese D.H. (ed) (1968). *Tobacco consumption in various countries,* 2nd edition. Tobacco Research Council, London. Research Paper 6.

Beese D.H. (ed) (1972). *Tobacco consumption in various countries,* 3rd edition. Tobacco Research Council, London. Research Paper 6.

Department of Statistics (1979). *1976 census of population and dwellings. Bulletin No. 24 Cigarette smoking.* Department of Statistics, Wellington. Cat No. 02.124.

Department of Statistics (1983). *New Zealand census of population and dwellings, 1981. Bulletin on cigarette smoking.* Department of Statistics, Wellington. Cat. No. 02.124.

Doll R. (1972). Cancers related to smoking. In: Richardson R.G. (ed) *The second world conference on smoking and health. Proceedings of a conference organised by the Health Education Council Imperial College London 20-24 September 1971.* Pitman Medical, Bath; 10-23.

Evans J.G., Prior I.A.M. and Cooke N.J. (1969). The Carterton Study: 4. Serum cholesterol levels of a sample of New Zealand European adults. *N Z Med J,* **69**, 346-50.

Flight R.J., McKenzie-Pollock M., Hamilton M.A., Salmond C.E. and Stokes Y.M. (1984). The health status of fourth form students in Northland. *N Z Med J,* **97**, 1-6.

Ford D.J., Scragg R., Weir J. and Gaiser J. (1995). A national survey of cigarette smoking in fourth-form school children in New Zealand. *N Z Med J,* **108**, 454-7.

Gardiner C.E., Taylor C.N.D. and Roberts L.D. (1961). *Smoking habits of school children. A survey of the smoking habits of New Zealand school children.* Medical Statistics Branch, Department of Health, Wellington. (Special Report No. 5.)

Hay D.R. (1976). Is it worth stopping smoking? *Modern Medicine of New Zealand,* **July 19**, 9-16.

Hay D.R. and Christmas B.W. (1976). The smoking habits of women doctors and doctors' wives in New Zealand. *Prev Med,* **5**, 78-88.

Hay D.R. and Foster F.H. (1984). Intercensal trends in cigarette smoking in New Zealand. 1: age, sex and ethnic status. *N Z Med J,* **97**, 283-5.

Jackson R. and Beaglehole R. (1985). Secular trends in underreporting of cigarette consumption. *Am J Epidemiol,* **122**, 341-4.

Laugesen M. (1996). *Tobacco statistics 1996.* Cancer Society of New Zealand (Inc.) and Ministry of Health, Wellington, New Zealand.

Laugesen M. and Scragg R. (1999). Trends in cigarette smoking in fourth-form students in New Zealand, 1992-1997. *N Z Med J,* **112**, 308-11.

Lee P.N. (ed) (1975). *Tobacco consumption in various countries,* 4th edition. Tobacco Research Council, London. Research Paper 6.

Maxwell J.C.Jr. (successive years). How the brands ranked. Maxwell International Estimates. *World Tobacco.*

Ministry of Health New Zealand (1999). *Tobacco facts 1999.* http://www.moh.govt.nz/.

Mitchell D.R. (1983). A comparison of high school students' smoking behaviours in 1968 and 1981. *N Z Med J,* **96**, 534-6.

National Research Bureau (1975). *Report to the Cancer Society of New Zealand.*§

Newman I.M., Ang J., Irwin R.P. and Smith J.M. (1970). Adolescent cigarette smoking. *N Z Med J,* **72**, 161-6.

Nye P.A., Haye K.L., McKenzie-Pollock J.B., Caughley B.L. and Housham R.W. (1980). What encourages and discourages children to smoke? Knowledge about health hazards and recommendations for health education. *N Z Med J,* **91**, 432-5.

Prior I.A.M., Evans J.G., Morrison R.B.I. and Davidson F. (1968). The Carterton Study: 1. Sampling methods and response rates. *N Z Med J,* **68**, 150-2.

Ree G.H. (1986). School health. Smoking habits and associated factors in school children. *N Z Med J,* **99**, 807-9.

Reeder A.I., Williams S., McGee R. and Glasgow H. (1999). Tobacco smoking among fourth form school students in Wellington, New Zealand, 1991-97. *Australian and New Zealand Journal of Public Health,* **23**, 494-500.

RP6, See Beese (ed) (1968), Beese (ed) (1972), Lee (ed) (1975)

Shaw R.A., Crane J. and O'Donnell T.V. (1991). The changes in smoking habits in a rural adolescent population, 1975-89. *N Z Med J,* **104**, 40-3.

Stanhope J.M. (1978). Social patterns of adolescent cigarette smoking in a rural community. *N Z Med J,* **87**, 343-8.

Stanhope J.M. and Prior I.A.M. (1975). Smoking behaviour and respiratory health in a teenage sample: the Rotorua Lake Study. 1. *N Z Med J,* **82**, 71-6.

Stanton W.R., McClelland M., Elwood C., Ferry D. and Silva P.A. (1996). Prevalence, reliability and bias of adolescents' reports of smoking and quitting. *Addiction,* **91**, 1705-14.

Stanton W.R., Silva P.A. and Oei T.P.S. (1989). Prevalence of smoking in a Dunedin sample followed from age 9 to 15 years. *N Z Med J,* **102**, 637-9.

WHO (1989). The WHO MONICA project: a worldwide monitoring system for cardiovascular diseases. In: *World health statistics annual 1989*. WHO, Geneva; 25-149.

WHO MONICA Project (1988). Geographical variation in the major risk factors of coronary heart disease in men and women aged 35-64 years. *World Health Stat Q,* **41**, 115-40.

§ Original paper not obtained, but information taken as quoted by another author

Norway 20

Sales data

See Tables 20.1-20.3.

From 1927 until the Second World War the consumption of manufactured cigarettes per adult was about 1 cigarette per day. After a drop during the war, consumption quickly rose to about 1.5-2 cigarettes per day and remained at this level until a further increase in the 1980s to 3 cigarettes per day. Estimates of hand-rolled cigarette consumption are available for 1939 and since 1946. Consumption per adult before the war was very low. It increased from 0.5 cigarettes per day in 1946 to nearly 4 cigarettes per day in the mid-1970s, and then declined to 2 cigarettes per day in 1995. Total cigarette consumption reached nearly 6 cigarettes per day in 1980. From the early 1960s to the late 1980s, more hand-rolled cigarettes were consumed than manufactured cigarettes.

The consumption of all tobacco products per adult was about 4 g per day until the war, when it fell to below 2 g. Since the late 1940s, consumption has remained about 5-6 g per day. In the 1920s-1930s about 20% of tobacco was consumed as manufactured cigarettes. This increased to about 30% from the 1940s to the early 1980s, and then to 50% by the mid-1990s. The percentage sold as pipe and hand-rolling tobacco was 32% in 1927, mainly used at that time for pipes (Lund *et al* (1995)). Usage in pipes has since declined to negligible levels, but with the increasing popularity of hand-rolled cigarettes, sales increased to nearly 70% in the mid-1970s, then declined to about 45%. Chewing tobacco and snuff were the predominant products before the 1930s (Lund *et al* (1995)), accounting for nearly 50% of sales. This decreased to about 5% since the early 1970s. Only about 1-3% of consumption has been in cigars.

These figures include estimates of purchases in Sweden and tax-free sales, which increased substantially in the 1980s (see Table 20.1.5, p. 484, and *Notes on sources of sales data*, p. 502).

Survey data

See Tables 20.4-20.8

According to a market research survey in the 1950s, the prevalence of smoking among men was 72% for all tobacco products and 53% for cigarettes. Among women it was 25%, with virtually no women smoking products other than cigarettes.

Two sources provide annual information on smoking in Norway: source 1, Norges Markedsdata, since 1960 and source 4, Statens Tobakksskaderåd (National Council on Smoking and Health, NCSH), since 1973. Both sources give the prevalence only for tobacco smoking. According to source 1, in 1960 the prevalence of tobacco smoking among those aged 15 years and over was 63% in men and 25% in women, decreasing among men to about 40% in the 1990s and increasing then levelling among women at nearly 40% since the late 1970s. Data presented by source 4, from 1973 onwards, are consistently lower by about 5% for men and 8% for women. Trends by age are difficult to assess owing to differences between the sources and different age groups used.

In school-based surveys, the prevalence of smoking among teenage boys was higher than among girls when first surveyed in 1957, but decreased thereafter, and since the 1970s has generally been similar to that among girls. For the youngest age group reported (15-24 for source 1 and 16-24 for source 4), the prevalence has been consistently higher among young women than among young men since the mid-1970s according to source 1, but this pattern is not clearly seen in source 4.

Comparison of survey and sales data, only possible for source 4, suggests that these surveys under-reported consumption by 5-25%. However this comparison should be regarded with caution due to the uncertainty in the sales data relating to cross border trade. For instance, in 1980, our estimate of understatement is about 25%, whereas according to Statens Tobakksskaderåd (NCSH) (1996) it was 15%. Between 1973 and 1985, the estimated number of cigarettes smoked per person per day (sales-adjusted) was 6-7 for men and 3-4 for women.

Table 20.1.1 Total annual sales of tobacco products, 1927-1973

Year	Cigarettes tonnes	Cigarettes millions	Cigars tonnes	Cigars millions	Pipe and hand-rolling tobacco tonnes	Chewing tobacco tonnes	Snuff tonnes	All tobacco products tonnes
1927	540	512	90	21	950	950	450	2990
1928	540	510	90	22	1000	950	450	3040
1929	640	545	90	21	1040	950	500	3220
1930	730	615	90	23	1090	910	450	3270
1931	640	551	50	20	1130	820	410	3040
1932	640	568	50	20	1130	770	410	2990
1933	680	583	50	20	1180	680	410	2990
1934	730	619	90	23	1220	680	410	3130
1935	730	651	90	25	1320	640	410	3180
1936	820	731	90	26	1410	640	410	3360
1937	950	841	90	30	1450	590	450	3540
1938	950	833	90	31	1500	590	450	3580
1939	1040	909	90	31	1680	590	450	3860
1940	1130	973	90	31	1720	540	540	4040
1941	820	725	50	21	1220	360	540	2990
1942	680	608	50	12	860	320	450	2360
1943	680	562	0	7	680	230	360	1950
1944	410	358	0	5	590	180	270	1450
1945	590	517	0	5	860	180	270	1910
1946	1500	1288	50	14	2130	540	500	4720
1947	1860	1548	50	22	2360	410	500	5170
1948	1810	1506	50	21	2360	450	540	5220
1949	1680	1396	50	22	2400	360	540	5030
1950	1540	1280	50	18	2400	320	540	4850
1951	1450	1232	50	16	2450	320	540	4810
1952	1630	1344	50	17	2590	270	540	5080
1953	1540	1305	50	21	2630	270	540	5030
1954	1590	1339	50	23	2540	270	540	4990
1955	1590	1427	50	21	2630	230	540	5030
1956	1450	1340	50	21	2590	230	540	4850
1957	1590	1441	50	24	2720	230	500	5080
1958	1540	1394	50	25	2860	230	500	5170
1959	1540	1420	50	26	2990	180	500	5260
1960	1630	1491	50	26	3130	180	450	5440
1961	1590	1424	90	34	3360	180	450	5670
1962	1630	1464	90	37	3490	180	450	5850
1963	1540	1403	90	41	3490	140	450	5720
1964	1450	1280	140	59	3540	140	450	5720
1965	1630	1462	90	50	3720	140	410	5990
1966	1680	1506	90	50	3900	140	410	6210
1967	1770	1624	140	55	3990	90	360	6350
1968	1950	1773	140	55	3990	90	410	6580
1969	2090	1917	140	55	4220	90	270	6800
1970	2000	1831	90	45	4040	90	320	6530
1971	1910	1752	90	55	3990	90	320	6400
1972	2040	1862	90	54	4310	90	320	6850
1973	2000	1842	90	53	4350	90	270	6800

Source: see *Notes on sources of sales data*, p. 502

Table 20.1.2 Total annual sales of tobacco products, 1974-1995

Year	Cigarettes tonnes	Cigarettes millions	Cigars tonnes	Pipe and hand-rolling tobacco tonnes	Chewing tobacco tonnes	Snuff tonnes	Tax-free and border sales tonnes	All tobacco products tonnes
1974	1735	1735	90	4493	85	283	140	6826
1975	1755	1755	98	4580	63	263	150	6909
1976	1720	1720	101	4397	69	267	160	6714
1977	1957	1957	91	4401	69	283	170	6971
1978	1851	1851	84	4188	59	268	190	6640
1979	2042	2042	79	4335	60	260	200	6976
1980	2232	2232	76	4427	57	263	220	7275
1981	1995	1995	70	4373	55	270	250	7013
1982	1750	1750	61	4066	48	248	595	6768
1983	1768	1768	61	4154	43	247	880	7153
1984	1950	1950	65	4062	42	274	940	7333
1985	2303	2303	64	3999	40	292	805	7503
1986	2627	2627	60	3770	36	279	940	7712
1987	2740	2740	57	3551	31	270	915	7564
1988	2849	2849	51	3494	30	279	920	7623
1989	2935	2935	49	3425	26	285	900	7620
1990	2948	2948	49	3483	24	286	825	7615
1991	3016	3016	48	3491	20	283	785	7643
1992	2682	2682	45	3167	19	263	965	7141
1993	2820	2820	45	3365	20	295	840	7385
1994	2588	2588	43	3048	18	301	940	6938
1995	2653	2653	40	2944	17	314	990	6958

Source : see *Notes on sources of sales data*, p. 502

Table 20.1.3 Manufactured cigarettes (i) percentage of total sales as filter cigarettes, 1961-1981, and (ii) sales-weighted average tar yield per cigarette (SWAT), 1970-1980

Year	% Filter	SWAT mg / cig
1961	25.0	
1962	28.0	
1963	30.0	
1964	35.0	
1967	42.0	
1968	44.0	
1969	49.4	
1970	52.0	27
1971	52.0	
1972	65.0	
1973	68.5	

Year	% Filter	SWAT mg / cig
1974	70.0	
1975	73.0	24
1976	73.0	23
1977		23
1978	75.0	22
1979	75.0	21
1979	75.0	21
1980	80.0	20
1981	82.0	

Source : see *Notes on sources of sales data*, p. 502

Table 20.1.4 Total annual sales of cigarette papers, 1939-1995

Year	Cigarette papers millions
1939	94
1946	360
1947	345
1948	271
1949	656
1950	735
1951	697
1952	822
1953	819
1954	917
1955	929
1956	971
1957	1032
1958	1050
1959	1132
1960	1323
1961	2129
1962	2519
1963	2758
1964	2513
1965	2938
1966	3161
1967	3260
1968	3417
1969	3742
1970	3549
1971	3612
1972	4120
1973	3950
1974	4621
1975	4701
1976	4451
1977	4420
1978	4365
1979	4401
1980	4654
1981	4757
1982	4419
1983	4663
1984	4275
1985	4179
1986	3950
1987	3911
1988	3626
1989	3579
1990	3652
1991	3664
1992	3457
1993	3527
1994	3418
1995	3284

Source : see *Notes on sources of sales data,* p. 502

Table 20.1.5 Total annual sales of tobacco products, 1960-1995, adjusted for cross-border sales

Year	Manufactured cigarettes millions	Tax-free and border sales tonnes	Pipe and hand-rolling tobacco, cross-border sales from Sweden tonnes	Estimated cross-border sales of cigarettes		Adjusted total manufactured cigarettes millions
				tonnes	millions	
1960	1491	0		0	0	1491
1961	1424	10		10	10	1434
1962	1464	20		20	20	1484
1963	1403	30		30	30	1433
1964	1280	40		40	40	1320
1965	1462	50		50	50	1512
1966	1506	60		60	60	1566
1967	1624	70		70	70	1694
1968	1773	80		80	80	1853
1969	1917	90		90	90	2007
1970	1831	100	34	66	66	1897
1971	1752	110	36	74	74	1826
1972	1862	120	40	80	80	1942
1973	1842	130	44	86	86	1928
1974	1735	140	46	94	94	1829
1975	1755	150	50	100	100	1855
1976	1720	160	54	106	106	1826
1977	1957	170	56	114	114	2071
1978	1851	190	64	126	126	1977
1979	2042	200	68	132	132	2174
1980	2232	220	74	146	146	2378
1981	1995	250	84	166	166	2161
1982	1750	595	200	395	395	2145
1983	1768	880	350	530	530	2298
1984	1950	940	350	590	590	2540
1985	2303	805	280	525	525	2828
1986	2627	940	350	590	590	3217
1987	2740	915	336	579	579	3319
1988	2849	920	318	602	602	3451
1989	2935	900	308	592	592	3527
1990	2948	825	237	588	588	3536
1991	3016	785	204	581	581	3597
1992	2682	965	272	693	693	3375
1993	2820	840	160	680	680	3500
1994	2588	940	189	751	751	3339
1995	2653	990	194	796	796	3449

Source : see *Notes on sources of sales data*, p. 502

Table 20.2 Consumption[1] of (i) cigarettes and (ii) all tobacco products, 1927-1995 sales-based data, including estimated hand-rolled cigarette consumption. Males and females aged 15 years and over

Year	Manufactured cigarettes		Hand-rolled cigarettes		Total cigarettes		All tobacco products	
	Total annual in millions	Number/ adult/day	Total annual in millions	Number/ adult/day	Total annual in millions	Number/ adult/day	Total annual in tonnes	Grams/ adult/day
1927	512	0.7			512	0.7	2990	4.1
1928	510	0.7			510	0.7	3040	4.2
1929	545	0.7			545	0.7	3220	4.4
1930	615	0.8			615	0.8	3270	4.5
1931	551	0.8			551	0.8	3040	4.2
1932	568	0.7			568	0.7	2990	3.9
1933	583	0.8			583	0.8	2990	3.9
1934	619	0.8			619	0.8	3130	4.1
1935	651	0.8			651	0.8	3180	4.0
1936	731	0.9			731	0.9	3360	4.2
1937	841	1.0			841	1.0	3540	4.4
1938	833	1.0			833	1.0	3580	4.3
1939	909	1.1	85	0.1	994	1.2	3860	4.6

Table 20.2 *(continued)*

Year	Manufactured cigarettes		Hand-rolled cigarettes		Total cigarettes		All tobacco products	
	Total annual in millions	Number/ adult/day	Total annual in millions	Number/ adult/day	Total annual in millions	Number/ adult/day	Total annual in tonnes	Grams/ adult/day
1940	973	1.2			973	1.2	4040	4.8
1941	725	0.9			725	0.9	2990	3.6
1942	608	0.7			608	0.7	2360	2.8
1943	562	0.6			562	0.6	1950	2.2
1944	358	0.4			358	0.4	1450	1.7
1945	517	0.6			517	0.6	1910	2.2
1946	1288	1.5	324	0.4	1612	1.8	4720	5.4
1947	1548	1.8	311	0.4	1859	2.1	5170	5.9
1948	1506	1.7	244	0.3	1750	1.9	5220	5.7
1949	1396	1.5	590	0.6	1986	2.2	5030	5.5
1950	1280	1.4	662	0.7	1942	2.2	4850	5.4
1951	1232	1.4	627	0.7	1859	2.1	4810	5.3
1952	1344	1.5	740	0.8	2084	2.3	5080	5.6
1953	1305	1.4	737	0.8	2042	2.2	5030	5.5
1954	1339	1.5	825	0.9	2164	2.3	4990	5.4
1955	1427	1.5	836	0.9	2263	2.4	5030	5.4
1956	1340	1.4	874	0.9	2214	2.4	4850	5.2
1957	1441	1.5	929	1.0	2370	2.5	5080	5.4
1958	1394	1.5	945	1.0	2339	2.5	5170	5.4
1959	1420	1.5	1019	1.1	2439	2.5	5260	5.5
1960	1491	1.5	1191	1.2	2682	2.8	5440	5.6
1961	1424	1.5	1916	2.0	3340	3.4	5670	5.8
1962	1464	1.5	2267	2.3	3731	3.8	5850	5.9
1963	1403	1.4	2482	2.5	3885	3.9	5720	5.7
1964	1280	1.3	2262	2.2	3542	3.5	5720	5.6
1965	1462	1.4	2644	2.6	4106	4.0	5990	5.9
1966	1506	1.5	2845	2.8	4351	4.2	6210	6.0
1967	1624	1.6	2934	2.8	4558	4.4	6350	6.1
1968	1773	1.7	3075	2.9	4848	4.6	6580	6.3
1969	1917	1.8	3368	3.2	5285	5.0	6800	6.4
1970	1831	1.7	3194	3.0	5025	4.7	6530	6.1
1971	1752	1.6	3251	3.0	5003	4.6	6400	5.9
1972	1862	1.7	3708	3.4	5570	5.1	6850	6.3
1973	1842	1.7	3555	3.2	5397	4.9	6800	6.2
1974	1829	1.7	4159	3.8	5988	5.4	6826	6.2
1975	1855	1.7	4231	3.8	6086	5.5	6909	6.2
1976	1826	1.6	4006	3.6	5832	5.2	6714	6.0
1977	2071	1.8	3978	3.5	6049	5.3	6971	6.2
1978	1977	1.7	3929	3.4	5906	5.2	6640	5.8
1979	2174	1.9	3961	3.4	6135	5.3	6976	6.1
1980	2378	2.0	4189	3.6	6567	5.7	7275	6.3
1981	2161	1.8	4281	3.7	6442	5.5	7013	6.0
1982	2145	1.8	3977	3.4	6122	5.2	6768	5.7
1983	2298	1.9	4197	3.5	6495	5.4	7153	6.0
1984	2540	2.1	3848	3.2	6388	5.3	7333	6.1
1985	2828	2.3	3761	3.1	6589	5.4	7503	6.2
1986	3217	2.6	3555	2.9	6772	5.5	7712	6.3
1987	3319	2.7	3520	2.9	6839	5.5	7564	6.1
1988	3451	2.8	3263	2.6	6714	5.4	7623	6.1
1989	3527	2.8	3221	2.6	6748	5.4	7620	6.1
1990	3536	2.8	3287	2.6	6823	5.4	7615	6.1
1991	3597	2.9	3298	2.6	6895	5.5	7643	6.1
1992	3375	2.7	3111	2.5	6486	5.1	7141	5.6
1993	3500	2.8	3174	2.5	6674	5.3	7385	5.8
1994	3339	2.6	3076	2.4	6415	5.0	6938	5.4
1995	3449	2.7	2956	2.3	6405	5.0	6958	5.4

1 Including estimated tax-free and border sales 1974-1995

Source : see *Notes on sources of sales data,* p. 502

Figure 20.1 Daily consumption of (i) manufactured and total number of cigarettes, and (ii) all tobacco products, 1927-1995.
Males and females aged 15 years and over. *Source:* see Table 20.2

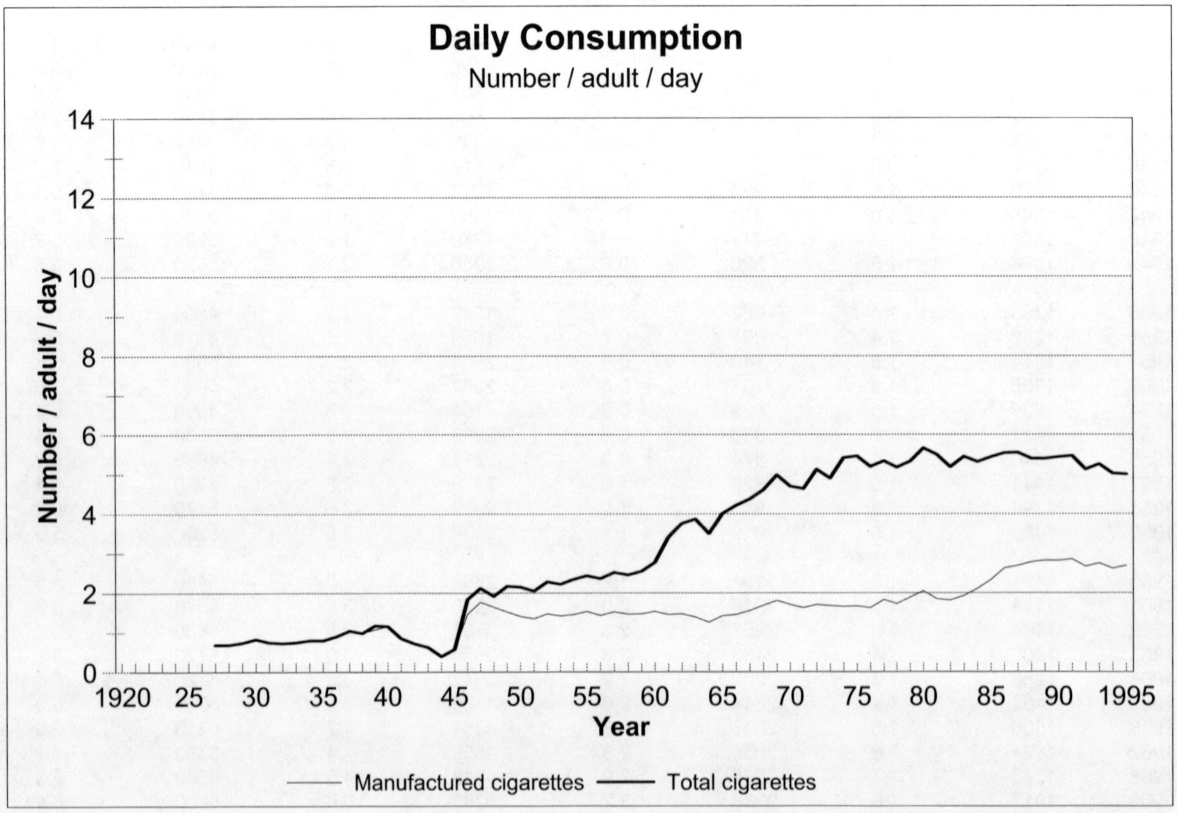

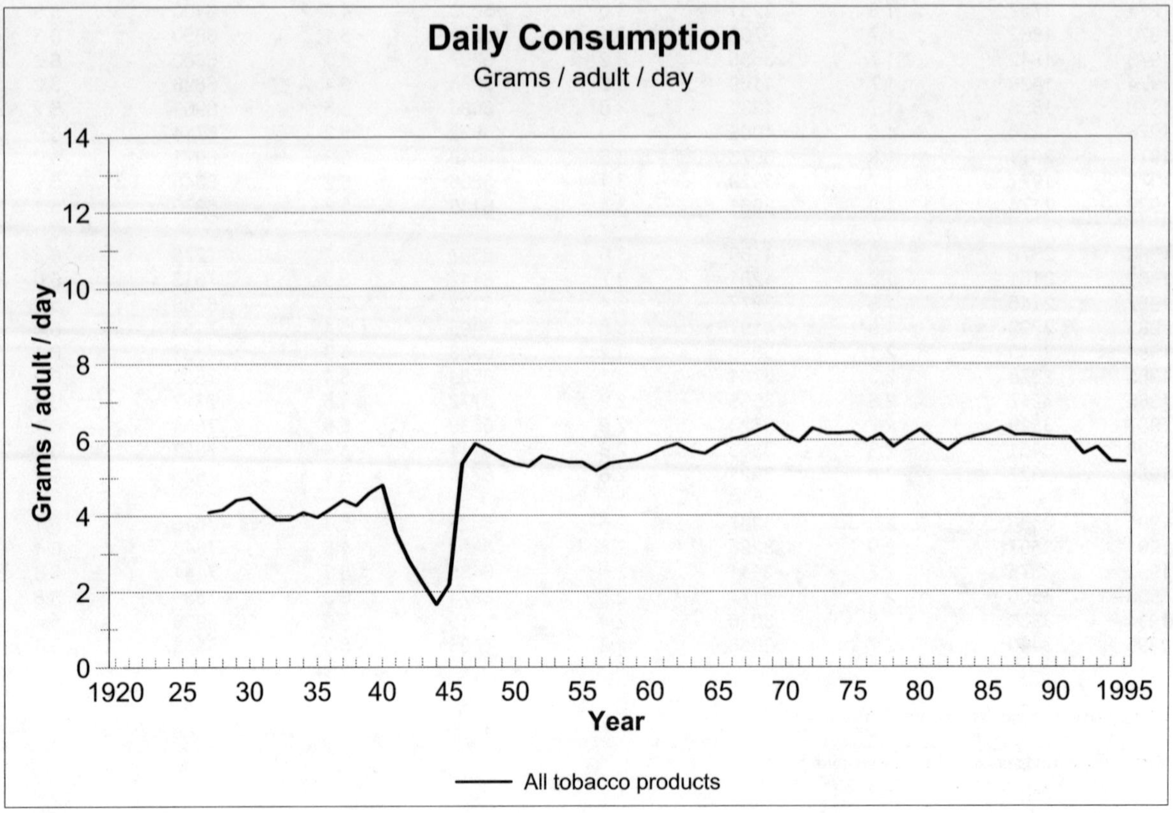

Table 20.3 Percentage sales[1] of tobacco in different forms (by weight), selected years 1927-1995

Year	Cigarettes (%)	Cigars (%)	Pipe and hand-rolling (%)	Chewing (%)	Snuff (%)
1927	18.1	3.0	31.8	31.8	15.1
1935	23.0	2.8	41.5	20.1	12.9
1945	30.9	0.0	45.0	9.4	14.1
1955	31.6	1.0	52.3	4.6	10.7
1965	24.4	1.5	62.1	2.3	6.8
1975	26.8	1.4	67.0	0.9	3.8
1985	37.7	0.9	57.0	0.5	3.9
1995	49.6	0.6	45.1	0.2	4.5

1 Including estimated tax free and border sales 1975-1995

Source : calculated from Tables 20.1.1, 20.1.2 & 20.1.5

Figure 20.2 Percentage sales of tobacco in different forms (by weight), selected years 1927-1995
Source: see Table 20.3

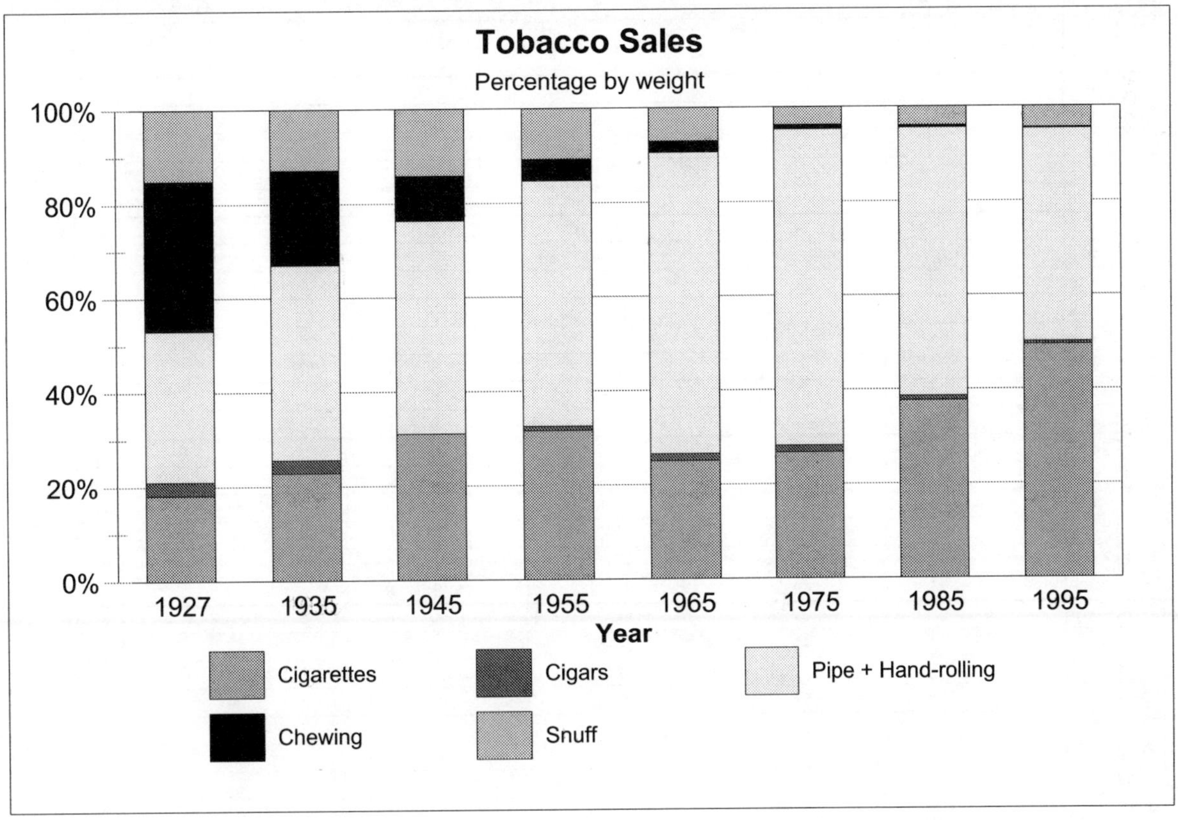

Table 20.4M Prevalence of smoking, males: some selected Norwegian surveys by age, 1954-1995 *(continues on p. 490)*

Frequency / Product / Source / Year	12	13	14	15	16	17	18	19	20-24	25-29	30-34	35-39	40-44	45-49	50-54	55-59	60-64	65-69	70-74	75-79	80+	All ages
54 2 TC U				53																		
54 2 A U				80							79			67			60					72
57 5 U R		3	7	13	24	35	38	35														
57 5 U A		57	58	60	62	62	64	63														
60 1 A R				64							73			66			45					64
61 1 A R				58							73			67			50					64
62 1 A R				55							72			66			49					63
62 11 TC U														56		51	40					
62 11 A U														71		67	58					
63 1 A R				55							72			65			49					62
63 5 U R	1	3	8	19																		
63 5 U A	47	47	50	58																		
64 1 A R				49							66			61			43					56
64 9 U U												67		62		54		42				
64 10 TC R												47				31						
64 10 A R												62				50						
65 1 A R				49							66			61			45					57
66 1 A R				53							68			64			48					59
67 1 A R				51							65			62				47				58
68 1 A R				54							66			63				44				58
69 1 A R				54							65			61				44				58
70 1 A R				54							59			62				44				56
71 1 A R				48							56			59				43				53
71 6 U R							5															
72 1 A R				50							55			58				42				53
72 6 U R							4															
72 12 UC R									46		46		46									
72 12 A R									51		51		56									
73 1 A R				50							58			57				42				54
73 3 UC R				46																		
73 4 A R					44					49		59		57		53		39				51
74 1 A R				50							56			54				39				52
74 4 A R					47					58		53		60		54		42				53
75 1 A R				45						55			57				44					52
75 4 A R					38					50		46		58		55		41				48
75 7 UC R	2	7	16	23																		15
75 7 UC A	28	35	46	47																		42
76 1 A R				47						56			56				46					51
76 4 A R					44					51		51		61		45		39				49
76 13 A U					47																	
77 1 A R				42						52			51				40					47
77 4 A R					36					48		49		48		48		35				44
78 1 A R				44						53			53				42					49
78 4 A R					39					52		46		47		44		41				45
79 1 A R				43						52			50				39					47
79 4 A R					33					50		45		46		45		39				43
79 14 U R		7																				
79 14 U A	18	17																				
80 1 A R				40						49			50				42					46
80 4 A R					35					42		42		44		50		40				42
80 7 UC R		6	13	22																		13
80 7 UC A		23	36	42																		34
81 1 A R				40						50			46				38					44
81 4 A R					34					45		43		47		34		35				40
82 1 A R				39						50			47				39					44
82 4 A R					33					42		45		38		41		39				40

Table 20.4F Prevalence of smoking, females: some selected Norwegian surveys by age, 1954-1995 *(continues on p. 491)*

Frequency Product Source Year	Age group																					
	12	13	14	15	16	17	18	19	20-24	25-29	30-34	35-39	40-44	45-49	50-54	55-59	60-64	65-69	70-74	75-79	80+	All ages
54 2 TC U				25																		
54 2 A U				33							32			17			6					25
57 5 U R		0	0	3	4	11	17	13														
57 5 U A		25	36	39	42	45	61	53														
60 1 A R				37							34			20			7					27
61 1 A R				40							34			22			6					28
62 1 A R				35							36			20			9					26
62 11 TC U																						
62 11 A U																						
63 1 A R				35							38			22			7					27
63 5 U R	0	1	3	7																		
63 5 U A	28	33	38	43																		
64 1 A R				34							35			21			6					26
64 9 U U												36		24		15		7				
64 10 TC R												27				11						
64 10 A R												27				11						
65 1 A R				33							35			21			7					26
66 1 A R				38							38			25			10					29
67 1 A R				38							39			23				8				30
68 1 A R				44							39			25				9				33
69 1 A R				47							43			25				11				36
70 1 A R				45							44			29				12				37
71 1 A R				45							42			26				9				35
71 6 U R																						
72 1 A R				48							43			30				10				38
72 6 U R																						
72 12 UC R																						
72 12 A R																						
73 1 A R				49							43			31				14				38
73 3 UC R				37																		
73 4 A R					42					46		42		33		19		13				32
74 1 A R				49							42			28				12				37
74 4 A R					43					47		37		37		20		9				32
75 1 A R				55						48			36				15					39
75 4 A R					39					45		39		34		27		7				33
75 7 UC R	2	7	17	28																		17
75 7 UC A	24	36	51	59																		48
76 1 A R				48						48			36				15					38
76 4 A R					40					39		38		38		22		12				32
76 13 A U													36									
77 1 A R				52						47			37				18					40
77 4 A R					37					42		33		34		21		11				30
78 1 A R				55						48			36				18					40
78 4 A R					36					42		35		37		21		11				31
79 1 A R				49						48			37				19					39
79 4 A R					37					40		39		32		28		13				33
79 14 U R		9																				
79 14 U A	8	27																				
80 1 A R				50						46			39				19					39
80 4 A R					36					41		36		30		21		11				30
80 7 UC R		4	11	21																		12
80 7 UC A		19	35	46																		33
81 1 A R				47						47			37				20					38
81 4 A R					33					39		34		38		25		10				31
82 1 A R				48						46			41				20					39
82 4 A R					37					48		35		33		28		15				34

Table 20.4M *(continued from p. 488, continued on p. 492)*
Prevalence of smoking, males

Frequency / Product / Source / Year	12	13	14	15	16	17	18	19	20-24	25-29	30-34	35-39	40-44	45-49	50-54	55-59	60-64	65-69	70-74	75-79	80+	All ages
83 1 A R				40						51			46				40					45
83 4 A R					29					43		46		44		51		41				42
83 15 U *		6		17																		
83 15 U R		9		23																		
83 15 U A		19		32																		
84 1 A R				36						50			50				39					44
84 4 A R					32					44		48		42		44		38				42
85 1 A R				39						49			49				38					44
85 4 A R					35					45		46		44		46		35				42
85 7 UC R		3	11	21																		12
85 7 UC A		18	28	43																		30
85 8 U U				38																		
85 15 U *		6		16																		
85 15 U R		10		20																		
85 15 U A		16		29																		
86 1 A R				37						51			48				38					44
86 4 A R					29					46		41		43		37		34				39
86 16 U R							51															
86 16 U A							62															
87 1 A R				39						52			48				40					45
87 4 A R					33					44		43		43		41		38				40
87 17 U R								44														
88 1 A R				36						46			46				37					42
88 4 A R					28					44		47		47		44		38				41
89 1 A R				36						47			46				36					42
89 4 A R					24					39		45		36		44		36				37
89 15 U *		3		17																		
89 15 U R		5		22																		
89 15 U A		9		29																		
89 18 U A								40														
90 1 A R				34						47			43				35					41
90 4 A R					26					42		41		39		35		35				36
90 7 U R		2	7	17																		9
90 7 U A		11	22	31																		22
90 19 U R		2																				
90 19 U A		3																				
91 1 A R				33						45			45				35					40
91 4 A R					31					41		42		38		32		23				36
91 19 U R			9																			
91 19 U A			12																			
92 1 A R				35						46			45				34					41
92 4 A R					29					40		42		46		36		27				37
92 19 U R				13																		
92 19 U A				18																		
92 20 UC *				16																		
92 20 UC R				20																		
92 20 UC A				35																		
93 1 A R				36						45			44				32					40
93 4 A R					32					39		41		42		40		28				38
93 15 UC R		5		20																		
93 19 U R					16																	
93 19 U A					19																	
94 1 A R				34						43			43				30					38
94 4 A R					32					41		42		30		33		25				35

Table 20.4F *(continued from p. 489, continued on p. 493)*
Prevalence of smoking, females

Frequency / Product / Source / Year	12	13	14	15	16	17	18	19	20-24	25-29	30-34	35-39	40-44	45-49	50-54	55-59	60-64	65-69	70-74	75-79	80+	All ages
83 1 A R				49						51			39				21					41
83 4 A R					31					43		39		32		26		11				32
83 15 U *		3		22																		
83 15 U R		6		28																		
83 15 U A		13		39																		
84 1 A R				45						49			40				22					40
84 4 A R					31					46		40		41		26		10				34
85 1 A R				42						49			40				20					39
85 4 A R					34					42		36		35		28		9				32
85 7 UC R		3	10	19																		11
85 7 UC A		17	27	39																		28
85 8 U U				40																		
85 15 U *		6		17																		
85 15 U R		8		24																		
85 15 U A		15		38																		
86 1 A R				43						49			40				23					39
86 4 A R					28					43		37		35		25		15				31
86 16 U R																						
86 16 U A																						
87 1 A R				48						52			41				25					42
87 4 A R					32					44		37		38		27		15				33
87 17 U R																						
88 1 A R				43						50			41				25					41
88 4 A R					28					44		40		36		34		26				35
89 1 A R				44						50			41				23					41
89 4 A R					35					41		44		35		21		14				34
89 15 U *		4		16																		
89 15 U R		6		22																		
89 15 U A		11		32																		
89 18 U A																						
90 1 A R				41						50			41				22					38
90 4 A R					30					44		43		30		32		15				33
90 7 U R		1	8	20																		10
90 7 U A		11	25	43																		26
90 19 U R		5																				
90 19 U A		7																				
91 1 A R				38						47			40				20					36
91 4 A R					28					39		41		34		28		19				33
91 19 U R			9																			
91 19 U A			14																			
92 1 A R				39						49			42				21					37
92 4 A R					28					43		36		35		28		12				32
92 19 U R				23																		
92 19 U A				30																		
92 20 UC *				25																		
92 20 UC R				37																		
92 20 UC A				46																		
93 1 A R				41						44			42				25					38
93 4 A R					29					45		42		33		33		23				36
93 15 UC R		4		21																		
93 19 U R					28																	
93 19 U A					34																	
94 1 A R				38						48			41				22					37
94 4 A R					23					36		35		36		30		25				31

Table 20.4M *(continued from p. 490)* Prevalence of smoking, males

Frequency Product Source Year	12	13	14	15	16	17	18	19	20-24	25-29	30-34	35-39	40-44	45-49	50-54	55-59	60-64	65-69	70-74	75-79	80+	All ages
95 1 A R				37						45			45				34					41
95 4 A R					29					36		37		35		33		26				33
95 7 U R		2	7	14																		8
95 7 U A		12	16	33																		23
95 21 UC R				17																		
95 21 UC A				33																		

Table 20.5M Number of cigarettes smoked per smoker per day, males: some selected Norwegian surveys by age, 1954-1995

Product Source Year	12	13	14	15	16	17	18	19	20-24	25-29	30-34	35-39	40-44	45-49	50-54	55-59	60-64	65-69	70-74	75-79	80+	All ages
54 2 A				9.8																		
57 5 UC		4.2	5.6	7.1	8.1	10	11	12														
62 11 TCE														12		11	11					
73 4 TC					12					16		14		14		12		9.1				13
74 4 TC					11					14		14		15		13		10				13
75 4 TC					11					15		16		13		12		11				13
75 7 UC	4.6	4.8	5.4	7.1																		
76 4 TC					12					15		14		12		12		9.7				13
77 4 TC					12					15		17		15		12		11				14
78 4 TC					11					15		15		12		12		11				13
79 4 TC					13					15		16		15		12		10				14
79 14 UC		5.6																				
80 4 TC					12					15		13		16		11		11				13
81 4 TC					12					15		18		14		14		12				14
82 4 TC					13					14		15		14		15		11				14
83 4 TC					14					15		17		15		15		11				15
84 4 TC					14					14		16		16		14		15				15
85 4 TC					15																	
86 4 TC					15																	
86 16 UCE							12															
87 4 TC					14																	
87 17 UCE								15														
88 4 TC					16																	
89 4 TC					15																	
89 18 UCE								16														
90 4 TC					15																	
91 4 TC					15																	
92 4 TC					15																	
92 20 UC				7																		
93 4 TC					15																	
94 4 TC					15																	
95 4 TC					15																	
95 21 UCE				9.6																		

Source see *Notes on sources of survey data*, p. 503
Frequency: A = all smokers (including occasional)
R = regular or daily smokers
All ages relevant to ages used and as given in original source
U = unspecified
* = refer to *Notes on sources of survey data*, p. 503

Product: MC = manufactured cigarettes
TC = total cigarettes (including hand-rolled)
UC = cigarettes (type unspecified)
A = all products
E indicates mean estimated from percentage distribution (see also *Consumption category estimation*, p. xxxiv, and Appendix III, p. 789)

Table 20.4F *(continued from p. 491)*
Prevalence of smoking, females

Year Source Product Frequency	12	13	14	15	16	17	18	19	20-24	25-29	30-34	35-39	40-44	45-49	50-54	55-59	60-64	65-69	70-74	75-79	80+	All ages
95 1 A R				39						46			43				21					37
95 4 A R					29					34		40		35		26		19				32
95 7 U R		3	9	17																		9
95 7 U A		16	29	42																		29
95 21 UC R				19																		
95 21 UC A				39																		

Table 20.5F Number of cigarettes smoked per smoker per day, females: some selected Norwegian surveys by age, 1954-1995

Year Source Product	12	13	14	15	16	17	18	19	20-24	25-29	30-34	35-39	40-44	45-49	50-54	55-59	60-64	65-69	70-74	75-79	80+	All ages
54 2 A																						
57 5 UC		4.5	8.8	5.6	7.2	6.3	6.5	8.0														
62 11 TCE																						
73 4 TC					9.4					11		9.7		10		10		8.6				9.9
74 4 TC					10					9.2		12		10		9.7		8.2				10
75 4 TC					9.7					11		11		12		11		6.9				11
75 7 UC	3.4	4.4	5.3	6.5																		
76 4 TC					9.7					11		11		11		10		8.3				10
77 4 TC					9.7					11		12		10		9.4		11				11
78 4 TC					10					12		12		11		9.7		11				11
79 4 TC					11					11		13		10		10		9.1				11
79 14 UC		2.1																				
80 4 TC					9.4					12		12		12		10		11				11
81 4 TC					12					10		13		12		11		8.5				11
82 4 TC					10					11		13		10		9.2		9.5				11
83 4 TC					11					12		12		13		11		8.1				11
84 4 TC					11					12		13		12		12		12				12
85 4 TC					12																	
86 4 TC					13																	
86 16 UCE																						
87 4 TC					12																	
87 17 UCE																						
88 4 TC					12																	
89 4 TC					12																	
89 18 UCE																						
90 4 TC					12																	
91 4 TC					12																	
92 4 TC					12																	
92 20 UC				7																		
93 4 TC					12																	
94 4 TC					12																	
95 4 TC					12																	
95 21 UCE				7.6																		

Source: see *Notes on sources of survey data*, p. 503
Frequency: A = all smokers (including occasional)
R = regular or daily smokers
All ages: relevant to ages used and as given in original source
U = unspecified
* = refer to *Notes on sources of survey data*, p. 503

Product: MC = manufactured cigarettes
TC = total cigarettes (including hand-rolled)
UC = cigarettes (type unspecified)
A = all products
E indicates mean estimated from percentage distribution (see also *Consumption category estimation*, p. xxxiv, and Appendix III, p. 789)

Table 20.6M Number of cigarettes smoked per person per day, males: some selected Norwegian surveys by age, 1954-1995, with percentage total sales

Product Source Year	12	13	14	15	16	17	18	19	20-24	25-29	30-34	35-39	40-44	45-49	50-54	55-59	60-64	65-69	70-74	75-79	80+	All ages	% Total sales
54 2 A				7.1																			**
57 5 UC		0.1	0.4	0.9	1.9	3.5	4.0	4.2															**
62 11 TC														7.0		5.7	4.2						**
73 4 TC					5.3					8.0		8.2		8.0		6.2		3.5				6.7	94%T
74 4 TC					5.4					8.2		7.6		9.1		6.7		4.3				7.0	88%T
75 4 TC					4.3					7.3		7.5		7.8		6.7		4.6				6.3	84%T
75 7 UC	0.1	0.3	0.9	1.6																			**
76 4 TC					5.4					7.5		7.2		7.4		5.3		3.8				6.3	85%T
77 4 TC					4.5					7.1		8.1		7.1		5.8		3.8				6.1	81%T
78 4 TC					4.3					8.0		6.9		5.7		5.3		4.6				5.9	83%T
79 4 TC					4.4					7.4		7.0		6.9		5.5		3.9				6.0	82%T
79 14 UC		0.4																					**
80 4 TC					4.1					6.2		5.4		7.1		5.7		4.4				5.5	72%T
81 4 TC					4.0					6.6		7.5		6.4		4.7		4.3				5.7	76%T
82 4 TC					4.2					5.8		6.9		5.4		6.2		4.3				5.6	81%T
83 4 TC					4.1					6.3		7.8		6.6		7.8		4.5				6.3	82%T
84 4 TC					4.5					6.1		7.9		6.8		6.0		5.5				6.3	86%T
85 4 TC					6.2																		85%T
86 4 TC					6.0																		82%T
86 16 UC							6.3																**
87 4 TC					5.8																		81%T
87 17 UC								7															**
88 4 TC					6.4																		89%T
89 4 TC					5.5																		81%T
89 18 UC								6.3															**
90 4 TC					5.4																		80%T
91 4 TC					5.3																		78%T
92 4 TC					5.5																		84%T
92 20 UC				1.1																			**
93 4 TC					5.8																		87%T
94 4 TC					5.1																		80%T
95 4 TC					4.9																		79%T
95 21 UC				1.6																			**

Source: see *Notes on sources of survey data*, p. 503

Product:
MC = manufactured cigarettes
TC = total cigarettes (including hand-rolled)
UC = cigarettes (type unspecified)
A = all products
U = unspecified

All ages: relevant to ages used and as given in original source

% Total sales: estimated % of total sales of M = manufactured or T = total cigarette consumption implied by survey, sexes combined

** = cannot be calculated

--- = adjusted by original author

* = refer to *Notes on sources of survey data*, p. 503

Table 20.6F Number of cigarettes smoked per person per day, females: some selected Norwegian surveys by age, 1954-1995, with percentage total sales

Product Source Year	12	13	14	15	16	17	18	19	20-24	25-29	30-34	35-39	40-44	45-49	50-54	55-59	60-64	65-69	70-74	75-79	80+	All ages	% Total sales
54 2 A																							**
57 5 UC		0.0	0.0	0.2	0.3	0.7	1.1	1.0															**
62 11 TC																							**
73 4 TC					3.9					4.8		4.1		3.3		2.0		1.1				3.2	94%T
74 4 TC					4.3					4.3		4.4		3.7		1.9		0.7				3.2	88%T
75 4 TC					3.8					4.9		4.1		3.9		2.8		0.5				3.5	84%T
75 7 UC	0.1	0.3	0.9	1.8																			**
76 4 TC					3.9					4.1		4.1		4.1		2.3		1.0				3.3	85%T
77 4 TC					3.6					4.8		3.9		3.5		2.0		1.2				3.2	81%T
78 4 TC					3.7					4.8		4.2		4.1		2.0		1.3				3.4	83%T
79 4 TC					3.9					4.3		5.0		3.3		2.8		1.2				3.6	82%T
79 14 UC		0.2																					**
80 4 TC					3.4					4.9		4.4		3.5		2.1		1.2				3.3	72%T
81 4 TC					3.9					4.1		4.3		4.4		2.8		0.9				3.5	76%T
82 4 TC					3.7					5.4		4.7		3.4		2.6		1.4				3.7	81%T
83 4 TC					3.3					5.2		4.5		4.0		2.7		0.9				3.6	82%T
84 4 TC					3.3					5.4		5.0		4.8		3.1		1.2				4.0	86%T
85 4 TC					3.8																		85%T
86 4 TC					4.0																		82%T
86 16 UC																							**
87 4 TC					4.0																		81%T
87 17 UC																							**
88 4 TC					4.2																		89%T
89 4 TC					4.0																		81%T
89 18 UC																							**
90 4 TC					4.1																		80%T
91 4 TC					4.1																		78%T
92 4 TC					3.9																		84%T
92 20 UC				1.8																			**
93 4 TC					4.3																		87%T
94 4 TC					3.7																		80%T
95 4 TC					3.7																		79%T
95 21 UC				1.4																			**

Source: see *Notes on sources of survey data*, p. 503

Product:
MC = manufactured cigarettes
TC = total cigarettes (including hand-rolled)
UC = cigarettes (type unspecified)
A = all products
U = unspecified

All ages: relevant to ages used and as given in original source

% Total sales: estimated % of total sales of M = manufactured or T = total cigarette consumption implied by survey, sexes combined
** = cannot be calculated
--- = adjusted by original author
* = refer to *Notes on sources of survey data*, p. 503

Table 20.7M Number of cigarettes smoked per person per day, sales-adjusted, males: some selected Norwegian surveys[1] by age, 1973-1995, with percentage total sales

Product Source Year	Age group 12	13	14	15	16	17	18	19	20-24	25-29	30-34	35-39	40-44	45-49	50-54	55-59	60-64	65-69	70-74	75-79	80+	All ages	% Total sales
73 4 TC					5.6					8.5		8.7		8.5		6.6		3.7				7.1	94%T
74 4 TC					6.1					9.3		8.6		10		7.6		4.9				7.9	88%T
75 4 TC					5.1					8.7		9.0		9.3		8.0		5.5				7.5	84%T
76 4 TC					6.3					8.8		8.4		8.7		6.2		4.5				7.4	85%T
77 4 TC					5.5					8.7		10		8.7		7.1		4.7				7.5	81%T
78 4 TC					5.2					9.6		8.3		6.8		6.4		5.5				7.1	83%T
79 4 TC					5.4					9.1		8.6		8.4		6.7		4.8				7.3	82%T
80 4 TC					5.7					8.6		7.5		9.9		7.9		6.1				7.6	72%T
81 4 TC					5.2					8.7		9.8		8.4		6.2		5.6				7.5	76%T
82 4 TC					5.2					7.1		8.5		6.6		7.6		5.3				6.9	81%T
83 4 TC					5.0					7.7		9.5		8.0		9.5		5.5				7.7	82%T
84 4 TC					5.2					7.1		9.1		7.9		6.9		6.4				7.3	86%T
85 4 TC					7.4																		85%T
86 4 TC					7.3																		82%T
87 4 TC					7.2																		81%T
88 4 TC					7.2																		89%T
89 4 TC					6.9																		81%T
90 4 TC					6.8																		80%T
91 4 TC					6.8																		78%T
92 4 TC					6.5																		84%T
93 4 TC					6.6																		87%T
94 4 TC					6.4																		80%T
95 4 TC					6.2																		79%T

1 Based on those surveys in Table 20.6 with data for both sexes and age range at least 21-64 (see *Cigarette consumption per person*, p. xxxv)

Source: See *Notes on sources of survey data*, p. 503

Product:
- MC = manufactured cigarettes
- TC = total cigarettes (including hand-rolled)
- UC = cigarettes (type unspecified)
- A = all products
- U = unspecified

All ages: relevant to ages used and as given in original source

% Total sales: Adjustment factor used, estimated % of total sales of M = manufactured or T = total cigarette consumption implied by survey, sexes combined

--- = adjusted by original author

* = refer to *Notes on sources of survey data*, p. 503

Table 20.7F Number of cigarettes smoked per person per day, sales-adjusted, females: some selected Norwegian surveys[1] by age, 1973-1995, with percentage total sales

Product Source Year	12	13	14	15	16	17	18	19	20-24	25-29	30-34	35-39	40-44	45-49	50-54	55-59	60-64	65-69	70-74	75-79	80+	All ages	% Total sales
73 4 TC					4.1					5.1		4.3		3.5		2.1		1.2				3.4	94%T
74 4 TC					4.9					4.9		5.0		4.2		2.1		0.8				3.6	88%T
75 4 TC					4.5					5.9		4.9		4.7		3.4		0.6				4.2	84%T
76 4 TC					4.6					4.8		4.8		4.8		2.7		1.2				3.9	85%T
77 4 TC					4.4					5.9		4.8		4.3		2.5		1.5				3.9	81%T
78 4 TC					4.4					5.8		5.0		4.9		2.4		1.6				4.1	83%T
79 4 TC					4.8					5.3		6.1		4.0		3.4		1.5				4.4	82%T
80 4 TC					4.7					6.8		6.1		4.9		2.9		1.7				4.6	72%T
81 4 TC					5.1					5.4		5.6		5.8		3.7		1.2				4.6	76%T
82 4 TC					4.5					6.6		5.8		4.2		3.2		1.7				4.5	81%T
83 4 TC					4.0					6.3		5.5		4.9		3.3		1.1				4.4	82%T
84 4 TC					3.8					6.3		5.8		5.6		3.6		1.4				4.6	86%T
85 4 TC					4.5																		85%T
86 4 TC					4.9																		82%T
87 4 TC					5.0																		81%T
88 4 TC					4.7																		89%T
89 4 TC					4.9																		81%T
90 4 TC					5.1																		80%T
91 4 TC					5.3																		78%T
92 4 TC					4.7																		84%T
93 4 TC					4.9																		87%T
94 4 TC					4.7																		80%T
95 4 TC					4.8																		79%T

1 Based on those surveys in Table 20.6 with data for both sexes and age range at least 21-64 (see *Cigarette consumption per person*, p. xxxv)

Source: See *Notes on sources of survey data*, p. 503
Product: MC = manufactured cigarettes
TC = total cigarettes (including hand-rolled)
UC = cigarettes (type unspecified)
A = all products
U = unspecified

All ages: relevant to ages used and as given in original source
% Total sales: Adjustment factor used, estimated % of total sales of M = manufactured or T = total cigarette consumption implied by survey, sexes combined
--- = adjusted by original author
* = refer to *Notes on sources of survey data*, p. 503

Table 20.8 Estimated[1] prevalence of smoking and estimated[1] number of cigarettes per person per day (unadjusted and sales-adjusted): summary of Tables 20.4, 20.6 and 20.7, 1954-1995.
Males and females aged 15 years and over

Year	Source[2]	Product[3]	Prevalence[4]						Number of cigarettes						
									Unadjusted[7]			Sales-adjusted[8]			
			Manufactured cigarettes		Total cigarettes[5]		All products[6]		Number/ person/day		Total sales %	Manufactured cigarettes number/ person/day		Total cigarettes[9] number/ person/day	
			M	F	M	F	M	F	M	F		M	F	M	F
1954	2	*TC+A*			53	25	73	23	7.1[10]					(3.4	1.3)
1960	1	A					63	25							
1961	1	A					63	26							
1962	1	A					61	25							
1963	1	A					61	26							
1964	1	A					55	24							
1965	1	A					55	24							
1966	1	A					58	28							
1967	1	A					57	28							
1968	1	A					58	30							
1969	1	A					57	32							
1970	1	A					56	33							
1971	1	A					52	32							
1972	1	A					52	34							
1973	1	A					53	35							
	3	UC			46	37								(6.0	3.9)
	4	TC+A					49	31	6.3	3.0	94			6.6	3.2
1974	1	A					51	34							
	4	TC+A					51	31	6.6	3.1	88			7.4	3.5
1975	1	A					51	37							
	4	TC+A					46	30	6.0	3.2	84			7.2	3.8
1976	1	A					52	35							
	4	TC+A					47	30	5.8	3.1	85			6.9	3.6
1977	1	A					47	37							
	4	TC+A					43	28	5.7	3.0	81			7.1	3.7
1978	1	A					49	38							
	4	TC+A					44	29	5.5	3.1	83			6.6	3.8
1979	1	A					47	37							
	4	TC+A					42	30	5.6	3.2	82			6.8	3.9
1980	1	A					46	37							
	4	TC+A					41	28	5.1	3.1	72			7.1	4.2
1981	1	A					44	36							
	4	TC+A					39	28	5.3	3.2	76			6.9	4.1

Table 20.8 (continued)

Year	Source[2]	Product[3]	Prevalence[4]						Number of cigarettes						
									Unadjusted[7]			Sales-adjusted[8]			
			Manufactured cigarettes		Total cigarettes[5]		All products[6]		Number/ person/day		Total sales %	Manufactured cigarettes number/ person/day		Total cigarettes[9] number/ person/day	
			M	F	M	F	M	F	M	F		M	F	M	F
1982	1	A					44	37							
	4	TC+A					39	31	5.1	3.3	81			6.3	4.1
1983	1	A					44	38							
	4	TC+A					41	28	5.8	3.2	82			7.0	3.9
1984	1	A					44	38							
	4	TC+A					40	30	5.7	3.5	86			6.6	4.1
1985	1	A					44	37							
	4	TC+A					41	29	5.8	3.4	85			6.8	4.1
1986	1	A					44	38							
	4	TC+A					37	29	5.6	3.6	82			6.8	4.4
1987	1	A					45	40							
	4	TC+A					39	30	5.4	3.6	81			6.7	4.5
1988	1	A					42	39							
	4	TC+A					40	32	5.9	3.7	89			6.7	4.2
1989	1	A					42	38							
	4	TC+A					36	30	5.2	3.6	80			6.4	4.4
1990	1	A					40	38							
	4	TC+A					35	31	5.1	3.6	80			6.4	4.5
1991	1	A					40	36							
	4	TC+A					34	30	4.9	3.6	78			6.3	4.7
1992	1	A					41	37							
	4	TC+A					36	29	5.1	3.5	84			6.1	4.2
1993	1	A					40	38							
	4	TC+A					36	32	5.4	3.8	87			6.2	4.4
1994	1	A					38	37							
	4	TC+A					34	29	4.7	3.3	80			5.9	4.2
1995	1	A					41	37							
	4	TC+A					32	29	4.6	3.3	79			5.8	4.2

1 Surveys covering an age range of at least 21-64 are included. Any gaps in the data for ages 15-20 and 65 years and over are filled in by assumed extensions to the age distribution, given in *Notes on sources of survey data*, p. 503. Method: see *Summary of adult smoking*, p. xxxvi
2 See *Notes on sources of survey data*, p. 503
3 Product: MC = manufactured cigarettes, TC = total cigarettes (including hand-rolled), UC = cigarettes (type unspecified), A = all products, U = unspecified. Frequency of smoking is indicated by: regular or daily smokers in normal type, all smokers (including occasional) in bold, unspecified in italics
4 From Table 20.4
5 This column includes prevalence of smoking classified as UC = cigarettes (type unspecified)
6 This column includes prevalence of smoking classified as U = unspecified product
7 From Table 20.6
8 From Table 20.7, except data in parentheses, which are derived from the prevalence of smoking from Table 20.4 as described in *Summary of adult smoking*, p. xxxvi
9 Number of cigarettes classified as UC = cigarettes (type unspecified) has been adjusted to total cigarette sales and included in this column
10 All tobacco products, grams/person/day

Figure 20.3 Estimated prevalence of smoking: of (i) total cigarettes and (ii) all tobacco products by year of survey, 1954-1995.
Males and females aged 15 years and over. *Source:* see Table 20.8

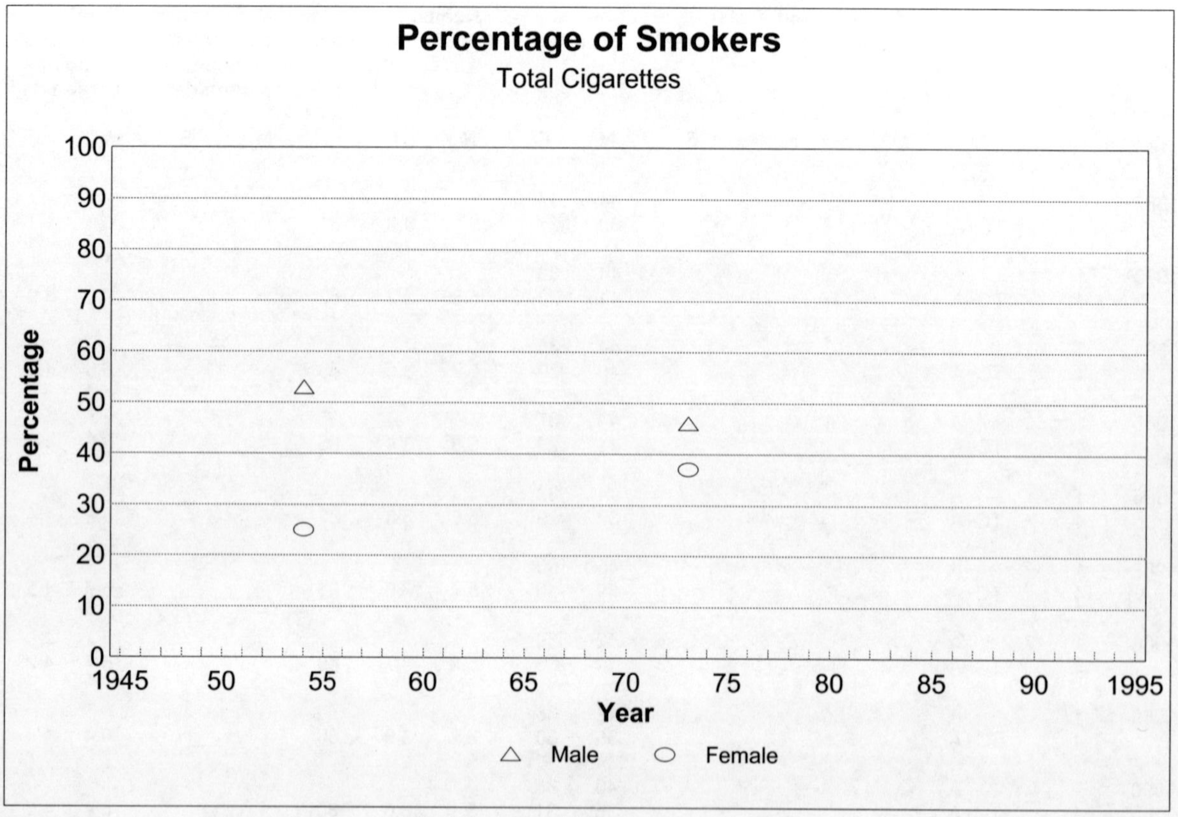

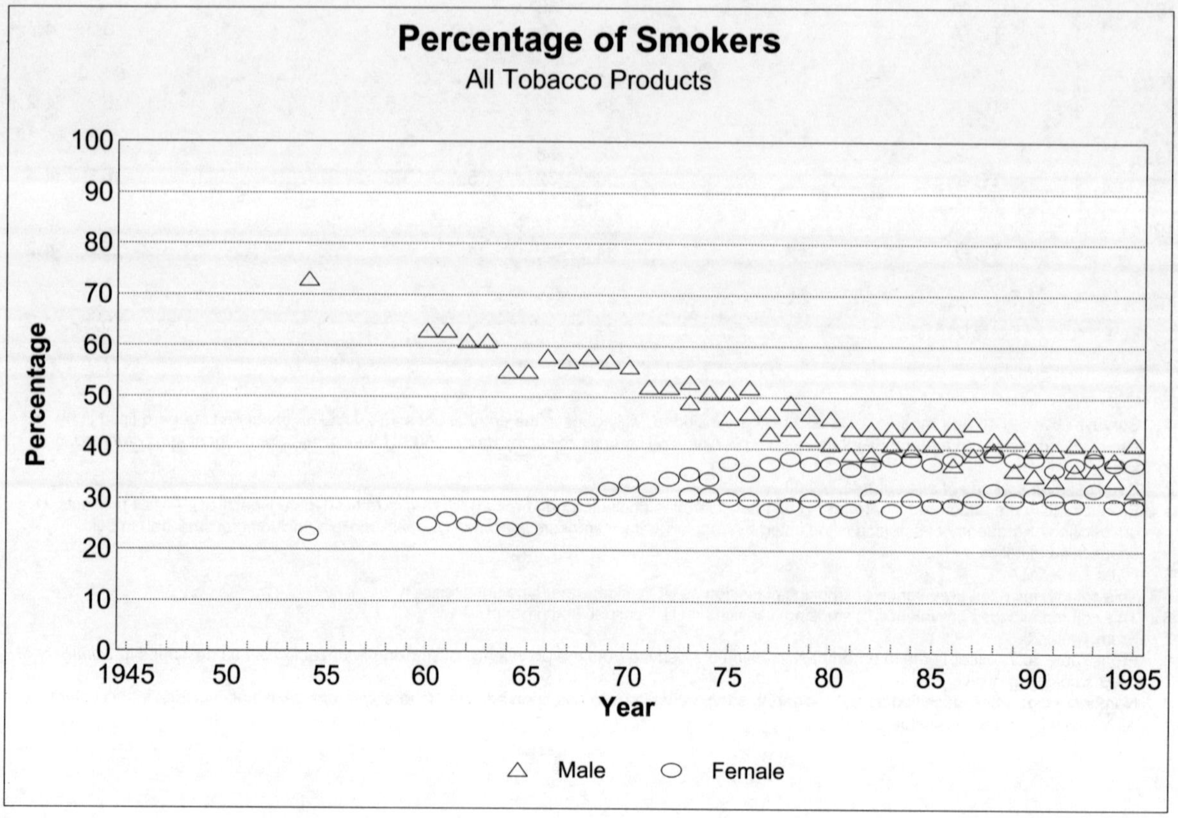

Figure 20.4 Estimated number of cigarettes smoked per person per day, sales-adjusted, 1954-1995.
Males and females aged 15 years and over. *Source:* see Table 20.8

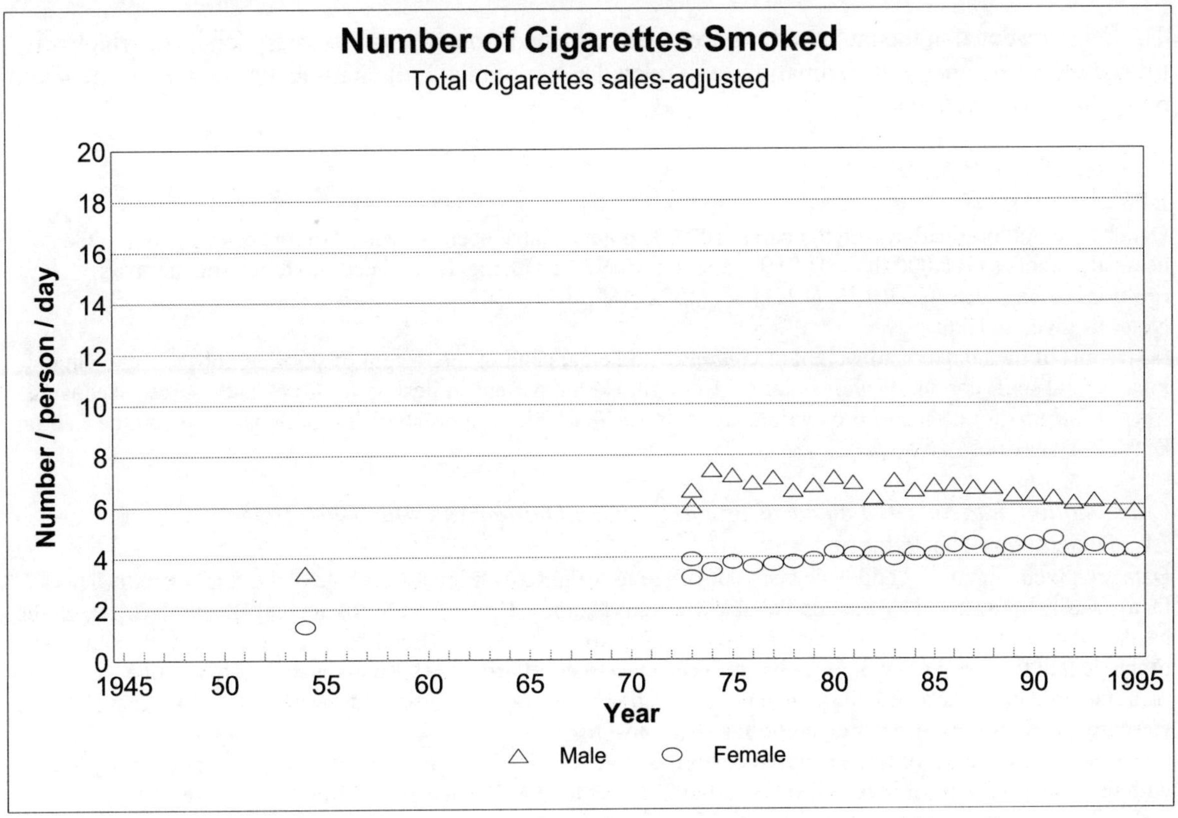

Notes on sources of sales data

The data presented in the tables and figures were obtained from several sources, details of which are given below, together with estimations and related assumptions. Full citations of the sources are given on p. 507 under *References*.

Consumption data before 1974
RP6
Data by weight, originally given to nearest 100 000 pounds, have been converted to tonnes and given to the nearest 10 tonnes (100 000 lbs = 45.359 tonnes). For 1970-1973, cigars included the following numbers (millions) of cigarlets: (1970) 30, (1971) 20, (1972) 18, (1973) 15.
Notes as given in RP6:
(a) Details of the number and weight of cigarettes and cigars and of the weight of smoking tobacco, chewing tobacco and snuff consumed were obtained from Tobakkindustriens Felleskontor, Oslo. The sources used were *Norges Industri* for details of production, and *Norges Handel* for import statistics, both published by the Central Bureau of Statistics of Norway.

Consumption data for 1974 onwards and tax-free and border sales for 1961-1995
J.L. Tiedemanns Tobaksfabrik
Data are given in numbers and have been converted to weight assuming an average of 1 g per cigarette. This factor was recommended by Statens Tobakkskaderåd (National Council on Smoking and Health, NCSH), on the basis of data on the weight of cigarettes around 1970. No more recent official data are available, although it is probable that the weight of cigarettes has reduced since then. Bjartveit (1990) gives the weight of one manufactured cigarette as not more than 0.8 g, based on their own measurements at the time of writing. (Data in RP6 imply a factor of 1.1 g per cigarette for 1955 onwards.)

Note that data for manufactured cigarettes from J.L. Tiedemanns for earlier years do not exactly agree with data from RP6 (quantities in RP6 are 20-30% lower in 1944-45 and 10-15% higher in 1948-52).

Following increases in excise duties in 1980 and 1981, many Norwegians started buying cigarettes and pipe and hand-rolling tobacco in Sweden where prices were much lower. Estimates from J.L. Tiedemanns of tax-free sales and border trade to Norwegians have been included in the totals given in Table 20.1.2. They are available only for all products combined. However, estimates of cross-border sales of pipe and hand-rolling tobacco are available from Wicklin (1998) and are shown in Table 20.1.5. We assumed in the calculations shown in this table that cross-border sales of cigars, chewing tobacco and snuff are negligible. The estimates of cross-border sales of pipe and hand-rolling tobacco are subtracted from the estimates of total tax-free and border sales (from J.L. Tiedemanns) to give our estimate of cross-border sales of manufactured cigarettes. This is added to domestic sales of manufactured cigarettes to give the adjusted total sales of manufactured cigarettes. These values are used in Table 20.2 for the years 1974-1995.

Joossens and Raw (1998) quoting Lund (1990) estimate the contraband market share in Norway as 2%. The J.L. Tiedemanns estimate of tax-free and border sales is approximately 12% for 1986-1989.

Plain/Filter cigarette consumption
1961-1981 Maxwell (successive years)
In 1997 the proportion of cigarette production which was filter cigarettes was 96% (United States Department of Agriculture (1999)).

Tar yield of cigarettes
1970-1980 Mørck *et al* (1982)
Smedslund and Götestam (1999) quoting Hauknes (1994) give the 'average yield' of Norwegian manufactured cigarettes as 13.86 mg of tar and 1.11 mg of nicotine. Their estimate for the yield of a hand-rolled cigarette is 34.09 mg of tar and 2.46 mg of nicotine.

From 1996, the tar content of cigarettes was limited to 15mg per cigarette (Harkin *et al* (1997)).

Cigarette paper sales
Statens Tobakkskaderåd (NCSH)

Estimates of hand-rolled cigarettes for 1939-1995

We have taken as our estimate of hand-rolled cigarette consumption 90% of cigarette paper sales These estimates (if taken with the further assumption of 1 g per cigarette) appear consistent with statements by Mørck *et al* (1982) that about 90% of pipe and hand-rolling tobacco is accounted for by hand-rolled cigarettes, and that hand-rolled cigarettes as a percentage of all cigarettes rose from 10% before the Second World War to 60-70% in 1982. They also agree with Kreyberg (1954) who implies the following proportions of hand-rolled tobacco out of pipe and hand-rolling tobacco combined:

Year	% hand-rolled of all loose tobacco
1939	5
1946	18
1947	19
1948	11
1949	28
1950	30
1951	28

Estimates of hand-rolled cigarette consumption in the latest available year were also given in the introductions to successive editions of RP6:

Year	Annual (millions)	Number/ adult/day
1966	2 908	2.8
1970	3 283	3.1
1973	3 470	3.2

These estimates are within 3% of those given in Table 20.2.

Dymond (1996) gives the weight of tobacco in one hand-rolled cigarette as 900 mg (range 800-1 000 mg).

Notes on sources of survey data

Each source of survey data—either an individual survey or a series of surveys repeated over a number of years—is cited by a source number. This number is shown in the tables and corresponds to the source numbers given below, where details of the source publication and of the survey methodology are given. Full citations of the sources are given on p. 507 under *References*.

Source number

1 **Norges Markedsdata and J.L. Tiedemanns Tobaksfabrik (personal communication) quoting AC Nielsen Norge**

a. Market analysis of smoking habits carried out by the public opinion institute Norges Markedsdata (Market Data of Norway) and Nielsen Norge. Sample size (males) about 7 000, (females) about 7 000. Results published twice a year, average presented here

2 **Kreyberg (1955) quoting Fakta**

a. Results of a market research survey. Year approximate, lower age limit unknown. Results presented here are averages over 4 urban/rural groups. Sample size (males) 1 969, (females) 2 096

b. Consumption per smoker and consumption per person are number of grams per day

c. Kreyberg (1954) also presented data collected in 1953 as controls in a study of lung cancer, in 7 groups of males and 5 groups of women. These data have not been presented in the Table 20.4 since they include ex-smokers. However they are of interest being of a very early date and some results for prevalence of smoking are presented here. One group consisted of all persons (patients and their accompanying friends or relatives) attending the Oslo First Aid Station. Sample size (males) 699, (females) 301. Other groups are not presented here individually as they were occupational groups, or had poor response rates or small sample sizes, but the aggregated results given by Kreyberg (1955) are shown. Sample size (males) 4 158 including 2 337 doctors, (females) 985 including 168 doctors. Only 3 women, all doctors, smoked products other than cigarettes.

Prevalence of smoking

Age	15-24	25-34	35-39	45-54	55-64	65-74
Oslo						
Male, TC A	72	81	82	66	55	25
Male, A A	75	89	90	84	81	71
Female	50	49	43	28	13	7
Aggregate		**<35**	**35-44**	**45-54**	**55-64**	**65-84**
Male		79	86	89	87	83
Female		41	39	31	13	10

TC, A defined as for Table 20.4

3 **Le Meitour-Kaplan (1977), quoting Nordic Research Association (1973)**

a. Survey conducted November-December 1973 in four Nordic countries. Total sample size 6 000. Age group unknown (see also Denmark source 3, Sweden source 4, and Finland source 8)

b. Smokers: smoked 'yesterday'

4 **Statens Tobakksskaderåd (NCSH) (1996, 1999 and personal communication), Wicklin (1998)**

a. Until 1991, part of the Manpower Survey (Arbeidskrafts Undersøkelse, AKU) carried out by Statistics Norway, about 3 000 persons interviewed annually (personal interviews to 1980, then telephone interviews). From 1992, part of the Statistic Norway omnibus, about 2 500 persons, reducing to 2 000 in 1995, primarily personal interviews. Question on tobacco prevalence remained same over the years. Non-response variable, but about 30%

b. Regular smokers: smoked daily. Percentage of occasional smokers remained stable at around 10% for both men and women (during 1973-1984)

c. Calculation of consumption per person based on percentage smokers of any product and number of cigarettes per smoker

d. Data for cigarette consumption per smoker from 1989 taken from chart

e. Assumed extension to age distribution for percentage smokers, age 15: males (1973-1976) 20%, (1977-1995) 15% and females (1973-1981) 20%, (1982-1995) 15%. Number of cigarettes/person/day: males 1.0 and females 0.8. For age 75+: males (1973-1985) 30%, (1986-1990) 25%, (1991-1995) 20% and females (1973-1985) 5%, (1986-1995) 10%. Number of cigarettes/person/day: males 1.0 and females 0.5

5 **Nilsen (1959), Aarø *et al* (1981), quoting Nilsen (1967)**

a. Surveys conducted by Norwegian Cancer Society. In 1957, anonymous questionnaire survey carried out in various types of school throughout the country (about 5% of rural schools, 10% of urban schools and 20% of Oslo schools). Aimed to be representative of the school population (although not of the total age group, e.g. only 10% of 19-year-olds still attended schools). Sample size (males) 4 967, (females) 4 324. No details available for 1963 survey

b. Regular smokers: smoked daily. All smokers: smoked daily or occasionally. Consumption per smoker relates to daily smokers

6 **Hermansen and Vellar (1974)**

a. Sample size (1971) 24 338, (1972) 24 162

b. Regular smokers: smoked daily.

7 **Aarø *et al* (1981), Bjartveit (1990), Statens Tobakksskaderåd (NCSH) (1996 and personal communication)**

a. National studies involving all Norwegian pupils of the relevant age groups. Attendance rate over 90%. Question on tobacco prevalence remained same over the years. Representative samples of questionnaires analysed. Sample size (1975) 6 968, (1980) 5 431, and (1985) 5 127

b. Regular smokers: smoked daily

c. Data shown in *All ages* column refers to age 13-15 only

8 **Geizerova and Masironi (1988)**

a. No original source

9,10 Zeiner-Henriksen (1976), Haenszel and Hougen (1972)

a. Study conducted 1964-1965. Results shown as source **9** are from a sample representative of the whole country; sample size (males) 6 713, (females) 8 206, response rate 80%. Results shown as source **10** include additional samples in four counties (Finmark, Avst-Agder, Vest-Agder and Rogaland) and a sample of siblings of Norwegian-born migrants to the USA; combined sample size (males) 12 521, (females) 14 626; response rate in sibling sample 66%

b. Among cigarette only smokers (source 10), the % distribution by type of cigarette was:

	Hand-rolled cigarettes only	Manufactured cigarettes only	Mixed
Males	70.0	15.8	14.2
Females	42.3	42.9	14.8

11 Pedersen *et al* (1969)

a. Baseline of a study of male lung cancer in Finland and Norway, May 1962-Feb 1963. See also Finland, source 3. Norwegian part of the study was conducted in 3 urban and 3 rural areas. Personal interviews at home or work. Sample size 4 092, response rate 87%. Results presented here are unweighted averages over region

b. The proportion of cigarette smokers (including ex-cigarette smokers) reporting smoking only manufactured was 5-50%, hand-rolled 30-90% and both types 3-15% in the different areas

c. Consumption category estimation based on 1-4, 5-9, 10-14, 15-19, 20-24, 25-29, 30+ cigarettes/smoker/day

12 Leren *et al* (1975)

a. Baseline of the Oslo study, health screening of 17 965 men (all Oslo men age 40-49 and a random sample age 20-39), 1972-1973.

Age	Sample size	Attendance rate (%)
20-24	382	33
24-29	591	43
30-34	393	49
35-39	397	62
40-44	7 427	65
45-49	8 775	65

13 Thürmer and Bjartveit (1990)

a. Based on methods of the Oslo study (source 12), all residents of 3 counties age 40-49 invited to attend National Health Screening Service, 1974-1978. Numbers attended (males) 16 963, (females) 16 148. Attendance rate (males) 90%, (females) 94%

14 Tell *et al* (1984)

a. Baseline of the Oslo Youth Study, conducted at six schools in Oslo. Anonymous questionnaire completed in class with teachers absent. Approximate ages corresponding to school grades 5 (not presented here), 6 and 7. Sample size 828 (after exclusion of non-Norwegians), response rate 82%

b. Regular smokers: smoked daily. Results for cigarettes per smoker and cigarettes per person are for daily smokers

15 Klepp *et al* (1991), King and Coles (1992), King *et al* (1996)

a. Part of the HBSC (Health Behaviour in School-Aged Children) Study, a collaborative cross-national research study sponsored by the WHO school classes or schools were randomly selected, targeting age groups 11 (not presented here), 13 and 15.

Year	Target age	Mean age	Sample size
1983	13	13.4	1 265
	15	15.4	1 061
1985	13	—	1 302
	15	—	1 291
1989	13	13.4	1 633
	15	15.4	1 648
1993	13	13.5	1 701
	15	15.5	1 637

c. Regular smokers: smoke once a week or more. Smokers marked as frequency *: smoked daily
d. There are minor discrepancies between the results presented here (Klepp *et al* (1991)) and those presented by other authors Nutbeam *et al* (1989), van Reek *et al* (1990), King and Coles (1992))

16-18 Twelve months military service is compulsory for males age 19 or 20, about 25% are excluded for medical or other reasons. Three months are spent at a training school in southern Norway, followed by 9 months service usually in Northern Norway near the Russian border (Schei *et al* (1990), Schei and Johanne Søgaard (1994))

16 Schei and Johanne Søgaard (1994)

a. Survey among conscripts during last 9 months of military service in Northern Norway. Mean age 20.6 years. Sample size (of useable questionnaires) 2 112, response rate 90.4%
b. Consumption category estimation based on 1-9, 10-19, 20+ cigarettes/smoker/day

17 Samdal *et al* (1991)

a. Survey among conscripts during last 9 months of military service, in Northern Norway. 98% were aged 19-22. Sample size 1 511
b. Consumption category estimation based on 1-10, 11-20, 21+ cigarettes/smoker/day

18 Bovim *et al* (1990)

a. Study of recruits interviewed at start of military service and after three months. Data presented here relate to start of service. Sample size 903. Year not stated
b. Age range 18-27, of whom 74% were age 19-20
c. Consumption category estimation based on 1-5, 6-10 and 11+ cigarettes/smoker/day

19 Friestad and Klepp (1996)

a. Representative sample in county Hordaland, followed up over four years. Sample size 1 195
b. Regular smokers: smoked every day. All smokers: smoked every day or every week. The categories reported were daily, weekly, occasionally and never, so do not appear to have allowed for ex-smokers

20 Lokeland *et al* (1993)

a. Anonymous questionnaire study pupils at 19 schools in Bergen municipality. Approximate age corresponding to school grade 9. Sample size (males) 318, (females) 323
b. Regular smokers: smoked every day or every week. Smokers marked as frequency *: smoked daily

21 Hibell *et al* (1997)

a. Nationally representative survey forming part of ESPAD (European School Survey Project on Alcohol and Other Drugs). Target was pupils born in 1979, thus age 15-16 at time of survey in March1995. Approximately 98% of this group still in school. Anonymous questionnaire completed and sealed in envelope by pupil, in class. Teachers present, but discouraged from walking round the classroom. Sample size (males) 1 979, (females) 1 931. Response rate 91%
b. Regular smokers: smoked 1 or more cigarettes per day in last 30 days. All smokers: smoked in last 30 days
c. Consumption category estimation based on 1-5, 6-10, 11-20, 21+ cigarettes/smoker/day

Additional information (not presented in tables)
Statens Tobakkskaderåd (NCSH) (2000)

In 1996-1998, among daily cigarette smokers, the % distribution by type of cigarette was:

Age	Males			Females		
	Hand-rolled only	Manufactured only	Mixed	Hand-rolled only	Manufactured only	Mixed
16-24	27	46	27	10	74	16
25-34	41	42	17	30	61	9
35-44	54	31	15	39	43	18
45-54	61	28	11	45	35	20
55-64	82	15	3	54	32	14
66-74	85	9	6	44	47	9

References

Aarø L.E., Hauknes A. and Berglund E.-L. (1981). Smoking among Norwegian schoolchildren 1975-1980. I. Extent of smoking in the age group 12-15 years, 1975. *Scand J Psychol,* **22**, 161-9.

Beese D.H. (ed) (1968). *Tobacco consumption in various countries,* 2nd edition. Tobacco Research Council, London. Research Paper 6.

Beese D.H. (ed) (1972). *Tobacco consumption in various countries,* 3rd edition. Tobacco Research Council, London. Research Paper 6.

Bjartveit K. (1990). Fifteen years of comprehensive legislation: results and conclusions. In: Durston B. and Jamrozik K. (eds) *Tobacco & health 1990. The global war. Seventh World Conference on Tobacco and Health, Perth, Western Australia, 1-5 April 1990.* Organising Committee of the Seventh World Conference on Tobacco and Health, 189 Royal Street, East Perth, Western Australia 6004; 71-80.

Bovim G., Aasland O.G. and Tyssedal J.S. (1990). Endring i bruk av alkohol og tobakk under rekruttskolen (Changes in the use of alcohol and tobacco during introductory military service). *Tidsskr Nor Laegeforen,* **110**, 1705-6.

Dymond H.F. (1996). A survey of roll-your-own tobacco use and practice and considerations for the analysis of smoking articles made from it. *Tobacco Science,* **40**, 82-6.

Friestad C. and Klepp K.I. (1996). Fra eksperimentering til vanerøyking. En tre års oppfølgingsundersøkelse av ungdoms røykevaner. (From experimentation to habitual smoking. A three-year follow-up study of adolescents' smoking behaviour). *Tidsskr Nor Laegeforen,* **116**, 635-8.

Geizerova H. and Masironi R. (1988). Cigarette smoking in children and adolescents: world review. In: Aoki M., Hisamichi S. and Tominaga S. (eds) *Smoking and health 1987. Proceedings of the 6th World Conference on Smoking and Health, Tokyo, 9-12 November 1987.* Elsevier Science Publishers B.V. (Biomedical Division), Amsterdam; 601-5. International Congress Series No. 780.

Haenszel W. and Hougen A. (1972). Prevalence of respiratory symptoms in Norway. *Journal of Chronic Diseases,* **25**, 519-44.

Harkin A.M., Anderson P. and Goos C. (1997). *Smoking, drinking and drug taking in the European Region.* Alcohol, Drugs and Tobacco Programme, WHO Regional Office for Europe, Copenhagen.

Hauknes A. (1994). *Analysis of hazardous substances in rolling tobacco.* Statens tobakksskaderåd (NCSH), Oslo.

Hermansen L. and Vellar O.D. (1974). Røkevaner hos unge norske menn 1971-1972. *Tidsskr Nor Laegeforen,* **94**, 1440-2.

Hibell B., Andersson B., Bjarnason T., Kokkevi A., Morgan M. and Narusk A. (1997). *The 1995 ESPAD report. The European school survey project on alcohol and other drugs. Alcohol and other drug use among students in 26 European countries.* The Swedish Council for Information on Alcohol and Other Drugs. Council of Europe (Pompidou Group).

Joossens L. and Raw M. (1998). Cigarette smuggling in Europe: who really benefits? *Tob Control,* **7** , 66-71.

King A., Wold B., Tudor-Smith C. and Harel Y. (1996). *The health of youth, a cross-national survey.* WHO Regional Publications, Europe, Copenhagen. European Series No. 69.

King A.J.C. and Coles B. (1992). *The health of Canada's youth. Views and behaviours of 11-, 13- and 15-year-olds from 11 countries.* Health and Welfare Canada, Ottawa.

Klepp K.-I., Wold B. and Aarø L.E. (1991). Røyking og bruk av alkohol blant norske skolebarn: tendenser i 1980-årene. (Smoking and alcohol use among Norwegian schoolchildren: trends in the 1980s). *Tidsskr Nor*

Laegeforen, **111**, 2859-63.

Kreyberg H.J.A. (1954). A study of tobacco smoking in Norway. *Br J Cancer,* **8**, 13-33.

Kreyberg L. (1955). Lung cancer and tobacco smoking in Norway. *Br J Cancer,* **9**, 495-510.

Le Meitour-Kaplan A. (1977). Situational Analysis: Profile of women's smoking habits in Continental Western Europe. In: Steinfeld J., Griffiths W., Ball K. and Taylor R.M. (eds) *Health consequences, education, cessation activities, and social action, Volume II. Proceedings of the Third World Conference on Smoking and Health, New York City, June 2-5, 1975.* US Department of Health, Education and Welfare, USA; 309-27. DHEW Publication No (NIH) 77-1413.

Lee P.N. (ed) (1975). *Tobacco consumption in various countries,* 4th edition. Tobacco Research Council, London. Research Paper 6.

Leren P., Askevold E.M., Foss O.P., Frøili A., *et al* (1975). The Oslo Study—cardiovascular disease in middle-aged and young Oslo men. *Acta Medica Scandinavica,* **Suppl 588**, 1-38. Almqvist & Wiksell Periodical Company, Stockholm.

Lokeland T., Nygard A.B., Salbu H.R., Salvesen I., *et al* (1993). Etablering av røykevaner blant ungdom. En undersøkelse blant elever i niendeklasse (Establishing smoking habits—a study among pupils in the 9th grade). *Tidsskr Nor Laegeforen,* **113**, 3259-61.

Lund K.E. (1990). *A note on the changes in tobacco use since 1970.* National Council on Tobacco and Health, Oslo. NCTH document 36/1990. [§]

Lund K.E., Rönneberg A. and Hafstad A. (1995). The social and demographic diffusion of the tobacco epidemic in Norway. In: Slama K. (ed) *Tobacco and Health, Ninth World Conference on Tobacco and Health, Paris, Oct 10-14 1994.* Plenum Press, New York and London; 565-70.

Maxwell J.C.Jr. (successive years). How the brands ranked. Maxwell International Estimates. *World Tobacco.*

Mørck H.I., Linde J., Agner E., Hein H.O., Gyntelberg F. and Nielsen P.E. (1982). Tobaksforbrug og rygevaner i Norden 1920-1980. (Tobacco consumption and smoking habits in the Nordic countries). *Nord Med,* **97**, 134-46.

Nilsen E. (1959). Smoking habits among school children in Norway. *British Journal of Preventive and Social Medicine,* **13**, 5-13.[§]

Nilsen E. (1967). *Forandringer i røykevaner over 10 år. (Change in smoking behaviour over 10 years).* Norwegian Cancer Society, Oslo.[§]

Nordic Research Association (1973). *1973 Survey. Antalet rökare i fyra nordiska länder i november-december 1973.*

Nutbeam D., Aar L. and Catford J. (1989). Understanding children's health behaviour: the implications for health promotion for young people. *Soc Sci Med,* **29**, 317-25.

Pedersen E., Magnus K., Mork T., Hougen A., *et al* (1969). Lung cancer in Finland and Norway, an epidemiological study. *Acta Pathologica et Microbiologica Scandinavica,* **Suppl 199**, 1-74. Munksgaard, Copenhagen.

RP6, See Beese (ed) (1968), Beese (ed) (1972), Lee (ed) (1975)

Samdal F., Haaverstad R., Almdahl S.M., Skogesal O., Sommerseth J. and Schei E. (1991). Bruk av alkohol og tobakk under militærtjenesten. En undersøkelse blant soldater i Brigaden i Nord-Norge (Use of alcohol and tobacco during military service. A study among soldiers in the brigade in northern Norway). *Tidsskr Nor*

Laegeforen, **111**, 2725-7.

Schei E., Fønnebø V. and Aarø L.-E. (1990). Use of smokeless tobacco among Norwegian army conscripts. In: Durston B. and Jamrozik K. (eds) *Tobacco & health 1990. The global war. Seventh World Conference on Tobacco and Health, Perth, Western Australia, 1-5 April 1990.* Organising Committee of the Seventh World Conference on Tobacco and Health, 189 Royal Street, East Perth, Western Australia 6004; 453-4.

Schei E. and Johanne Søgaard A. (1994). The impact of military service on young men's smoking behavior. *Prev Med,* **23**, 242-8.

Smedslund G. and Götestam K.G. (1999). Effects of handrolled unfiltered cigarettes versus manufactured filter cigarettes on symptoms and diseases in current smokers. *European Journal of Psychiatry,* **13**, 47-57.

Statens Tobakkskaderåd (NCSH) (1999). *Statistikk og undersøkelser.* www.tobakk.no/statistikk/statistikk.htm.

Statens Tobakkskaderåd (NCSH) (2000). *Tobakksprodukter.* Statens Tobakkskaderåd, Norway. http://www/tobakk.no/statistikk/tot2.htm.

Statens Tobakksskaderåd (NCSH) (1996). *Tobakksbruk og holdninger i Norge—utviklingen 1973-95. (Tobacco consumption and attitudes in Norway—the development 1973-95)* . Statens Tobakksskaderåd, Oslo.

Tell G.S., Klepp K.-I., Vellar O.D. and McAlister A. (1984). Preventing the onset of cigarette smoking in Norwegian adolescents: The Oslo Youth Study. *Prev Med,* **13**, 256-75.

Thürmer H. and Bjartveit K. (1990). Socio-economic characteristics of female vs. male smokers in Norway. In: Durston B. and Jamrozik K. (eds) *Tobacco & health 1990. The global war. Seventh World Conference on Tobacco and Health, Perth, Western Australia, 1-5 April 1990.* Organising Committee of the Seventh World Conference on Tobacco and Health, 189 Royal Street, East Perth, Western Australia 6004; 253-4.

United States Department of Agriculture (1999). *Norway, Tobacco annual, 1999.* (Foreign Agriculture Service GAIN Report (Global Agriculture Information Network) .) GAIN Report #NO9004. http://www.fas.usda.gov/webmap.html.

van Reek J., Adriaanse H. and Aarø L.E. (1990). Smoking by schoolchildren in eleven European countries. In: Durston B. and Jamrozik K. (eds) *Tobacco & health 1990. The global war. Seventh world conference on tobacco and health, 1st-5th April 1990, Perth, Western Australia.* Organising committee of the Seventh World Conference on Tobacco and Health, 189 Royal Street, East Perth, Western Australia 6004; 301-2.

Wicklin B. (ed) (1998). *Tobaksstatistik 1970-1997. Konsumtion av tobaksvaror, priser, inkomster, rökvanor, handel och illegala tillförseln mm i Sverige, Norge, Danmark och Finland (Tobacco statistics 1970-1997. Consumption of tobacco products prices income, smoking habits, trade and attempted smuggling etc. in Sweden, Norway, Denmark and Finland).* Svenska tobaksbranschföreningar, Örebro, Sweden.

Zeiner-Henriksen T. (1976). Røkevaner i den norske befolkning. (Smoking habits in the Norwegian population). *Tidsskr Nor Laegeforen,* **96**, 617-20.

§ Original paper not obtained, but information taken as quoted by another author

Poland 21

Sales data

See Tables 21.1-21.3

In the 1920s and 1930s, consumption of manufactured cigarettes per adult was less than 1 cigarette per day. After the Second World War, consumption rose rapidly, virtually doubling from 3 cigarettes per day in 1949 to 6 in 1960. It continued to rise, until about 1980 when it levelled at around 10 cigarettes per day.

The consumption of all tobacco products per adult was 2-3 g per day before the Second World War. About 35% was consumed as manufactured cigarettes.The remainder was mainly smoked in hand-made cigarettes (in cigarette tubes or rolled in tissue paper). Pipes were smoked only in western Poland (Staszewski (1960a)). By 1949, consumption had risen to 3.5 g, of which 95% was consumed as manufactured cigarettes. Products other than cigarettes virtually disappeared by the mid-1950s.

Survey data

See Tables 21.4-21.8

Based on non-representative surveys in the 1950s and the 1960s, the prevalence of smoking among those aged 15 years and over was 60-80% among men and 10-20% among women. Nationally representative surveys are available from 1974, at which time the estimated prevalence of regular smoking was 58% in men and 17% in women. By 1995, it had fallen to 47% in men. Among women, estimates fluctuate, but were generally 25-30% in the 1980s, and 22-25% in the 1990s. A further 2-6% of both sexes were occasional smokers. More men than women smoke at all ages. A decline in smoking prevalence with increasing age is more marked in women than in men.

Few data are available on smoking among teenagers. A series of surveys between 1979 and 1985 among pupils in Lódź showed some decline in prevalence, more marked in boys than girls, but nationally based surveys showed an increase between 1990 and 1994. A survey in Lubin showed substantially higher prevalence in vocational school students than in general schools. All surveys reported that more boys than girls smoked.

Comparison between survey and sales data suggest that surveys under-reported by 10-40%. Between 1957 and 1995, the estimated number of cigarettes smoked per person per day (sales-adjusted) for men increased from 12 to 15, and then decreased to 13. For women, it increased from 1 to 6.

Table 21.1.1 Total annual sales of tobacco products, 1925-1957

Year	Cigarettes				Cigars		Other tobacco tonnes	Snuff tonnes	All tobacco products tonnes
	Total tonnes	With mouthpiece millions	Without mouthpiece millions	Total millions	tonnes	millions			
1925	6203			7754	287	52	11242	390	18122
1929	8152			10190	429	78	13011	446	22038
1933	6108	3843	3792	7635	201	36	10927	314	17550
1937	6159	3951	3748	7699	159	29	12583	253	19154
1949	20691	810	19881	20691	137	25	973	93	21894
1953	30517	428	30088	30517	124	22	343	95	31079
1957	42551	1012	41539	42551	172	31			42723

Source : see *Notes on sources of sales data*, p. 528

Table 21.1.2 Total annual sales of tobacco products, 1960-1995

Year	Cigarettes	
	tonnes	millions
1960	44286	44286
1961	49982	49982
1962	53079	53079
1963	53440	53440
1964	47300	47300
1965	53377	53377
1966	59829	59829
1967	58781	58781
1968	64418	64418
1969	68733	68733
1970	69183	69183
1971	67832	67832
1972	81757	81757
1973	76230	76230
1974	81403	81403
1975	83875	83875
1976	89468	89468
1977	90600	90600
1978	91786	91786
1979	92920	92920
1980	94851	94851
1981	90104	90104
1982	91741	91741
1983	85717	85717
1984	88276	88276
1985	92744	92744
1986	99038	99038
1987	103268	103268
1988	95071	95071
1989	96073	96073
1990	102944	102944
1991	112667	112667
1992	95878	95878
1993	103767	103767
1994	95487	95487
1995	101117	101117

Source : see *Notes on sources of sales data,* p. 528

Table 21.1.3 Manufactured cigarettes (i) percentage of total sales as filter cigarettes, 1967-1995, and (ii) tar and nicotine yield per cigarette (popular brands), 1980-1995

Year	% Filter	Tar mg / cig	Nicotine mg / cig
1967	4.8		
1968	5.9		
1969	9.4		
1970	11.8		
1971	14.1		
1972	17.8		
1973	22.8		
1974	30.7		
1975	30.9		
1976	33.7		
1977	36.9		
1978	40.9		
1979	43.1		
1980	44.8	17.1 - 23.6	0.9 - 2.05
1983		19.5 - 24.4	1.04 - 1.88
1984	44	20.1 - 28.4	1.49 - 2.24
1985		18.9 - 31.9	1.13 - 2.63
1986		18.0 - 26.3	0.92 - 2.12
1987		17.2 - 25.7	0.69 - 1.94
1988		20.2 - 25.4	0.97 - 1.50
1990	56.3	17.0 - 20.3	1.17 - 1.44
1991	62.4	15.3 - 21.6	0.97 - 1.44
1992	71.7	14.1 - 21.2	0.92 - 1.39
1993	80.2	16.7 - 18.6	1.06 - 1.81
1994	80.3	14.5 - 16.9	1.13 - 1.52
1995	80.2	13.9 - 16.1	1.17 - 1.55

Source : see *Notes on sources of sales data*, p. 528

Table 21.2 Consumption of (i) cigarettes and (ii) all tobacco products, 1925-1995 sales-based data, including estimated hand-rolled cigarette consumption. Males and females aged 15 years and over

Year	Manufactured cigarettes		Hand-rolled cigarettes		Total cigarettes		All tobacco products	
	Total annual in millions	Number/ adult/day	Total annual in millions	Number/ adult/day	Total annual in millions	Number/ adult/day	Total annual in tonnes	Grams/ adult/day
1925	7754	1.0					18122	2.4
1929	10190	1.3					22038	2.9
1933	7635	0.9					17550	2.1
1937	7699	0.9					19154	2.1
1949	20691	3.2					21894	3.4
1953	30517	4.6					31079	4.6
1957	42551	6.1					42723	6.1
1960	44286	6.2					44286	6.2
1961	49982	6.9					49982	6.9
1962	53079	7.2					53079	7.2
1963	53440	7.1					53440	7.1
1964	47300	6.1					47300	6.1
1965	53377	6.7					53377	6.7
1966	59829	7.4					59829	7.4
1967	58781	7.1					58781	7.1
1968	64418	7.6					64418	7.6
1969	68733	8.0					68733	8.0
1970	69183	8.0					69183	8.0
1971	67832	7.7					67832	7.7
1972	81757	9.1					81757	9.1
1973	76230	8.3					76230	8.3
1974	81403	8.7					81403	8.7
1975	83875	8.8					83875	8.8
1976	89468	9.4					89468	9.4
1977	90600	9.4					90600	9.4
1978	91786	9.4					91786	9.4
1979	92920	9.5					92920	9.5
1980	94851	9.6					94851	9.6
1981	90104	9.1					90104	9.1
1982	91741	9.2					91741	9.2
1983	85717	8.6					85717	8.6
1984	88276	8.8					88276	8.8
1985	92744	9.2					92744	9.2
1986	99038	9.7					99038	9.7
1987	103268	10.1					103268	10.1
1988	95071	9.2					95071	9.2
1989	96073	9.3					96073	9.3
1990	102944	9.9					102944	9.9
1991	112667	10.7					112667	10.7
1992	95878	9.1					95878	9.1
1993	103767	9.7					103767	9.7
1994	95487	8.9					95487	8.9
1995	101117	9.3					101117	9.3

Source : see *Notes on sources of sales data*, p. 528

Figure 21.1 Daily consumption of (i) manufactured and total number of cigarettes, and (ii) all tobacco products, 1925-1995.
Males and females aged 15 years and over. *Source:* see Table 21.2

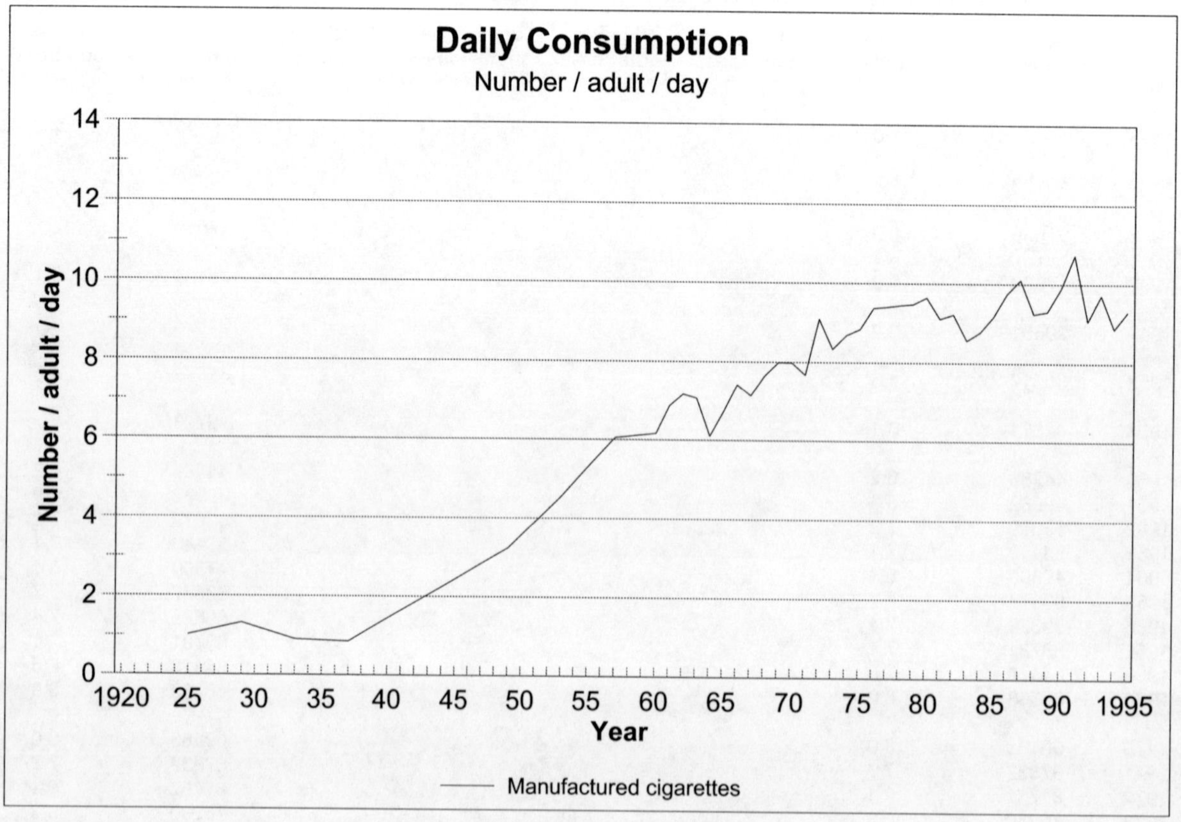

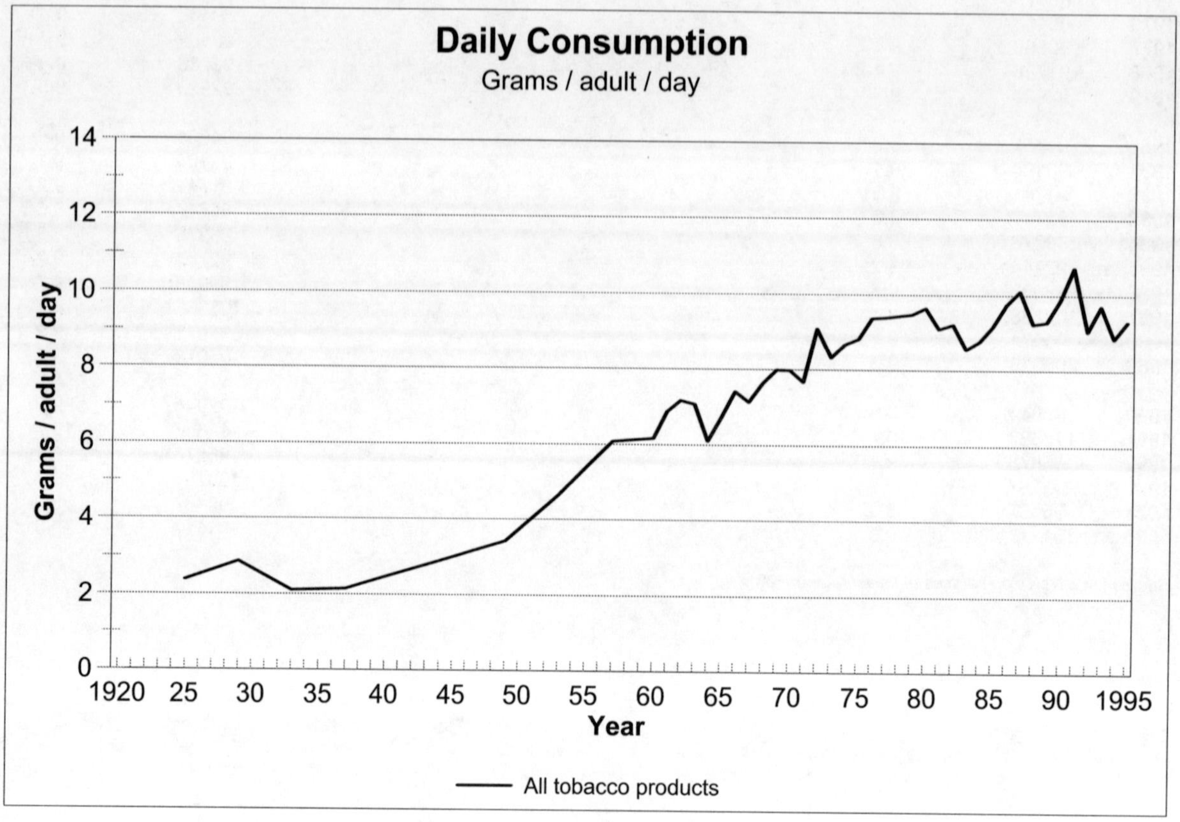

Table 21.3 Percentage sales of tobacco in different forms (by weight), selected years 1925-1995

Year	Cigarettes (%)	Cigars (%)	Other tobacco (%)	Snuff (%)
1925	34.2	1.6	62.0	2.2
1933	34.8	1.1	62.3	1.8
1949	94.5	0.6	4.4	0.4
1957	99.6	0.4	0.0	0.0
1965	100.0	0.0	0.0	0.0
1975	100.0	0.0	0.0	0.0
1985	100.0	0.0	0.0	0.0
1995	100.0	0.0	0.0	0.0

Source : calculated from Table 21.1.1, assumed to be 100% cigarettes from 1960 onwards

Figure 21.2 Percentage sales of tobacco in different forms (by weight), selected years 1925-1995
Source: see Table 21.3

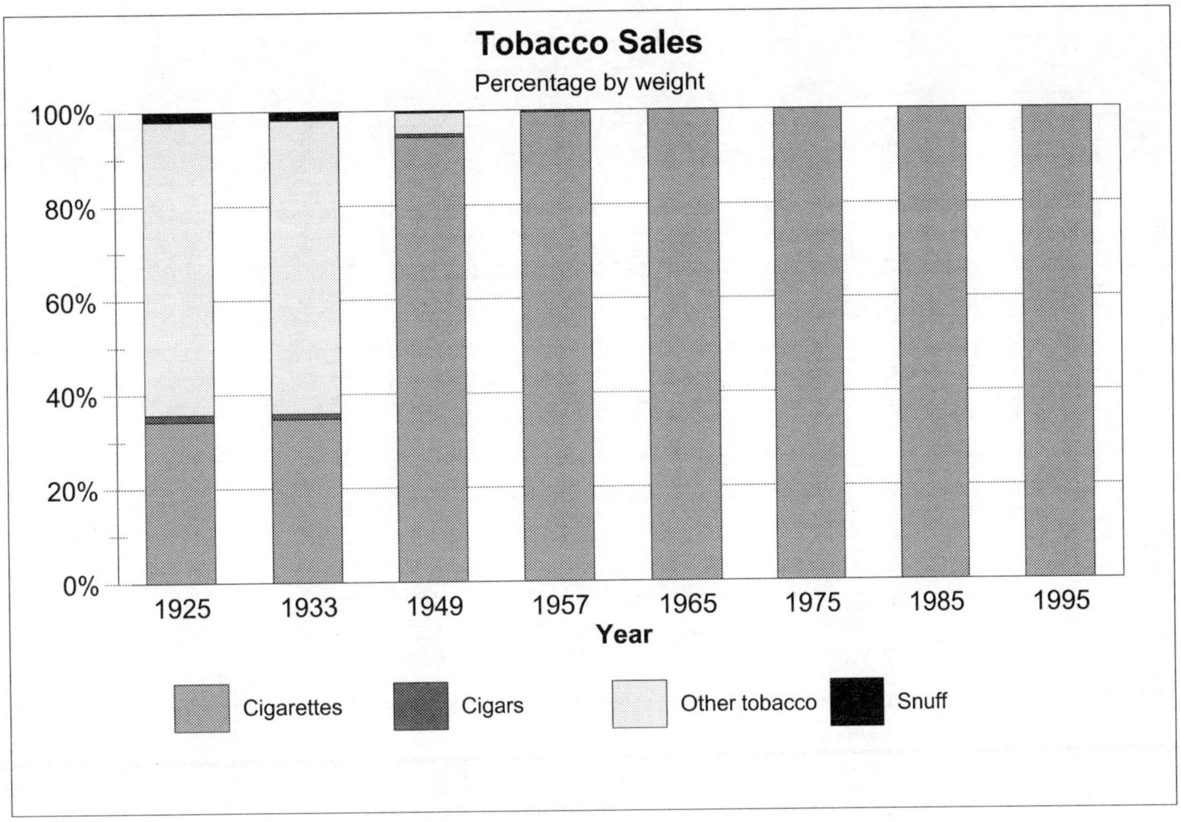

Table 21.4M Prevalence of smoking, males: some selected Polish surveys by age, 1957-1995

Frequency / Product / Source / Year	Age group																					
	12	13	14	15	16	17	18	19	20-24	25-29	30-34	35-39	40-44	45-49	50-54	55-59	60-64	65-69	70-74	75-79	80+	All ages
57 2 U A									83													
68 3 A R								67		70		65		67		47		46				65
70 4 UC U				49																		
73 3 A R									63													
73 5 U A				75																		
74 1 A R									64		66		69		65		48					59
74 1 A A					64																	
75 6 UC R					59																	
75 6 UC A										72												64
76 8 UC U					69					77			75				65					73
79 9 U *		29																				
80 1 A R									70		67		70		59		44					53
80 1 A A					63																	
81 3 A R											67		60		50		45		29		31	53
82 1 A R									63		74		70		65		50					62
82 10 UC U					31				67	61	81	69	69		66		50					
82 11 UC U			21	15			67															
82 12 UC U				60		81																
83 9 U *		19																				
83 13 U U					63																	
84 14 UC R												61		62		48						58
84 14 A A												63		63		48						59
84 15 UC R												67		57		48						59
84 15 A A												69		58		49						60
85 1 A R									60	58	62	55	58		51		49					55
85 1 A A							60															
85 9 UC *			13																			
85 9 UC R			17																			
85 9 UC A			24																			
86 1 A R									51		61		60		46		38					54
86 1 A A					60																	
86 8 UC U					49					70			66				45					61
87 1 A R									61		55		64		54		29					53
87 1 A A					57																	
87 16 UC *				4	12		32															16
88 1 A R									67		60		47		55		41					52
88 1 A A					56																	
89 17 UC U																						
90 1 A R									60		62		61		48		34					52
90 1 A A					55																	
90 8 UC U					40					81			53				35					55
90 18 UC R		5		20																		
90 18 UC A		15		31																		
91 1 A R									56		58		46		55		27					48
91 1 A A					56																	
92 1 A R									50		61		66		50		38					53
92 1 A A					55																	
93 1 A R									45		63		55		44		39					48
93 1 A A					51																	
94 1 A R									45		63		63		50		39					50
94 1 A A					52																	
94 18 UC R		8		23																		
95 1 A R									53		59		56		51		33					47
95 1 A A					50																	
95 7 UC R				23																		
95 7 UC A				34																		

See footnotes on p. 520

Table 21.4F Prevalence of smoking, females: some selected Polish surveys by age, 1957-1995

Year	Source	Product	Frequency	12	13	14	15	16	17	18	19	20-24	25-29	30-34	35-39	40-44	45-49	50-54	55-59	60-64	65-69	70-74	75-79	80+	All ages
57	2	U	A									8													
68	3	A	R								30		23		28		25		13		3				24
70	4	UC	U				22																		
73	3	A	R										27												
73	5	U	A				40																		
74	1	A	R									27		18		23		18		6					18
74	1	A	A					21																	
75	6	UC	R					18																	
75	6	UC	A									35													21
76	8	UC	U							37			35			20				7					25
79	9	U	*		13																				
80	1	A	R									50		44		23		16		10					20
80	1	A	A					29																	
81	3	A	R											43		26		25		17		8		0	25
82	1	A	R									47		47		24		24		6					30
82	10	UC	U					14				40	54	57	34	24		24		5					
82	11	UC	U			0	4			23															
82	12	UC	U				24		56																
83	9	U	*		8																				
83	13	U	U					29																	
84	14	UC	R												19		9		2						11
84	14	A	A												20		10		2						12
84	15	UC	R												42		27		30						34
84	15	A	A												44		28		30						35
85	1	A	R									36	42	48	33	29		18		9					28
85	1	A	A							34															
85	9	UC	*			5																			
85	9	UC	R			9																			
85	9	UC	A			15																			
86	1	A	R									36		40		37		11		11					27
86	1	A	A					33																	
86	8	UC	U							34			43			25				4					28
87	1	A	R									27		41		19		20		9					22
87	1	A	A					26																	
87	16	UC	*																						
88	1	A	R									36		47		31		14		4					25
88	1	A	A					30																	
89	17	UC	U				35																		
90	1	A	R									28		46		35		16		6					25
90	1	A	A					29																	
90	8	UC	U							20			45			25				7					28
90	18	UC	R		1		10																		
90	18	UC	A		3		16																		
91	1	A	R									39		32		36		16		7					25
91	1	A	A					31																	
92	1	A	R									26		31		38		14		9					23
92	1	A	A					26																	
93	1	A	R									22		42		38		23		7					25
93	1	A	A					29																	
94	1	A	R									30		45		34		23		7					23
94	1	A	A					27																	
94	18	UC	R		2		13																		
95	1	A	R									21		42		40		24		8					23
95	1	A	A					25																	
95	7	UC	R				12																		
95	7	UC	A				23																		

See footnotes on p. 521

Table 21.5M Number of cigarettes smoked per smoker per day, males: some selected Polish surveys by age, 1957-1995

<table>
<tr><th rowspan="2">Product
Source
Year</th><th colspan="21">Age group</th><th rowspan="2">All ages</th></tr>
<tr><th>12</th><th>13</th><th>14</th><th>15</th><th>16</th><th>17</th><th>18</th><th>19</th><th>20-24</th><th>25-29</th><th>30-34</th><th>35-39</th><th>40-44</th><th>45-49</th><th>50-54</th><th>55-59</th><th>60-64</th><th>65-69</th><th>70-74</th><th>75-79</th><th>80+</th></tr>
<tr><td>57 2 A</td><td colspan="8"></td><td colspan="13">13</td><td></td></tr>
<tr><td>68 3 A</td><td colspan="7"></td><td colspan="11">18</td><td colspan="3"></td><td></td></tr>
<tr><td>73 3 A</td><td colspan="9"></td><td colspan="10">20</td><td colspan="2"></td><td></td></tr>
<tr><td>74 10 UCE</td><td colspan="3"></td><td colspan="18">17</td><td></td></tr>
<tr><td>75 6 UCE</td><td colspan="4"></td><td colspan="17">16</td><td></td></tr>
<tr><td>76 8 UCE</td><td colspan="4"></td><td colspan="5">18</td><td colspan="3">21</td><td colspan="4">20</td><td colspan="5">20</td><td></td></tr>
<tr><td>80 10 UCE</td><td colspan="3"></td><td colspan="18">18</td><td></td></tr>
<tr><td>82 10 UCE</td><td colspan="3"></td><td colspan="18">17</td><td></td></tr>
<tr><td>84 14 UC</td><td colspan="11"></td><td colspan="6">19</td><td colspan="4"></td><td></td></tr>
<tr><td>84 15 UC</td><td colspan="11"></td><td colspan="6">19</td><td colspan="4"></td><td></td></tr>
<tr><td>85 1 UC</td><td colspan="8"></td><td>16</td><td>19</td><td>22</td><td>20</td><td colspan="2">21</td><td colspan="2">21</td><td colspan="5">18</td><td>19</td></tr>
<tr><td>85 9 UC</td><td colspan="2"></td><td>7.5</td><td colspan="18"></td><td></td></tr>
<tr><td>86 8 UCE</td><td colspan="4"></td><td colspan="5">13</td><td colspan="3">19</td><td colspan="4">19</td><td colspan="5">19</td><td></td></tr>
<tr><td>90 8 UCE</td><td colspan="4"></td><td colspan="5">15</td><td colspan="3">18</td><td colspan="4">19</td><td colspan="5">16</td><td></td></tr>
<tr><td>95 7 UCE</td><td colspan="3"></td><td colspan="2">10</td><td colspan="16"></td><td></td></tr>
</table>

Source: see *Notes on sources of survey data*, p. 529
Frequency: A = all smokers (including occasional)
R = regular or daily smokers
All ages: relevant to ages used and as given in original source
U = unspecified
* = refer to *Notes on sources of survey data*, p. 529

Product: MC = manufactured cigarettes
TC = total cigarettes (including hand-rolled)
UC = cigarettes (type unspecified)
A = all products
E indicates mean estimated from percentage distribution (see also *Consumption category estimation*, p. xxxiv, and Appendix III, p. 789)

Table 21.5F Number of cigarettes smoked per smoker per day, females: some selected Polish surveys by age, 1957-1995

<table>
<tr><th rowspan="2">Product
Source
Year</th><th colspan="21">Age group</th><th rowspan="2">All ages</th></tr>
<tr><th>12</th><th>13</th><th>14</th><th>15</th><th>16</th><th>17</th><th>18</th><th>19</th><th>20-24</th><th>25-29</th><th>30-34</th><th>35-39</th><th>40-44</th><th>45-49</th><th>50-54</th><th>55-59</th><th>60-64</th><th>65-69</th><th>70-74</th><th>75-79</th><th>80+</th></tr>
<tr><td>57 2 A</td><td colspan="8"></td><td colspan="13">8.5</td><td></td></tr>
<tr><td>68 3 A</td><td colspan="7"></td><td colspan="11">13</td><td colspan="3"></td><td></td></tr>
<tr><td>73 3 A</td><td colspan="9"></td><td colspan="10">14</td><td colspan="2"></td><td></td></tr>
<tr><td>74 10 UCE</td><td colspan="3"></td><td colspan="18">12</td><td></td></tr>
<tr><td>75 6 UCE</td><td colspan="4"></td><td colspan="17">11</td><td></td></tr>
<tr><td>76 8 UCE</td><td colspan="4"></td><td colspan="5">15</td><td colspan="3">15</td><td colspan="4">17</td><td colspan="5">13</td><td></td></tr>
<tr><td>80 10 UCE</td><td colspan="3"></td><td colspan="18">12</td><td></td></tr>
<tr><td>82 10 UCE</td><td colspan="3"></td><td colspan="18">13</td><td></td></tr>
<tr><td>84 14 UC</td><td colspan="11"></td><td colspan="6">14</td><td colspan="4"></td><td></td></tr>
<tr><td>84 15 UC</td><td colspan="11"></td><td colspan="6">13</td><td colspan="4"></td><td></td></tr>
<tr><td>85 1 UC</td><td colspan="8"></td><td>10</td><td>14</td><td>15</td><td>16</td><td colspan="2">19</td><td colspan="2">14</td><td colspan="5">17</td><td>15</td></tr>
<tr><td>85 9 UC</td><td colspan="2"></td><td>7.8</td><td colspan="18"></td><td></td></tr>
<tr><td>86 8 UCE</td><td colspan="4"></td><td colspan="5">11</td><td colspan="3">13</td><td colspan="4">15</td><td colspan="5">13</td><td></td></tr>
<tr><td>90 8 UCE</td><td colspan="4"></td><td colspan="5">11</td><td colspan="3">14</td><td colspan="4">14</td><td colspan="5">14</td><td></td></tr>
<tr><td>95 7 UCE</td><td colspan="3"></td><td colspan="2">8.1</td><td colspan="16"></td><td></td></tr>
</table>

Source see *Notes on sources of survey data*, p. 529
Frequency: A = all smokers (including occasional)
R = regular or daily smokers
All ages relevant to ages used and as given in original source
U = unspecified
* = refer to *Notes on sources of survey data*, p. 529

Product: MC = manufactured cigarettes
TC = total cigarettes (including hand-rolled)
UC = cigarettes (type unspecified)
A = all products
E indicates mean estimated from percentage distribution (see also *Consumption category estimation*, p. xxxiv, and Appendix III, p. 789)

Table 21.6M Number of cigarettes smoked per person per day, males: some selected Polish surveys by age, 1957-1995, with percentage total sales

<table>
<tr><th rowspan="2">Product
Source
Year</th><th colspan="21">Age group</th><th rowspan="2">All ages</th><th rowspan="2">% Total sales</th></tr>
<tr><th>12</th><th>13</th><th>14</th><th>15</th><th>16</th><th>17</th><th>18</th><th>19</th><th>20-24</th><th>25-29</th><th>30-34</th><th>35-39</th><th>40-44</th><th>45-49</th><th>50-54</th><th>55-59</th><th>60-64</th><th>65-69</th><th>70-74</th><th>75-79</th><th>80+</th></tr>
<tr><td>57 2 A</td><td colspan="8"></td><td colspan="13">10</td><td></td><td>79%m</td></tr>
<tr><td>68 3 A</td><td colspan="7"></td><td colspan="11">12</td><td colspan="3"></td><td></td><td>83%m</td></tr>
<tr><td>73 3 A</td><td colspan="9"></td><td colspan="10">12</td><td colspan="2"></td><td></td><td>**</td></tr>
<tr><td>75 6 UC</td><td colspan="4"></td><td colspan="17">9.3</td><td></td><td>60%m</td></tr>
<tr><td>76 8 UC</td><td colspan="4"></td><td colspan="5">13</td><td colspan="3">16</td><td colspan="4">15</td><td colspan="5">13</td><td></td><td>93%m</td></tr>
<tr><td>84 14 UC *</td><td colspan="11"></td><td colspan="6">11</td><td colspan="4"></td><td></td><td>**</td></tr>
<tr><td>84 15 UC *</td><td colspan="11"></td><td colspan="6">11</td><td colspan="4"></td><td></td><td>**</td></tr>
<tr><td>85 1 UC</td><td colspan="8"></td><td>9.8</td><td>11</td><td>13</td><td>11</td><td colspan="2">12</td><td colspan="2">11</td><td colspan="5">8.6</td><td></td><td>75%m</td></tr>
<tr><td>85 9 UC</td><td colspan="2"></td><td>0.9</td><td colspan="18"></td><td></td><td>**</td></tr>
<tr><td>86 8 UC</td><td colspan="4"></td><td colspan="5">6.6</td><td colspan="3">13</td><td colspan="4">12</td><td colspan="5">8.5</td><td></td><td>72%m</td></tr>
<tr><td>90 8 UC</td><td colspan="4"></td><td colspan="5">6.0</td><td colspan="3">15</td><td colspan="4">10</td><td colspan="5">5.7</td><td></td><td>67%m</td></tr>
<tr><td>95 19 UC</td><td colspan="3"></td><td colspan="2">2.3</td><td colspan="16"></td><td></td><td>**</td></tr>
</table>

Table 21.7M Number of cigarettes smoked per person per day, sales-adjusted, males: some selected Polish surveys[1] by age, 1957-1990, with percentage total sales

<table>
<tr><th rowspan="2">Product
Source
Year</th><th colspan="21">Age group</th><th rowspan="2">All ages</th><th rowspan="2">% Total sales</th></tr>
<tr><th>12</th><th>13</th><th>14</th><th>15</th><th>16</th><th>17</th><th>18</th><th>19</th><th>20-24</th><th>25-29</th><th>30-34</th><th>35-39</th><th>40-44</th><th>45-49</th><th>50-54</th><th>55-59</th><th>60-64</th><th>65-69</th><th>70-74</th><th>75-79</th><th>80+</th></tr>
<tr><td>57 2 A</td><td colspan="8"></td><td colspan="13">13</td><td></td><td>79%m</td></tr>
<tr><td>68 3 A</td><td colspan="7"></td><td colspan="11">14</td><td colspan="3"></td><td></td><td>83%m</td></tr>
<tr><td>75 6 UC</td><td colspan="4"></td><td colspan="17">15</td><td></td><td>60%m</td></tr>
<tr><td>76 8 UC</td><td colspan="4"></td><td colspan="5">14</td><td colspan="3">17</td><td colspan="4">16</td><td colspan="5">14</td><td></td><td>93%m</td></tr>
<tr><td>85 1 UC</td><td colspan="8"></td><td>13</td><td>15</td><td>18</td><td>15</td><td colspan="2">16</td><td colspan="2">14</td><td colspan="5">12</td><td></td><td>75%m</td></tr>
<tr><td>86 8 UC</td><td colspan="4"></td><td colspan="5">9.1</td><td colspan="3">19</td><td colspan="4">17</td><td colspan="5">12</td><td></td><td>72%m</td></tr>
<tr><td>90 8 UC</td><td colspan="4"></td><td colspan="5">8.9</td><td colspan="3">22</td><td colspan="4">15</td><td colspan="5">8.5</td><td></td><td>67%m</td></tr>
</table>

1 Based on those surveys in Table 21.6 with data for both sexes and age range at least 21-64 (see *Cigarette consumption per person*, p. xxxv)

Source: see *Notes on sources of survey data*, p. 529
All ages: relevant to ages used and as given in original source
% Total sales: estimated % of total sales of M = manufactured or T = total cigarette consumption implied by survey, sexes combined, used as adjustment factor in Table 21.7
** = cannot be calculated
--- = adjusted by original author

Product: MC = manufactured cigarettes
TC = total cigarettes (including hand-rolled)
UC = cigarettes (type unspecified)
A = all products
U = unspecified
* = refer to *Notes on sources of survey data*, p. 529

Table 21.6F Number of cigarettes smoked per person per day, females: some selected Polish surveys by age, 1957-1995, with percentage total sales

Product Source Year	12	13	14	15	16	17	18	19	20-24	25-29	30-34	35-39	40-44	45-49	50-54	55-59	60-64	65-69	70-74	75-79	80+	All ages	% Total sales
57 2 A									0.7														79%m
68 3 A								3.2															83%m
73 3 A									3.8														**
75 6 UC					2.0																		60%m
76 8 UC					5.5					5.3			3.5				0.9						93%m
84 14 UC *												1.6											**
84 15 UC *												4.4											**
85 1 UC									3.7	5.7	7.1	5.2	5.4		2.5		1.6						75%m
85 9 UC			0.4																				**
86 8 UC					3.8					5.6			3.6				0.5						72%m
90 8 UC					2.2					6.1			3.5				1.0						67%m
95 19 UC				1.0																			**

Table 21.7F Number of cigarettes smoked per person per day, sales-adjusted, females: some selected Polish surveys[1] by age, 1957-1990, with percentage total sales

Product Source Year	12	13	14	15	16	17	18	19	20-24	25-29	30-34	35-39	40-44	45-49	50-54	55-59	60-64	65-69	70-74	75-79	80+	All ages	% Total sales
57 2 A									0.9														79%m
68 3 A								3.8															83%m
75 6 UC					3.3																		60%m
76 8 UC					5.9					5.7			3.8				1.0						93%m
85 1 UC									4.9	7.6	9.5	7.0	7.2		3.4		2.1						75%m
86 8 UC					5.3					7.7			5.0				0.7						72%m
90 8 UC					3.3					9.1			5.2				1.5						67%m

1 Based on those surveys in Table 21.6 with data for both sexes and age range at least 21-64 (see *Cigarette consumption per person*, p. xxxv)

Source: see *Notes on sources of survey data*, p. 529
All ages: relevant to ages used and as given in original source
% Total sales: estimated % of total sales of M = manufactured or T = total cigarette consumption implied by survey, sexes combined, used as adjustment factor in Table 21.7
** = cannot be calculated
--- = adjusted by original author

Product: MC = manufactured cigarettes
TC = total cigarettes (including hand-rolled)
UC = cigarettes (type unspecified)
A = all products
U = unspecified
* = refer to *Notes on sources of survey data*, p. 529

Table 21.8 Estimated[1] prevalence of smoking and estimated[1] number of cigarettes per person per day (unadjusted and sales-adjusted): summary of Tables 21.4, 21.6 and 21.7, 1957-1995.
Males and females aged 15 years and over

Year	Source[2]	Product[3]	Prevalence[4]						Number of cigarettes						
									Unadjusted[7]			Sales-adjusted[8]			
			Manufactured cigarettes		Total cigarettes[5]		All products[6]		Number/ person/day		Total sales %	Manufactured cigarettes[9] number/ person/day		Total cigarettes number/ person/day	
			M	F	M	F	M	F	M	F		M	F	M	F
1957	2	**U+A**					76	9	9.4[10]	0.7[10]	79	12.0	0.9		
1968	3	A					57	21	10.4[10]	2.7[10]	83	12.5	3.3		
1970	4	*UC*			49	22						(12.0	4.4)		
1973	5	**U**					75	40				(11.9	5.1)		
1974	1	A					58	17				(14.4	3.5)		
	1	**A**					63	20							
1975	6	UC			58	18			9.0	1.9	60	14.9	3.2		
	6	**UC**			63	21									
1976	8	*UC*			71	25			14.1	3.8	93	15.1	4.1		
1980	1	A					53	19				(15.3	4.5)		
	1	**A**					62	28							
1982	1	A					61	30				(13.5	5.3)		
	10	*UC*			62	29						(13.7	5.1)		
1983	13	*U*					62	29				(12.7	4.7)		
1985	1	UC+A					53	27	10.2	3.8	75	13.6	5.1		
	1	**A**					58	33							
1986	8	*UC*			60	27			10.9	3.5	72	15.0	4.9		
	1	A					53	27				(14.2	5.7)		
	1	**A**					59	32							
1987	1	A					52	22				(15.5	5.1)		
	1	**A**					56	26							
1988	1	A					51	25				(13.5	5.3)		
	1	**A**					55	29							
1989	17	*UC*				35									
1990	1	A					51	24				(14.6	5.6)		
	1	**A**					55	28							
	8	*UC*			56	26			10.1	3.5	67	15.0	5.2		
1991	1	A					47	24				(15.5	6.4)		
	1	**A**					55	31							
1992	1	A					52	22				(13.7	4.7)		
	1	**A**					54	25							
1993	1	A					47	25				(13.9	5.9)		
	1	**A**					50	29							
1994	1	A					50	23				(13.2	4.9)		
	1	**A**					51	27							
1995	1	A					47	23				(13.6	5.3)		
	1	**A**					49	25							

See footnotes on next page

Table 21.8 *(continued)*

1 Surveys covering an age range of at least 21-64 are included. Any gaps in the data for ages 15-20 and 65 years and over are filled in by assumed extensions to the age distribution, given in *Notes on sources of survey data*, p. 529. Method: see *Summary of adult smoking*, p. xxxvi
2 See *Notes on sources of survey data*, p. 529
3 Product: MC = manufactured cigarettes, TC = total cigarettes (including hand-rolled), UC = cigarettes (type unspecified), A = all products, U = unspecified. Frequency of smoking is indicated by: regular or daily smokers in normal type, all smokers (including occasional) in bold, unspecified in italics
4 From Table 21.4
5 This column includes prevalence of smoking classified as UC = cigarettes (type unspecified)
6 This column includes prevalence of smoking classified as U = unspecified product
7 From Table 21.6
8 From Table 21.7, except data in parentheses, which are derived from the prevalence of smoking from Table 21.4 as described in *Summary of adult smoking*, p. xxxvi
9 Number of cigarettes classified as UC = cigarettes (type unspecified), A = all products or U = product unspecified has been adjusted to manufactured cigarette sales and included in this column
10 All tobacco products, grams

Figure 21.3 Estimated prevalence of smoking of (i) cigarettes and (ii) all tobacco products: by year of survey, 1957-1995.
Males and females aged 15 years and over. *Source:* see Table 21.8

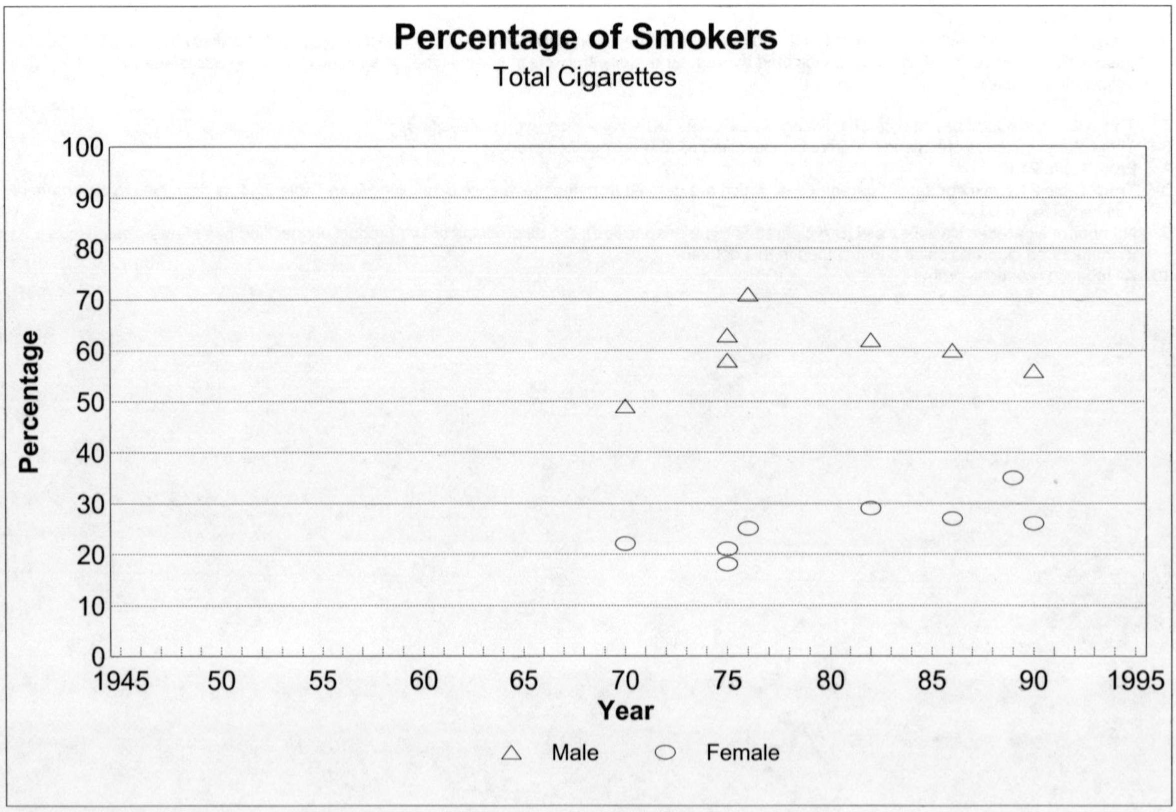

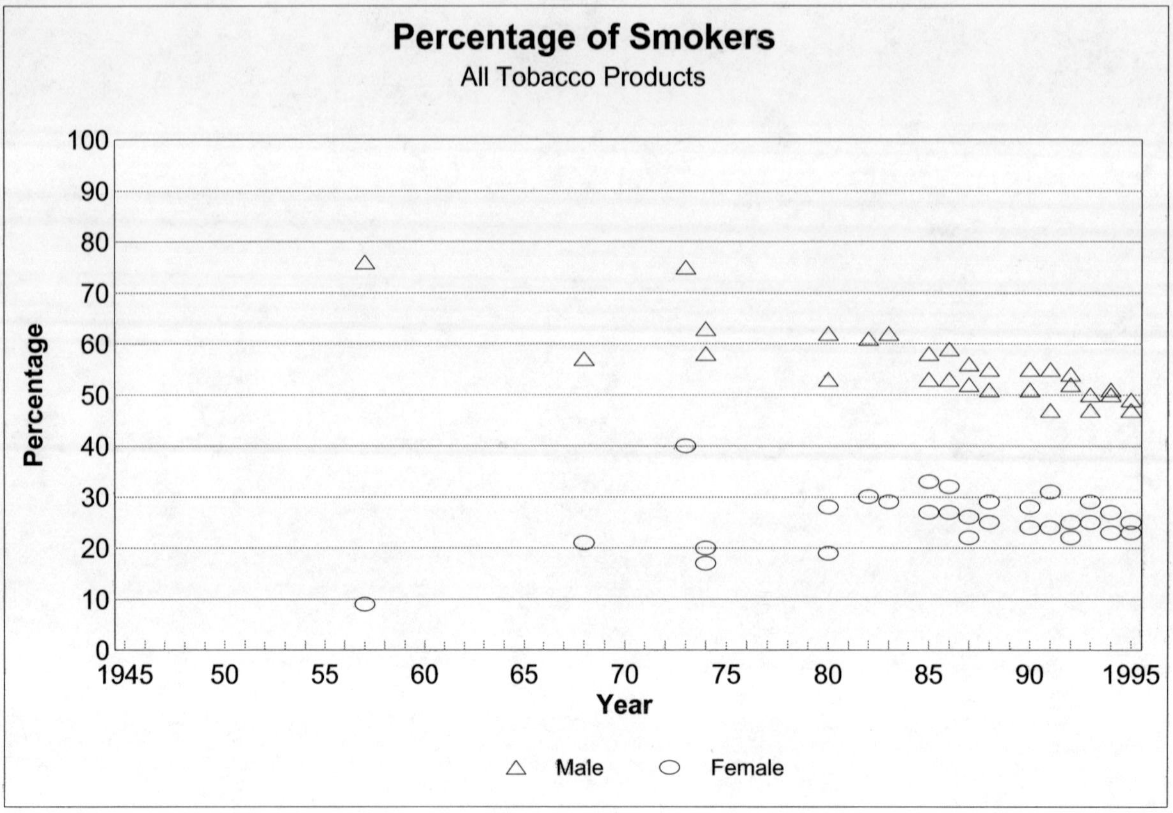

Figure 21.4 Estimated number of cigarettes smoked per person per day, sales-adjusted, 1957-1995.
Males and females aged 15 years and over. *Source:* see Table 21.8

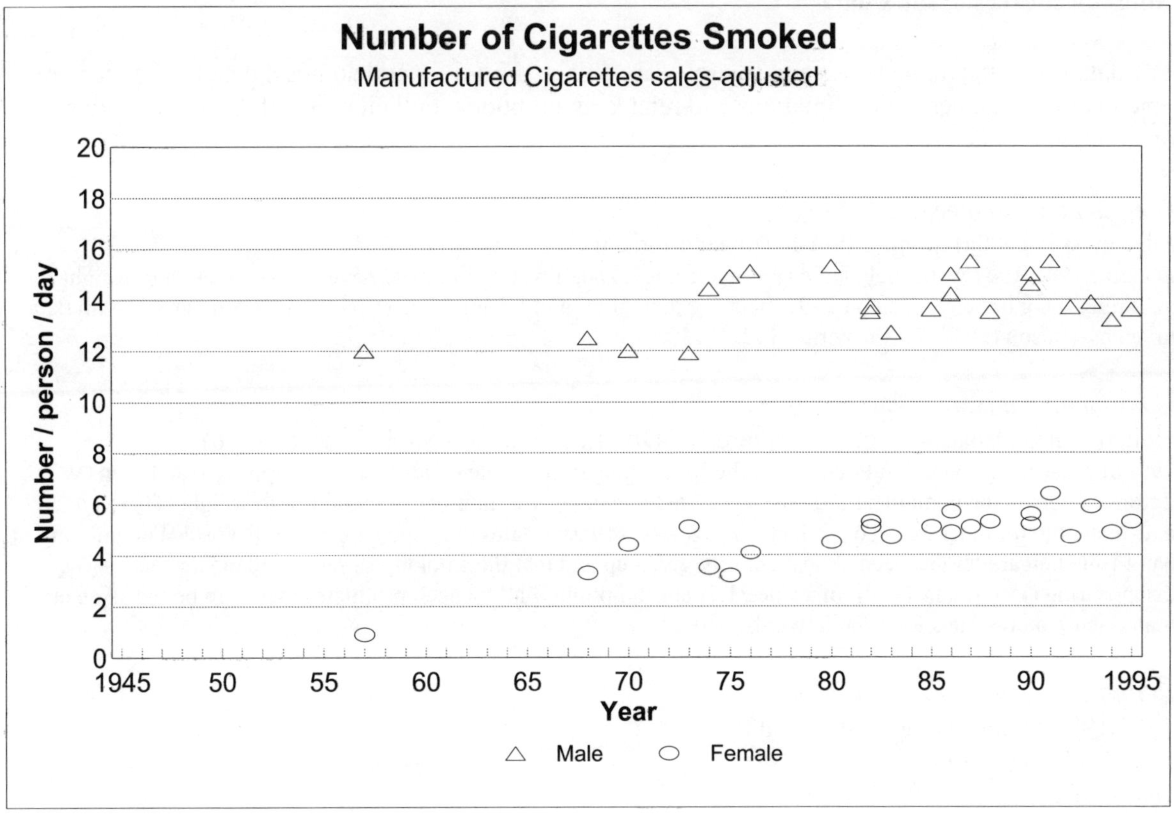

Notes on sources of sales data

The data presented in the tables and figures were obtained from several sources, details of which are given below, together with estimations and related assumptions. Full citations of the sources are given on p. 532 under *References*.

Consumption data before 1960

Staszewski (1960a) quoting Polish Tobacco Industry

Data for 1945-1947 were excluded due to inaccuracy. Data given in numbers have been converted to weight assuming 0.8 g per cigarette up to 1937 and 1 g thereafter, and 5.5 g per cigar, based on a comparison with data given by Hutson (1937) for the period 1922-1935.

Consumption data for 1960 onwards

United States Department of Agriculture (USDA) Economic Research Service (1996)

99% of tobacco consumed in Poland is in the form of cigarettes. One cigarette weighs approximately 1 g (W. Zatoński, personal communication). We have used this to convert number of cigarettes to weight. There are no data available for other tobacco products. Staszewski (1960a) states that since the Second World War smoking of hand-rolled cigarettes has been almost entirely given up and that the smoking of pipes and cigars was disappearing (i.e. around 1960). In Table 21.2, consumption of all tobacco products is taken to be the same as manufactured cigarettes for 1960 onwards.

Plain/Filter cigarette consumption

1967-1980 Maxwell (successive years)
1984 Boddewyn (1986)
1990-1992 Magier (1993)
1993-1995 USDA Economic Research Service (1996)

For 1990 onwards the data represent percentage of production rather than of sales.

Tar and nicotine yield of cigarettes

1980 Bednarzewski *et al* (1984)
1983-1995 Florek *et al* (1996)

These data give the range of yields of several of the most popular brands. Each brand varies considerably and irregularly over time, with none being consistently low yielding or high yielding across the years tested. Details of two brands are shown below. These brands have been tested over many years and are often the highest or lowest yielding for a year (indicated by + or - respectively in the table).

Year	Popularne				Carmen			
	Tar (mg/cig)		Nicotine (mg/cig)		Tar (mg/cig)		Nicotine (mg/cig)	
1980	17.1	-	1.23		23.6	+	1.96	
1983	19.7		1.04	-	19.5	-	1.88	+
1984	20.1	-	1.56		27.9		2.24	+
1985	18.9	-	1.13	-	31.9	+	2.63	+
1986	18.0	-	0.92	-	26.2		2.12	+
1987	18.5		1.18		25.7	+	1.94	+
1988	20.2	-	0.97	-	25.4	+	1.50	+
1990	17.0	-	1.18		17.8		1.44	+
1991	15.3	-	0.97	-				
1992	15.6		1.12		14.1	-	0.92	-
1993	18.6	+	1.50		16.7	-	1.34	
1994	16.9	+	1.52	+				
1995	15.4		1.55	+				

The tar yield per cigarette is limited to 20 mg; nicotine yield is limited to 1.8 mg (Harkin *et al* (1997)).

Estimates of hand-rolled cigarette consumption
Hand-rolled cigarette consumption has been assumed to be zero in calculations.

Notes on sources of survey data

Each source of survey data—either an individual survey or a series of surveys repeated over a number of years—is cited by a source number. This number is shown in the tables and corresponds to the source numbers given below, where details of the source publication and of the survey methodology are given. Full citations of the sources are given on p. 532 under *References*.

Source number

1 **Przewoźniak and Zatoński (1996), Zatoński *et al* (1988)**

a. A series of surveys representative of the Polish population. Carried out by Ośrodek Badania Opinii Publicznej (OBOP) in Warsaw except for the 1991 survey which was carried out by Centrum Badania Opinii Społecznej (CBOS)
b. Target sample sizes (1974-1991) 1 000, (1992-1995) 1 500. Actual sample sizes not stated
c. Percentages of smokers smoking various tobacco products were given, as follows:

Year	Men				Women			
	Cigarettes		Other	No data	Cigarettes		Other	No data
	filter	non-filter			filter	non-filter		
1982	28	70	2	0	74	26	0	0
1985	40	57	2	1	75	23	1	1
1986	53	43	4	1	82	17	2	0
1987	50	49	1	0	85	13	2	0
1988	51	48	1	0	81	15	4	0
1990	57	43	1	0	92	8	0	0
1991	61	40	0	0	72	28	0	0
1992	70	30	0	0	86	14	0	0
1993	70	29	0	0	90	9	1	0
1994	71	29	0	0	92	8	0	0
1995	71	29	0	0	93	7	0	0

d. Results in *All ages* column of Table 21.4 relate to age 16+ (except 1985, age 18+)
e. Assumed extension to age distribution for percentage smokers, age 15: males (regular) 15%, (all) 20%; females (regular) 5%, (all) 10%. For age 15-17 (1985 only): males (regular) 20%, (all) 25%; females (regular) 10%, (all) 15%. Number of cigarettes/person/day, age 15-19 (1985 only): males 3.0 and females 1.0

2 **Staszewski (1960a, 1960b), WHO (1975)**

a. According to WHO (1975), a randomized sample of the population of Upper Silesia in 1960, but same data given by Staszewski (1960a) as ever smokers among the control group in a study at the Oncology Institute in Gliwice 1955-1958
b. Sample size (males) 912, (females) 1 813
c. Smokers: consume at least 1 gram of tobacco a day. Cigarettes per smoker based on total tobacco consumed, using 1 cigarette = 1 g, 1 cigar = 4 g of tobacco
d. 68% of male smokers smoked only cigarettes. Women smoked cigarettes only
e. Assumed extension to age distribution for percentage smokers, age 15-19: males 30% and females 10%. Number of cigarettes/person/day: males 3.0 and females 0.5

3 **Sawicki and Lawrence (1977), Jedrychowski *et al* (1985)**

a. A longitudinal survey of permanent residents of Cracow (1 779 dwellings). Of the 667 not re-interviewed in 1973, 131 had died. Age-specific results for 1968 are based only on those successfully followed up in 1981

Year	Sample size		
	Males	Females	Total
1968	1 925	2 430	
1973	1 581	2 107	
1981	—	—	2 968

b. Cigarettes per smoker results include an 'insignificant' proportion of subjects reporting pipe-smoking, calculating 1 g of the smoked tobacco as equivalent to one cigarette

c. Assumed extension to age distribution for percentage smokers (1968 only), age 15-18: males 30% and females 2%. Number of cigarettes/person/day, age 15-18: males 2.0 and females 0.5. For age 71+: males 2.0 and females 0.5

4 Czyżyk and Królewski (1976) quoting Mró (1976)

a. Representative sample of the population of Warsaw

5 WHO (1975)

a. An estimate of the prevalence in the whole population

6 Otawska (1975)

a. Representative of Polish population. Sample size 1 000

b. Prevalence of regular smoking deduced from % occasional smokers among all smokers

c. Consumption category estimation based on <10, 10-20, >20 cigarettes/smoker/day

d. Assumed extension to age distribution for percentage smokers, age 15: males (regular) 15%, (all) 20%; females (regular) 5%, (all) 10%. Number of cigarettes/person/day: males 1.0 and females 0.5

7 Hibell *et al* (1997)

a. Nationally representative survey forming part of ESPAD (European School Survey Project on Alcohol and Other Drugs). Target was pupils born in 1979, thus age 15-16 at time of survey in May 1995. Approximately 93% of this group still in school. Anonymous questionnaire completed and sealed in envelope by pupil, in class. Teachers absent. Sample size (males) 4 494, (females) 4 349. Response rate (males) 81%, (females) 85%

b. Regular smokers: smoked 1 or more cigarettes per day in last 30 days. All smokers: smoked in last 30 days

c. Consumption category estimation based on 1-5, 6-10, 11-20, 21+ cigarettes/smoker/day

8 Jokiel (1989, 1996)

a. Representative samples of the Polish population. Surveys conducted in collaboration with Osrodkiem Badania Opinii Publicznej w Warszawie (Warsaw Public Opinion Research Centre).

Year	Sample size	
	Males	Females
1976	939	1 037
1986	418	460
1990	408	455

b. Consumption category estimation based on <1 packet, 1 packet and >1 packet, assuming 1 packet=20 cigarettes

c. Assumed extension to age distribution for percentage smokers, age 15: males 20% and females 10%. Number of cigarettes/person/day: males 1.0 and females 0.5

9 Wijatkowski (1983), Wijatkowski *et al* (1990)

a. Anonymous surveys in Lódź schools

b. Sample sizes (1979) unknown, (1983) 378, (1985) 1 082

c. Smokers marked as frequency *: smoked daily. Regular smokers: smoked once a week or more. All smokers: smoked once a week or more, or has smoked less than weekly for at least 3 months

10 Zatoński *et al* (1986)

a. Details of survey unknown

b. Consumption category estimation based on 1-10, 11-20, >20 cigarettes/smoker/day

c. Assumed extension to age distribution for percentage smokers, age 15: males 20% and females 10%

11-12 Bednarzewski *et al* (1984)

a. Survey, using an anonymous inquiry form, in elementary, secondary and vocational schools in the City of Lubin. Sample size 635 boys and 635 girls

b. Data given as source **11** are for primary and general schools. Data given as source **12** are for vocational schools

13 Masironi and Rothwell (1988)

a. No original source. Age group not stated

b. Assumed extension to age distribution for percentage smokers, age 15: males 20% and females 10%

14-15 WHO (1989), WHO MONICA Project (1988)

a. Two regional surveys forming part of WHO MONICA project:

	Region	Population size	Sample size	Participation rate (%)	Sample used		Date
					Males	Females	
14	Tarnobrzeg (Krakow)	185 600	3 373	81	1 250	1 472	Jun 1983-Nov 1984
15	Warsaw	180 100	3 600	74	1 309	1 337	Dec 1983-Jan 1985

All figures are for age 35-64 only

b. *All ages* column is standardized to world population

c. Regular cigarette smokers: smoked cigarettes daily. All smokers: smoked cigarettes daily or occasionally, or smoked 1 g pipe tobacco or 1 cigar per week. Cigarettes per smoker refers to regular and occasional cigarette smokers

d. Calculation for cigarettes per person based on % regular cigarette smokers and cigarettes per regular or occasional cigarette smoker, so may underestimate

16 Baszczyński *et al* (1988)

a. Survey of 1 483 schoolboys. Year not stated

b. Smoking marked as frequency *: 5 or more cigarettes a day

17 Chollat-Traquet (1992)

a. No original source

18 King and Coles (1992), King *et al* (1996)

a. Part of the HBSC (Health Behaviour in School-Aged Children) Study, a collaborative cross-national research study sponsored by the WHO. School classes or schools were randomly selected, targeting age groups 11 (not presented here), 13 and 15. The target sample size was 1 300 in each age group

Year	Total sample size	Target age 13		Target age 15	
		Mean age	Sample size	Mean age	Sample size
1990	4 613	13.6	—	15.7	—
1994	—	13.7	1 514	15.7	1 540

b. Regular smokers: smoke once a week or more

Additional information (not presented in tables)

Staszewski (1960a) states that it is estimated that before the Second World War, smokers constituted about 20% of the entire population and that after the war the percentage increased mainly by a greater number of women smokers (personal communication from the Polish Tobacco Industry).

References

Boddewyn J.J. (ed) (1986). *Tobacco advertising bans and consumption in 16 countries*. International Advertising Association, New York.

Baszczyński J., Sordyl E. and Karpisński E. (1988). Kierunki zapobiegania miażdżycy naczyń i chorobie niedokrwiennej serca w orkresie młodzieńczym (Methods of arteriosclerosis and ischemic heart disease prevention in young age). *Wiad Lek,* **41**, 273-7.

Bednarzewski J., Wróbel J., Kulesza J., Wojtaszek L. and Wydro D. (1984). Nałóg palenia tytoniu wśród uczącej się młodzieży Lublina. (Tobacco smoking habit in the adolescents in Lubin schools). *Wiad Lek,* **37**, 1159-66.

Chollat-Traquet C. (1992). *Women and tobacco* . WHO, Geneva.

Czyżyk A. and Królewski A.S. (1976). Is cigarette smoking more frequent among insulin-treated diabetics? *Diabetes,* **25**, 717-8.

Florek E., Przewoźniak K. and Zatoński W. (1996). Wybrane substancje toksyczne i kancerogenne w papierosach sprzedawanych w Polsce w latach 1983-1995. In: Zatoński W. and Przewoźniak K. (eds) *Palenie tytoniu w Polsce: postawy, nastepstwa zdrowotne i profilaktyka.* Centrum Onkologii-Instytut im. Marii Skłodowskiej-Curie, Warsaw; 89-110.

Harkin A.M., Anderson P. and Goos C. (1997). *Smoking, drinking and drug taking in the European Region.* Alcohol, Drugs and Tobacco Programme, WHO Regional Office for Europe, Copenhagen.

Hibell B., Andersson B., Bjarnason T., Kokkevi A., Morgan M. and Narusk A. (1997). *The 1995 ESPAD report. The European school survey project on alcohol and other drugs. Alcohol and other drug use among students in 26 European countries.* The Swedish Council for Information on Alcohol and Other Drugs. Council of Europe (Pompidou Group).

Hutson J.B. (1937). *Consumption and production of tobacco in Europe.* USDA, Washington DC. Technical bulletin No. 587.

Jedrychowski W., Soroka W., Wysocki M. and Krzyżanowski M. (1985). Longitudinal monitoring of changes in individual smoking habit over 13-year period among adults. *Tokai J Exp Clin Med,* **10**, 315-21.

Jokiel M. (1989). Zmiany w strukturze palenia papierósow w Polsce w latach 1976-1986. (Changes in the pattern of cigarette smoking in Poland 1976-1986). *Nowotwory,* **39**, 76-82.

Jokiel M. (1996). Zmiany w strukturze palenia tytoniu w Polsce w latach 1976, 1986 i 1990 (Changes in tobacco smoking patterns in Poland in the years 1976, 1986 and 1990). *Przegl Epidemiol,* **50**, 299-307.

King A., Wold B., Tudor-Smith C. and Harel Y. (1996). *The health of youth, a cross-national survey.* WHO Regional Publications, Europe, Copenhagen. European Series No. 69.

King A.J.C. and Coles B. (1992). *The health of Canada's youth. Views and behaviours of 11-, 13- and 15-year-olds from 11 countries.* Health and Welfare Canada, Ottawa.

Magier T. (1993). *The Polish tobacco industry 1990-1993 (presented at the world tobacco symposium, Sovincentr, Moscow, 22-24 September 1993).* World Tobacco.

Masironi R. and Rothwell K. (1988). Tendances et effets du tabagisme dans le monde (Smoking trends and effects worldwide). *World Health Stat Q,* **41**, 228-41.

Maxwell J.C.Jr. (successive years). How the brands ranked. Maxwell International Estimates. *World Tobacco.*

Mró E. (1976). Skala zdrownia ludnosci Warszawy. *Przegl Epidemiol,* **30**. §

Otawska E. (1975). Palić—nie palić. *Aktualnosci Radiowo-Telewizyjne,* **8**, 14-9.

Przewoźniak K. and Zatoński W. (1996). Palenie tytoniu w dorosłej populacji polski latach 1974-1995. In: Zatoński W. and Przewoźniak K. (eds) *Palenie tytoniu w Polsce: postawy, nastepstwa zdrowotne i profilaktyka*. Centrum Onkologii-Instytut im. Marii Skłodowskiej-Curie, Warsaw; 127-62.

Sawicki F. and Lawrence P.S. (1977). *Chronic nonspecific respiratory disease in the city of Cracow*. National Institute of Hygiene, Warsaw.

Staszewski J. (1960b). Palenie tytoniu a choroby narządów oddechowych i układu krążenia (Tobacco smoking and some diseases of the respiratory and circulatory system). *Polish Medical Weekly,* **15**, 1106-10.

Staszewski J. (1960a). Smoking and cancer in Poland. *Br J Cancer,* **14**, 419-35.

USDA Economic Research Service (1996). *Tobacco statistics*. Albert R. Mann Library, Cornell University, Ithaca, New York. ERS 94012. (With supplementary material from Tobacco Annual Reports.). http://usda.mannlib.cornell.edu/data-sets/specialty/94012.

WHO (1989). The WHO MONICA project: a worldwide monitoring system for cardiovascular diseases. In: *World health statistics annual 1989*. WHO, Geneva; 25-149.

WHO MONICA Project (1988). Geographical variation in the major risk factors of coronary heart disease in men and women aged 35-64 years. *World Health Stat Q,* **41**, 115-40.

Wijatkowski S. (1983). Anti-tobacco educational film in the light of receivers' opinion: 13-15-year-old youths. In: Forbes W.F., Frecker R.C. and Nostbakken D. (eds) *Proceedings of the Fifth World Conference on Smoking and Health, Winnipeg, Canada, 1983, Volume 1*. Canadian Council on Smoking and Health, Ottawa, Ontario; 367-70.

Wijatkowski S., Forgays D.G., Wrzesniewski K. and Gorski T. (1990). Smoking behavior and personality characteristics in Polish adolescents. *International Journal of the Addictions,* **25**, 363-73.

WHO (1975). Survey on smoking and health in the European Region, 1974-75: preliminary data as at 1 May 1975. *Presented at the Third World Conference on Smoking and Health, New York, 2-5 June 1975*. WHO; 1-55.

Zatoński W., Przewoźniak K. and Gottesman K. (1988). Czestość palenia tytoniu w Polsce 1985 roku. (Frequency of smoking in Poland in 1985). *Zdrowie Publiczne,* **3**, 151-6.

Zatoński W., Przewoźniak K. and Grottesman K. (1986). Zakres i nastepstwa zdrowotne palenia tytoniu w Polsce. In: Strzelecki Z. (ed) *Alkohol, narkotyki, tytoń. Skutki demograficzne w Polsce*. PAX, Warsaw; 169-200.

§ Original paper not obtained, but information taken as quoted by another author

Portugal 22

Sales data

See Tables 22.1-22.3.

Sales data have been available since 1940, but data since 1974 are incomplete and the different sources are not consistent.

From 1940 until the mid-1970s the consumption of manufactured cigarettes per adult increased from about 1 cigarette per day, levelled out at about 5 cigarettes in the 1980s and then increased again to 6 cigarettes by the mid-1990s. We estimate that consumption of hand-rolled cigarettes per adult decreased from 1 cigarette per day in 1950 to virtually none in the 1990s.

The consumption of tobacco products per adult increased slowly from 2 g per day in 1940 to 6 g in the 1990s. In the early 1940s, about 45% of tobacco was consumed as manufactured cigarettes. This increased rapidly, reaching 90% by 1960 and has been about 99% since 1980. The remaining consumption was nearly all as pipe and hand-rolling tobacco, predominantly for hand-rolling.

Survey data

See Tables 22.4-22.8

No survey data on smoking habits are available until the mid-1970s. There is little difference for men, and no difference for women, between the reported prevalence of smoking cigarettes and of smoking any product, since cigarettes were the predominant product used by that time. In the 1970s, the prevalence of smoking among those aged 15 years and over was 45-48% in men. By the 1990s this had decreased to 30-40%. Among women, estimates varied considerably, but have generally risen, from 1-10% in the 1970s to 7-17% in the 1990s.

Data on adult smoking by age are available mainly from National Health Surveys in 1987 and 1995, although the smoking definitions used were not identical in the two surveys. More men than women smoked at all ages, and very few women aged over about 50 smoked. Data on smoking by teenagers are not available until 1990. Most surveys showed that the prevalence of smoking was slightly higher among boys than among girls.

Comparison of survey and sales data was possible for the two national and one regional health survey, which under-reported consumption by 30-35%. Between 1983 and 1995 the estimated number of cigarettes smoked per person per day (sales-adjusted) was 8-10 for men and 1-3 for women.

Table 22.1.1 Total annual sales of tobacco products, 1940-1972

Year	Cigarettes		Cigars and cigarillos		Pipe and hand-rolling tobacco tonnes	Snuff tonnes	All tobacco products tonnes
	tonnes	millions	tonnes	millions			
1940	1430	1428	30	6	1770	50	3280
1941	1720	1716	30	6	1910	50	3700
1942	2170	2170	50	9	2000	50	4260
1943	2250	2251	50	10	1910	50	4260
1944	2310	2305	50	10	2090	50	4490
1945	2410	2411	40	7	2180	50	4670
1946	2630	2626	20	3	2180	50	4870
1947	3160	3161	10	2	1770	50	4990
1948	3340	3343	10	1	2040	50	5440
1949	3570	3573	10	2	1630	50	5260
1950	3630	3633	10	1	1450	50	5140
1951	3800	3802	10	1	1450	50	5300
1952	4180	4183	10	1	1450	50	5690
1953	4220	4215	10	1	1320	50	5580
1954	4320	4317	10	2	1180	0	5510
1955	4670	4674	10	2	1090	0	5770
1956	5100	5100	10	2	950	0	6060
1957	5090	5088	10	2	820	0	5920
1958	5510	5510	10	2	820	0	6340
1959	5780	5778	10	2	770	0	6560
1960	6290	6287	10	1	730	0	7020
1961	5570	5570	10	1	680	0	6260
1962	5830	5827	10	2	730	0	6560
1963	6760	6757	10	1	730	0	7490
1964	7030	7029	10	1	820	0	7850
1965	7480	7482	10	1	540	0	8030
1966	8030	7989	10	1	540	0	8580
1967	8260	8237	10	2	500	0	8770
1968	8850	8820	10	2	450	0	9310
1969	8690	8689	10	1	450	0	9150
1970	8930	8924	10	1	360	0	9290
1971	9080	9082	10	1	360	0	9450
1972	9410	9406	10	1	320	0	9730

Source: see *Notes on sources of sales data*, p. 549

Table 22.1.2 Total annual sales of tobacco products, 1973-1995

Year	Cigarettes		Cigars and cigarillos		Hand-rolling tobacco	Pipe tobacco	All tobacco products
	tonnes	millions	tonnes	millions	tonnes	tonnes	tonnes
1973		10203					
1974		11052					
1975		12043					
1976		11834					
1977		12564					
1978		12537					
1979	11986	11986			184	14	12184
1980	11988	11988			155	14	12157
1981	12606	12606			144	12	12762
1982	12990	12990			129	13	13132
1983	13635	13635			131	15	13781
1984	13507	13507			139	15	13661
1985	13594	13594			137	15	13746
1986	13660	13660					
1987	14934	14934					
1988	14537	14537					
1989	14541	14541	31	14	126		14698
1990	15486	15486	32	15	123		15641
1991	15930	15930	36	16	130		16096
1992	16700	16700	37	17	139		16876
1993	17022	17022	53	13			
1994	17594	17594	75	19			
1995	16247	16247	82	21			

Source : see *Notes on sources of sales data*, p. 549

Table 22.1.3 Manufactured cigarettes, percentage of total sales as filter cigarettes, 1961-1994

Year	% Filter
1961	19.1
1962	22.2
1963	22.6
1964	24.7
1965	28.1
1966	33.3
1967	38.0
1968	42.6
1969	46.4
1970	51.0
1971	56.7
1972	56.6
1973	73.2
1974	76.4
1975	77.5
1976	76.1
1977	77.6
1978	76.7
1979	78.3
1980	80.8
1981	83.5
1982	84.7
1983	85.4
1984	85.4
1985	86.7
1993	95.5
1994	95.4

Source : see *Notes on sources of sales data*, p. 549

Table 22.2 Consumption of (i) cigarettes and (ii) all tobacco products, 1940-1995 sales-based data, including estimated hand-rolled cigarette consumption. Males and females aged 15 years and over

Year	Manufactured cigarettes		Hand-rolled cigarettes		Total cigarettes		All tobacco products	
	Total annual in millions	Number/ adult/day	Total annual in millions	Number/ adult/day	Total annual in millions	Number/ adult/day	Total annual in tonnes	Grams/ adult/day
1940	1428	0.7					3280	1.7
1941	1716	0.9					3700	1.9
1942	2170	1.1					4260	2.2
1943	2251	1.1					4260	2.2
1944	2305	1.1					4490	2.2
1945	2411	1.2					4670	2.3
1946	2626	1.3					4870	2.3
1947	3161	1.5					4990	2.4
1948	3343	1.6					5440	2.6
1949	3573	1.7					5260	2.4
1950	3633	1.7	1852	0.9	5485	2.5	5140	2.4
1951	3802	1.7	1852	0.8	5654	2.6	5300	2.4
1952	4183	1.9	1852	0.8	6035	2.7	5690	2.6
1953	4215	1.9	1686	0.8	5901	2.6	5580	2.5
1954	4317	1.9	1507	0.7	5824	2.6	5510	2.4
1955	4674	2.0	1392	0.6	6066	2.7	5770	2.5
1956	5100	2.2	1213	0.5	6313	2.7	6060	2.6
1957	5088	2.2	1047	0.5	6135	2.6	5920	2.6
1958	5510	2.4	1047	0.5	6557	2.8	6340	2.7
1959	5778	2.5	983	0.4	6761	2.9	6560	2.8
1960	6287	2.7	932	0.4	7219	3.1	7020	3.1
1961	5570	2.4	868	0.4	6438	2.8	6260	2.7
1962	5827	2.5	932	0.4	6759	2.9	6560	2.8
1963	6757	2.9	932	0.4	7689	3.3	7490	3.2
1964	7029	3.0	1047	0.4	8076	3.4	7850	3.3
1965	7482	3.2	690	0.3	8172	3.5	8030	3.4
1966	7989	3.4	690	0.3	8679	3.7	8580	3.6
1967	8237	3.5	638	0.3	8875	3.8	8770	3.7
1968	8820	3.7	575	0.2	9395	4.0	9310	3.9
1969	8689	3.7	575	0.2	9264	3.9	9150	3.9
1970	8924	4.0	460	0.2	9384	4.2	9290	4.1
1971	9082	4.0	460	0.2	9542	4.2	9450	4.2
1972	9406	4.2	409	0.2	9815	4.4	9730	4.3
1973	10203	4.5						
1974	11052	4.7						
1975	12043	4.8						
1976	11834	4.6						
1977	12564	4.9						
1978	12537	4.9						
1979	11986	4.6	184	0.1	12170	4.7	12184	4.7
1980	11988	4.5	155	0.1	12143	4.5	12157	4.5
1981	12606	4.7	144	0.1	12750	4.7	12762	4.8
1982	12990	4.8	129	0.0	13119	4.8	13132	4.8
1983	13635	5.0	131	0.0	13766	5.0	13781	5.0
1984	13507	4.9	139	0.1	13646	4.9	13661	4.9
1985	13594	4.9	137	0.0	13731	4.9	13746	4.9
1986	13660	4.9						
1987	14934	5.3						
1988	14537	5.1						
1989	14541	5.1	126	0.0	14667	5.1	14698	5.1
1990	15486	5.4	123	0.0	15609	5.4	15641	5.4
1991	15930	5.5	130	0.0	16060	5.6	16096	5.6
1992	16700	5.7	139	0.0	16839	5.8	16876	5.8
1993	17022	5.8						
1994	17594	6.0						
1995	16247	5.5						

Source : see *Notes on sources of sales data,* p. 549

Figure 22.1 Daily consumption of (i) manufactured and total number of cigarettes, and (ii) all tobacco products, 1940-1995.
Males and females aged 15 years and over. *Source:* see Table 22.2

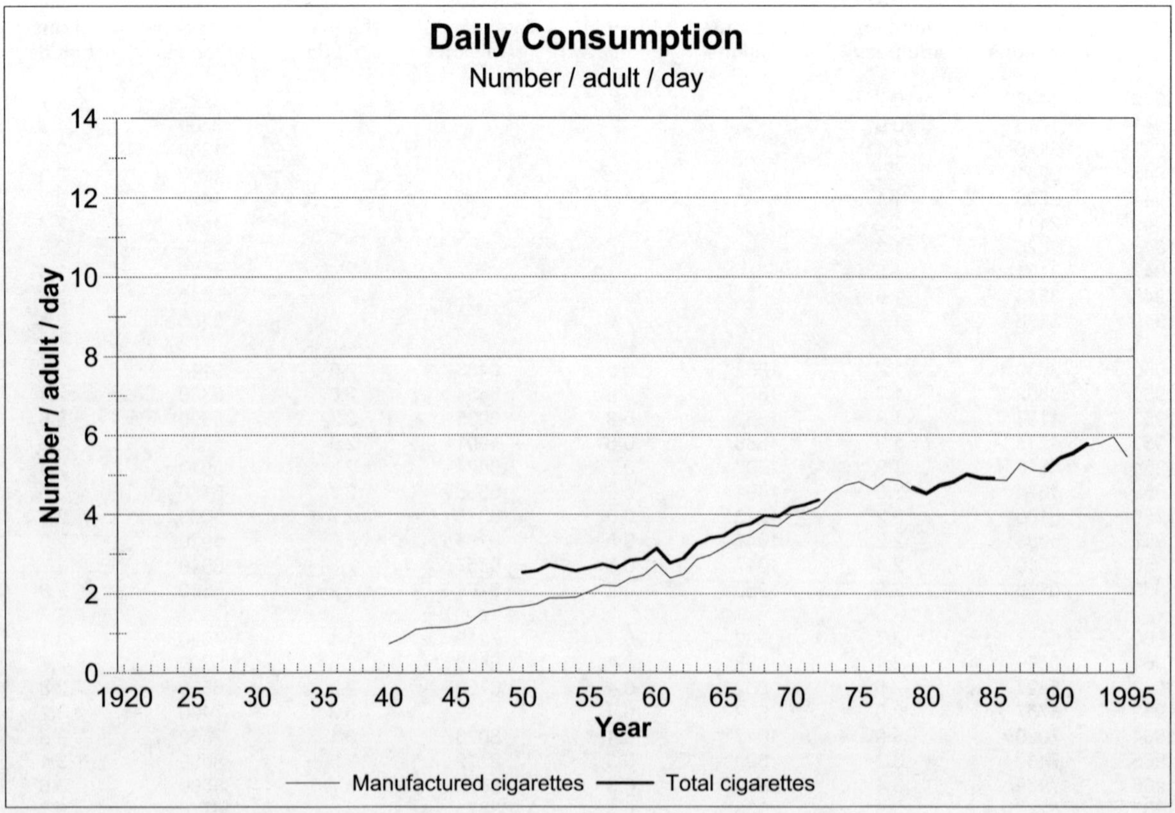

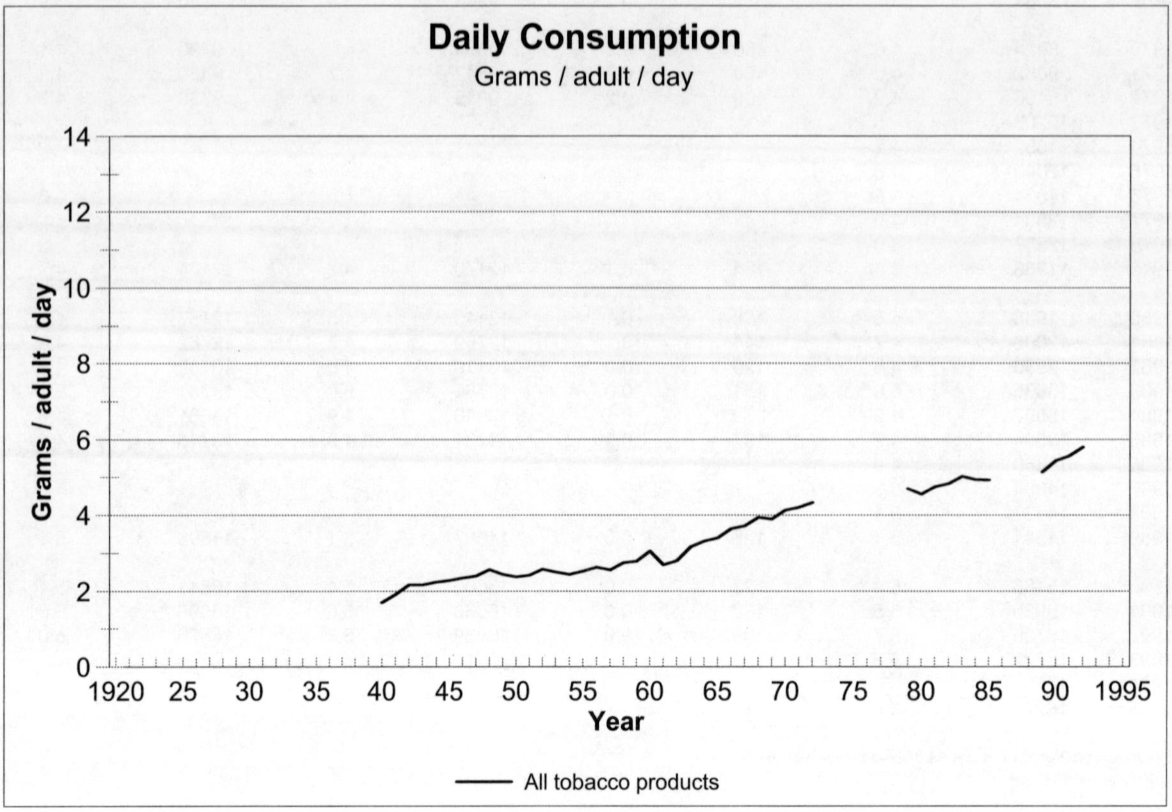

Table 22.3 Percentage sales of tobacco[1] in different forms (by weight), selected years 1940-1990

Year	Cigarettes (%)	Cigars and cigarillos (%)	Other tobacco (%)
1940	43.6	0.9	55.5
1950	70.6	0.2	29.2
1960	89.6	0.1	10.4
1970	96.1	0.1	3.9
1980	98.6	0.0	1.4
1990	99.0	0.2	0.8

1 No data for cigars and cigarillos 1980, no data for pipe tobacco 1990

Source : calculated from Tables 22.1.1 & 22.1.2

Figure 22.2 Percentage sales of tobacco in different forms (by weight), selected years 1940-1990
Source: see Table 22.3

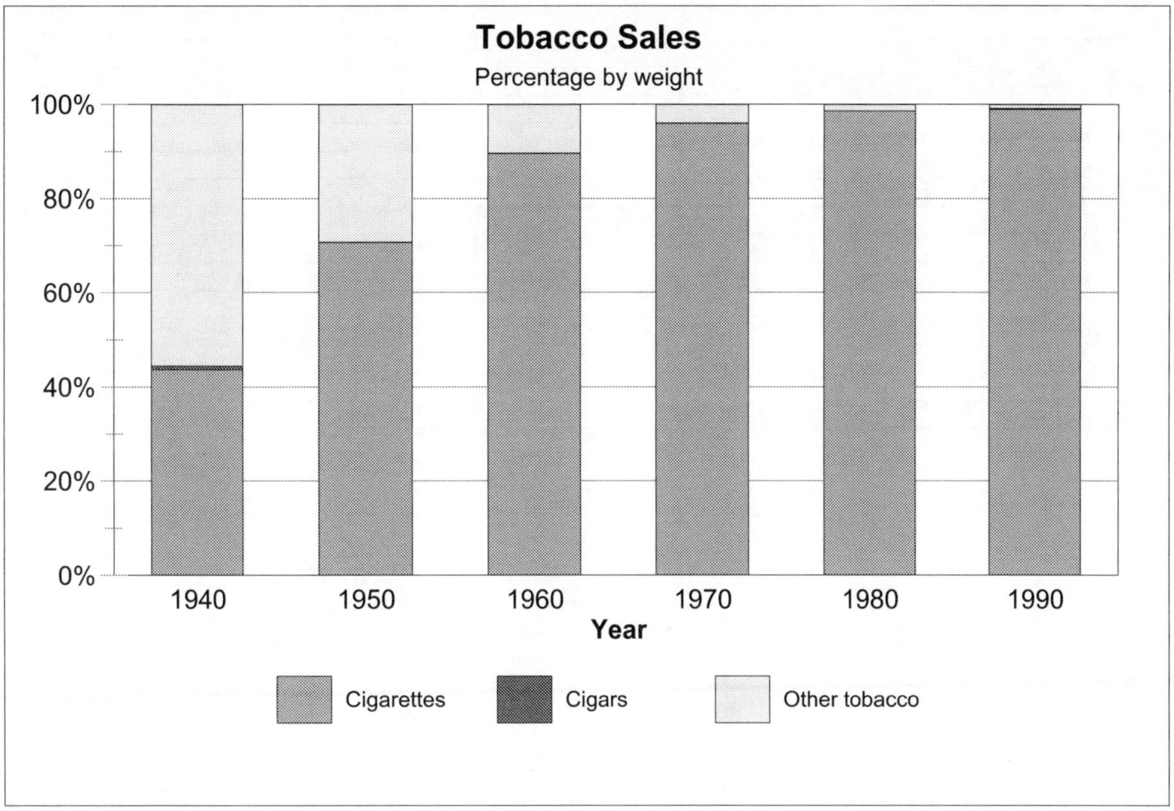

Table 22.4M Prevalence of smoking, males: some selected Portuguese surveys by age, 1975-1995

<table>
<tr><th rowspan="2">Frequency
Product
Source
Year</th><th colspan="21">Age group</th><th rowspan="2">All ages</th></tr>
<tr><th>12</th><th>13</th><th>14</th><th>15</th><th>16</th><th>17</th><th>18</th><th>19</th><th>20-24</th><th>25-29</th><th>30-34</th><th>35-39</th><th>40-44</th><th>45-49</th><th>50-54</th><th>55-59</th><th>60-64</th><th>65-69</th><th>70-74</th><th>75-79</th><th>80+</th></tr>
<tr><td>75 1 U U</td><td colspan="3"></td><td colspan="18">45</td><td></td></tr>
<tr><td>77 2 U U</td><td colspan="3"></td><td colspan="6">55</td><td colspan="12"></td><td>48</td></tr>
<tr><td>80 2 U U</td><td colspan="3"></td><td colspan="18">46</td><td></td></tr>
<tr><td>83 2 U U</td><td colspan="3"></td><td colspan="18">41</td><td></td></tr>
<tr><td>83 3 UC U</td><td></td><td colspan="20">35</td><td></td></tr>
<tr><td>83 4 U U</td><td colspan="8"></td><td>62</td><td colspan="12"></td><td></td></tr>
<tr><td>83 5 U R</td><td colspan="3"></td><td colspan="18">45</td><td></td></tr>
<tr><td>84 2 U U</td><td colspan="3"></td><td colspan="6">40</td><td colspan="12"></td><td>38</td></tr>
<tr><td>85 2 U U</td><td colspan="3"></td><td colspan="6">35</td><td colspan="12"></td><td>36</td></tr>
<tr><td>85 5 U R</td><td colspan="3"></td><td colspan="18">42</td><td></td></tr>
<tr><td>87 2 U U</td><td colspan="3"></td><td colspan="18">34</td><td></td></tr>
<tr><td>87 5 U R</td><td colspan="3"></td><td colspan="18">34</td><td></td></tr>
<tr><td>87 6 UC U</td><td colspan="3"></td><td colspan="18">52</td><td></td></tr>
<tr><td>87 7 UC U</td><td colspan="3"></td><td colspan="5">18</td><td colspan="4">48</td><td colspan="4">32</td><td colspan="5">20</td><td>33</td></tr>
<tr><td>87 7 A U</td><td colspan="3"></td><td colspan="5">18</td><td colspan="4">49</td><td colspan="4">33</td><td colspan="5">21</td><td>34</td></tr>
<tr><td>88 2 U U</td><td colspan="3"></td><td colspan="6">45</td><td colspan="12"></td><td>46</td></tr>
<tr><td>88 6 U U</td><td colspan="21"></td><td></td></tr>
<tr><td>89 6 U U</td><td colspan="21"></td><td></td></tr>
<tr><td>90 8 U R</td><td colspan="2"></td><td>5</td><td>13</td><td colspan="17"></td><td></td></tr>
<tr><td>90 8 U A</td><td>2</td><td colspan="3">7</td><td colspan="17"></td><td></td></tr>
<tr><td>90 9 U U</td><td colspan="3"></td><td colspan="18">43</td><td></td></tr>
<tr><td>90 10 U U</td><td colspan="9"></td><td colspan="3">40</td><td colspan="9"></td><td></td></tr>
<tr><td>92 9 U U</td><td colspan="3"></td><td colspan="18">40</td><td></td></tr>
<tr><td>94 9 U U</td><td colspan="3"></td><td colspan="18">38</td><td></td></tr>
<tr><td>95 7 UC R</td><td colspan="3">0</td><td colspan="3">8</td><td colspan="2">25</td><td>39</td><td colspan="2">49</td><td colspan="2">42</td><td colspan="2">31</td><td colspan="2">21</td><td colspan="2">15</td><td colspan="2">8</td><td>27</td></tr>
<tr><td>95 7 A R</td><td colspan="3">0</td><td colspan="3">8</td><td colspan="2">25</td><td>39</td><td colspan="2">49</td><td colspan="2">42</td><td colspan="2">32</td><td colspan="2">21</td><td colspan="2">16</td><td colspan="2">9</td><td>27</td></tr>
<tr><td>95 7 A A</td><td colspan="3">1</td><td colspan="3">12</td><td colspan="2">29</td><td>44</td><td colspan="2">54</td><td colspan="2">46</td><td colspan="2">35</td><td colspan="2">24</td><td colspan="2">18</td><td colspan="2">11</td><td>30</td></tr>
<tr><td>95 11 UC R</td><td colspan="3"></td><td colspan="2">12</td><td colspan="16"></td><td></td></tr>
<tr><td>95 11 UC A</td><td colspan="3"></td><td colspan="2">22</td><td colspan="16"></td><td></td></tr>
<tr><td>95 12 U U</td><td colspan="8"></td><td colspan="2">35</td><td colspan="2">33</td><td colspan="2">20</td><td colspan="2">13</td><td colspan="2">8</td><td colspan="2">10</td><td>13</td><td>16</td></tr>
<tr><td>95 13 U U</td><td colspan="6"></td><td colspan="14">40</td><td></td><td></td></tr>
<tr><td>95 14 U U</td><td>2</td><td>2</td><td>5</td><td>10</td><td>15</td><td>22</td><td>31</td><td>36</td><td colspan="13"></td><td>15</td></tr>
</table>

Source: see *Notes on sources of survey data*, p. 550
Product: MC = manufactured cigarettes
TC = total cigarettes (including hand-rolled)
UC = cigarettes (type unspecified)
A = all products

Frequency: A = all smokers (including occasional)
R = regular or daily smokers
All ages: relevant to ages used and as given in original source
U = unspecified
* = refer to *Notes on sources of survey data*, p. 550

Table 22.4F Prevalence of smoking, females: some selected Portuguese surveys by age, 1975-1995

Year Source Product Frequency	Age group 12	13	14	15	16	17	18	19	20-24	25-29	30-34	35-39	40-44	45-49	50-54	55-59	60-64	65-69	70-74	75-79	80+	All ages
75 1 U U				10																		
77 2 U U				14																		3
80 2 U U				1																		
83 2 U U				9																		
83 3 UC U		10																				
83 4 U U									30													
83 5 U R				10																		
84 2 U U				17																		10
85 2 U U				17																		9
85 5 U R				10																		
87 2 U U				5																		
87 5 U R				5																		
87 6 UC U				14																		
87 7 UC U				6					13				3				1					5
87 7 A U				6					13				3				1					5
88 2 U U				31																		12
88 6 U U				12																		
89 6 U U				12																		
90 8 U R			0	7																		
90 8 U A	0	3																				
90 9 U U				11																		
90 10 U U				20									6									
92 9 U U				12																		
94 9 U U				15																		
95 7 UC R	0			3			9		16	17		11		4		1		1		1		6
95 7 A R	0			3			9		16	17		11		4		1		1		1		6
95 7 A A	1			5			12		18	20		13		5		2		1		1		7
95 11 UC R				12																		
95 11 UC A				25																		
95 12 U U									17		17		5		0		0		1		0	5
95 13 U U							18															
95 14 U U	1	1	4	7	12	17	22	23														11

Source: see *Notes on sources of survey data*, p. 550

Product: MC = manufactured cigarettes
TC = total cigarettes (including hand-rolled)
UC = cigarettes (type unspecified)
A = all products

Frequency: A = all smokers (including occasional)
R = regular or daily smokers

All ages: relevant to ages used and as given in original source

U = unspecified

* = refer to *Notes on sources of survey data*, p. 550

Table 22.5M Number of cigarettes smoked per smoker per day, males: some selected Portuguese surveys by age, 1987-1995

Product Source Year	Age group 12	13	14	15	16	17	18	19	20-24	25-29	30-34	35-39	40-44	45-49	50-54	55-59	60-64	65-69	70-74	75-79	80+	All ages
87 7 UC				14					20				22				17					20
95 7 UC	8.3			14			14		17	21		23		24		21		18		15		21
95 11 UCE				11																		
95 13 UCE*							14															

Table 22.6M Number of cigarettes smoked per person per day, males: some selected Portuguese surveys by age, 1987-1995, with percentage total sales

Product Source Year	Age group 12	13	14	15	16	17	18	19	20-24	25-29	30-34	35-39	40-44	45-49	50-54	55-59	60-64	65-69	70-74	75-79	80+	All ages	% Total sales
87 7 UC				2.4					9.4				7.1				3.5					6.5	68%T
95 7 UC	0.0			1.2			3.5		6.8	10		9.7		7.6		4.5		2.8		1.3		5.6	67%T
95 11 UC				1.4																			**
95 13 UC *							5.6																64%T

Table 22.7M Number of cigarettes smoked per person per day, sales-adjusted, males: some selected Portuguese surveys[1] by age, 1987-1995, with percentage total sales

Product Source Year	Age group 12	13	14	15	16	17	18	19	20-24	25-29	30-34	35-39	40-44	45-49	50-54	55-59	60-64	65-69	70-74	75-79	80+	All ages	% Total sales
87 7 UC				3.6					14				10				5.2					9.6	68%T
95 7 UC	0.0			1.8			5.3		10	15		15		11		6.8		4.2		2.0		8.4	67%T
95 13 UC *							8.7																64%T

1 Based on those surveys in Table 22.6 with data for both sexes and age range at least 21-64 (see *Cigarette consumption per person*, p. xxxv)

Source: see *Notes on sources of survey data*, p. 550
All ages: relevant to ages used and as given in original source
% Total sales: estimated % of total sales of M = manufactured or T = total cigarette consumption implied by survey, sexes combined, used as adjustment factor in Table 22.7
** = cannot be calculated
--- = adjusted by original author
* = refer to *Notes on sources of survey data*, p. 550

Product: MC = manufactured cigarettes
TC = total cigarettes (including hand-rolled)
UC = cigarettes (type unspecified)
A = all products
U = unspecified
E indicates mean estimated from percentage distribution (see also *Consumption category estimation*, p. xxxiv, and Appendix III, p. 789)

Table 22.5F Number of cigarettes smoked per smoker per day, females: some selected Portuguese surveys by age, 1987-1995

<table>
<tr><th rowspan="2">Product
Source
Year</th><th colspan="21">Age group</th><th rowspan="2">All ages</th></tr>
<tr><th>12</th><th>13</th><th>14</th><th>15</th><th>16</th><th>17</th><th>18</th><th>19</th><th>20-24</th><th>25-29</th><th>30-34</th><th>35-39</th><th>40-44</th><th>45-49</th><th>50-54</th><th>55-59</th><th>60-64</th><th>65-69</th><th>70-74</th><th>75-79</th><th>80+</th></tr>
<tr><td>87 7 UC</td><td colspan="3"></td><td colspan="5">9.8</td><td colspan="3">13</td><td colspan="4">16</td><td colspan="6">12</td><td>13</td></tr>
<tr><td>95 7 UC</td><td colspan="3">5.0</td><td colspan="3">11</td><td colspan="2">12</td><td>13</td><td colspan="2">14</td><td colspan="2">15</td><td colspan="2">15</td><td colspan="2">17</td><td colspan="2">16</td><td colspan="2">11</td><td>14</td></tr>
<tr><td>95 11 UCE</td><td colspan="3"></td><td colspan="2">9.2</td><td colspan="16"></td><td></td></tr>
<tr><td>95 13 UCE*</td><td colspan="6"></td><td colspan="14">12</td><td></td><td></td></tr>
</table>

Table 22.6F Number of cigarettes smoked per person per day, females: some selected Portuguese surveys by age, 1987-1995, with percentage total sales

<table>
<tr><th rowspan="2">Product
Source
Year</th><th colspan="21">Age group</th><th rowspan="2">All ages</th><th rowspan="2">% Total sales</th></tr>
<tr><th>12</th><th>13</th><th>14</th><th>15</th><th>16</th><th>17</th><th>18</th><th>19</th><th>20-24</th><th>25-29</th><th>30-34</th><th>35-39</th><th>40-44</th><th>45-49</th><th>50-54</th><th>55-59</th><th>60-64</th><th>65-69</th><th>70-74</th><th>75-79</th><th>80+</th></tr>
<tr><td>87 7 UC</td><td colspan="3"></td><td colspan="5">0.5</td><td colspan="3">1.7</td><td colspan="4">0.5</td><td colspan="6">0.1</td><td>0.7</td><td>68%T</td></tr>
<tr><td>95 7 UC</td><td colspan="3">0.0</td><td colspan="3">0.3</td><td colspan="2">1.1</td><td>2.0</td><td colspan="2">2.4</td><td colspan="2">1.7</td><td colspan="2">0.6</td><td colspan="2">0.2</td><td colspan="2">0.1</td><td colspan="2">0.1</td><td>0.9</td><td>67%T</td></tr>
<tr><td>95 11 UC</td><td colspan="3"></td><td colspan="2">1.1</td><td colspan="16"></td><td></td><td>**</td></tr>
<tr><td>95 13 UC *</td><td colspan="6"></td><td colspan="14">2.1</td><td></td><td></td><td>64%T</td></tr>
</table>

Table 22.7F Number of cigarettes smoked per person per day, sales-adjusted, females: some selected Portuguese surveys[1] by age, 1987-1995, with percentage total sales

<table>
<tr><th rowspan="2">Product
Source
Year</th><th colspan="21">Age group</th><th rowspan="2">All ages</th><th rowspan="2">% Total sales</th></tr>
<tr><th>12</th><th>13</th><th>14</th><th>15</th><th>16</th><th>17</th><th>18</th><th>19</th><th>20-24</th><th>25-29</th><th>30-34</th><th>35-39</th><th>40-44</th><th>45-49</th><th>50-54</th><th>55-59</th><th>60-64</th><th>65-69</th><th>70-74</th><th>75-79</th><th>80+</th></tr>
<tr><td>87 7 UC</td><td colspan="3"></td><td colspan="5">0.8</td><td colspan="3">2.5</td><td colspan="4">0.7</td><td colspan="6">0.1</td><td>1.0</td><td>68%T</td></tr>
<tr><td>95 7 UC</td><td colspan="3">0.0</td><td colspan="3">0.5</td><td colspan="2">1.7</td><td>3.0</td><td colspan="2">3.6</td><td colspan="2">2.6</td><td colspan="2">0.9</td><td colspan="2">0.3</td><td colspan="2">0.2</td><td colspan="2">0.2</td><td>1.4</td><td>67%T</td></tr>
<tr><td>95 13 UC *</td><td colspan="6"></td><td colspan="14">3.3</td><td></td><td></td><td>64%T</td></tr>
</table>

1 Based on those surveys in Table 22.6 with data for both sexes and age range at least 21-64 (see *Cigarette consumption per person*, p. xxxv)

Source: see *Notes on sources of survey data*, p. 550
All ages: relevant to ages used and as given in original source
% Total sales: estimated % of total sales of M = manufactured or T = total cigarette consumption implied by survey, sexes combined, used as adjustment factor in Table 22.7
** = cannot be calculated
--- = adjusted by original author
* = refer to *Notes on sources of survey data*, p. 550

Product:
MC = manufactured cigarettes
TC = total cigarettes (including hand-rolled)
UC = cigarettes (type unspecified)
A = all products
U = unspecified
E indicates mean estimated from percentage distribution (see also *Consumption category estimation*, p. xxxiv, and Appendix III, p. 789)

Table 22.8 Estimated[1] prevalence of smoking and estimated[1] number of cigarettes per person per day (unadjusted and sales-adjusted): summary of Tables 22.4, 22.6 and 22.7, 1975-1995.
Males and females aged 15 years and over

Year	Source[2]	Product[3]	Prevalence[4]						Number of cigarettes						
									Unadjusted[7]			Sales-adjusted[8]			
			Manufactured cigarettes		Total cigarettes[5]		All products[6]		Number/ person/day		Total sales %	Manufactured cigarettes number/ person/day		Total cigarettes[9] number/ person/day	
			M	F	M	F	M	F	M	F		M	F	M	F
1975	1	*U*					45	10							
1977	2	*U*					48	3							
1980	2	*U*					46	1							
1983	2	*U*					41	9							
	3	*UC*			35	10								(8.4	2.0)
	5	U					45	10							
1984	2	*U*					38	10							
1985	2	*U*					36	9							
	5	U					42	10							
1987	2	*U*					34	5							
	5	U					34	5							
	6	*UC*			52	14								(9.1	2.0)
	7	*UC+A*			34	6	35	6	6.8	0.8	68			9.9	1.2
1988	2	*U*					46	12							
	6	*U*						11							
1989	6	*U*						12							
1990	9	*U*					43	11							
1992	9	*U*					40	12							
1994	9	*U*					38	15							
1995	7	UC+A			29	7	29	7	6.5	1.1	67			9.8	1.6
	7	**A**					32	8							
	12	*U*					23	9							
	13	UC+*U*					38	17	5.3	2.0	64			8.2	3.1

1 Surveys covering an age range of at least 21-64 are included. Any gaps in the data for ages 15-20 and 65 years and over are filled in by assumed extensions to the age distribution, given in *Notes on sources of survey data*, p. 550. Method: see *Summary of adult smoking*, p. xxxvi
2 See *Notes on sources of survey data*, p. 550
3 Product: MC = manufactured cigarettes, TC = total cigarettes (including hand-rolled), UC = cigarettes (type unspecified), A = all products, U = unspecified. Frequency of smoking is indicated by: regular or daily smokers in normal type, all smokers (including occasional) in bold, unspecified in italics
4 From Table 22.4
5 This column includes prevalence of smoking classified as UC = cigarettes (type unspecified)
6 This column includes prevalence of smoking classified as U = unspecified product
7 From Table 22.6
8 From Table 22.7, except data in parentheses, which are derived from the prevalence of smoking from Table 22.4 as described in *Summary of adult smoking*, p. xxxvi
9 Number of cigarettes classified as UC = cigarettes (type unspecified) has been adjusted to total cigarette sales and included in this column. For adjustment to sales of total cigarettes, estimates of hand-rolled cigarettes in 1985 were used for 1987, and 1992 for 1995

Figure 22.3 Estimated prevalence of smoking: by year of survey, 1975-1995. Males and females aged 15 years and over. *Source:* see Table 22.8

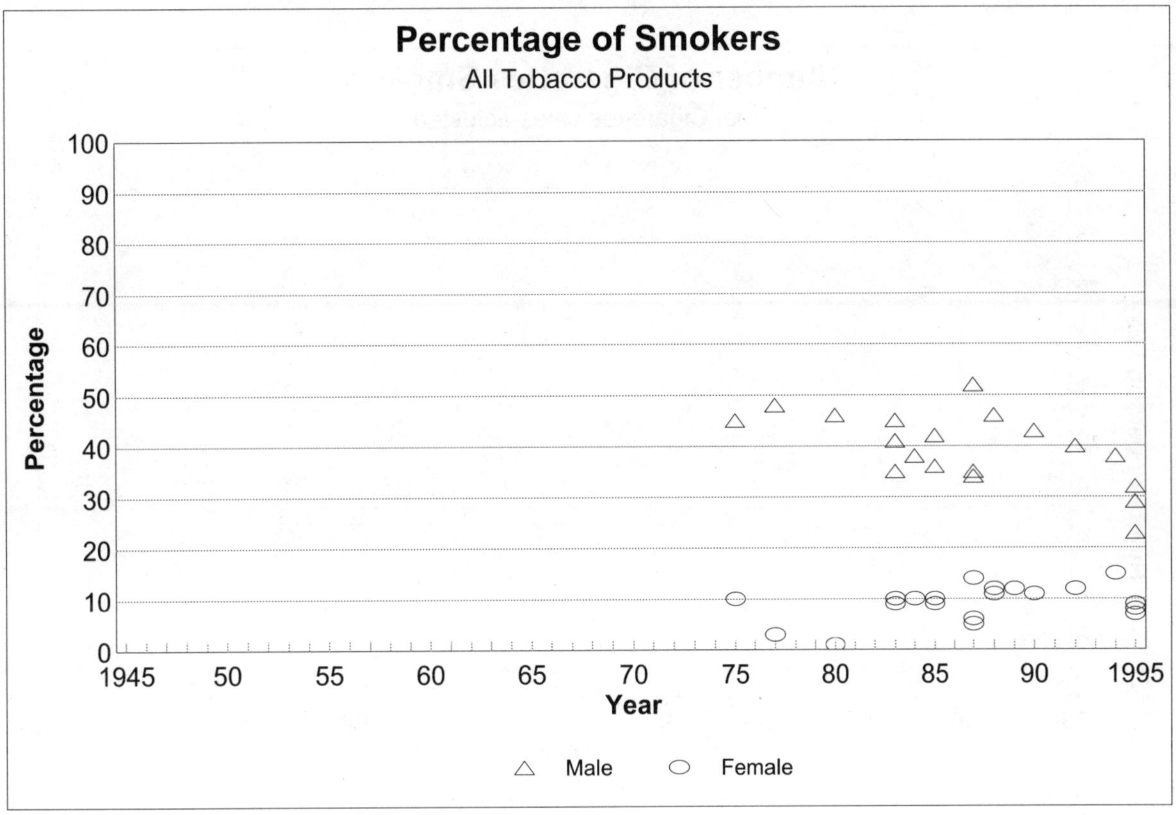

Note: Since cigarettes were the predominant product in this period, results for cigarettes and for all products have been combined here.

Figure 22.4 Estimated number of cigarettes smoked per person per day, sales-adjusted, 1983-1995.
Males and females aged 15 years and over. *Source:* see Table 22.8

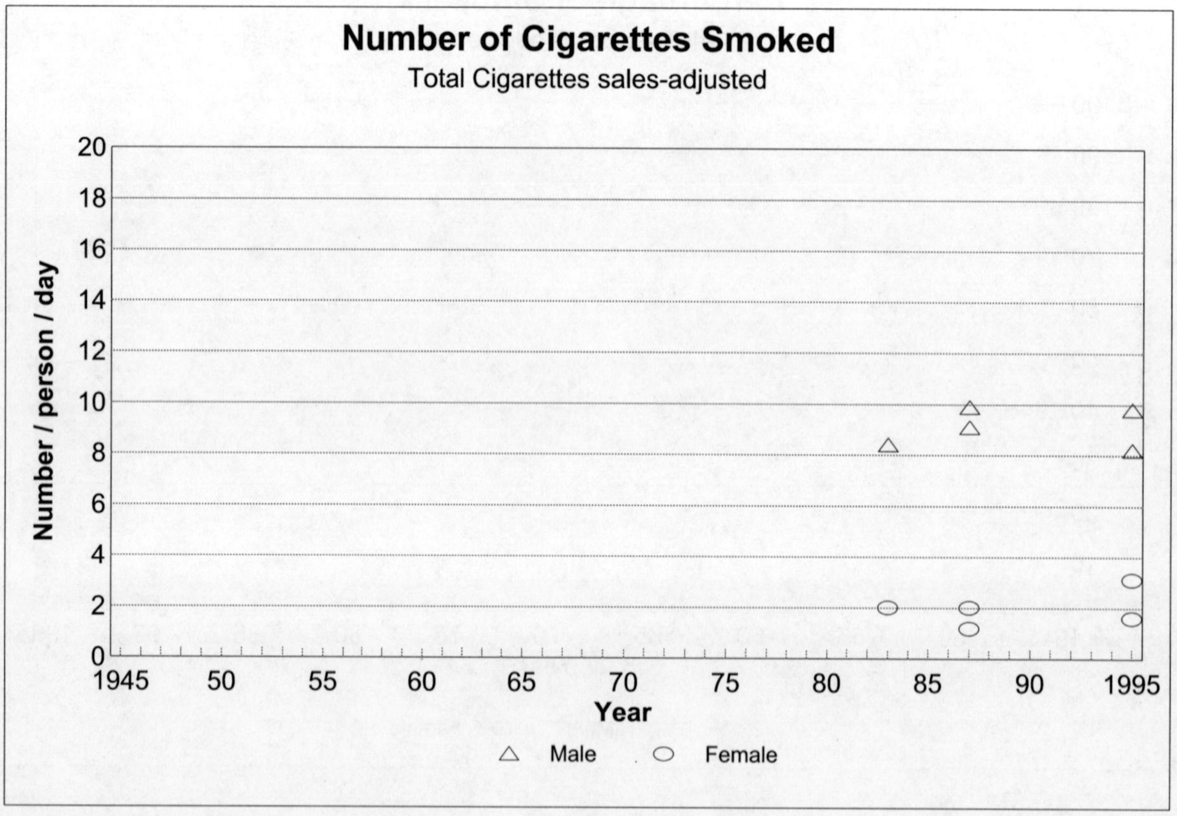

Notes on sources of sales data

The data presented in the tables and figures were obtained from several sources, details of which are given below, together with estimations and related assumptions. Full citations of the sources are given on p. 552 under *References*.

Consumption data before 1973

RP6

Data by weight, originally given to nearest 100 000 pounds, have been converted to tonnes and given to the nearest 10 tonnes (100 000 lbs = 45.359 tonnes). Where weight conversion factors have been quoted in RP6, the weights have been calculated without rounding and then converted to tonnes.

Notes as given in RP6:

(a) Details of the weight of tobacco consumed by products were obtained from *Estatistica Industrial* published by the National Institute of Statistics, Lisbon, and from trade sources.

(b) The number of cigarettes consumed have been estimated from the cigarette consumption in pounds weight by using a conversion factor of 2.205 lbs per 1 000. The conversion factor used for cigars and cigarillos was 12 lbs per 1 000.

Consumption data for 1973-1985

1973-1978 Maxwell International Estimates

1979-1985 Tabaqueira

Data from Tabaqueira were given in numbers and have been converted to weight assuming 1 g per cigarette (based on values in RP6).

The calculation for total tobacco consumption for 1979-1985 excludes cigars and cigarillos, as data were not available in those years but were low in earlier years.

The Anuário Estatístico gives cigarette production, in tonnes, for Portugal including Açores and Madeira for 1974-1987. The National Statistical Institute (INE) gives data for imports and exports of cigarettes and other products for 1970-1985. From these we have calculated total sales of cigarettes as follows:

Year	Production, tonnes	Net exports, tonnes	Sales, tonnes
1974	11 572	-31	11 603
1975	12 233	47	12 186
1976	12 409	125	12 284
1977	13 352	118	13 234
1978	13 583	247	13 336
1979	13 507	200	13 307
1980	13 281	228	13 053
1981	13 605	193	13 412
1982	14 864	-1	14 865
1983	15 531	152	15 379
1984	14 798	160	14 638
1985	14 593	155	14 438

These figures are consistently higher than those given by Tabaqueira, possibly because of the inclusion of the autonomous regions of Açores and Madeira.

Consumption data for 1986 onwards

United States Department of Agriculture (USDA) Economic Research Service (1996), Joossens *et al* (1994)

Data for cigarettes, cigars and cigarillos were given in millions and have been converted to weight assuming 1 g per cigarette, 6 g per cigar, 2 g per cigarillo and 4 g per cigar or cigarillo.

The calculation for total tobacco consumption for 1989-1992 excludes pipe tobacco, as data were not available in those years but were low in other years.

Plain/Filter cigarette consumption
1961-1978 Maxwell (successive years)
1979-1985 Tabaqueira
1993-1994 USDA Economic Research Service (1996)
For 1993 and 1994 the data represent the percentage of production rather than of sales.

Tar yield of cigarettes
The tar yield per cigarette was limited by EC directive (Directive 90/239/EEC) to 15 mg by the end of 1992, and to 12 mg by the end of 1997 (Harkin *et al* (1997)). The nicotine yield per cigarette has been limited to 1.3 mg since the end of 1992 (USDA Economic Research Service (1996)).

Estimates of hand-rolled cigarette consumption for 1950-1995
We have taken as our estimate of hand-rolled cigarette consumption 83% of pipe and hand-rolling tobacco sales up to 1973, and all hand-rolling tobacco sales from 1979 onwards, at 0.65 g per cigarette
RP6 gave hand-rolled cigarette consumption in 1966 as 1.0 million pounds (450 tonnes) equivalent to 697 million cigarettes, out of a total tobacco consumption of 1.2 million pounds (540 tonnes). These quantities imply 0.65 g per hand-rolled cigarette, and 83% of loose tobacco used for hand-rolling. The data from Tabaqueira show hand-rolling tobacco as 90-93% of all loose tobacco consumption in the period 1979-1985.

Notes on sources of survey data

Each source of survey data—either an individual survey or a series of surveys repeated over a number of years—is cited by a source number. This number is shown in the tables and corresponds to the source numbers given below, where details of the source publication and of the survey methodology are given. Full citations of the sources are given on p. 552 under *References*.

Source number

1 **Benjamin (1978)**
  a. No original source

2 **Joossens *et al* (1994)**
  a. Conselho de Prevenção do Tabagismo
  b. Results shown in *All ages* column of Table 22.4 relate to age 15+

3 **Tabaqueira, Lisbon (personal communication)**

4 **Geizerova and Masironi (1988)**
  a. No original source

5 **Organisation for Economic Co-operation and Development (1993)**
  a. No original source

6 **Karaoglou and Naett (1991) quoting Europe against Cancer Programme (no details), and Hill (1992) quoting Commission des Communautés Européennes (1987)**

7 **Cavelaars *et al* (2000) and P Santana (personal communication)**
  a. National health survey. Representative sample of the population excluding institutionalized persons. Personal interviews.
  1987: Sample size (males) 18 056, (females) 18 171. Response rate 74%.
  1995: Lower age limit 10. Sample size (males) 21 633, (females) 23 804
  b. Regular smokers: (1987) smoked regularly in last 2 weeks, (1995) smoked daily

8 **van Reek *et al* (1992), van Reek and Adriaanse (1995)**

a. A series of surveys of Young Europeans. About 800 children aged 11-15 years interviewed in each EC country except Luxembourg (where only 250 interviewed). Lowest age group 11-12. Interviews conducted at home, with parents absent

b. Regular smokers: smoked daily. All smokers: smoked at least once a week

9 **Joossens *et al* (1994)**

a. Eurobarometer, a series of surveys by the Member States at the request of the EU Commission in the framework of the 'Europe against Cancer' Programme. Conducted 1989/1990, 1991/1992 and 1994

10 **WHO (1997)**

a. No original source. Data presented as 1990 represent approximated results for 1989-1992

11 **Hibell *et al* (1997)**

a. Nationally representative survey forming part of ESPAD (European School Survey Project on Alcohol and Other Drugs). Target was pupils born in 1979, thus age 15-16 at time of survey in March1995. Percentage of this group still in school is not stated. Anonymous questionnaire completed and sealed in envelope by pupil, in class. Teachers present, but discouraged from walking round the classroom. Sample size (males) 852, (females) 1 182. Response rate 92%

b. Regular smokers: smoked 1 or more cigarettes per day in last 30 days. All smokers: smoked in last 30 days

c. Consumption category estimation based on 1-5, 6-10, 11-20, 21+ cigarettes/smoker/day

12 **Nunes *et al* (1997)**

a. Screening for cardiovascular risk factors in Viseu municipality. Subjects volunteered in response to radio and poster campaign. Sample size (males) 679 and (females) 1 173, comprising 3% of the population

b. Assumed extension to age distribution for percentage smokers, age 15-19: males 25% and females 20%

13 **Ramos and Barros (1998)**

a. Health survey in Porto. Random sample using electoral lists. Sample size (males) 535, (females) 653. Response rate 80%

b. Consumption category estimation based on two categories, 1-19 and >20 (assume 20+) cigarettes/smoker/day, and resulting figures should be regarded with caution

c. Assumed extension to age distribution for percentage smokers, age 15-17: males 15% and females 12%. For age 81+: males 12% and females 0.5%. Number of cigarettes/person/day, age 15-17: males 1.5 and females 1.0. For age 81+: males 3.0 and females 0.1

14 **Manninen (1997) quoting Barros *et al* (1995) (no details)**

a. Secondary school from each district. Sample size 16 013

References

Beese D.H. (ed) (1968). *Tobacco consumption in various countries,* 2nd edition. Tobacco Research Council, London. Research Paper 6.

Beese D.H. (ed) (1972). *Tobacco consumption in various countries,* 3rd edition. Tobacco Research Council, London. Research Paper 6.

Benjamin B. (1978). *Tobacco smoking in the world. Report of the WHO Expert Committee on Smoking Control, Geneva 23-28 October 1978*

Cavelaars A.E.J.M., Kunst A.E., Geurts J.J.M., Crialesi R., *et al* (2000). Educational differences in smoking: international comparison. *BMJ,* **320**, 1102-7.

Commission des Communautés Européennes (1987). *Les Européens et la prévention du cancer: une étude d'opinion publique.* Commission des Communautés Européennes, Brussels.

Geizerova H. and Masironi R. (1988). Cigarette smoking in children and adolescents: world review. In: Aoki M., Hisamichi S. and Tominaga S. (eds) *Smoking and health 1987. Proceedings of the 6th World Conference on Smoking and Health, Tokyo, 9-12 November 1987.* Elsevier Science Publishers B.V. (Biomedical Division), Amsterdam; 601-5. International Congress Series No. 780.

Harkin A.M., Anderson P. and Goos C. (1997). *Smoking, drinking and drug taking in the European Region.* Alcohol, Drugs and Tobacco Programme, WHO Regional Office for Europe, Copenhagen.

Hibell B., Andersson B., Bjarnason T., Kokkevi A., Morgan M. and Narusk A. (1997). *The 1995 ESPAD report. The European school survey project on alcohol and other drugs. Alcohol and other drug use among students in 26 European countries.* The Swedish Council for Information on Alcohol and Other Drugs. Council of Europe (Pompidou Group).

Hill C. (1992). Trends in tobacco use in Europe. *Journal of the National Cancer Institute Monographs,* **12**, 21-4.

Joossens L., Naett C., Howie C. and Muldoon A. (1994). *Tobacco and health in the European Union. An overview.* European Bureau for Action on Smoking Prevention (BASP), Brussels.

Karaoglou A. and Naett C. (1991). *Is she still a smoker?* BASP, Brussels. (European Bureau for Action on Smoking Prevention.)

Lee P.N. (ed) (1975). *Tobacco consumption in various countries,* 4th edition. Tobacco Research Council, London. Research Paper 6.

Manninen J. (ed) (1997). *Smoking prevalence and tobacco policies in the member states of the European Union. A summary of the overviews by country.* National Public Health Institute, Helsinki. http://www.ktl.fi/enypat/data/smokprev_eu.htm.

Maxwell J.C.Jr. (successive years). How the brands ranked. Maxwell International Estimates. *World Tobacco.*

Nunes L., Pipa J., Nascimento C., Costa A., *et al* (1997). Prevalência de alguns factores de risco cardiovascular numa população do concelho de Viseu. (Prevalence of several cardiovascular risk factors in a population in the municipality of Viseu). *Rev Port Cardiol,* **16**, 703-7.

Organisation for Economic Co-operation and Development (1993). *OECD health systems. Facts and trends 1960-1991. Health policy studies no 3.* OECD, Paris. (Health policy studies, Volume 1.)

Ramos E. and Barros H. (1998). Diet and smoking in Spain and Portugal: a comment [Letter]. *European Journal of Public Health,* **8**, 89-90.

RP6, See Beese (ed) (1968), Beese (ed) (1972), Lee (ed) (1975)

USDA Economic Research Service (1996). *Tobacco statistics.* Albert R. Mann Library, Cornell University,

Ithaca, New York. ERS 94012. (With supplementary material from Tobacco Annual Reports.). http://usda.mannlib.cornell.edu/data-sets/specialty/94012.

van Reek J. and Adriaanse H. (1995). Daily smoking among adolescents in the European Community. *Rev Epidemiol Sante Publique,* **43**, 281-2.

van Reek J., Adriaanse H. and Karaoglou A. (1992). Smoking among children in the European Community. *J Public Health Med,* **14**, 93-4.

WHO (1997). *Tobacco or health: A global status report.* WHO, Geneva. www.cdc.gov/nccdphp/osh/who/whoampro.htm.

Romania 23

Sales data

See Tables 23.1-23.3

Consumption of manufactured cigarettes per adult was 0.5-1 cigarette per day during the 1920s and 1930s. By 1960 it had increased to 4 cigarettes per day and, apart from a dip due to shortages in the late 1980s, it continued to rise slowly, reaching 6 cigarettes per day by 1995.

Consumption of all tobacco products per adult was about 4 g per day in the 1920s, falling to 2.5 g in the 1930s. At that period, around 20-25% of tobacco was used in manufactured cigarettes, with most of the remainder used in hand-made cigarettes and in pipes. Although data on other products are not available for recent years, consumption is reported to have been almost exclusively of manufactured cigarettes.

Consumption data from the mid 1980s onwards should be regarded with caution because of the size of illegal trade (see *Notes on sources of sales data,* p. 567).

Survey data

See Tables 23.4-23.8

Much of the survey data presented here comes from individual regional epidemiological studies, mainly of respiratory diseases, and the results may not be representative of the population generally. Between 1969 and 1995, estimates of the prevalence of smoking among those aged 15 years and over were in the range 30-55% for men. For women, estimates were in the range 1-16%, showing some increasing trend. At all age groups more men than women smoke.

Comparison of sales and survey data was possible in one case, where consumption from a local survey scaled up by the whole population under-reported by over 40%. Between 1970 and 1995, the estimated number of cigarettes smoked per person per day (sales-adjusted) was about 9-10 for men. For women it increased from 0.5 to 2.5 in the same period.

Table 23.1.1 Total annual sales of tobacco products, 1920-1935

Year	Cigarettes tonnes	Cigarettes millions	Cigars tonnes	Smoking mixtures tonnes	All tobacco products tonnes
1920	819	819	193	7965	8977
1921	1763	1763	204	9662	11629
1922	2239	2239	282	15483	18004
1923	2722	2722	145	12701	15568
1924	3889	3889	177	11503	15569
1925	3826	3826	157	11863	15846
1926	4077	4077	174	12217	16468
1927	4255	4255	177	10529	14961
1928	3907	3907	188	12969	17064
1929	4042	4042	123	9631	13796
1930	3015	3015	98	9250	12363
1931	2597	2597	72	8174	10843
1932	2404	2404	64	8698	11166
1933	2349	2349	66	8692	11107
1934	2179	2179	73	8337	10589
1935	2297	2297	77	8775	11149

Source : see *Notes on sources of sales data*, p. 567

Table 23.1.3 Manufactured cigarettes, percentage of total sales as filter cigarettes, 1972-1997

Year	% Filter
1972	22
1973	24
1974	29
1975	33
1976	35
1977	34
1978	35
1979	36
1993	44.2
1994	54.5
1995	56.1
1996	63.4
1997	82.0

Source : see *Notes on sources of sales data*, p. 567

Table 23.2 Consumption of (i) cigarettes and (ii) all tobacco products, 1920-1995 sales-based data, including estimated hand-rolled cigarette consumption. Males and females aged 15 years and over

Year	Manufactured cigarettes		Hand-rolled cigarettes		Total cigarettes		All tobacco products	
	Total annual in millions	Number/ adult/day	Total annual in millions	Number/ adult/day	Total annual in millions	Number/ adult/day	Total annual in tonnes	Grams/ adult/day
1920	819	0.2					8977	2.2
1921	1763	0.5					11629	3.0
1922	2239	0.6					18004	4.6
1923	2722	0.7					15568	3.9
1924	3889	1.0					15569	3.9
1925	3826	0.9					15846	3.6
1926	4077	1.0					16468	4.0
1927	4255	1.0					14961	3.5
1928	3907	0.9					17064	4.0
1929	4042	0.9					13796	3.2
1930	3015	0.7					12363	2.8
1931	2597	0.6					10843	2.4
1932	2404	0.5					11166	2.4
1933	2349	0.5					11107	2.4
1934	2179	0.5					10589	2.3
1935	2297	0.5					11149	2.4
1960	20733	4.3					20733	4.3
1961	21870	4.5					21870	4.5
1962	22098	4.5					22098	4.5
1963	21209	4.3					21209	4.3
1964	22399	4.4					22399	4.4
1965	23000	4.5					23000	4.5
1966	25000	4.9					25000	4.9
1967	24500	4.7					24500	4.7
1968	25200	4.7					25200	4.7
1969	25700	4.8					25700	4.8
1970	26000	4.7					26000	4.7
1971	26200	4.7					26200	4.7
1972	27000	4.8					27000	4.8
1973	28000	4.9					28000	4.9
1974	29000	5.0					29000	5.0
1975	30000	5.2					30000	5.2
1976	31000	5.3					31000	5.3
1977	32000	5.4					32000	5.4
1978	33000	5.6					33000	5.6
1979	33500	5.6					33500	5.6
1980	34000	5.7					34000	5.7
1981	35000	5.9					35000	5.9
1982	36000	6.0					36000	6.0
1983	35800	5.9					35800	5.9
1984	35800	5.8					35800	5.8
1985	36000	5.8					36000	5.8
1986	35750	5.7					35750	5.7
1987	29400	4.6					29400	4.6
1988	31525	4.9					31525	4.9
1989	32100	5.0					32100	5.0
1990	32100	5.0					32100	5.0
1991	23500	3.6					23500	3.6
1992	27500	4.3					27500	4.3
1993	36040	5.5					36040	5.5
1994	37000	5.7					37000	5.7
1995	41300	6.3					41300	6.3

Source : see *Notes on sources of sales data*, p. 567

Figure 23.1 Daily consumption of (i) manufactured cigarettes, and (ii) all tobacco products, 1920-1995
Males and females aged 15 years and over. *Source:* see Table 23.2

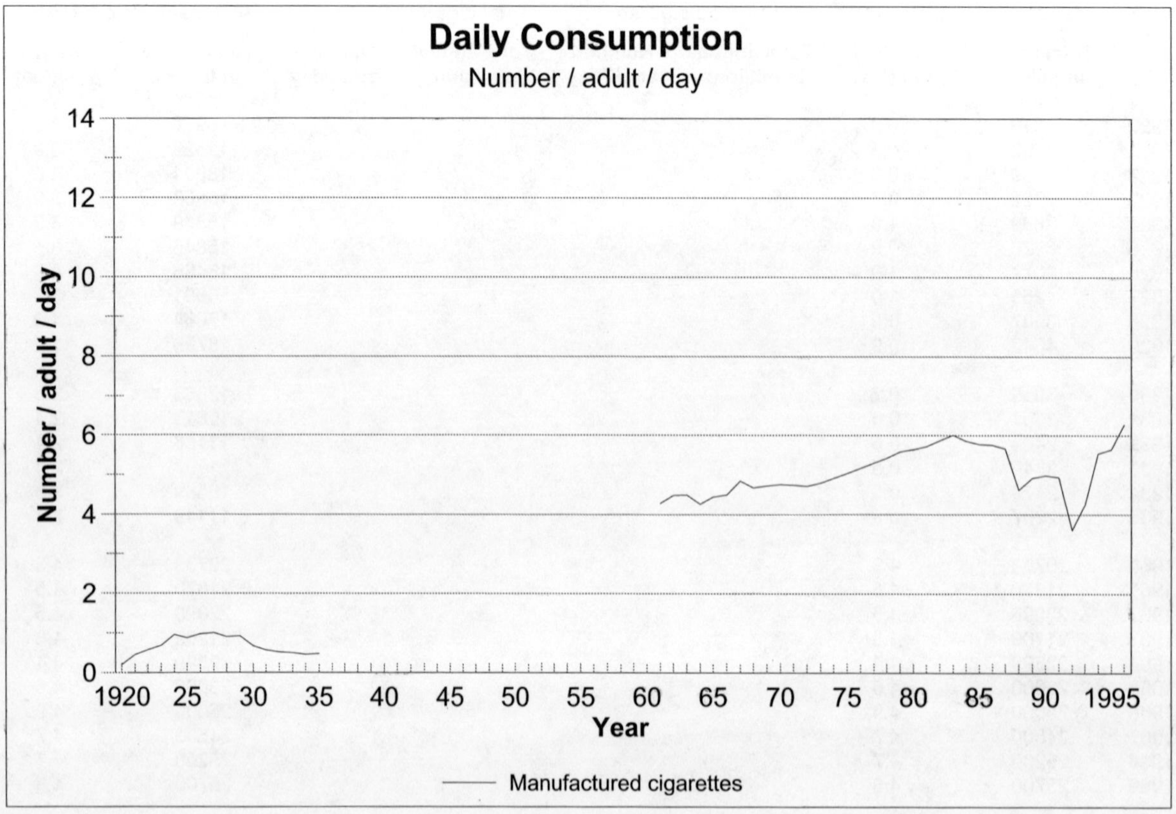

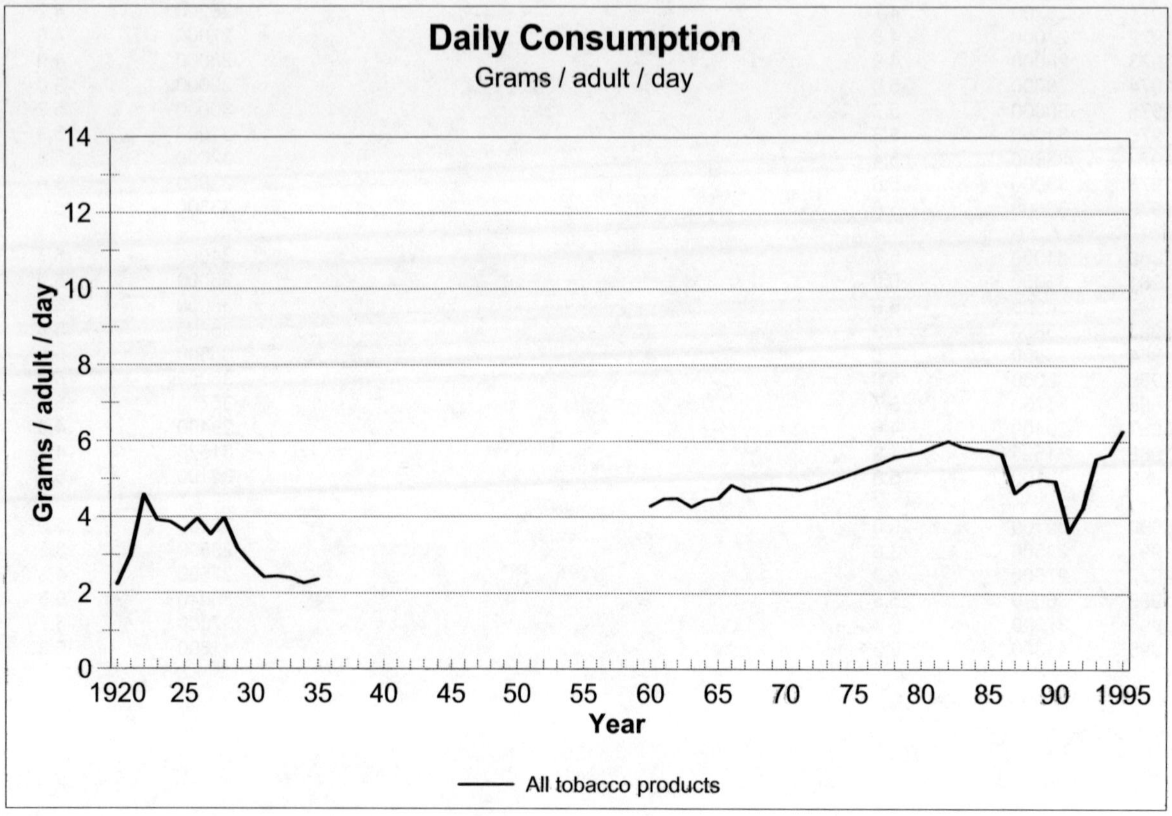

Table 23.3 Percentage sales of tobacco in different forms (by weight), selected years 1925-1995

Year	Cigarettes (%)	Cigars (%)	Smoking mixtures (%)
1925	24.1	1.0	74.9
1935	20.6	0.7	78.7
1965	100.0	0.0	0.0
1975	100.0	0.0	0.0
1985	100.0	0.0	0.0
1995	100.0	0.0	0.0

Source : calculated from Table 23.1.1, assumed to be 100% cigarettes from 1960 onwards

Figure 23.2 Percentage sales of tobacco in different forms (by weight), selected years 1925-1995
Source: see Table 21.3

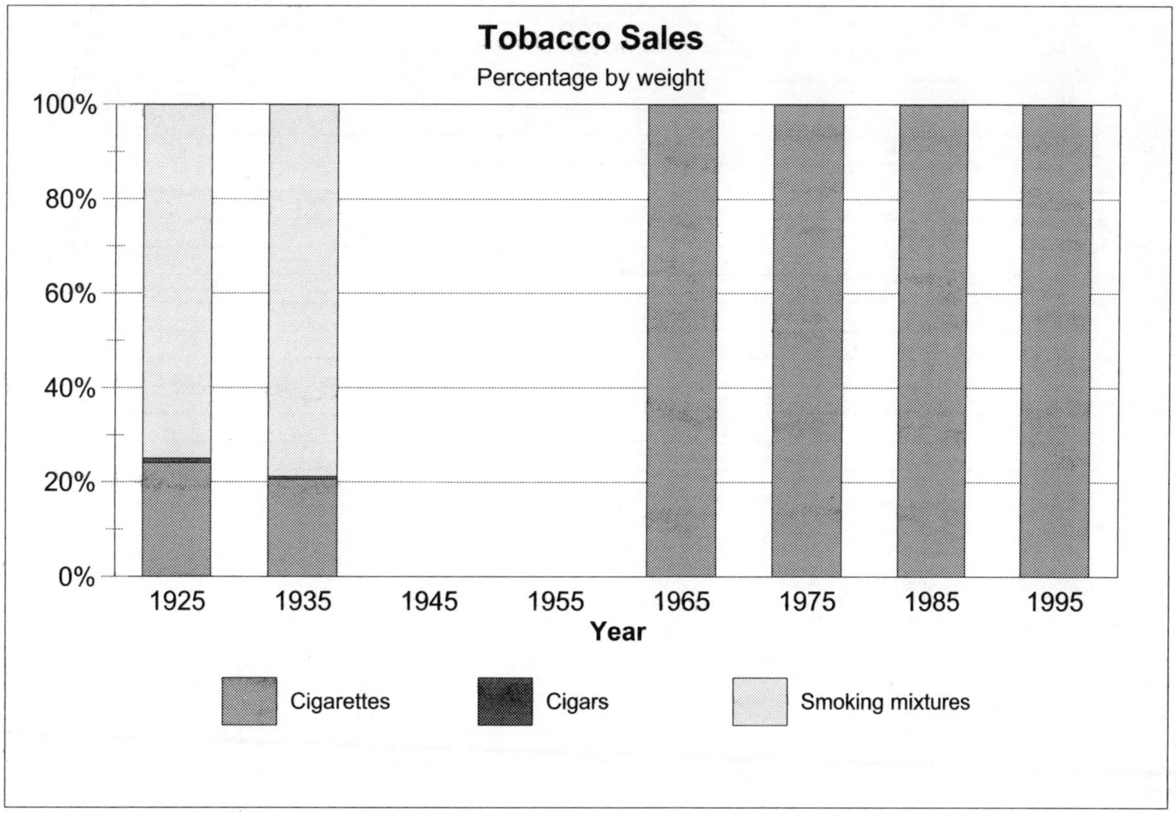

Table 23.4M Prevalence of smoking, males: some selected Romanian surveys by age, 1968-1995

<table>
<tr><th rowspan="2">Frequency
Product
Source
Year</th><th colspan="21">Age group</th><th rowspan="2">All ages</th></tr>
<tr><th>12</th><th>13</th><th>14</th><th>15</th><th>16</th><th>17</th><th>18</th><th>19</th><th>20-24</th><th>25-29</th><th>30-34</th><th>35-39</th><th>40-44</th><th>45-49</th><th>50-54</th><th>55-59</th><th>60-64</th><th>65-69</th><th>70-74</th><th>75-79</th><th>80+</th></tr>
<tr><td>68 1 U U</td><td colspan="10"></td><td colspan="11">37</td><td></td></tr>
<tr><td>69 2 U U</td><td colspan="8"></td><td colspan="9">52</td><td colspan="4"></td><td></td></tr>
<tr><td>69 3 U U</td><td colspan="8">3</td><td colspan="13">41</td><td></td></tr>
<tr><td>70 4 UC R</td><td colspan="3"></td><td colspan="5">10</td><td colspan="2">47</td><td colspan="2">44</td><td colspan="2">34</td><td colspan="2">37</td><td colspan="5">25</td><td>33</td></tr>
<tr><td>71 5 U U</td><td colspan="3"></td><td colspan="18">41</td><td></td></tr>
<tr><td>71 6 UC *</td><td colspan="12"></td><td colspan="4">33</td><td colspan="5"></td><td></td></tr>
<tr><td>71 8 UC R</td><td colspan="12"></td><td>44</td><td>41</td><td>41</td><td>31</td><td>33</td><td colspan="4">23</td><td></td></tr>
<tr><td>71 9 U U</td><td colspan="12"></td><td colspan="2">53</td><td colspan="2">52</td><td colspan="5"></td><td></td></tr>
<tr><td>71 10 U U</td><td colspan="12"></td><td colspan="4">46</td><td colspan="5"></td><td></td></tr>
<tr><td>76 7 UC *</td><td colspan="12"></td><td colspan="4">28</td><td colspan="5"></td><td></td></tr>
<tr><td>80 11 U U</td><td colspan="6">26</td><td colspan="3">68</td><td colspan="2">70</td><td colspan="2">54</td><td colspan="4">47</td><td colspan="4">39</td><td>56</td></tr>
<tr><td>80 12 U U</td><td colspan="6">28</td><td colspan="3">58</td><td colspan="2">72</td><td colspan="2">69</td><td colspan="4">50</td><td colspan="4">42</td><td>55</td></tr>
<tr><td>80 13 U U</td><td colspan="6">28</td><td colspan="3">53</td><td colspan="2">57</td><td colspan="2">51</td><td colspan="4">49</td><td colspan="4">39</td><td>49</td></tr>
<tr><td>80 14 U U</td><td colspan="6">19</td><td colspan="3">32</td><td colspan="2">36</td><td colspan="2">34</td><td colspan="4">33</td><td colspan="4">31</td><td>34</td></tr>
<tr><td>80 15 U U</td><td colspan="6">32</td><td colspan="3">57</td><td colspan="2">53</td><td colspan="2">47</td><td colspan="4">42</td><td colspan="4">40</td><td>47</td></tr>
<tr><td>80 16 U R</td><td colspan="3">3</td><td colspan="18"></td><td></td></tr>
<tr><td>80 16 U A</td><td colspan="3">30</td><td colspan="18"></td><td></td></tr>
<tr><td>80 18 MC R</td><td colspan="3"></td><td colspan="18">48</td><td></td></tr>
<tr><td>82 17 UC R</td><td colspan="3">11</td><td colspan="18"></td><td></td></tr>
<tr><td>84 19 U U</td><td colspan="3"></td><td colspan="18">31</td><td></td></tr>
<tr><td>87 20 U U</td><td colspan="9"></td><td colspan="8">45</td><td colspan="4"></td><td></td></tr>
<tr><td>87 21 U R</td><td colspan="4"></td><td>14</td><td></td><td>34</td><td colspan="14"></td><td></td></tr>
<tr><td>89 22 U A</td><td colspan="3"></td><td colspan="18">44</td><td></td></tr>
<tr><td>92 23 U U</td><td colspan="4">21</td><td colspan="17"></td><td></td></tr>
<tr><td>94 22 U A</td><td colspan="3"></td><td colspan="6"></td><td colspan="4">62</td><td colspan="8"></td><td>43</td></tr>
<tr><td>95 24 U U</td><td colspan="2"></td><td colspan="5">38</td><td colspan="14"></td><td></td></tr>
<tr><td>95 25 U U</td><td colspan="3"></td><td colspan="18">46</td><td></td></tr>
<tr><td>95 26 U U</td><td colspan="8"></td><td colspan="5">49</td><td colspan="8"></td><td></td></tr>
<tr><td>95 27 U U</td><td colspan="3"></td><td colspan="5">44</td><td colspan="13"></td><td></td></tr>
<tr><td>95 28 U U</td><td colspan="3"></td><td colspan="5">39</td><td colspan="13"></td><td></td></tr>
</table>

Source: see *Notes on sources of survey data*, p. 567

Product: MC = manufactured cigarettes
TC = total cigarettes (including hand-rolled)
UC = cigarettes (type unspecified)
A = all products

Frequency: A = all smokers (including occasional)
R = regular or daily smokers

All ages: relevant to ages used and as given in original source
U = unspecified
* = refer to *Notes on sources of survey data*, p. 567

Table 23.4F Prevalence of smoking, females: some selected Romanian surveys by age, 1968-1995

<table>
<tr><th>Year</th><th>Source</th><th>Product</th><th>Frequency</th><th colspan="21">Age group</th><th rowspan="2">All ages</th></tr>
<tr><th></th><th></th><th></th><th></th><th>12</th><th>13</th><th>14</th><th>15</th><th>16</th><th>17</th><th>18</th><th>19</th><th>20-24</th><th>25-29</th><th>30-34</th><th>35-39</th><th>40-44</th><th>45-49</th><th>50-54</th><th>55-59</th><th>60-64</th><th>65-69</th><th>70-74</th><th>75-79</th><th>80+</th></tr>
<tr><td>68</td><td>1</td><td>U</td><td>U</td><td colspan="10"></td><td colspan="11">12</td><td></td></tr>
<tr><td>69</td><td>2</td><td>U</td><td>U</td><td colspan="8"></td><td colspan="9">9</td><td colspan="4"></td><td></td></tr>
<tr><td>69</td><td>3</td><td>U</td><td>U</td><td colspan="8"></td><td colspan="13">1</td><td></td></tr>
<tr><td>70</td><td>4</td><td>UC</td><td>R</td><td colspan="3"></td><td colspan="5">0</td><td colspan="2">3</td><td colspan="2">5</td><td colspan="2">4</td><td colspan="2">9</td><td colspan="5">4</td><td>4</td></tr>
<tr><td>71</td><td>5</td><td>U</td><td>U</td><td colspan="3"></td><td colspan="18">3</td><td></td></tr>
<tr><td>71</td><td>6</td><td>UC</td><td>*</td><td colspan="21"></td><td></td></tr>
<tr><td>71</td><td>8</td><td>UC</td><td>R</td><td colspan="12"></td><td>10</td><td>11</td><td>9</td><td>11</td><td>8</td><td colspan="4">7</td><td></td></tr>
<tr><td>71</td><td>9</td><td>U</td><td>U</td><td colspan="21"></td><td></td></tr>
<tr><td>71</td><td>10</td><td>U</td><td>U</td><td colspan="21"></td><td></td></tr>
<tr><td>76</td><td>7</td><td>UC</td><td>*</td><td colspan="21"></td><td></td></tr>
<tr><td>80</td><td>11</td><td>U</td><td>U</td><td colspan="6">6</td><td colspan="3">13</td><td colspan="2">14</td><td colspan="2">10</td><td colspan="4">7</td><td colspan="4">4</td><td>10</td></tr>
<tr><td>80</td><td>12</td><td>U</td><td>U</td><td colspan="6">7</td><td colspan="3">21</td><td colspan="2">24</td><td colspan="2">17</td><td colspan="4">9</td><td colspan="4">7</td><td>18</td></tr>
<tr><td>80</td><td>13</td><td>U</td><td>U</td><td colspan="6">7</td><td colspan="3">15</td><td colspan="2">16</td><td colspan="2">10</td><td colspan="4">8</td><td colspan="4">6</td><td>13</td></tr>
<tr><td>80</td><td>14</td><td>U</td><td>U</td><td colspan="6">0</td><td colspan="3">6</td><td colspan="2">8</td><td colspan="2">5</td><td colspan="4">3</td><td colspan="4">3</td><td>4</td></tr>
<tr><td>80</td><td>15</td><td>U</td><td>U</td><td colspan="6">10</td><td colspan="3">24</td><td colspan="2">22</td><td colspan="2">17</td><td colspan="4">15</td><td colspan="4">9</td><td>18</td></tr>
<tr><td>80</td><td>16</td><td>U</td><td>R</td><td colspan="3">3</td><td colspan="18"></td><td></td></tr>
<tr><td>80</td><td>16</td><td>U</td><td>A</td><td colspan="3">25</td><td colspan="18"></td><td></td></tr>
<tr><td>80</td><td>18</td><td>MC</td><td>R</td><td colspan="3"></td><td colspan="18">13</td><td></td></tr>
<tr><td>82</td><td>17</td><td>UC</td><td>R</td><td colspan="3">4</td><td colspan="18"></td><td></td></tr>
<tr><td>84</td><td>19</td><td>U</td><td>U</td><td colspan="3"></td><td colspan="18">7</td><td></td></tr>
<tr><td>87</td><td>20</td><td>U</td><td>U</td><td colspan="9"></td><td colspan="8">19</td><td colspan="4"></td><td></td></tr>
<tr><td>87</td><td>21</td><td>U</td><td>R</td><td colspan="4"></td><td>6</td><td></td><td>12</td><td colspan="14"></td><td></td></tr>
<tr><td>89</td><td>22</td><td>U</td><td>A</td><td colspan="3"></td><td colspan="18">11</td><td></td></tr>
<tr><td>92</td><td>23</td><td>U</td><td>U</td><td colspan="4">8</td><td colspan="17"></td><td></td></tr>
<tr><td>94</td><td>22</td><td>U</td><td>A</td><td colspan="3"></td><td colspan="6"></td><td colspan="4">25</td><td colspan="8"></td><td>15</td></tr>
<tr><td>95</td><td>24</td><td>U</td><td>U</td><td colspan="2"></td><td colspan="5">22</td><td colspan="14"></td><td></td></tr>
<tr><td>95</td><td>25</td><td>U</td><td>U</td><td colspan="3"></td><td colspan="18">15</td><td></td></tr>
<tr><td>95</td><td>26</td><td>U</td><td>U</td><td colspan="8"></td><td colspan="5">16</td><td colspan="8"></td><td></td></tr>
<tr><td>95</td><td>27</td><td>U</td><td>U</td><td colspan="3"></td><td colspan="5">28</td><td colspan="13"></td><td></td></tr>
<tr><td>95</td><td>28</td><td>U</td><td>U</td><td colspan="3"></td><td colspan="5">41</td><td colspan="13"></td><td></td></tr>
</table>

Source: see *Notes on sources of survey data*, p. 567
Product: MC = manufactured cigarettes
TC = total cigarettes (including hand-rolled)
UC = cigarettes (type unspecified)
A = all products

Frequency: A = all smokers (including occasional)
R = regular or daily smokers
All ages: relevant to ages used and as given in original source
U = unspecified
* = refer to *Notes on sources of survey data*, p. 567

Table 23.5M Number of cigarettes smoked per smoker per day, males: selected Romanian survey by age, 1970

<table>
<tr><th rowspan="2">Product
Source
Year</th><th colspan="21">Age group</th><th rowspan="2">All ages</th></tr>
<tr><th>12</th><th>13</th><th>14</th><th>15</th><th>16</th><th>17</th><th>18</th><th>19</th><th>20-24</th><th>25-29</th><th>30-34</th><th>35-39</th><th>40-44</th><th>45-49</th><th>50-54</th><th>55-59</th><th>60-64</th><th>65-69</th><th>70-74</th><th>75-79</th><th>80+</th></tr>
<tr><td>70 4 UC</td><td colspan="3"></td><td colspan="5">11</td><td colspan="2">15</td><td colspan="2">17</td><td colspan="2">17</td><td colspan="2">20</td><td colspan="5">18</td><td>18</td></tr>
</table>

Table 23.6M Number of cigarettes smoked per person per day, males: selected Romanian survey by age, 1970, with percentage total sales

<table>
<tr><th rowspan="2">Product
Source
Year</th><th colspan="21">Age group</th><th rowspan="2">All ages</th><th rowspan="2">% Total sales</th></tr>
<tr><th>12</th><th>13</th><th>14</th><th>15</th><th>16</th><th>17</th><th>18</th><th>19</th><th>20-24</th><th>25-29</th><th>30-34</th><th>35-39</th><th>40-44</th><th>45-49</th><th>50-54</th><th>55-59</th><th>60-64</th><th>65-69</th><th>70-74</th><th>75-79</th><th>80+</th></tr>
<tr><td>70 4 UC</td><td colspan="3"></td><td colspan="5">1.0</td><td colspan="2">7.2</td><td colspan="2">7.5</td><td colspan="2">5.8</td><td colspan="2">7.1</td><td colspan="5">4.5</td><td>5.8</td><td>64%m</td></tr>
</table>

Table 23.7M Number of cigarettes smoked per person per day, sales-adjusted, males: selected Romanian survey[1] by age, 1970, with percentage total sales

<table>
<tr><th rowspan="2">Product
Source
Year</th><th colspan="21">Age group</th><th rowspan="2">All ages</th><th rowspan="2">% Total sales</th></tr>
<tr><th>12</th><th>13</th><th>14</th><th>15</th><th>16</th><th>17</th><th>18</th><th>19</th><th>20-24</th><th>25-29</th><th>30-34</th><th>35-39</th><th>40-44</th><th>45-49</th><th>50-54</th><th>55-59</th><th>60-64</th><th>65-69</th><th>70-74</th><th>75-79</th><th>80+</th></tr>
<tr><td>70 4 UC</td><td colspan="3"></td><td colspan="5">1.6</td><td colspan="2">11</td><td colspan="2">12</td><td colspan="2">9.0</td><td colspan="2">11</td><td colspan="5">7.1</td><td>9.0</td><td>64%m</td></tr>
</table>

1 Based on those surveys in Table 23.6 with data for both sexes and age range at least 21-64 (see *Cigarette consumption per person*, p. xxxv)

Source: see *Notes on sources of survey data*, p. 567
All ages: relevant to ages used and as given in original source
% Total sales: estimated % of total sales of M = manufactured or T = total cigarette consumption implied by survey, sexes combined, used as adjustment factor in Table 23.7
** = cannot be calculated
--- = adjusted by original author
* = refer to *Notes on sources of survey data*, p. 567

Product: MC = manufactured cigarettes
TC = total cigarettes (including hand-rolled)
UC = cigarettes (type unspecified)
A = all products
U = unspecified
E indicates mean estimated from percentage distribution (see also *Consumption category estimation*, p. xxxiv, and Appendix III, p. 789)

Table 23.5F Number of cigarettes smoked per smoker per day, females: selected Romanian survey by age, 1970

Product Source Year	12	13	14	15	16	17	18	19	20-24	25-29	30-34	35-39	40-44	45-49	50-54	55-59	60-64	65-69	70-74	75-79	80+	All ages
70 4 UC				2.0					14		11		11		16		7.3					13

Table 23.6F Number of cigarettes smoked per person per day, females: selected Romanian survey by age, 1970, with percentage total sales

Product Source Year	12	13	14	15	16	17	18	19	20-24	25-29	30-34	35-39	40-44	45-49	50-54	55-59	60-64	65-69	70-74	75-79	80+	All ages	% Total sales
70 4 UC				0.0					0.5		0.6		0.4		1.4		0.3					0.5	64%m

Table 23.7F Number of cigarettes smoked per person per day, sales-adjusted, females: selected Romanian survey[1] by age, 1970, with percentage total sales

Product Source Year	12	13	14	15	16	17	18	19	20-24	25-29	30-34	35-39	40-44	45-49	50-54	55-59	60-64	65-69	70-74	75-79	80+	All ages	% Total sales
70 4 UC				0.0					0.7		0.9		0.7		2.1		0.5					0.8	64%m

1 Based on those surveys in Table 23.6 with data for both sexes and age range at least 21-64 (see *Cigarette consumption per person*, p. xxxv)

Source: see *Notes on sources of survey data*, p. 567
All ages: relevant to ages used and as given in original source
% Total sales: estimated % of total sales of M = manufactured or T = total cigarette consumption implied by survey, sexes combined, used as adjustment factor in Table 23.7
** = cannot be calculated
--- = adjusted by original author
* = refer to *Notes on sources of survey data*, p. 567

Product: MC = manufactured cigarettes
TC = total cigarettes (including hand-rolled)
UC = cigarettes (type unspecified)
A = all products
U = unspecified
E indicates mean estimated from percentage distribution (see also *Consumption category estimation*, p. xxxiv, and Appendix III, p. 789)

Table 23.8 Estimated[1] prevalence of smoking and estimated[1] number of cigarettes per person per day (unadjusted and sales-adjusted): summary of Tables 23.4, 23.6 and 23.7, 1969-1995.
Males and females aged 15 years and over

Year	Source[2]	Product[3]	Prevalence[4]						Number of cigarettes						
									Unadjusted[7]			Sales-adjusted[8]			
			Manufactured cigarettes		Total cigarettes[5]		All products[6]		Number/ person/day		Total sales %	Manufactured cigarettes[9] number/ person/day		Total cigarettes number/ person/day	
			M	F	M	F	M	F	M	F		M	F	M	F
1969	2	*U*					44	8							
	3	*U*					34	1							
1970	4	UC			34	4			5.8	0.5	64	9.0	0.8		
1971	5	*U*					41	3				(9.2	0.5)		
1980	11	*U*					52	9				(10.3	1.4)		
	12	*U*					55	14				(9.7	2.0)		
	13	*U*					48	10				(10.0	1.7)		
	14	*U*					31	4				(10.6	1.1)		
	15	*U*					46	16				(9.0	2.6)		
	18	MC	48	13								(9.6	2.1)		
1984	19	*U*					31	7				(10.0	1.8)		
1989	22	**U**					44	11				(8.4	1.7)		
1994	22	**U**					43	15				(8.9	2.5)		
1995	25	*U*					46	15				(10.1	2.6)		

1 Surveys covering an age range of at least 21-64 are included. Any gaps in the data for ages 15-20 and 65 years and over are filled in by assumed extensions to the age distribution, given in *Notes on sources of survey data*, p. 567. Method: see *Summary of adult smoking*, p. xxxvi
2 See *Notes on sources of survey data*, p. 567
3 Product: MC = manufactured cigarettes, TC = total cigarettes (including hand-rolled), UC = cigarettes (type unspecified), A = all products, U = unspecified. Frequency of smoking is indicated by: regular or daily smokers in normal type, all smokers (including occasional) in bold, unspecified in italics
4 From Table 23.4
5 This column includes prevalence of smoking classified as UC = cigarettes (type unspecified)
6 This column includes prevalence of smoking classified as U = unspecified product
7 From Table 23.6
8 From Table 23.7, except data in parentheses, which are derived from the prevalence of smoking from Table 23.4 as described in *Summary of adult smoking*, p. xxxvi
9 Number of cigarettes classified as UC = cigarettes (type unspecified) or U = product unspecified has been adjusted to manufactured cigarette sales and included in this column

Figure 23.3 Estimated prevalence of smoking of (i) cigarettes and (ii) all tobacco products: by year of survey, 1969-1995.
Males and females aged 15 years and over. *Source:* see Table 23.8

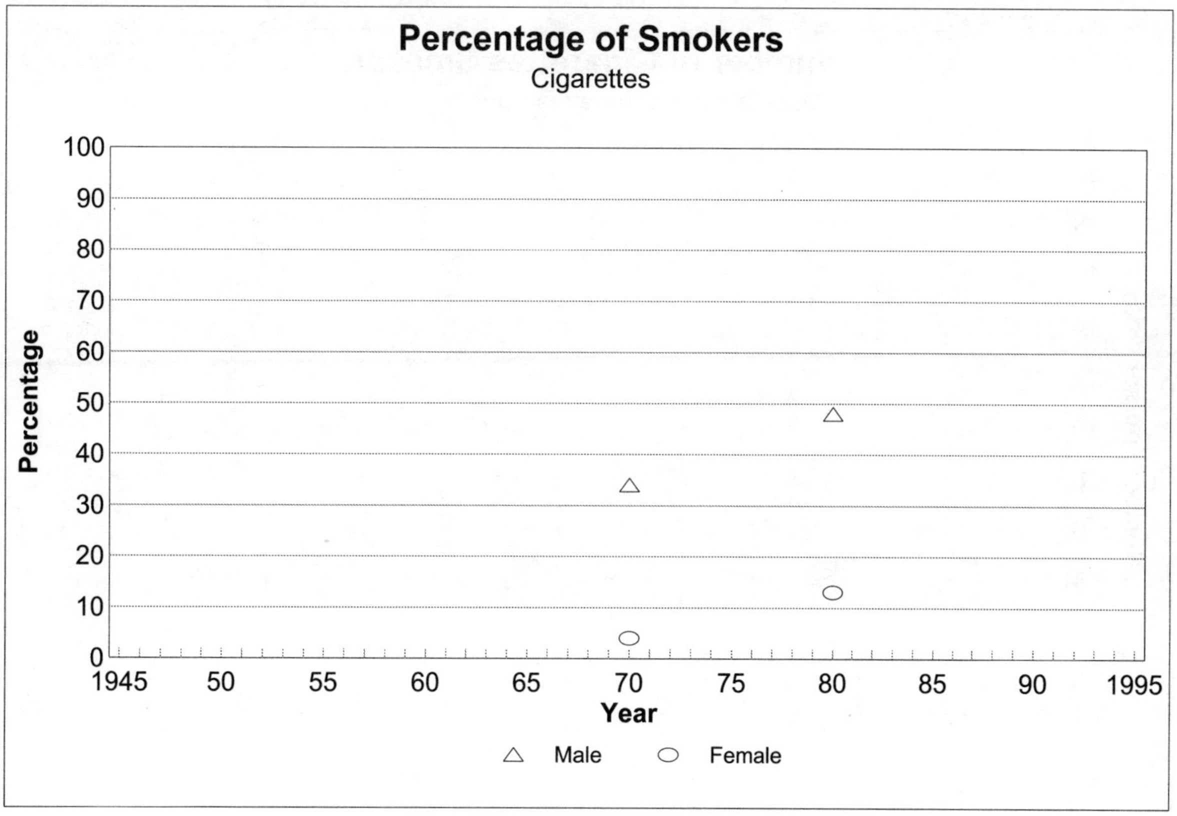

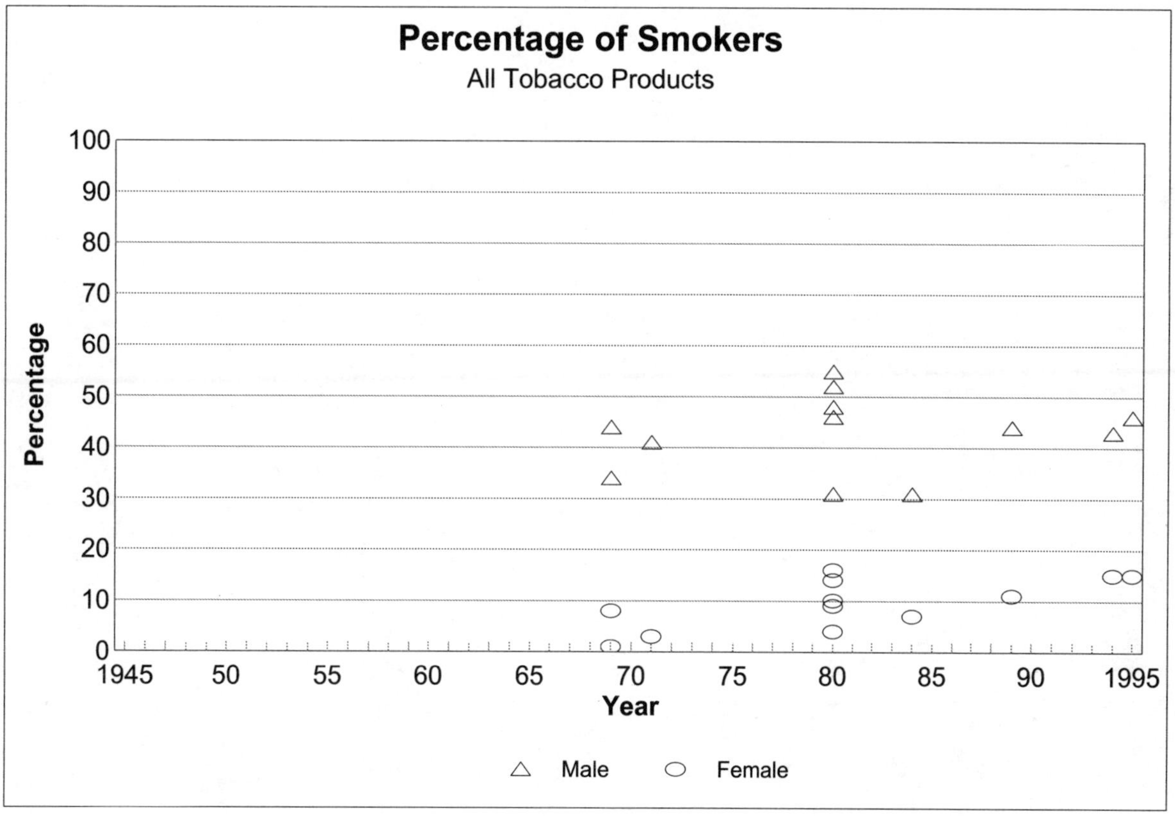

Figure 23.4 Estimated number of cigarettes smoked per person per day, sales-adjusted, 1970-1995.
Males and females aged 15 years and over. *Source:* see Table 23.8

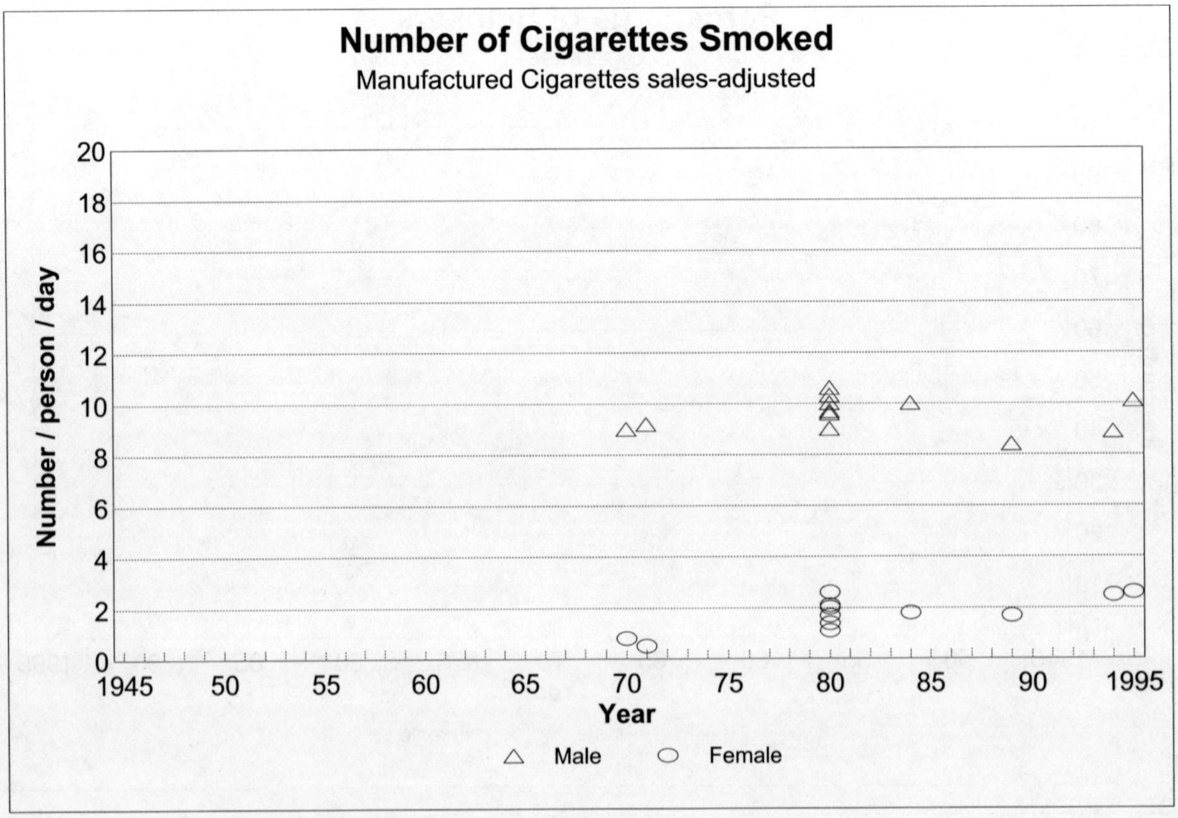

Notes on sources of sales data

The data presented in the tables and figures were obtained from several sources, details of which are given below, together with estimations and related assumptions. Full citations of the sources are given on p. 570 under *References*.

Consumption data for 1920-1935

Hutson (1937)

Data, originally given to the nearest 1 000 pounds, have been converted to tonnes and given to the nearest tonne (1 000 lbs = 0.45359 tonnes). No information is available on the average weight of cigarettes. For conversion from weight to numbers we assumed an average cigarette weight of 1 g.

Consumption data for 1960 onwards (Table 23.2)

United States Department of Agriculture (USDA) Economic Research Service (1996)

Information is available for cigarettes only. Barnea and Barnea (1983) state that in modern times tobacco consumption has been almost exclusively of ready-made cigarettes, the consumption of other forms of tobacco having been abandoned. In Table 23.2, consumption of all tobacco products is taken to be the same as manufactured cigarettes for 1960 onwards. No information is available on the average weight of cigarettes. For conversion from numbers to weights we assumed an average cigarette weight of 1 g.

Zatonski (1991) states that during 1987 few cigarettes at all were available. Cigarette consumption was said to be being held at an artificially low level because production could not satisfy demand.

John (1993) quotes a director of the Romanian Tobacco Monopoly as saying that of approximately 8 000 million imported cigarettes, around 5 000 million are legal imports, the rest being illegal trade. Prislopeanu (1998) quotes estimates of between 3 000 million and 5 000 million smuggled cigarettes being sold per year.

Plain/Filter cigarette consumption

1972-1979 Barnea and Barnea (1983)

1993-1997 USDA Economic Research Service (1996)

These data represent percentage of production rather than of sales. The later years are included to show the recent rapid increase. The recent increase in imports of international brands, which are mainly filter cigarettes, will have tended to increase the percentage of filter cigarettes smoked (USDA Economic Research Service (1996)).

Boddewyn (1986) gives a figure of 65% for 1984. No other information is given.

Tar yield of cigarettes

Barnea *et al* (1974) give the tar yields of the six most popular brands in Romania. These had a range of 16.2-25.5 mg tar per cigarette and a nicotine content (not yield) of 1.60-2.40% of the weight of tobacco in the cigarette. Barnea and Barnea (1983) give the nicotine content of Romanian cigarettes as in the range 1.37-1.60%. Didilescu (1994) gives the tar yields and nicotine contents of two popular cigarette brands (1990) as:

Brand	**Carpaţi**	**Snagov**
Quality*	common	superior
Tar (mg)	16	14
Nicotine content	1.53%	1.55%

*as described by Barnea and Barnea (1983)

Estimates of hand-rolled cigarette consumption

Hand-rolled cigarette consumption has been assumed to be zero in calculations.

Notes on sources of survey data

Each source of survey data—either an individual survey or a series of surveys repeated over a number of years—is cited by a source number. This number is shown in the tables and corresponds to the source numbers given below, where details of the source publication and of the survey methodology are given. Full citations of the sources are given on p. 570 under *References*.

Source number

1 **Manu *et al* (1970)**

a. Part of a study of chronic bronchitis in a district of Bucharest 1968-1969. Sample size (males) 380, (females) 620, which was 25% of the population aged 30+ in the district. Response rate 74%

2 **Racoveanu *et al* (1970)**

a. Study of bronchitis in 3 districts. Year not stated.

Location	Description	Sample size
Bucharest	Capital city, clerical workers	197
Sf Gheorghe	Fishing village in Danube delta	180
Fundata	Mountain village, principally shepherds and forestry workers	216

b. Assumed extension to age distribution for percentage smokers, age 15-19: males 10% and females 1%. For age 66+: males 20% and females 3%

3 **Barnea *et al* (1974)**

a. Study of chronic bronchitis in 12 districts, which differed in geography, customs and occupation. Lower age limit not stated. Sample size 37 050, of which 30 262 and 24 910 were age 10+ and 20+ respectively

b. Assumed extension to age distribution for percentage smokers, age 15-19: females only 1%

4 **Golli (1971)**

a. Survey in the suburban district of Craiova. Sample size (males) 1 329, (females) 1 613, which was 93% of the adult population

5 **Benjamin (1978) quoting Barnea *et al* (1972) (no details)**

6-7 **Steinbach *et al* (1982)**

a. The Bucharest Multifactorial Prevention Trial of Coronary Heart Disease. Results shown as source **6** are from initial screening of a random sample of 5 000 men from 4 districts of Bucharest, response rate 80%; source **7** from a randomly selected control group of 5 000 men from a 5th district, first examined 5 years later

b. Smokers: smoked 15+ cigarettes per day

8 **Duţu *et al* (1972)**

a. Study of respiratory symptoms in a district of Bucharest. Sample size (males) 780, (females) 1 024

b. There were no pipe or cigar smokers

9 **Racoveanu *et al* (1975) quoting Nicolaescu *et al* (1972)**

a. Study of general population in Bucharest. Year not stated. Sample size (males only) 1 685

10 **Racoveanu *et al* (1975) quoting Racoveanu *et al* (1973)**

a. Study in the general population in Hunedoara, a highly industrialized city. Year not stated. Sample size (males only) 636

11-15 **Barnea and Barnea (1983) quoting Barnea *et al* (1980)**

a. Study in 5 towns.

	Town	Description	Sample size	
			Males	Females
11	Hunedoara	Old industrial town	2 899	1 043
12	Petroşani	Old industrial town	1 024	1 015
13	Piteşti	Recently developed town	1 431	1 473
14	Slatina	Recently developed town	1 207	1 239
15	Bucharest	Capital city	2 003	2 165

16 Barnea and Barnea (1983)

a. Study in school pupils in two provincial towns, Oradea and Craiova. Lower age limit 10. Sample size 1 075

b. Regular smokers: 'steady smokers'. All smokers: 'attempted to smoke'

c. There is a discrepancy with results presented by Barnea (1981)

17 Barnea and Barnea (1983)

a. Study of school pupils in Bucharest. Lower age limit 10

b. Regular smokers: smoked at least 4 cigarettes per week

18 Mackay (1994)

a. No original source. Age group not stated

19 Zatonski (1991)

a. No original source. Age group not stated (adults)

20 Marin-Tarlea *et al* (1998)

a. Part of the WHO MONICA project. Sample size (males) 701, (females) 876

21 Mihăilescu (1994)

a. Study at 3 high schools in Bucharest. Approximate ages corresponding to school grades X and XII. Sample size (grade X) 246, (grade XII) 284

b. Regular smokers: smoked daily

22 Didilescu (1996), Didilescu *et al* (1997)

a. Results from Centrul de Calcul, Statistică Sanitară and Documentare Medicală al Ministerului Sănătăţii

b. Results in the *All ages* column relate to age 15+

23 WHO (1997)

a. No original source. A secondary school in Bucharest, age group not stated

24 Didilescu (1996), Didilescu and Marica (2000)

a. Study by Institutul de Pneumoftiziologie in 1995-1996 on pupils in 10 crowded towns. Approximate ages (14, 16, 18) corresponding to school grades VIII, X, XII. Sample size 8 817

25 Toma (1997)

a. No original source. Age group and year not stated

26 USDA (1996)

a. Market survey

b. It is also reported that smoking prevalence is higher in urban areas (35%) than rural (27%)

27-28 Ciufecu *et al* (1997a, 1997b)

a. Studies of smoking knowledge and behaviour among grade 9-12 pupils at a two high schools. Year not stated. Sample size (males) 69, (females) 59

	Location	Sample size	
		Males	Females
27	Sebeş, Alba	69	59
28	Bucharest	44	79

References

Boddewyn J.J. (ed) (1986). *Tobacco advertising bans and consumption in 16 countries*. International Advertising Association, New York.

Barnea E. (1981). Rolul fumatului in cancerul broncopulmonar. Situaţia in Románia. Necesitatea măsurilor profilactice. Studiu Sinteză (The role of smoking and the frequency of bronchopulmonary cancer. The situation in Romania. The need for prophylactic measures. Synoptic study). *Oncologia,* **20**, 137-52.

Barnea M. and Barnea E. (1983). Reasons grounding tobacco campaigns. Remarks on the situation in SR Romania. *Sante Publique,* **26**, 267-80.

Barnea M., Diaconescu L., Barnea E., Ianuli C. and Sabau A. (1980). *Studii fizico-chimice si epidemiologice in vederea evaluarii fumatului ca factor de risc cancerigen la populatia tarii noastre.* Comunicare la sesiunea stiintifica IMF, Bucuresti.

Barnea M., Zamfirescu M., Eremia D., Cotta S., *et al* (1974). Fumatul şi prevalenţa bronşitei cronice la populaţia din 12 localităţi din R.S.R. (Smoking and the prevalence of chronic bronchitis in 12 communities in Romania). *Viata Medicala,* **21**, 121-5.

Benjamin B. (1978). *Tobacco smoking in the world. Report of the WHO Expert Committee on Smoking Control, Geneva 23-28 October 1978*

Ciufecu C., Haber G. and Vrînceanu L. (1997a). Educaţia pentru sănătate—tabagism—Testarea cunoştinţelor şi a comportamentelor unor grupuri socio-profesionale—elevi, părinţi, profesori—de la colegiul 'Lucian Blaba'—Sebeş, Alba. (Education for health—smoking—testing the knowledge and behavior of some socio-occupational groups—students, parents, professors from Lucian Blaga High School in Sebes, Alba). *Bacteriol Virusol Parazitol Epidemiol,* **42**, 135-42.

Ciufecu C., Vrânceanu L. and Mita N. (1997b). Educaţia pentru sănătate—tabagism—Testarea cunoştinţelor si a comportamentelor unor grupuri socio-profesionale—elevi, părinţi, profesori. (Education for health—smoking. Testing the knowledge and behavior of some socio-professional groups—students, parents and teachers). *Pneumoftiziologia,* **46**, 229-32.

Didilescu C. (1994). Aspecte economice ale fumatului. *Pneumoftiziologia,* **43**, 237-9.

Didilescu C. (1996). Consumul de tutun, între tragismul datelor şi indiferenţă (Tobacco consumption, between the tragedy of the data and indifference). *Pneumoftiziologia,* **45**, 191-2.

Didilescu C. and Marica C. (2000). Socio-epidemiological data underlying the programme for control of tobacco use in Romania, 1997-2000. In: Lu R., Mackay J., Niu S. and Peto R. (eds) *Tobacco: The Growing Epidemic. Proceedings of the Tenth World Conference on Tobacco or Health, 24-28 August 1997, Beijing, China.* Springer-Verlag, London; 691

Didilescu C., Micu E. and Munteanu I. (1997). Aspecte epidemiologice ale tabagismului în Europa. (The epidemiological aspects of tobacco use disorder in Europe). *Pneumoftiziologia,* **46**, 67-71.

Duţu Şt., Bungeţianu Gh. and Jienescu Z. (1972). Studiu epidemiologic al bronhopneumopatiei obstructive cronice într-un teritoriu al oraşului Bucureşti. (Epidemiologic study of chronic obstructive bronchopneumopathy within a district of the town of Bucharest). *Ftiziologia,* **21**, 261-82.

Golli V. (1971). Studiu asupra obiceiului de a fuma (A study of smoking habits). *Igiena,* **20**, 167-78.

Hutson J.B. (1937). *Consumption and production of tobacco in Europe*. USDA, Washington DC. Technical bulletin No. 587.

John G.A. (1993). RTM faces the hard, cold facts of freedom. *Tobacco International,* **195**, 31-4.

Mackay J.L. (1994). The fight against tobacco in developing countries. *Tuber Lung Dis,* **75**, 8-24.

Manu P., Dumitriu M., Ghişe O. and Comănescu C. (1970). Cercetări epidemiologice privind bronşita conică la un lot din populaţia generalăa oraşului Bucureşti (Epidemiological study of chronic bronchitis in a general population group in Bucharest). *Med Interna,* **22**, 1123-34.

Marin-Tarlea M., Carp C., Apetrei E., Serban I., *et al* (1998). Trends in the prevalence of risk factors. A ten-year survey—MONICA programme [Abstract]. Meeting of Working Group on Epidemiology & Prevention of the European Society of Cardiology, Shannon, Ireland, May 14-17 1998. *Ir J Med Sci,* **167(Sup 7)**, 25-6.

Mihăilescu P. (1994). Problema fumatului în România (The smoking problem in Romania). *Pneumoftiziologia,* **43**, 233-6.

Nicolaescu V., Racoveanu C., Manicatide M. and Stanciu M. (1972). Prevalence of respiratory symptoms and of chronic bronchitis in a group of Bucharest city dwellers. *Viata Medicala,* **19**, 515.§

Prislopeanu I. (1998). Privatisation rolls on after late start. *Tobacco Journal International,* **May 1**, 106, 108.

Racoveanu C., Cretescu R., Manicatide M., Nicolaescu V. and Stanciu M. (1973). Prevalence of respiratory symptoms and chronic bronchitis in a population 'at risk' in Hunedoara. In: *Scientific Session, 'N.Gh.Lupu' Institute of Internal Medicine,Bucharest, February 1973.*§

Racoveanu C., Nicolaescu V., Manicatide M., Răiciulescu N., Drăgulescu I. and Olaru C. (1970). Cercetări epidemiologice în bronşita cronică (Epidemiological studies on chronic bronchitis). *Studii si Cercetari Med Interna,* **11**, 219-24.

Racoveanu C., Teculescu D., Manicatide M. and Nicolaescu V. (1975). Smoking habits in Romania. *Int J Epidemiol,* **4**, 25-9.

Steinbach M., Constantineanu M., Harnagea P., Theodorini S., *et al* (1982). The Bucharest multifactorial prevention trial of coronary heart disease. General methodology and risk factor correction after five year follow-up (1971-1977). *Revue Roumaine de Medecine,* **20**, 117-36.

Toma T.P. (1997). Romania plans tough antismoking laws. *BMJ,* **314**, 1506.

USDA (1996). *Tobacco annual report (Romania)*. USDA, Washington DC. AGR Number RO6010. http://www.fas.usda.gov.

USDA Economic Research Service (1996). *Tobacco statistics*. Albert R. Mann Library, Cornell University, Ithaca, New York. ERS 94012. (With supplementary material from Tobacco Annual Reports.). http://usda.mannlib.cornell.edu/data-sets/specialty/94012.

WHO (1997). *Tobacco or health: A global status report*. WHO, Geneva. www.cdc.gov/nccdphp/osh/who/whoampro.htm.

Zatonski W. (1991). Country reports. *World Smoking and Health,* **16**, 12-21.

§ Original paper not obtained, but information taken as quoted by another author

Spain 24

Sales data

See Tables 24.1-24.3.

Data on consumption of tobacco products are available since 1927, except for the years of the Spanish Civil War (1936-1939). From 1927 until 1950 the consumption of manufactured cigarettes per adult remained fairly stable at about 1 cigarette per day. Consumption rose to 7 cigarettes per day by the late 1970s and remained at that level through to the 1990s. Filter cigarettes became popular quite early, forming 10% of all cigarettes by 1961 and exceeding 80% since the mid 1970s. In 1957, when estimates were first available, consumption of hand-rolled cigarettes per adult was about 1.5 cigarettes per day. It has since decreased, and by the 1980s only very few hand-rolled cigarettes were consumed. Cigarettes made with dark tobacco were popular until the mid 1970s, constituting around 90% of all cigarettes. Blond cigarettes then increased steadily in popularity, exceeding sales of dark cigarettes around 1988 (Tabacalera (1989)).

The consumption of tobacco products per adult was about 4.5 g per day until 1935. In 1942, a minimum of 2 g per day was reached, but there was a return to pre-war levels by 1946 and this level continued until about 1960. Consumption rose to nearly 8 g per day by the late 1970s. In 1927, 20% of tobacco was consumed in manufactured cigarettes, increasing to 94% in 1993. Consumption of pipe and hand-rolling tobacco declined from 72% in 1927 to very low levels by the 1970s. The proportion of cigars fluctuated somewhat since 1927, but accounted for 5% of sales in the 1990s.

Survey data

See Tables 24.4-24.8

Few survey data are available for Spain before 1978 when the first nationally based survey was carried out.

Around 1970, the prevalence of tobacco smoking among those aged 15 years and over was 65% in men and 10% in women. By the 1990s, the prevalence among men had fallen about 45% while among women it had increased to about 25%.

The prevalence of smoking is higher among men than among women at all ages, although some surveys in the 1990s show little difference for younger adults, below about age 25. Very few elderly women smoke. Although comparisons are difficult due to different smoking definitions reported, between 1978 and 1993 the prevalence of smoking decreased in younger (below 25) and older (over 50) men. Conversely among women, prevalence altered little in those age groups but increased among the middle age groups. When first reported in 1978 (source 3) the prevalence of smoking among teenage boys was higher than among girls, but other surveys since 1986 have shown prevalence either similar, or higher among girls than among boys.

Comparison between survey and sales data suggests that a survey carried out in 1978 (source 3) overestimated sales by 5%, while one national and three regional surveys in the 1990s under-reported by 10-20%. The estimated number of cigarettes smoked per person per day (sales-adjusted) for men was about 11-12 between 1970 and 1985, falling to 9 by 1995. For women, it increased from 1 to 3 over the same period.

Table 24.1.1 Total annual sales of tobacco products, 1927-1973

Year	Cigarettes		Cigars		Smoking tobacco	All tobacco products
	tonnes	millions	tonnes	millions	tonnes	tonnes
1927	5400	5416	2130	315	19230	26760
1928	6580	6592	1950	287	19050	27580
1929	7350	7367	1860	275	18140	27350
1930	7800	7822	1810	266	17960	27580
1931	7620	7611	1860	272	18330	27810
1932	8210	8198	1950	284	17640	27810
1933	7760	7775	1950	285	15970	25670
1934	7120	7117	1810	268	17600	26540
1935	6710	6718	1720	250	18960	27400
1940	6760	6756	730	110	11840	19320
1941	7210	7198	680	98	7260	15150
1942	7440	7440	640	93	5850	13930
1943	9160	9160	450	69	6490	16100
1944	8800	8813	500	73	9570	18870
1945	9210	9192	450	69	13790	23450
1946	10250	10261	450	68	18190	28890
1947	10930	10927	410	62	15380	26720
1948	9800	9783	410	63	14700	24900
1949	10020	10010	410	61	18780	29210
1950	8850	8825	540	80	19370	28760
1951	9660	9682	590	89	16280	26540
1952	11520	11538	590	89	20590	32700
1953	12700	12707	590	88	12470	25760
1954	13830	13839	640	90	14970	29440
1955	15560	15554	680	98	14420	30660
1956	15100	15109	950	144	13020	29080
1957	18230	18222	1180	175	11930	31340
1958	21860	21872	1320	193	12020	35200
1959	22820	22839	1320	193	10210	34340
1960	24900	24892	1220	180	9210	35330
1961	27260	27220	1360	199	8530	37150
1962	30300	30294	1450	210	6990	38740
1963	33930	33915	1860	276	5260	41050
1964	36560	36570	2310	337	4220	43090
1965	40100	40087	2720	397	4080	46900
1966	42320	42324	3130	461	3580	49030
1967	45000	44999	3360	493	2950	51300
1968	47170	47174	3490	515	2540	53210
1969	47310	47287	3400	502	2310	53020
1970	50080	50084	3810	560	1950	55840
1971	50850	50843	4130	606	1770	56740
1972	53250	53234	4580	671	1590	59420
1973	56650	56623	5170	763	1500	63320

Source: see *Notes on sources of sales data*, p. 588

Table 24.1.2 Total annual sales of tobacco products, 1965-1995

Year	Cigarettes		Cigars		Picadura tonnes	All tobacco products tonnes
	tonnes	millions	tonnes	millions		
1965	40550	40550	2706	398	4026	47282
1974	60378	60378	6400	941	1397	68175
1975	58321	58321	7463	1098	1189	66973
1976	63205	63205	6931	1019	1078	71214
1977	66869	66869	6775	996	993	74637
1978	63490	63490	5825	857	709	70024
1979	70508	70508	6063	892	667	77238
1980	70437	70437	6146	904	705	77288
1981	64256	64256	6227	916	628	71111
1982	68739	68739	6045	889	546	75330
1983	71190	71190	5612	825	488	77290
1984	74205	74205	5688	836	435	80328
1985	79137	79137	5601	824	404	85142
1986	77827	77827	5433	799	360	83620
1987	79955	79955	5304	780	364	85623
1988	77310	77310	5080	747	537	82927
1989	79360	79360	4957	729		
1990	81920	81920	4957	729		
1991	84460	84460	4937	726		
1992	80320	80320	4719	694		
1993	74400	74400	4318	635	418	79136
1994	80180	80180	4508	663		
1995	75380	75380	4712	693		

Source : see *Notes on sources of sales data,* p. 588

Table 24.1.3 Manufactured cigarettes, percentage of total sales as filter cigarettes, 1961-1981

Year	% Filter
1961	10.0
1962	13.0
1963	15.0
1964	17.0
1966	31.5
1967	37.3
1968	42.9
1969	47.2
1970	48.8
1971	52.5
1974	81.0
1975	84.1
1976	87.1
1977	88.8
1978	91.2
1979	93.2
1980	94.0
1981	93.8

Source : see *Notes on sources of sales data,* p. 588

Table 24.2 Consumption of (i) cigarettes and (ii) all tobacco products, 1927-1995 sales-based data, including estimated hand-rolled cigarette consumption. Males and females aged 15 years and over

Year	Manufactured cigarettes		Hand-rolled cigarettes		Total cigarettes		All tobacco products	
	Total annual in millions	Number/ adult/day	Total annual in millions	Number/ adult/day	Total annual in millions	Number/ adult/day	Total annual in tonnes	Grams/ adult/day
1927	5416	1.0					26760	4.7
1928	6592	1.2					27580	4.8
1929	7367	1.3					27350	4.7
1930	7822	1.3					27580	4.7
1931	7611	1.3					27810	4.6
1932	8198	1.4					27810	4.6
1933	7775	1.3					25670	4.2
1934	7117	1.2					26540	4.3
1935	6718	1.1					27400	4.4
1940	6756	1.0					19320	2.9
1941	7198	1.1					15150	2.3
1942	7440	1.1					13930	2.1
1943	9160	1.4					16100	2.4
1944	8813	1.3					18870	2.8
1945	9192	1.3					23450	3.4
1946	10261	1.5					28890	4.2
1947	10927	1.6					26720	3.8
1948	9783	1.4					24900	3.6
1949	10010	1.4					29210	4.0
1950	8825	1.2					28760	3.9
1951	9682	1.3					26540	3.5
1952	11538	1.5					32700	4.3
1953	12707	1.7					25760	3.4
1954	13839	1.8					29440	3.8
1955	15554	2.0					30660	4.0
1956	15109	1.9					29080	3.7
1957	18222	2.3	12766	1.6	30988	4.0	31340	4.0
1958	21872	2.8	13084	1.7	34956	4.4	35200	4.5
1959	22839	2.9	11211	1.4	34050	4.3	34340	4.3
1960	24892	3.1	10090	1.3	34982	4.4	35330	4.4
1961	27220	3.4	9525	1.2	36745	4.5	37150	4.6
1962	30294	3.7	7594	0.9	37888	4.6	38740	4.7
1963	33915	4.1	5652	0.7	39567	4.8	41050	5.0
1964	36570	4.4	4527	0.5	41097	4.9	43090	5.2
1965	40087	4.8	4376	0.5	44463	5.3	46900	5.6
1966	42324	5.0	3819	0.4	46143	5.4	49030	5.8
1967	44999	5.3	3152	0.4	48151	5.6	51300	6.0
1968	47174	5.4	2713	0.3	49887	5.7	53210	6.1
1969	47287	5.4	2508	0.3	49795	5.7	53020	6.0
1970	50084	5.6	2059	0.2	52143	5.9	55840	6.3
1971	50843	5.7	1868	0.2	52711	5.9	56740	6.3
1972	53234	5.9	1553	0.2	54787	6.0	59420	6.6
1973	56623	6.2	1444	0.2	58067	6.4	63320	6.9
1974	60378	6.6	1397	0.2	61775	6.7	68175	7.4
1975	58321	6.3	1189	0.1	59510	6.4	66973	7.2
1976	63205	6.6	1078	0.1	64283	6.7	71214	7.4
1977	66869	6.9	993	0.1	67862	7.0	74637	7.7
1978	63490	6.4	709	0.1	64199	6.5	70024	7.1
1979	70508	7.1	667	0.1	71175	7.1	77238	7.7

Table 24.2 *(continued)*

Year	Manufactured cigarettes		Hand-rolled cigarettes		Total cigarettes		All tobacco products	
	Total annual in millions	Number/ adult/day	Total annual in millions	Number/ adult/day	Total annual in millions	Number/ adult/day	Total annual in tonnes	Grams/ adult/day
1980	70437	6.9	705	0.1	71142	7.0	77288	7.6
1981	64256	6.3	628	0.1	64884	6.3	71111	6.9
1982	68739	6.6	546	0.1	69285	6.7	75330	7.2
1983	71190	6.7	488	0.0	71678	6.8	77290	7.3
1984	74205	6.9	435	0.0	74640	7.0	80328	7.5
1985	79137	7.3	404	0.0	79541	7.4	85142	7.9
1986	77827	7.1	360	0.0	78187	7.2	83620	7.7
1987	79955	7.2	364	0.0	80319	7.3	85623	7.7
1988	77310	6.9	537	0.0	77847	7.0	82927	7.4
1989	79360	7.0						
1990	81920	7.2						
1991	84460	7.3						
1992	80320	6.9						
1993	74400	6.3	418	0.0	74818	6.4	79136	6.7
1994	80180	6.8						
1995	75380	6.3						

Source : see *Notes on sources of sales data*, p. 588

Figure 24.1 Daily consumption of (i) manufactured and total number of cigarettes, and (ii) all tobacco products, 1927-1995.
Males and females aged 15 years and over. *Source:* see Table 24.2

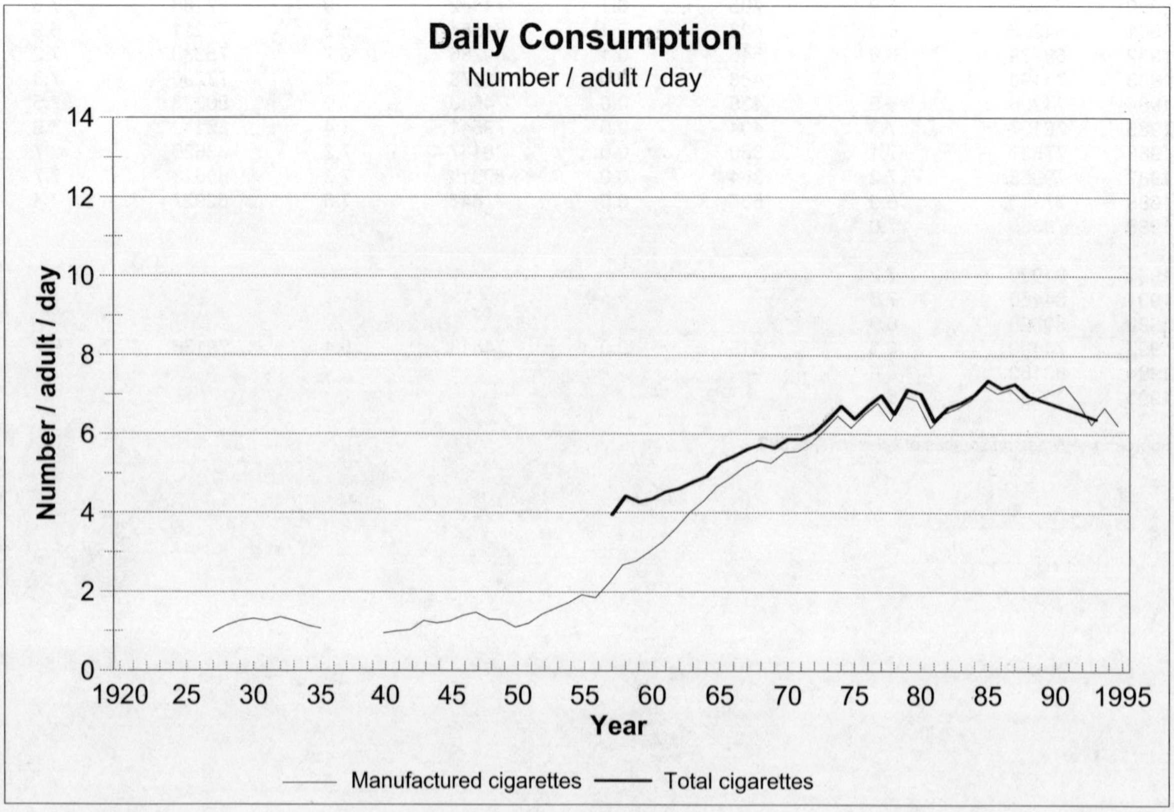

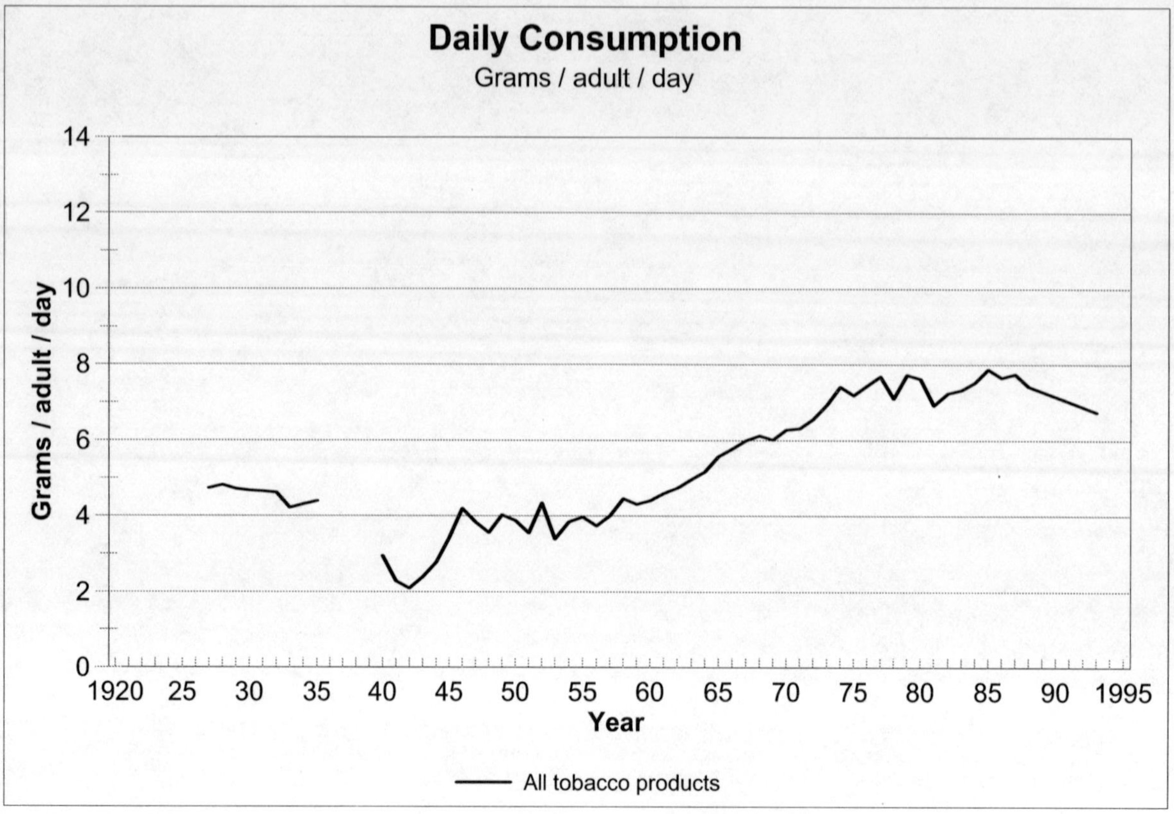

Table 24.3 Percentage sales of tobacco in different forms (by weight), selected years 1927-1993

Year	Cigarettes (%)	Cigars (%)	Smoking tobacco (%)
1927	20.2	8.0	71.9
1935	24.5	6.3	69.2
1945	39.3	1.9	58.8
1955	50.8	2.2	47.0
1965	85.5	5.8	8.7
1975	87.1	11.1	1.8
1985	92.9	6.6	0.5
1993	94.0	5.5	0.5

Source : calculated from Tables 24.1.1 & 24.1.2

Figure 24.2 Percentage sales of tobacco in different forms (by weight), selected years 1927-1993
Source: see Table 24.3

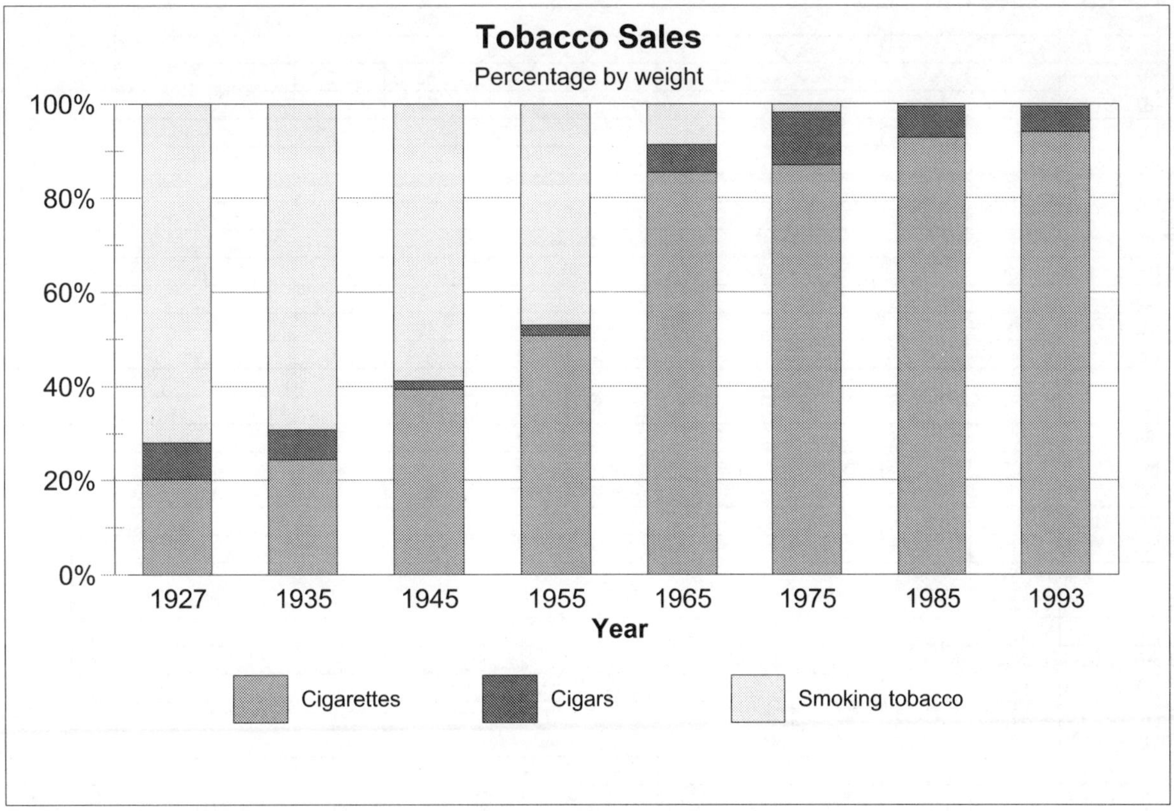

Table 24.4M Prevalence of smoking, males: some selected Spanish surveys by age, 1968-1995

Frequency / Product / Source / Year	12	13	14	15	16	17	18	19	20-24	25-29	30-34	35-39	40-44	45-49	50-54	55-59	60-64	65-69	70-74	75-79	80+	All ages
68 4 UC *											35		42		41							38
68 4 UC A											65		67		72							67
70 1 U U					66																	
78 3 UC U	14		23		62				72	66					65			46				54
78 15 U U					65																	
81 16 UC R										56												
81 16 A R										63												
81 17 UC R										41												
81 17 A R										50												
82 2 A A				59						67		61		61		48						58
82 2 A A				63																		
83 18 A A				46						64		67		58		52		40				55
85 5 U U				59																		
86 2 A A				54						69		61		57		47						58
86 8 U *		3																				
86 8 U R		7																				
86 8 U A		25																				
86 14 U R				54																		
86 19 U U					51																	
87 6 UC R										63		53		42		43						47
87 6 A A										66		63		54		52						47
87 7 UC R					52																	
87 7 A A					54					64				54				34				55
87 10 A *		3																				
87 10 A R		9																				
87 10 A A		13																				
87 13 UC R					23					40				30				13				30
89 7 U U					55																	
89 11 U R												56		46		45						49
89 11 U A												58		52		56						55
89 12 U R												48		37		31						39
89 12 U A												56		45		37						47
89 14 U R				52																		
89 19 U U					53																	
90 2 A A				39						53		57		65		48		34				47
90 8 UC R		7		18																		
90 8 UC A		18		27																		
90 9 U R			3	15																		
90 9 U A	0	10																				
90 10 A A	3																					
90 19 UC U									72		70		50		45		41					59
90 20 A A					49					60		64		53		47		40		37		52
92 10 A *		2	9	18	25	29	36															
92 10 A R		6	14	27	38	41	44															
92 18 A A				43						60		55		51		46		26				46
92 21 A R			28						54		56		64		47		29					47
92 21 A A			46						62		64		69		53		32					55
93 7 A R					39					57				44				23		17		44
93 7 U U					55					63				46				29				48
94 2 A R				35						55		52		43		34		21				39
94 2 A A				39						58		54		46		37		23				42
94 8 UC *		1		15		24	27															
94 8 UC R		3		20		30	35															
94 8 UC A		9		28		37	40															
94 10 A *		5																				
94 10 A A		10																				
95 7 A R					44																	
95 7 A A					47																	
95 22 U U	2	14	15	12	22																	

See footnotes on next page

Table 24.4F Prevalence of smoking, females: some selected Spanish surveys by age, 1968-1995

Frequency Product Source Year	Age group 12	13	14	15	16	17	18	19	20-24	25-29	30-34	35-39	40-44	45-49	50-54	55-59	60-64	65-69	70-74	75-79	80+	All ages
68 4 UC *																						
68 4 UC A																						
70 1 U U					10																	
78 3 UC U	3		4		48				48	16					5			3				17
78 15 U U					17																	
81 16 UC R										15												
81 16 A R										15												
81 17 UC R										9												
81 17 A R										9												
82 2 A A				48						35		12		9		4						20
82 2 A A				60																		
83 18 A A				42						39		25		14		9		5				21
85 5 U U				20																		
86 2 A A				50						39		15		14		3						23
86 8 U *		3																				
86 8 U R		6																				
86 8 U A		24																				
86 14 U R				22																		
86 19 U U					20																	
87 6 UC R										37		12		4		2						7
87 6 A A										41		14		5		4						8
87 7 UC R					22																	
87 7 A A					49					33				5				2				23
87 10 A *		4																				
87 10 A R		8																				
87 10 A A		13																				
87 13 UC R					11					10				2				0				6
89 7 U U					23																	
89 11 U R												21		5		4						10
89 11 U A												23		6		6						12
89 12 U R												33		12		4						17
89 12 U A												36		14		4						19
89 14 U R				21																		
89 19 U U					25																	
90 2 A A				37						45		19		11		6		1				22
90 8 UC R		5		27																		
90 8 UC A		12		35																		
90 9 U R			3	11																		
90 9 U A	0	11																				
90 10 A A	2																					
90 19 UC U									58		32		15		3		1					23
90 20 A A					21					50		21		6		2		0		0		18
92 10 A *		1	12	16	30	30	30															
92 10 A R		6	25	20	38	37	34															
92 18 A A				42						54		36		16		9		4				25
92 21 A R			33						56		47		24		17		6					32
92 21 A A			52						62		55		31		19		8					39
93 7 A R					33					34				9				1		2		21
93 7 U U					45					32				6				2				25
94 2 A R				30						41		29		10		3		1				19
94 2 A A				34						45		30		11		3		2				21
94 8 UC *		3		19		29	37															
94 8 UC R		6		27		38	46															
94 8 UC A		9		37		44	52															
94 10 A *		4																				
94 10 A A		8																				
95 7 A R					25																	
95 7 A A					27																	
95 22 U U	1	17	20	22	23																	

See footnotes on next page

Table 24.5M Number of cigarettes smoked per smoker per day, males: some selected Spanish surveys by age, 1968-1995

<table>
<tr><th rowspan="2">Product
Source
Year</th><th colspan="21">Age group</th><th rowspan="2">All ages</th></tr>
<tr><th>12</th><th>13</th><th>14</th><th>15</th><th>16</th><th>17</th><th>18</th><th>19</th><th>20-24</th><th>25-29</th><th>30-34</th><th>35-39</th><th>40-44</th><th>45-49</th><th>50-54</th><th>55-59</th><th>60-64</th><th>65-69</th><th>70-74</th><th>75-79</th><th>80+</th></tr>
<tr><td>68 4 UC</td><td colspan="10"></td><td colspan="2">15</td><td colspan="2">17</td><td colspan="2">16</td><td colspan="5"></td><td>16</td></tr>
<tr><td>78 3 UCE*</td><td colspan="2"></td><td colspan="2">12</td><td colspan="4">13</td><td>18</td><td colspan="5">20</td><td colspan="3">19</td><td colspan="4">18</td><td></td></tr>
<tr><td>87 6 UC</td><td colspan="11"></td><td colspan="6">17</td><td colspan="4"></td><td></td></tr>
<tr><td>87 7 UCE</td><td colspan="8"></td><td colspan="9">20</td><td colspan="4"></td><td></td></tr>
<tr><td>89 11 UCE</td><td colspan="11"></td><td colspan="2">21</td><td colspan="2">20</td><td colspan="2">18</td><td colspan="4"></td><td>20</td></tr>
<tr><td>89 12 UCE</td><td colspan="11"></td><td colspan="2">20</td><td colspan="2">21</td><td colspan="2">18</td><td colspan="4"></td><td>20</td></tr>
<tr><td>90 19 UCE</td><td colspan="8"></td><td colspan="2">19</td><td colspan="2">18</td><td colspan="2">20</td><td colspan="2">17</td><td colspan="2">15</td><td colspan="3"></td><td>18</td></tr>
<tr><td>90 20 UC</td><td colspan="4"></td><td colspan="17">19</td><td></td></tr>
<tr><td>92 21 UC</td><td colspan="2"></td><td colspan="16">19</td><td colspan="3"></td><td></td></tr>
<tr><td>94 2 UC</td><td colspan="3"></td><td colspan="10">19</td><td colspan="4">20</td><td colspan="4"></td><td>19</td></tr>
<tr><td>95 7 UCE</td><td colspan="4"></td><td colspan="17">18</td><td></td></tr>
</table>

Table 24.6M Number of cigarettes smoked per person per day, males: some selected Spanish surveys by age, 1968-1995, with percentage total sales

<table>
<tr><th rowspan="2">Product
Source
Year</th><th colspan="21">Age group</th><th rowspan="2">All ages</th><th rowspan="2">% Total sales</th></tr>
<tr><th>12</th><th>13</th><th>14</th><th>15</th><th>16</th><th>17</th><th>18</th><th>19</th><th>20-24</th><th>25-29</th><th>30-34</th><th>35-39</th><th>40-44</th><th>45-49</th><th>50-54</th><th>55-59</th><th>60-64</th><th>65-69</th><th>70-74</th><th>75-79</th><th>80+</th></tr>
<tr><td>68 4 UC</td><td colspan="10"></td><td colspan="2">9.8</td><td colspan="2">11</td><td colspan="2">11</td><td colspan="5"></td><td>11</td><td>**</td></tr>
<tr><td>78 3 UC *</td><td colspan="2"></td><td colspan="2">2.7</td><td colspan="4">7.9</td><td>13</td><td colspan="5">13</td><td colspan="3">13</td><td colspan="4">8.3</td><td></td><td>104%T</td></tr>
<tr><td>87 6 UC *</td><td colspan="11"></td><td colspan="6">7.9</td><td colspan="4"></td><td></td><td>**</td></tr>
<tr><td>87 7 UC</td><td colspan="8"></td><td colspan="9">12</td><td colspan="4"></td><td></td><td>**</td></tr>
<tr><td>89 11 UC</td><td colspan="11"></td><td colspan="2">12</td><td colspan="2">9.0</td><td colspan="2">7.9</td><td colspan="4"></td><td>9.7</td><td>**</td></tr>
<tr><td>89 12 UC</td><td colspan="11"></td><td colspan="2">9.5</td><td colspan="2">7.6</td><td colspan="2">5.4</td><td colspan="4"></td><td>7.7</td><td>**</td></tr>
<tr><td>90 19 UC</td><td colspan="8"></td><td colspan="2">13</td><td colspan="2">13</td><td colspan="2">12</td><td colspan="2">7.8</td><td colspan="2">6.0</td><td colspan="3"></td><td>11</td><td>84%T</td></tr>
<tr><td>90 20 UC</td><td colspan="4"></td><td colspan="17">9.9</td><td></td><td>79%T</td></tr>
<tr><td>92 21 UC</td><td colspan="2"></td><td colspan="16">8.7</td><td colspan="3"></td><td></td><td>88%T</td></tr>
<tr><td>95 7 UC</td><td colspan="4"></td><td colspan="17">7.2</td><td></td><td>78%T</td></tr>
</table>

Source: see *Notes on sources of survey data*, p. 589
All ages: relevant to ages used and as given in original source
% Total sales: estimated % of total sales of M = manufactured or T = total cigarette consumption implied by the survey, sexes combined
** = cannot be calculated
--- = adjusted by original author
Frequency A = all smokers (including occasional)
R = regular or daily smokers

Product: MC = manufactured cigarettes
TC = total cigarettes (including hand-rolled)
UC = cigarettes (type unspecified)
A = all products
E indicates mean estimated from percentage distribution (see also *Consumption category estimation*, p. xxxiv, and Appendix III, p. 789)
U = unspecified
* = refer to *Notes on sources of survey data*, p. 589

Table 24.5F Number of cigarettes smoked per smoker per day, females: some selected Spanish surveys by age, 1968-1995

<table>
<tr><th rowspan="2">Product
Source
Year</th><th colspan="22">Age group</th><th rowspan="2">All ages</th></tr>
<tr><th>12</th><th>13</th><th>14</th><th>15</th><th>16</th><th>17</th><th>18</th><th>19</th><th>20-24</th><th>25-29</th><th>30-34</th><th>35-39</th><th>40-44</th><th>45-49</th><th>50-54</th><th>55-59</th><th>60-64</th><th>65-69</th><th>70-74</th><th>75-79</th><th>80+</th></tr>
<tr><td>68 4 UC</td><td colspan="22"></td><td></td></tr>
<tr><td>78 3 UCE*</td><td colspan="2"></td><td colspan="2">9.7</td><td colspan="4">11</td><td>13</td><td colspan="5">14</td><td colspan="3">13</td><td colspan="4">12</td><td></td></tr>
<tr><td>87 6 UC</td><td colspan="11"></td><td colspan="6">9</td><td colspan="4"></td><td></td></tr>
<tr><td>87 7 UCE</td><td colspan="8"></td><td colspan="9">13</td><td colspan="4"></td><td></td></tr>
<tr><td>89 11 UCE</td><td colspan="11"></td><td colspan="2">14</td><td colspan="2">11</td><td colspan="2">10</td><td colspan="4"></td><td>13</td></tr>
<tr><td>89 12 UCE</td><td colspan="11"></td><td colspan="2">15</td><td colspan="2">15</td><td colspan="2">13</td><td colspan="4"></td><td>15</td></tr>
<tr><td>90 19 UCE</td><td colspan="8"></td><td colspan="2">10</td><td colspan="2">11</td><td colspan="2">11</td><td colspan="2">11</td><td colspan="2">15</td><td colspan="3"></td><td>10</td></tr>
<tr><td>90 20 UC</td><td colspan="4"></td><td colspan="18">12</td><td></td></tr>
<tr><td>92 21 UC</td><td colspan="2"></td><td colspan="16">14</td><td colspan="3"></td><td></td></tr>
<tr><td>94 2 UC</td><td colspan="3"></td><td colspan="10">14</td><td colspan="4">14</td><td colspan="4"></td><td>14</td></tr>
<tr><td>95 7 UCE</td><td colspan="4"></td><td colspan="18">13</td><td></td></tr>
</table>

Table 24.6F Number of cigarettes smoked per person per day, females: some selected Spanish surveys by age, 1968-1995, with percentage total sales

<table>
<tr><th rowspan="2">Product
Source
Year</th><th colspan="22">Age group</th><th rowspan="2">All ages</th><th rowspan="2">% Total sales</th></tr>
<tr><th>12</th><th>13</th><th>14</th><th>15</th><th>16</th><th>17</th><th>18</th><th>19</th><th>20-24</th><th>25-29</th><th>30-34</th><th>35-39</th><th>40-44</th><th>45-49</th><th>50-54</th><th>55-59</th><th>60-64</th><th>65-69</th><th>70-74</th><th>75-79</th><th>80+</th></tr>
<tr><td>68 4 UC</td><td colspan="22"></td><td></td><td>**</td></tr>
<tr><td>78 3 UC *</td><td colspan="2"></td><td colspan="2">0.4</td><td colspan="4">5.3</td><td>6.3</td><td colspan="5">2.1</td><td colspan="3">0.6</td><td colspan="4">0.4</td><td></td><td>104%T</td></tr>
<tr><td>87 6 UC *</td><td colspan="11"></td><td colspan="6">6.0</td><td colspan="4"></td><td></td><td>**</td></tr>
<tr><td>87 7 UC</td><td colspan="8"></td><td colspan="9">3.3</td><td colspan="4"></td><td></td><td>**</td></tr>
<tr><td>89 11 UC</td><td colspan="11"></td><td colspan="2">2.9</td><td colspan="2">0.1</td><td colspan="2">0.4</td><td colspan="4"></td><td>1.4</td><td>**</td></tr>
<tr><td>89 12 UC</td><td colspan="11"></td><td colspan="2">4.8</td><td colspan="2">1.9</td><td colspan="2">0.5</td><td colspan="4"></td><td>2.5</td><td>**</td></tr>
<tr><td>90 19 UC</td><td colspan="8"></td><td colspan="2">5.9</td><td colspan="2">3.4</td><td colspan="2">1.7</td><td colspan="2">0.4</td><td colspan="2">0.1</td><td colspan="3"></td><td>2.4</td><td>84%T</td></tr>
<tr><td>90 20 UC</td><td colspan="4"></td><td colspan="18">2.0</td><td></td><td>79%T</td></tr>
<tr><td>92 21 UC</td><td colspan="2"></td><td colspan="16">4.5</td><td colspan="3"></td><td></td><td>88%T</td></tr>
<tr><td>95 7 UC</td><td colspan="4"></td><td colspan="18">3.0</td><td></td><td>78%T</td></tr>
</table>

Source: see *Notes on sources of survey data*, p. 589
All ages: relevant to ages used and as given in original source
% Total sales: estimated % of total sales of M = manufactured or T = total cigarette consumption implied by the survey, sexes combined
** = cannot be calculated
--- = adjusted by original author
Frequency A = all smokers (including occasional)
R = regular or daily smokers

Product: MC = manufactured cigarettes
TC = total cigarettes (including hand-rolled)
UC = cigarettes (type unspecified)
A = all products
E indicates mean estimated from percentage distribution (see also *Consumption category estimation*, p. xxxiv, and Appendix III, p. 789)
U = unspecified
* = refer to *Notes on sources of survey data*, p. 589

Table 24.7M Number of cigarettes smoked per person per day, sales-adjusted, males: some selected Spanish surveys[1] by age, 1978-1995, with percentage total sales

<table>
<tr><th rowspan="2">Product
Source
Year</th><th colspan="21">Age group</th><th rowspan="2">All ages</th><th rowspan="2">% Total sales</th></tr>
<tr><th>12</th><th>13</th><th>14</th><th>15</th><th>16</th><th>17</th><th>18</th><th>19</th><th>20-24</th><th>25-29</th><th>30-34</th><th>35-39</th><th>40-44</th><th>45-49</th><th>50-54</th><th>55-59</th><th>60-64</th><th>65-69</th><th>70-74</th><th>75-79</th><th>80+</th></tr>
<tr><td>78 3 UC *</td><td colspan="2"></td><td colspan="2">2.6</td><td colspan="4">7.6</td><td>12</td><td colspan="5">13</td><td colspan="3">12</td><td colspan="4">8.0</td><td></td><td>104%T</td></tr>
<tr><td>90 19 UC</td><td colspan="8"></td><td colspan="2">16</td><td colspan="2">15</td><td colspan="2">14</td><td colspan="2">9.2</td><td colspan="2">7.1</td><td colspan="3"></td><td>13</td><td>84%T</td></tr>
<tr><td>90 20 UC</td><td colspan="4"></td><td colspan="17">12</td><td></td><td>79%T</td></tr>
<tr><td>92 21 UC</td><td colspan="2"></td><td colspan="16">9.8</td><td colspan="3"></td><td></td><td>88%T</td></tr>
<tr><td>95 7 UC</td><td colspan="4"></td><td colspan="17">9.1</td><td></td><td>78%T</td></tr>
</table>

Table 24.7F Number of cigarettes smoked per person per day, sales-adjusted, females: some selected Spanish surveys[1] by age, 1978-1995, with percentage total sales

<table>
<tr><th rowspan="2">Product
Source
Year</th><th colspan="21">Age group</th><th rowspan="2">All ages</th><th rowspan="2">% Total sales</th></tr>
<tr><th>12</th><th>13</th><th>14</th><th>15</th><th>16</th><th>17</th><th>18</th><th>19</th><th>20-24</th><th>25-29</th><th>30-34</th><th>35-39</th><th>40-44</th><th>45-49</th><th>50-54</th><th>55-59</th><th>60-64</th><th>65-69</th><th>70-74</th><th>75-79</th><th>80+</th></tr>
<tr><td>78 3 UC *</td><td colspan="2"></td><td colspan="2">0.4</td><td colspan="4">5.1</td><td>6.0</td><td colspan="5">2.0</td><td colspan="3">0.6</td><td colspan="4">0.4</td><td></td><td>104%T</td></tr>
<tr><td>90 19 UC</td><td colspan="8"></td><td colspan="2">7.0</td><td colspan="2">4.0</td><td colspan="2">2.0</td><td colspan="2">0.5</td><td colspan="2">0.1</td><td colspan="3"></td><td>2.8</td><td>84%T</td></tr>
<tr><td>90 20 UC</td><td colspan="4"></td><td colspan="17">2.5</td><td></td><td>79%T</td></tr>
<tr><td>92 21 UC</td><td colspan="2"></td><td colspan="16">5.1</td><td colspan="3"></td><td></td><td>88%T</td></tr>
<tr><td>95 7 UC</td><td colspan="4"></td><td colspan="17">3.9</td><td></td><td>78%T</td></tr>
</table>

1 Based on those surveys in Table 24.6 with data for both sexes and age range at least 21-64 (see *Cigarette consumption per person*, p. xxxv)

Source: See *Notes on sources of survey data*, p. 589

Product:
MC = manufactured cigarettes
TC = total cigarettes (including hand-rolled)
UC = cigarettes (type unspecified)
A = all products
U = unspecified

All ages: relevant to ages used and as given in original source

% Total sales: Adjustment factor used, estimated % of total sales of M = manufactured or T = total cigarette consumption implied by survey, sexes combined
--- = adjusted by original author

* = refer to *Notes on sources of survey data*, p. 589

Table 24.8 Estimated[1] prevalence of smoking and estimated[1] number of cigarettes per person per day (unadjusted and sales-adjusted): summary of Tables 24.4, 24.6 and 24.7, 1970-1995.
Males and females aged 15 years and over

Year	Source[2]	Product[3]	Prevalence[4]						Number of cigarettes						
									Unadjusted[7]			Sales-adjusted[8]			
			Manufactured cigarettes		Total cigarettes[5]		All products[6]		Number/ person/day		Total sales %	Manufactured cigarettes number/ person/day		Total cigarettes[9] number/ person/day	
			M	F	M	F	M	F	M	F		M	F	M	F
1970	1	*U*					65	10							
1978	3	*UC*			54	15			11.7	2.2	104			11.3	2.1
	15	*U*					64	16							
1982	2	**A**					57	21							
1983	18	**A**					55	24							
1985	5	*U*					59	20							
1986	2	**A**					56	23							
	14	U					54	22							
	19	*U*					50	20							
1987	7	UC+**A**			51	22	54	22						(11.0	3.8)
	13	UC			30	6								(12.8	2.1)
1989	7	*U*					54	23							
	14	U					52	21							
	19	*U*					53	25							
1990	2	**A**					49	21							
	19	*UC*			54	23			9.9	2.5	84			11.7	3.0
	20	UC+**A**					52	18	9.7	2.0	79			12.2	2.5
1992	18	**A**					47	28							
	21	UC+A					46	29	8.4	4.0	88			9.5	4.5
	21	**A**					54	35							
1993	7	A					44	20							
	7	*U*					51	21							
1994	2	A					41	20							
	2	**A**					44	22							
1995	7	UC+A					43	24	7.1	3.0	78			9.0	3.9
	7	**A**					47	27							

1 Surveys covering an age range of at least 21-64 are included. Any gaps in the data for ages 15-20 and 65 years and over are filled in by assumed extensions to the age distribution, given in *Notes on sources of survey data*, p. 589. Method: see *Summary of adult smoking*, p. xxxvi
2 See *Notes on sources of survey data*, p. 589
3 Product: MC = manufactured cigarettes, TC = total cigarettes (including hand-rolled), UC = cigarettes (type unspecified), A = all products, U = unspecified. Frequency of smoking is indicated by: regular or daily smokers in normal type, all smokers (including occasional) in bold, unspecified in italics
4 From Table 24.4
5 This column includes prevalence of smoking classified as UC = cigarettes (type unspecified)
6 This column includes prevalence of smoking classified as U = unspecified product
7 From Table 24.6
8 From Table 24.7, except data in parentheses, which are derived from the prevalence of smoking from Table 24.4 as described in *Summary of adult smoking*, p. xxxvi
9 Number of cigarettes classified as UC = cigarettes (type unspecified) has been adjusted to total cigarette sales and included in this column

Figure 24.3 Estimated prevalence of smoking of (i) cigarettes and (ii) all tobacco products: by year of survey, 1970-1995.
Males and females aged 15 years and over. *Source:* see Table 24.8

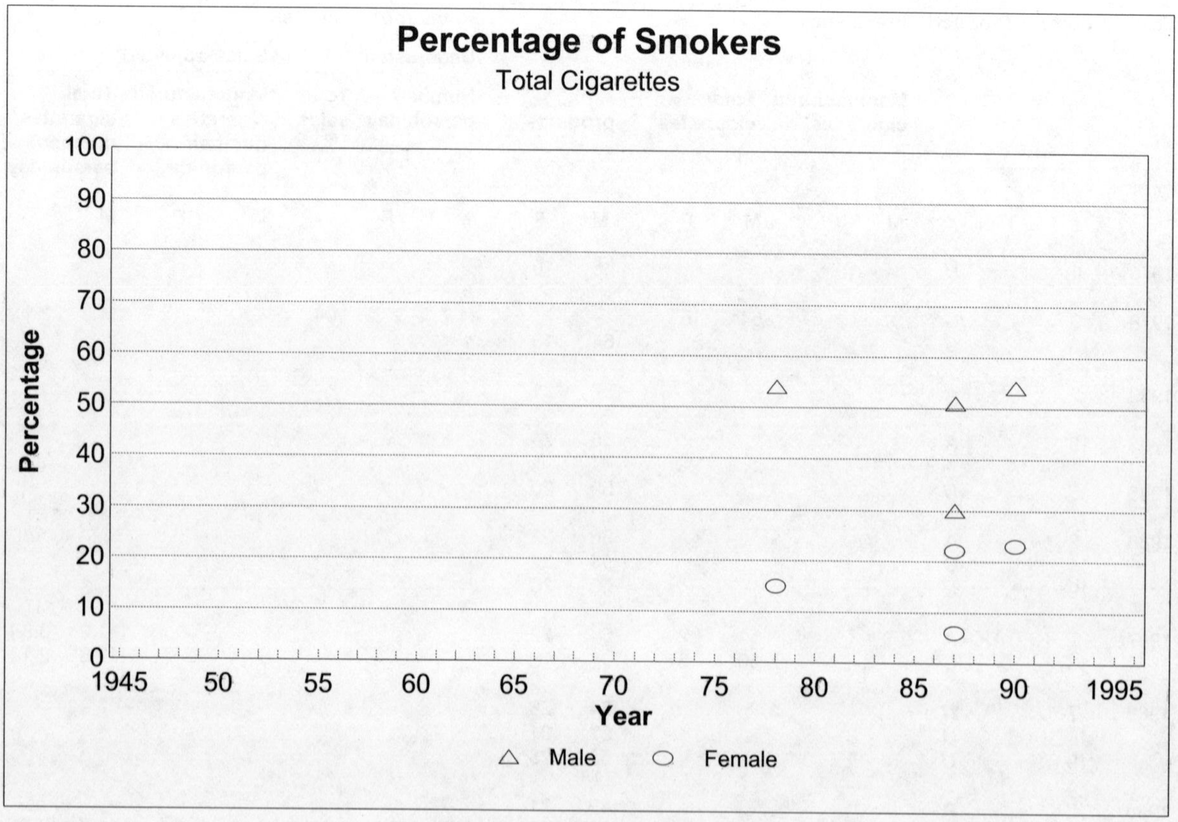

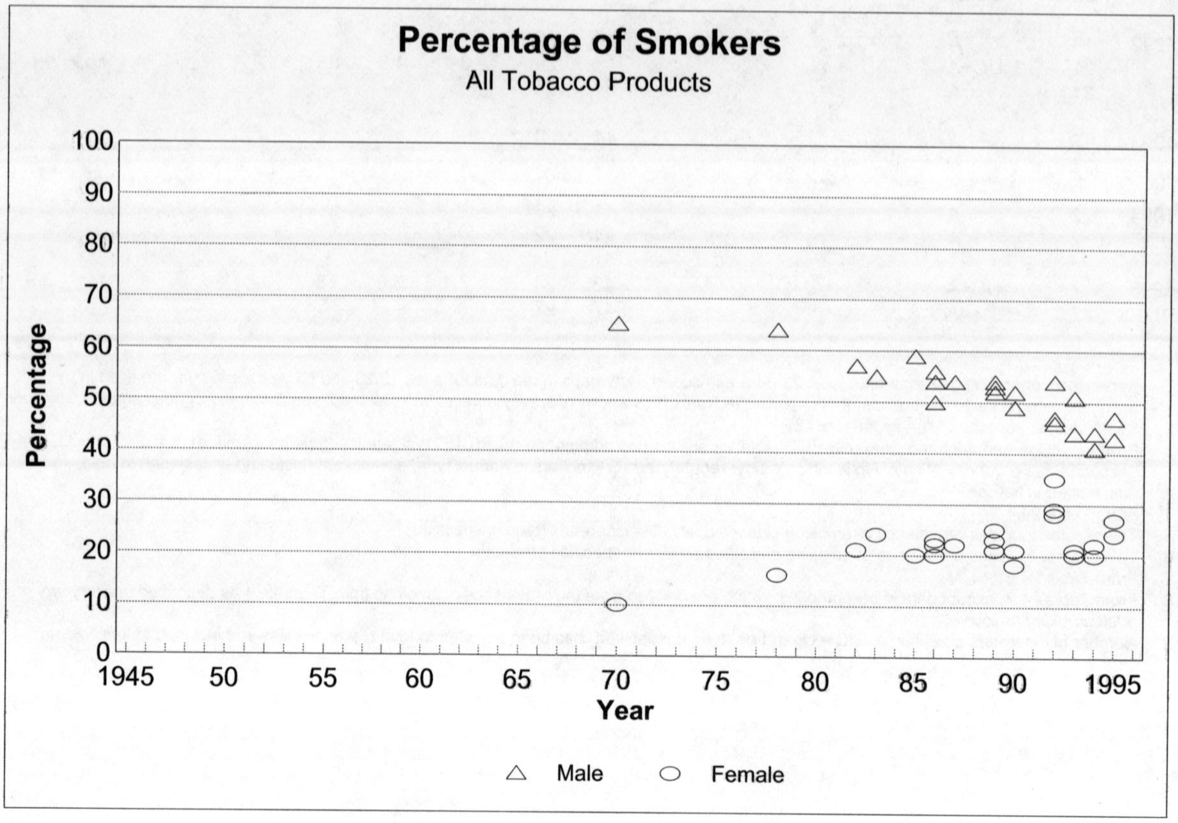

Figure 24.4 Estimated number of cigarettes smoked per person per day, sales-adjusted, 1978-1995.
Males and females aged 15 years and over. *Source:* see Table 24.8

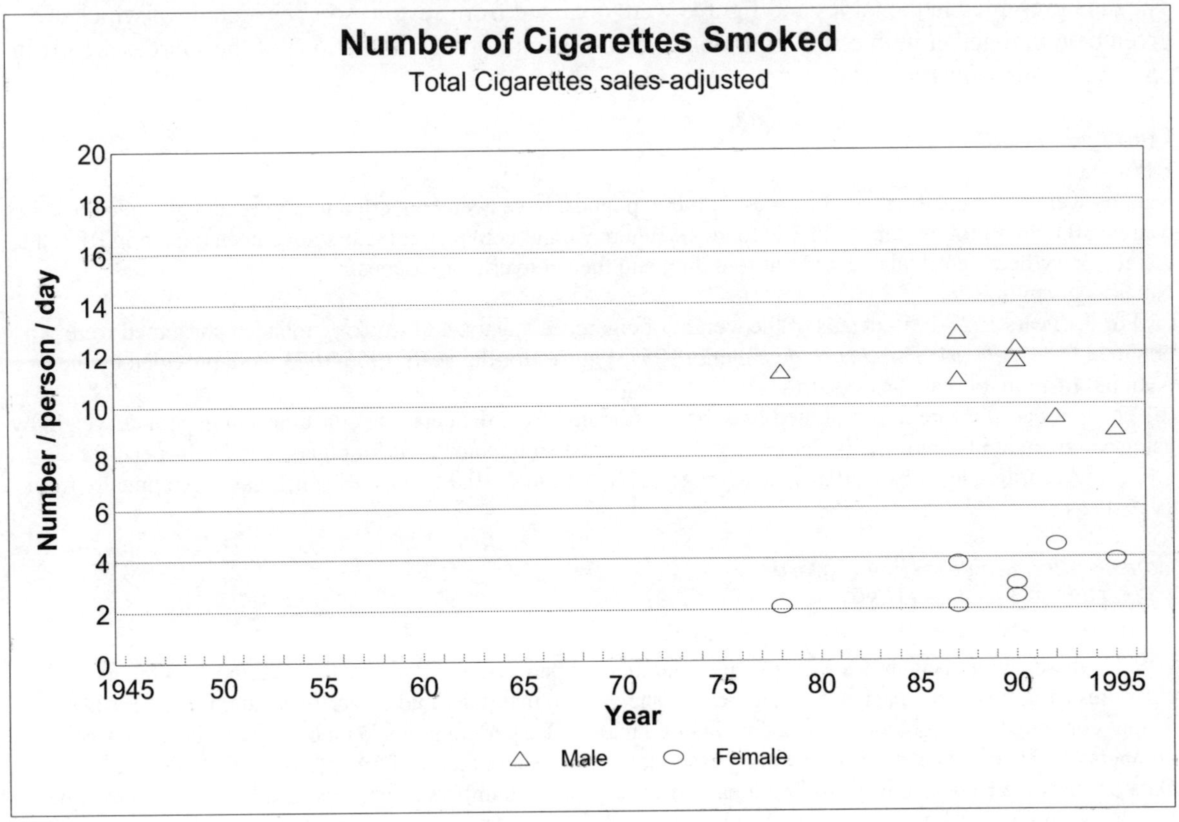

Notes

Notes on sources of sales data

The data presented in the tables and figures were obtained from several sources, details of which are given below, together with estimations and related assumptions. Full citations of the sources are given on p. 592 under *References*.

Consumption data before 1974
RP6

Data by weight, originally given to nearest 100 000 pounds, have been converted to tonnes and given to the nearest 10 tonnes (100 000 lbs = 45.359 tonnes). Where weight conversion factors have been quoted in RP6, the weights have been re-calculated without rounding and then converted to tonnes.

Notes as given in RP6:

(a) For the years 1927-1955 details of the weight of cigarettes, cigars, and smoking tobacco consumed were obtained from *Annuario Estadistico de Espana*, 1957. Figures for the years 1956-1973 were provided by the National Institute of Statistics, Madrid.

(b) The number of cigarettes consumed have been estimated from the cigarette consumption in pounds weight by using a conversion factor of 2.205 lbs per 1 000. The conversion factor used for cigars was 15 lbs per 1 000.

According to Hutson (1937), an average of 2 000 pounds (0.9 tonnes) of snuff was used annually from 1926-1934

Consumption data for 1974 onwards
1974-1988 Tabacalera (1989)
1989-1995 Tabacalera (1999), Crescenti (1994)

Data for manufactured cigarettes were given as numbers of packets, and have been converted to numbers of cigarettes assuming that 1 packet = 20 cigarettes. The data on manufactured cigarette consumption have been further converted to weight assuming a conversion factor of 1 g per cigarette. Data on cigars were given as numbers and have been converted to weight assuming a conversion factor of 6.8 g (based on values used in RP6). Data on Picadura (pipe and hand-rolling tobacco) were given as numbers of packets, and have been converted to weight assuming that 1 packet = 25 g. Data for pipe and fine-cut tobacco separately are available only for 1993: pipe 97 tonnes, fine-cut 321 tonnes (Crescenti (1994)).

Note that comparison between data from RP6 and Tabacalera (1989) in the overlapping years 1957-1973 suggests an average weight of about 23 g per packet of smoking tobacco up to 1970 and 25 g thereafter. There are minor discrepancies between the two sources for the other products—data for 1965 from Tabacalera (1989) are shown in Table 24.1.2 (for comparison with Table 24.1.1) as an example.

Recent assessments of cigarette smuggling suggest that about 10% of the market (Joossens *et al* (1994)) or about 10 000 million cigarettes a year (Barford (1994)) were being smuggled in the years before 1994. Effective anti-smuggling measures were introduced at the end of 1993. 1994 cigarette sales figures were also affected by buying in advance of price increases in January 1995 (Crescenti (1995)).

Plain/Filter cigarette consumption
Maxwell (successive years)

Tar yield of cigarettes

The tar yield per cigarette was limited by EC directive (Directive 90/239/EEC) to 15 mg by the end of 1992, and to 12 mg by the end of 1997; nicotine yield is limited to 1.3 mg (Harkin *et al* (1997)).

Estimates of hand-rolled cigarette consumption

We have estimated hand-rolled cigarette consumption as all Picadura sales, assuming 1g per cigarette. This follows Tabacalera (1989) where Picadura sales are shown in a table headed 'cigarillos negros' (dark cigarettes). However, these estimates may be too high as they ignore usage in pipe, e.g. 23% of Picadura sales were pipe tobacco in 1993 (Crescenti (1994)).

Notes on sources of survey data

Each source of survey data—either an individual survey or a series of surveys repeated over a number of years—is cited by a source number. This number is shown in the tables and corresponds to the source numbers given below, where details of the source publication and of the survey methodology are given. Full citations of the sources are given on p. 592 under *References*.

Source number

1 **WHO (1975)**

a. Age and year not stated

b. Assumed extension to age distribution for percentage smokers, age 15: males 20% and females 10%

2 **Salto *et al* (1993), Pardell *et al* (1997), Fernandez *et al* (1999)**

a. Series of surveys for the Departamento de Sanidad y Seguridad Social de la Generalitat de Cataluña. Cross-sectional representative surveys of the non-institutionalized adult population of Cataluña (Catalonia). The 1994 survey formed part of the Catalan Health Interview Survey.

Year	Sample size			Response rate (%)
	Total	Males	Females	
1982	1 487	695	791	93
1986	1 500			94
1990	1 556			97
1994	9 941			95

b. Assumed extension to age distribution for percentage smokers, age 65+ (1982, 1986 only): males 40% and females 5%

3 **Vioque and Bolumar (1987)**

a. Sample-based survey by National Institute for Statistics. Lowest age group 6-13. High level of non-response for cigarettes/smoker/day at ages <15 and 65+

b. Consumption category estimation based on two categories, 0-20 (assumed 1-19) and 20+ cigarettes/smoker/day, and resulting figures should be regarded with caution. Alternative allocation of smokers of 20 cigarettes/day could have a large effect

4 **Tomás-Abadal *et al* (1994)**

a. Survey of healthy male workers in a factory in Manresa, Catalonia. Sample size 1 059

5 **Adriaanse *et al* (1986), quoting WHO (1985)**

a. Age group not stated

6 **WHO (1989), WHO MONICA Project (1988)**

a. Regional survey forming part of WHO MONICA Project:

Region	Population size	Sample size	Participation rate (%)	Sample used*		Date
				Males	Females	
Catalonia	367 300	2 629	76	1 276	1 293	Apr 1986-July 1988

* 'Sample used' includes age 25-34; all other figures are for age 35-64 only

b. *All ages* column relates only to age 35-64 and is standardized to world population

c. Regular smokers: smoked cigarettes daily. All smokers: smoked cigarettes daily or occasionally, or 1 g pipe tobacco or 1 cigar per week. Cigarettes per smoker refers to regular and occasional cigarette smokers

d. Calculation for cigarettes per person based on % regular cigarette smokers and cigarettes per regular or occasional cigarette smoker, so may underestimate

7 De Onis and Villar (1991), Cordoba Garcia *et al* (1992), Joossens *et al* (1994), Gutiérrez-Fisac and Artalejo (1995), Ministerio de Sanidad y Consumo (1996, 2000), Statistika Centralbyrån (1995)

a. Encuesta Nacional de Salud de España (ENSE). Nationwide representative sample.

Year	Sample size		Response
	Males	Females	rate (%)
1987	13 311	14 445	90
1989	4 136		—
1993	21 120		99
1995	3 136	3 344	—

b. Smokers: smoked habitually, any quantity. Regular smoker: smoked daily

c. For 1987, consumption category estimation based on 1-9, 10-19 and 20+ cigarettes/smoker/day. The first of these categories may include those who smoke less than one cigarette per day as there is no category reported for those smoking occasionally. This would mean that our estimates of cigarettes per smoker and per person are slightly higher than they should be

d. For 1995, consumption category estimation based on 1-10, 11-20, 21-40 and 41+ cigarettes/smoker/day

e. Assumed extension to age distribution for percentage smokers, age 15: males 20%; females (1987, 1989) 15%, (1993) 20%, (1995) 25%. Number of cigarettes/person/day (1995 only): males and females 2.0

8 Nutbeam and Aarø (1990), King and Coles (1992), King *et al* (1996), Mendoza Berjano *et al* (1998)

a. Part of the HBSC (Health Behaviour in School-Aged Children) Study, a collaborative cross-national research study sponsored by the WHO. School classes or schools were randomly selected, targeting age groups 11 (not presented here), 13 and 15. The target sample size was 1 300 in each age group. The 1994 survey also included 17- and 18-year-olds, for whom schooling is not compulsory. Sample sizes, 1986-1987: (boys) 619, (girls) 554; 1990: 3 372; 1994:

Target age	Sample size
13	1 576
15	1 487
17	1 405
18	726

For 1990 and 1994, the mean ages of the samples were:

Target age	Mean age	
	1990	1994
13	13.8	13.5
15	15.8	15.6

b. Smokers marked as frequency *: smoked daily. Regular smokers: smoke once a week or more

9 van Reek *et al* (1992), van Reek and Adriaanse (1995)

a. A series of surveys of Young Europeans. About 800 children aged 11-15 years interviewed in each EC country except Luxembourg (where only 250 interviewed). Lowest age group 11-12. Interviews conducted at home, with parents absent

b. Regular smokers: smoked daily. All smokers: smoked at least once a week

10 Comín Beltran *et al* (1989), Aubà and Villalbí (1993), Ariza i Cardenal and Nebot i Adell (1995), Villalbi *et al* (1999)

a. Surveys for the Institut Municipal de la Salut de Barcelona using representative samples of schoolchildren in the city. Approximately age groups corresponding to school year groups, except 1992 when data by age are presented.

Year	Sample size	Response rate (%)
1987	1 113	94
1990	1 011	92
1992	2 140	85
1994	840	99

b. Smokers marked as frequency *: smoked daily. Regular smokers: smoked each week. Smokers: smoked habitually

11-12 Banegas *et al* (1993)

a. A nationwide cross-sectional study of cardiovascular risk factors. Sample size 2 021. Participation rate 73%. Results shown as **11** represent the rural population, those shown as **12** the urban population

b. Smokers: includes those who had given up less than six months before interview and those who smoked occasionally, including special occasion only smokers

c. Consumption category estimation based on 1-9, 10-19 and 20+ cigarettes/smoker/day

13 Regidor and Gutiérrez-Fisac (1999)

a. Evaluations in Spain of Health Indicators for the WHO European Region Health for All Programme. Implemented as National Health Survey by the Ministerio de Sanidad y Consumo

b. Assumed extension to age distribution for percentage smokers, age 15: males 20% and females 15%

14 Organisation for Economic Co-operation and Development (1993)

a. No original source

15 Joossens *et al* (1994) quoting the Spanish Ministry of Health

a. Assumed extension to age distribution for percentage smokers, age 15: males 20% and females 10%

16-17 Berrino *et al* (1988)

a. International study of smoking habits as part of a project on the etiology of laryngeal cancer. Surveys carried out between 1978 and 1984 (shown against 1981 in Table 24.4). Upper age limit 85.

	Region	Sample size	
		Males	**Females**
16	Zaragoza	341	362
17	Navarra	525	135

b. Regular smokers: smoked more than a gram of tobacco per day for at least the last six months

18 Nebot *et al* (1996)

a. Encuesta de Salud de Barcelona. Sample size: (1983) 3 134, (1992) 5 004

b. Smokers: smoked any amount of cigarettes, cigars or pipes at the time of the interview

19 Cordoba Garcia *et al* (1992)

a. Various cross-sectional surveys of the adult population of Aragon. Sample sizes (1986) 1 800, (1989) 906, (1990) 2 781

b. Consumption category estimation based on 1-9, 10-19 and 20+ cigarettes/smoker/day

c. Assumed extension to age distribution for percentage smokers, age 15 (1986, 1989): males 20% and females 15%. For age 15-19 (1990): males 35% and females 30%. For age 70+ (1990): males 35% and females 0.5%. Number of cigarettes/person/day, age 15-19 (1990): males 8.0 and females 5.0. For age 70+ (1990): males 3.0 and females 0.1

20 Bueno Cavanillas *et al* (1993)

a. Survey of the province of Granada. Sample size 1 537 adults

b. Assumed extension to age distribution for percentage smokers, age 15: males and females 20%. Number of cigarettes/person/day: males and females 2.0

21 del Río and Alvarez (1994)

a. Survey representative of the population of the region of Castille and Leon. Sample size 2 500

b. Assumed extension to age distribution for percentage smokers, age 71+: males (regular) 25%, (all) 30%; females (regular) 3%, (all) 5%. Number of cigarettes/person/day: males 3.0 and females 0.1

22 Segura *et al* (2000)

a. Survey representative of school pupils in Gran Canaria. Year not stated. Sample size 1 369, response rate 99%

References

Adriaanse H., van Reek J. and van Zutphen W.M. (1986). Rookgewoonten van atrsen wereldwijd; een overzicht van 100 onderzoekinge naar tabaksgebruik onder artsen in 31 landen in de periode 1951-1985 (Worldwide physicians' smoking habits; a review of 100 surveys into physicians' tobacco consumption in 31 countries in the period 1951-1985. *Ned Tijdschr Geneeskd,* **130**, 2224-9.

Ariza i Cardenal C. and Nebot i Adell M. (1995). Factores asociados al consumo de tabaco en una muestra de escolares de enseñanza primaria y secundaria (Associated factors to smoking in a sample of schoolchildren at primary and secondary levels). *Gac Sanit,* **9**, 101-9.

Aubà J. and Villalbí J.R. (1993). Tabaco y adolescentes: influencia del entorno personal (Smoking and teens: influence of the personal environment). *Med Clin,* **100**, 506-9.

Banegas J.R.B., Villar F.V., Pérez de Andrés C., García-Pascual R.J., *et al* (1993). Estudio epidemiológico de los factores de riesgo cardiovascular en la población española de 35 a 64 años. (Epidemiological study on cardiovascular risk factors in 35-64 years old population in Spain). *Rev Sanid Hig Publica,* **67**, 419-45.

Barford M.F. (1994). Targeting the cigarette smugglers. *Tobacco Journal International,* **5**, 54-6.

Beese D.H. (ed) (1968). *Tobacco consumption in various countries,* 2nd edition. Tobacco Research Council, London. Research Paper 6.

Beese D.H. (ed) (1972). *Tobacco consumption in various countries,* 3rd edition. Tobacco Research Council, London. Research Paper 6.

Berrino F., Merletti F., Zubiri A., Del Moral A., *et al* (1988). A comparative study of smoking, drinking and dietary habits in population samples in France, Italy, Spain and Switzerland. II. Tobacco smoking. *Rev Epidemiol Sante Publique,* **36**, 166-76.

Bueno Cavanillas A., Ramos Cuadra A.M., Rodríguez Tapioles R., Pérez Huertas M.A. and Gálvez Vargas R. (1993). Hábito tabáquico de la población de la provincia de Granada (The tobacco habit of the population of the province of Granada). *Gac Sanit,* **7**, 221-7.

Comín Beltran E., Nebot Adell M. and Villalbi Hereter J.R. (1989). Exercici i consum de tabac i alcohol dels escolars de Barcelona (Physical exercise and tobacco and alcohol consumption of the schoolchildren in Barcelona). *Gac Sanit,* **3**, 355-65.

Cordoba Garcia R., Sanz Andres C., Martinez Rodes P., Martinez-Berganza Asensio A. and Cia Gomez P. (1992). Estudio del hábito tabáquico en población adulta aragonesa (Study of smoking habit among the adult population of Aragon). *An Med Interna,* **9**, 433-8.

Crescenti M.G. (1994). The new face of Europe. *Tobacco Journal International,* **5**, 81-7.

Crescenti M.G. (1995). Setback for smugglers gives room for optimism in Spain. *Tobacco Journal International,* **3**, 30-34.

De Onis M. and Villar J. (1991). La consommation de tabac chez la femme espagnole. *World Health Stat Q,* **44**, 80-8.

del Río M.C. and Alvarez F.J. (1994). Patterns of smoking in Spain. Results from a regional general population survey. *Eur J Epidemiol,* **10**, 595-8.

Fernandez E., Schiaffino A., La Vecchia C., Borràs J.M., *et al* (1999). Age at starting smoking and number of cigarettes smoked in Catalonia, Spain. *Prev Med,* **28**, 361-6.

Gutiérrez-Fisac J.L. and Artalejo F.R. (1995). Relación entre obesidad, hábito tabáquico y actividad física en el tiempo libre en la población española de 20 a 64 años (The relationship between obesity, smoking habit and physical activity during leisure time in the 20 to 64-year-old Spanish population). *Med Clin,* **104**, 293-7.

Harkin A.M., Anderson P. and Goos C. (1997). *Smoking, drinking and drug taking in the European Region.* Alcohol, Drugs and Tobacco Programme, WHO Regional Office for Europe, Copenhagen.

Hutson J.B. (1937). *Consumption and production of tobacco in Europe.* USDA, Washington DC. Technical bulletin No. 587.

Joossens L., Naett C., Howie C. and Muldoon A. (1994). *Tobacco and health in the European Union. An overview.* European Bureau for Action on Smoking Prevention (BASP), Brussels.

King A., Wold B., Tudor-Smith C. and Harel Y. (1996). *The health of youth, a cross-national survey.* WHO Regional Publications, Europe, Copenhagen. European Series No. 69.

King A.J.C. and Coles B. (1992). *The health of Canada's youth. Views and behaviours of 11-, 13- and 15-year-olds from 11 countries.* Health and Welfare Canada, Ottawa.

Lee P.N. (ed) (1975). *Tobacco consumption in various countries,* 4th edition. Tobacco Research Council, London. Research Paper 6.

Maxwell J.C.Jr. (successive years). How the brands ranked. Maxwell International Estimates. *World Tobacco.*

Mendoza Berjano R., Batista Foguet J.M., Sanchez Garcia M. and Carrasco Gonzalez A.M. (1998). El consumo de tabaco, alcohol y otras drogas en los adolescentes escolarizados españoles (The consumptio of tobacco, alcohol and other drugs by adolescent Spanish students). *Gac Sanit,* **12**, 263-71.

Ministerio de Sanidad y Consumo (1996). *Encuesta nacional de salud de España 1995.* Centro de publicaciones, Madrid.

Ministerio de Sanidad y Consumo (2000). *Encuesta nacional de salud de España.* http://www.msc.es/.

Nebot M., Borrell C., Ballestín M. and Villalbí J.R. (1996). Prevalencia y caracteristícas asociadas al consumo de tabaco en población general en Barcelona entre 1983 y 1992 (Prevalence and features associated with smoking in the general population in Barcelona from 1983 to 1992). *Rev Clin Esp,* **196**, 359-64.

Nutbeam D. and Aarø L.E. (1990). Smoking and alienation from school: the implications for health education with young people. Results from the WHO study of health behaviour in schoolchildren. In: Durston B. and Jamrozik K. (eds) *Tobacco & health 1990. The global war. Seventh World Conference on Tobacco and Health, Perth, Western Australia, 1-5 April 1990.* Organising Committee of the Seventh World Conference on Tobacco and Health, 189 Royal Street, East Perth, Western Australia 6004; 539-44.

Organisation for Economic Co-operation and Development (1993). *OECD health systems. Facts and trends 1960-1991. Health policy studies no 3.* OECD, Paris. (Health policy studies, Volume 1.)

Pardell H., Saltó E., Tresserras R., Juncà S., *et al* (1997). La evoluciân del hábito tabáquico en Cataluña. (Smoking prevalence trends in Catalonia (Spain), 1982-1994). *Med Clin,* **109**, 125-9.

Regidor E. and Gutiérrez-Fisac J.L. (1999). *Health indicators. Fourth evaluation in Spain of the European regional health for all programme.* Ministerio de Sanidad y Consumo, Madrid.

RP6, See Beese (ed) (1968), Beese (ed) (1972), Lee (ed) (1975)

Salto E., Plans P., Fuentes M., Pardell H. and Salleras L. (1993). Epidemiología del hábito tabáquico entre los escolares y jóvenes de Cataluña (Smoking epidemiology among students and youngsters in Catalonia). *Anales Espanoles de Pediatria,* **39 Suppl 55**, 146-8.

Segura J.M., Calvo J.R., Navarro M.C., Torres M., *et al* (2000). Tobacco use among adolescents aged 10-16 in Gran Canaria, Canary Islands, Spain. In: Lu R., Mackay J., Niu S. and Peto R. (eds) *Tobacco: The Growing Epidemic. Proceedings of the Tenth World Conference on Tobacco or Health, 24-28 August 1997, Beijing,*

China. Springer-Verlag, London; 263-4.

Statistika Centralbyrån (1995). *Tobacco consumption 1970-1994 in the member states of the European Union and in Norway and Iceland*. European Commission.

Tabacalera (1989). *Series historicas de consumo de tabaco elaborado, 1957-1988*. Ediciones Tabapress,S.A., Madrid.

Tabacalera (1999). *Annual report 1998*. Tabapress, S.A., Madrid.

Tomás-Abadal L., Varas-Lorenzo C., Bernades-Bernat E. and Balaguer-Vintró I. (1994). Coronary risk factors and a 20-year incidence of coronary heart disease and mortality in a Mediterranean industrial population. The Manresa study, Spain. *Eur Heart J,* **15**, 1028-36.

van Reek J. and Adriaanse H. (1995). Daily smoking among adolescents in the European Community. *Rev Epidemiol Sante Publique,* **43**, 281-2.

van Reek J., Adriaanse H. and Karaoglou A. (1992). Smoking among children in the European Community. *J Public Health Med,* **14**, 93-4.

Villalbi J.R., Barniol J., Nebot M., Diez E. and Ballestin M. (1999). Tendencias en el tabaquismo de los escolares: Barcelona, 1987-1996 (Trends in smoking among school children: Barcelona, 1978-1996). *Aten Primaria,* **23**, 359-62.

Vioque J. and Bolumar F. (1987). Trends in mortality from lung cancer in Spain, 1951-80. *J Epidemiol Community Health,* **41**, 74-8.

WHO (1989). The WHO MONICA project: a worldwide monitoring system for cardiovascular diseases. In: *World health statistics annual 1989*. WHO, Geneva; 25-149.

WHO MONICA Project (1988). Geographical variation in the major risk factors of coronary heart disease in men and women aged 35-64 years. *World Health Stat Q,* **41**, 115-40.

WHO (1985). Smoking survey among health professionals in Catalunya 1985. *Paper presented at WHO Meeting Southern European Action on Smoking, Barcelona.* WHO/Euro and Dept Sanitat i Seg Soc. §

WHO (1975). Survey on smoking and health in the European Region, 1974-75: preliminary data as at 1 May 1975. *Presented at the Third World Conference on Smoking and Health, New York, 2-5 June 1975*. WHO.

§ Original paper not obtained, but information taken as quoted by another author

Sweden 25

Sales data

See Tables 25.1-25.3.

From 1920 until 1945 the consumption of manufactured cigarettes per adult was about 1 cigarette per day. Consumption rose steadily until the mid-1970s when it levelled at 5 cigarettes per day. It then fell to 3 cigarettes per day. Between 1950 and 1980, our estimates for hand-rolled cigarettes suggest that consumption, always much lower than that of manufactured cigarettes, was about 0.2 to 0.3 cigarettes per adult per day; there may have been some rise in consumption in the 1980s, but this is uncertain as cross-border sales of hand-rolling tobacco to Norway were high at that period.

Smokeless tobacco has been used orally in Sweden for centuries. Snuff manufacturing in Sweden started in the early 18th century. Initially it was inhaled through the nose. The practice known as 'snuff dipping' was widespread in Sweden in the late 19th century. The snuff consists of very finely ground tobacco with high (about 50%) moisture content, of which a 'pinch' is placed between the cheek and the gum (Ramström (1990)). Around 1980 portion-bag-packed snuff was introduced on the Swedish market (Axéll (1993)). In 1920 the consumption of snuff per adult was about 4 g per day. Consumption fell to 1 g per day about 1970, then increased to 2 g per day by 1995.

The consumption of all tobacco products per adult was about 4.5 g per day before the Second World War and thereafter about 5.5 g per day. In the 1920s, the largest proportion of tobacco was used for snuff, while consumption of manufactured cigarettes accounted for only 8%. The proportion of manufactured cigarettes increased to over 60% in the 1960s and 1970s, but decreased again to 44% in 1995. The proportion of tobacco used as snuff correspondingly decreased to below 20%, then increased in recent decades, to 45% in 1995. Since the 1950s, the proportion used as pipe and hand-rolling tobacco has been slowly decreasing, to below 10% since the late 1970s. Consumption of cigars and cigarillos declined from 8% in 1925 to 1% in 1995.

Survey data

See Tables 25.4-25.8

In the late nineteenth century, smoking was largely restricted to men. Smoking by women was generally considered immoral, but was permitted for independent women (Haglund (1988), Hyllienmark (1983)).

In 1946, the prevalence of tobacco smoking among those aged 15 years and over was 50% in men and about 10% in women. Survey data are available annually from industry sources (sources 1 and 2) from 1969, but a discrepancy in the age range covered by the two sources leads to an apparent difference in prevalence for females (aged 15 years and over) of about 5% in Table 25.8; for males, one cannot distinguish how much of the difference of 15-20% is due to this discrepancy and how much to the difference in prevalence between cigarette smokers and smokers of all products. Since 1977, survey data are also available from Statistics Sweden (source 8).

The prevalence of cigarette smoking among men fell from about 40% in the late 1960s to 23% in the late-1980s. Over the same period the additional percentage smoking other products probably fell from 15 to 3%, so that the prevalence of smoking fell from about 55% to 26%; it continued to decrease to 22% by 1995. The prevalence among women rose to 30% (source 1) or 35% (source 2) by the mid-1970s, but then fell again to 23% by 1995; virtually no women smoke products other than cigarettes. In the 1990s, the estimated prevalence was similar or slightly higher among women than among men.

Data on adult smoking by age are available since 1963. In that year, more men than women smoked at all ages. Since the 1970s most surveys have shown that considerably more women than men smoked up to about age 30 (or age 40 in the 1990s) and that the prevalence was about equal among those aged 30-50 (or 40-60 in the 1990s); the prevalence continued to be quite low among older women. The prevalence of smoking decreased among young men and young women, but this was more marked for young men.

Comparison between survey and sales data suggests that the survey under-reported consumption by 25-35%. In 1963, the estimated number of cigarettes smoked per person per day (sales-adjusted) was 5 for men and 2.5 for women; from 1969 onwards, it was estimated to be about 6 for men decreasing to 5 by 1987, and about 4 for women.

Table 25.1.1 Total annual sales of tobacco products, 1920-1973

Year	Cigarettes		Cigars		Cigarillos		Smoking tobacco	Chewing tobacco	Snuff	All tobacco products
	tonnes	millions	tonnes	millions	tonnes	millions	tonnes	tonnes	tonnes	
1920	820	1559	540	89	320	118	770	360	6530	9340
1921	730	1345	360	58	320	117	820	320	6080	8620
1922	640	1123	360	62	320	118	910	270	5670	8160
1923	590	1058	230	40	360	120	950	270	5490	7890
1924	640	1089	230	39	360	128	1000	230	5350	7800
1925	640	1085	270	39	410	137	1040	230	5310	7890
1926	680	1204	270	41	410	141	1040	230	5260	7890
1927	730	1284	270	40	410	141	1000	180	5130	7710
1928	860	1446	270	39	410	146	1000	180	4990	7710
1929	950	1640	270	37	450	160	1000	180	4850	7710
1930	1090	1864	230	36	500	174	950	140	4850	7760
1931	1270	1999	230	32	500	171	910	140	4850	7890
1932	1360	2012	180	31	500	171	1000	140	4850	8030
1933	1320	1894	180	29	450	170	1000	140	4760	7850
1934	1500	1878	180	29	450	174	1000	90	4580	7800
1935	1630	1843	180	27	500	179	1000	90	4490	7890
1936	1770	1806	180	26	500	187	1040	90	4400	7980
1937	1910	1822	180	26	500	193	1040	90	4400	8120
1938	2040	1889	140	25	540	196	1090	90	4350	8260
1939	2180	1976	140	23	540	197	1090	90	4260	8300
1940	2400	2126	140	20	450	176	1360	90	3900	8350
1941	2310	2191	140	25	450	204	1540	90	3860	8390
1942	1500	2235	140	24	410	171	1680	50	3400	7170
1943	1680	2237	180	34	360	158	1680	50	3270	7210
1944	2360	2307	180	30	410	160	2000	50	3490	8480
1945	2810	2468	180	28	410	154	1950	50	3490	8890
1946	3720	3141	180	30	410	157	1720	50	3490	9570
1947	4310	3670	180	27	360	146	1540	50	3450	9890
1948	4490	3809	140	26	360	144	1630	50	3360	10020
1949	4670	3984	140	23	320	134	1540	50	3220	9930

Table 25.1.1 *(continued)*

Year	Cigarettes tonnes	Cigarettes millions	Cigars tonnes	Cigars millions	Cigarillos tonnes	Cigarillos millions	Smoking tobacco tonnes	Chewing tobacco tonnes	Snuff tonnes	All tobacco products
1950	4850	4352	140	23	320	133	1500	50	3130	9980
1951	4850	4416	140	20	230	104	1410	50	2900	9570
1952	5530	5121	140	21	270	114	1500	50	2950	10430
1953	5580	5248	140	20	270	115	1500	50	2900	10430
1954	5530	5289	140	23	270	129	1500	50	2900	10390
1955	5760	5548	140	23	270	135	1450	50	2860	10520
1956	5940	5714	140	21	270	130	1360	50	2770	10520
1957	6080	5903	140	21	270	134	1320	50	2720	10570
1958	6210	6066	90	20	270	137	1450	50	2680	10750
1959	6530	6240	90	19	270	142	1500	50	2630	11070
1960	7080	6740	140	21	360	197	1590	50	2680	11880
1961	7530	7216	90	29	360	188	1540	50	2590	12160
1962	7760	7498	90	29	360	195	1540	50	2540	12340
1963	7980	7860	450	223	Included with cigars for 1963 to 1973		1540	0	2540	12520
1964	7940	7810	640	310			1720	0	2540	12840
1965	8160	8300	590	311			1720	0	2490	12970
1966	8620	8700	590	318			1720	0	2490	13430
1967	8350	8927	680	331			1720	0	2400	13150
1968	8620	9679	680	333			1680	0	2360	13340
1969	8660	10147	640	334			1590	0	2400	13290
1970	8350	10269	640	326			1590	0	2490	13060
1971	7760	9957	540	282			1540	0	2630	12470
1972	8710	11243	500	254			1410	0	2680	13290
1973	7080	9265	450	249			1450	0	2720	11700

Source: see *Notes on sources of sales data,* p. 616

Table 25.1.2 Total annual sales of tobacco products, 1974-1995

Year	Cigarettes tonnes	Cigarettes millions	Cigars tonnes	Cigars millions	Pipe and hand-rolling tobacco: Home tonnes	Pipe and hand-rolling tobacco: Cross-border [1] tonnes	Chewing tobacco tonnes	Snuff tonnes	All tobacco products tonnes
1974	7196	11070	474	252	1308	46	15	2812	11805
1975	7587	11673	465	250	1237	50	14	2943	12246
1976	7792	11988	443	241	1184	54	14	3189	12622
1977	7382	11357	378	210	1103	56	15	3361	12239
1978	7623	11727	325	179	1055	64	15	3442	12460
1979	7782	11973	301	167	1019	68	18	3550	12670
1980	7741	11909	280	155	1055	74	18	3665	12759
1981	7464	11483	249	142	1040	84	22	3759	12534
1982	7840	12062	236	138	1113	200	23	3929	13141
1983	7514	11560	200	125	1160	350	24	4029	12927
1984	7476	11502	192	119	1397	350	22	4332	13419
1985	7249	11152	175	111	1400	280	20	4560	13404
1986	7287	11211	169	108	1236	350	19	4673	13384
1987	7219	11106	156	102	1145	336	18	4695	13233
1988	7278	11197	143	94	1101	318	16	4594	13132
1989	7116	10948	150	102	1107	308	15	4606	12994
1990	6899	10614	183	134	1158	237	14	4632	12886
1991	6852	10541	184	139	1155	204	13	4836	13040
1992	7128	10966	174	134	1184	272	13	5007	13506
1993	5670	8723	144	111	1145	160	13	5034	12006
1994	5662	8710	129	100	1130	189	13	5238	12172
1995	5280	8123	117	90	1097	194	12	5407	11913

1 Cross-border sales to Norway. Additional to Home tonnes. Not included in All tobacco products column

Source : see *Notes on sources of sales data,* p. 616

Table 25.1.3 Manufactured cigarettes (i) percentage of total sales as filter cigarettes, 1960-1981, (ii) sales-weighted average tar yield per cigarette (SWAT), 1964-1980, and (iii) sales-weighted average nicotine yield per cigarette (SWAN), 1964-1974

Year	% Filter	SWAT mg / cig	SWAN mg / cig
1960	10.3		
1961	12.8		
1962	17.0		
1963	21.0		
1964	29.0	31.0	1.80
1965		29.0	1.75
1966	48.1	27.0	1.70
1967	54.5	28.0	2.00
1968	62.0	26.0	1.75
1969	67.0	25.0	1.70
1970	70.0	23.0	1.60
1971	74.9	23.0	1.60
1972	77.8	22.0	1.55
1973	80.4	21.0	1.55
1974	82.3	22.0	1.60
1975	82.0	21.4	
1976	85.4	20.8	
1977	87.6	18.7	
1978		17.0	
1979	89.0	15.7	
1980	90.0	15.1	
1981	91.0		

Source : see *Notes on sources of sales data*, p. 616

Table 25.2 Consumption of (i) cigarettes and (ii) all tobacco products, 1920-1995 sales-based data, including estimated hand-rolled cigarette consumption. Males and females aged 15 years and over

Year	Manufactured cigarettes		Hand-rolled cigarettes		Total cigarettes		All tobacco products	
	Total annual in millions	Number/ adult/day	Total annual in millions	Number/ adult/day	Total annual in millions	Number/ adult/day	Total annual in tonnes	Grams/ adult/day
1920	1559	1.0					9340	6.1
1921	1345	0.9					8620	5.6
1922	1123	0.7					8160	5.3
1923	1058	0.7					7890	5.0
1924	1089	0.7					7800	5.0
1925	1085	0.7					7890	4.9
1926	1204	0.7					7890	4.8
1927	1284	0.8					7710	4.7
1928	1446	0.9					7710	4.7
1929	1640	1.0					7710	4.6
1930	1864	1.1					7760	4.6
1931	1999	1.2					7890	4.6
1932	2012	1.2					8030	4.7
1933	1894	1.1					7850	4.5
1934	1878	1.1					7800	4.5
1935	1843	1.0					7890	4.4
1936	1806	1.0					7980	4.5
1937	1822	1.0					8120	4.5
1938	1889	1.0					8260	4.5
1939	1976	1.1					8300	4.5
1940	2126	1.1					8350	4.5
1941	2191	1.2					8390	4.5
1942	2235	1.2					7170	3.9
1943	2237	1.2					7210	3.9
1944	2307	1.2					8480	4.5
1945	2468	1.3					8890	4.7
1946	3141	1.7					9570	5.0
1947	3670	1.9					9890	5.1
1948	3809	2.0					10020	5.2
1949	3984	2.0					9930	5.0

Table 25.2 *(continued)*

Year	Manufactured cigarettes		Hand-rolled cigarettes		Total cigarettes		All tobacco products	
	Total annual in millions	Number/ adult/day	Total annual in millions	Number/ adult/day	Total annual in millions	Number/ adult/day	Total annual in tonnes	Grams/ adult/day
1950	4352	2.2	675	0.3	5027	2.6	9980	5.1
1951	4416	2.2	634	0.3	5050	2.6	9570	4.8
1952	5121	2.6	675	0.3	5796	2.9	10430	5.3
1953	5248	2.6	675	0.3	5923	3.0	10430	5.2
1954	5289	2.6	675	0.3	5964	3.0	10390	5.2
1955	5548	2.7	652	0.3	6200	3.1	10520	5.2
1956	5714	2.8	612	0.3	6326	3.1	10520	5.2
1957	5903	2.9	594	0.3	6497	3.2	10570	5.1
1958	6066	2.9	652	0.3	6718	3.2	10750	5.2
1959	6240	3.0	675	0.3	6915	3.3	11070	5.3
1960	6740	3.2	716	0.3	7456	3.5	11880	5.6
1961	7216	3.4	693	0.3	7909	3.7	12160	5.7
1962	7498	3.5	693	0.3	8191	3.8	12340	5.7
1963	7860	3.6	693	0.3	8553	3.9	12520	5.7
1964	7810	3.5	774	0.4	8584	3.9	12840	5.8
1965	8300	3.7	774	0.3	9074	4.1	12970	5.8
1966	8700	3.9	774	0.3	9474	4.2	13430	6.0
1967	8927	3.9	774	0.3	9701	4.3	13150	5.8
1968	9679	4.2	756	0.3	10435	4.6	13340	5.8
1969	10147	4.4	716	0.3	10862	4.7	13290	5.8
1970	10269	4.4	716	0.3	10984	4.7	13060	5.6
1971	9957	4.3	693	0.3	10650	4.5	12470	5.3
1972	11243	4.8	634	0.3	11878	5.1	13290	5.7
1973	9265	3.9	652	0.3	9918	4.2	11700	5.0
1974	11070	4.7	589	0.2	11659	4.9	11805	5.0
1975	11673	4.9	557	0.2	12230	5.2	12246	5.2
1976	11988	5.0	533	0.2	12521	5.3	12622	5.3
1977	11357	4.7	496	0.2	11853	5.0	12239	5.1
1978	11727	4.9	475	0.2	12202	5.1	12460	5.2
1979	11973	4.9	459	0.2	12432	5.1	12670	5.2
1980	11909	4.9	475	0.2	12384	5.1	12759	5.2
1981	11483	4.7	437	0.2	11920	4.9	12534	5.1
1982	12062	4.9	534	0.2	12596	5.1	13141	5.3
1983	11560	4.7	615	0.2	12175	4.9	12927	5.2
1984	11502	4.6	894	0.4	12396	5.0	13419	5.4
1985	11152	4.5	980	0.4	12132	4.9	13404	5.4
1986	11211	4.5	865	0.3	12076	4.8	13384	5.3
1987	11106	4.4	802	0.3	11908	4.7	13233	5.3
1988	11197	4.4	771	0.3	11968	4.7	13132	5.2
1989	10948	4.3	775	0.3	11723	4.6	12994	5.1
1990	10614	4.1	811	0.3	11425	4.5	12886	5.0
1991	10541	4.1	808	0.3	11350	4.4	13040	5.1
1992	10966	4.2	829	0.3	11795	4.6	13506	5.2
1993	8723	3.4	802	0.3	9524	3.7	12006	4.6
1994	8710	3.3	791	0.3	9501	3.6	12172	4.7
1995	8123	3.1	768	0.3	8891	3.4	11913	4.6

Source : see *Notes on sources of sales data*, p. 616

Figure 25.1 Daily consumption of (i) manufactured and total number of cigarettes, and (ii) all tobacco products, 1920-1995.
Males and females aged 15 years and over. *Source:* see Table 25.2

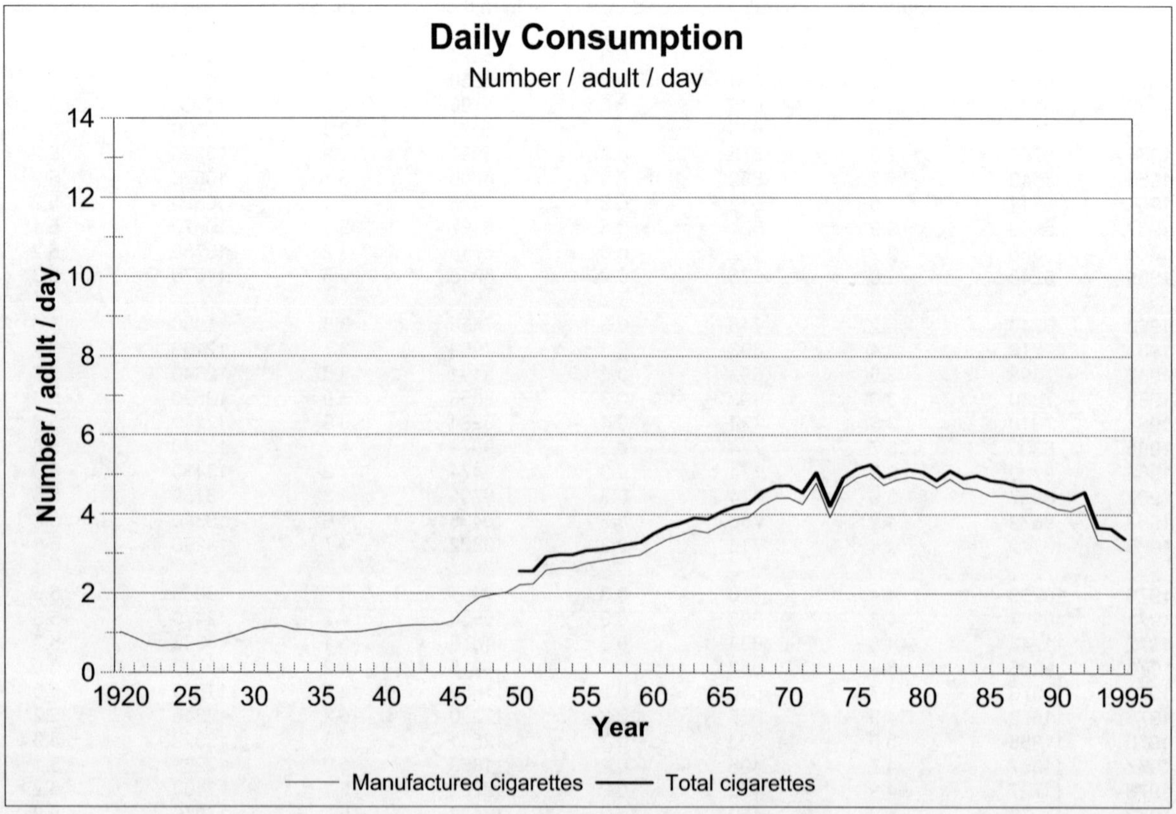

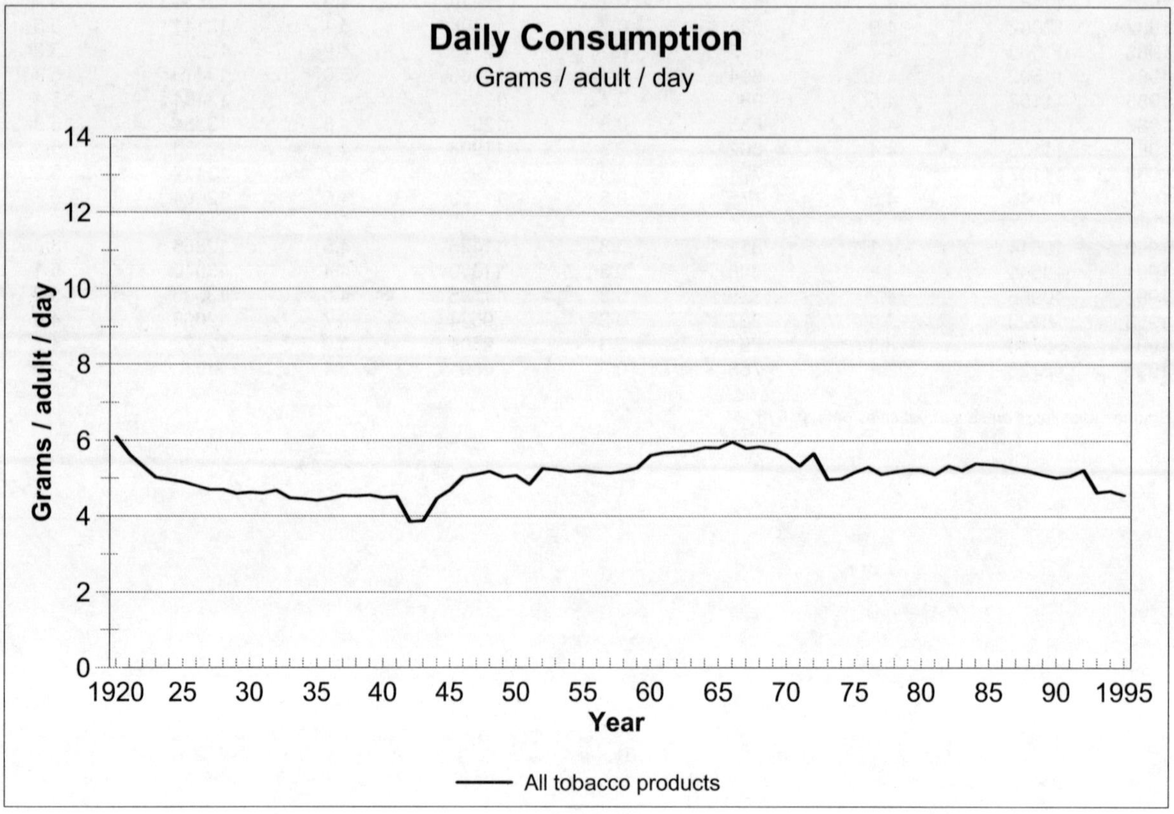

Table 25.3 Percentage sales of tobacco in different forms (by weight), selected years 1925-1995

Year	Cigarettes (%)	Cigars and cigarillos (%)	Pipe and hand-rolling (%)	Chewing (%)	Snuff (%)
1925	8.1	8.6	13.2	2.9	67.3
1935	20.7	8.6	12.7	1.1	56.9
1945	31.6	6.6	21.9	0.6	39.3
1955	54.8	3.9	13.8	0.5	27.2
1965	62.9	2.4	13.3	0.0	19.2
1975	62.0	3.8	10.1	0.1	24.0
1985	54.1	1.3	10.4	0.1	34.0
1995	44.3	1.0	9.2	0.1	45.4

Source : calculated from Tables 25.1.1 & 25.1.2

Figure 25.2 Percentage sales of tobacco in different forms (by weight), selected years 1925-1995
Source: see Table 25.3

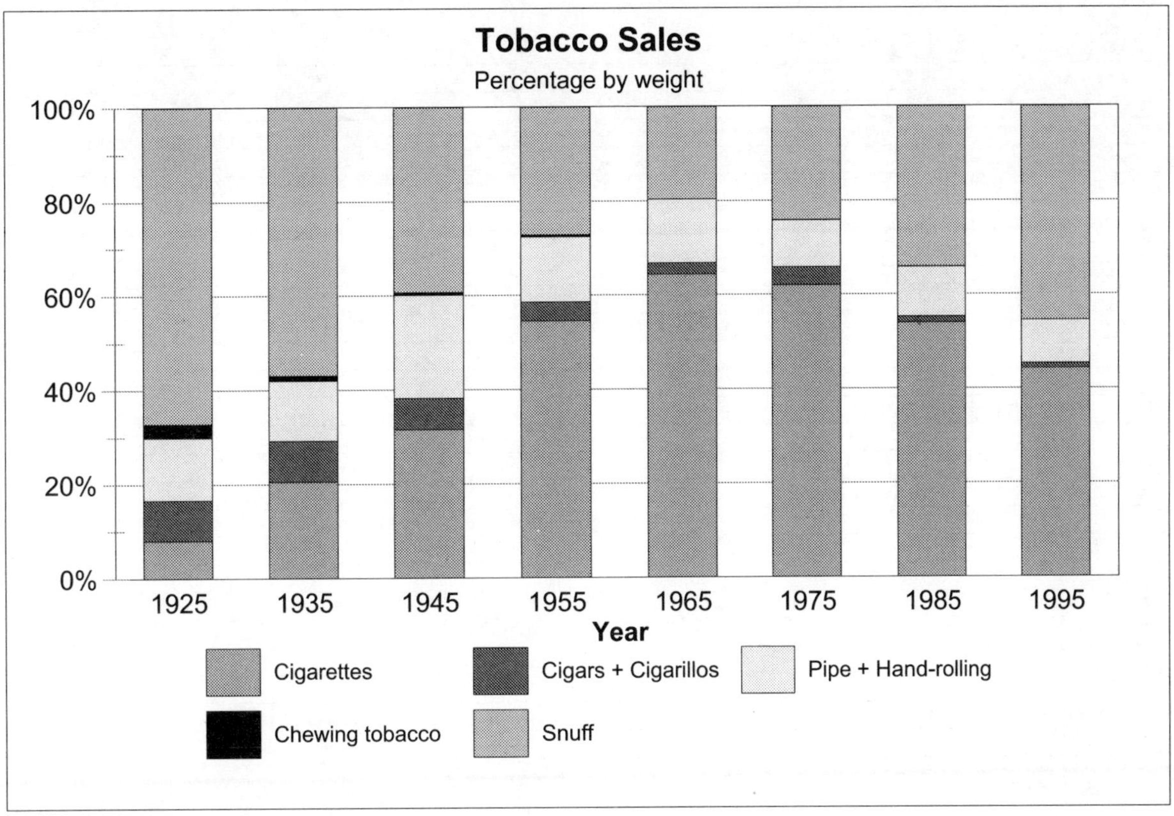

Table 25.4M Prevalence of smoking, males: some selected Swedish surveys by age, 1946-1995 *(continues on p. 604)*

Frequency / Product / Source / Year	12	13	14	15	16	17	18	19	20-24	25-29	30-34	35-39	40-44	45-49	50-54	55-59	60-64	65-69	70-74	75-79	80+	All ages
46 9 U U							50															
63 6 UC R							44			42		36			26							35
63 6 UC A							60			60		57			49							
63 6 A R							51			54		53			46							49
63 6 A A							62			64		62			58							62
67 5 UC U													35		28		23		14			
68 10 U U																						
68 18 A R	0																					
68 18 A A	8																					
69 1 UC U				43																		
69 12 U U				54																		
70 1 UC U				42																		
71 1 UC U				40																		
71 2 A R				55																		
71 3 UC U				44					48		43		39		37		33					42
71 7 U U		14			41																	
71 18 A R				22																		
71 18 A A				35																		
72 1 UC U				40																		
72 2 A R				55																		
72 5 UC U			28						41		34		30									
72 7 U U		10			35																	
72 12 U U				49																		
72 18 A R					32																	
72 18 A A					37																	
73 1 UC U				40																		
73 2 A R				56																		
73 4 UC R				38																		
73 7 U U		10			31																	
73 18 A R						32																
73 18 A A						40																
74 1 UC U				39																		
74 2 A R				55																		
74 7 U U		10			31																	
74 18 A R							38															
74 18 A A							56															
75 1 UC U				41							41				33							39
75 2 A R				54																		
75 7 U U		12			32																	
76 1 UC U				36							40				29							35
76 2 A R				52																		
76 7 U U		11			27																	
76 14 UC R							36															
76 14 A R							43															
76 14 A A							51															
77 1 UC U				33							41				29							34
77 2 A R				50																		
77 7 U U		9			25																	
77 8 U R					35					49		43		42		40		32				41
77 12 U U				39																		
77 14 A R							39															
77 14 A A							48															
77 18 A R									⟨35⟩													
77 18 A A									⟨38⟩													

Table 25.4F Prevalence of smoking, females: some selected Swedish surveys by age, 1946-1995 *(continues on p. 605)*

Frequency / Product / Source / Year	12	13	14	15	16	17	18	19	20-24	25-29	30-34	35-39	40-44	45-49	50-54	55-59	60-64	65-69	70-74	75-79	80+	All ages
46 9 U U							9															
63 6 UC R							36			32		25			11							23
63 6 UC A							51			43		34			17							
63 6 A R							36			32		25			11							23
63 6 A A							51			43		34			17							32
67 5 UC U													28		17		8		2			
68 10 U U												⟨47⟩		⟨44⟩	⟨37⟩	⟨38⟩	⟨20⟩					
68 18 A R	5																					
68 18 A A	10																					
69 1 UC U				33																		
69 12 U U				32																		
70 1 UC U				35																		
71 1 UC U				34																		
71 2 A R				34																		
71 3 UC U				43					49		38		33		23		12					35
71 7 U U		16			47																	
71 18 A R				43																		
71 18 A A				60																		
72 1 UC U				34																		
72 2 A R				34																		
72 5 UC U			35						45		34		28									
72 7 U U		12			47																	
72 12 U U				33																		
72 18 A R					49																	
72 18 A A					57																	
73 1 UC U				34																		
73 2 A R				35																		
73 4 UC R				34																		
73 7 U U		10			45																	
73 18 A R						54																
73 18 A A						60																
74 1 UC U				36																		
74 2 A R				36																		
74 7 U U		12			45																	
74 18 A R							57															
74 18 A A							72															
75 1 UC U				46							38				21							35
75 2 A R				36																		
75 7 U U		13			45																	
76 1 UC U				49							38				23							37
76 2 A R				38																		
76 7 U U		12			40																	
76 14 UC R							34															
76 14 A R							34															
76 14 A A							41															
77 1 UC U				43							36				21							33
77 2 A R				34																		
77 7 U U		11			40																	
77 8 U R					47					46		33		27		22		12				32
77 12 U U				21																		
77 14 A R							31															
77 14 A A							39															
77 18 A R									⟨56⟩													
77 18 A A									⟨59⟩													

Table 25.4M (continued from p. 602, continues on p. 606)
Prevalence of smoking, males

Frequency / Product / Source / Year	12	13	14	15	16	17	18	19	20-24	25-29	30-34	35-39	40-44	45-49	50-54	55-59	60-64	65-69	70-74	75-79	80+	All ages
78 1 UC U				34							37				27							33
78 2 A R				47																		
78 7 U U		10			25																	
78 14 A R							38															
78 14 A A							49															
79 1 UC U				28							37				29							32
79 2 A R				47																		
79 7 U U		6			21																	
79 14 UC R							31															
79 14 A R							37															
79 14 A A							46															
80 1 UC U				20							34				28							29
80 7 U U		5			21																	
80 8 A R					28					43				37				32		25		36
80 14 UC R							26															
80 14 A R							31															
80 14 A A							41															
81 1 UC U				28							34				25							29
81 8 A R					25					38				35				33		28		34
81 11 U R			18																			
81 11 U A	0		22																			
81 14 A R							30															
81 14 A A							38															
81 18 A R										⟨30⟩												
81 18 A A										⟨34⟩												
81 19 A R	2			13																		
82 1 UC U				29							33				27							30
82 8 A R					24					40				35				30		24		34
82 12 U U				30																		
82 14 A R							17			29		34				34						30
82 14 A A							42			48		45				37						42
82 19 A R	1			12																		
83 1 UC U				24							36				24							29
83 8 A R					22					38				34				25		25		32
83 14 A R							17					36										30
83 14 A A							40															
83 15 A R							32															
83 19 A R	2			11																		
84 8 A R					22					38				38				28		23		33
84 13 U U					16																	
84 15 A R					22					35		31				27						28
84 15 A A					37					47		38				30						37
84 19 A R				11																		
85 8 A R					23					33				34				25		21		30
85 15 UC R					14					28		31				18						24
85 15 A R					14					31		36				22						27
85 15 A A					29					46		44				28						37
85 16 UC R										26		35		34		27						32
85 16 A R										30		37		35		28						32
85 16 A A										42		44		40		36						41
85 19 A R	1			11																		
86 8 A R					17					34				34				22		21		29
86 17 UC R										21		24		24		23						24
86 17 A A										37		37		34		31						34
86 19 A R				12																		
86 21 U *		1		9																		
86 21 U R		4		15																		
86 21 U A		6		22																		

Table 25.4F *(continued from p. 603, continues on p. 607)*
Prevalence of smoking, females

<table>
<tr><th rowspan="2">Frequency
Product
Source
Year</th><th colspan="21">Age group</th><th rowspan="2">All ages</th></tr>
<tr><th>12</th><th>13</th><th>14</th><th>15</th><th>16</th><th>17</th><th>18</th><th>19</th><th>20-24</th><th>25-29</th><th>30-34</th><th>35-39</th><th>40-44</th><th>45-49</th><th>50-54</th><th>55-59</th><th>60-64</th><th>65-69</th><th>70-74</th><th>75-79</th><th>80+</th></tr>
<tr><td>78 1 UC U</td><td colspan="3"></td><td colspan="7">41</td><td colspan="4">38</td><td colspan="3">23</td><td colspan="4"></td><td>34</td></tr>
<tr><td>78 2 A R</td><td colspan="3"></td><td colspan="18">35</td><td></td></tr>
<tr><td>78 7 U U</td><td></td><td>10</td><td colspan="2"></td><td>38</td><td colspan="16"></td><td></td></tr>
<tr><td>78 14 A R</td><td colspan="6"></td><td colspan="12">34</td><td colspan="3"></td><td></td></tr>
<tr><td>78 14 A A</td><td colspan="6"></td><td colspan="12">44</td><td colspan="3"></td><td></td></tr>
<tr><td>79 1 UC U</td><td colspan="3"></td><td colspan="7">39</td><td colspan="4">38</td><td colspan="3">23</td><td colspan="4"></td><td>33</td></tr>
<tr><td>79 2 A R</td><td colspan="3"></td><td colspan="18">34</td><td></td></tr>
<tr><td>79 7 U U</td><td></td><td>8</td><td colspan="2"></td><td>34</td><td colspan="16"></td><td></td></tr>
<tr><td>79 14 UC R</td><td colspan="6"></td><td colspan="12">32</td><td colspan="3"></td><td></td></tr>
<tr><td>79 14 A R</td><td colspan="6"></td><td colspan="12">32</td><td colspan="3"></td><td></td></tr>
<tr><td>79 14 A A</td><td colspan="6"></td><td colspan="12">39</td><td colspan="3"></td><td></td></tr>
<tr><td>80 1 UC U</td><td colspan="3"></td><td colspan="7">37</td><td colspan="4">36</td><td colspan="3">20</td><td colspan="4"></td><td>31</td></tr>
<tr><td>80 7 U U</td><td></td><td>6</td><td colspan="2"></td><td>33</td><td colspan="16"></td><td></td></tr>
<tr><td>80 8 A R</td><td colspan="4"></td><td colspan="5">37</td><td colspan="4">40</td><td colspan="4">24</td><td colspan="2">14</td><td colspan="2">4</td><td>29</td></tr>
<tr><td>80 14 UC R</td><td colspan="6"></td><td colspan="12">26</td><td colspan="3"></td><td></td></tr>
<tr><td>80 14 A R</td><td colspan="6"></td><td colspan="12">26</td><td colspan="3"></td><td></td></tr>
<tr><td>80 14 A A</td><td colspan="6"></td><td colspan="12">33</td><td colspan="3"></td><td></td></tr>
<tr><td>81 1 UC U</td><td colspan="3"></td><td colspan="7">37</td><td colspan="4">36</td><td colspan="3">25</td><td colspan="4"></td><td>32</td></tr>
<tr><td>81 8 A R</td><td colspan="4"></td><td colspan="5">36</td><td colspan="4">35</td><td colspan="4">25</td><td colspan="2">12</td><td colspan="2">6</td><td>27</td></tr>
<tr><td>81 11 U R</td><td colspan="2"></td><td colspan="2">7</td><td colspan="17"></td><td></td></tr>
<tr><td>81 11 U A</td><td colspan="2">0</td><td colspan="2">14</td><td colspan="17"></td><td></td></tr>
<tr><td>81 14 A R</td><td colspan="6"></td><td colspan="12">31</td><td colspan="3"></td><td></td></tr>
<tr><td>81 14 A A</td><td colspan="6"></td><td colspan="12">37</td><td colspan="3"></td><td></td></tr>
<tr><td>81 18 A R</td><td colspan="21">⟨48⟩</td><td></td></tr>
<tr><td>81 18 A A</td><td colspan="21">⟨48⟩</td><td></td></tr>
<tr><td>81 19 A R</td><td colspan="2">1</td><td></td><td colspan="2">23</td><td colspan="16"></td><td></td></tr>
<tr><td>82 1 UC U</td><td colspan="3"></td><td colspan="7">35</td><td colspan="4">33</td><td colspan="3">23</td><td colspan="4"></td><td>31</td></tr>
<tr><td>82 8 A R</td><td colspan="4"></td><td colspan="5">32</td><td colspan="4">38</td><td colspan="4">27</td><td colspan="2">12</td><td colspan="2">3</td><td>28</td></tr>
<tr><td>82 12 U U</td><td colspan="3"></td><td colspan="18">30</td><td></td></tr>
<tr><td>82 14 A R</td><td colspan="6"></td><td colspan="3">34</td><td>39</td><td colspan="4">29</td><td colspan="4">20</td><td colspan="3"></td><td>30</td></tr>
<tr><td>82 14 A A</td><td colspan="6"></td><td colspan="3">50</td><td>55</td><td colspan="4">39</td><td colspan="4">23</td><td colspan="3"></td><td>41</td></tr>
<tr><td>82 19 A R</td><td colspan="2">1</td><td></td><td colspan="2">19</td><td colspan="16"></td><td></td></tr>
<tr><td>83 1 UC U</td><td colspan="3"></td><td colspan="7">35</td><td colspan="4">35</td><td colspan="3">19</td><td colspan="4"></td><td>30</td></tr>
<tr><td>83 8 A R</td><td colspan="4"></td><td colspan="5">29</td><td colspan="4">37</td><td colspan="4">25</td><td colspan="2">10</td><td colspan="2">8</td><td>26</td></tr>
<tr><td>83 14 A R</td><td colspan="6"></td><td colspan="3">29</td><td></td><td colspan="4">30</td><td colspan="4"></td><td colspan="3"></td><td>28</td></tr>
<tr><td>83 14 A A</td><td colspan="6"></td><td colspan="12">36</td><td colspan="3"></td><td></td></tr>
<tr><td>83 15 A R</td><td colspan="6"></td><td colspan="12">27</td><td colspan="3"></td><td></td></tr>
<tr><td>83 19 A R</td><td colspan="2">2</td><td></td><td colspan="2">18</td><td colspan="16"></td><td></td></tr>
<tr><td>84 8 A R</td><td colspan="4"></td><td colspan="5">31</td><td colspan="4">37</td><td colspan="4">29</td><td colspan="2">14</td><td colspan="2">5</td><td>28</td></tr>
<tr><td>84 13 U U</td><td colspan="4"></td><td>22</td><td colspan="16"></td><td></td></tr>
<tr><td>84 15 A R</td><td colspan="4"></td><td colspan="5">28</td><td>42</td><td colspan="4">33</td><td colspan="4">18</td><td colspan="3"></td><td>29</td></tr>
<tr><td>84 15 A A</td><td colspan="4"></td><td colspan="5">45</td><td>55</td><td colspan="4">38</td><td colspan="4">23</td><td colspan="3"></td><td>37</td></tr>
<tr><td>84 19 A R</td><td colspan="3"></td><td colspan="2">16</td><td colspan="16"></td><td></td></tr>
<tr><td>85 8 A R</td><td colspan="4"></td><td colspan="5">30</td><td colspan="4">37</td><td colspan="4">27</td><td colspan="2">13</td><td colspan="2">6</td><td>27</td></tr>
<tr><td>85 15 UC R</td><td colspan="4"></td><td colspan="5">27</td><td>40</td><td colspan="4">33</td><td colspan="4">12</td><td colspan="3"></td><td>27</td></tr>
<tr><td>85 15 A R</td><td colspan="4"></td><td colspan="5">28</td><td>41</td><td colspan="4">34</td><td colspan="4">13</td><td colspan="3"></td><td>29</td></tr>
<tr><td>85 15 A A</td><td colspan="4"></td><td colspan="5">40</td><td>51</td><td colspan="4">41</td><td colspan="4">15</td><td colspan="3"></td><td>36</td></tr>
<tr><td>85 16 UC R</td><td colspan="9"></td><td>41</td><td colspan="2">37</td><td colspan="2">38</td><td colspan="2">27</td><td colspan="5"></td><td>35</td></tr>
<tr><td>85 16 A R</td><td colspan="9"></td><td>41</td><td colspan="2">37</td><td colspan="2">38</td><td colspan="2">27</td><td colspan="5"></td><td>36</td></tr>
<tr><td>85 16 A A</td><td colspan="9"></td><td>44</td><td colspan="2">42</td><td colspan="2">42</td><td colspan="2">30</td><td colspan="5"></td><td>39</td></tr>
<tr><td>85 19 A R</td><td colspan="2">1</td><td></td><td colspan="2">14</td><td colspan="16"></td><td></td></tr>
<tr><td>86 8 A R</td><td colspan="4"></td><td colspan="5">26</td><td colspan="4">37</td><td colspan="4">24</td><td colspan="2">16</td><td colspan="2">7</td><td>27</td></tr>
<tr><td>86 17 UC R</td><td colspan="9"></td><td>29</td><td colspan="2">35</td><td colspan="2">24</td><td colspan="2">18</td><td colspan="5"></td><td>27</td></tr>
<tr><td>86 17 A A</td><td colspan="9"></td><td>35</td><td colspan="2">40</td><td colspan="2">28</td><td colspan="2">20</td><td colspan="5"></td><td>31</td></tr>
<tr><td>86 19 A R</td><td colspan="3"></td><td colspan="2">15</td><td colspan="16"></td><td></td></tr>
<tr><td>86 21 U *</td><td></td><td>2</td><td></td><td>11</td><td colspan="17"></td><td></td></tr>
<tr><td>86 21 U R</td><td></td><td>5</td><td></td><td>17</td><td colspan="17"></td><td></td></tr>
<tr><td>86 21 U A</td><td></td><td>6</td><td></td><td>24</td><td colspan="17"></td><td></td></tr>
</table>

Table 25.4M *(continued from p. 604)*
Prevalence of smoking, males

Year	Source	Product	Frequency	12	13	14	15	16	17	18	19	20-24	25-29	30-34	35-39	40-44	45-49	50-54	55-59	60-64	65-69	70-74	75-79	80+	All ages
87	8	A	R					17					32				35				28		22		29
87	15	UC	R					15					28		28				21						23
87	15	A	R					14					29		30				29						27
87	15	A	A					29					42		40				33						37
87	19	A	R	3			10																		
88	8	A	R					17					32				31				27		18		28
88	19	A	R				10																		
88	20	U	U				17																		
89	8	A	R					16					28				30				20		21		25
89	19	A	R	10			12																		
89	20	U	U				23																		
89	21	UC	R		5		15																		
89	21	UC	A		10		24																		
90	8	A	R					14					29				32				25		15		26
90	16	A	R										24		39		31		34						32
90	17	UC	R										17		26		24		25						23
90	19	A	R				13																		
90	22	U	R				20																		
91	8	A	R					17					30				29				25		12		26
91	19	A	R	4			13																		
91	22	U	R				19																		
92	8	A	R					14					28				31				23		17		25
92	18	A	R												29										
92	18	A	A												32										
92	19	A	R				16																		
92	22	U	R				22																		
93	8	A	R					14					25				30				19		14		23
93	19	A	R	4			14																		
93	21	UC	R		3		15																		
93	22	U	R				20																		
94	8	A	R					15					21				29				16		15		22
94	17	UC	R										11		26		17		20						19
94	19	A	R				12																		
94	22	U	R				17																		
95	8	A	R					14					22				28				21		15		22
95	16	A	R										20		24		30		28						26
95	19	A	R	4			13																		
95	22	U	R				27																		
95	23	UC	R				14																		
95	23	UC	A				28																		

Source: see *Notes on sources of survey data*, p. 617
Product: MC = manufactured cigarettes
TC = total cigarettes (including hand-rolled)
UC = cigarettes (type unspecified)
A = all products

Frequency: A = all smokers (including occasional)
R = regular or daily smokers
All ages: relevant to ages used and as given in original source
U = unspecified
* = refer to *Notes on sources of survey data*, p. 617

Table 25.4F *(continued from p. 605)*
Prevalence of smoking, females

<table>
<tr><th rowspan="2">Year</th><th rowspan="2">Source</th><th rowspan="2">Product</th><th rowspan="2">Frequency</th><th colspan="21">Age group</th><th rowspan="2">All ages</th></tr>
<tr><th>12</th><th>13</th><th>14</th><th>15</th><th>16</th><th>17</th><th>18</th><th>19</th><th>20-24</th><th>25-29</th><th>30-34</th><th>35-39</th><th>40-44</th><th>45-49</th><th>50-54</th><th>55-59</th><th>60-64</th><th>65-69</th><th>70-74</th><th>75-79</th><th>80+</th></tr>
<tr><td>87</td><td>8</td><td>A</td><td>R</td><td colspan="4"></td><td colspan="5">27</td><td colspan="4">35</td><td colspan="4">28</td><td colspan="2">13</td><td colspan="2">7</td><td>26</td></tr>
<tr><td>87</td><td>15</td><td>UC</td><td>R</td><td colspan="4"></td><td colspan="5">30</td><td colspan="2">37</td><td colspan="4">29</td><td colspan="4">14</td><td colspan="2"></td><td>27</td></tr>
<tr><td>87</td><td>15</td><td>A</td><td>R</td><td colspan="4"></td><td colspan="5">30</td><td colspan="2">37</td><td colspan="4">29</td><td colspan="4">14</td><td colspan="2"></td><td>27</td></tr>
<tr><td>87</td><td>15</td><td>A</td><td>A</td><td colspan="4"></td><td colspan="5">41</td><td colspan="2">47</td><td colspan="4">36</td><td colspan="4">16</td><td colspan="2"></td><td>34</td></tr>
<tr><td>87</td><td>19</td><td>A</td><td>R</td><td colspan="2">3</td><td></td><td colspan="2">15</td><td colspan="16"></td><td></td></tr>
<tr><td>88</td><td>8</td><td>A</td><td>R</td><td colspan="4"></td><td colspan="5">28</td><td colspan="4">36</td><td colspan="4">27</td><td colspan="2">13</td><td colspan="2">6</td><td>26</td></tr>
<tr><td>88</td><td>19</td><td>A</td><td>R</td><td colspan="3"></td><td colspan="2">15</td><td colspan="16"></td><td></td></tr>
<tr><td>88</td><td>20</td><td>U</td><td>U</td><td colspan="3"></td><td>24</td><td colspan="17"></td><td></td></tr>
<tr><td>89</td><td>8</td><td>A</td><td>R</td><td colspan="4"></td><td colspan="5">26</td><td colspan="4">35</td><td colspan="4">27</td><td colspan="2">16</td><td colspan="2">7</td><td>26</td></tr>
<tr><td>89</td><td>19</td><td>A</td><td>R</td><td colspan="2">8</td><td></td><td colspan="2">17</td><td colspan="16"></td><td></td></tr>
<tr><td>89</td><td>20</td><td>U</td><td>U</td><td colspan="3"></td><td>30</td><td colspan="17"></td><td></td></tr>
<tr><td>89</td><td>21</td><td>UC</td><td>R</td><td></td><td>5</td><td></td><td>20</td><td colspan="17"></td><td></td></tr>
<tr><td>89</td><td>21</td><td>UC</td><td>A</td><td></td><td>9</td><td></td><td>29</td><td colspan="17"></td><td></td></tr>
<tr><td>90</td><td>8</td><td>A</td><td>R</td><td colspan="4"></td><td colspan="5">22</td><td colspan="4">34</td><td colspan="4">28</td><td colspan="2">17</td><td colspan="2">7</td><td>26</td></tr>
<tr><td>90</td><td>16</td><td>A</td><td>R</td><td colspan="9"></td><td colspan="2">28</td><td colspan="2">33</td><td colspan="2">32</td><td colspan="2">27</td><td colspan="4"></td><td>30</td></tr>
<tr><td>90</td><td>17</td><td>UC</td><td>R</td><td colspan="9"></td><td colspan="2">24</td><td colspan="2">34</td><td colspan="2">26</td><td colspan="2">20</td><td colspan="4"></td><td>26</td></tr>
<tr><td>90</td><td>19</td><td>A</td><td>R</td><td colspan="3"></td><td colspan="2">19</td><td colspan="16"></td><td></td></tr>
<tr><td>90</td><td>22</td><td>U</td><td>R</td><td colspan="3"></td><td colspan="5">31</td><td colspan="13"></td><td></td></tr>
<tr><td>91</td><td>8</td><td>A</td><td>R</td><td colspan="4"></td><td colspan="5">23</td><td colspan="4">31</td><td colspan="4">28</td><td colspan="2">14</td><td colspan="2">5</td><td>24</td></tr>
<tr><td>91</td><td>19</td><td>A</td><td>R</td><td colspan="2">5</td><td></td><td colspan="2">18</td><td colspan="16"></td><td></td></tr>
<tr><td>91</td><td>22</td><td>U</td><td>R</td><td colspan="3"></td><td colspan="5">27</td><td colspan="13"></td><td></td></tr>
<tr><td>92</td><td>8</td><td>A</td><td>R</td><td colspan="4"></td><td colspan="5">21</td><td colspan="4">34</td><td colspan="4">30</td><td colspan="2">18</td><td colspan="2">9</td><td>27</td></tr>
<tr><td>92</td><td>18</td><td>A</td><td>R</td><td colspan="21">⟨36⟩</td><td></td></tr>
<tr><td>92</td><td>18</td><td>A</td><td>A</td><td colspan="21">⟨40⟩</td><td></td></tr>
<tr><td>92</td><td>19</td><td>A</td><td>R</td><td colspan="3"></td><td colspan="2">18</td><td colspan="16"></td><td></td></tr>
<tr><td>92</td><td>22</td><td>U</td><td>R</td><td colspan="3"></td><td colspan="5">27</td><td colspan="13"></td><td></td></tr>
<tr><td>93</td><td>8</td><td>A</td><td>R</td><td colspan="4"></td><td colspan="5">19</td><td colspan="4">28</td><td colspan="4">28</td><td colspan="2">18</td><td colspan="2">6</td><td>23</td></tr>
<tr><td>93</td><td>19</td><td>A</td><td>R</td><td colspan="2">5</td><td></td><td colspan="2">18</td><td colspan="16"></td><td></td></tr>
<tr><td>93</td><td>21</td><td>UC</td><td>R</td><td></td><td>4</td><td></td><td>19</td><td colspan="17"></td><td></td></tr>
<tr><td>93</td><td>22</td><td>U</td><td>R</td><td colspan="3"></td><td colspan="5">26</td><td colspan="13"></td><td></td></tr>
<tr><td>94</td><td>8</td><td>A</td><td>R</td><td colspan="4"></td><td colspan="5">20</td><td colspan="4">29</td><td colspan="4">28</td><td colspan="2">13</td><td colspan="2">7</td><td>24</td></tr>
<tr><td>94</td><td>17</td><td>UC</td><td>R</td><td colspan="9"></td><td colspan="2">24</td><td colspan="2">29</td><td colspan="2">32</td><td colspan="2">21</td><td colspan="4"></td><td>27</td></tr>
<tr><td>94</td><td>19</td><td>A</td><td>R</td><td colspan="3"></td><td colspan="2">20</td><td colspan="16"></td><td></td></tr>
<tr><td>94</td><td>22</td><td>U</td><td>R</td><td colspan="3"></td><td colspan="5">29</td><td colspan="13"></td><td></td></tr>
<tr><td>95</td><td>8</td><td>A</td><td>R</td><td colspan="4"></td><td colspan="5">21</td><td colspan="4">29</td><td colspan="4">27</td><td colspan="2">15</td><td colspan="2">7</td><td>24</td></tr>
<tr><td>95</td><td>16</td><td>A</td><td>R</td><td colspan="9"></td><td colspan="2">25</td><td colspan="2">33</td><td colspan="2">26</td><td colspan="2">22</td><td colspan="4"></td><td>26</td></tr>
<tr><td>95</td><td>19</td><td>A</td><td>R</td><td colspan="2">4</td><td></td><td colspan="2">17</td><td colspan="16"></td><td></td></tr>
<tr><td>95</td><td>22</td><td>U</td><td>R</td><td colspan="3"></td><td colspan="5">19</td><td colspan="13"></td><td></td></tr>
<tr><td>95</td><td>23</td><td>UC</td><td>R</td><td colspan="3"></td><td colspan="2">18</td><td colspan="16"></td><td></td></tr>
<tr><td>95</td><td>23</td><td>UC</td><td>A</td><td colspan="3"></td><td colspan="2">33</td><td colspan="16"></td><td></td></tr>
</table>

Source: see *Notes on sources of survey data*, p. 617
Product: MC = manufactured cigarettes
TC = total cigarettes (including hand-rolled)
UC = cigarettes (type unspecified)
A = all products

Frequency: A = all smokers (including occasional)
R = regular or daily smokers
All ages: relevant to ages used and as given in original source
U = unspecified
* = refer to *Notes on sources of survey data*, p. 617

Table 25.5M Number of cigarettes smoked per smoker per day, males: some selected Swedish surveys by age, 1963-1995

Year Source Product	12	13	14	15	16	17	18	19	20-24	25-29	30-34	35-39	40-44	45-49	50-54	55-59	60-64	65-69	70-74	75-79	80+	All ages
63 6 UCE								8.4		13			12			10						12
67 5 UC														11		9.8		7.9		6.6		
68 18 AE	0																					
71 18 AE				8																		
72 5 UC						11				13		14	14									
72 18 AE					8																	
73 18 AE						10																
74 18 AE							14															
77 18 AE									⟨15⟩													
81 18 AE										⟨15⟩												
83 14 UC													15									
85 15 UC							14			15			17					14				15
85 16 UC															18							
85 16 AE*										19		19		21		16						19
86 17 UC															14							
87 15 UC							16			19			18					16				17
90 16 AE*										15		19		19		17						18
92 18 AE												⟨17⟩										
95 16 AE*										15		18		18		18						18
95 23 UCE				11																		

Source: see *Notes on sources of survey data*, p. 617

Product:
MC = manufactured cigarettes
TC = total cigarettes (including hand-rolled)
UC = cigarettes (type unspecified)
A = all products
U = unspecified

Product (cont): E indicates mean estimated from percentage distribution (see also *Consumption category estimation*, p. xxxiv, and Appendix III, p. 789)

All ages: relevant to ages used and as given in original source

* = refer to *Notes on sources of survey data*, p. 617

Table 25.5F Number of cigarettes smoked per smoker per day, females: some selected Swedish surveys by age, 1963-1995

<table>
<tr><th rowspan="2">Product
Source
Year</th><th colspan="21">Age group</th><th rowspan="2">All ages</th></tr>
<tr><th>12</th><th>13</th><th>14</th><th>15</th><th>16</th><th>17</th><th>18</th><th>19</th><th>20-24</th><th>25-29</th><th>30-34</th><th>35-39</th><th>40-44</th><th>45-49</th><th>50-54</th><th>55-59</th><th>60-64</th><th>65-69</th><th>70-74</th><th>75-79</th><th>80+</th></tr>
<tr><td>63 6 UCE</td><td colspan="6"></td><td colspan="3">8.3</td><td colspan="2">8.9</td><td colspan="3">9.1</td><td colspan="4">7.9</td><td colspan="3"></td><td>8.7</td></tr>
<tr><td>67 5 UC</td><td colspan="12"></td><td colspan="2">9.3</td><td colspan="2">8.8</td><td colspan="2">8.3</td><td colspan="3">5.8</td><td></td></tr>
<tr><td>68 18 AE</td><td>3</td><td colspan="20"></td><td></td></tr>
<tr><td>71 18 AE</td><td colspan="3"></td><td>8</td><td colspan="17"></td><td></td></tr>
<tr><td>72 5 UC</td><td colspan="2"></td><td colspan="6">9.3</td><td colspan="2">12</td><td colspan="2">11</td><td>12</td><td colspan="8"></td><td></td></tr>
<tr><td>72 18 AE</td><td colspan="4"></td><td>10</td><td colspan="16"></td><td></td></tr>
<tr><td>73 18 AE</td><td colspan="5"></td><td>11</td><td colspan="15"></td><td></td></tr>
<tr><td>74 18 AE</td><td colspan="6"></td><td>13</td><td colspan="14"></td><td></td></tr>
<tr><td>77 18 AE</td><td colspan="8"></td><td>⟨16⟩</td><td colspan="12"></td><td></td></tr>
<tr><td>81 18 AE</td><td colspan="9"></td><td>⟨15⟩</td><td colspan="11"></td><td></td></tr>
<tr><td>83 14 UC</td><td colspan="6"></td><td colspan="12">13</td><td colspan="3"></td><td></td></tr>
<tr><td>85 15 UC</td><td colspan="4"></td><td colspan="5">13</td><td colspan="2">14</td><td colspan="4">15</td><td colspan="4">14</td><td colspan="2"></td><td>14</td></tr>
<tr><td>85 16 UC</td><td colspan="11"></td><td colspan="6">14</td><td colspan="4"></td><td></td></tr>
<tr><td>85 16 AE*</td><td colspan="9"></td><td colspan="2">15</td><td colspan="2">15</td><td colspan="2">16</td><td colspan="2">13</td><td colspan="4"></td><td>15</td></tr>
<tr><td>86 17 UC</td><td colspan="11"></td><td colspan="6">11</td><td colspan="4"></td><td></td></tr>
<tr><td>87 15 UC</td><td colspan="4"></td><td colspan="5">13</td><td colspan="2">15</td><td colspan="4">14</td><td colspan="4">11</td><td colspan="2"></td><td>13</td></tr>
<tr><td>90 16 AE*</td><td colspan="9"></td><td colspan="2">16</td><td colspan="2">16</td><td colspan="2">16</td><td colspan="2">15</td><td colspan="4"></td><td>16</td></tr>
<tr><td>92 18 AE</td><td colspan="11"></td><td>⟨14⟩</td><td colspan="9"></td><td></td></tr>
<tr><td>95 16 AE*</td><td colspan="9"></td><td colspan="2">15</td><td colspan="2">15</td><td colspan="2">17</td><td colspan="2">15</td><td colspan="4"></td><td>15</td></tr>
<tr><td>95 23 UCE</td><td colspan="3"></td><td colspan="2">9.3</td><td colspan="16"></td><td></td></tr>
</table>

Source: see *Notes on sources of survey data*, p. 617
Product: MC = manufactured cigarettes
TC = total cigarettes (including hand-rolled)
UC = cigarettes (type unspecified)
A = all products
U = unspecified

Product (cont): E indicates mean estimated from percentage distribution (see also *Consumption category estimation*, p. xxxiv, and Appendix III, p. 789)
All ages: relevant to ages used and as given in original source
* = refer to *Notes on sources of survey data*, p. 617

Table 25.6M Number of cigarettes smoked per person per day, males: some selected Swedish surveys by age, 1963-1995, with percentage total sales

<table>
<tr><th rowspan="2">Product Source Year</th><th colspan="21">Age group</th><th rowspan="2">All ages</th><th rowspan="2">% Total sales</th></tr>
<tr><th>12</th><th>13</th><th>14</th><th>15</th><th>16</th><th>17</th><th>18</th><th>19</th><th>20-24</th><th>25-29</th><th>30-34</th><th>35-39</th><th>40-44</th><th>45-49</th><th>50-54</th><th>55-59</th><th>60-64</th><th>65-69</th><th>70-74</th><th>75-79</th><th>80+</th></tr>
<tr><td>63 6 UC</td><td colspan="6"></td><td colspan="3">3.7</td><td colspan="2">5.3</td><td colspan="3">4.4</td><td colspan="4">2.6</td><td colspan="3"></td><td>4.0</td><td>65%T</td></tr>
<tr><td>67 5 UC</td><td colspan="12"></td><td colspan="2">4.0</td><td colspan="2">2.8</td><td colspan="2">1.8</td><td colspan="3">0.9</td><td></td><td>**</td></tr>
<tr><td>68 18 A</td><td>0</td><td colspan="20"></td><td></td><td>**</td></tr>
<tr><td>71 18 A</td><td colspan="3"></td><td>2</td><td colspan="17"></td><td></td><td>**</td></tr>
<tr><td>72 5 UC</td><td colspan="2"></td><td colspan="6">2.9</td><td colspan="2">5.3</td><td colspan="2">4.7</td><td>4.2</td><td colspan="8"></td><td></td><td>**</td></tr>
<tr><td>72 18 A</td><td colspan="4"></td><td>3</td><td colspan="16"></td><td></td><td>**</td></tr>
<tr><td>73 18 A</td><td colspan="5"></td><td>3</td><td colspan="15"></td><td></td><td>**</td></tr>
<tr><td>74 18 A</td><td colspan="6"></td><td>5</td><td colspan="14"></td><td></td><td>**</td></tr>
<tr><td>77 18 A</td><td colspan="8"></td><td>⟨5⟩</td><td colspan="12"></td><td></td><td>**</td></tr>
<tr><td>81 18 A</td><td colspan="9"></td><td>⟨4⟩</td><td colspan="11"></td><td></td><td>**</td></tr>
<tr><td>83 14 UC</td><td colspan="6"></td><td colspan="13">4.8</td><td colspan="2"></td><td></td><td>76%T</td></tr>
<tr><td>85 15 UC</td><td colspan="4"></td><td colspan="5">2</td><td colspan="2">4</td><td colspan="4">5</td><td colspan="4">3</td><td colspan="2"></td><td>4</td><td>72%T</td></tr>
<tr><td>85 16 UC *</td><td colspan="21">5.8</td><td></td><td>**</td></tr>
<tr><td>85 16 A *</td><td colspan="9"></td><td colspan="2">5.6</td><td colspan="2">6.8</td><td colspan="2">7.5</td><td colspan="2">4.8</td><td colspan="4"></td><td>6.1</td><td>**</td></tr>
<tr><td>86 17 UC *</td><td colspan="21">3.3</td><td></td><td>**</td></tr>
<tr><td>87 15 UC</td><td colspan="4"></td><td colspan="5">2</td><td colspan="2">5</td><td colspan="4">5</td><td colspan="4">3</td><td colspan="2"></td><td>4</td><td>75%T</td></tr>
<tr><td>90 16 A *</td><td colspan="9"></td><td colspan="2">3.5</td><td colspan="2">7.3</td><td colspan="2">5.9</td><td colspan="2">5.8</td><td colspan="4"></td><td>5.9</td><td>**</td></tr>
<tr><td>92 18 A</td><td colspan="11"></td><td>⟨5⟩</td><td colspan="9"></td><td></td><td>**</td></tr>
<tr><td>95 16 A *</td><td colspan="9"></td><td colspan="2">3.1</td><td colspan="2">4.3</td><td colspan="2">5.5</td><td colspan="2">5.2</td><td colspan="4"></td><td>4.7</td><td>**</td></tr>
<tr><td>95 23 UC</td><td colspan="3"></td><td colspan="2">1.5</td><td colspan="16"></td><td></td><td>**</td></tr>
</table>

Table 25.7M Number of cigarettes smoked per person per day, sales-adjusted, males: some selected Swedish surveys[1] by age, 1963-1987, with percentage total sales

<table>
<tr><th rowspan="2">Product Source Year</th><th colspan="21">Age group</th><th rowspan="2">All ages</th><th rowspan="2">% Total sales</th></tr>
<tr><th>12</th><th>13</th><th>14</th><th>15</th><th>16</th><th>17</th><th>18</th><th>19</th><th>20-24</th><th>25-29</th><th>30-34</th><th>35-39</th><th>40-44</th><th>45-49</th><th>50-54</th><th>55-59</th><th>60-64</th><th>65-69</th><th>70-74</th><th>75-79</th><th>80+</th></tr>
<tr><td>63 6 UC</td><td colspan="6"></td><td colspan="3">5.7</td><td colspan="2">8.1</td><td colspan="3">6.8</td><td colspan="4">4.0</td><td colspan="3"></td><td>6.1</td><td>65%T</td></tr>
<tr><td>83 14 UC</td><td colspan="6"></td><td colspan="13">6.3</td><td colspan="2"></td><td></td><td>76%T</td></tr>
<tr><td>85 15 UC</td><td colspan="4"></td><td colspan="5">3</td><td colspan="2">6</td><td colspan="4">7</td><td colspan="4">3</td><td colspan="2"></td><td>5</td><td>72%T</td></tr>
<tr><td>87 15 UC</td><td colspan="4"></td><td colspan="5">3</td><td colspan="2">7</td><td colspan="4">7</td><td colspan="4">5</td><td colspan="2"></td><td>5</td><td>75%T</td></tr>
</table>

1 Based on those surveys in Table 25.6 with data for both sexes and age range at least 21-64 (see *Cigarette consumption per person*, p. xxxv)

Source: see *Notes on sources of survey data*, p. 617
All ages: relevant to ages used and as given in original source
% Total sales: estimated % of total sales of M = manufactured or T = total cigarette consumption implied by survey, sexes combined, used as adjustment factor in Table 25.7
** = cannot be calculated
--- = adjusted by original author

Product: MC = manufactured cigarettes
TC = total cigarettes (including hand-rolled)
UC = cigarettes (type unspecified)
A = all products
U = unspecified
* = refer to *Notes on sources of survey data*, p. 617

Table 25.6F Number of cigarettes smoked per person per day, females: some selected Swedish surveys by age, 1963-1995, with percentage total sales

Product Source Year	12	13	14	15	16	17	18	19	20-24	25-29	30-34	35-39	40-44	45-49	50-54	55-59	60-64	65-69	70-74	75-79	80+	All ages	% Total sales
63 6 UC								3.0		2.8			2.3			0.8						2.0	65%T
67 5 UC														2.6		1.5		0.7		0.1			**
68 18 A	0																						**
71 18 A				3																			**
72 5 UC						3.3				5.2		3.8	3.2										**
72 18 A					5																		**
73 18 A						6																	**
74 18 A							8																**
77 18 A									〈9〉														**
81 18 A										〈7〉													**
83 14 UC													3.5										76%T
85 15 UC							4			6			5					2				4	72%T
85 16 UC *														4.8									**
85 16 A *										6.1		5.6		6.1		3.6						5.4	**
86 17 UC *														2.9									**
87 15 UC							4			6			4					2				4	75%T
90 16 A *										4.4		5.2		5.0		4.2						4.7	**
92 18 A												〈5〉											**
95 16 A *										3.9		5.1		4.4		3.4						4.2	**
95 23 UC				1.7																			**

Table 25.7F Number of cigarettes smoked per person per day, sales-adjusted, females: some selected Swedish surveys[1] by age, 1963-1987, with percentage total sales

Product Source Year	12	13	14	15	16	17	18	19	20-24	25-29	30-34	35-39	40-44	45-49	50-54	55-59	60-64	65-69	70-74	75-79	80+	All ages	% Total sales
63 6 UC								4.6		4.3			3.5			1.2						3.1	65%T
83 14 UC													4.6										76%T
85 15 UC							5			8			7					2				5	72%T
87 15 UC							5			7			5					2				5	75%T

1 Based on those surveys in Table 25.6 with data for both sexes and age range at least 21-64 (see *Cigarette consumption per person*, p. xxxv)

Source: see *Notes on sources of survey data*, p. 617
All ages: relevant to ages used and as given in original source
% Total sales: estimated % of total sales of M = manufactured or T = total cigarette consumption implied by survey, sexes combined, used as adjustment factor in Table 25.7
** = cannot be calculated
--- = adjusted by original author

Product:
MC = manufactured cigarettes
TC = total cigarettes (including hand-rolled)
UC = cigarettes (type unspecified)
A = all products
U = unspecified
* = refer to *Notes on sources of survey data*, p. 617

Table 25.8 Estimated[1] prevalence of smoking and estimated[1] number of cigarettes per person per day (unadjusted and sales-adjusted): summary of Tables 25.4, 25.6 and 25.7, 1946-1995.
Males and females aged 15 years and over

Year	Source[2]	Product[3]	Prevalence[4]						Number of cigarettes						
									Unadjusted[7]			Sales-adjusted[8]			
			Manufactured cigarettes		Total cigarettes[5]		All products[6]		Number/ person/day		Total sales %	Manufactured cigarettes number/ person/day		Total cigarettes[9] number/ person/day	
			M	F	M	F	M	F	M	F		M	F	M	F
1946	9	*U*					48	9							
1963	6	UC+A			32	20	46	20	3.4	1.7	65			5.2	2.6
	6	**UC+A**			50	28	56	28							
1969	1	*UC*			40	29								(6.0	3.5)
	12	*U*					54	32							
1970	1	*UC*			39	30								(5.8	3.7)
1971	1	*UC*			37	29								(5.6	3.6)
	2	A					55	34							
	3	*UC*			38	29								(5.6	3.5)
1972	1	*UC*			37	29								(6.2	3.9)
	2	A					55	34							
	12	*U*					49	33							
1973	1	*UC*			37	29								(5.2	3.3)
	2	A					56	35							
	4	UC			38	34								(4.9	3.5)
1974	1	*UC*			36	31								(5.9	4.0)
	2	A					55	36							
1975	1	*UC*			35	30								(6.2	4.2)
	2	A					54	36							
1976	1	*UC*			33	31								(6.0	4.6)
	2	A					52	38							
	14	UC+A			34	30	40	30						(6.2	4.4)
	14	**A**					48	36							
1977	1	*UC*			32	28								(5.8	4.1)
	2	A					50	34							
	8	U					39	30							
	12	*U*					39	21							
	14	A					37	27							
	14	**A**					45	34							
1978	1	*UC*			31	29								(5.8	4.4)
	2	A					47	35							
	14	A					36	30							
	14	**A**					46	38							
1979	1	*UC*			29	28								(5.8	4.5)
	2	A					47	34							
	14	UC			29	28									
	14	A					35	28							
	14	**A**					43	34							
1980	1	*UC*			26	26								(5.6	4.6)
	8	A					36	28							
	14	UC+A			25	23	29	23						(5.9	4.3)
	14	**A**					39	29							

Table 25.8 *(continued)*

Year	Source[2]	Product[3]	Prevalence[4]						Number of cigarettes						
									Unadjusted[7]			Sales-adjusted[8]			
			Manufactured cigarettes		Total cigarettes[5]		All products[6]		Number/ person/day		Total sales %	Manufactured cigarettes number/ person/day		Total cigarettes[9] number/ person/day	
			M	F	M	F	M	F	M	F		M	F	M	F
1981	1	*UC*			27	28								(5.4	4.3)
	8	A					33	26							
	14	A					29	27							
	14	**A**					36	32							
1982	1	*UC*			28	26								(5.9	4.3)
	8	A					33	27							
	12	*U*					30	30							
	14	A					29	25							
	14	**A**					40	34							
1983	1	*UC*			27	25								(5.6	4.2)
	8	A					31	26							
	14	UC+A					28	24	4.4	3.0	76			5.9	4.0
	14	**A**					37	31							
	15	A					30	23							
1984	8	A					33	27							
	15	A					28	26							
	15	**A**					36	34							
1985	8	A					29	26							
	15	UC+A			23	24	27	25	3.6	3.4	72			4.9	4.8
	15	**A**					36	32							
1986	8	A					28	26							
1987	8	A					29	25							
	15	UC+A			23	24	26	24	4.0	3.2	75			5.2	4.2
	15	**A**					35	30							
1988	8	A					27	25							
1989	8	A					25	25							
1990	8	A					25	25							
1991	8	A					25	23							
1992	8	A					25	26							
1993	8	A					23	23							
1994	8	A					21	23							
1995	8	A					22	23							

1 Surveys covering an age range of at least 21-64 are included. Any gaps in the data for ages 15-20 and 65 years and over are filled in by assumed extensions to the age distribution, given in *Notes on sources of survey data*, p. 617. Method: see *Summary of adult smoking*, p. xxxvi
2 See *Notes on sources of survey data*, p. 617
3 Product: MC = manufactured cigarettes, TC = total cigarettes (including hand-rolled), UC = cigarettes (type unspecified), A = all products, U = unspecified. Frequency of smoking is indicated by: regular or daily smokers in normal type, all smokers (including occasional) in bold, unspecified in italics
4 From Table 25.4
5 This column includes prevalence of smoking classified as UC = cigarettes (type unspecified)
6 This column includes prevalence of smoking classified as U = unspecified product
7 From Table 25.6
8 From Table 25.7, except data in parentheses, which are derived from the prevalence of smoking from Table 25.4 as described in *Summary of adult smoking*, p. xxxvi
9 Number of cigarettes classified as UC = cigarettes (type unspecified) has been adjusted to total cigarette sales and included in this column

Figure 25.3 Estimated prevalence of smoking of (i) cigarettes and (ii) all tobacco products: by year of survey, 1946-1995.
Males and females aged 15 years and over. *Source:* see Table 25.8

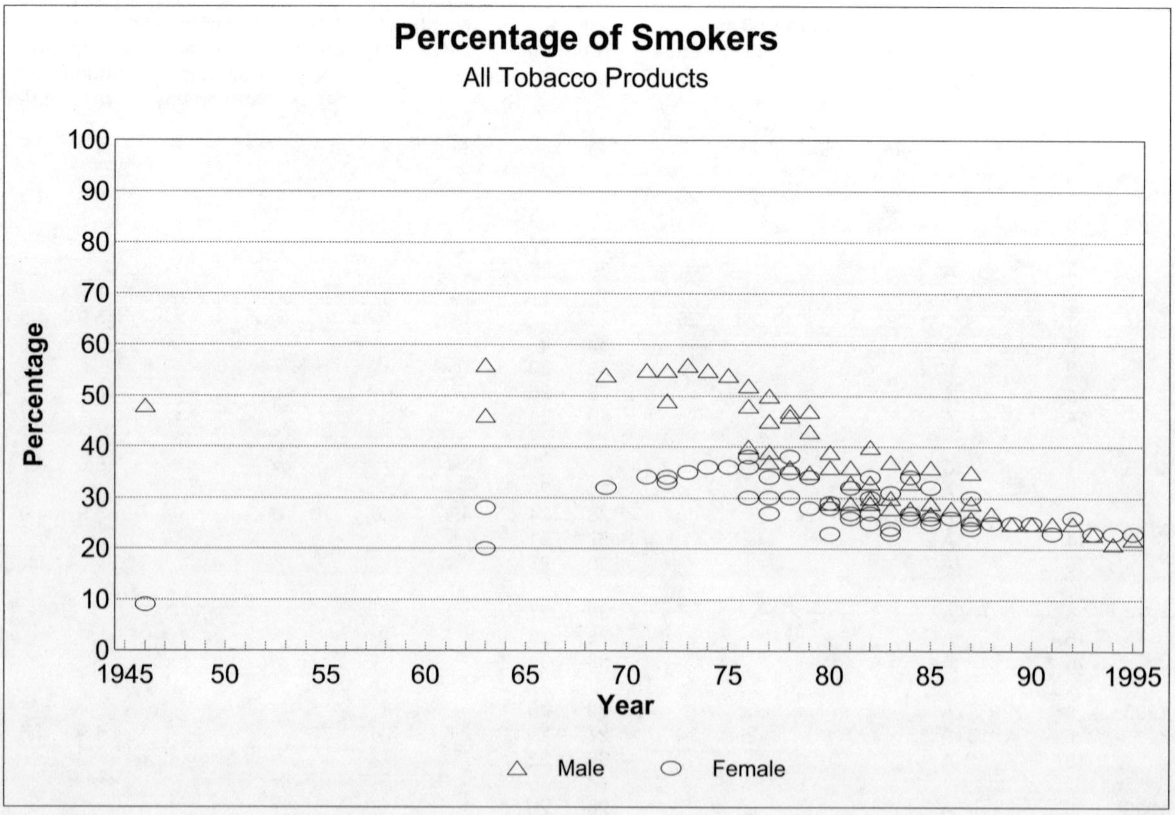

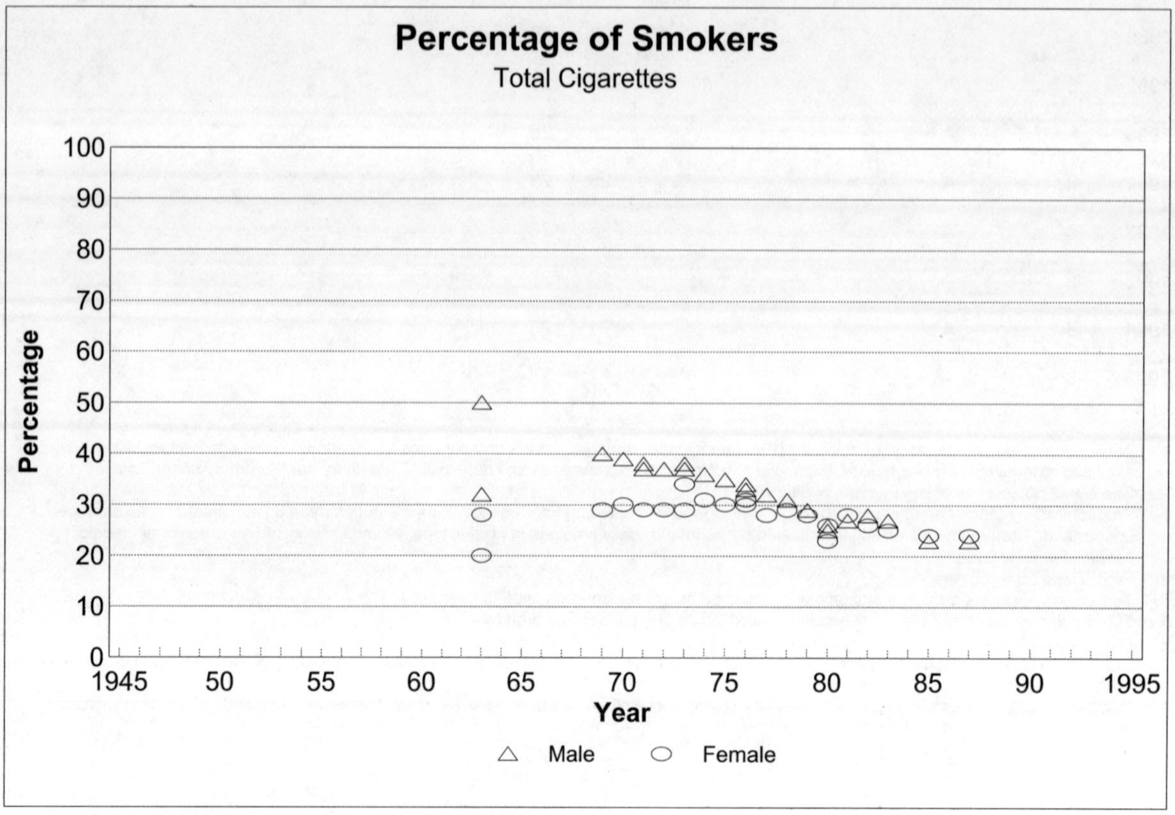

Figure 25.4 Estimated number of cigarettes smoked per person per day, sales-adjusted, 1963-1987.
Males and females aged 15 years and over. *Source:* see Table 25.8

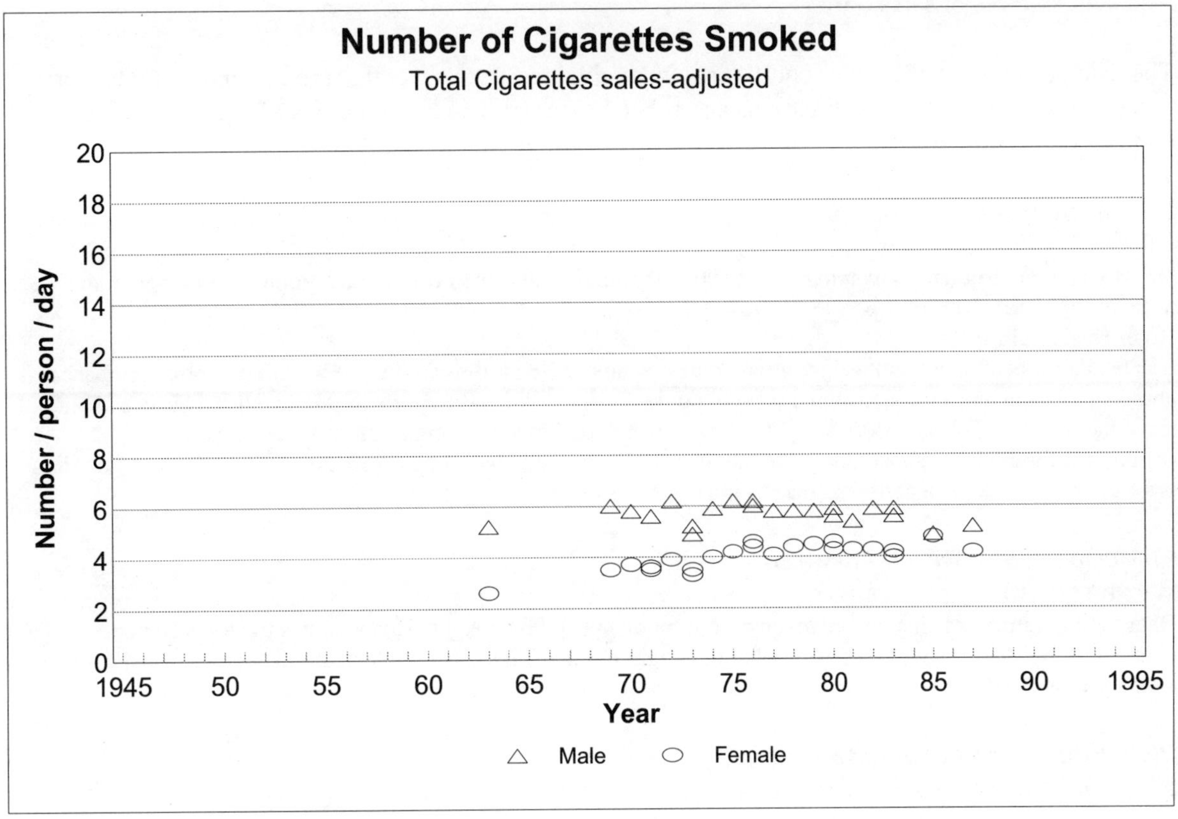

Notes on sources of sales data

The data presented in the tables and figures were obtained from several sources, details of which are given below, together with estimations and related assumptions. Full citations of the sources are given on p. 621 under *References*.

Consumption data before 1974

RP6

Data by weight, originally given to nearest 100 000 pounds, have been converted to tonnes and given to the nearest 10 tonnes (100 000 lbs = 45.359 tonnes).

Notes as given in RP6:

(a) Details of the number and weight of cigarettes, cigars and cigarillos and of the weight of smoking tobacco, chewing tobacco and snuff consumed were obtained from the Annual Reports of the Swedish Tobacco Monopoly (now the Swedish Tobacco Company). Cigarillos were combined with cigars from 1963 onwards.

(b) Figures for cigarette consumption per adult in 1972 and 1973 have been corrected for the effect of hoarding prior to an increase in cigarette tax on 1st January, 1973.

Consumption data for 1974 onwards

Wicklin (1998)

Data for cigarettes and cigars were given both in numbers and by weight. This assumes the tobacco content of a cigarette to be an average of 0.65 g and that of a cigar or cigarillo to be 2 g which are the conventional conversion rates used by WHO.

Plain/Filter cigarette consumption

1960-1981 Maxwell (successive years)

Tar and nicotine yield of cigarettes

1964-1974 Hjern (1976)

1975-1980 Mørck *et al* (1982)

Hjern (1976) gives the sales-weighted mean of domestic brands which made up 80-85 % of the total cigarette market. Mørck *et al* (1982) quote the Swedish tobacco industry.

Lundh *et al* (1977) give details of ten popular cigarette brands in 1975: tar range 12-25 mg, nicotine range 1.0-1.9 mg, weight range 0.61-0.91 g.

The tar yield per cigarette was limited by EC directive (Directive 90/239/EEC) to 15 mg by the end of 1992, and to 12 mg by the end of 1997; nicotine yield is limited to 1.3 mg (Harkin *et al* (1997)).

Estimates of hand-rolled cigarette consumption for 1950-1995

We have taken as our estimate of hand-rolled cigarette consumption 45% of pipe and hand-rolling tobacco sales before 1980, an increasing proportion for 1981-1985 (see table below) and 70% for 1986 onwards, at 1 g per cigarette

There is little evidence on which to base estimates of hand-rolled cigarette consumption before 1980. Mørck *et al* (1982) stated that 'hand-rolled cigarettes account for only 4-5% of the overall cigarette market in 1980'. Assuming l g per hand-rolled cigarette, this represented approximately 45% of pipe and hand-rolling tobacco. This agrees with data from Svenska Tobaks AB for hand-rolling tobacco and pipe tobacco separately, available from 1981-1985, but these data, and data for cigarette papers and filters from 1984, show that consumption of hand-rolled cigarettes rose during the 1980s, both absolutely and relative to other smoking products. In 1985, for instance, they represented 10% of total cigarettes and 74% of pipe and hand-rolling tobacco. However, these data may give a distorted picture since they include border trade to Norway where hand-rolled cigarettes are a major product. To avoid this problem, we use the Svenska Tobaks AB sales data and the estimates in Wicklin (1998) for border trade, and we assume that the border trade consists entirely of hand-rolling tobacco (rather than pipe tobacco), to calculate the following proportions:

Year	% hand-rolling tobacco among pipe and hand-rolling tobacco
1981	42
1982	48
1983	53
1984	64
1985	69

Notes on sources of survey data

Each source of survey data—either an individual survey or a series of surveys repeated over a number of years—is cited by a source number. This number is shown in the tables and corresponds to the source numbers given below, where details of the source publication and of the survey methodology are given. Full citations of the sources are given on p. 621 under *References*.

Source number

1 **Svenska Tobaks AB**
 a. Year given as 1969 represents 1969-1970 etc.
 b. Assumed extension to age distribution for percentage smokers, age 68+: males 15% and females 5%

2 **Mørck *et al* (1982), based on data from Svenska Tobaks**
 a. Smokers: smoked daily

3 **Le Meitour-Kaplan (1977), quoting Swedish Tobacco Company**
 a. Assumed extension to age distribution for percentage smokers, age 68+: males 15% and females 5%

4 **Le Meitour-Kaplan (1977), quoting Nordic Research Association (1973)**
 a. Survey conducted November-December 1973 in four Nordic countries. Total sample size 6 000. Age group not stated (see also Denmark source 3, Norway source 3, and Finland source 8)
 b. Smokers: smoked 'yesterday'

5 **Dr B. Floderus-Myrhed (personal communication)**
 a. Data from Swedish part of Swedish-Finnish twin cohort study. Data for 1967 based on all like-sexed twin pairs born in Sweden 1886-1925 provided that both in a pair were alive in 1967 and that both answered a questionnaire in that year. Corresponding criteria applied to younger cohort born 1926-1958 and where both were alive in 1972

6 **Statistiska Centralbyrån (Central Bureau of Statistics) (1965)**
 a. Representative postal survey. Sample size 55 074. Response rate 89%, increased to 94% by telephone and personal interviews
 b. Consumption category estimation based on 1-3, 4-7, 8-15, 16-25, and 26+ cigarettes/smoker/day
 c. Assumed extension to age distribution for percentage smokers, age 15-17: males (UC/R) 20%, (UC/A) 22%, (A/R) 25%, (A/A) 30%; females 20%. Number of cigarettes/person/day: males 1.0 and females 0.8. For age 70+: males (UC/R) 15%, (UC/A) 20%, (A/R) 25%, (A/A) 30%; females (regular) 2%, (all) 4%. Number of cigarettes/person/day: males 1.0 and females 0.5

7 **Hibell and Jonsson (1977), Nordgren (1980), Ramström (1982a, 1982b)**
 a. Annual survey by Swedish National Board of Education on alcohol, drugs, tobacco and sniffing practices. Random samples of students age 13 and 16 at 187 schools. Anonymous questionnaires completed in class and sealed in envelope, with teachers present.

Year	Sample size			
	Males		Females	
	Age 13	Age 16	Age 13	Age 16
1971	2 521	1 914	2 346	1 921
1972	3 840	3 089	3 697	2 996
1973	2 838	2 789	2 796	2 805
1974	2 720	2 352	2 586	2 282

Response rate in 1972 (age 13 and 16) 88%, other years (age 13) approximately 93%, (age 16) 85%

b. Results for 18-year-olds according to type of course being studied given by Hibell and Jonsson (1977) are not presented here

8 Rosén *et al* (1987), Wicklin (1998), Wersäll and Eklund (1998), Statistika Centralbyrån (1995)

a. Surveys of Living Conditions (Undersknigar on levnadsförhållanden). Annual interview survey of random sample of Swedish population, conducted by Statistics Sweden. Sample size 7 000-15 000 per year. Response rate about 80%

b. There are some minor discrepancies in results presented by the different sources

c. Assumed extension to age distribution for percentage smokers, age 15: males (1977) 20%, (1980-1995) 12% and females (1977) 25%, (1980-1995) 17%. For age 75+ (1977 only): males 20%, and females 5%. For age 85+: males (1980-1982) 20%, (1983-1989) 15%, (1990-1995) 12%; females 3%

9 Nordlund (1998) quoting Swedish Gallup Institute

a. Markedly different estimates of prevalence are given by Hyllienmark (1983), who reports that in the 1940s 75-80% of men and 52% of women smoked

b. Assumed extension to age distribution for percentage smokers, age 15-17: males 20% and females 5%

10 Noppa and Bengtsson (1980)

a. Survey in Göteberg. Population sample 1 462 women, response rate 90%. Ages 38, 46, 50, 54, and 60

11 Holmqvist (1985)

a. Survey in two secondary modern schools in Lund. Sample size (males) 203, (females) 201

12 Adriaanse *et al* (1986), quoting Ramström (1985)

a. Age group no stated

13 Geizerova and Masironi (1988)

a. No original source

14-15 Anonymous (1983, 1984, 1985), Ramström (1986), Ramström and Tibblin (1988), Wersäll and Eklund (1998)

a. Representative survey by NTS (Nationalfoereningen foer upplysning om tobakens skadeverknignar, Swedish National Smoking and Health Association)
Source 14, 1976-1983: Conducted by SIFO. Personal interviews. Response rate 75-80%
Source 15, 1983-1988: Conducted by SCB. Postal questionnaire. Response rate (1983) 83%
Both methods were used in 1983 to compare results. Sample size 2 000-2 500 per year

b. Assumed extension to age distribution for percengage smokers, age 15-17: males UC/R and A/R (1976) 25%, (1977-1979) 20%, (1980-1983) 15%; males A/A (1976) 30%, (1977-1979) 25%, (1980-1983) 20%; females UC/R and A/R (1976) 30%, (1977-1979), 25% (1980-1983) 20%; females A/A (1976) 35%, (1977-1979) 30%, (1980-1983) 25%. For age (1984-1987): males (UC/R and A/R) 12%, (A/A) 15%; females (UC/R and A/R) 17%, (A/A) 20%. For age 71+ or age 75+: males UC/R (1976-1982) 20%, (1983-1987) 15%; males A/R (1976-1982) 25%, (1983-1987) 20%; males A/A (1976-1982) 30%, (1983-1987) 25%; females (UC/R and A/R) 5%, (A/A) 8%. Number of cigarettes/person/day, age 15-17: males 2.0 and females 3.0. For age 71+: males 3.0 and females 0.5. For age 15: males 1.0 and females 2.0. For age 75+: males 2.0 and females 1.0

16-17 WHO (1989), WHO MONICA Project (1988), Wilhelmsen *et al* (1997), Peltonen *et al* (1998)

a. Regional surveys forming part of WHO MONICA project:

	Region	Population size	Sample size	Participation rate (%)	Sample used*		Date
					Male	Female	
16	Göteborg	153 400	1 461	75	685	726	Feb 1985-Nov 1986
17	Northern Sweden	189 700	1 501	84	935	923	Jan 1986-Apr 1986

* 'Sample used' includes age 25-34; all other figures are for age 35-64 only

b. Further surveys were carried out in later years:

	Region	Year	Sample size		Participation rate (%)	
			Males	Females	Males	Females
16	Göteborg	1990	786	789	67	69
16		1995	746	872	64	63
17	Northern Sweden	1990	776	807	78	81
17		1994	748	786	75	79

c. For 1985-1986, *All ages* column relates only to age 35-64 and is standardized to world population. For 1990 on, *All ages* column relates to age 25-64 and (source 17 only) is standardized to the 1990 population in northern Sweden

d. Regular cigarette smokers: smoked cigarettes daily. All regular smokers (source 16): smoked 1 g of tobacco per day (counting 1 cigarette = 1 g, 1 cheroot = 2 g, 1 cigar = 5 g). All smokers (1985-1986): smoked cigarettes daily or occasionally, or smoked 1 g pipe tobacco or 1 cigar per week. Cigarettes per smoker (1985-1986) refers to regular and occasional cigarette smokers

e. Calculation for cigarettes per person (1985-1986) based on % regular cigarette smokers and cigarettes per regular or occasional cigarette smoker, so may underestimate. Consumption category estimation (all products, source 16) based on two categories 1-14 and 15+ g/smoker/day, and resulting figures should be regarded with caution.

f. There are some discrepancies in the results presented by the different sources for Northern Sweden in 1986

18 Janson (1999)

a. Longitudinal study of a cohort recruited in 1955-1957 at the Solna ante-natal clinic. Considered representative of Swedish urban communities. Original participation rate 97%. Response rate at each followup around 80% of survivors, except at age 12 when it dropped to 65% for administrative reasons. Sample size (males) 122, (females) 90

b. Followup interviews were conducted at single years of age, and are shown in Tables 25.4-6 for the midpoint year

c. Regular smokers: smoked daily. All smokers: smoked daily or not daily. Pipe and cigar smoking were included, but are reported to have been infrequent at all ages

d. Consumption category estimation based on 1-2, 3-6, 7-10,11-16, 17-20, >20 cigarette equivalents/smoker/day, counting 1 g tobacco equivalent to 1 cigarette

19 Wicklin (1998) quoting Central Association for Information on Alcohol and Drugs (CAN) (1997)

20 Silfverforsen *et al* (1990) quoting Andersson and Hibell (1989)

a. Nationally representative survey of schoolchildren

21 Nutbeam and Aarø (1990), King and Coles (1992), King *et al* (1996)

a. Part of the HBSC (Health Behaviour in School-Aged Children) Study, a collaborative cross-national research study sponsored by the WHO. School classes or schools were randomly selected, targeting age groups 11 (not presented here), 13 and 15. The target sample size was 1 300 in each age group.

Year	Sample size		Mean age	
	Target age 13	Target age 15	Target Age 13	Target age 15
1986-7	—	1 062	—	—
1989	3 553		13.4	15.4
1993	1 208	1 151	13.5	15.5

c. Smokers marked as frequency *: smoked daily. Regular smokers: smoke once a week or more

22 United States Department of Agriculture (USDA) (1999)

a. No original source. Age group not stated (boys/girls)

23 Hibell *et al* (1997)

a. Nationally representative survey forming part of ESPAD (European School Survey Project on Alcohol and Other Drugs). Target was pupils born in 1979, thus age 15-16 at time of survey in March1995. Approximately 99% of this group still in school. Anonymous questionnaire completed and sealed in envelope by pupil, in class. Teachers present, but discouraged from walking round the classroom. Sample size (males) 1 746, (females) 1 725. Response rate (males) 84%, (females) 87%

b. Regular smokers: smoked 1 or more cigarettes per day in last 30 days. All smokers: smoked in last 30 days

c. Consumption category estimation based on 1-5, 6-10, 11-20, 21+ cigarettes/smoker/day

References

Adriaanse H., van Reek J. and van Zutphen W.M. (1986). Rookgewoonten van atrsen wereldwijd; een overzicht van 100 onderzoekinge naar tabaksgebruik onder artsen in 31 landen in de periode 1951-1985 (Worldwide physicians' smoking habits; a review of 100 surveys into physicians' tobacco consumption in 31 countries in the period 1951-1985. *Ned Tijdschr Geneeskd,* **130**, 2224-9.

Andersson B. and Hibell B. (1989). *Schoolchildren's Drug Habits 1989.* Central Association for Information on Alcohol and Drugs (CAN), Stockholm.§

Anonymous (1983). Tobaksvanor i Sverige 1982. Några resultat från NTS rökvaneundersökning. (Tobacco habits in Sweden, 1982. Some results from the study on smoking habits carried out by the NTS). *Tobaken Och Vi,* **28**, 16-20.

Anonymous (1984). Tobaksvanor i Sverige 1983. (Smoking habits in Sweden 1983). *Tobaken Och Vi,* **29** , 17-9.

Anonymous (1985). Svenska folkets rökvanor 1984. *Tobaken Och Vi,* **30**, 15-7.

Axéll T.E. (1993). Oral mucosal changes related to smokeless tobacco usage: research findings in Scandinavia. *Eur J Cancer,* **29B**, 299-302.

Beese D.H. (ed) (1968). *Tobacco consumption in various countries,* 2nd edition. Tobacco Research Council, London. Research Paper 6.

Beese D.H. (ed) (1972). *Tobacco consumption in various countries,* 3rd edition. Tobacco Research Council, London. Research Paper 6.

Central Association for Information on Alcohol and Drugs (CAN) (1997). *Skolelevers drogvanor.* CAN.§

Geizerova H. and Masironi R. (1988). Cigarette smoking in children and adolescents: world review. In: Aoki M., Hisamichi S. and Tominaga S. (eds) *Smoking and health 1987. Proceedings of the 6th World Conference on Smoking and Health, Tokyo, 9-12 November 1987.* Elsevier Science Publishers B.V. (Biomedical Division), Amsterdam; 601-5. International Congress Series No. 780.

Haglund M. (1988). Development trends in smoking among women in Sweden—an analysis. In: Aoki M., Hisamichi S. and Tominaga S. (eds) *Smoking and health 1987. Proceedings of the 6th World Conference on Smoking and Health, Tokyo, 9-12 November 1987.* Elsevier Science Publishers B.V. (Biomedical Division), Amsterdam; 525-9. International Congress Series No. 780.

Harkin A.M., Anderson P. and Goos C. (1997). *Smoking, drinking and drug taking in the European Region.* Alcohol, Drugs and Tobacco Programme, WHO Regional Office for Europe, Copenhagen.

Hibell B., Andersson B., Bjarnason T., Kokkevi A., Morgan M. and Narusk A. (1997). *The 1995 ESPAD report. The European school survey project on alcohol and other drugs. Alcohol and other drug use among students in 26 European countries.* The Swedish Council for Information on Alcohol and Other Drugs. Council of Europe (Pompidou Group).

Hibell B. and Jonsson E. (1977). Alcohol, drug, tobacco and sniffing practices among Swedish schoolchildren 1971-1974. *British Journal of Addiction,* **72**, 117-27.

Hjern L. (1976). Cigarette smoke tar and nicotine levels in Sweden during the decade 1964-1974. In: Wynder E.L., Hoffmann D. and Gori G.B. (eds) *Modifying the risk for the smoker, Volume I. Proceedings of the Third World Conference on Smoking and Health, New York City, June 2-5, 1975.* US Department of Health, Education and Welfare, USA; 97-102. DHEW Publication No (NIH) 76-1221.

Holmqvist P. (1985). Smoking habits in school-children with 2 years follow-up. *Child Care Health Dev,* **11**, 151-8.

Hyllienmark G. (1983). Rökning, rökfrihet och Könsroller. (Smoking, freedom from smoking and sex roles). *Tobaken Och Vi,* **28**, 16-22.

Janson H. (1999). Longitudinal patterns of tobacco smoking from childhood to middle age. *Addict Behav,* **24**, 239-49.

King A., Wold B., Tudor-Smith C. and Harel Y. (1996). *The health of youth, a cross-national survey.* WHO Regional Publications, Europe, Copenhagen. European Series No. 69.

King A.J.C. and Coles B. (1992). *The health of Canada's youth. Views and behaviours of 11-, 13- and 15-year-olds from 11 countries.* Health and Welfare Canada, Ottawa.

Le Meitour-Kaplan A. (1977). Situational Analysis: Profile of women's smoking habits in Continental Western Europe. In: Steinfeld J., Griffiths W., Ball K. and Taylor R.M. (eds) *Health consequences, education, cessation activities, and social action, Volume II. Proceedings of the Third World Conference on Smoking and Health, New York City, June 2-5, 1975.* US Department of Health, Education and Welfare, USA; 309-27. DHEW Publication No (NIH) 77-1413.

Lee P.N. (ed) (1975). *Tobacco consumption in various countries,* 4th edition. Tobacco Research Council, London. Research Paper 6.

Lundh B., Ohlin P. and Westling H. (1977). Starka och svaga cigarretter—med och utan filter. *Lakartidningen,* **74**, 2356-8.

Maxwell J.C.Jr. (successive years). How the brands ranked. Maxwell International Estimates. *World Tobacco.*

Mørck H.I., Linde J., Agner E., Hein H.O., Gyntelberg F. and Nielsen P.E. (1982). Tobaksforbrug og rygevaner i Norden 1920-1980. (Tobacco consumption and smoking habits in the Nordic countries). *Nord Med,* **97**, 134-46.

Noppa H. and Bengtsson C. (1980). Obesity in relation to smoking: a population study of women in Göteborg, Sweden. *Prev Med,* **9**, 534-43.

Nordgren P. (1980). The Swedish programme: activities in schools and youth organizations. In: Ramström L.M. (ed) *The smoking epidemic, a matter of worldwide concern. Proceedings of the fourth world conference on smoking and health, Stockholm, 1979.* Almqvist & Wiskell International, Stockholm; 287-92.

Nordic Research Association (1973). *1973 Survey. Antalet rökare i fyra nordiska länder i november-december 1973.*[§]

Nordlund L.A. (1998). Trends in smoking habits and lung cancer in Sweden. *Eur J Cancer Prev,* **7**, 109-16.

Nutbeam D. and Aarø L.E. (1990). Smoking and alienation from school: the implications for health education with young people. Results from the WHO study of health behaviour in schoolchildren. In: Durston B. and Jamrozik K. (eds) *Tobacco & health 1990. The global war. Seventh World Conference on Tobacco and Health, Perth, Western Australia, 1-5 April 1990.* Organising Committee of the Seventh World Conference on Tobacco and Health, 189 Royal Street, East Perth, Western Australia 6004; 539-44.

Peltonen M., Huhtasaari F., Stegmayr B., Lundberg V. and Asplund K. (1998). Secular trends in social patterning of cardiovascular risk factor levels in Sweden. The Northern Sweden MONICA Study 1986-1994. *J Intern Med,* **244**, 1-9.

Ramström L. (1985). Extrapolations of several studies on smoking in Sweden. *Norske Statens Tobakskarderet.*[§]

Ramström L.M. (1982a). Fortschritte gegen das Rauchen in Schweden. In: *Rauchen oder Gesundheit. Politische, präventive und therapeutische Aspekte. Kongress zum Weltgesundheitstag 1980 in Bonn-Bad Godesberg.* Neuland-Verlagsgesellschaft mbH, Hamburg; 17-23.

Ramström L.M. (1982b). National action in Sweden. In: Fontana F. (ed) *Tabacco e giovani (Tobacco and youth), International conference, Venice 9-11 November 1981.* ATTI, Venice; 119-22.

Ramström L.M. (1986). *Tobaksvanor i Sverige 1985. Resultat från NTS-Undersökningen 1985. (Tobacco habits in Sweden 1985. Results from an NTS study 1985).* NTS, Stockholm. Tema Tobak Nr. 3.

Ramström L.M. (1990). Smokeless tobacco—a potential gateway to smoking. In: Durston B. and Jamrozik K. (eds) *Tobacco & health 1990. The global war. Seventh World Conference on Tobacco and Health, Perth, Western Australia, 1-5 April 1990.* Organising Committee of the Seventh World Conference on Tobacco and Health, 189 Royal Street, East Perth, Western Australia 6004; 451-2.

Ramström L.M. and Tibblin H. (1988). *Tobaksvanor i Sverige 1987. Resultat från NTS-undersökning 1987. (Tobacco habits in Sweden 1987. Results from study of National Association against Tobacco Damage 1987).* NTS, Stockholm. Tema Tobak Nr. 7.

Rosén M., Wall S., Hanning M., Lindberg G. and Nyström L. (1987). Smoking habits and their confounding effects among occupational groups in Sweden. *Scand J Soc Med,* **15**, 233-40.

RP6, See Beese (ed) (1968), Beese (ed) (1972), Lee (ed) (1975)

Silfverforsen L., Nygren A. and Bolinder G. (1990). The Swedish Society of Medicine's and the Folksam Group's action programme against the use of tobacco. In: Durston B. and Jamrozik K. (eds) *Tobacco & health 1990. The global war. Seventh World Conference on Tobacco and Health, Perth, Western Australia, 1-5 April 1990.* Organising Committee of the Seventh World Conference on Tobacco and Health, 189 Royal Street, East Perth, Western Australia 6004; 324-6.

Statistika Centralbyrån (1995). *Tobacco consumption 1970-1994 in the member states of the European Union and in Norway and Iceland.* European Commission.

Statistiska Centralbyrån (Central Bureau of Statistics) (1965). *Rökvanor i Sverige. En postenkätundersökning våren 1963. (Smoking habits in Sweden. A mail survey—spring 1963).* Statistiska Centralbyrån, Utredningsinstitutet, Stockholm.

USDA (1999). *Tobacco annual report for Sweden 1999.* (Foreign Agriculture Service GAIN Report (Global Agriculture Information Network) .) GAIN Report #SW9007. http://www.fas.usda.gov/webmap.html then 'Attache Reports'.

Wersäll J.P. and Eklund G. (1998). The decline of smoking among Swedish men. *Int J Epidemiol,* **27**, 20-6.

WHO (1989). The WHO MONICA project: a worldwide monitoring system for cardiovascular diseases. In: *World health statistics annual 1989.* WHO, Geneva; 25-149.

WHO MONICA Project (1988). Geographical variation in the major risk factors of coronary heart disease in men and women aged 35-64 years. *World Health Stat Q,* **41**, 115-40.

Wicklin B. (ed) (1998). *Tobaksstatistik 1970-1997. Konsumtion av tobaksvaror, priser, inkomster, rökvanor, handel och illegala tillförseln mm i Sverige, Norge, Danmark och Finland (Tobacco statistics 1970-1997. Consumption of tobacco products prices income, smoking habits, trade and attempted smuggling etc. in Sweden, Norway, Denmark and Finland).* Svenska tobaksbranschföreninger, Örebro, Sweden.

Wilhelmsen L., Johansson S., Rosengren A., Wallin I., Dotevall A. and Lappas G. (1997). Risk factors for cardiovascular disease during the period 1985-1995 in Göteborg, Sweden. The GOT-MONICA Project. *J Intern Med,* **242**, 199-211.

§ Original paper not obtained, but information taken as quoted by another author

Switzerland 26

Sales data

See Tables 26.1-26.3.
Data are available since 1934, but from 1974 they are incomplete and conflicting. They include sales to tourists and frontier zone traffic but, at least from the main source, exclude imports.

From 1934 until 1972 the consumption of manufactured cigarettes per adult increased, with some fluctuations, reaching a peak of nearly 11 cigarettes per day. Thereafter consumption decreased to 8 cigarettes per day in the 1980s. No information on smoking of hand-rolled cigarettes is available.

The consumption of tobacco products per adult increased, with some fluctuations, from 6 g per day in 1934 to 12-13 g at the beginning of the 1970s. Thereafter we have not been able to estimate the total tobacco consumption. In the mid-1930s, 25% of all tobacco was consumed in manufactured cigarettes. This proportion increased to about 80% in the early 1970s; consumption of both cigars and smoking tobacco was higher than cigarettes before the war, but decreased to 17% and 4% respectively.

Trümpy (1983) summarized the development of smoking in Switzerland as follows: 'According to Swiss documents, a resistance initially arose against smoking, which was imported from America and propagated mainly among soldiers, but it eventually became increasingly tolerated. Outdoor smoking was disapproved of up to the mid-nineteenth century, and women were not allowed to indulge in cigarette smoking before 1918; since 1945, it has increased in both sexes. Medical warning began extensively only after 1970'.

Survey data

See Tables 26.4-26.8
Apart from a survey in a rural area in the 1950s, no data on adult smoking are available before the 1970s. Nationally based surveys generally showed that the prevalence of tobacco smoking among men aged 15 years and over fell from about 50-60% in the mid-1970s to 35-40% in the 1990s. The prevalence of cigarette smoking was about 8 percentage points lower when reported separately (source 1). Over the same period, the prevalence among women fell from about 30-40% to 25-30%. Very few women smoke products other than cigarettes.

In general, more men smoked than women at all ages, but from the mid-1970s some surveys show that there were more young women who smoked than young men. A lower percentage of smokers in older age groups was more marked in women than in men. The prevalence of smoking other products but not cigarettes increased with age, for instance in 1975, other products were smoked by 2% of men under age 25, but by 15% over age 55.

Comparison of survey and sales data suggests that surveys under-reported consumption by 30-55%. Between 1972 and 1993, the estimated number of cigarettes smoked per person per day (sales-adjusted) decreased for men from about 15 to 10, while for women it remained around 6. However, these sales-adjusted figures may overestimate consumption by the Swiss population.

Table 26.1.1 Total annual sales of tobacco products, 1920-1973

Year	Cigarettes		Cigars		Smoking tobacco	All tobacco products
	tonnes	millions	tonnes	millions	tonnes	tonnes
1934-1937	1720	1728	2400	481	2630	6760
1938-1940	2270	2262	2490	500	2540	7300
1941	2720	2746	3040	611	2770	8530
1942	2720	2715	2860	573	2770	8350
1943	3180	3167	2860	567	2590	8620
1944	3450	3444	2490	499	2310	8260
1945	3950	3964	2360	473	2090	8390
1946	4400	4416	2860	569	2950	10210
1947	4990	5009	2990	597	2490	10480
1948	4990	4989	2810	559	2180	9980
1949	5130	5143	2180	437	2130	9430
1950	5400	5405	2220	440	2220	9840
1951	5400	5672	2360	470	2220	9980
1952	6210	6222	2400	477	2130	10750
1953	5900	6191	2450	489	2130	10480
1954	5940	6236	2400	478	2040	10390
1955	6300	6625	2540	504	2000	10840
1956	6760	7081	2400	477	1950	11110
1957	6800	7488	2270	454	1860	10930
1958	7480	8248	2490	502	1860	11840
1959	7760	8557	2450	492	1860	12070
1960	8850	9751	2400	478	1680	12930
1961	9840	10866	2590	517	1720	14150
1962	10610	11691	2950	588	1680	15240
1963	11970	11986	2900	582	1720	16600
1964	11570	11550	3180	639	1630	16370
1965	13740	13728	3080	620	1590	18420
1966	11070	11051	3130	624	1360	15560
1967	12700	12715	3180	634	1410	17280
1968	13610	13603	3310	661	1320	18230
1969	15420	15427	3270	650	1270	19960
1970	16280	16300	3310	662	1220	20820
1971	17870	17900	3360	679	1000	22230
1972	18690	18700	3670	744	1000	23360
1973	16470	16500	3580	727	910	20960

Source: see *Notes on sources of sales data*, p. 640

Table 26.1.2 Total annual sales of Swiss produced tobacco products, 1974-1995

Year	Cigarettes sales millions	Cigars production millions	Pipe and hand-rolling tobacco production tonnes	Tessin specialities (cigars)[1]	
				Toscani production millions	Brissago production millions
1974	16479	597	983	20	37
1975	15493	468	880	17	34
1976	15317	438	821	15	34
1977	15906	430	807	14	34
1978	15369	393	739	11	31
1979	15038	339	679	10	30
1980	15381	360	707	10	29
1981	15689	353	647	9	27
1982	15991	334	621	8	26
1983	16305	266	573	8	23
1984	16163	260	532	8	23
1985	15793	262	497	7	22
1986	15823	250	432	7	21
1987	15886	241	403	6	20
1988	15855	219	348	6	17
1989	15964	219	354	6	17
1990	15890	208	299	5	17
1991	16050	197	294	5	16
1992	16926	197	272	6	15
1993	15929	177	255	6	14
1994	15592	155	214	5	14
1995	15507	158	189	4	14

1 The column headed 'Cigars' excludes these products

Source : see *Notes on sources of sales data,* p. 640

Table 26.1.3 Total annual production, import, export and sales of tobacco products, 1974-1989

Year	Cigarettes (millions)				Cigars (millions)				Pipe tobacco (tonnes)			
	prod'n	import	export	sales	prod'n	import	export	sales	prod'n	import	export	sales
1971	30935	993	12287	19641	762	27			1017	2058		
1972	32026	1014	15000	18040	771	24			1007	2616		
1973	31075	759	14000	17834	750	27			904	3627		
1974	27995	175	11000	17170	666	31			983	2160		
1975	26726	145	10624	16247	529	41			880	2250		
1976	27788	338	12761	15365	493	46			821	2063		
1977	30537	328	14213	16652	483	57			807	2328		
1978	29734	268	14432	15570	441	57			739	2210		
1979	29281	215	14002	15494	389	79			678	2377		
1980	31264	199	15125	16338	407	111			707	2543		
1981	27569	208	12498	15279	394	120			647	2690		
1982	26497	188	10293	16392	373	115			621	2654		
1983	25681	210	9465	16426	300	80			573	2718		
1984	25449	230	9150	16529	294	79	16	357	531	2740	598	2673
1985	23150	228	6940	16438	294	77	15	356	497	2726	702	2521
1986	23556	185	7739	16002	281	79	13	347	432	2588	605	2415
1987	24863	197	8660	16400	270	71	14	327	403	2710	508	2605
1988	27074	297	11065	16306	245	75	11	309	348	2441	574	2215
1989	28059	359	12290	16128	244	79	12	311	354	2580	388	2546

Source : see *Notes on sources of sales data,* p. 640

Table 26.1.4 Manufactured cigarettes (i) percentage of total sales as filter cigarettes, 1945-1991 and (ii) sales-weighted average tar yield per cigarette (SWAT), 1970-1978

Year	% Filter	SWAT mg / cig	Year	% Filter	SWAT mg / cig
1945	5.5		1975	94.0	15.6
1950	23.8		1976	96.1	14
1955	49.9		1977	96.6	13
			1978	96.8	13
1960	74.7		1979	96.9	
1961	77.4				
1962	78.7		1980	97.3	
1963	81.3		1981	97.0	
1964	83.8		1982	96.8	
1965	85.3		1983	97.1	
1966	86.5		1984	97.2	
1967	87.9		1985	97.2	
1968	89.2		1986	97.5	
1969	90.8		1987	97.8	
			1988	98.1	
1970	92.9	24.3	1989	98.3	
1971	94.4	20.1			
1972	94.7	18.8	1990	98.6	
1973	94.7	18.4	1991	98.8	
1974	93.0	17.4			

Source : see *Notes on sources of sales data*, p. 640

Table 26.2 Consumption of (i) cigarettes and (ii) all tobacco products, 1920-1995 sales-based data, including estimated hand-rolled cigarette consumption. Males and females aged 15 years and over

Year	Manufactured cigarettes		Hand-rolled cigarettes		Total cigarettes		All tobacco products	
	Total annual in millions	Number/ adult/day	Total annual in millions	Number/ adult/day	Total annual in millions	Number/ adult/day	Total annual in tonnes	Grams/ adult/day
1934-1937	1728	1.5					6760	5.8
1938-1940	2262	1.9					7300	6.1
1941	2746	2.3					8530	7.1
1942	2715	2.3					8350	6.9
1943	3167	2.6					8620	6.9
1944	3444	2.8					8260	6.7
1945	3964	3.2					8390	6.8
1946	4416	3.5					10210	8.0
1947	5009	3.9					10480	8.2
1948	4989	3.9					9980	7.8
1949	5143	3.9					9430	7.2
1950	5405	4.1					9840	7.5
1951	5672	4.3					9980	7.6
1952	6222	4.7					10750	8.0
1953	6191	4.6					10480	7.8
1954	6236	4.6					10390	7.6
1955	6625	4.8					10840	7.9
1956	7081	5.1					11110	8.0
1957	7488	5.3					10930	7.7
1958	8248	5.8					11840	8.3
1959	8557	5.9					12070	8.3

Table 26.2 *(continued)*

Year	Manufactured cigarettes		Hand-rolled cigarettes		Total cigarettes		All tobacco products	
	Total annual in millions	Number/ adult/day	Total annual in millions	Number/ adult/day	Total annual in millions	Number/ adult/day	Total annual in tonnes	Grams/ adult/day
1960	9751	6.6					12930	8.8
1961	10866	7.2					14150	9.4
1962	11691	7.6					15240	9.9
1963	11986	7.6					16600	10.5
1964	11550	7.2					16370	10.2
1965	13728	8.5					18420	11.4
1966	11051	6.7					15560	9.5
1967	12715	7.7					17280	10.4
1968	13603	8.1					18230	10.8
1969	15427	9.0					19960	11.7
1970	16300	9.5					20820	12.1
1971	17900	10.3					22230	12.8
1972	18700	10.7					23360	13.3
1973	16500	9.3					20960	11.8
1974	16479	9.2						
1975	15493	8.6						
1976	15317	8.5						
1977	15906	8.8						
1978	15369	8.5						
1979	15038	8.2						
1980	15381	8.3						
1981	15689	8.4						
1982	15991	8.4						
1983	16305	8.5						
1984	16163	8.4						
1985	15793	8.1						
1986	15823	8.1						
1987	15886	8.0						
1988	15855	7.9						
1989	15964	7.9						
1990	15890	7.8						
1991	16050	7.8						
1992	16926	8.2						
1993	15929	7.6						
1994	15592	7.4						
1995	15507	7.4						

Source : see *Notes on sources of sales data*, p. 640

Figure 26.1 Daily consumption of (i) manufactured and total number of cigarettes, and (ii) all tobacco products, 1934-1995.
Males and females aged 15 years and over. *Source:* see Table 26.2

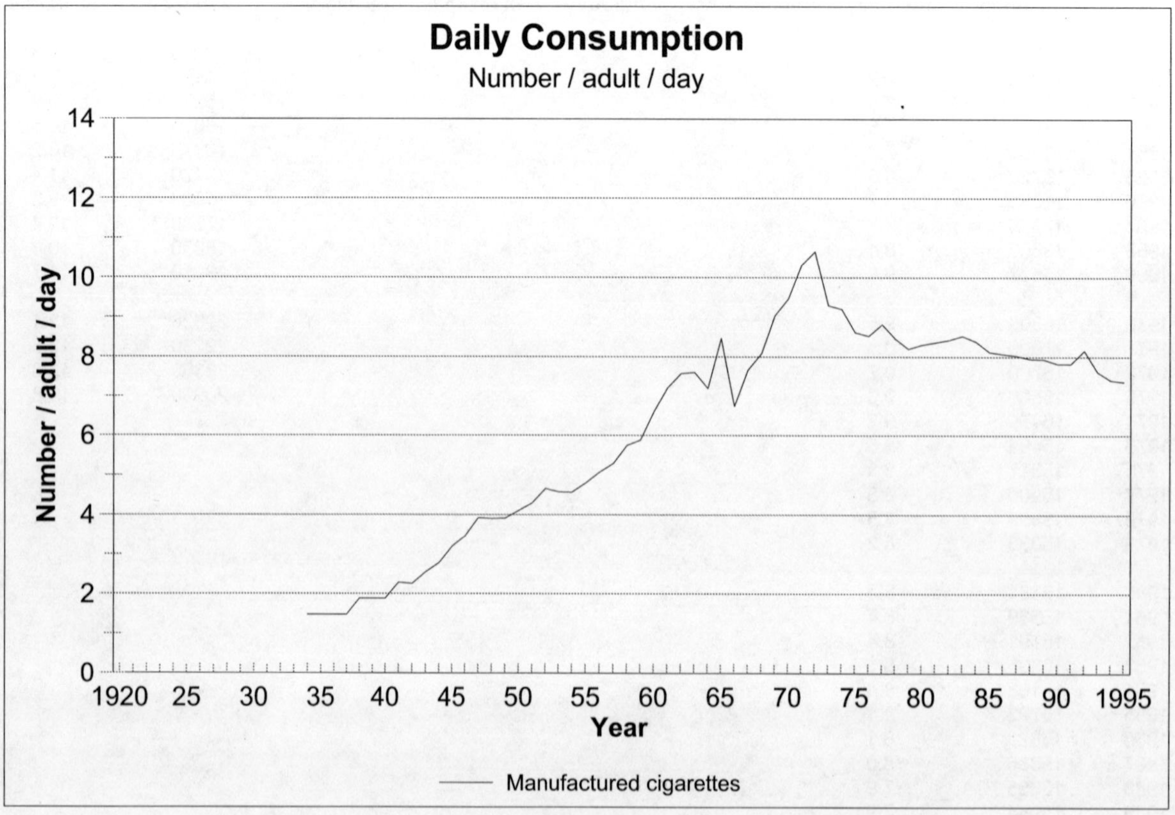

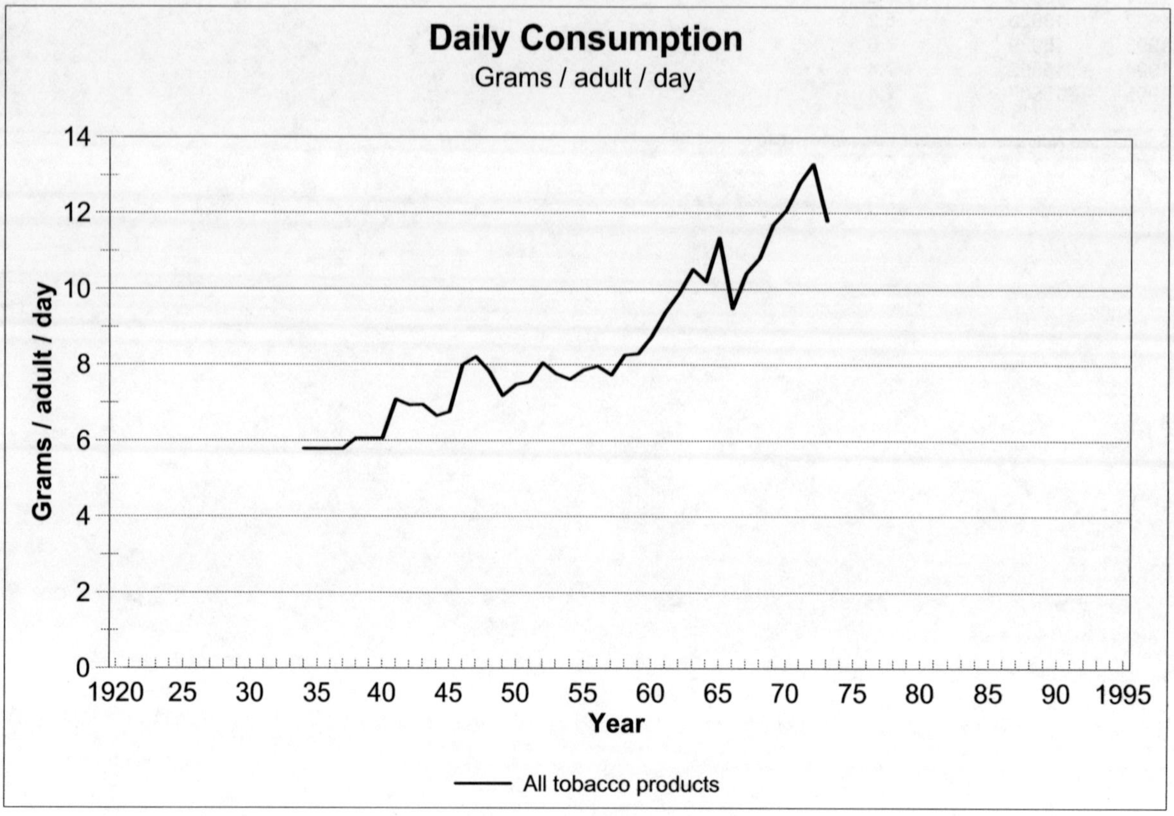

Table 26.3 Percentage sales of tobacco in different forms (by weight), selected years 1935-1973

Year	Cigarettes (%)	Cigars (%)	Smoking tobacco (%)
1935	25.4	35.5	38.9
1945	47.1	28.1	24.9
1955	58.1	23.4	18.5
1965	74.6	16.7	8.6
1973	78.6	17.1	4.3

Source : calculated from Table 26.1.1

Figure 26.2 Percentage sales of tobacco in different forms (by weight), selected years 1925-1995
Source: see Table 26.3

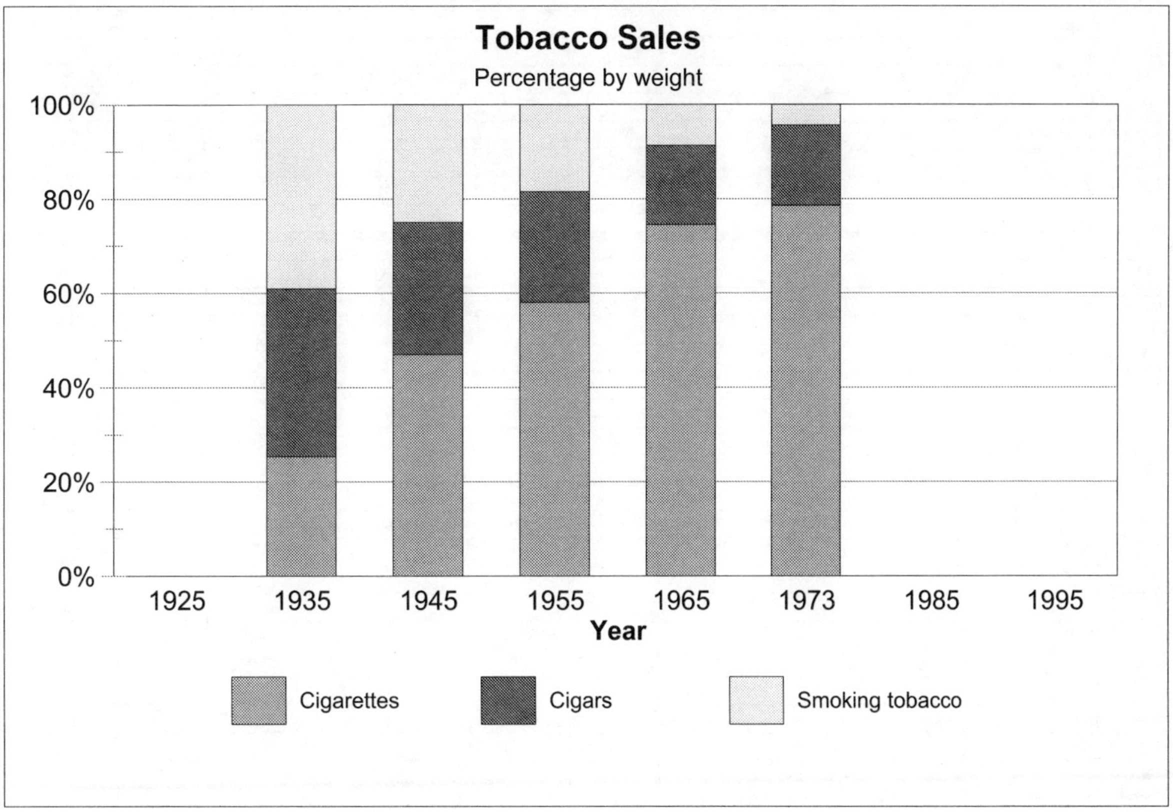

Table 26.4M Prevalence of smoking, males: some selected Swiss surveys by age, 1956-1994

Frequency / Product / Source / Year	12	13	14	15	16	17	18	19	20-24	25-29	30-34	35-39	40-44	45-49	50-54	55-59	60-64	65-69	70-74	75-79	80+	All ages
56 13 UC R								42				37			19				4			28
56 13 A R								50				60			62				48			55
71 3 UC R								55														
71 6 U U													44									
71 14 UC R																						
71 14 UC A																						
73 5 A R								60														
74 2 U U						58				69				62				52				61
75 1 UC *						27				41			37					32				35
75 1 UC R						34				49			44					36				42
75 1 A R						36				55			57					51				52
77 2 U U						46				51				54				34				48
77 4 A R							43				51					47						
78 3 UC R								43														
78 15 UC R																33						
78 15 A R																40						
79 16 UC U										39			34			30						35
79 16 A U										52			50			50						51
80 2 U U						48				59				53				33				50
80 4 A R							47				45					46						
81 1 UC *						36				45			33					18				33
81 1 UC R						40				53			38					20				38
81 1 A R						40				58			49					31				46
81 8 U U						30																
82 7 UC U									41		44		39			33		28		26		37
83 2 U A						43				46				43				34				42
85 9 UC R										38		34			34		28					32
85 9 A A										49		47			50		45					47
85 10 UC R												43			37		33					38
85 10 A A												53			46		40					47
86 2 U A						31				42				36				23				34
86 11 U *		2		10																		
86 11 U R		3		13																		
86 11 U A		13		22																		
86 17 U R		2		13																		
87 2 U U						30				46			40					38				41
89 2 U A						37				50				43				30				41
89 9 UC R										44		38			31		31		15			
89 9 A A										52		50			45		42		33			
89 10 UC R												33			30		27					
89 10 A A												40			38		31					
90 2 U A						35				50				41				30				39
91 2 U A						33				45				43				30				39
92 2 U A						32				44				37				28				36
92 2 U A						24			43	43	46	44	41			37		29				37
92 12 U A						29			42	45	41	42	42			33		26				37
93 2 U A											41											
94 11 UC R		5		17																		
94 17 UC *				11																		
94 17 UC R		4		16																		

Source: see *Notes on sources of survey data*, p. 641

Product: MC = manufactured cigarettes
TC = total cigarettes (including hand-rolled)
UC = cigarettes (type unspecified)
A = all products

Frequency: A = all smokers (including occasional)
R = regular or daily smokers

All ages: relevant to ages used and as given in original source

U = unspecified

* = refer to *Notes on sources of survey data*, p. 641

Table 26.4F Prevalence of smoking, females: some selected Swiss surveys by age, 1956-1994

<table>
<tr><th rowspan="2">Frequency
Product
Source
Year</th><th colspan="22">Age group</th></tr>
<tr><th>12</th><th>13</th><th>14</th><th>15</th><th>16</th><th>17</th><th>18</th><th>19</th><th>20-24</th><th>25-29</th><th>30-34</th><th>35-39</th><th>40-44</th><th>45-49</th><th>50-54</th><th>55-59</th><th>60-64</th><th>65-69</th><th>70-74</th><th>75-79</th><th>80+</th><th>All ages</th></tr>
<tr><td>56 13 UC R</td><td></td><td></td><td></td><td></td><td></td><td></td><td></td><td></td><td></td><td></td><td></td><td></td><td></td><td></td><td></td><td></td><td></td><td></td><td></td><td></td><td></td><td></td></tr>
<tr><td>56 13 A R</td><td></td><td></td><td></td><td></td><td></td><td></td><td></td><td></td><td></td><td></td><td></td><td></td><td></td><td></td><td></td><td></td><td></td><td></td><td></td><td></td><td></td><td></td></tr>
<tr><td>71 3 UC R</td><td></td><td></td><td></td><td></td><td></td><td></td><td></td><td>41</td><td></td><td></td><td></td><td></td><td></td><td></td><td></td><td></td><td></td><td></td><td></td><td></td><td></td><td></td></tr>
<tr><td>71 6 U U</td><td></td><td></td><td></td><td></td><td colspan="17">26</td><td></td></tr>
<tr><td>71 14 UC R</td><td></td><td></td><td></td><td></td><td></td><td>36</td><td>26</td><td>25</td><td>18></td><td></td><td></td><td></td><td></td><td></td><td></td><td></td><td></td><td></td><td></td><td></td><td></td><td>26</td></tr>
<tr><td>71 14 UC A</td><td></td><td></td><td></td><td></td><td></td><td colspan="3">42</td><td></td><td></td><td></td><td></td><td></td><td></td><td></td><td></td><td></td><td></td><td></td><td></td><td></td><td></td></tr>
<tr><td>73 5 A R</td><td></td><td></td><td></td><td></td><td></td><td></td><td></td><td></td><td></td><td></td><td></td><td></td><td></td><td></td><td></td><td></td><td></td><td></td><td></td><td></td><td></td><td></td></tr>
<tr><td>74 2 U U</td><td></td><td></td><td></td><td colspan="6">49</td><td colspan="2">49</td><td colspan="5">40</td><td colspan="3">14</td><td></td><td></td><td>40</td></tr>
<tr><td>75 1 UC *</td><td></td><td></td><td></td><td colspan="6">46</td><td colspan="2">46</td><td colspan="4">26</td><td colspan="4">14</td><td></td><td></td><td>29</td></tr>
<tr><td>75 1 UC R</td><td></td><td></td><td></td><td colspan="6">46</td><td colspan="2">46</td><td colspan="4">26</td><td colspan="4">14</td><td></td><td></td><td>29</td></tr>
<tr><td>75 1 A R</td><td></td><td></td><td></td><td colspan="6">46</td><td colspan="2">46</td><td colspan="4">26</td><td colspan="4">14</td><td></td><td></td><td>29</td></tr>
<tr><td>77 2 U U</td><td></td><td></td><td></td><td colspan="6">46</td><td colspan="2">48</td><td colspan="5">33</td><td colspan="3">17</td><td></td><td></td><td>37</td></tr>
<tr><td>77 4 A R</td><td></td><td></td><td></td><td></td><td colspan="5">41</td><td colspan="4">29</td><td colspan="5">15</td><td></td><td></td><td></td><td></td></tr>
<tr><td>78 3 UC R</td><td></td><td></td><td></td><td></td><td></td><td></td><td></td><td>44</td><td></td><td></td><td></td><td></td><td></td><td></td><td></td><td></td><td></td><td></td><td></td><td></td><td></td><td></td></tr>
<tr><td>78 15 UC R</td><td></td><td></td><td></td><td></td><td></td><td></td><td></td><td></td><td></td><td colspan="12">25</td><td></td></tr>
<tr><td>78 15 A R</td><td></td><td></td><td></td><td></td><td></td><td></td><td></td><td></td><td></td><td colspan="12">25</td><td></td></tr>
<tr><td>79 16 UC U</td><td></td><td></td><td></td><td></td><td></td><td></td><td></td><td></td><td colspan="3">36</td><td colspan="3">22</td><td colspan="3">11</td><td></td><td></td><td></td><td></td><td>25</td></tr>
<tr><td>79 16 A U</td><td></td><td></td><td></td><td></td><td></td><td></td><td></td><td></td><td colspan="3">36</td><td colspan="3">23</td><td colspan="3">11</td><td></td><td></td><td></td><td></td><td>26</td></tr>
<tr><td>80 2 U U</td><td></td><td></td><td></td><td colspan="6">45</td><td colspan="2">40</td><td colspan="5">36</td><td colspan="3">13</td><td></td><td></td><td>35</td></tr>
<tr><td>80 4 A R</td><td></td><td></td><td></td><td></td><td colspan="5">41</td><td colspan="4">28</td><td colspan="5">17</td><td></td><td></td><td></td><td></td></tr>
<tr><td>81 1 UC *</td><td></td><td></td><td></td><td colspan="6">42</td><td colspan="2">46</td><td colspan="4">28</td><td colspan="4">11</td><td></td><td></td><td>28</td></tr>
<tr><td>81 1 UC R</td><td></td><td></td><td></td><td colspan="6">42</td><td colspan="2">46</td><td colspan="4">28</td><td colspan="4">11</td><td></td><td></td><td>28</td></tr>
<tr><td>81 1 A R</td><td></td><td></td><td></td><td colspan="6">42</td><td colspan="2">46</td><td colspan="4">28</td><td colspan="4">11</td><td></td><td></td><td>28</td></tr>
<tr><td>81 8 U U</td><td></td><td></td><td></td><td colspan="6">43</td><td></td><td></td><td></td><td></td><td></td><td></td><td></td><td></td><td></td><td></td><td></td><td></td><td></td></tr>
<tr><td>82 7 UC U</td><td></td><td></td><td></td><td></td><td></td><td></td><td></td><td></td><td colspan="2">37</td><td colspan="2">28</td><td colspan="2">21</td><td colspan="2">16</td><td colspan="2">11</td><td colspan="3">5</td><td>22</td></tr>
<tr><td>83 2 U A</td><td></td><td></td><td></td><td colspan="6">38</td><td colspan="2">39</td><td colspan="5">26</td><td colspan="3">12</td><td></td><td></td><td>30</td></tr>
<tr><td>85 9 UC R</td><td></td><td></td><td></td><td></td><td></td><td></td><td></td><td></td><td></td><td colspan="2">33</td><td colspan="2">31</td><td colspan="2">15</td><td colspan="2">13</td><td></td><td></td><td></td><td></td><td>21</td></tr>
<tr><td>85 9 A A</td><td></td><td></td><td></td><td></td><td></td><td></td><td></td><td></td><td></td><td colspan="2">41</td><td colspan="2">40</td><td colspan="2">26</td><td colspan="2">16</td><td></td><td></td><td></td><td></td><td>29</td></tr>
<tr><td>85 10 UC R</td><td></td><td></td><td></td><td></td><td></td><td></td><td></td><td></td><td></td><td></td><td></td><td colspan="2">28</td><td colspan="2">25</td><td colspan="2">17</td><td></td><td></td><td></td><td></td><td>24</td></tr>
<tr><td>85 10 A A</td><td></td><td></td><td></td><td></td><td></td><td></td><td></td><td></td><td></td><td></td><td></td><td colspan="2">34</td><td colspan="2">29</td><td colspan="2">18</td><td></td><td></td><td></td><td></td><td>28</td></tr>
<tr><td>86 2 U A</td><td></td><td></td><td></td><td colspan="6">30</td><td colspan="2">40</td><td colspan="5">27</td><td colspan="3">10</td><td></td><td></td><td>28</td></tr>
<tr><td>86 11 U *</td><td></td><td>2</td><td></td><td>12</td><td></td><td></td><td></td><td></td><td></td><td></td><td></td><td></td><td></td><td></td><td></td><td></td><td></td><td></td><td></td><td></td><td></td><td></td></tr>
<tr><td>86 11 U R</td><td></td><td>3</td><td></td><td>16</td><td></td><td></td><td></td><td></td><td></td><td></td><td></td><td></td><td></td><td></td><td></td><td></td><td></td><td></td><td></td><td></td><td></td><td></td></tr>
<tr><td>86 11 U A</td><td></td><td>9</td><td></td><td>27</td><td></td><td></td><td></td><td></td><td></td><td></td><td></td><td></td><td></td><td></td><td></td><td></td><td></td><td></td><td></td><td></td><td></td><td></td></tr>
<tr><td>86 17 U R</td><td></td><td>2</td><td></td><td>14</td><td></td><td></td><td></td><td></td><td></td><td></td><td></td><td></td><td></td><td></td><td></td><td></td><td></td><td></td><td></td><td></td><td></td><td></td></tr>
<tr><td>87 2 U U</td><td></td><td></td><td></td><td colspan="6">33</td><td colspan="2">44</td><td colspan="4">23</td><td colspan="4">13</td><td></td><td></td><td>29</td></tr>
<tr><td>89 2 U A</td><td></td><td></td><td></td><td colspan="6">33</td><td colspan="2">42</td><td colspan="5">29</td><td colspan="3">13</td><td></td><td></td><td>30</td></tr>
<tr><td>89 9 UC R</td><td></td><td></td><td></td><td></td><td></td><td></td><td></td><td></td><td></td><td colspan="2">36</td><td colspan="2">33</td><td colspan="2">20</td><td colspan="2">16</td><td colspan="2">10</td><td></td><td></td><td></td></tr>
<tr><td>89 9 A A</td><td></td><td></td><td></td><td></td><td></td><td></td><td></td><td></td><td></td><td colspan="2">41</td><td colspan="2">37</td><td colspan="2">27</td><td colspan="2">19</td><td colspan="2">13</td><td></td><td></td><td></td></tr>
<tr><td>89 10 UC R</td><td></td><td></td><td></td><td></td><td></td><td></td><td></td><td></td><td></td><td></td><td></td><td colspan="2">31</td><td colspan="2">29</td><td colspan="2">16</td><td></td><td></td><td></td><td></td><td></td></tr>
<tr><td>89 10 A A</td><td></td><td></td><td></td><td></td><td></td><td></td><td></td><td></td><td></td><td></td><td></td><td colspan="2">34</td><td colspan="2">31</td><td colspan="2">16</td><td></td><td></td><td></td><td></td><td></td></tr>
<tr><td>90 2 U A</td><td></td><td></td><td></td><td colspan="6">30</td><td colspan="2">43</td><td colspan="5">29</td><td colspan="3">11</td><td></td><td></td><td>29</td></tr>
<tr><td>91 2 U A</td><td></td><td></td><td></td><td colspan="6">35</td><td colspan="2">39</td><td colspan="5">29</td><td colspan="3">14</td><td></td><td></td><td>29</td></tr>
<tr><td>92 2 U A</td><td></td><td></td><td></td><td colspan="6">27</td><td colspan="2">35</td><td colspan="5">26</td><td colspan="3">14</td><td></td><td></td><td>26</td></tr>
<tr><td>92 2 U A</td><td></td><td></td><td></td><td colspan="5">20</td><td>37</td><td>38</td><td>39</td><td>36</td><td colspan="2">32</td><td colspan="2">23</td><td colspan="3">13</td><td></td><td></td><td>29</td></tr>
<tr><td>92 12 U A</td><td></td><td></td><td></td><td colspan="5">18</td><td>33</td><td>34</td><td>33</td><td>33</td><td colspan="2">28</td><td colspan="2">21</td><td colspan="3">11</td><td></td><td></td><td>24</td></tr>
<tr><td>93 2 U A</td><td></td><td></td><td></td><td colspan="16">32</td><td></td><td></td><td></td></tr>
<tr><td>94 11 UC R</td><td></td><td>4</td><td></td><td>18</td><td></td><td></td><td></td><td></td><td></td><td></td><td></td><td></td><td></td><td></td><td></td><td></td><td></td><td></td><td></td><td></td><td></td><td></td></tr>
<tr><td>94 17 UC *</td><td></td><td></td><td></td><td>14</td><td></td><td></td><td></td><td></td><td></td><td></td><td></td><td></td><td></td><td></td><td></td><td></td><td></td><td></td><td></td><td></td><td></td><td></td></tr>
<tr><td>94 17 UC R</td><td></td><td>5</td><td></td><td>19</td><td></td><td></td><td></td><td></td><td></td><td></td><td></td><td></td><td></td><td></td><td></td><td></td><td></td><td></td><td></td><td></td><td></td><td></td></tr>
</table>

Source: see *Notes on sources of survey data*, p. 641
Product: MC = manufactured cigarettes
TC = total cigarettes (including hand-rolled)
UC = cigarettes (type unspecified)
A = all products

Frequency: A = all smokers (including occasional)
R = regular or daily smokers
All ages: relevant to ages used and as given in original source
U = unspecified
* = refer to *Notes on sources of survey data*, p. 641

Table 26.5M Number of cigarettes smoked per smoker per day, males: some selected Swiss surveys by age, 1956-1985

<table>
<tr><th rowspan="2">Product
Source
Year</th><th colspan="21">Age group</th><th rowspan="2">All ages</th></tr>
<tr><th>12</th><th>13</th><th>14</th><th>15</th><th>16</th><th>17</th><th>18</th><th>19</th><th>20-24</th><th>25-29</th><th>30-34</th><th>35-39</th><th>40-44</th><th>45-49</th><th>50-54</th><th>55-59</th><th>60-64</th><th>65-69</th><th>70-74</th><th>75-79</th><th>80+</th></tr>
<tr><td>56 13 UCE</td><td colspan="10"></td><td colspan="11">16</td><td></td></tr>
<tr><td>56 13 AE</td><td colspan="10"></td><td colspan="11">16</td><td></td></tr>
<tr><td>71 3 UCE</td><td colspan="7"></td><td>16</td><td colspan="13"></td><td></td></tr>
<tr><td>71 6 UC</td><td colspan="4"></td><td colspan="17">16</td><td></td></tr>
<tr><td>71 14 UC</td><td colspan="21"></td><td></td></tr>
<tr><td>75 1 UCE*</td><td colspan="3"></td><td colspan="6">14</td><td colspan="2">22</td><td colspan="4">18</td><td colspan="4">16</td><td colspan="2"></td><td>18</td></tr>
<tr><td>77 4 A</td><td colspan="4"></td><td colspan="5">20</td><td colspan="4">21</td><td colspan="5">16</td><td colspan="3"></td><td></td></tr>
<tr><td>78 3 UCE</td><td colspan="7"></td><td>16</td><td colspan="13"></td><td></td></tr>
<tr><td>79 16 UCE</td><td colspan="8"></td><td colspan="3">19</td><td colspan="3">21</td><td colspan="3">16</td><td colspan="4"></td><td>19</td></tr>
<tr><td>80 4 A</td><td colspan="4"></td><td colspan="5">22</td><td colspan="4">21</td><td colspan="5">18</td><td colspan="3"></td><td></td></tr>
<tr><td>81 1 UCE*</td><td colspan="3"></td><td colspan="6">17</td><td colspan="2">20</td><td colspan="4">21</td><td colspan="4">21</td><td colspan="2"></td><td>20</td></tr>
<tr><td>82 7 UCE</td><td colspan="8"></td><td colspan="2">21</td><td colspan="2">22</td><td colspan="2">21</td><td colspan="2">22</td><td colspan="2">18</td><td colspan="3">14</td><td>20</td></tr>
<tr><td>85 9 UC</td><td colspan="11"></td><td colspan="6">20</td><td colspan="4"></td><td></td></tr>
<tr><td>85 10 UC</td><td colspan="11"></td><td colspan="6">20</td><td colspan="4"></td><td></td></tr>
</table>

Table 26.6M Number of cigarettes smoked per person per day, males: some selected Swiss surveys by age, 1956-1985, with percentage total sales

<table>
<tr><th rowspan="2">Product
Source
Year</th><th colspan="21">Age group</th><th rowspan="2">All ages</th><th rowspan="2">% Total sales</th></tr>
<tr><th>12</th><th>13</th><th>14</th><th>15</th><th>16</th><th>17</th><th>18</th><th>19</th><th>20-24</th><th>25-29</th><th>30-34</th><th>35-39</th><th>40-44</th><th>45-49</th><th>50-54</th><th>55-59</th><th>60-64</th><th>65-69</th><th>70-74</th><th>75-79</th><th>80+</th></tr>
<tr><td>56 13 UC</td><td colspan="10"></td><td colspan="11">3.7</td><td></td><td>**</td></tr>
<tr><td>56 13 A</td><td colspan="10"></td><td colspan="11">9.3</td><td></td><td>**</td></tr>
<tr><td>71 3 UC</td><td colspan="7"></td><td>8.6</td><td colspan="13"></td><td></td><td>**</td></tr>
<tr><td>71 6 UC *</td><td colspan="4"></td><td colspan="17">6.9</td><td></td><td>46%m</td></tr>
<tr><td>71 14 UC</td><td colspan="21"></td><td></td><td>**</td></tr>
<tr><td>75 1 UC *</td><td colspan="3"></td><td colspan="6">4.9</td><td colspan="2">11</td><td colspan="4">8.0</td><td colspan="4">5.9</td><td colspan="2"></td><td>7.7</td><td>62%m</td></tr>
<tr><td>77 4 A</td><td colspan="4"></td><td colspan="5">8.6</td><td colspan="4">11</td><td colspan="5">7.5</td><td colspan="3"></td><td></td><td>**</td></tr>
<tr><td>78 3 UC</td><td colspan="7"></td><td>6.7</td><td colspan="13"></td><td></td><td>**</td></tr>
<tr><td>79 16 UC</td><td colspan="8"></td><td colspan="3">7.5</td><td colspan="3">7.1</td><td colspan="3">4.9</td><td colspan="4"></td><td>6.7</td><td>55%m</td></tr>
<tr><td>80 4 A</td><td colspan="4"></td><td colspan="5">10</td><td colspan="4">9.3</td><td colspan="5">8.1</td><td colspan="3"></td><td></td><td>**</td></tr>
<tr><td>81 1 UC *</td><td colspan="3"></td><td colspan="6">6.8</td><td colspan="2">11</td><td colspan="4">8.0</td><td colspan="4">4.2</td><td colspan="2"></td><td>7.6</td><td>68%m</td></tr>
<tr><td>82 7 UC</td><td colspan="8"></td><td colspan="2">8.5</td><td colspan="2">9.8</td><td colspan="2">8.1</td><td colspan="2">7.2</td><td colspan="2">4.9</td><td colspan="3">3.7</td><td>7.4</td><td>62%m</td></tr>
<tr><td>85 9 UC *</td><td colspan="11"></td><td colspan="6">6.4</td><td colspan="4"></td><td></td><td>**</td></tr>
<tr><td>85 10 UC *</td><td colspan="11"></td><td colspan="6">7.6</td><td colspan="4"></td><td></td><td>**</td></tr>
</table>

Source: see *Notes on sources of survey data*, p. 641
All ages: relevant to ages used and as given in original source
% Total sales: estimated % of total sales of M = manufactured or T = total cigarette consumption implied by the survey, sexes combined
** = cannot be calculated
--- = adjusted by original author
* = refer to *Notes on sources of survey data*, p. 641

Product: MC = manufactured cigarettes
TC = total cigarettes (including hand-rolled)
UC = cigarettes (type unspecified)
A = all products
U = unspecified
E indicates mean estimated from percentage distribution (see also *Consumption category estimation*, p. xxxiv, and Appendix III, p. 789)

Table 26.5F Number of cigarettes smoked per smoker per day, females: some selected Swiss surveys by age, 1956-1985

<table>
<tr><th rowspan="2">Product
Source
Year</th><th colspan="21">Age group</th><th rowspan="2">All ages</th></tr>
<tr><th>12</th><th>13</th><th>14</th><th>15</th><th>16</th><th>17</th><th>18</th><th>19</th><th>20-24</th><th>25-29</th><th>30-34</th><th>35-39</th><th>40-44</th><th>45-49</th><th>50-54</th><th>55-59</th><th>60-64</th><th>65-69</th><th>70-74</th><th>75-79</th><th>80+</th></tr>
<tr><td>56 13 UCE</td><td colspan="21"></td><td></td></tr>
<tr><td>56 13 AE</td><td colspan="21"></td><td></td></tr>
<tr><td>71 3 UCE</td><td colspan="7"></td><td>10</td><td colspan="13"></td><td></td></tr>
<tr><td>71 6 UC</td><td colspan="4"></td><td colspan="17">11</td><td></td></tr>
<tr><td>71 14 UC</td><td colspan="5"></td><td colspan="3">9.8</td><td colspan="13"></td><td></td></tr>
<tr><td>75 1 UCE*</td><td colspan="3"></td><td colspan="6">13</td><td colspan="2">11</td><td colspan="4">12</td><td colspan="4">13</td><td colspan="2"></td><td>12</td></tr>
<tr><td>77 4 A</td><td colspan="4"></td><td colspan="5">13</td><td colspan="4">18</td><td colspan="5">12</td><td colspan="3"></td><td></td></tr>
<tr><td>78 3 UCE</td><td colspan="7"></td><td>12</td><td colspan="13"></td><td></td></tr>
<tr><td>79 16 UCE</td><td colspan="8"></td><td colspan="3">14</td><td colspan="3">13</td><td colspan="3">12</td><td colspan="4"></td><td>14</td></tr>
<tr><td>80 4 A</td><td colspan="4"></td><td colspan="5">15</td><td colspan="4">18</td><td colspan="5">14</td><td colspan="3"></td><td></td></tr>
<tr><td>81 1 UCE*</td><td colspan="3"></td><td colspan="6">15</td><td colspan="2">15</td><td colspan="4">16</td><td colspan="4">14</td><td colspan="2"></td><td>15</td></tr>
<tr><td>82 7 UCE</td><td colspan="8"></td><td colspan="2">15</td><td colspan="2">17</td><td colspan="2">17</td><td colspan="2">16</td><td colspan="2">14</td><td colspan="3">14</td><td>16</td></tr>
<tr><td>85 9 UC</td><td colspan="11"></td><td colspan="6">13</td><td colspan="4"></td><td></td></tr>
<tr><td>85 10 UC</td><td colspan="11"></td><td colspan="6">15</td><td colspan="4"></td><td></td></tr>
</table>

Table 26.6F Number of cigarettes smoked per person per day, females: some selected Swiss surveys by age, 1956-1985, with percentage total sales

<table>
<tr><th rowspan="2">Product
Source
Year</th><th colspan="21">Age group</th><th rowspan="2">All ages</th><th rowspan="2">% Total sales</th></tr>
<tr><th>12</th><th>13</th><th>14</th><th>15</th><th>16</th><th>17</th><th>18</th><th>19</th><th>20-24</th><th>25-29</th><th>30-34</th><th>35-39</th><th>40-44</th><th>45-49</th><th>50-54</th><th>55-59</th><th>60-64</th><th>65-69</th><th>70-74</th><th>75-79</th><th>80+</th></tr>
<tr><td>56 13 UC</td><td colspan="21"></td><td></td><td>**</td></tr>
<tr><td>56 13 A</td><td colspan="21"></td><td></td><td>**</td></tr>
<tr><td>71 3 UC</td><td colspan="7"></td><td>4.1</td><td colspan="13"></td><td></td><td>**</td></tr>
<tr><td>71 6 UC *</td><td colspan="4"></td><td colspan="17">2.9</td><td></td><td>46%m</td></tr>
<tr><td>71 14 UC</td><td colspan="5"></td><td colspan="3">4.1</td><td colspan="13"></td><td></td><td>**</td></tr>
<tr><td>75 1 UC *</td><td colspan="3"></td><td colspan="6">5.8</td><td colspan="2">5.3</td><td colspan="4">3.2</td><td colspan="4">1.8</td><td colspan="2"></td><td>3.5</td><td>62%m</td></tr>
<tr><td>77 4 A</td><td colspan="4"></td><td colspan="5">5.2</td><td colspan="4">5.2</td><td colspan="5">1.9</td><td colspan="3"></td><td></td><td>**</td></tr>
<tr><td>78 3 UC</td><td colspan="7"></td><td>5.1</td><td colspan="13"></td><td></td><td>**</td></tr>
<tr><td>79 16 UC</td><td colspan="8"></td><td colspan="3">5.0</td><td colspan="3">3.0</td><td colspan="3">1.2</td><td colspan="4"></td><td>3.4</td><td>55%m</td></tr>
<tr><td>80 4 A</td><td colspan="4"></td><td colspan="5">6.2</td><td colspan="4">5.1</td><td colspan="5">2.2</td><td colspan="3"></td><td></td><td>**</td></tr>
<tr><td>81 1 UC *</td><td colspan="3"></td><td colspan="6">6.4</td><td colspan="2">7.0</td><td colspan="4">4.3</td><td colspan="4">1.6</td><td colspan="2"></td><td>4.3</td><td>68%m</td></tr>
<tr><td>82 7 UC</td><td colspan="8"></td><td colspan="2">5.5</td><td colspan="2">4.6</td><td colspan="2">3.5</td><td colspan="2">2.5</td><td colspan="2">1.6</td><td colspan="3">0.7</td><td>3.4</td><td>62%m</td></tr>
<tr><td>85 9 UC *</td><td colspan="11"></td><td colspan="6">2.7</td><td colspan="4"></td><td></td><td>**</td></tr>
<tr><td>85 10 UC *</td><td colspan="11"></td><td colspan="6">3.6</td><td colspan="4"></td><td></td><td>**</td></tr>
</table>

Source: see *Notes on sources of survey data*, p. 641
All ages: relevant to ages used and as given in original source
% Total sales: estimated % of total sales of M = manufactured or T = total cigarette consumption implied by the survey, sexes combined
** = cannot be calculated
--- = adjusted by original author
* = refer to *Notes on sources of survey data*, p. 641

Product: MC = manufactured cigarettes
TC = total cigarettes (including hand-rolled)
UC = cigarettes (type unspecified)
A = all products
U = unspecified
E indicates mean estimated from percentage distribution (see also *Consumption category estimation*, p. xxxiv, and Appendix III, p. 789)

Table 26.7M Number of cigarettes smoked per person per day, sales-adjusted, males: some selected Swiss surveys[1] by age, 1971-1982, with percentage total sales

Product Source Year	12	13	14	15	16	17	18	19	20-24	25-29	30-34	35-39	40-44	45-49	50-54	55-59	60-64	65-69	70-74	75-79	80+	All ages	% Total sales
71 6 UC *					15																		46%m
75 1 UC *				7.9						17		13				9.5						12	62%m
79 16 UC									14			13			8.9							12	55%m
81 1 UC *				10						16		12				6.2						11	68%m
82 7 UC									14		16		13		12		7.8		5.9			12	62%m

Table 26.7F Number of cigarettes smoked per person per day, sales-adjusted, females: some selected Swiss surveys[1] by age, 1971-1982, with percentage total sales

Product Source Year	12	13	14	15	16	17	18	19	20-24	25-29	30-34	35-39	40-44	45-49	50-54	55-59	60-64	65-69	70-74	75-79	80+	All ages	% Total sales
71 6 UC *					6.2																		46%m
75 1 UC *				9.3						8.5		5.1				2.9						5.6	62%m
79 16 UC									9.1			5.5			2.2							6.2	55%m
81 1 UC *				9.5						10		6.4				2.4						6.4	68%m
82 7 UC									8.8		7.4		5.6		4.0		2.6		1.1			5.4	62%m

1 Based on those surveys in Table 26.6 with data for both sexes and age range at least 21-64 (see *Cigarette consumption per person*, p. xxxv)

Source: See *Notes on sources of survey data*, p. 641

Product:
MC = manufactured cigarettes
TC = total cigarettes (including hand-rolled)
UC = cigarettes (type unspecified)
A = all products
U = unspecified

All ages: relevant to ages used and as given in original source

% Total sales: Adjustment factor used, estimated % of total sales of M = manufactured or T = total cigarette consumption implied by survey, sexes combined

--- = adjusted by original author

* = refer to *Notes on sources of survey data*, p. 641

Table 26.8 Estimated[1] prevalence of smoking and estimated[1] number of cigarettes per person per day (unadjusted and sales-adjusted): summary of Tables 26.4, 26.6 and 26.7, 1956-1993.
Males and females aged 15 years and over

Year	Source[2]	Product[3]	Prevalence[4]						Number of cigarettes						
									Unadjusted[7]			Sales-adjusted[8]			
			Manufactured cigarettes		Total cigarettes[5]		All products[6]		Number/ person/day		Total sales %	Manufactured cigarettes[9] number/ person/day		Total tobacco grams/ person/day	
			M	F	M	F	M	F	M	F		M	F	M	F
1956	13	UC+A			28		54								
1971	6	UC+*U*					43	25	6.8	2.9	46	14.7	6.2		
1974	2	*U*					60	37				(12.5	6.1)		
1975	1	UC*			34	30			7.3	3.6	62	11.8	5.7		
	1	UC+A			41	30	50	30							
1977	2	*U*					47	34				(11.4	6.5)		
	4	A					47	24	8.7	3.5	[10]				
1979	16	*UC+A*			34	22	46	23	6.3	2.9	55	11.4	5.2		
1980	2	*U*					49	32				(11.0	5.8)		
	4	A					45	23	8.5	3.7	[10]				
1981	1	UC*			32	28			7.2	4.2	68	10.7	6.2		
	1	UC+A			36	28	44	28							
1982	7	*UC*			36	21			7.3	3.4	62	11.7	5.4		
1983	2	**U**					41	27				(11.4	5.9)		
1986	2	**U**					33	25				(10.1	6.2)		
1987	2	*U*					38	25				(10.6	5.6)		
1989	2	**U**					40	28				(10.3	5.7)		
1990	2	**U**					39	27				(10.2	5.6)		
1991	2	**U**					38	27				(10.1	5.7)		
1992	2	**U**					35	24				(10.6	5.8)		
	12	**U**					36	24				(10.9	5.6)		
1993	2	**U**					40	30				(9.6	5.8)		

1 Surveys covering an age range of at least 21-64 are included. Any gaps in the data for ages 15-20 and 65 years and over are filled in by assumed extensions to the age distribution, given in *Notes on sources of survey data*, p. 641. Method: see *Summary of adult smoking*, p. xxxvi
2 See *Notes on sources of survey data*, p. 641
3 Product: MC = manufactured cigarettes, TC = total cigarettes (including hand-rolled), UC = cigarettes (type unspecified), A = all products, U = unspecified. Frequency of smoking is indicated by: regular or daily smokers in normal type, all smokers (including occasional) in bold, unspecified in italics
4 From Table 26.4
5 This column includes prevalence of smoking classified as UC = cigarettes (type unspecified)
6 This column includes prevalence of smoking classified as U = unspecified product
7 From Table 26.6
8 From Table 26.7, except data in parentheses, which are derived from the prevalence of smoking from Table 26.4 as described in *Summary of adult smoking*, p. xxxvi
9 Number of cigarettes classified as UC = cigarettes (type unspecified) has been adjusted to manufactured cigarette sales and included in this column
10 All tobacco products, grams/person/day. Not adjusted due to lack of suitable sales data

Figure 26.3 Estimated prevalence of smoking of (i) cigarettes and (ii) all tobacco products: by year of survey, 1956-1993.
Males and females aged 15 years and over. *Source:* see Table 26.8

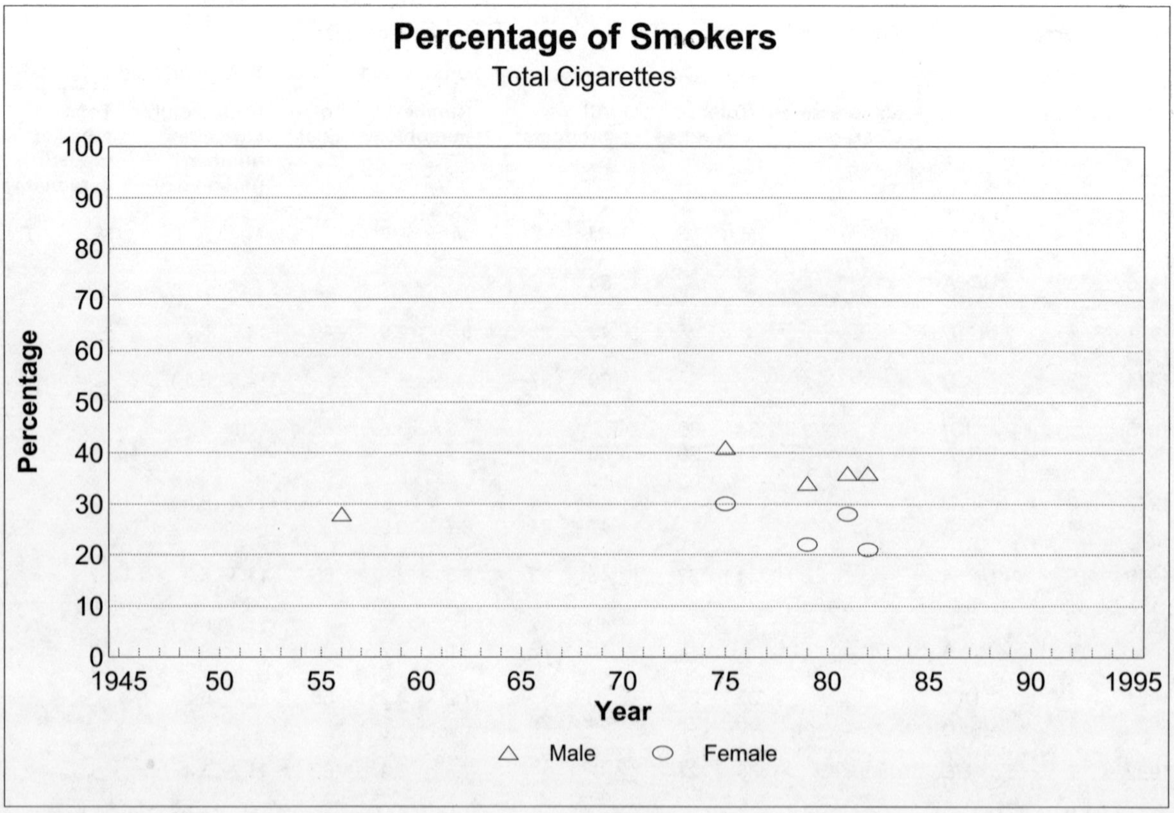

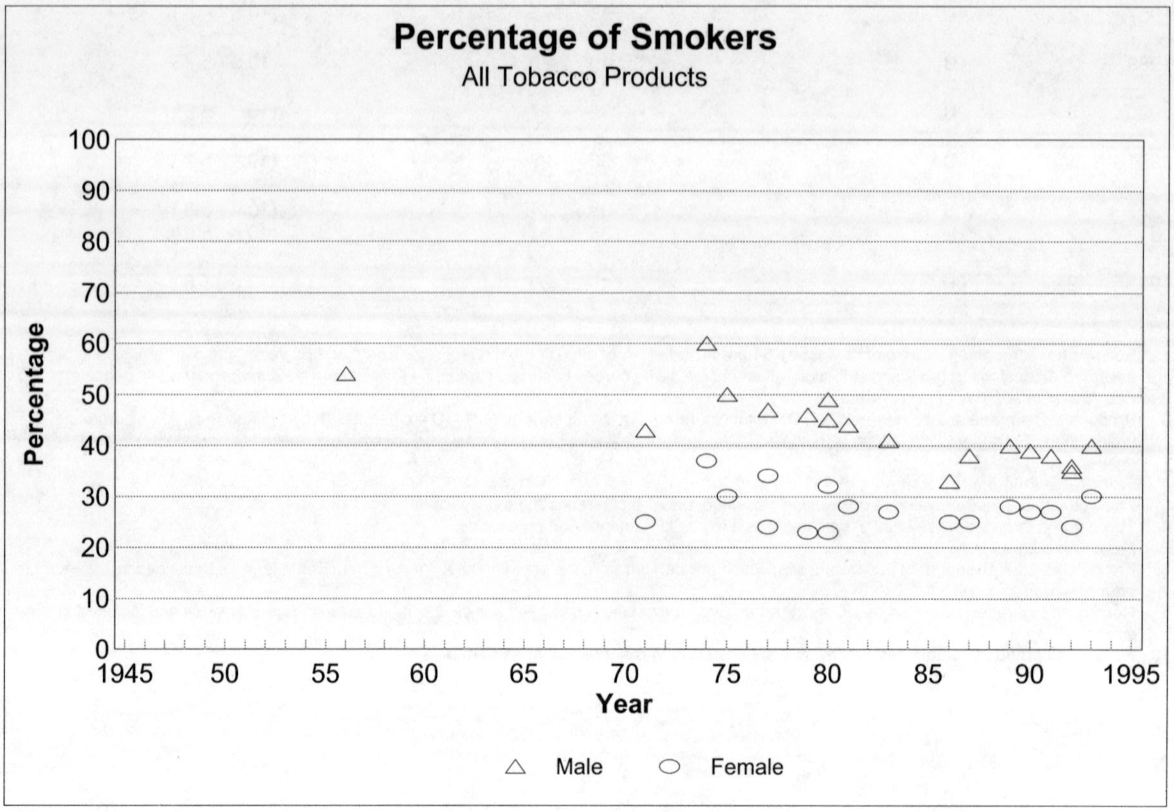

Figure 26.4 Estimated number of cigarettes smoked per person per day, sales-adjusted, 1971-1993.
Males and females aged 15 years and over. *Source:* see Table 26.8

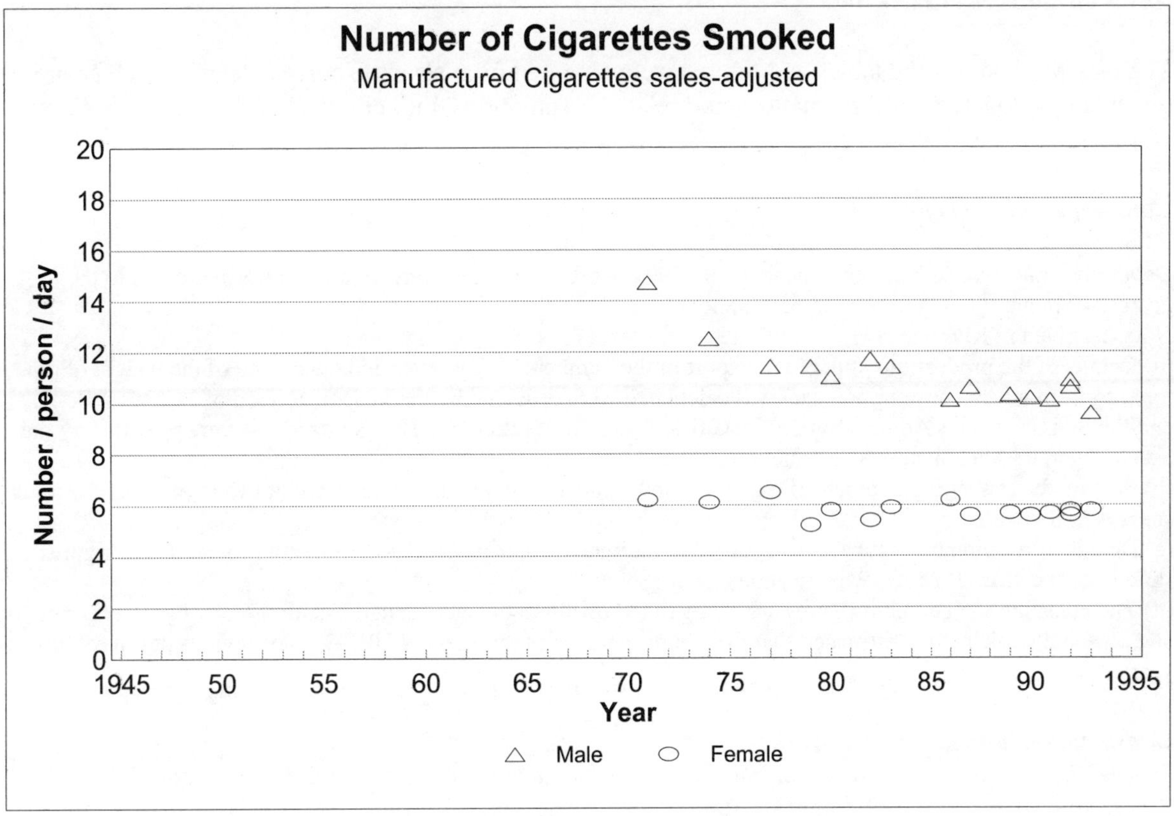

Notes on sources of sales data

The data presented in the tables and figures were obtained from several sources, details of which are given below, together with estimations and related assumptions. Full citations of the sources are given on p. 645 under *References*.

Consumption data before 1974

RP6

Data by weight, originally given to nearest 100 000 pounds, have been converted to tonnes and given to the nearest 10 tonnes (100 000 lbs = 45.359 tonnes).

Notes as given in RP6:

(a) Details of the production, import and export of the numbers of cigarettes and cigars and of the weight of pipe tobacco from which consumption data was calculated were provided by the Federal Bureau of Statistics, Berne and the Swiss Customs Administration. Statistics of sales of tobacco goods in Switzerland were provided by the Swiss Cigarette Manufacturers Association.

(b) Factors for converting numbers of cigarettes and cigars consumed into pounds weight were provided by trade sources in Switzerland.

(c) Details of the amount of tobacco consumed in individual years before 1941 were not provided. The figures shown for the years 1934 to 1940 are annual averages.

(d) The consumption per adult figures are exaggerated owing to the increasing consumption by borderers, tourists, and seasonal workers. It is estimated that these three categories represented 30%-35% of Swiss sales in recent years.

Consumption data for 1974 onwards

Tables 26.1.2 and 26.2: Association Suisse des Fabricants de Cigarettes (ASFC), Verband Schweiz. Zigarrenfabrikanten, Verein Schweiz. Rauchtabak-Fabrikanten, Körner (1992), Glass (1997)

Table 26.1.3: Schweizerische Fachstelle für Alkoholprobleme (SFA)

Estimates of cigarette consumption in Switzerland based on different sources vary considerably, for instance for the years 1971-1975

Year	**RP6**	**ASFC**[1]	**SFA**[2]	**Maxwell International Estimates**[3]	
				Series A	**Series B**
1971	17 900	17 857	19 640	30 900	—
1972	18 700	18 685	18 039	32 000	—
1973	16 500	18 455	17 834	31 076	—
1974	—	16 479	17 170	28 000	17 600
1975	—	15 492	16 247	—	15 500

1 Sales in Switzerland of Swiss production

2 Production plus imports less exports

3 Maxwell gives no explanation of the two series, but series A is equivalent to SFA production data; series B is believed to exclude sales in Italy of Swiss-made cigarettes

The ASFC estimates have been used in Table 26.2. However, these do not relate directly to consumption by the Swiss population as they do not take account of imports, sales to tourists or frontier zone traffic. Tourist and cross-border sales are estimated as 1.7% of the cigarette market in 1995 (Glass (1997)).

We have not been able to estimate the total tobacco consumption, since production figures for cigars differ between the two sources and import/export figures for cigars and pipe and hand-rolling tobacco are not available for all years. Imports of smoking tobacco are estimated as 50% of sales in 1990 (thus doubling the figure given for sales of Swiss production) and imports of cigars constituted 15% of total cigar sales in 2000 (Mäder (1991), Verband Schweiz. Zigarrenfabrikaten).

Swiss-made cigars are of several types known as stumpen or bouts (a type of cheroot), Kopfzigarren or bouts tournés, Toscani and Brissago, these last two being specialities of the Italian canton of Tessin (Ticino). According to Hutson (1937) stumpen are short cigars, rather small, clipped at both ends and wrapped in Java tobacco; Brissago are long slender cigars made entirely from Kentucky-Tennessee and dark Virginia tobacco; Toscani are short cigars of conical shape manufactured almost entirely from Kentucky tobacco. According to Abelin and Gsell (1967) Swiss cigar products generally are drier and burn more easily than American types.

Plain/Filter cigarette consumption
ASFC

Tar yield of cigarettes
1970-1975 Weber (1976)
1976-1978 Gubéran (1980)
The maximum tar yield of cigarettes was set at 15 mg from 1995 (Harkin *et al* (1997)). In 1996, cigarettes with between 1 and 5 mg of tar accounted for 32% of the market, and those over 10 mg for 31% (Glass (1997)).

Estimates of hand-rolled cigarette consumption
No information on smoking of hand-rolled cigarettes is available.

Notes on sources of survey data

Each source of survey data—either an individual survey or a series of surveys repeated over a number of years—is cited by a source number. This number is shown in the tables and corresponds to the source numbers given below, where details of the source publication and of the survey methodology are given. Full citations of the sources are given on p. 645 under *References*.

Source number

1 Abelin and Wüthrich (1976), Abelin and Müller (1983)

a. Surveys by Schweizerische Fachstelle für Alkoholprobleme (SFA/ISPA) in French and German speaking regions.

Year	Sample size	
	Males	Females
1975	417	480
1981	562	749

b. Smokers: smoked at least one cigarette per day or equivalent weight of pipe or cigar tobacco. Percentage of smokers shown as frequency * and the consumption per smoker are for smokers of cigarettes only (i.e. excluding smokers of cigarettes plus another form of tobacco). Calculation of consumption per person for males assumes that consumption by 'cigarette and other' smokers is the same as by 'cigarette only' smokers

c. Consumption category estimation based on 1-9, 10-19, and 20+ cigarettes/smoker/day

d. Assumed extension to age distribution for percentage smokers, age 75+: (A) males (1975) 30%, (1981) 25%; (UC) males (1975) 25%, (1981) 15%; (UC*) males (1975) 20%, (1981) 15%; females 10%. Number of cigarettes/person/day: males (1975) 4.0, (1980) 3.0 and females 0.5

2 Gmel (1995)

a. Various surveys, presented together by Gmel (1995) to show trends in consumption.

Year	Study name	Sample size	Source reference
1974	PKS	2 060	Demoscope (1989)
1977	PKS	2 003	Demoscope (1989)
1980	PKS	2 041	Demoscope (1989)
1983	Perma-Umfrage	10 307	Demoscope (1989)
1986	Perma-Umfrage	12 842	Demoscope (1989)
1987	SFA/ISPA	1 115	Fahrenkrug and Müller (1989)
1989	Enquête Perma	12 885	Demoscope (1989)
1990	Enquête Perma	12 848	Demoscope
1991	Enquête Perma	13 031	Demoscope
1992	Enquête Perma	13 198	Demoscope
1993	Enquête Perma	12 855	Demoscope

Other surveys quoted by Gmel (1995) are presented separately in this chapter. The PKS and 'Perma' studies were carried out by l'institut Demoscope (an opinion poll organization). The 'Perma' studies were carried out for l'Office fédéral de la santé publique using a random quota sampling method

b. For 1992, alternative results from Gmel (2000) using narrower age groups are also shown in Table 26.4. There are some minor discrepancies between the results (and also in results by Schmid *et al* (1999), not shown)

c. Assumed extension to age distribution for percentage smokers, age 75+: males (1974-1982) 25%, (1986-1993) 20%; females 10%

3 Binder *et al* (1979)

a. Surveys in Canton of Zurich, representative samples.

	Sample size	
	Males	Females
1971	6 033	1 376
1978	3 579	2 296

b. Consumption category estimation based on 1-2, 3-7, 8-14, 15-21, and 22+ cigarettes/smoker/day

4 Nater *et al* (1985)

a. Survey in two cities in 1977-1978, controls in community intervention programme, and follow-up in 1980-1981. Sample size 1 358

b. Consumption data per smoker and per person are for all tobacco types, in grams

c. Assumed extension to age distribution for percentage smokers, age 15: males and females 15%. For age 70+: males 40% and females 10%. Number of cigarettes/person/day, age 15: males 2.0 and females 1.0. For age 70+: males 5.0 and females 1.0

5 Battegay *et al* (1975)

a. Survey among military recruits. Sample size 4 056 men. Age group not stated

6 Le Meitour-Kaplan (1977), quoting Anonymous (1972)

a. A survey by a commercial firm (Konsonanz). Year not stated

b. Calculation of consumption per person based on percentage (unspecified product) smokers and number of (unspecified) cigarettes per smoker

c. Assumed extension to age distribution for percentage smokers, age 15: males and females 15%. Number of cigarettes/person/day: males 2.0 and females 1.0

7 Swiss National Health Survey SOMIPOPS, quoted by La Vecchia *et al* (1988)

a. Questionnaire mailed to randomly selected sample, representative of population age 20 years and over. Personal interviews were then arranged with each person in the sample. 1981-1983. Sample size 4 255, of whom 836 foreign residents. Response rate 73%

b. Consumption category estimation (age-specific only) based on <5, 5-14, 15-24, and 25+ cigarettes/smoker/day. Estimation for overall age group by original authors

c. Assumed extension to age distribution for percentage smokers, age 15-19: males 30% and females 25%. Number of cigarettes/person/day: males 5.0 and females 4.0

8 WHO Tobacco or Health Programme, quoted by Geizerova and Masironi (1988)

a. No original source

9-10 WHO MONICA Project (1988), WHO (1989), Rickenbach *et al* (1993)

a. Two regional surveys forming part of WHO MONICA project:

	Region	Population size	Sample size	Participation rate (%)	Sample used* Males	Sample used* Females	Date
9	Vaud/Fribourg	280 200	1 966	62	851	778	Oct 1984-June 1985
			2 011	61	1 034	975	Oct 1988-June 1989
10	Ticino	110 900	1 948	78	781	769	Nov 1985-May 1986
			1 455	73	749	709	Oct 1988-Apr 1989

* Vaud/Fribourg 'sample used' includes age 25-34; all other figures are for age 35-64 only

b. *All ages* column relates only to age 35-64 and is standardized to world population

c. Regular cigarette smokers: smoked cigarettes daily. All smokers: smoked cigarettes daily or occasionally, or smoked 1 g pipe tobacco or 1 cigar per week. Cigarettes per smoker refers to regular and occasional cigarette smokers

d. Calculation for cigarettes per person based on % regular cigarette smokers and cigarettes per regular or occasional cigarette smoker, so may underestimate

11 Nutbeam and Aarø (1990), King *et al* (1996)

a. Part of the HBSC (Health Behaviour in School-Aged Children) Study, a collaborative cross-national research study sponsored by the WHO. School classes or schools were randomly selected, targeting age groups 11 (not presented here), 13 and 15. The target sample size was 1 300 in each age group

b. 1985-1986: sample size (age 13) 820, (age 15) 816.
1994:

Target age	Mean age	Sample size
13	13.5	3 438
15	15.4	3 251

c. Regular smokers: smoke once a week or more. Smokers marked as frequency *: smoked daily

12 Enquête suisse sur la santé/Schweizerische Gesundheitsbafragung (ESS/SGB) quoted by Institut suisse de prévention de l'alcoolisme et autres toxicomanies (SFA/ISPA) (1999), Schmid *et al* (1999), Gmel (2000), Cavelaars *et al* (2000)

a. Telephone surveys representative of the Swiss population. Four stage sampling, 3 stages in 1992 and the fourth in 1993. Total sample size 15 282. Response rate 71%

b. Consumption category estimation based on two categories, 1-9 and 10+ cigarette equivalents/smoker/day and resulting figures should be regarded with caution. Cigarette equivalents were based on a pipe or cigarillo = 2.5 cigarettes, and a cigar = 5 cigarettes

c. Assumed extension to age distribution for percentage smokers, age 75+: males 20% and females 10%

13 Abelin and Gsell (1967)

a. A survey of a rural town. Sample included 98% of all inhabitants, but only results for males are available. Sample size (males) 824

b. Cigarette smokers: smoked one cigarette per day. All smokers: smoked one cigarette per day or 30 units per month, where units were defined as a cigarette = 1 unit, a Brissago or Toscani cigar = 5 units, a Stumpen = 4 units, a pipe = 2.5 units

c. Consumption category estimation based on 1-9, 10-19, 20-34 and 35+ units/cigarette smoker/day or units/smoker/day

d. Assumed extension to age distribution for percentage smokers (males only), age 15-16: 15%

14 Le Meitour-Kaplan (1977)

a. Survey of young women in the Canton of Zurich. Sample size 1 381

15 Berrino *et al* (1988)

a. A survey of the Canton of Geneva. Upper age limit 85

b Smokers: smoked more than a gram of tobacco/day for at least the last six months

16 Schüler *et al* (1980)

a. A study of two rural communities in the Canton of Zurich. Year not stated. Sample size (males) 1 754, (females) 1 628
b. Prevalence values presented have been adjusted to exclude subjects who did not answer the question
c. Consumption category estimation based on categories described as <10, 10-20, 20 exactly, 20-40 and >40 cigarettes/smoker/day (1-9, 10-19, 20, 21-40 and >40 cigarettes/smoker/day assumed)
d. Assumed extension to age distribution for percentage smokers, age 15-19: males and females, 35%. For age 65+: males (UC) 25%, (A) 30%; females 10%. Number of cigarettes/person/day, age 15-19: males and females 5.0. For age 65+: males 5.0 and females 0.5

17 Consommation de psychotropes chez les écoliers quoted by Institut suisse de prévention de l'alcoolisme et autres toxicomanies (SFA/ISPA) (1999)

a. Four-yearly surveys of Swiss school children. Sample size (1986) 1 984, (1994) 2 790
b. Smokers marked as frequency *: smoked every day. Regular smokers: smoked at least weekly

References

Abelin T. and Gsell O.R. (1967). Relative risk of pulmonary cancer in cigar and pipe smokers. *Cancer,* **20**, 1288-96.

Abelin Th. and Müller R. (1983). Trend der Rauchgewohnheiten in der Schweiz 1975-1981. (Trends in smoking habits in Switzerland 1975-1981). *Soz Praventivmed,* **28**, 185-95.

Abelin Th. and Wüthrich P. (1976). Repräsentativerhebung über die Rauchgewohnheiten in der deutsch-, französisch- und romanischsprachigen Schweiz 1975. (Sample survey of smoking habits in the German, French and Romansh speaking parts of Switzerland). *Soz Praventivmed,* **21**, 17-23.

Anonymous (1972). *Konsonanz.* No 35.[§]

Battegay R., Mühlemann R., Zehnder R. and Dillinger A. (1975). Konsumverhalten einer repräsentativen Stichprobe von 4082 gesunden 20jährigen Schweizer Männern in bezug auf Alkohol, Drogen und Rauchwaren (The consumption of alcohol, drugs and the smoking habits of 4 082 healthy young Swiss men as evidenced by a random study). *Schweiz Med Wochenschr,* **105**, 180-7.

Beese D.H. (ed) (1968). *Tobacco consumption in various countries,* 2nd edition. Tobacco Research Council, London. Research Paper 6.

Beese D.H. (ed) (1972). *Tobacco consumption in various countries,* 3rd edition. Tobacco Research Council, London. Research Paper 6.

Berrino F., Merletti F., Zubiri A., Del Moral A., *et al* (1988). A comparative study of smoking, drinking and dietary habits in population samples in France, Italy, Spain and Switzerland. II. Tobacco smoking. *Rev Epidemiol Sante Publique,* **36**, 166-76.

Binder J., Sieber M. and Angst J. (1979). Entwicklung des Suchtmittelkonsums bei 19/20jährigen Jugenlichen. *Schweiz Med Wochenschr,* **109**, 1298-305.

Cavelaars A.E.J.M., Kunst A.E., Geurts J.J.M., Crialesi R., *et al* (2000). Educational differences in smoking: international comparison. *BMJ,* **320**, 1102-7.

Demoscope *Rauchergewohnheiten.* Perma-Umfrage-System.[§]

Demoscope (1989). *Trendauswertung über die Jahre 1974-1989.* Perma-Umfrage-System.[§]

Fahrenkrug H. and Müller R. (1989). *Alkohol und Gesundheit in der Schweiz—Bericht über eine Umfrage aus dem Jahre 1987.* Schweizerische Fachstelle für Alkohol- und andere Drogenprobleme (SFA), Lausanne.[§]

Geizerova H. and Masironi R. (1988). Cigarette smoking in children and adolescents: world review. In: Aoki M., Hisamichi S. and Tominaga S. (eds) *Smoking and health 1987. Proceedings of the 6th World Conference on Smoking and Health, Tokyo, 9-12 November 1987.* Elsevier Science Publishers B.V. (Biomedical Division), Amsterdam; 601-5. International Congress Series No. 780.

Glass C. (1997). Getting lighter: Swiss smokers are enjoying more and more lights. *Tobacco Reporter,* **September**, 48-9.

Gmel G. (1995). Le nombre de fumeurs et de fumeuses serait-il à nouveau en progression? Des chiffres déconcertants concernant la fumée. *Bulletin de l'office fédéral de la santé publique,* **20**, 38-47.

Gmel G. (2000). Prävalenz des Tabakkonsums in der Schweiz der 1990er Jahre—Schätzung der Konsumtrends aufgrund zweier Methoden. (Prevalence of tobacco consumption in Switzerland of the 1990s—trend estimation based on two methods). *Soz Praventivmed,* **45**, 64-72.

Gubéran E. (1980). Tendances de la mortalité en Suisse. 3. Tumeurs: 1921-1978. *Schweiz.Med.Wochenschr.,* **110 Suppl 11**, 1-18. Schwabe & Co AG, Basel.

Harkin A.M., Anderson P. and Goos C. (1997). *Smoking, drinking and drug taking in the European Region.* Alcohol, Drugs and Tobacco Programme, WHO Regional Office for Europe, Copenhagen.

Hutson J.B. (1937). *Consumption and production of tobacco in Europe.* USDA, Washington DC. Technical bulletin No. 587.

Institut suisse de prévention de l'alcoolisme et autres toxicomanies (SFA/ISPA) (1999). *Chiffres et donnees sur l'alcool et les autres drogues 1999*. SFA/ISPA, Lausanne.

King A., Wold B., Tudor-Smith C. and Harel Y. (1996). *The health of youth, a cross-national survey*. WHO Regional Publications, Europe, Copenhagen. European Series No. 69.

Körner M. (1992). Swiss cigarette market saturated. *Tobacco International,* **194**, 27-8.

La Vecchia C., Levi F., Decarli A., Wietlisbach V., Negri E. and Gutzwiller F. (1988). Trends in smoking and lung cancer mortality in Switzerland. *Prev Med,* **17**, 712-24.

Le Meitour-Kaplan A. (1977). Situational Analysis: Profile of women's smoking habits in Continental Western Europe. In: Steinfeld J., Griffiths W., Ball K. and Taylor R.M. (eds) *Health consequences, education, cessation activities, and social action, Volume II. Proceedings of the Third World Conference on Smoking and Health, New York City, June 2-5, 1975*. US Department of Health, Education and Welfare, USA; 309-27. DHEW Publication No (NIH) 77-1413.

Lee P.N. (ed) (1975). *Tobacco consumption in various countries,* 4th edition. Tobacco Research Council, London. Research Paper 6.

Mäder R. (1991). Swiss market for smoking tobacco drops again. *Tobacco Journal International,* **November/December**, 46.

Nater B., Gutzwiller F., Abelin Th., Degiampietro P., Junod B. and Groupe d'Etude du Programme National Suisse de Recherche 1A (1985). Evolution de la consommation de tabac dans 2 villes d'intervention et 2 villes témoins suisses. (Changes in tobacco consumption during a community oriented primary prevention program in Switzerland). *Rev Epidemiol Sante Publique,* **33**, 80-9.

Nutbeam D. and Aarø L.E. (1990). Smoking and alienation from school: the implications for health education with young people. Results from the WHO study of health behaviour in schoolchildren. In: Durston B. and Jamrozik K. (eds) *Tobacco & health 1990. The global war. Seventh World Conference on Tobacco and Health, Perth, Western Australia, 1-5 April 1990*. Organising Committee of the Seventh World Conference on Tobacco and Health, 189 Royal Street, East Perth, Western Australia 6004; 539-44.

Rickenbach M., Wietlisbach V., Beretta-Piccoli C., Moccetti T. and Gutzwiller F. (1993). Tabakkonsum, Blutdruck und Körpergewicht in der Schweizer Bevölkerung: MONICA-Studie 1988-89 (Smoking, blood pressure and body weight in the Swiss population: MONICA study 1988-89). *Schweiz Med Wochenschr,* **123(Suppl 48)**, 21-8.

RP6, See Beese (ed) (1968), Beese (ed) (1972), Lee (ed) (1975)

Schmid H., Gmel G. and Janin Jaquat B. (1999). Neue epidemiologische befunde zum rauchen in der Schweiz. *Suchtmagazin,* **5**, 3-13.

Schüler G., Stransky M., Schwarzenbach F.H., Epstein F.H. and Schär M. (1980). Rauchgewohnheiten in zwei Zürcher Landgemeinden (Smoking habits in two rural communities in the Canton of Zurich, Switzerland). *Schweiz Rundsch Med Prax,* **69**, 1661-70.

Trümpy H. (1983). Volkskundliche Überlegungen zum Rauchen. (Smoking in history). *Ther Umsch,* **40**, 165-8.

Weber K.H. (1976). Recent changes in tobacco products and their acceptance by the consumer. In: *Proceedings of the 6th International Tobacco Science Congress, Tokyo*. 15-30.

WHO (1989). The WHO MONICA project: a worldwide monitoring system for cardiovascular diseases. In: *World health statistics annual 1989*. WHO, Geneva; 25-149.

WHO MONICA Project (1988). Geographical variation in the major risk factors of coronary heart disease in men and women aged 35-64 years. *World Health Stat Q,* **41**, 115-40.

§ Original paper not obtained, but information taken as quoted by another author

United Kingdom 27

Much of the data presented in this chapter are available in the book UK Smoking Statistics (second edition), which includes more detailed information on smoking in the UK (full citation is given on p. 685 under *References*).

Sales data

See Tables 27.1-27.3.

Data on consumption of tobacco products cover the period since 1880. Production of manufactured cigarettes started in 1856, but during the nineteenth century tobacco for pipes and chewing, and tobacco for cigars and snuff, accounted for virtually all the tobacco sold. By 1905 consumption of manufactured cigarettes per adult had reached 1 cigarette per day and increased steadily, apart from a brief dip following the Second World War, to nearly 9 cigarettes per day during the 1970s. Consumption then declined to 4 cigarettes per day in 1995. Consumption of hand-rolled cigarettes has always been low, with a maximum consumption per adult of about 0.7 cigarettes per day during the 1960s and 1970s.

The consumption of tobacco products per adult was about 4 g per day between 1905 and 1915 after which it increased to nearly 9 g per day by the end of the Second World War. After recovery from a post-war dip, consumption declined again after 1960 to 4 g per day in 1995. This decline, predominantly in tobacco sold as cigarettes, was initially due to the introduction of filters, reducing the amount of tobacco used in each cigarette.

By 1925 more tobacco was used for manufactured cigarettes than all for other forms of tobacco combined, accounting for 57% of all sales. This proportion increased to 84% in 1946 and to 91% in 1995. The switch from plain to filter cigarettes began in the late 1950s, with filter cigarettes reaching 16% of manufactured cigarettes by 1960, and then rising rapidly to about 80% in 1980. Consumption of cigars and cigarillos increased to 3% of tobacco sales in the mid-1970s and decreased somewhat thereafter. Sales of pipe tobacco have been in continuous decline since the 1920s. Tobacco for hand-rolling accounted for about 5-6% of all tobacco sales from the 1950s to the 1980s but decreased somewhat in the 1990s.

The smuggling of tobacco products, especially hand-rolling tobacco, into the UK has grown during the 1990s. Anonymous (1995) points out that between 1992 and 1994, taxed sales of hand-rolling tobacco fell by 20% while sales of cigarette papers increased by 20%. Cole (1996) states that one of the most popular brands of hand-rolling tobacco in the UK (Drum) was not officially on sale there. The Tobacco Manufacturers' Association estimates that between 1992 and 1995 the proportion of sales which were untaxed rose from 4% to 6% for manufactured cigarettes and from 6% to 49% for hand-rolling tobacco.

Survey data

See Tables 27.4-27.8

Survey data have been available annually from the TAC (source 1) from 1948 to 1987, and at two-yearly intervals from the GHS (source 2) since 1972, although there are some difficulties in interpretation due to differing definitions used.

Limited data for the pre-war period show that the prevalence of smoking was very high among men, 90%, and that it increased among women from 15% in 1928 to 33% in 1938. In 1948, the prevalence of tobacco smoking among those aged 15 years and over was about 80% in men, decreasing to 35% in 1985. The prevalence of manufactured cigarette smoking among men fell from about 65% in 1948 to 33% in 1987 (source 1). The GHS data (source 2) also show a decline in cigarette smoking (manufactured and hand-rolled) from 1972 onwards, to about 30% in 1995. For women the prevalence of tobacco smoking remained at about 40% from 1948 until the late 1970s, when it started to decline to 27% in 1995. Very few women smoked products other than cigarettes.

Among men, the prevalence of tobacco smoking was about equal for all age groups (over age 20) until the 1980s, when a decrease in prevalence appeared among those aged 65 years and over. The prevalence of cigarette smoking has always been lower at older ages, due to a greater proportion of older men than younger men smoking tobacco in a form other than manufactured cigarettes. The prevalence of smoking among women age 60 or 65 years and over has also always been lower than among younger age groups.

In the early surveys, both for surveys conducted in schools and for the youngest reported age group of the adult surveys, the prevalence of smoking was higher among teenage boys than girls. Smoking among girls increased, and by the mid-1980s the difference in prevalence was no longer present.

Comparison of survey and sales data suggests that the GHS surveys under-reported consumption by 20-30%. Survey data provided by the TAC were already sales-adjusted, but the understatement was reported to be an average of 5%. Between 1949 and 1960, the estimated number of manufactured cigarettes smoked per person per day (sales-adjusted) for men rose from 8 to 11. Consumption remained fairly stable until the mid-1970s, and then declined to 6 in 1987. For women, consumption increased between 1948 and the mid-1970s, from about 3 to 7 cigarettes per person per day, and declined thereafter to 5 in 1987. Between 1974 and 1995 the total number of cigarettes per person per day (including hand-rolled) for men declined from 12 to 6, and for women from 7 to 4.

Table 27.1.1 Total annual sales of tobacco products, 1880-1967

Year	Manufactured cigarettes tonnes	Tobacco, cigars and snuff tonnes	All tobacco products tonnes
1880-84	0	29400	29400
1885-89	0	30800	30800
1890-94	500	34100	34600
1895-99	2800	35700	38500
1900-04	7200	34500	41700
1905-09	13300	30400	43700
1910-14	19400	27300	46700
1915	24600	28500	53100
1916	24100	26500	50600
1917	25000	26900	51900
1918	25800	27500	53300
1919	36200	35100	71300

Table 27.1.1 *(continued)*

Year	Cigarettes		Cigars and cigarillos		Snuff tonnes	Pipe tobacco tonnes	Hand-rolling tobacco tonnes	All tobacco products tonnes
	tonnes	millions	tonnes	millions				
1920	36420	36240	1180			31890		69490
1921	35430	35185	1180		Included	31300		67900
1922	34020	33730	1180		with	30440		65630
1923	34060	33725	1180		cigars	28620		63870
1924	34060	33835	1220		1920-1927	26310		61600
1925	36330	36030	1180			26350		63870
1926	37690	37435	1180			25450		64320
1927	40410	40030	1180			24990		66590
1928	43320	43035	640	135	450	24860		69260
1929	45950	45535	640	135	450	24180		71210
1930	48530	48335	640	140	410	23360		72940
1931	49310	49235	590	150	410	21860	730	72890
1932	49580	49630	500	135	410	19780	1630	71890
1933	51980	52130	500	135	410	18280	2400	73570
1934	53930	53625	540	145	410	17460	3360	75700
1935	57520	57330	590	155	450	17150	3270	78970
1936	62050	61635	590	165	450	16780	3270	83140
1937	66680	65835	640	170	450	16420	3180	87360
1938	70670	69740	590	170	450	16330	3180	91220
1939	73840	73810	500	175	450	15560	3310	93670
1940	73070	74805	360	125	450	18230		92120
1941	81330	82760	410	155	500	19460		101690
1942	85410	86110	450	150	540	19910		106320
1943	85860	85475	450	155	500	17600		104420
1944	86090	84525	410	130	540	16960		104010
1945	94800	93300	410	120	500	17420		113130
1946	100700	99015	360	100	450	14830	4080	120430
1947	87630	87525	540	125	360	12520	4540	105600
1948	83460	84180	410	110	360	13380	5220	102830
1949	80690	81950	360	105	320	12200	6350	99930
1950	82420	85145	360	115	320	11480	5900	100470
1951	86540	89335	360	120	320	10390	5900	103510
1952	88000	90400	410	125	320	10390	6260	105370
1953	90080	92695	360	130	360	10070	6170	107050
1954	92530	95230	410	140	320	9890	6120	109270
1955	95750	98670	410	150	320	9340	5990	111810
1956	97750	99560	450	180	320	8850	5810	113170
1957	100380	102250	540	210	320	8890	5990	116120
1958	102100	104020	590	250	320	8620	6620	118250
1959	104460	106600	680	290	270	8300	6990	120700
1960	108500	110900	730	315	270	7940	7120	124560
1961	110270	113400	730	315	270	7440	7260	125960
1962	104730	109900	860	390	270	7800	7170	120840
1963	107860	115200	950	445	230	7300	7570	123920
1964	104690	114400	1220	590	230	7080	7670	120880
1965	100110	112000	1320	700	230	6580	7350	115570
1966	101290	117600	1590	900	230	6350	7120	116570
1967	100380	119100	1810	1135	230	6300	7120	115850

Source: see *Notes on sources of sales data*, p. 678

Table 27.1.2 Total annual sales of tobacco products, 1968-1995

Year	Cigarettes		Cigars		Cigarillos		Pipe tobacco tonnes	Hand-roll tobacco tonnes	Snuff tonnes	All tobacco products tonnes
	tonnes	millions	tonnes	millions	tonnes	millions				
1968	99880	121800	1590	835	270	345	5990	6990	230	114940
1969	98200	124900	1630	845	230	290	5940	6850	230	113080
1970	97700	127900	1860	975	180	215	5760	6530	180	112220
1971	92580	122400	2590	1360	140	195	5990	5940	180	107410
1972	98070	130500	2770	1410	140	165	5670	6170	180	112990
1973	103830	137400	3130	1545	140	170	5580	6120	180	118980
1974	102330	137000	3080	1600	140	165	5400	6120	180	117250
1975	96410	132600	3220	1640	140	160	5030	6440	180	111420
1976	93150	130600	3130	1580	90	145	4990	6530	140	108030
1977	89700	125900	2950	1570	90	120	4940	6480	140	104300
1978	98910	125200	3080	1610	40	120	4620	6080	180	112910
1979	98590	124300	3080	1650	90	105	4220	5710	90	111780
1980	97180	121500	2900	1610	90	85	3990	5620	90	109870
1981	89380	110300	2810	1540	90	70	3810	6210	90	102390
1982	82600	102000	2700	1465	0	55	3500	6200	100	95100
1983	83000	101600	2600	1445	0	50	3300	5800	100	94800
1984	81600	99000	2700	1400	0	45	3200	5300	100	92900
1985	81100	97750	2600	1380	0	40	3000	5000	100	91800
1986	76088	95110	2547	1415	30	30	2710	4840	0	86215
1987	78704	98380	2700	1500	26	26	2520	4800	0	88750
1988	77840	97300	2718	1510	23	23	2290	4550	0	87421
1989	77840	97300	2691	1495	14	14	2080	4310	0	86935
1990	78660	98325	2664	1480	0	0	1975	4170	0	87469
1991	76720	95900	2601	1445	0	0	1805	4095	0	85221
1992	71640	89550	2349	1305	0	0	1600	3840	0	79429
1993	72520	90650	2304	1280	0	0	1500	3515	0	79839
1994	69800	87250	2142	1190	0	0	1310	3050	0	76302
1995	63648	79560	1926	1070	0	0	1090	2570	0	69234

Source : see *Notes on sources of sales data*, p. 678

Table 27.1.3 Manufactured cigarettes (i) percentage of total sales as filter cigarettes, 1921-1987, (ii) sales-weighted average tar yield per cigarette (SWAT), 1921-1995, (iii) sales-weighted average nicotine yield per cigarette (SWAN), 1921-1995, and (iv) sales-weighted average carbon monoxide (CO) yield per cigarette (SWACO), 1921-1990

Year	% Filter	SWAT mg / cig	SWAN mg / cig	SWACO mg / cig
1921-1928	0.0	34.0	1.90	22.0
1929	0.1	34.0	1.90	22.0
1930	0.2	34.0	1.90	22.0
1931	0.4	32.0	2.10	20.0
1932	0.4	32.0	2.10	20.0
1933	0.4	32.0	2.10	20.0
1934	0.4	32.0	2.10	20.0
1935	0.4	32.0	2.10	20.0
1936	0.6	32.0	2.10	20.0
1937	0.6	32.0	2.10	20.0
1938	0.7	32.0	2.10	20.0
1939	0.8	32.0	2.10	20.0

Table 27.1.3 *(continued)*

Year	% Filter	SWAT mg / cig	SWAN mg / cig	SWACO mg / cig
1940	0.7	32.0	2.10	20.0
1941	0.7	32.0	2.10	20.0
1942	0.7	32.0	2.10	20.0
1943	0.7	32.0	2.10	20.0
1944	0.8	32.0	2.10	20.0
1945	0.7	32.0	2.10	20.0
1946	0.7	32.0	2.10	20.0
1947	0.6	32.0	2.10	20.0
1948	0.8	32.0	2.10	20.0
1949	1.3	32.0	2.10	20.0
1950	2.0	32.0	2.10	20.0
1951	1.0	31.0	2.00	21.0
1952	1.0	31.0	2.00	21.0
1953	1.1	31.0	2.00	21.0
1954	1.6	31.0	2.00	21.0
1955	1.9	31.0	2.00	21.0
1956	3.1	31.0	2.00	21.0
1957	5.3	31.0	2.00	21.0
1958	9.3	31.0	2.00	21.0
1959	12.1	31.0	2.00	21.0
1960	15.8	31.0	2.00	21.0
1961	19.5	29.0	1.95	19.5
1962	26.0	29.0	1.95	19.5
1963	32.8	29.0	1.95	19.5
1964	41.8	29.0	1.95	19.5
1965	53.0	29.0	1.95	19.5
1966	60.6	25.0	1.70	18.5
1967	65.9	25.0	1.70	18.5
1968	70.7	25.0	1.70	18.5
1969	75.5	25.0	1.70	18.5
1970	78.3	25.0	1.70	18.5
1971	79.8	22.2	1.44	17.1
1972	81.7	21.0	1.35	17.0
1973	83.0	19.9	1.29	
1974	84.5	19.3	1.28	
1975	86.6	18.8	1.32	
1976	88.1	17.9	1.33	16.0
1977	90.0	17.6	1.28	16.1
1978	90.4	17.5	1.40	16.5
1979	91.5	16.8	1.39	16.6
1980	92.8	16.4	1.32	16.0
1981	93.6	15.9	1.34	15.3
1982	94.4	15.4	1.31	15.2
1983	95.1	15.1	1.30	14.7
1984	95.7	14.7	1.30	14.2
1985	96.3	14.4	1.32	14.6
1986	96.8	13.9	1.30	14.7
1987	97.2	13.5	1.21	14.3
1988		13.3	1.17	14.3
1989		12.9	1.17	14.2
1990		12.8	1.15	14.6
1991		11.6	0.90	
1992		11.3	0.90	
1993		11.0	0.90	
1994		11.1	0.90	
1995		10.7	0.90	

Source : see *Notes on sources of sales data,* p. 678

Table 27.2 Consumption of (i) cigarettes and (ii) all tobacco products, 1905-1995 sales-based data, including estimated hand-rolled cigarette consumption. Males and females aged 15 years and over

Year	Manufactured cigarettes		Hand-rolled cigarettes		Total cigarettes		All tobacco products	
	Total annual in millions	Number/ adult/day	Total annual in millions	Number/ adult/day	Total annual in millions	Number/ adult/day	Total annual in tonnes	Grams/ adult/day
1905	11200	1.0					42800	4.1
1906	12400	1.2					43100	4.1
1907	13600	1.2					44500	4.1
1908	14400	1.3					44500	4.1
1909	14800	1.3					43500	3.8
1910	16400	1.5					44600	4.1
1911	18200	1.6					46000	4.1
1912	19500	1.7					46000	4.1
1913	20700	1.8					47300	4.1
1914	22400	1.9					49600	4.1
1915	24600	2.1					53100	4.7
1916	24100	2.1					50600	4.4
1917	25100	2.2					51900	4.7
1918	25800	2.3					53300.	4.7
1919	36200	3.1					71300	6.0
1920	36240	3.0					69490	5.7
1921	35185	2.8					67900	5.4
1922	33730	2.7					65630	5.2
1923	33725	2.7					63870	5.0
1924	33835	2.8					61600	5.1
1925	36030	3.0					63870	5.3
1926	37435	3.1					64320	5.2
1927	40030	3.2					66590	5.4
1928	43035	3.5					69260	5.6
1929	45535	3.6					71210	5.7
1930	48335	3.8					72940	5.8
1931	49235	3.9	896	0.1	50131	3.9	72890	5.7
1932	49630	3.9	2016	0.2	51646	4.0	71890	5.6
1933	52130	4.0	2968	0.2	55098	4.3	73570	5.7
1934	53625	4.1	4144	0.3	57769	4.4	75700	5.8
1935	57330	4.4	4040	0.3	61370	4.7	78970	6.0
1936	61635	4.6	4030	0.3	65665	4.9	83140	6.3
1937	65835	4.9	3900	0.3	69735	5.2	87360	6.5
1938	69740	5.2	3940	0.3	73680	5.4	91220	6.7
1939	73810	5.4	4088	0.3	77898	5.7	93670	6.9
1940	74805	5.5					92120	6.8
1941	82760	6.1					101690	7.5
1942	86110	6.4					106320	7.9
1943	85475	6.4					104420	7.8
1944	84525	6.5					104010	8.0
1945	93300	7.1					113130	8.6
1946	99015	7.1	5040	0.4	104055	7.5	120430	8.7
1947	87525	6.2	5600	0.4	93125	6.6	105600	7.5
1948	84180	5.9	6624	0.5	90804	6.4	102830	7.3
1949	81950	5.8	8064	0.6	90014	6.3	99930	7.0
1950	85145	6.0	7488	0.5	92633	6.5	100470	7.0
1951	89335	6.3	7696	0.5	97031	6.8	103510	7.3
1952	90400	6.4	8170	0.6	98570	6.9	105370	7.4
1953	92695	6.5	8051	0.6	100746	7.1	107050	7.5
1954	95230	6.7	8424	0.6	103654	7.3	109270	7.6
1955	98670	6.9	8237	0.6	106907	7.5	111810	7.8
1956	99560	6.9	8192	0.6	107752	7.5	113170	7.9
1957	102250	7.1	8448	0.6	110698	7.7	116120	8.1
1958	104020	7.2	9344	0.6	113364	7.8	118250	8.2
1959	106600	7.3	9856	0.7	116456	8.0	120700	8.3

Table 27.2 *(continued)*

Year	Manufactured cigarettes		Hand-rolled cigarettes		Total cigarettes		All tobacco products	
	Total annual in millions	Number/ adult/day	Total annual in millions	Number/ adult/day	Total annual in millions	Number/ adult/day	Total annual in tonnes	Grams/ adult/day
1960	110900	7.6	10299	0.7	121199	8.3	124560	8.5
1961	113400	7.7	10496	0.7	123896	8.4	125960	8.5
1962	109900	7.3	11300	0.8	121200	8.1	120840	8.1
1963	115200	7.6	11169	0.7	126369	8.4	123920	8.2
1964	114400	7.5	11546	0.8	125946	8.3	120880	8.0
1965	112000	7.3	11742	0.8	123742	8.1	115570	7.6
1966	117600	7.7	11178	0.7	128778	8.4	116570	7.6
1967	119100	7.8	11103	0.7	130203	8.5	115850	7.6
1968	121800	7.9	11359	0.7	133159	8.7	114940	7.5
1969	124900	8.1	11165	0.7	136065	8.8	113080	7.3
1970	127900	8.3	10875	0.7	138775	9.0	112220	7.3
1971	122400	7.9	9915	0.6	132315	8.6	107410	7.0
1972	130500	8.4	10698	0.7	141198	9.1	112990	7.3
1973	137400	8.8	10383	0.7	147783	9.5	118980	7.7
1974	137000	8.8	10088	0.6	147088	9.4	117250	7.5
1975	132600	8.5	10924	0.7	143524	9.2	111420	7.1
1976	130600	8.3	11500	0.7	142100	9.0	108030	6.9
1977	125900	8.0	11100	0.7	137000	8.7	104300	6.6
1978	125200	7.9	10550	0.7	135750	8.5	112910	7.1
1979	124300	7.8	9500	0.6	133800	8.4	111780	7.0
1980	121500	7.5	9400	0.6	130900	8.1	109870	6.8
1981	110300	6.8	11500	0.7	121800	7.5	102390	6.3
1982	102000	6.2	11700	0.7	113700	6.9	95100	5.8
1983	101600	6.2	11200	0.7	112800	6.8	94800	5.7
1984	99000	6.0	9850	0.6	108850	6.6	92900	5.6
1985	97750	5.9	9500	0.6	107250	6.4	91800	5.5
1986	95110	5.7	9680	0.6	104790	6.2	86215	5.1
1987	98380	5.8	9600	0.6	107980	6.4	88750	5.3
1988	97300	5.8	9100	0.5	106400	6.3	87421	5.2
1989	97300	5.7	8620	0.5	105920	6.3	86935	5.1
1990	98325	5.8	8340	0.5	106665	6.3	87469	5.2
1991	95900	5.6	8190	0.5	104090	6.1	85221	5.0
1992	89550	5.2	7680	0.4	97230	5.7	79429	4.6
1993	90650	5.3	7030	0.4	97680	5.7	79839	4.7
1994	87250	5.1	6100	0.4	93350	5.4	76302	4.4
1995	79560	4.6	5140	0.3	84700	4.9	69234	4.0

Source : see *Notes on sources of sales data*, p. 678

Figure 27.1 Daily consumption of (i) manufactured and total number of cigarettes, and (ii) all tobacco products, 1920-1995.
Males and females aged 15 years and over. *Source:* see Table 27.2

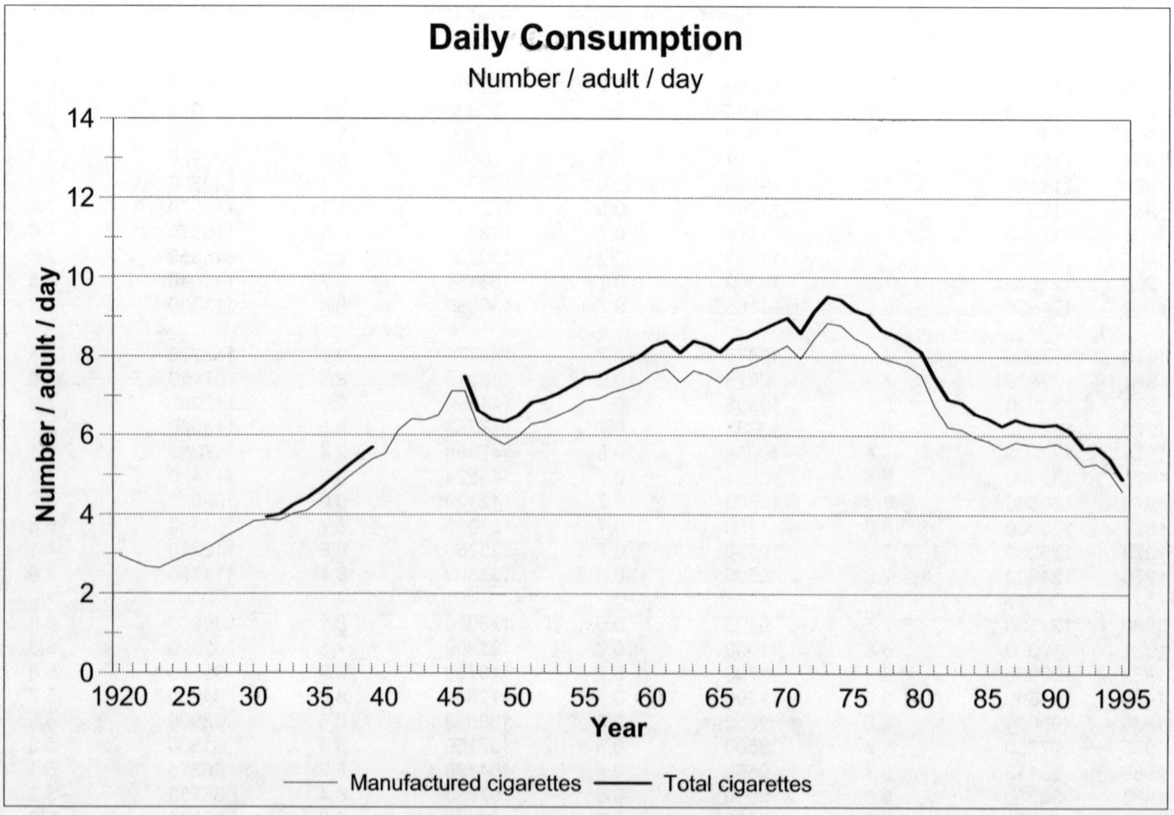

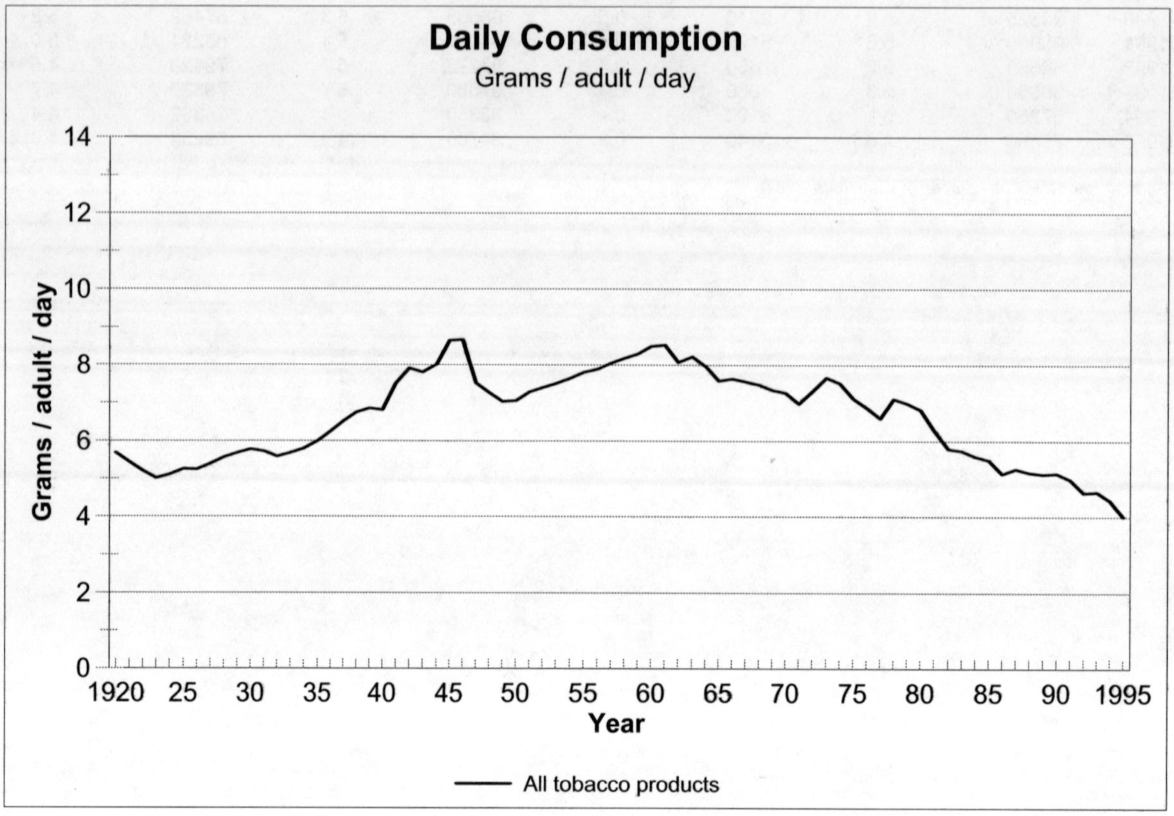

Table 27.3 Percentage sales of tobacco in different forms (by weight), selected years 1925-1995

Year	Cigarettes (%)	Cigars and cigarillos (%)	Pipe tobacco (%)	Hand-rolling tobacco (%)	Snuff (%)
1925	56.9	1.8	41.3	(With Pipe)	(With Cigars)
1935	72.8	0.7	21.7	4.1	0.6
1946	83.6	0.3	12.3	3.4	0.4
1955	85.6	0.4	8.4	5.4	0.3
1965	86.6	1.1	5.7	6.4	0.2
1975	86.5	3.0	4.5	5.8	0.2
1985	88.3	2.8	3.3	5.4	0.1
1995	91.9	2.8	1.6	3.7	0.0

Source : calculated from Tables 27.1.1 & 27.1.2

Figure 27.2 Percentage sales of tobacco in different forms (by weight), selected years 1925-1995
Source: see Table 27.3

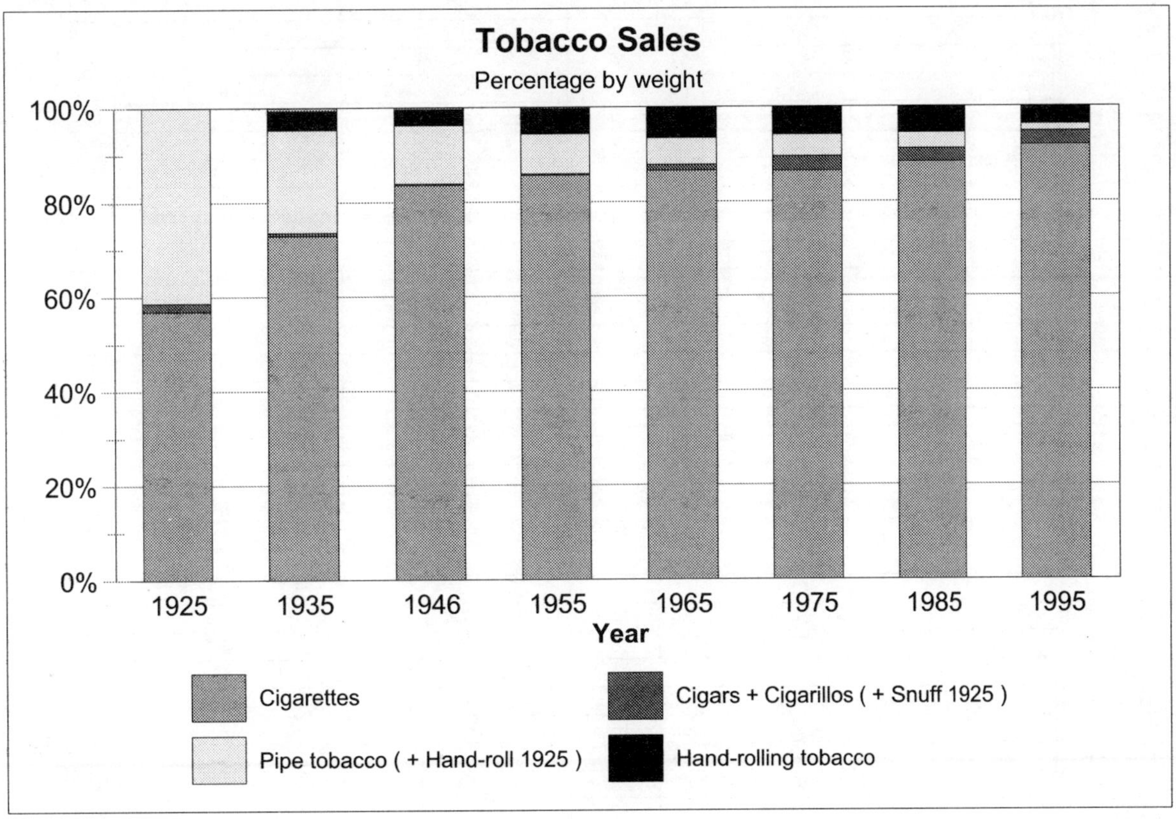

Table 27.4M Prevalence of smoking, males: some selected British surveys by age, 1928-1995 *(continues on p. 658)*

Year Source Product Frequency	12	13	14	15	16	17	18	19	20-24	25-29	30-34	35-39	40-44	45-49	50-54	55-59	60-64	65-69	70-74	75-79	80+	All ages
28 37 U U					90																	
38 37 U U					90																	
48 1 MC U					61				74	76		70					39					65
48 1 A U					62				79	84		84					85					82
49 1 MC U					54				73	71		68					38					63
49 1 A U					56				78	81		84					82					81
50 1 MC U					51				68	70		66					38					62
50 1 A U					52				71	79		81					78					77
51 1 MC U					51				68	70		66					42					62
51 1 A U					52				71	80		81					81					78
52 1 MC U					47				62	67		64					40					59
52 1 A U					49				67	77		80					79					76
53 1 MC U					47				61	67		64					42					59
53 1 A U					48				66	76		79					78					75
54 1 MC U					46				63	66		63					42					59
54 1 A U					47				67	75		79					80					75
55 1 MC U					47				59	67		62					39					58
55 1 A U					49				63	76		78					79					74
56 1 MC U					52				65	67		65					45					61
56 1 A U					55				67	74		79					79					75
56 21 UC R	28	25	44	47																		
57 1 MC U					59				61	66		63					45					60
57 1 A U					60				65	74		77					79					75
57 22 UC R	19	33	38	39	36																	
58 1 MC U					54				63	65		63					42					58
58 1 A U					56				66	68		77					72					72
58 23 UC R	6	14	24	29																		
59 1 MC U					60				62	65		63					48					60
59 1 A U					62				65	73		74					76					73
59 24 UC A	26																					
60 1 MC U					65				67	64		64					46					61
60 1 A U					65				70	73		78					69					74
61 1 MC U					61				67	60		61					46					59
61 1 A U					62				71	68		75					71					72
62 1 MC U					61				62	59		60					44					57
62 1 A U					63				67	67		74					69					70
63 1 MC U					56				65	60		54					42					54
63 1 A U					58				69	69		71					64					68
63 25 UC U									59													
63 25 A U									67													
64 1 MC U					56				61	55		57					45					54
64 1 A U					58				66	64		73					69					69
65 1 MC U					50				63	56		56					44					54
65 1 A U					52				68	67		71					69					68
65 5 UC R	19		27																			
66 1 MC U					54				60	59		56					44					54
66 1 A U					57				66	69		71					69					68
66 3 UC R	9	17	27	38																		
66 4 UC R	4	5	16	22																		
66 5 UC R	17		29																			
66 26 UC U			30																			
67 1 MC U					52				61	56		56					45					54
67 1 A U					55				68	65		73					67					68
68 1 MC U					57				59	57		57					46					55
68 1 A U					58				65	67		72					68					69
69 1 MC U					53				62	60		54					44					54
69 1 A U					55				68	70		72					66					68

Table 27.4F Prevalence of smoking, females: some selected British surveys by age, 1928-1995 *(continues on p. 659)*

Frequency Product Source Year	Age group																					All ages
	12	13	14	15	16	17	18	19	20-24	25-29	30-34	35-39	40-44	45-49	50-54	55-59	60-64	65-69	70-74	75-79	80+	
28 37 U U					15																	
38 37 U U					33																	
48 1 MC U					43				54	52		41					23					41
48 1 A U																						
49 1 MC U					33				53	55		43					24					41
49 1 A U																						
50 1 MC U					36				48	53		38					23					38
50 1 A U																						
51 1 MC U					28				43	52		39					21					38
51 1 A U																						
52 1 MC U					29				45	52		40					20					38
52 1 A U																						
53 1 MC U					26				43	49		40					23					37
53 1 A U																						
54 1 MC U					25				42	49		40					21					36
54 1 A U																						
55 1 MC U					26				39	51		41					22					37
55 1 A U																						
56 1 MC U					33				43	52		44					29					41
56 1 A U					33				44	47	57	48			37		29					42
56 21 UC R																						
57 1 MC U					40				46	55		46					28					44
57 1 A U																						
57 22 UC R	4	7	12	16	18																	
58 1 MC U					32				45	48		45					19					39
58 1 A U					32				45	46	51	50			38		19					40
58 23 UC R	0	3	4	5																		
59 1 MC U					33				47	55		49					19					42
59 1 A U																						
59 24 UC A	8																					
60 1 MC U					45				48	53		47					22					42
60 1 A U																						
61 1 MC U					45				51	50		50					24					43
61 1 A U					45				52	51		54			42		24					44
62 1 MC U					46				51	49		49					23					42
62 1 A U																						
63 1 MC U					39				50	49		51					24					43
63 1 A U					40				50	49		56			44		24					43
63 25 UC U									37													
63 25 A U									38													
64 1 MC U					40				49	51		48					22					41
64 1 A U																						
65 1 MC U					40				51	50		50					23					42
65 1 A U					40				51	50		54			46		23					43
65 5 UC R	5		18																			
66 1 MC U					47				53	50		52					26					45
66 1 A U																						
66 3 UC R																						
66 4 UC R																						
66 5 UC R	4		20																			
66 26 UC U			31																			
67 1 MC U					43				52	49		51					26					44
67 1 A U																						
68 1 MC U					46				53	47		51					24					43
68 1 A U					46				53	48		54			48		24					43
69 1 MC U					53				53	53		50					25					44
69 1 A U																						

Table 27.4M *(continued from p. 656, continues on p. 660)*
Prevalence of smoking, males

Frequency / Product / Source / Year	Age group: 12	13	14	15	16	17	18	19	20-24	25-29	30-34	35-39	40-44	45-49	50-54	55-59	60-64	65-69	70-74	75-79	80+	All ages
70 1 MC U					55				58	60		55					46					55
70 1 A U					56				65	70		71					68					68
71 1 MC U					53				57	55		50					43					51
71 1 A U					55				62	67		66					64					65
72 1 MC U					51				60	54		51					42					51
72 1 A U					54				65	65		70					63					66
72 2 UC A					43				55	56		55			54		47					52
73 1 MC U					49				62	53		49					41					49
73 1 A U					51				69	65		68					65					66
74 1 MC U					48				55	55		51					40					49
74 1 A U					48				61	66		69					61					64
74 2 UC A					42				52	56		55			53		44					51
74 7 UC R	6																					
74 27 UC R					38																	
75 1 MC U					49				53	46		49					41					47
75 1*MC U					51					46		47			49			38				47
75 1 A U					52				62	59		65					61					62
75 1* A U					57					59		62			67			60				62
75 6 UC *	5	7	6	6	5																	
75 6 UC R	8	15	19	26	24																	
75 7 UC R	9																					
76 1 MC U					48					48		46			47			32				45
76 1 A U					51					60		62			65			51				59
76 2 UC A					39				47	48		50			49		40					46
76 7 UC R		16																				
77 1 MC U					47					46		43			41			32				42
77 1 A U					52					59		61			61			56				58
77 7 UC R			21																			
78 1 MC U					46					44		43			40			30				41
78 1 A U					49					54		58			59			50				55
78 2 UC A					35				45	48		48			48		38					45
78 7 UC R				26																		
78 28 UC R	7																					
79 1 MC U					48					46		43			39			30				42
79 1 A U					51					58		58			56			51				55
79 6 UC R	4	9	16	21	22																	
79 8 UC R	10	29	21	33																		
79 9 UC R	0	5	8	23																		
80 1 MC U					44					47		43			43			28				42
80 1 A U					48					58		58			60			48				55
80 2 UC A					32				44	47		45			47		36					42
80 28 UC R	7																					
81 1 MC U					41					42		39			35			26				37
81 1 A U					44					53		53			53			45				50
81 10 UC R	7	24	24	23																		
82 1 MC U					42					38		37			33			27				36
82 1 A U					46					50		52			52			44				49
82 2 UC A					31				41	40		40			42		33					38
82 11 UC R	2	8	18	24	26																	
82 11 UC A	7	16	26	34	31																	
82 12 UC R	6	8	21	29																		
82 12 UC A	12	17	29	37																		
82 28 UC R		14																				
83 1 MC U					41					36		37			33			25				35
83 1 A U					45					48		50			48			43				47
83 16 U R		11		23																		
83 29 UC A		23	26																			

Table 27.4F *(continued from p. 657, continues on p. 661)*
Prevalence of smoking, females

<table>
<tr><th rowspan="2">Frequency / Product / Source / Year</th><th colspan="21">Age group</th><th rowspan="2">All ages</th></tr>
<tr><th>12</th><th>13</th><th>14</th><th>15</th><th>16</th><th>17</th><th>18</th><th>19</th><th>20-24</th><th>25-29</th><th>30-34</th><th>35-39</th><th>40-44</th><th>45-49</th><th>50-54</th><th>55-59</th><th>60-64</th><th>65-69</th><th>70-74</th><th>75-79</th><th>80+</th></tr>
<tr><td>70 1 MC U</td><td colspan="4"></td><td colspan="4">52</td><td>54</td><td colspan="2">51</td><td colspan="5">50</td><td colspan="5">26</td><td>44</td></tr>
<tr><td>70 1 A U</td><td colspan="21"></td><td></td></tr>
<tr><td>71 1 MC U</td><td colspan="4"></td><td colspan="4">48</td><td>50</td><td colspan="2">49</td><td colspan="5">49</td><td colspan="5">24</td><td>42</td></tr>
<tr><td>71 1 A U</td><td colspan="4"></td><td colspan="4">49</td><td>50</td><td colspan="2">49</td><td colspan="3">51</td><td colspan="2">46</td><td colspan="5">24</td><td>42</td></tr>
<tr><td>72 1 MC U</td><td colspan="4"></td><td colspan="4">46</td><td>48</td><td colspan="2">51</td><td colspan="5">48</td><td colspan="5">25</td><td>42</td></tr>
<tr><td>72 1 A U</td><td colspan="4"></td><td colspan="4">46</td><td>48</td><td colspan="2">51</td><td colspan="3">51</td><td colspan="2">44</td><td colspan="5">25</td><td>42</td></tr>
<tr><td>72 2 UC A</td><td colspan="4"></td><td colspan="4">39</td><td>48</td><td colspan="2">49</td><td colspan="3">48</td><td colspan="2">47</td><td colspan="5">25</td><td>41</td></tr>
<tr><td>73 1 MC U</td><td colspan="4"></td><td colspan="4">49</td><td>54</td><td colspan="2">47</td><td colspan="5">52</td><td colspan="5">25</td><td>43</td></tr>
<tr><td>73 1 A U</td><td colspan="4"></td><td colspan="4">49</td><td>54</td><td colspan="2">48</td><td colspan="3">54</td><td colspan="2">51</td><td colspan="5">25</td><td>44</td></tr>
<tr><td>74 1 MC U</td><td colspan="4"></td><td colspan="4">47</td><td>50</td><td colspan="2">52</td><td colspan="5">52</td><td colspan="5">26</td><td>44</td></tr>
<tr><td>74 1 A U</td><td colspan="4"></td><td colspan="4">47</td><td>51</td><td colspan="2">52</td><td colspan="3">55</td><td colspan="2">49</td><td colspan="5">27</td><td>44</td></tr>
<tr><td>74 2 UC A</td><td colspan="4"></td><td colspan="4">38</td><td>44</td><td colspan="2">46</td><td colspan="3">49</td><td colspan="2">48</td><td colspan="5">26</td><td>41</td></tr>
<tr><td>74 7 UC R</td><td>3</td><td colspan="20"></td><td></td></tr>
<tr><td>74 27 UC R</td><td colspan="4"></td><td>34</td><td colspan="16"></td><td></td></tr>
<tr><td>75 1 MC U</td><td colspan="4"></td><td colspan="4">46</td><td>53</td><td colspan="2">49</td><td colspan="5">49</td><td colspan="5">27</td><td>43</td></tr>
<tr><td>75 1*MC U</td><td colspan="4"></td><td colspan="5">50</td><td colspan="2">49</td><td colspan="3">50</td><td colspan="3">46</td><td colspan="4">23</td><td>43</td></tr>
<tr><td>75 1 A U</td><td colspan="4"></td><td colspan="4">46</td><td>53</td><td colspan="2">49</td><td colspan="3">51</td><td colspan="2">49</td><td colspan="5">28</td><td>43</td></tr>
<tr><td>75 1* A U</td><td colspan="4"></td><td colspan="5">50</td><td colspan="2">49</td><td colspan="3">51</td><td colspan="3">46</td><td colspan="4">24</td><td>43</td></tr>
<tr><td>75 6 UC *</td><td>3</td><td>5</td><td>8</td><td>6</td><td>5</td><td colspan="16"></td><td></td></tr>
<tr><td>75 6 UC R</td><td>5</td><td>12</td><td>20</td><td>23</td><td>22</td><td colspan="16"></td><td></td></tr>
<tr><td>75 7 UC R</td><td colspan="2">6</td><td colspan="19"></td><td></td></tr>
<tr><td>76 1 MC U</td><td colspan="4"></td><td colspan="5">51</td><td colspan="2">47</td><td colspan="3">48</td><td colspan="3">45</td><td colspan="4">21</td><td>42</td></tr>
<tr><td>76 1 A U</td><td colspan="4"></td><td colspan="5">52</td><td colspan="2">48</td><td colspan="3">49</td><td colspan="3">45</td><td colspan="4">21</td><td>42</td></tr>
<tr><td>76 2 UC A</td><td colspan="4"></td><td colspan="4">34</td><td>45</td><td colspan="2">43</td><td colspan="3">45</td><td colspan="2">46</td><td colspan="5">24</td><td>38</td></tr>
<tr><td>76 7 UC R</td><td></td><td colspan="2">13</td><td colspan="18"></td><td></td></tr>
<tr><td>77 1 MC U</td><td colspan="4"></td><td colspan="5">47</td><td colspan="2">46</td><td colspan="3">47</td><td colspan="3">45</td><td colspan="4">23</td><td>41</td></tr>
<tr><td>77 1 A U</td><td colspan="4"></td><td colspan="5">47</td><td colspan="2">47</td><td colspan="3">47</td><td colspan="3">46</td><td colspan="4">23</td><td>41</td></tr>
<tr><td>77 7 UC R</td><td colspan="2"></td><td colspan="2">19</td><td colspan="17"></td><td></td></tr>
<tr><td>78 1 MC U</td><td colspan="4"></td><td colspan="5">45</td><td colspan="2">47</td><td colspan="3">47</td><td colspan="3">40</td><td colspan="4">21</td><td>40</td></tr>
<tr><td>78 1 A U</td><td colspan="4"></td><td colspan="5">45</td><td colspan="2">48</td><td colspan="3">47</td><td colspan="3">41</td><td colspan="4">22</td><td>40</td></tr>
<tr><td>78 2 UC A</td><td colspan="4"></td><td colspan="4">33</td><td>43</td><td colspan="2">42</td><td colspan="3">43</td><td colspan="2">42</td><td colspan="5">24</td><td>37</td></tr>
<tr><td>78 7 UC R</td><td colspan="3"></td><td colspan="2">23</td><td colspan="16"></td><td></td></tr>
<tr><td>78 28 UC R</td><td>2</td><td colspan="20"></td><td></td></tr>
<tr><td>79 1 MC U</td><td colspan="4"></td><td colspan="5">46</td><td colspan="2">45</td><td colspan="3">44</td><td colspan="3">43</td><td colspan="4">21</td><td>39</td></tr>
<tr><td>79 1 A U</td><td colspan="4"></td><td colspan="5">47</td><td colspan="2">45</td><td colspan="3">45</td><td colspan="3">44</td><td colspan="4">22</td><td>40</td></tr>
<tr><td>79 6 UC R</td><td>5</td><td>12</td><td>17</td><td>23</td><td>19</td><td colspan="16"></td><td></td></tr>
<tr><td>79 8 UC R</td><td>13</td><td>16</td><td>16</td><td>26</td><td colspan="17"></td><td></td></tr>
<tr><td>79 9 UC R</td><td>0</td><td>9</td><td>14</td><td>20</td><td colspan="17"></td><td></td></tr>
<tr><td>80 1 MC U</td><td colspan="4"></td><td colspan="5">40</td><td colspan="2">45</td><td colspan="3">44</td><td colspan="3">46</td><td colspan="4">21</td><td>39</td></tr>
<tr><td>80 1 A U</td><td colspan="4"></td><td colspan="5">40</td><td colspan="2">46</td><td colspan="3">44</td><td colspan="3">47</td><td colspan="4">21</td><td>39</td></tr>
<tr><td>80 2 UC A</td><td colspan="4"></td><td colspan="4">32</td><td>40</td><td colspan="2">44</td><td colspan="3">43</td><td colspan="2">44</td><td colspan="5">24</td><td>37</td></tr>
<tr><td>80 28 UC R</td><td>2</td><td colspan="20"></td><td></td></tr>
<tr><td>81 1 MC U</td><td colspan="4"></td><td colspan="5">40</td><td colspan="2">42</td><td colspan="3">43</td><td colspan="3">40</td><td colspan="4">19</td><td>36</td></tr>
<tr><td>81 1 A U</td><td colspan="4"></td><td colspan="5">40</td><td colspan="2">43</td><td colspan="3">43</td><td colspan="3">41</td><td colspan="4">20</td><td>37</td></tr>
<tr><td>81 10 UC R</td><td>9</td><td>37</td><td>35</td><td>38</td><td colspan="17"></td><td></td></tr>
<tr><td>82 1 MC U</td><td colspan="4"></td><td colspan="5">38</td><td colspan="2">38</td><td colspan="3">41</td><td colspan="3">41</td><td colspan="4">21</td><td>35</td></tr>
<tr><td>82 1 A U</td><td colspan="4"></td><td colspan="5">38</td><td colspan="2">38</td><td colspan="3">41</td><td colspan="3">42</td><td colspan="4">22</td><td>36</td></tr>
<tr><td>82 2 UC A</td><td colspan="4"></td><td colspan="4">30</td><td>40</td><td colspan="2">37</td><td colspan="3">38</td><td colspan="2">40</td><td colspan="5">23</td><td>33</td></tr>
<tr><td>82 11 UC R</td><td>1</td><td>6</td><td>14</td><td>25</td><td>25</td><td colspan="16"></td><td></td></tr>
<tr><td>82 11 UC A</td><td>8</td><td>17</td><td>24</td><td>37</td><td>36</td><td colspan="16"></td><td></td></tr>
<tr><td>82 12 UC R</td><td>5</td><td>10</td><td>21</td><td>26</td><td colspan="17"></td><td></td></tr>
<tr><td>82 12 UC A</td><td>10</td><td>24</td><td>32</td><td>39</td><td colspan="17"></td><td></td></tr>
<tr><td>82 28 UC R</td><td></td><td colspan="2">9</td><td colspan="18"></td><td></td></tr>
<tr><td>83 1 MC U</td><td colspan="4"></td><td colspan="5">42</td><td colspan="2">40</td><td colspan="3">39</td><td colspan="3">39</td><td colspan="4">20</td><td>35</td></tr>
<tr><td>83 1 A U</td><td colspan="4"></td><td colspan="5">42</td><td colspan="2">41</td><td colspan="3">40</td><td colspan="3">39</td><td colspan="4">20</td><td>36</td></tr>
<tr><td>83 16 U R</td><td></td><td>20</td><td></td><td>27</td><td colspan="17"></td><td></td></tr>
<tr><td>83 29 UC A</td><td></td><td>36</td><td>36</td><td colspan="18"></td><td></td></tr>
</table>

Table 27.4M *(continued from p. 658, continues on p. 662)*
Prevalence of smoking, males

Frequency Product Source Year	12	13	14	15	16	17	18	19	20-24	25-29	30-34	35-39	40-44	45-49	50-54	55-59	60-64	65-69	70-74	75-79	80+	All ages
84 1 MC U					38					42		35			35			24				35
84 1 A U					41					52		51			52			39				47
84 2 UC A					29				40	40		39			39		30					36
84 11 UC R	2	10	16	28	29																	
84 11 UC A	8	21	27	38	37																	
84 12 UC R	8	10	22	29																		
84 12 UC A	17	17	31	36																		
84 13 UC *	5	13	21	28																		
84 14 UC R										35		37		32		33						34
84 14 A A										39		49		44		43						46
85 1 MC U					42					40		36			29			24				35
85 1 A U					46					50		51			45			39				46
85 13 UC *	8	12	17	25																		
85 13 UC R	10	15	21	30																		
86 1 MC U					42					36		35			31			20				33
86 1 A U					43					43		48			44			33				43
86 2 UC A					30				41	37		37			35		29					35
86 11 UC R	2	5	6	18																		
86 11 UC A	7	9	13	24																		
86 12 UC R	2	7	11	24																		
86 12 UC A	5	12	15	27																		
86 13 UC *	3	10	16	20																		
86 13 UC R	5	12	18	24																		
86 15 UC R										39		54		54		47						52
86 15 A A										45		67		60		59						62
86 17 U *		5		13																		
86 17 U R		7		16																		
86 17 U A		12		20																		
86 18 U *		3		17																		
86 18 U R		5		19																		
86 18 U A		6		21																		
87 1 MC U					42					38		35			29			21				34
87 1 A U					43					45		50			42			35				44
87 13 UC *	4	6	12	20																		
87 13 UC R	4	8	15	25																		
88 2 UC A					28				37	37		37			33		26					33
88 11 UC R	2	5	8	17																		
88 11 UC A	4	10	15	24																		
90 2 UC A					28				38	36		34			28		24					31
90 11 UC R	2	6	10	25																		
90 11 UC A	6	11	18	35																		
90 12 UC R	4	8	16	22																		
90 12 UC A	10	17	26	30																		
90 17 U *		5		11																		
90 17 U R		8		15																		
90 17 U A		11		20																		
90 18 UC R		8		16																		
90 18 UC A		12		20																		
90 30 U R			4	8																		
90 30 U A	0		6																			
91 20 UC A					34					31		32		32		30		27		14		30
92 2 UC A					29				39	34		32			28		21					29
92 11 UC R	2	6	14	21																		
92 11 UC A	7	11	24	30																		
92 12 UC R	2	9	14	22																		
92 12 UC A	8	15	20	30																		
92 20 UC A					43					38		35		32		27		26		15		33

Table 27.4F *(continued from p.659, continues on p. 663)*
Prevalence of smoking, females

Frequency Product Source Year	Age group																					
	12	13	14	15	16	17	18	19	20 - 24	25 - 29	30 - 34	35 - 39	40 - 44	45 - 49	50 - 54	55 - 59	60 - 64	65 - 69	70 - 74	75 - 79	80+	All ages
84 1 MC U					38					39		37			39			20				34
84 1 A U					38					40		37			40			20				35
84 2 UC A					32				36	36		36			39		23					32
84 11 UC R	2	9	19	28	30																	
84 11 UC A	8	22	30	37	45																	
84 12 UC R	3	12	22	34																		
84 12 UC A	11	22	34	41																		
84 13 UC *	5	14	23	26																		
84 14 UC R										38		35		30		35						33
84 14 A A										40		37		33		36						35
85 1 MC U					40					42		38			37			19				34
85 1 A U					40					42		39			37			19				35
85 13 UC *	7	13	21	25																		
85 13 UC R	11	17	25	29																		
86 1 MC U					41					37		40			34			17				33
86 1 A U					41					38		40			35			17				34
86 2 UC A					30				38	35		34			35		22					31
86 11 UC R	2	5	16	27																		
86 11 UC A	4	12	22	35																		
86 12 UC R	3	8	21	26																		
86 12 UC A	6	16	28	34																		
86 13 UC *	4	13	21	21																		
86 13 UC R	6	16	25	25																		
86 15 UC R										50		57		49		42						50
86 15 A A										51		59		51		43						52
86 17 U *		9		15																		
86 17 U R		12		20																		
86 17 U A		18		25																		
86 18 U *		4		20																		
86 18 U R		5		24																		
86 18 U A		7		28																		
87 1 MC U					42					38		37			35			20				34
87 1 A U					42					39		37			36			21				34
87 13 UC *	2	10	15	20																		
87 13 UC R	4	13	20	25																		
88 2 UC A					28				37	35		35			34		21					30
88 11 UC R	0	4	12	22																		
88 11 UC A	1	9	19	31																		
90 2 UC A					32				39	34		33			29		20					29
90 11 UC R	2	9	16	25																		
90 11 UC A	5	15	24	37																		
90 12 UC R	3	10	18	28																		
90 12 UC A	8	21	30	36																		
90 17 U *		6		16																		
90 17 U R		11		22																		
90 17 U A		20		29																		
90 18 UC R		8		18																		
90 18 UC A		14		23																		
90 30 U R			11	13																		
90 30 U A	1	11																				
91 20 UC A					35					37		30		43		24		17		15		30
92 2 UC A					25				37	34		30			29		19					28
92 11 UC R	2	9	15	25																		
92 11 UC A	7	15	24	36																		
92 12 UC R	2	9	23	28																		
92 12 UC A	8	18	31	40																		
92 20 UC A					37					37		32		30		28		18		16		29

Table 27.4M (continued from p.660)
Prevalence of smoking, males

Frequency / Product / Source / Year	12	13	14	15	16	17	18	19	20-24	25-29	30-34	35-39	40-44	45-49	50-54	55-59	60-64	65-69	70-74	75-79	80+	All ages
93 11 UC R	3	3	14	19																		
93 11 UC A	6	12	22	28																		
93 20 UC A					32					34		32		28		25		20		13		28
94 2 UC A	28								40	34		31			27		18					28
94 11 UC R	2	4	14	26																		
94 11 UC A	7	16	24	39																		
94 12 UC R	2	11	15	20																		
94 17 UC R		8		18																		
94 18 UC R		7		21																		
94 19 UC R		10		23																		
94 20 UC A					35					36		31		30		22		21		12		29
94 20 A A					36					40		38		39		31		29		22		35
95 20 UC A					36					39		31		30		24		18		11		29
95 20 A A					38					43		37		38		32		26		20		35
95 31 UC R				23																		
95 31 UC A				32																		
95 32 UC R				6																		
95 32 UC A				33																		
95 33 UC R				6																		
95 33 UC A				29																		
95 34 UC R				6																		
95 34 UC A				27																		
95 35 UC R				4																		
95 35 UC A				34																		
95 36 UC R				6																		
95 36 UC A				32																		

Source: see *Notes on sources of survey data*, p. 679
Product: MC = manufactured cigarettes
TC = total cigarettes (including hand-rolled)
UC = cigarettes (type unspecified)
A = all products

Frequency: A = all smokers (including occasional)
R = regular or daily smokers
All ages: relevant to ages used and as given in original source
U = unspecified
* = refer to *Notes on sources of survey data*, p. 679

Table 27.4F (continued from p. 661)
Prevalence of smoking, females

Frequency / Product / Source / Year	12	13	14	15	16	17	18	19	20-24	25-29	30-34	35-39	40-44	45-49	50-54	55-59	60-64	65-69	70-74	75-79	80+	All ages
93 11 UC R	3	5	18	26																		
93 11 UC A	10	15	31	35																		
93 20 UC A					32					32		30		27		25		18		11		26
94 2 UC A					27				38	30		28			26		17					26
94 11 UC R	3	8	20	30																		
94 11 UC A	8	19	33	42																		
94 12 UC R	3	10	21	23																		
94 17 UC R		13		27																		
94 18 UC R		12		26																		
94 19 UC R		13		25																		
94 20 UC A					34					33		28		29		24		19		11		27
94 20 A A					34					33		29		30		24		19		11		27
95 20 UC A					37					32		27		30		24		19		10		27
95 20 A A					37					32		27		30		25		19		10		27
95 31 UC R				29																		
95 31 UC A				40																		
95 32 UC R				7																		
95 32 UC A				40																		
95 33 UC R				2																		
95 33 UC A				31																		
95 34 UC R				6																		
95 34 UC A				38																		
95 35 UC R				3																		
95 35 UC A				37																		
95 36 UC R				7																		
95 36 UC A				40																		

Source: see *Notes on sources of survey data*, p. 679
Product: MC = manufactured cigarettes
TC = total cigarettes (including hand-rolled)
UC = cigarettes (type unspecified)
A = all products

Frequency: A = all smokers (including occasional)
R = regular or daily smokers
All ages: relevant to ages used and as given in original source
U = unspecified
* = refer to *Notes on sources of survey data*, p. 679

Table 27.5M Number of cigarettes smoked per smoker per day, males: some selected British surveys by age, 1949-1995.
(continues on p. 666)

Product Source Year	Age group																					
	12	13	14	15	16	17	18	19	20 - 24	25 - 29	30 - 34	35 - 39	40 - 44	45 - 49	50 - 54	55 - 59	60 - 64	65 - 69	70 - 74	75 - 79	80+	All ages
49 1 MC					8.9				13	13	15	16					11					14
50 1 MC					9.7				14	16	15	17					15	9.6				15
51 1 MC					10				15	16	17	17					14	10				16
52 1 MC					9.3				16	17	18	19					16	13				17
53 1 MC					11				16	17	19	19					17	12				17
54 1 MC					10				16	18	19	20					16	11				18
55 1 MC					12				17	19	19	21					17	13				19
56 1 MC					11				16	17	17	19			20		16	12				17
57 1 MC					11				16	17	18	21			19		18	14				18
57 22 UCE*	1.0	1.2	1.6	1.8	2.3																	
58 1 MC					12				18	17	19	21			20		19	12				19
58 23 UCE*	14		17																			
59 1 MC					13				17	17	20	21			20		18	13				18
60 1 MC					13				18	18	19	21			21		18	12				19
61 1 MC					13				17	18	19	20			21		19	16				19
62 1 MC					15				19	19	19	20			20		17	13				19
63 1 MC					14				19	20	20	22			21		17					20
64 1 MC					14				19	19	19	21			21		17					19
65 1 MC					14				19	19	20	20			19		16					18
66 1 MC					14				18	19	17	20			19		16					18
67 1 MC					15				18	20	18	20			20		16					19
68 1 MC					16				19	18	19	20			20		14					18
69 1 MC					16				19	20	19	21			20		15					19
70 1 MC					16				19	20	20	21			20		16					19
71 1 MC					17				21	21	21	22			22		17					20
72 1 MC					18				21	22	23	23			22		17					21
72 2 UC					15				18	18		19			18		14					17
73 1 MC					19				22	24	24	25			23		18					22
74 1 MC					19				22	21	22	24			22		18					21
74 2 UC					16				19	19		20			18		14					18
74 27 UCE*					4.3																	
75 1 MC					19				22	22	23	23			24		23	14				22
75 6 UCE*	7	10	10	13	12																	
76 1 MC					19				23	24		23			23			15				22
76 2 UC					15				19	20		20			19		15					18
77 1 MC					19				22	23		23			23			16				22
78 1 MC					19				23	23		24			23			15				22
78 2 UC					14				17	19		20			20		15					18
79 1 MC					18				21	23		23			22			17				22
80 1 MC					18				20	21		24			22			17				21
80 2 UC					14				16	19		20			19		15					18
81 1 MC					16				21	20		22			20			17				20
82 1 MC					16				19	20		22			21			17				20
82 2 UC					12				16	17		20			18		16					17
82 11 UC	7.1																					
82 12 UC	7.4																					
83 1 MC					16				18	22		22			22			15				20
84 1 MC					15				18	20		22			20			16				20
84 2 UC					12				15	16		19			18		15					16
84 11 UC	7.0																					
84 12 UC	7.3																					
84 14 UC												19										
85 1 MC					16				18	19		22			20			15				19

Table 27.5F Number of cigarettes smoked per smoker per day, females: some selected British surveys by age, 1949-1995.
(continues on p. 667)

Year Source Product	12	13	14	15	16	17	18	19	20-24	25-29	30-34	35-39	40-44	45-49	50-54	55-59	60-64	65-69	70-74	75-79	80+	All ages
49 1 MC					4.7				6.7	6.9	7.7	7.4					4.7					6.9
50 1 MC					5.3				7.9	7.4	9.3	8.9					6.3					8.0
51 1 MC					5.3				7.3	9.1	8.9	8.9					5.6					8.1
52 1 MC					6.1				7.9	9.6	9.3	9.3					5.4					8.6
53 1 MC					6.1				8.3	9.3	10	10					5.7					9.1
54 1 MC					6.7				8.9	9.9	11	11					6.0					9.6
55 1 MC					7.4				9.6	11	9.9	11					5.9					10
56 1 MC					6.6				8.6	10	11	12			10		6.6					10
57 1 MC					6.7				8.4	11	11	11			11		7.1					10
57 22 UCE*	0.6	1.0	0.9	0.8	1.3																	
58 1 MC					7.4				9.7	11	12	13			12		8.0					11
58 23 UCE*																						
59 1 MC					6.7				8.9	11	12	12			12		7.3					11
60 1 MC					7.3				9.6	9.4	12	12			11		8.1					11
61 1 MC					7.7				9.1	12	11	12			12		7.7					11
62 1 MC					9.3				11	12	12	12			12		8.4					11
63 1 MC					9.3				12	12	13	14			12		9.7					12
64 1 MC					9.9				11	12	14	14			13		9.3					12
65 1 MC					9.1				12	13	13	13			13		8.9					12
66 1 MC					9.7				12	14	13	14			12		8.4					12
67 1 MC					11				12	12	12	14			13		9.9					12
68 1 MC					11				13	13	13	14			13		9.1					12
69 1 MC					12				15	15	15	14			14		11					14
70 1 MC					13				15	15	14	15			14		10					14
71 1 MC					13				16	15	15	16			14		11					14
72 1 MC					14				16	17	17	17			14		11					15
72 2 UC					11				13	14		13			12		8.6					12
73 1 MC					15				18	18	18	17			16		13					16
74 1 MC					16				18	18	19	17			17		12					16
74 2 UC					12				14	15		15			13		9.7					13
74 27 UCE*					3.3																	
75 1 MC					16				17	18	18	17			15		13	10				16
75 6 UCE*	4	6	8	9	9																	
76 1 MC					17				18	19		18			17			12				17
76 2 UC					13				16	16		16			15		11					14
77 1 MC					15				17	19		19			16			12				17
78 1 MC					15				17	19		19			16			12				17
78 2 UC					13				14	16		16			14		11					14
79 1 MC					15				18	19		19			15			12				17
80 1 MC					14				17	17		18			17			12				16
80 2 UC					12				15	16		16			15		10					15
81 1 MC					14				17	17		19			17			12				16
82 1 MC					13				16	17		18			16			12				16
82 2 UC					11				14	16		15			14		11					14
82 11 UC	6.3																					
82 12 UC	6.2																					
83 1 MC					13				16	17		18			16			11				16
84 1 MC					12				16	16		19			15			11				15
84 2 UC					11				13	15		15			14		11					14
84 11 UC	7.0																					
84 12 UC	6.7																					
84 14 UC												16										
85 1 MC					13				15	16		18			16			12				16

Table 27.5M *(continued from p.664)*
Number of cigarettes smoked per smoker per day, males

Product Source Year	12	13	14	15	16	17	18	19	20-24	25-29	30-34	35-39	40-44	45-49	50-54	55-59	60-64	65-69	70-74	75-79	80+	All ages
86 1 MC					16				18	20		21			20			18				19
86 2 UC					12				15	16		19			17		15					16
86 11 UC	7.6																					
86 12 UC	8.0																					
86 15 UC												22										
87 1 MC					17				18	19		20			20			16				19
88 2 UC					12				16	17		19			19		15					17
88 11 UC	7.4																					
90 2 UC					13				16	16		19			17		15					17
90 11 UC	8.0																					
90 12 UC	7.7																					
91 20 UCE					15					16		19		19		18		15		14		17
92 2 UC					12				13	14		19			18		15					16
92 11 UC	8.3																					
92 12 UC	8.6																					
92 20 UCE					13					16		18		18		20		14		9.9		16
93 11 UC	7.3																					
93 20 UC					13					15		17		18		18		14		11		16
94 2 UC					10				13	15		18			20		14					16
94 11 UC	7.7																					
94 12 UC	8.0																					
94 20 UCE					12					16		17		19		17		14		10		16
95 20 UC					13					15		17		19		17		15		11		16
95 31 UCE				10																		

Source: see *Notes on sources of survey data*, p. 679
Product: MC = manufactured cigarettes
TC = total cigarettes (including hand-rolled)
UC = cigarettes (type unspecified)
A = all products
U = unspecified

Product (cont): E indicates mean estimated from percentage distribution (see also *Consumption category estimation*, p. xxxiv, and Appendix III, p. 789)
All ages: relevant to ages used and as given in original source
* = refer to *Notes on sources of survey data*, p. 679

Table 27.5F *(continued from p.665)*
Number of cigarettes smoked per smoker per day, females

Product Source Year	12	13	14	15	16	17	18	19	20-24	25-29	30-34	35-39	40-44	45-49	50-54	55-59	60-64	65-69	70-74	75-79	80+	All ages
86 1 MC					13				15	16		19			16			11				16
86 2 UC					11				12	14		16			14		12					14
86 11 UC	6.4																					
86 12 UC	6.6																					
86 15 UC												18										
87 1 MC					13				14	16		18			16			11				15
88 2 UC					11				14	15		16			15		12					14
88 11 UC	5.9																					
90 2 UC					11				13	15		15			15		12					14
90 11 UC	7.0																					
90 12 UC	6.6																					
91 20 UCE					11					16		17		16		13		11		11		14
92 2 UC					10				13	14		16			15		12					14
92 11 UC	6.3																					
92 12 UC	6.9																					
92 20 UCE					11					13		17		15		13		11		6.6		13
93 11 UC	6.3																					
93 20 UC					12					13		14		16		14		12		10		13
94 2 UC					10				13	14		15			15		13					14
94 11 UC	6.7																					
94 12 UC	6.6																					
94 20 UCE					11					13		15		15		14		11		11		13
95 20 UC					12					13		15		15		14		13		9.3		13
95 31 UCE				9.1																		

Source: see *Notes on sources of survey data*, p. 679
Product: MC = manufactured cigarettes
TC = total cigarettes (including hand-rolled)
UC = cigarettes (type unspecified)
A = all products
U = unspecified

Product (cont): E indicates mean estimated from percentage distribution (see also *Consumption category estimation*, p. xxxiv, and Appendix III, p. 789)
All ages: relevant to ages used and as given in original source
* = refer to *Notes on sources of survey data*, p. 679

Table 27.6M Number of cigarettes smoked per person per day, males: some selected British surveys[1] by age, 1957-1995, with percentage total sales

Product Source Year	12	13	14	15	16	17	18	19	20-24	25-29	30-34	35-39	40-44	45-49	50-54	55-59	60-64	65-69	70-74	75-79	80+	All ages	% Total sales
57 22 UC *	0.2	0.4	0.6	0.7	0.8																		**
72 2 UC					6.3				9.7	10		10			9.6		6.4					8.9	74%T
74 2 UC					6.6				9.8	11		11			9.6		6.3					9.1	75%T
74 27 UC *					1.6																		**
75 6 UC *	0	1	1	1	1																		**
76 2 UC					5.9				9.1	9.5		10			9.1		6.2					8.5	75%T
78 2 UC					4.9				7.8	9.2		9.5			9.4		5.7					8.2	76%T
80 2 UC					4.5				7.1	9.1		9.0			8.7		5.2					7.4	77%T
82 2 UC					3.9				6.7	6.9		7.8			7.7		5.1					6.6	79%T
82 11 UC	0.9																						**
82 12 UC	1.1																						**
84 2 UC					3.6				6.1	6.5		7.2			7.0		4.4					5.9	78%T
84 11 UC	1.0																						**
84 12 UC	1.3																						**
84 14 UC *												6.5											**
86 2 UC					3.7				6.3	5.8		7.0			6.0		4.3					5.8	78%T
86 11 UC	0.6																						**
86 12 UC	0.9																						**
86 15 UC *												12											**
88 2 UC					3.4				5.8	6.3		7.2			6.2		3.8					5.7	78%T
88 11 UC	0.6																						**
90 2 UC					3.6				6.0	5.9		6.6			4.8		3.6					5.2	73%T
90 11 UC	0.9																						**
90 12 UC	1.0																						**
91 20 UC					4.9					4.9		6.1		6.0		5.3		4.0		1.9		5.0	75%T
92 2 UC					3.4				5.1	4.9		5.9			5.2		3.1					4.6	74%T
92 11 UC	0.7																						**
92 12 UC	0.7																						**
92 20 UC					5.6					6.2		6.2		5.9		5.3		3.5		1.5		5.3	79%T
93 11 UC	0.7																						**
93 20 UC					4.2					5.1		5.4		5.0		4.5		2.8		1.4		4.5	69%T
94 2 UC					2.8				5.4	5.2		5.6			5.5		2.5					4.6	74%T
94 11 UC	0.9																						**
94 12 UC	0.9																						**
94 20 UC					4.2					5.4		5.3		5.5		3.8		2.9		1.1		4.6	72%T
95 20 UC					4.5					5.7		5.2		5.7		4.1		2.6		1.2		4.5	82%T
95 31 UC				2.4																			**

1 Data from source 1 are not presented here. They are adjusted by the original author to match total sales, and are included in Table 27.7

Source: see *Notes on sources of survey data*, p. 679
All ages: relevant to ages used and as given in original source
% Total sales: estimated % of total sales of M = manufactured or T = total cigarette consumption implied by survey, sexes combined, used as adjustment factor in Table 27.7
** = cannot be calculated
--- = adjusted by original author

Product: MC = manufactured cigarettes
TC = total cigarettes (including hand-rolled)
UC = cigarettes (type unspecified)
A = all products
U = unspecified
* = refer to *Notes on sources of survey data*, p. 679

Table 27.6F Number of cigarettes smoked per person per day, females: some selected British surveys[1] by age, 1957-1995, with percentage total sales

Year Source Product	12	13	14	15	16	17	18	19	20-24	25-29	30-34	35-39	40-44	45-49	50-54	55-59	60-64	65-69	70-74	75-79	80+	All ages	% Total sales
57 22 UC *	0.0	0.1	0.2	0.3	0.4																		**
72 2 UC					4.2				6.2	6.8		6.5			5.8		2.1					5.1	74%T
74 2 UC					4.7				6.2	7.1		7.3			6.2		2.5					5.5	75%T
74 27 UC *					1.1																		**
75 6 UC *	0	0	1	1	0																		**
76 2 UC					4.3				7.1	6.7		7.2			6.8		2.6					5.5	75%T
78 2 UC					4.2				6.2	6.8		6.7			6.1		2.7					5.3	76%T
80 2 UC					3.8				5.8	7.0		7.1			6.6		2.5					5.4	77%T
82 2 UC					3.3				5.7	5.8		5.9			5.8		2.5					4.6	79%T
82 11 UC	0.7																						**
82 12 UC	1.0																						**
84 2 UC					3.7				4.7	5.4		5.5			5.5		2.6					4.4	78%T
84 11 UC	1.0																						**
84 12 UC	1.1																						**
84 14 UC *												5.3											**
86 2 UC					3.3				4.6	5.0		5.4			5.0		2.6					4.3	78%T
86 11 UC	0.9																						**
86 12 UC	1.0																						**
86 15 UC *												9.0											**
88 2 UC					3.2				5.0	5.2		5.7			5.0		2.4					4.2	78%T
88 11 UC	0.6																						**
90 2 UC					3.7				5.1	5.0		5.0			4.4		2.3					4.0	73%T
90 11 UC	0.7																						**
90 12 UC	0.9																						**
91 20 UC					3.9					5.6		5.1		6.8		3.2		1.7		1.7		4.2	75%T
92 2 UC					2.5				4.7	4.7		4.8			4.3		2.2					3.9	74%T
92 11 UC	0.6																						**
92 12 UC	0.9																						**
92 20 UC					3.9					4.7		5.4		4.5		3.6		1.9		0.9		3.8	79%T
93 11 UC	0.7																						**
93 20 UC					3.8					4.2		4.2		4.3		3.5		2.2		1.1		3.4	69%T
94 2 UC					2.7				4.9	4.2		4.2			3.9		2.2					3.6	74%T
94 11 UC	0.9																						**
94 12 UC	0.9																						**
94 20 UC					3.6					4.2		4.3		4.3		3.4		2.2		1.3		3.5	72%T
95 20 UC					4.3					4.0		4.0		4.6		3.4		2.4		0.9		3.6	82%T
95 31 UC				2.6																			**

1 Data from source 1 are not presented here. They are adjusted by the original author to match total sales, and are included in Table 27.7

Source: see *Notes on sources of survey data*, p. 679
All ages: relevant to ages used and as given in original source
% Total sales: estimated % of total sales of M = manufactured or T = total cigarette consumption implied by survey, sexes combined, used as adjustment factor in Table 27.7
** = cannot be calculated
--- = adjusted by original author

Product: MC = manufactured cigarettes
TC = total cigarettes (including hand-rolled)
UC = cigarettes (type unspecified)
A = all products
U = unspecified
* = refer to *Notes on sources of survey data*, p. 679

Table 27.7M Number of cigarettes smoked per person per day, sales-adjusted, males: some selected British surveys[1] by age, 1949-1995, with percentage total sales

Product Source Year	Age group 12	13	14	15	16	17	18	19	20-24	25-29	30-34	35-39	40-44	45-49	50-54	55-59	60-64	65-69	70-74	75-79	80+	All ages	% Total sales
49 1 MC					4.8				9.5	9.9		11					4.1					8.9	---M
50 1 MC					5.0				9.6	11		11					4.3					9.5	---M
51 1 MC					5.2				9.9	11		11					4.9					9.7	---M
52 1 MC					4.4				9.7	12		12					5.5					10	---M
53 1 MC					5.2				9.8	12		12					5.8					10	---M
54 1 MC					4.7				10	12		13					5.4					11	---M
55 1 MC					5.6				9.8	13		13					5.5					11	---M
56 1 MC					5.7				10	11		13					5.9					11	---M
57 1 MC					6.5				9.6	12		13					6.8					11	---M
58 1 MC					6.6				11	11		13					5.9					11	---M
59 1 MC					7.7				11	12		13					6.9					11	---M
60 1 MC					8.4				12	12		14					6.3					11	---M
61 1 MC					8.0				11	11		13					7.9					11	---M
62 1 MC					9.3				12	11		12					6.3					11	---M
63 1 MC					8.0				12	12		12					7.1					11	---M
64 1 MC					8.1				12	11		12					7.5					10	---M
65 1 MC					7.1				12	11		11					6.9					10	---M
66 1 MC					7.3				11	12	10	12	11	11	11	9.6	9.3	6.7	4.8	6.0	1.4	10	---M
67 1 MC					8.0				12	12	10	12	12	11	9.9	10	9.0	6.7	5.6	3.6	3.3	10	---M
68 1 MC					9.2				11	10	11	12	12	12	11	10	8.1	7.8	5.5	3.4	1.9	11	---M
69 1 MC					8.5				12	12	12	12	13	11	12	10	8.2	7.4	4.9	3.6	2.6	10	---M
70 1 MC					8.4				12	12	12	13	13	12	11	9.6	9.6	8.0	4.5	4.1	3.1	11	---M
71 1 MC					8.8				12	11	12	11	11	14	12	8.6	9.2	6.7	7.0	3.0	3.6	10	---M
72 1 MC					9.4				12	12	12	12	12	13	11	10	8.9	7.1	5.9	5.8	2.6	11	---M
72 2 UC					8.4				13	14		14			13		8.7					12	74%T
73 1 MC					9.4				14	13	13	14	12	11	12	9.0	9.9	7.3	5.1	3.4	4.1	11	---M
74 1 MC					8.8				12	12	12	13	11	14	11	11	8.1	9.0	5.8	4.4	2.9	11	---M
74 2 UC					8.8				13	14		14			13		8.3					12	75%T
75 1 MC					9.2				12	10	10	11	11	10	13	11	11	8.1	4.7	4.2	1.9	10	---M
76 1 MC					8.8				11	11	11	11	10	11	12	9.7	10	6.2	4.5	3.0	2.5	9.7	---M
76 2 UC					7.9				12	13		13			12		8.2					11	75%T
77 1 MC					8.4				11	11	9.9	9.7	10	9.9	9.9	10	7.4	6.4	4.2	3.8	4.8	9.1	---M
78 1 MC					8.1				11	9.9	10	10	12	8.8	12	7.7	7.8	6.6	4.4	4.5	1.4	9.1	---M
78 2 UC					6.5				10	12		13			12		7.5					11	76%T
79 1 MC					7.8				11	9.9	12	9.6	9.7	11	9.6	7.7	8.6	6.2	4.7	5.6	2.7	9.0	---M
80 1 MC					7.3				9.0	9.9	10	11	10	9.7	11	8.8	8.8	4.9	4.8	4.8	2.6	8.8	---M
80 2 UC					5.9				9.2	12		12			11		6.8					9.7	77%T
81 1 MC					6.2				8.9	9.2	8.4	9.3	8.0	8.5	7.8	8.2	5.6	4.5	5.1	2.7	1.8	7.6	---M
82 1 MC					6.3				8.2	7.1	8.2	8.2	7.7	8.5	8.2	6.7	5.5	6.2	3.7			7.0	---M
82 2 UC					4.9				8.5	8.8		9.9			9.8		6.5					8.3	79%T
83 1 MC					6.2				7.7	7.5	8.1	8.0	8.8	7.0	8.0	7.3	6.4	4.5	3.3			6.8	---M
84 1 MC					5.9				7.0	8.8	8.4	8.1	7.1	8.2	6.8	8.6	5.6	4.7	3.1			6.8	---M
84 2 UC					4.6				7.9	8.4		9.3			9.1		5.7					7.6	78%T
85 1 MC					6.7				7.7	8.2	7.0	8.6	7.8	7.4	5.9	6.2	4.9	4.7	3.1			6.5	---M
86 1 MC					6.3				7.5	6.6	8.1	7.4	7.7	6.8	7.1	5.6	5.9	4.4	2.9			6.4	---M
86 2 UC					4.7				8.1	7.5		9.0			7.7		5.5					7.4	78%T
87 1 MC					6.3				8.0	7.8	6.8	7.7	6.8	7.0	6.6	5.6	5.8	4.1	3.0			6.4	---M
88 2 UC					4.3				7.4	8.2		9.3			8.0		4.9					7.3	78%T
90 2 UC					4.9				8.2	8.1		9.0			6.6		5.0					7.2	73%T
91 20 UC					6.6					6.6		8.2		8.0		7.1		5.3		2.5		6.7	75%T
92 2 UC					4.6				7.0	6.6		8.1			7.0		4.2					6.3	74%T
92 20 UC					7.1					7.9		7.8		7.4		6.7		4.5		1.9		6.7	79%T
93 20 UC					6.1					7.4		7.9		7.4		6.6		4.1		2.1		6.5	69%T
94 2 UC					3.9				7.3	7.1		7.6			7.4		3.5					6.2	74%T
94 20 UC					5.8					7.5		7.3		7.7		5.3		4.0		1.5		6.4	72%T
95 20 UC					5.5					6.9		6.4		6.9		5.0		3.2		1.5		5.5	82%T

1 Based on surveys from source 1 and those surveys in Table 27.6 with data for both sexes and age range at least 21-64 (see also *Cigarette consumption per person* p. xxxv)

2 For other footnotes see Table 27.6

Table 27.7F Number of cigarettes smoked per person per day, sales-adjusted, females: some selected British surveys[1] by age, 1949-1995, with percentage total sales

Product Source Year	Age group 12	13	14	15	16	17	18	19	20-24	25-29	30-34	35-39	40-44	45-49	50-54	55-59	60-64	65-69	70-74	75-79	80+	All ages	% Total sales
49 1 MC					1.6				3.6	4.0		3.2					1.1					2.8	---M
50 1 MC					1.9				3.8	4.6		3.4					1.4					3.0	---M
51 1 MC					1.5				3.1	4.7		3.5					1.2					3.1	---M
52 1 MC					1.8				3.5	4.9		3.7					1.1					3.3	---M
53 1 MC					1.6				3.6	4.8		4.1					1.3					3.4	---M
54 1 MC					1.7				3.7	5.1		4.3					1.3					3.5	---M
55 1 MC					1.9				3.7	5.3		4.7					1.3					3.7	---M
56 1 MC					2.2				3.7	5.4		4.8					1.9					4.2	---M
57 1 MC					2.7				3.9	5.9		5.1					2.0					4.4	---M
58 1 MC					2.4				4.4	5.6		5.5					1.5					4.3	---M
59 1 MC					2.2				4.2	6.3		6.0					1.4					4.6	---M
60 1 MC					3.3				4.6	5.7		5.5					1.8					4.4	---M
61 1 MC					3.5				4.7	5.8		6.1					2.9					4.7	---M
62 1 MC					4.3				5.8	5.9		5.9					1.9					4.7	---M
63 1 MC					3.6				6.0	6.0		6.7					2.3					5.3	---M
64 1 MC					3.9				5.5	6.6		6.3					2.0					5.0	---M
65 1 MC					3.7				6.2	6.5		6.5					2.0					5.1	---M
66 1 MC					4.4				7.0	6.8	6.7	7.1	7.8	8.0	5.5	5.2	3.6	2.0	2.0	0.6	0.1	5.6	---M
67 1 MC					4.7				6.6	6.4	5.9	7.1	7.3	7.0	6.7	5.6	3.4	3.0	1.6	0.7	0.7	5.5	---M
68 1 MC					5.3				6.7	6.6	5.8	6.4	7.5	7.4	6.4	5.6	3.0	2.6	1.8	1.0	0.4	5.6	---M
69 1 MC					6.4				8.1	8.5	7.7	7.0	8.1	7.3	6.6	5.8	4.5	2.3	2.3	1.0	0.8	6.1	---M
70 1 MC					6.6				8.5	7.3	7.3	7.4	8.2	7.0	6.4	6.8	3.7	3.4	2.0	1.1	1.2	6.2	---M
71 1 MC					6.2				8.2	7.3	7.3	6.3	9.7	8.4	7.0	6.2	4.1	2.6	1.9	1.0	0.6	6.0	---M
72 1 MC					6.4				7.7	8.5	8.5	8.5	8.4	8.5	8.0	4.7	4.5	3.0	1.5	1.2	0.8	6.3	---M
72 2 UC					5.7				8.4	9.1		8.7			7.9		2.9					6.9	74%T
73 1 MC					7.5				9.2	8.5	8.6	7.8	8.9	10	8.6	7.4	5.2	3.3	2.3	1.5	1.0	7.0	---M
74 1 MC					7.5				8.8	9.0	9.6	9.2	8.4	11	9.6	6.7	5.5	4.0	2.3	1.4	0.8	7.2	---M
74 2 UC					6.2				8.3	9.4		9.7			8.3		3.3					7.3	75%T
75 1 MC					7.3				8.8	9.0	8.0	8.2	9.0	9.0	7.3	7.1	5.5	3.7	2.3	1.5	1.2	6.8	---M
76 1 MC					8.4				9.6	8.5	8.8	9.4	8.1	8.6	9.7	7.7	4.9	4.0	2.2	1.2	1.2	7.1	---M
76 2 UC					5.7				9.4	8.9		9.6			9.0		3.4					7.3	75%T
77 1 MC					6.8				8.8	8.2	8.2	9.2	8.4	8.5	9.2	8.0	6.0	4.0	3.1	1.0	0.8	7.0	---M
78 1 MC					6.4				8.0	8.6	9.0	8.8	8.1	9.3	8.2	6.3	4.9	3.4	2.7	1.6	0.7	6.7	---M
78 2 UC					5.6				8.2	9.0		8.9			8.0		3.6					7.1	76%T
79 1 MC					6.2				8.8	7.4	9.3	8.2	7.7	8.6	7.3	7.1	5.1	3.0	2.6	2.3	1.2	6.6	---M
80 1 MC					5.2				7.4	7.8	7.5	8.2	7.4	8.0	9.3	8.0	5.8	3.7	2.5	1.6	1.0	6.4	---M
80 2 UC					5.0				7.6	9.1		9.2			8.6		3.3					7.0	77%T
81 1 MC					5.3				7.0	7.1	7.0	7.3	8.0	8.2	7.0	7.0	5.1	3.0	2.5	2.3	1.0	6.0	---M
82 1 MC					4.7				6.4	5.9	6.8	7.5	8.0	6.4	7.7	6.8	5.2	3.7	1.8			5.6	---M
82 2 UC					4.1				7.3	7.3		7.4			7.3		3.2					5.9	79%T
83 1 MC					5.2				7.1	6.6	6.7	7.0	7.0	7.5	7.4	6.2	5.6	3.1	1.6			5.5	---M
84 1 MC					4.4				6.0	6.0	6.7	7.1	7.7	5.5	5.8	6.7	4.9	3.6	1.6			5.2	---M
84 2 UC					4.7				6.0	7.0		7.1			7.0		3.4					5.7	78%T
85 1 MC					5.5				5.8	7.0	6.3	6.0	7.1	7.4	5.8	6.3	5.3	4.1	1.4			5.3	---M
86 1 MC					5.2				6.4	6.0	5.9	7.4	7.5	7.1	5.2	6.6	4.4	2.5	1.4			5.2	---M
86 2 UC					4.2				5.9	6.5		7.0			6.4		3.4					5.5	78%T
87 1 MC					5.5				5.8	5.9	6.7	6.4	6.6	6.7	5.9	5.6	5.3	4.0	1.5			5.2	---M
88 2 UC					4.1				6.5	6.6		7.3			6.4		3.1					5.5	78%T
90 2 UC					5.0				7.0	6.9		6.9			6.1		3.2					5.5	73%T
91 20 UC					5.2					7.5		6.8		9.0		4.3		2.3		2.3		5.6	75%T
92 2 UC					3.4				6.3	6.4		6.5			5.9		3.0					5.3	74%T
92 20 UC					5.0					6.0		6.8		5.7		4.5		2.4		1.2		4.8	79%T
93 20 UC					5.6					6.1		6.1		6.3		5.1		3.2		1.6		4.9	69%T
94 2 UC					3.7				6.6	5.6		5.6			5.3		2.9					4.9	74%T
94 20 UC					5.0					5.8		6.0		5.9		4.7		3.1		1.8		4.8	72%T
95 20 UC					5.2					4.9		4.9		5.6		4.1		2.9		1.1		4.4	82%T

1 Based on surveys from source 1 and those surveys in Table 27.6 with data for both sexes and age range at least 21-64 (see also *Cigarette consumption per person* p. xxxv)

2 For other footnotes see Table 27.6

Table 27.8 Estimated[1] prevalence of smoking and estimated[1] number of cigarettes per person per day (unadjusted and sales-adjusted): summary of Tables 27.4, 27.6 and 27.7, 1928-1995.
Males and females aged 15 years and over

Year	Source[2]	Product[3]	Prevalence[4]						Number of cigarettes						
									Unadjusted[7]			Sales-adjusted[8]			
			Manufactured cigarettes		Total cigarettes[5]		All products[6]		Number/ person/day		Total sales %	Manufactured cigarettes number/ person/day		Total cigarettes[9] number/ person/day	
			M	F	M	F	M	F	M	F		M	F	M	F
1928	37	*U*					89	15							
1938	37	*U*					89	33							
1948	1	*MC+A*	65	40			81					(8.1	4.0)		
1949	1	*MC+A*	62	41			80		8.8	2.8	---	8.8	2.8		
1950	1	*MC+A*	60	38			76		9.1	3.1	---	9.1	3.1		
1951	1	*MC+A*	61	37			77		9.5	3.0	---	9.5	3.0		
1952	1	*MC+A*	58	37			75		9.9	3.1	---	9.9	3.1		
1953	1	*MC+A*	59	37			74		10.1	3.3	---	10.1	3.3		
1954	1	*MC+A*	58	36			74		10.3	3.5	---	10.3	3.5		
1955	1	*MC+A*	57	37			74		10.5	3.7	---	10.5	3.7		
1956	1	*MC+A*	60	41			74	41	10.3	3.9	---	10.3	3.9		
1957	1	*MC+A*	59	42			74		10.5	4.2	---	10.5	4.2		
1958	1	*MC+A*	58	38			71	38	10.6	4.2	---	10.6	4.2		
1959	1	*MC+A*	60	41			72		10.8	4.5	---	10.8	4.5		
1960	1	*MC+A*	60	41			73		11.2	4.3	---	11.2	4.3		
1961	1	*MC+A*	58	43			71	43	10.8	4.8	---	10.8	4.8		
1962	1	*MC+A*	56	42			69		10.4	4.7	---	10.4	4.7		
1963	1	*MC+A*	53	42			67	42	10.4	5.1	---	10.4	5.1		
	25	*UC+A*			58	37	66	38						(11.3	5.7)
1964	1	*MC+A*	54	41			68		10.2	4.9	---	10.2	4.9		
1965	1	*MC+A*	53	42			67	42	9.8	5.0	---	9.8	5.0		
1966	1	*MC+A*	54	44			68		9.7	5.2	---	9.7	5.2		
1967	1	*MC+A*	53	43			68		9.9	5.2	---	9.9	5.2		
1968	1	*MC+A*	54	42			68	43	10.0	5.2	---	10.0	5.2		
1969	1	*MC+A*	53	44			68		10.2	5.9	---	10.2	5.9		
1970	1	*MC+A*	54	40			67		10.3	5.9	---	10.3	5.9		
1971	1	*MC+A*	50	40			64	42	10.2	5.9	---	10.2	5.9		
1972	1	*MC+A*	50	40			65	41	10.5	6.1	---	10.5	6.1		
	2	**UC**			52	40			8.8	4.9	74			11.9	6.6

Table 27.8 *(continued)*

Year	Source[2]	Product[3]	Prevalence[4]						Number of cigarettes						
									Unadjusted[7]			Sales-adjusted[8]			
			Manufactured cigarettes		Total cigarettes[5]		All products[6]		Number/ person/day		Total sales %	Manufactured cigarettes number/ person/day		Total cigarettes[9] number/ person/day	
			M	F	M	F	M	F	M	F		M	F	M	F
1973	1	*MC+A*	49	43			65	43	10.7	6.9	---	10.7	6.9		
1974	1	*MC+A*	49	43			63	44	10.4	7.1	---	10.4	7.1		
	2	**UC**			50	40			9.0	5.4	75			12.0	7.1
1975	1	*MC+A*	47	42			61	43	9.9	6.7	---	9.9	6.7		
	1	*MC+A*	46	43			61	43							
1976	1	*MC+A*	44	41			58	42	9.6	7.0	---	9.6	7.0		
	2	**UC**			45	37			8.3	5.4	75			11.1	7.2
1977	1	*MC+A*	42	41			57	41	8.9	6.8	---	8.9	6.8		
1978	1	*MC+A*	41	39			54	40	8.9	6.5	---	8.9	6.5		
	2	**UC**			44	36			7.9	5.2	76			10.4	6.8
1979	1	*MC+A*	41	39			54	40	8.8	6.4	---	8.8	6.4		
1980	1	*MC+A*	41	38			54	39	8.6	6.2	---	8.6	6.2		
	2	**UC**			42	36			7.4	5.2	77			9.6	6.8
1981	1	*MC+A*	37	36			49	37	7.3	5.8	---	7.3	5.8		
1982	1	*MC+A*	35	35			48	36	6.9	5.5	---	6.9	5.5		
	2	**UC**			38	33			6.4	4.6	79			8.2	5.8
1983	1	*MC+A*	34	35			46	36	6.8	5.5	---	6.8	5.5		
1984	1	*MC+A*	35	34			47	34	6.8	5.2	---	6.8	5.2		
	2	**UC**			36	32			5.9	4.3	78			7.6	5.6
1985	1	*MC+A*	34	34			46	35	6.5	5.3	---	6.5	5.3		
1986	1	*MC+A*	33	33			42	33	6.3	5.1	---	6.3	5.1		
	2	**UC**			34	31			5.6	4.2	78			7.2	5.4
1987	1	*MC+A*	33	34			43	34	6.3	5.1	---	6.3	5.1		
1988	2	**UC**			33	30			5.6	4.2	78			7.2	5.5
1990	2	**UC**			31	29			5.2	4.0	73			7.1	5.5
1991	20	**UC**			30	30			5.0	4.2	75			6.7	5.6
1992	2	**UC**			30	28			4.6	3.8	74			6.3	5.1
	20	**UC**			33	29			5.3	3.7	79			6.7	4.7
1993	20	**UC**			28	26			4.4	3.5	69			6.4	5.0
1994	2	**UC**			29	26			4.6	3.5	74			6.2	4.7
	20	**UC+A**			29	26	35	27	4.4	3.5	72			6.1	4.8
1995	20	**UC+A**			30	27	35	27	4.6	3.5	82			5.6	4.3

See footnotes on next page

1 Surveys covering an age range of at least 21-64 are included. Any gaps in the data for ages 15-20 and 65 years and over are filled in by assumed extensions to the age distribution, given in *Notes on sources of survey data*, p. 679. Method: see *Summary of adult smoking*, p. xxxvi
2 See *Notes on sources of survey data*, p. 679
3 Product: MC = manufactured cigarettes, TC = total cigarettes (including hand-rolled), UC = cigarettes (type unspecified), A = all products, U = unspecified. Frequency of smoking is indicated by: regular or daily smokers in normal type, all smokers (including occasional) in bold, unspecified in italics
4 From Table 27.4
5 This column includes prevalence of smoking classified as UC = cigarettes (type unspecified)
6 This column includes prevalence of smoking classified as U = unspecified product
7 From Table 27.6
8 From Table 27.7, except data in parentheses, which are derived from the prevalence of smoking from Table 27.4 as described in *Summary of adult smoking*, p. xxxvi. Sales-adjustment is to UK sales, although most surveys relate to GB, see *Notes on sources of survey data*, p.679
9 Number of cigarettes classified as UC = cigarettes (type unspecified) has been adjusted to total cigarette sales and included in this column

Figure 27.3 Estimated prevalence of smoking of (i) manufactured cigarettes, (ii) total cigarettes and (iii) all tobacco products: by year of survey, 1948-1995.
Males and females aged 15 years and over. *Source:* see Table 27.8

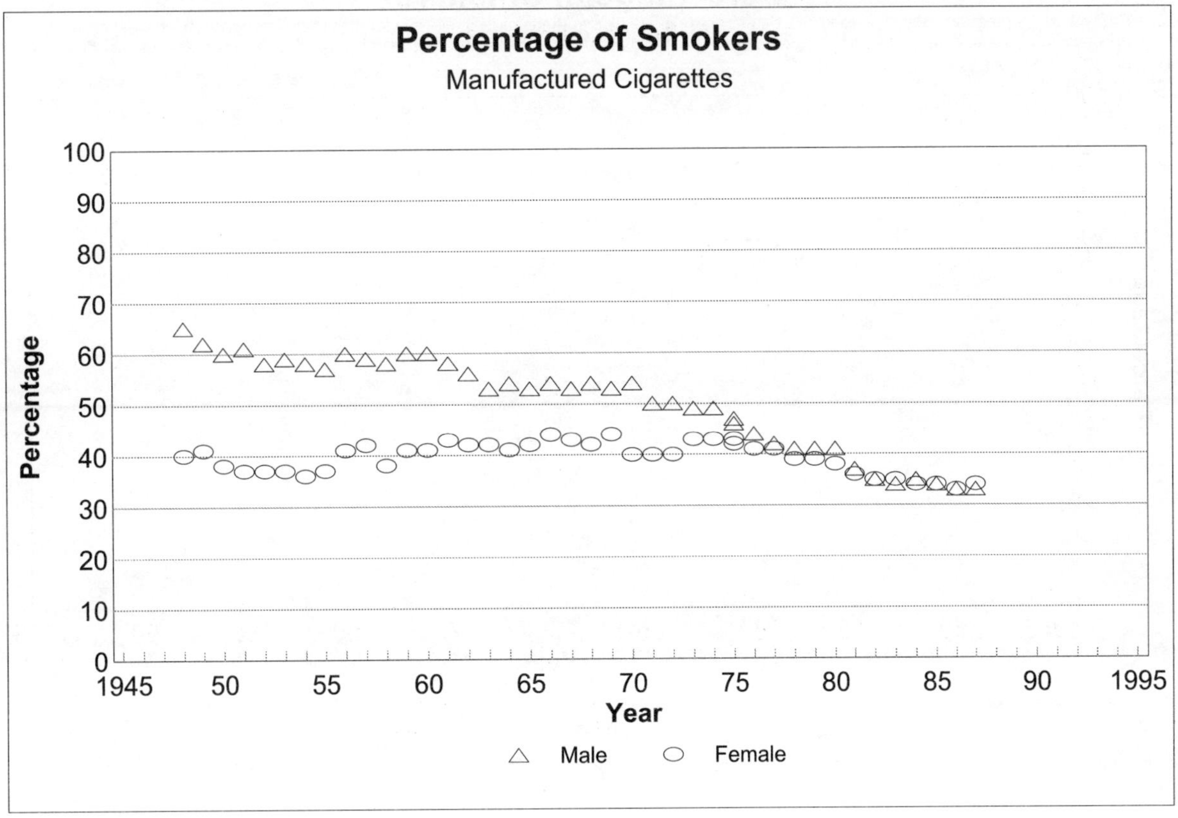

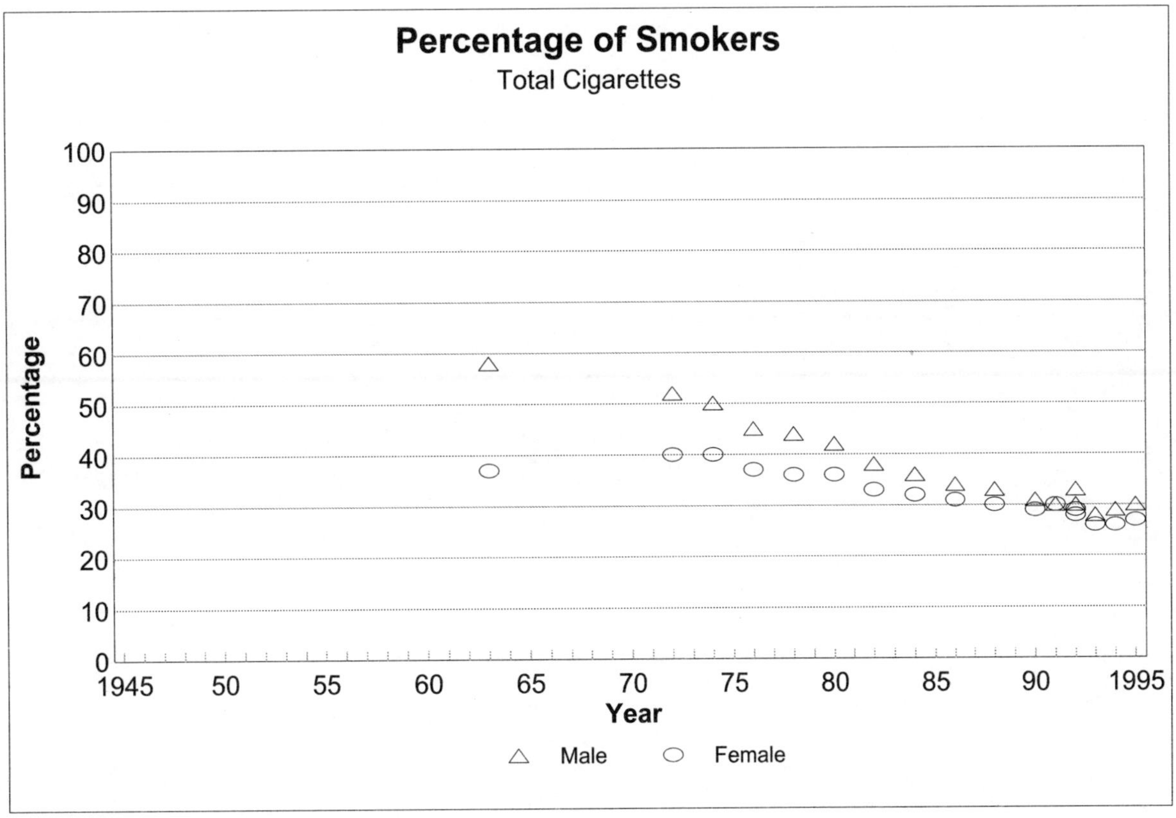

Figure 27.3 *(continued)*

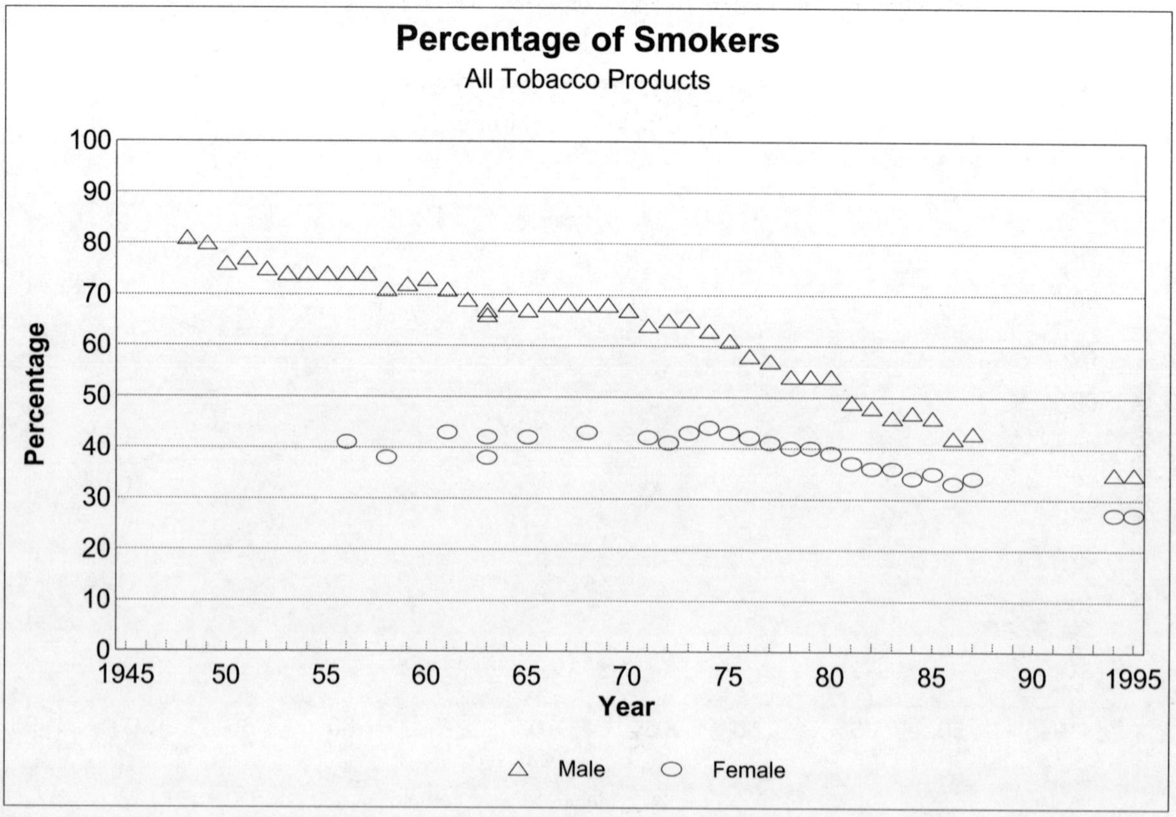

Figure 27.4 Estimated number of (i) manufactured cigarettes and (ii) total cigarettes smoked per person per day, sales-adjusted, 1948-1995.
Males and females aged 15 years and over. *Source:* see Table 27.8

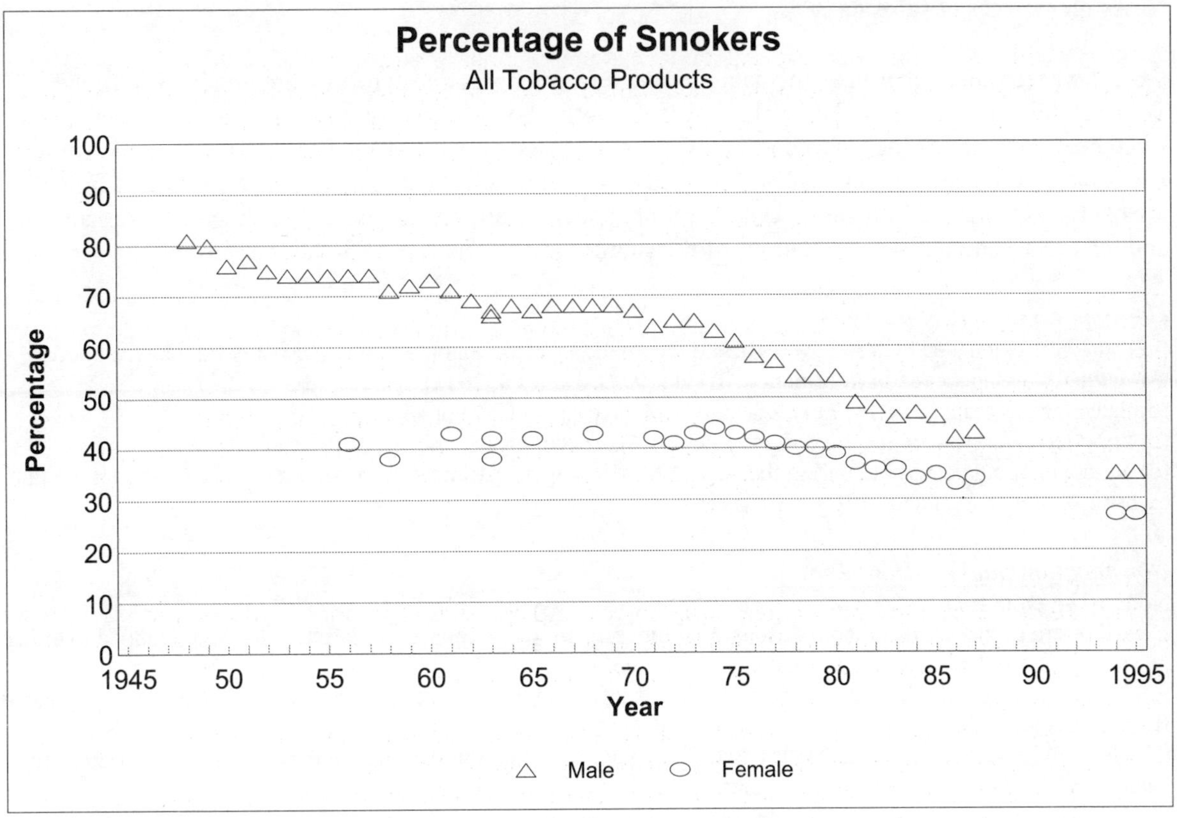

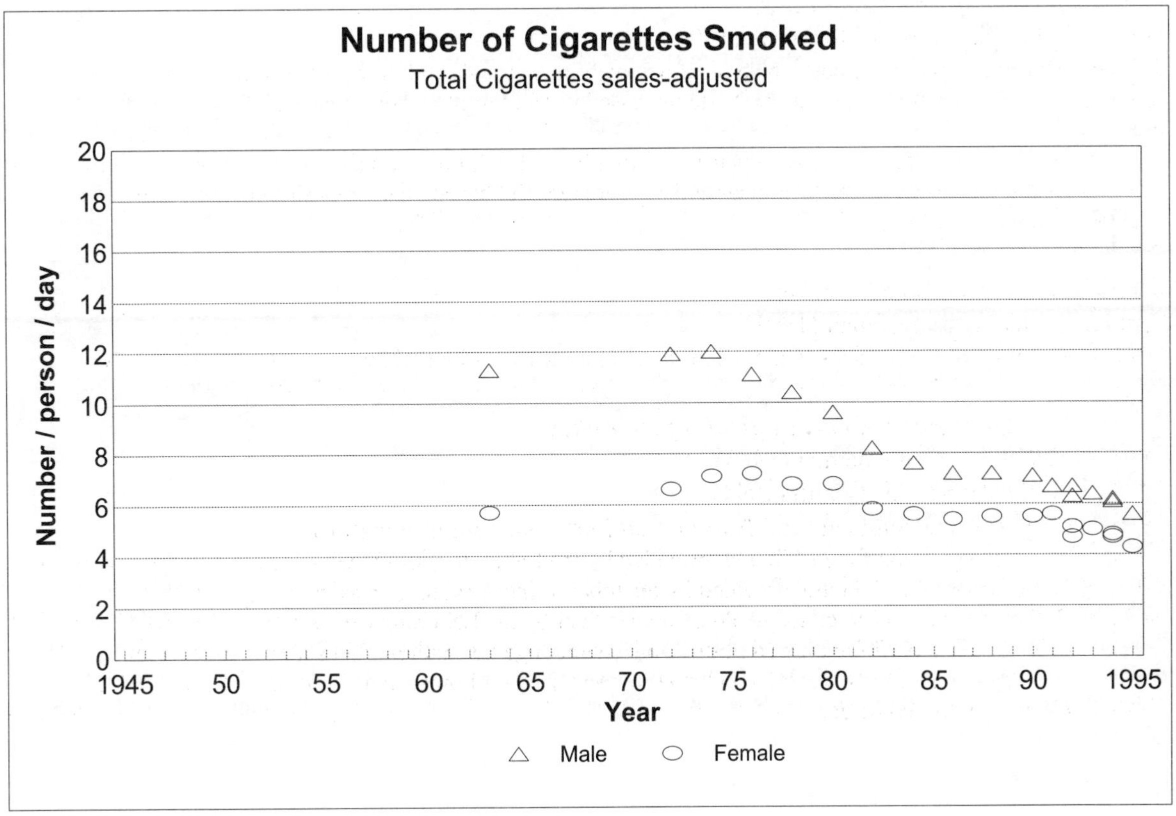

Notes on sources of sales data

Except where stated otherwise, the data presented in the tables and figures were obtained from the Tobacco Advisory Council (TAC). TAC was formerly the Tobacco Research Council (TRC) and has since been renamed as the Tobacco Manufacturers' Association (TMA). The data relate to the United Kingdom (UK), i.e. England, Wales, Scotland and Northern Ireland. Sales in the Republic of Ireland are excluded from 1924 onwards. Details of other sources are given below, together with estimations and related assumptions. Full citations of the sources are given on p. 685 under *References*.

Consumption data before 1920

(a) Data were calculated by TAC from sales to the public of home-manufactured and imported tobacco goods using the following source of information: Todd (1947), Tables 9, 26 (a), (b), (c), (d).
(b) Sales for the years 1914-1919 exclude duty-free supplies to HM Forces.
(c) Imported cigarettes are included in the category 'Tobacco, cigars, and snuff' prior to 1900.
(d) Numbers of cigarettes sold during the years 1905-1919 were estimated from cigarette sales in pounds weight by using a conversion factor of 1 g = 1 cigarette.

Consumption data for 1920-1985

Notes as given in RP6:
Cigarillos are products manufactured from cigar tobacco, are approximately cigarette sized and wrapped in either paper or processed tobacco sheet of natural tobacco colour.
(a) The weights of manufactured cigarettes, cigars, snuff and other tobacco sold to the public have been estimated from trade sources.
(b) The conversion factors for cigarettes and cigars have been estimated by the trade and include allowances for changes in the ratio of large to small cigarettes and for the growth of filter cigarettes.

Before 1982 data by weight, originally given to nearest 100 000 pounds, have been converted to tonnes and given to the nearest 10 tonnes (100 000 lbs = 45.359 tonnes). For 1982-1985 data were given in thousands of tonnes.

Consumption data for 1986 onwards

Tobacco Manufacturers' Association (1999)
Sales of tobacco goods to the trade. The basis of estimation is broadly in line with consumption except for the timing of sales. For example, sales to the trade increased in 1987 prior to pre-budget restrictions by HM Customs in 1988.

Data for cigarettes, cigars and cigarillos were given in millions and have been converted to tonnes assuming 0.8 g per cigarette, 1.8 g per cigar and 1 g per cigarillo, based on averages calculated from Wald and Nicolaides-Bouman (1991).

Plain/Filter cigarette consumption

Wald and Nicolaides-Bouman (1991)
Data given in this source are sales of plain and filter cigarettes as estimated by Imperial Tobacco Limited.

Tar, nicotine and carbon monoxide yields of cigarettes

1921-1971 Government Chemist (1981)
1972-1990 Department of Health (1994)
1991-1995 Tobacco Manufacturers' Association (personal communication)
These sources use yield data for each brand, provided by the Laboratory of the Government Chemist, together with the market share of each brand, provided by the tobacco industry, to give sales-weighted averages. The yield data for 1920-1972 were measured using old cigarettes kept by the Laboratory or donated to them. Jarvis and Russell (1986) used yield information from the same source together with market shares derived from non-industry sources (National Opinion Polls on behalf of the Office of Population Censuses and Surveys (OPCS)) to give the following average yields:

Year	Tar	Nicotine	CO
1972	20.5	1.33	
1973	18.7	1.22	
1974	18.7	1.25	
1975	18.6	1.30	
1976	17.7	1.27	
1977	17.2	1.31	
1978	17.1	1.36	16.1
1979	16.5	1.35	16.2
1980	16.0	1.28	16.1
1981	15.6	1.31	14.9
1982	15.4	1.32	15.4
1983	15.0	1.29	14.5
1984	14.6	1.28	13.9
1985	14.0	1.26	14.1

These are generally lower than, but within 6% of, the quoted average yields.

In a study in 1995 of hand-rolled cigarettes produced by volunteers who habitually smoked hand-rolled cigarettes, Darrall and Figgins (1999) found average values per cigarette to be: tar 15.7 mg (range 9.9-21.0 mg), nicotine 1.3 mg (range 0.9-1.8 mg) and carbon monoxide 10.9 mg (range 5.5-14.1 mg).

The tar yield per cigarette was limited by EC directive (Directive 90/239/EEC) to 15 mg by the end of 1992, and to 12 mg by the end of 1997 (Harkin *et al* (1997)).

Estimates of hand-rolled cigarette consumption for 1931-1985

The weight of tobacco sold has been divided into pipe tobacco and hand-rolling tobacco according to estimates of the amounts actually used in these ways. Numbers of hand-rolled cigarettes have been estimated from sales of tobacco and consumer survey findings.

Estimates of hand-rolled cigarette consumption for 1986 onwards

We have taken as our estimate of hand-rolled cigarette consumption all sales of hand-rolling tobacco, assuming an average weight per cigarette of 0.5 g.

The assumed weight per cigarette was based on averages calculated from Wald and Nicolaides-Bouman (1991). This is supported in Dymond (1996) (estimate of mean weight 490 mg) and in a study by Darrall and Figgins (1999) (average weight of tobacco per cigarette 0.505 g) but Crescenti (1994) suggests that the use of king-sized cigarette papers can give a hand-rolled cigarette weighing more than 1 g.

Notes on sources of survey data

Each source of survey data—either an individual survey or a series of surveys repeated over a number of years—is cited by a source number. This number is shown in the tables and corresponds to the source numbers given below, where details of the source publication and of the survey methodology are given. Full citations of the sources are given on p. 685 under *References*.

Many of the main sources of survey data (notably sources 1 and 2) relate to Great Britain (GB), i.e. England, Wales and Scotland. Since sales data relate to the whole UK (including Northern Ireland), we have used the UK population for all calculations related to sales-adjustment, i.e. effectively assuming that consumption in Northern Ireland is the same as in the rest of the UK.

Source number

1 TAC

a. Annual surveys carried out by Research Service Ltd., a market research company, in GB. Sample size usually about 10 000

b. Smokers: by self definition. Consumption per smoker based on amount smoked 'yesterday'

c. Survey results were adjusted (by TAC) against UK sales figures for under-reporting. For manufactured cigarettes, adjustment was applied only to consumption per smoker until 1969, after which adjustment was split between consumption and prevalence. Understatement averaged 5%, and the adjustment only increased the overall prevalence of manufactured cigarette smoking by around 1%, and average consumption by about half a cigarette per day. Hand-rolling tobacco was adjusted in the same way. Pipe tobacco and cigars were not adjusted. (By our method of calculation on consumption per person, surveys represent 95-102% of manufactured cigarette consumption)

d. The age groups used by the TAC changed in 1976; data for 1975 are presented according to both old and new age groupings

e. Consumption per smoker converted from weekly. Consumption per person for 1966 onwards converted from annual; before 1966 calculated by multiplying prevalence and consumption per smoker (where age groups not equivalent, population-weighted averages calculated)

f. Assumed extension to age distribution for percentage smokers, age 15: males (before 1970) 30%, (1970-1979) 25%, (1980 onwards) 20%; females (before 1969) 20%, (1969-1979) 23%, (1980 onwards) 25%. Number of cigarettes/person/day: males (before 1957) 2.0, (1957-1979) 3.0, (1980 onwards) 2.0; females (before 1956) 0.5, (1956-1965) 1.0, (1966-1968) 2.0, (1969-1979) 3.0, (1980 onwards) 2.0

2 OPCS (1989), Office for National Statistics (ONS) (1998)

a. General Household Survey (GHS). Conducted in GB. Sample size until 1982 about 14 000 households, thereafter about 12 000; response rate 83% of households (number of persons interviewed approximately equal to twice number of households responding). Proxy interviews occurred in approximately 5% of households

b. Cigarette smoker: smokes cigarettes at all nowadays. Consumption per smoker is based on numbers usually smoked on weekdays and at weekends

c. Assumed extension to age distribution for percentage smokers, age 15: males (1972-1978) 25%, (1980 onwards) 20%; females (before 1980) 23%, (1980 onwards) 25%. Number of cigarettes/person/day: males and females (1972-1978) 2.0, (1980 onwards) 1.0

3 Bynner (1969)

a. Study in England and Wales. Total sample size (from age 11) 5 601, boys only

b. It is also reported that 4% of 11-year-olds were smokers

4 TRC

a. Study in southeast England, 1965-1966. Total sample size (from age 10) 1 944, boys only

b. It is also reported that 5% of 10-11-year-olds were smokers

5 Holland and Elliot (1968)

a. Study in southeast England. Lower age limit 11. Sample size 9 786

6 Rawbone *et al* (1979, 1982)

a. Studies in secondary schools in Hounslow, an outer-London borough. Total sample size (from age 11) (1975) 10 498, (1979) 12 002

b. Smokers marked as frequency *: smoked daily. Regular smokers: smoked at least one cigarette per week

c. It is also reported that 11-year-olds included 5% male and 3% female smokers in 1975, and 4% male and 3% female smokers in 1979

d. Consumption category estimation based on 7-40 and 40+ cigarettes/smoker/week (1-5 and 6+ cigarettes/smoker/day assumed), and resulting figures should be regarded with caution

7 Murray *et al* (1983)

a. Medical Research Council/Derbyshire longitudinal smoking study. Study in secondary schools in Derbyshire. Sample size 6 000

b. Regular smokers: smoked at least once a week

8, 9 McKennell (1980)

a. Methodological study in 48 British secondary schools designed to show differences of reported smoking for different places and methods of interview. Year not stated. Total sample size (from age

11) 4 000. Results presented here were selected as the most widely differing results among those from a range of situations. Source **8**: group self-completion questionnaires in school. Source **9**: oral interviews at home

b. Regular smokers: smoked one cigarette or more a week

c. It is also reported that 11-year-olds included (source **8**) 9% male and 5% female smokers; (source **9**) 6%male and 0% female smokers

10 Ledwith and Osman (1984)

a. Study in Lothian. Total sample size (from age 11) 2 045

b. It is also reported that 11-year-olds included 7% male and 5% female smokers

11, 12 Dobbs and Marsh (1983, 1985), Goddard and Ikin (1987, 1989), Thomas *et al* (1993), Bolling (1994), Diamond and Goddard (1995), Department of Health (1998)

a. Surveys by OPCS/ONS of Smoking among Secondary School Children.
11 England and Wales. **12** Scotland.

Year	England and Wales[1]			Scotland		
	Sample size		Response	Sample size		Response
	Males	Females	rate (%)	Males	Females	rate (%)
1982	1 460	1 514	87	1 190	1 095	87
1984	1 928	1 689	82	1 365	1 408	80
1986	1 676	1 508	77	1 169	1 190	78
1988	1 489	1 529	87			
1990	1 643	1 478	82	1 359	1 317	88
1992	1 662	1 626	89	1 489	1 411	86
1993	1 613	1 527	80			
1994	1 522	1 523	78	1 350	1 375	83

[1] The 1988 survey was of England only. For 1990 onwards, England only reported

b. Regular smokers: usually smoked 1 or more cigarettes a week

c. Consumption figures derived from average cigarettes/regular smoker/week

13 Balding (1988)

a. Based on the annual data banks from the General Health Related Behaviour Questionnaire in schools in Great Britain. Results shown as 1984 are for 1983/1984.

Year	Sample size
1983/1984	20 061
1985	12 488
1986	17 678
1987	16 663

b. Smokers marked as frequency *: had smoked since yesterday. Regular smokers: had smoked in the past 7 days

c. The following results for smoking among 11-year-olds were also reported:

Year	Regular smoking (%)	
	Males	Females
1985	3	2
1986	2	2
1987	3	2

14,15 WHO (1989)

a. Regional surveys forming part of WHO MONICA project:

	Region	Population size	Sample size	Participation rate (%)	Sample used*		Date
					Males	Females	
14	Belfast	157 300	2 649	70	1 193	1 193	Oct 1983-Sept 1984
15	Glasgow	135 100	1 536	64	647	607	Feb 1986-July 1986

* age 25-34; all other figures are for age 35-64 only

b. *All ages* column relates only to age 35-64 and is standardized to world population

c. Regular cigarette smokers: smoked cigarettes daily. All smokers: smoked cigarettes daily or occasionally, or smoked 1 g pipe tobacco or 1 cigar per week. Cigarettes per smoker refers to regular and occasional cigarette smokers

d. Calculation for cigarettes per person based on % regular cigarette smokers and cigarettes per regular or occasional cigarette smoker, so may underestimate

16-19 Aarø *et al* (1986), Nutbeam and Aarø (1990), Smith (1991), King and Coles (1992), King *et al* (1996)

a. Part of the HBSC (Health Behaviour in School-Aged Children) Study, a collaborative cross-national research study sponsored by the WHO. School classes or schools were randomly selected, targeting age groups 11 (not presented here), 13 and 15. The target sample size was 1 300 in each age group. **16** England; **17** Wales; **18** Scotland; **19** Northern Ireland

b. 1983-1984: England (cities of Nottingham and Salford). Total sample size 3 398.

	Mean age	
Target age	**Boys**	**Girls**
13	14.1	14.2
15	16.1	16.1

c. 1986-1987: Wales and Scotland (Lothian region). Total sample size (Wales) 6 356. Sample size for 15-year-olds (Scotland) 1 482

d. 1989-1990: Wales and Scotland. Sample size (Wales) 6 724, (Scotland) 3 934.

	Mean age	
Target age	**Wales**	**Scotland**
13	14	13.7
15	16	15.6

e. 1993-1994: Wales, Scotland and Northern Ireland.

	Wales		Scotland		Northern Ireland	
Target age	**Mean age**	**Sample size**	**Mean age**	**Sample size**	**Mean age**	**Sample size**
13	13.9	1332	13.5	1 579	13.9	1 355
15	15.9	1266	15.6	1 373	15.9	1 269

f. Smokers marked as frequency *: smoked daily. Regular smokers: smoke once a week or more

20 OPCS (1993, 1994, 1995, 1996, 1997)

a. Health Survey for England. Series of surveys linked with the government Health of the Nation initiative. Smoking questions were the same as those used on the GHS, however the samples were smaller and the context of these surveys (which concentrate on health issues) may result in less frank responses. England only. Stratified sample of private households.

Year	Sample size (smoking questions)		Response rate (%)	Date of survey
	Males	**Females**		
1991	1 482	1 744	85	September-December
1992	1 865	2 149	82	September-December
1993	7 678	8 873	76	January-December
1994	7 160	8 613	77	January-December
1995	7 321	8 706	78	January-December

b. Cigarette smoker: smokes cigarettes at all nowadays. Consumption per smoker is based on number usually smoked on weekdays and at weekends

c. Consumption category estimation based on 0-9, 10-19 and 20+ cigarettes/smoker/day. Inclusion of non-regular smokers (<1 cigarette/day) in the estimation process will result in a slightly high estimate of cigarettes per smoker

d. Assumed extension to age distribution for percentage smokers, age 15: males 20% and females 25%. Number of cigarettes/person/day: males and females 1.0

21 Jones (1957)

a. Survey of 307 boys in a school in a working class area. Questions asked in the presence of fellow pupils and class teacher. Year not stated

b Regular smoking was self-defined. Number of cigarettes smoked weekly is given by groupings: most boys smoked less than 5 cigarettes per week

c. It was also reported that at age 11 there was 1 regular smoker out of 32 boys

22 Bothwell (1959)

a. Survey of secondary schools in Oxfordshire using anonymous questionnaires. Sample size (boys) 4 270, (girls) 4 044, response rate 90%

b. Regular smokers: smoked at least one cigarette a week

c. Consumption category estimation based on 1-5, 6-10, 11-15, 16-20, 21-30, 31-40 and 41+ cigarettes/smoker/week. As this is based on weekly rather than daily consumption, the resulting figures should be regarded with caution

23 London School of Hygiene and Tropical Medicine Study Group of the Public Health Department (1959)

a. Survey of six secondary schools (two grammar schools and four secondary modern schools) in an industrial county borough near London. Confidential questionnaire completed by the subject with a teacher in the room. Year not stated. Sample size (boys) 1 797, (girls) 1 682, response rate 90%

b. Regular smokers: smoked five or more cigarettes per week

c. Consumption category estimation based on 5-9, 10-19, 20-30 and 40+ cigarettes/smoker/week. As this is based on weekly rather than daily consumption, the resulting figures should be regarded with caution

24 Cartwright and Thomson (1960)

a. Survey in four Edinburgh senior schools using an anonymous self-completed questionnaire with no teacher present. Sample size (boys) 1 578, (girls) 1 568, response rate 77%

b. Smokers: smoked in the last four weeks

25 Readers Digest (1963)

a. Series of surveys conducted in European countries using identical questionnaires. British survey conducted by BMRB. Random sample of about 2 000 people

b. It is also reported that 13% of men (8% age <40 and 16% age 40+) smoke a pipe, and that 4% of men (2% age <40 and 5% age 40+) smoke cigars

c. Assumed extension to age distribution for percentage smokers, age 15-20: males (cigarettes) 55%, (all products) 57%; females 38%

26 Lemin (1967)

a. Survey in six Aberdeen schools using an anonymous self-completed questionnaire with a health visitor or teacher in the room. Year not stated. Sample size (boys) 482, (girls) 436

b. Smokers: self-defined

27 Pearson and Richardson (1978)

a. Results of the third follow-up of the National Child Development Study. Nationally representative (England, Scotland and Wales). Individual confidential questionnaires completed in school. Sample size (boys) 6 115, (girls) 5 857

b. Regular smokers: smoked at least one cigarette per week

c. Consumption category estimation based on 1-9, 10-29, 30-49 and 50+ cigarettes/smoker/week. As this is based on weekly rather than daily consumption, the resulting figures should be regarded with caution

28 Murray *et al* (1982, 1984)

a. Health Education Council's 'My Body' project. Results presented here are for the control group only.

	Sample size		Response
	Boys	Girls	rate (%)
1978	275	281	96
1980	130	111	90
1982	533		87

b. Regular smokers: smoked at least one cigarette in the last week

29 Ledwith and Osman (1984)

a. Survey in primary and secondary schools in Lothian Region. Group self-completion questionnaires in school (see source 8). Year not stated. Total sample size (from age 10) 2 983

b. Smokers: includes those who 'have smoked but not as often as one a week'

c. The following results for prevalence of smoking (%) were also reported for 10-11-year-olds:

Age	Boys	Girls
10	12.2	5.3
11	6.9	6.0

30 van Reek *et al* (1992), van Reek and Adriaanse (1995)

a. A series of surveys of Young Europeans. About 800 children aged 11-15 years interviewed in each EC country except Luxembourg (where only 250 interviewed). Lowest age group 11-12. Interviews conducted at home, with parents absent

b. Regular smokers: smoked daily. All smokers: smoked at least once a week

31 Hibell *et al* (1997)

a. Nationally representative survey forming part of ESPAD (European School Survey Project on Alcohol and Other Drugs). Target was pupils born in 1979, thus age 15-16 at time of survey in March1995. Approximately 90% of this group still in school. Anonymous questionnaire completed and sealed in envelope by pupil, in class. Teachers present, but discouraged from walking round the classroom. Sample size (males) 3 630, (females) 4 092. Response rate (males) 84%, (females) 84%

b. Regular smokers: smoked 1 or more cigarettes per day in last 30 days. All smokers: smoked in last 30 days

c. Consumption category estimation based on 1-5, 6-10, 11-20, 21+ cigarettes/smoker/day

32-36 Miller and Plant (1996)

a. Part of an international study initiated by the Pompidou Group of the Council of Europe. Survey representative of Great Britain and Northern Ireland, representing both state and independent secondary schools. Sample size 7 722

32 England; **33** Northern Ireland; **34** Scotland; **35** Wales; **36** United Kingdom, all regions

b. Regular smokers: smoked 11 or more cigarettes in the previous 30 days. Smokers: smoked in the previous 30 days

37 Stone (1945)

a. No original source

b. Assumed extension to age distribution for percentage smokers, age 15: males 30% and females 10%

References

Aarø L.E., Wold B., Kannas L. and Rimpelä M. (1986). Health behaviour in school children. A WHO cross-national survey. *Health Promotion,* **1**, 17-33.

Anonymous (1995). Rolling tobacco—an unbalanced situation. *Tobacco,* **May/Jun**, 10-2.

Balding J. (1988). Teenage smoking: the levels are falling at last! *Education and Health,* **6**, 68-70.

Beese D.H. (ed) (1968). *Tobacco consumption in various countries,* 2nd edition. Tobacco Research Council, London. Research Paper 6.

Beese D.H. (ed) (1972). *Tobacco consumption in various countries,* 3rd edition. Tobacco Research Council, London. Research Paper 6.

Bolling K. (1994). *Smoking among secondary school children in England in 1993. An enquiry carried out by Social Survey Division of OPCS on behalf of the Department of Health.* HMSO, London.

Bothwell P.W. (1959). The epidemiology of cigarette smoking in rural school children. *Medical Officer,* **102**, 125-32.

Bynner J.M. (1969). *The young smoker.* OPCS, HMSO, London. SS383.

Cartwright A. and Thomson J.G. (1960). Young smokers, an attitude study among schoolchildren, touching also on parental influence. *British Journal of Preventive and Social Medicine,* **14**, 28-34.

Cole J. (1996). Hand-rolling havens. *World Tobacco,* **153**, 56-60.

Crescenti M.G. (1994). A motley market for cigarette papers and filter tubes in Europe. *Tobacco Journal International,* **3**, 50-4.

Darrall K.G. and Figgins J.A. (1999). Roll-your-own smoke yields: theoretical and practical aspects. *Tob Control,* **7**, 168-75.

Department of Health (1994). *Statistics on smoking: England 1974 to 1993.* Department of Health, London. Statistical Bulletin 1994/14.

Department of Health (1998). *Statistics on smoking: England, 1976 to 1996.* Department of Health, London. Statistical Bulletin 1998/25.

Diamond A. and Goddard E. (1995). *Smoking among secondary school children in 1994. An enquiry carried out by Social Survey Division of OPCS on behalf of the Department of Health, the Welsh Office, and the Scottish Home and Health Department.* HMSO, London.

Dobbs J. and Marsh A. (1983). *Smoking among secondary school children.* OPCS, HMSO, London.

Dobbs J. and Marsh A. (1985). *Smoking among secondary school children in 1984.* OPCS, HMSO, London. SS1215.

Dymond H.F. (1996). A survey of roll-your-own tobacco use and practice and considerations for the analysis of smoking articles made from it. *Tobacco Science,* **40**, 82-6.

Goddard E. (1989). *Smoking among secondary school children in England in 1988.* OPCS, HMSO, London.

Goddard E. and Ikin C. (1987). *Smoking among secondary school children in 1986.* OPCS, HMSO, London.

Government Chemist (1981). Smoking and health. In: *1980 report of the Government Chemist.* HMSO; 67-85.

Harkin A.M., Anderson P. and Goos C. (1997). *Smoking, drinking and drug taking in the European Region.* Alcohol, Drugs and Tobacco Programme, WHO Regional Office for Europe, Copenhagen.

Hibell B., Andersson B., Bjarnason T., Kokkevi A., Morgan M. and Narusk A. (1997). *The 1995 ESPAD report. The European school survey project on alcohol and other drugs. Alcohol and other drug use among students in 26 European countries*. The Swedish Council for Information on Alcohol and Other Drugs. Council of Europe (Pompidou Group).

Holland W.W. and Elliot A. (1968). Cigarette smoking, respiratory symptoms, and anti-smoking propaganda. *Lancet,* **i**, 41-3.

Jarvis M. and Russell M.A.H. (1986). Data note-4. Sales-weighted tar, nicotine and carbon monoxide yields of UK cigarettes: 1985. *British Journal of Addiction,* **81**, 579-81.

Jones A.P. (1957). Cigarette smoking at school. *Lancet,* **i**, 631.

King A., Wold B., Tudor-Smith C. and Harel Y. (1996). *The health of youth, a cross-national survey*. WHO Regional Publications, Europe, Copenhagen. European Series No. 69.

King A.J.C. and Coles B. (1992). *The health of Canada's youth. Views and behaviours of 11-, 13- and 15-year-olds from 11 countries*. Health and Welfare Canada, Ottawa.

Ledwith F. and Osman L. (1984). The concomitants of smoking in primary and secondary school children in Scotland. In: *Health Education and Youth*. Falmer Press, London; 160-6.

Lee P.N. (ed) (1975). *Tobacco consumption in various countries,* 4th edition. Tobacco Research Council, London. Research Paper 6.

Lemin B. (1967). Smoking in 14-year-old school children. *Int J Nurs Stud,* **4**, 301-9.

London School of Hygiene and Tropical Medicine Study Group of the Public Health Department (1959). The smoking habits of school children. *British Journal of Preventive and Social Medicine,* **13**, 1-4.

McKennell A.C. (1980). Bias in the reported incidence of smoking by children. *Int J Epidemiol,* **9**, 167-77.

Miller P.M. and Plant M. (1996). Drinking, smoking, and illicit drug use among 15- and 16-year-olds in the United Kingdom. *BMJ,* **313**, 394-7.

Murray M., Swan A.V., Bewley B.R. and Johnson M.R.D. (1983). The development of smoking during adolescence—the MRC/Derbyshire smoking study. *Int J Epidemiol,* **12**, 185-92.

Murray M., Swan A.V. and Clarke G. (1984). Long term effect of a school based antismoking programme. *J Epidemiol Community Health,* **38**, 247-52.

Murray M., Swan A.V., Enock C., Johnson M.R.D., Banks M.H. and Reid D.J. (1982). The effectiveness of the Health Education Council's 'My Body' school health education project. *Health Education Journal,* **41**, 126-30.

Nutbeam D. and Aarø L.E. (1990). Smoking and alienation from school: the implications for health education with young people. Results from the WHO study of health behaviour in schoolchildren. In: Durston B. and Jamrozik K. (eds) *Tobacco & health 1990. The global war. Seventh World Conference on Tobacco and Health, Perth, Western Australia, 1-5 April 1990*. Organising Committee of the Seventh World Conference on Tobacco and Health, 189 Royal Street, East Perth, Western Australia 6004; 539-44.

Office for National Statistics (ONS) (1998). *Living in Britain. Results from the 1996 General Household Survey*. The Stationery Office, London.

Office of Population Censuses and Surveys (OPCS) (1989). *General household survey 1986*. HMSO, London. Series GHS no. 16.

OPCS (1993). *Health survey for England 1991*. HMSO, London. Series HS no. 1.

OPCS (1994). *Health survey for England 1992*. HMSO, London. Series HS no. 2.

OPCS (1995). *Health survey for England 1993*. HMSO, London. Series HS no. 3.

OPCS (1996). *Health survey for England 1994. Volume I: findings. Volume II: survey methodology and documentation*. HMSO, London. Series HS no. 4.

OPCS (1997). *Health survey for England 1995. Volume I: findings. Volume II: survey methodology and documentation*. HMSO, London. Series HS no. 5.

Pearson R. and Richardson K. (1978). The smoking habits of 16-year-olds in the National Child Development Study. *Public Health,* **92**, 136-44.

Rawbone R.G. and Guz A. (1982). Cigarette smoking among secondary schoolchildren 1975-79. *Arch Dis Child,* **57**, 352-8.

Rawbone R.G., Keeling C.A., Jenkins A. and Guz A. (1979). Cigarette smoking among secondary school children in 1975: its prevalence and some of the factors that promote smoking. *Health Education Journal,* **38**, 92-9.

Readers Digest (1963). *Products and people. A digest of the marketing survey of the European Common Market and Britain, 1963* . Reader's Digest Association Limited, London.

Smith C. (1991). Smoking among young people: some recent developments in Wales. *Health Education Journal,* **50**, 8-11.

Stone R. (1945). The analysis of market demand. Read before Royal Statistical Society, April 24th 1945. *Journal of the Royal Statistical Society.*

Thomas M., Holroyd S. and Goddard E. (1993). *Smoking among secondary school children in 1992. A survey carried out by Social Survey Division of OPCS on behalf of the Department of Health, the Welsh Office and the Scottish Office Home and Health Department.* HMSO, London.

Tobacco Manufacturers' Association (1999). *Statistics*. http://www.thetma.org.uk/statistics.htm and linked pages.

Todd G.F. (1947). *The statistical history of the tobacco trade 1870-1920*. Imperial Tobacco Co (of Great Britain and Ireland) Ltd, Bristol.

van Reek J. and Adriaanse H. (1995). Daily smoking among adolescents in the European Community. *Rev Epidemiol Sante Publique,* **43**, 281-2.

van Reek J., Adriaanse H. and Karaoglou A. (1992). Smoking among children in the European Community. *J Public Health Med,* **14**, 93-4.

Wald N. and Nicolaides-Bouman A. (eds) (1991). *UK Smoking Statistics,* 2nd edition. Wolfson Institute of Preventive Medicine and Oxford University Press, London and Oxford.

WHO (1989). The WHO MONICA project: a worldwide monitoring system for cardiovascular diseases. In: *World health statistics annual 1989*. WHO, Geneva; 25-149.

§ Original paper not obtained, but information taken as quoted by another author

United States of America 28

Sales data

See Tables 28.1-28.3.

From 1920 until 1963 the consumption of manufactured cigarettes per adult increased, with some fluctuations, from nearly 2 to 11 cigarettes per day. Consumption then decreased slowly to 6.5 cigarettes per day by 1995. The smoking of hand-rolled cigarettes has been relatively unimportant since the Second World War.

The consumption of tobacco products per adult was about 11 g per day through the 1920s, and then fell to 9 g by 1933. Thereafter it rose steadily and in the 1950s and early 1960s, consumption was about 13-14 g per day. It had fallen to 6 g per day by 1995. In 1925, 25% of all tobacco was consumed in manufactured cigarettes. This proportion increased and has been around 80% since the mid 1960s. Consumption of pipe and hand-rolling tobacco and chewing tobacco could not be calculated separately before 1949. Since then, pipe and hand-rolling tobacco has decreased to low levels, but chewing tobacco and also snuff have tended to increase; in 1995 they made up 12% of consumption. Consumption of cigars has decreased to 4%.

Survey data

See Tables 28.4-28.8

In the 1940s, the prevalence of cigarette smoking among those aged 15 years and over was about 50% in men and 30% in women. According to a regional sample of whites only, the prevalence of smoking of all products was 70% among men. The prevalence of cigarette smoking among men has reduced steadily since then to about 27-30% in 1995. The prevalence among women remained around 30% until about 1980, then fell to about 22-26%. Data on percentages of men and women who smoke products other than cigarettes are scarce; in 1985 (source 4) 7% of men and 1% of women used other products but not cigarettes (including smokeless tobacco).

Data on adult smoking by age are available since the 1940s. In general, more men than women smoked at all ages. From the late 1960s, the prevalence of smoking decreased in men at all ages, but less so above age 65; in women some decrease was seen below age 45, but until the mid 1980s there was an increase above age 65. However, a lower percentage of smokers in older age groups continued to be more marked in women than in men.

The prevalence of teenage smoking among girls was lower than among boys when first surveyed in 1968, but increased until the mid-1970s, and most surveys indicate that the prevalence among girls has been higher than among boys since the end of the 1970s.

Comparison of survey and sales data suggests that surveys under-reported consumption by 25-40%. The estimated number of cigarettes smoked per person per day (sales-adjusted) peaked for men in the mid-1960s at 14 and declined to 8 by 1995. For women it reached 8 cigarettes per day in the mid-1970s, and declined to 5 by 1995.

Table 28.1.1 Total annual sales of tobacco products, 1920-1973

Year	Cigarettes		Cigars		Pipe and hand-rolling tobacco tonnes	Chewing tobacco tonnes	Snuff tonnes	All tobacco products tonnes
	tonnes	millions	tonnes	millions				
1920	44660	44656	72630	8609	164970		16370	298640
1921	50910	50899	62730	7435	159120		16190	288950
1922	53590	53582	63500	7527	173320		17330	307740
1923	64480	64469	63320	7505	169050		17870	314720
1924	71040	71024	60650	7189	169640		31300	332630
1925	79990	79976	58630	6949	168920		17150	324680
1926	89470	89460	59120	7008	168740		17280	334620
1927	97200	97188	59120	7008	160530		18230	335090
1928	105940	105927	57990	6874	155810		18460	338210
1929	119070	119049	58820	6972	153180		18140	349210
1930	119650	119632	52920	6272	149140		18190	339900
1931	113470	113455	47720	5656	148780		17920	327890
1932	103610	103589	39860	4724	141660		16510	301630
1933	111780	111766	38410	4553	138300		16470	304960
1934	125720	125700	40650	4818	139300		16870	322540
1935	134630	134610	41700	4943	138030		17280	331640
1936	153190	153169	45240	5362	140430		16370	355240
1937	162660	162629	46540	5516	136490		16740	362420
1938	163790	163761	44660	5294	138750		16920	364120
1939	172500	172469	46140	5469	137350		17240	373220
1940	180690	180664	46330	5491	138030		17190	382240
1941	206470	206432	50060	5933	135490		17960	409970
1942	235880	235841	53480	6339	127230		18690	435280
1943	257790	257743	45140	5350	119070		19600	441580
1944	239330	239287	41150	4878	114210		19050	413750
1945	267700	267652	42410	5027	122560		19780	452440
1946	321530	321475	50020	5929	95750		18010	485310
1947	336020	335965	48140	5706	90360		17830	492340
1948	348790	348731	49440	5860	90580		18640	507450
1949	351870	351809	47460	5625	47990	39690	18600	505600
1950	360260	360199	47310	5608	47310	38960	18140	511990
1951	379790	379725	48750	5778	44180	38240	17780	528730
1952	394170	394109	50930	6037	42140	37560	17600	542400
1953	386890	386826	51520	6107	38240	37190	17640	531490
1954	368790	368725	50820	6024	36830	35970	17510	509920
1955	382120	382061	51280	6078	35290	35150	17690	521540
1956	393220	393154	50950	6039	31750	33660	17050	526630
1957	409500	409436	52260	6194	31250	32110	16370	541500
1958	436040	436354	53770	6586	33750	30840	15780	570180
1959	446200	453681	60230	7377	32610	30250	15240	584540
1960	452820	470136	57940	7097	32750	28940	15740	588190
1961	476500	488119	57830	7083	32980	29210	15290	611800
1962	474910	494463	57990	7103	31660	28940	15010	608520
1963	515730	509588	60700	7434	31620	29260	14470	651770
1964	495770	497447	72180	9899	37060	29710	14200	648920
1965	510290	511464	68080	8949	31660	28980	13380	652390
1966	502120	522533	65380	8610	31120	29120	13380	641120
1967	495320	527800	63770	8403	30120	29170	13110	631480
1968	491690	523008	62700	8331	31570	29660	12560	628190
1969	470370	510531	63120	8579	30980	31430	12200	608110
1970	471280	532769	64400	8881	33570	30930	12110	612290
1971	460390	528858	62720	8830	31520	32570	12070	599270
1972	490330	551017	61550	11125	30300	32890	11660	626720
1973	508020	590300	59610	11225	26990	33790	11570	639980

Source: see *Notes on sources of sales data*, p. 712

Table 28.1.2 Total annual sales of tobacco products, 1974-1995

Year	Cigarettes[1]		Large cigars[2,3]		Small cigars[4]		Pipe and hand-rolling tobacco[2,5]	Chewing tobacco[6]	Snuff[6]	All tobacco products
	tonnes[7]	millions	tonnes[7]	millions	tonnes	millions	tonnes	tonnes	tonnes	
1974	518340	599000	46116	6356	3986	3066	27220	35920	11340	642922
1975	516370	607200	42173	5804	3760	2892	24360	36560	11430	634653
1976	499840	613500	38994	5373	2811	2162	24360	38100	11700	615805
1977	498110	617000	37698	4994	2410	1854	21450	40230	11070	610968
1978	485290	616000	35322	4702	2025	1558	20050	41910	11020	595617
1979	511100	621500	32073	4304	1873	1441	17830	45770	10840	619486
1980	504570	631500	29833	4001	1834	1411	16920	48040	10840	612037
1981	493420	640000	29250	3893	1773	1364	16560	48310	11570	600883
1982	496090	634000	27231	3667	1645	1265	15290	39920	19910	600086
1983	482980	600000	26880	3605	1734	1334	15100	39280	20730	586704
1984	465480	600400	25927	3471	1604	1234	12470	39600	21640	566721
1985	471710	594000	23722	3197	1583	1218	12250	38560	22040	569865
1986	462640	583800	22837	3055	1256	966	11070	35700	21180	554683
1987	448700	575000	20298	2728	1500	1154	10700	34610	20460	536268
1988	443370	562500	18542	2531	1508	1160	10210	33880	21680	529190
1989	410180	540000	20078	2470	1482	1140	8750	33070	22320	495880
1990	412900	525000	16116	2345	1578	1214	8120	32070	23270	494054
1991	408230	510000	16235	2246	1680	1292	7440	32340	24220	490145
1992	395020	500000	16433	2219	1693	1302	7210	30710	25170	476236
1993	406590	485000	16577	2138	1652	1271	6940	28940	25760	486459
1994	366830	486000	16451	2294	1790	1377	6670	28030	26580	446351
1995	370370	487000	20766	2518	1816	1397	6440	28210	26940	454542

1 Taxable removals, overseas forces, inventory change and imports
2 Total removals (or sales) from US and Puerto Rican factories, plus imports, minus exports
3 Includes cigarillos
4 Taxable removals
5 1991-1995 adjusted (by USDA) to reflect estimated re-exports to Canada
6 US manufactured and invoiced to domestic customers
7 Weights of cigarettes and large cigars derived from USDA tables of per capita consumption
8 US output (virtually all sold domestically)

Source : see *Notes on sources of sales data,* p. 712

Table 28.1.3 Manufactured cigarettes (i) percentage of total sales as filter cigarettes, 1946-1994 (ii) sales-weighted average tar yield per cigarette (SWAT), 1954-1995, and (iii) sales-weighted average nicotine yield per cigarette (SWAN), 1954-1995

Year	% Filter	SWAT mg / cig	SWAN mg / cig
1946	0.1		
1947	0.2		
1948	0.3		
1949	0.3		
1950	0.6		
1951	0.7		
1952	1.3		
1953	2.9		
1954	9.2	37.0	2.60
1955	18.7	38.0	2.70
1956	27.6	34.0	2.70
1957	38.1	35.0	2.50
1958	45.3	31.0	2.00
1959	48.7	29.0	1.80
1960	50.9	27.0	1.60
1961	52.5	26.0	1.60
1962	54.6	26.0	1.50
1963	58.0	25.0	1.40
1964	60.9	23.0	1.30
1965	64.4	22.0	1.40
1966	68.3	23.0	1.50
1967	72.4	21.0	1.40
1968	74.9	21.6	1.35
1969	77.5	20.7	1.38
1970	80.1	20.0	1.31
1971	82.4	20.2	1.32
1972	83.7	19.9	1.39
1973	85.4	19.3	1.32
1974	86.7	18.4	1.24
1975	87.7	18.6	1.21
1976	88.5	18.1	1.16
1977	89.4	16.8	1.12
1978	90.9	16.1	1.11
1979	91.8	15.1	1.07
1980	92.5	14.1	1.04
1981	92.7	13.2	0.92
1982	93.2	13.5	0.89
1983	93.6	13.4	0.88
1984	94.2	13.0	0.89
1985	94.6	13.0	0.95
1986	95.0	13.4	0.93
1987	95.7	13.3	0.94
1988	96.0	13.3	0.94
1989	96.5	13.1	0.96
1990	96.8	12.5	0.93
1991	97.2	12.6	0.94
1992	97.5	12.4	0.92
1993	97.7	12.4	0.90
1994	97.9	12.1	0.90
1995		12.0	0.87

Source : see *Notes on sources of sales data*, p. 712

Table 28.1.4 Proportions of sales (i) of smokeless tobacco, 1982-1995, and (ii) of pipe & hand-rolling tobacco, 1968-1995, in various forms

Year	Smokeless tobacco						Pipe and hand-rolling tobacco	
	Chewing tobacco				Snuff		Hand rolling %	Pipe %
	Plug, firm %	Plug, moist %	Twist %	Loose leaf %	Dry %,	Moist %		
1968							24	76
1969							27	73
1970							32	68
1971							31	69
1972							23	77
1973							29	71
1974							25	75
1975							22	78
1976							22	78
1977							15	85
1978							18	82
1979							21	79
1980							22	78
1981							22	78
1982	7.7	3.9	1.4	53.8	8.5	24.8	24	76
1983	7.3	3.3	1.3	53.6	8.1	26.5	29	71
1984	6.4	3.0	1.2	54.1	7.6	27.8	30	70
1985	6.0	2.8	1.1	53.7	7.1	29.3	30	70
1986	5.5	2.6	1.1	53.5	7.0	30.2	29	71
1987	5.5	2.5	1.2	53.7	6.8	30.4	26	74
1988	4.8	2.1	1.1	53.0	6.3	32.7	23	77
1989	4.5	2.2	1.1	52.0	5.9	34.4	25	75
1990	4.1	1.8	1.0	51.1	5.6	36.5	22	78
1991	3.5	1.6	1.0	51.1	5.1	37.7	29	71
1992	3.2	1.4	1.0	49.4	5.0	40.1	34	66
1993	3.0	1.2	0.9	47.9	4.6	42.5	36	64
1994	2.6	1.0	0.9	46.8	4.5	44.2	38	62
1995	2.5	0.9	0.9	46.9	4.4	44.5	39	61

Source : see *Notes on sources of sales data*, p. 712

Table 28.2 Consumption of (i) cigarettes and (ii) all tobacco products, 1920-1995 sales-based data, including estimated hand-rolled cigarette consumption. Males and females aged 15 years and over

Year	Manufactured cigarettes		Hand-rolled cigarettes		Total cigarettes		All tobacco products	
	Total annual in millions	Number/ adult/day	Total annual in millions	Number/ adult/day	Total annual in millions	Number/ adult/day	Total annual in tonnes	Grams/ adult/day
1920	44656	1.7					298640	11.3
1921	50899	1.9					288950	10.7
1922	53582	1.9					307740	11.2
1923	64469	2.3					314720	11.2
1924	71024	2.5					332630	11.6
1925	79976	2.7					324680	11.1
1926	89460	3.0					334620	11.3
1927	97188	3.2					335090	11.1
1928	105927	3.4					338210	11.0
1929	119049	3.8					349210	11.2
1930	119632	3.8					339900	10.7
1931	113455	3.5					327890	10.2
1932	103589	3.2					301630	9.3
1933	111766	3.4					304960	9.2
1934	125700	3.8					322540	9.6
1935	134610	4.0					331640	9.8
1936	153169	4.5					355240	10.3
1937	162629	4.7					362420	10.4
1938	163761	4.6					364120	10.3
1939	172469	4.8					373220	10.5
1940	180664	5.0					382240	10.6
1941	206432	5.6					409970	11.2
1942	235841	6.4					435280	11.8
1943	257743	6.9					441580	11.8
1944	239287	6.3					413750	11.0
1945	267652	7.0					452440	11.9
1946	321475	8.4					485310	12.6
1947	335965	8.6					492340	12.6
1948	348731	8.9					507450	12.9
1949	351809	8.9	13300	0.3	365109	9.3	505600	12.8
1950	360199	9.0	12700	0.3	372899	9.3	511990	12.7
1951	379725	9.4	12200	0.3	391925	9.7	528730	13.0
1952	394109	9.7	11700	0.3	405809	9.9	542400	13.3
1953	386826	9.4	10600	0.3	397426	9.7	531490	12.9
1954	368725	8.9	10200	0.2	378925	9.1	509920	12.2
1955	382061	9.1	9800	0.2	391861	9.3	521540	12.4
1956	393154	9.2	8800	0.2	401954	9.4	526630	12.3
1957	409436	9.5	8700	0.2	418136	9.7	541500	12.5
1958	436354	9.9	9400	0.2	445754	10.2	570180	13.0
1959	453681	10.2	9000	0.2	462681	10.4	584540	13.1
1960	470136	10.4	9100	0.2	479236	10.6	588190	13.0
1961	488119	10.7	9100	0.2	497219	10.9	611800	13.4
1962	494463	10.6	8800	0.2	503263	10.8	608520	13.1
1963	509588	10.8	8800	0.2	518388	10.9	651770	13.8
1964	497447	10.3	10300	0.2	507747	10.5	648920	13.5
1965	511464	10.5	8800	0.2	520264	10.6	652390	13.3
1966	522533	10.5	8600	0.2	531133	10.7	641120	12.9
1967	527800	10.5	8300	0.2	536100	10.7	631480	12.5
1968	523008	10.2	9200	0.2	532208	10.4	628190	12.3
1969	510531	9.8	10400	0.2	520931	10.0	608110	11.7

Table 28.2 *(continued)*

Year	Manufactured cigarettes		Hand-rolled cigarettes		Total cigarettes		All tobacco products	
	Total annual in millions	Number/ adult/day	Total annual in millions	Number/ adult/day	Total annual in millions	Number/ adult/day	Total annual in tonnes	Grams/ adult/day
1970	532769	10.0	13200	0.2	545969	10.3	612290	11.5
1971	528858	9.7	12000	0.2	540858	10.0	599270	11.0
1972	551017	10.0	8700	0.2	559717	10.1	626720	11.3
1973	590300	10.5	9800	0.2	600100	10.7	639980	11.4
1974	599000	10.5	8500	0.1	607500	10.6	642922	11.2
1975	607200	10.3	6600	0.1	613800	10.4	634653	10.8
1976	613500	10.2	6800	0.1	620300	10.4	615805	10.3
1977	617000	10.1	3900	0.1	620900	10.2	610968	10.0
1978	616000	9.9	4500	0.1	620500	10.0	595617	9.6
1979	621500	9.8	4600	0.1	626100	9.9	619486	9.8
1980	631500	9.8	4400	0.1	635900	9.9	612037	9.5
1981	640000	9.8	4600	0.1	644600	9.9	600883	9.2
1982	634000	9.6	4700	0.1	638700	9.7	600086	9.1
1983	600000	9.0	5500	0.1	605500	9.1	586704	8.8
1984	600400	8.9	5600	0.1	606000	9.0	566721	8.4
1985	594000	8.7	4800	0.1	598800	8.8	569865	8.4
1986	583800	8.5	4500	0.1	588300	8.5	554683	8.0
1987	575000	8.2	4100	0.1	579100	8.3	536268	7.7
1988	562500	8.0	3600	0.1	566100	8.0	529190	7.5
1989	540000	7.6	3300	0.0	543300	7.7	495880	7.0
1990	525000	7.4	3000	0.0	528000	7.4	494054	6.9
1991	510000	7.1	3100	0.0	513100	7.1	490145	6.8
1992	500000	6.9	3400	0.0	503400	6.9	476236	6.6
1993	485000	6.6	3400	0.0	488400	6.7	486459	6.6
1994	486000	6.6	3300	0.0	489300	6.6	446351	6.0
1995	487000	6.5	3200	0.0	490200	6.6	454542	6.1

Source : see *Notes on sources of sales data*, p. 712

Figure 28.1 Daily consumption of (i) manufactured and total number of cigarettes, and (ii) all tobacco products, 1920-1995.
Males and females aged 15 years and over. *Source:* see Table 28.2

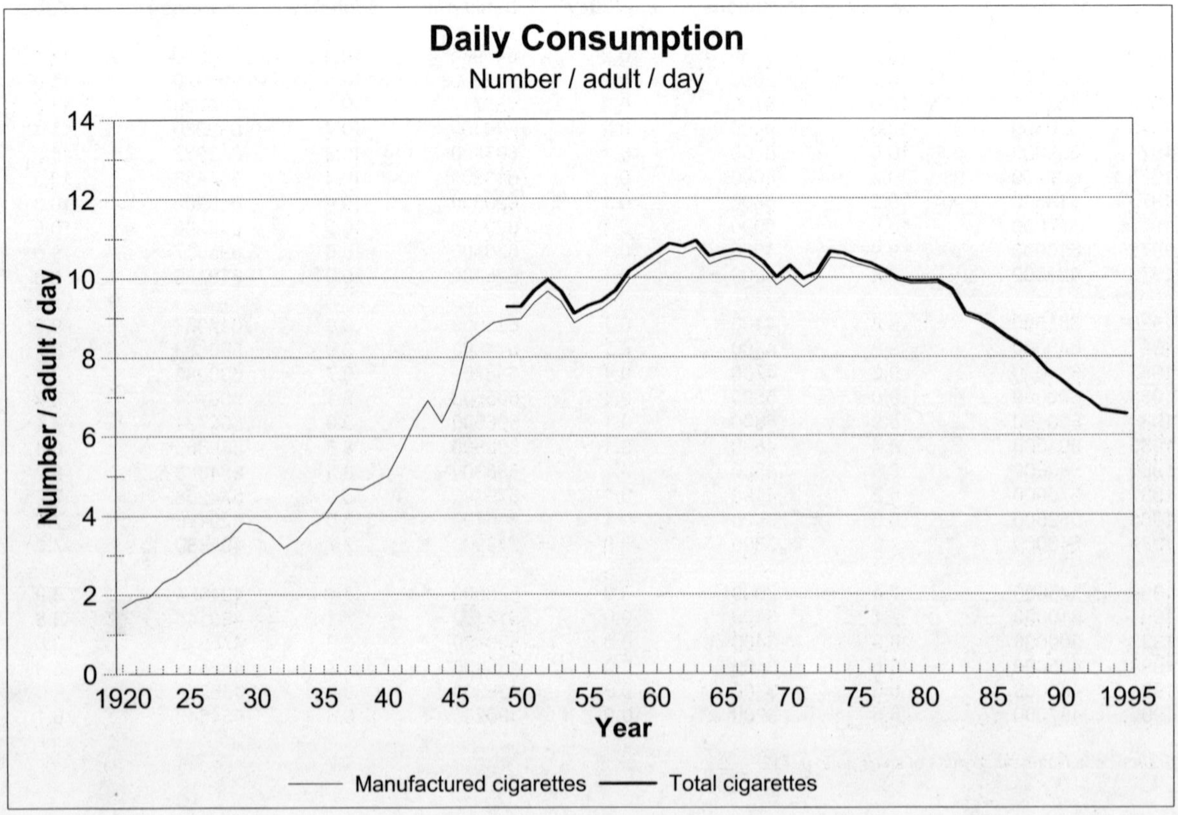

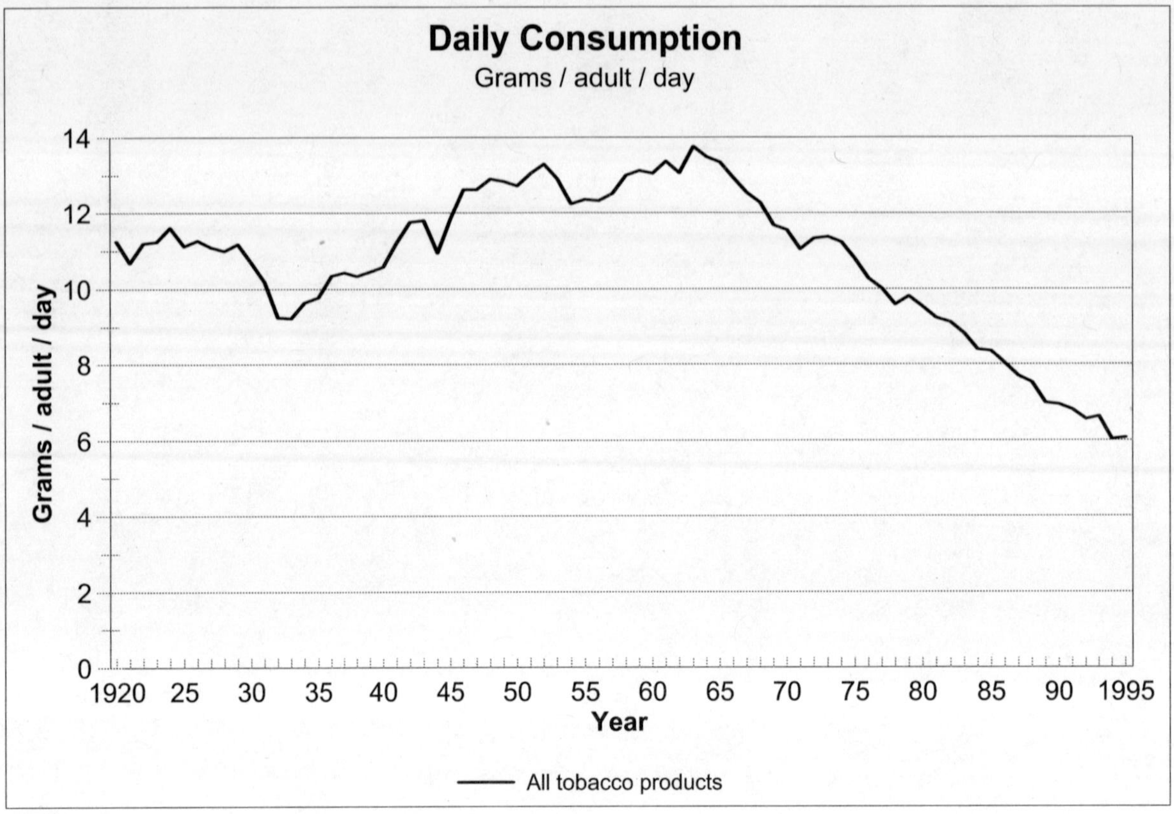

Table 28.3 Percentage sales of tobacco in different forms (by weight), selected years 1925-1995

<table>
<tr><th>Year</th><th>Cigarettes (%)</th><th>Cigars (%)</th><th>Snuff (%)</th><th>Pipe and hand-rolling tobacco (%)</th><th>Chewing tobacco (%)</th></tr>
<tr><td>1925</td><td>24.6</td><td>18.1</td><td>5.3</td><td colspan="2">52.0</td></tr>
<tr><td>1935</td><td>40.6</td><td>12.6</td><td>5.2</td><td colspan="2">41.6</td></tr>
<tr><td>1945</td><td>59.2</td><td>9.4</td><td>4.4</td><td colspan="2">27.1</td></tr>
<tr><td>1955</td><td>73.3</td><td>9.8</td><td>3.4</td><td>6.8</td><td>6.7</td></tr>
<tr><td>1965</td><td>78.2</td><td>10.4</td><td>2.1</td><td>4.9</td><td>4.4</td></tr>
<tr><td>1975</td><td>81.4</td><td>7.2</td><td>1.8</td><td>3.8</td><td>5.8</td></tr>
<tr><td>1985</td><td>82.8</td><td>4.2</td><td>3.9</td><td>2.1</td><td>6.8</td></tr>
<tr><td>1995</td><td>81.5</td><td>5.0</td><td>5.9</td><td>1.4</td><td>6.2</td></tr>
</table>

Source : calculated from Tables 28.1.1 & 28.1.2

Figure 28.2 Percentage sales of tobacco in different forms (by weight), selected years 1925-1995
Source: see Table 28.3

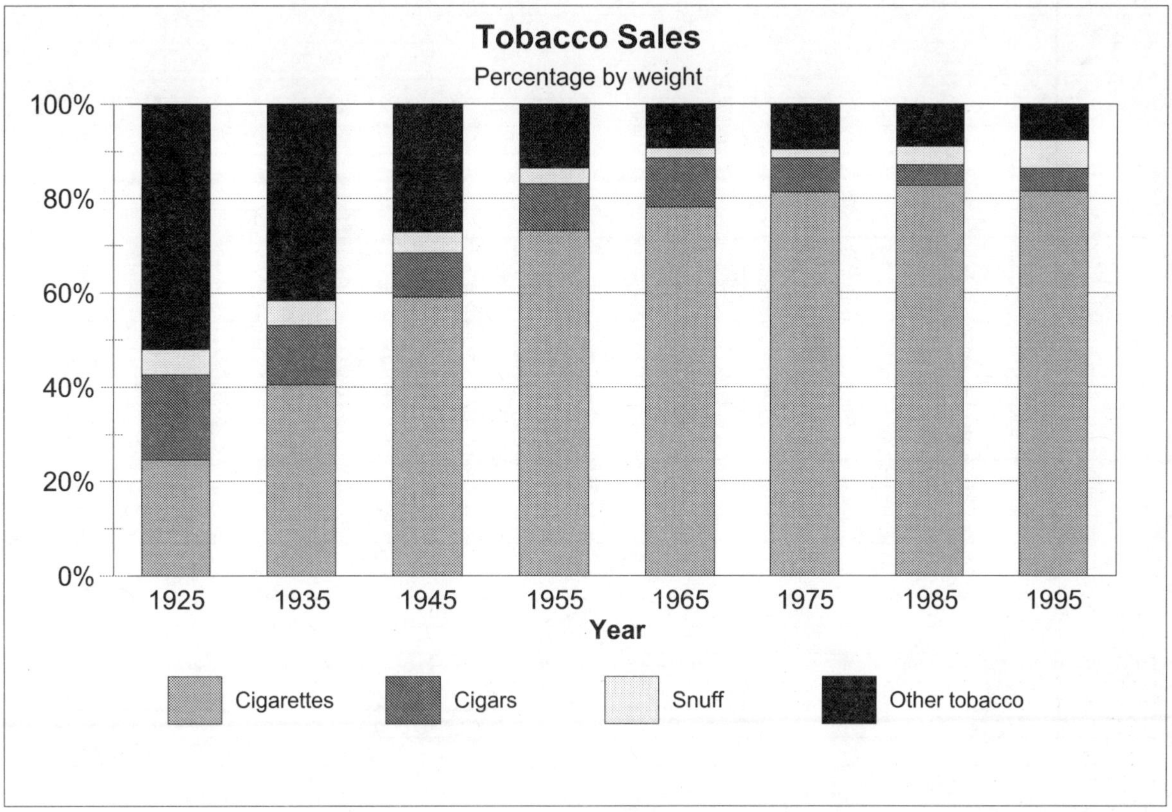

Table 28.4M Prevalence of smoking, males: some selected American surveys by age, 1935-1995 *(continues on p. 700)*

Frequency Product Source Year	Age group																					All ages
	12	13	14	15	16	17	18	19	20-24	25-29	30-34	35-39	40-44	45-49	50-54	55-59	60-64	65-69	70-74	75-79	80+	
35 11 UC U									66			40										
44 5 UC U							48															
47 10 UC U									67		61		61		51		35		11			
47 10 A U									78		79		82		71		65		45			
49 5 UC U							54															
55 4 UC R							48			60		58		54		41		22				50
55 4 UC A							53			64		62		58		46		26				54
58 13 UC R			15	25	31	35																26
58 13 UC A			18	30	36	40																30
59 9 UC R											60	58	57	55	51	46	39	32	25	18	12	46
59 9*UC R											59		55		50		36		23		10	47
59 9* A R											67		65		61		52		41		33	59
59 9* A A											67		65		61		53		43		34	59
59 14 UC A	7	15	20	38	46	46																27
64 3 UC U									67	60		60		53		51		35				53
65 2 UC U									59	61		58		56		47		33		21		52
66 3 UC U									62	60		59		54		48		33				52
66 4 UC R							48			59		57		53		46		24				49
66 4 UC A							48			59		57		53		46		25				49
67 4 UC U						44				56				50				26				48
68 1 UC *	0	1	4	11	17	20	31															12
68 1 UC R	1	2	6	14	20	26	36															15
68 1 UC A	2	3	8	15	23	30	39															17
68 4 UC U						41				55				47				25				46
70 1 UC *	2	3	6	11	16	23	35															14
70 1 UC R	2	4	11	17	22	32	43															19
70 1 UC A	2	4	11	17	23	33	43															19
70 2 UC U						44																
70 3 UC U									50	47		49		43		37		23				42
72 1 UC *	0	4	6	12	14	23	30															13
72 1 UC R	1	5	8	18	18	28	33															16
72 1 UC A	1	5	10	20	19	29	34															17
74 1 UC *	4			16		29																14
74 1 UC R	4			18		31																16
74 1 UC A	4			18		33																16
74 2 UC U									44	51				43				25				43
74 2 UC A							37															
74 15 UC A						48																
75 3 UC U									41	44		47		41		34		24				39
75 6 UC U																						
75 7 UC R						27																
75 7 UC A						37																
76 2 UC U									46	49		48		41				23				42
76 7 UC R						28																
76 7 UC A						38																
76 15 UC A						35																
77 2 UC U									40	48				41				23				41
77 7 UC R						28																
77 7 UC A						38																
77 15 UC A						39																
78 2 UC U									39	42				41				23				39
78 2 UC A							31															
78 7 UC R						26																
78 7 UC A						35																

Table 28.4F Prevalence of smoking, females: some selected American surveys by age, 1935-1995 *(continues on p. 701)*

Frequency / Product / Source / Year	12	13	14	15	16	17	18	19	20-24	25-29	30-34	35-39	40-44	45-49	50-54	55-59	60-64	65-69	70-74	75-79	80+	All ages
35 11 UC U									26				9									
44 5 UC U							36															
47 10 UC U									40		42		26		16		12		3			
47 10 A U									40		42		26		16		12		3			
49 5 UC U							33															
55 4 UC R							28			34		31		22		11		3				24
55 4 UC A							33			39		35		26		13		5				27
58 13 UC R			5	11	16	26																14
58 13 UC A			6	13	20	31																17
59 9 UC R											44	42	40	37	30	22	15	11	7	5	3	28
59 9*UC R											42		37		26		13		7		3	27
59 9* A R											42		37		26		13		7		3	27
59 9* A A											43		39		27		14		8		3	28
59 14 UC A	1	5	11	28	42	55																21
64 3 UC U									42	41		39		36		21		8				32
65 2 UC U									42	44		44		37		25		12		5		34
66 3 UC U									49	45		41		42		21		8				34
66 4 UC R							34			43		41		37		23		8				32
66 4 UC A							35			43		41		37		23		8				32
67 4 UC U						31				41				31				9				31
68 1 UC *	0	1	1	6	8	12	17															6
68 1 UC R	0	1	1	7	12	16	21															8
68 1 UC A	1	1	3	10	14	19	23															10
68 4 UC U						29				40				31				10				31
70 1 UC *	1	1	5	8	12	14	23															9
70 1 UC R	1	2	6	12	16	18	28															12
70 1 UC A	1	2	8	12	17	18	30															13
70 2 UC U						31																
70 3 UC U									32	40		39		36		24		10				31
72 1 UC *	0	3	3	12	14	23	22															11
72 1 UC R	1	4	4	13	20	26	25															13
72 1 UC A	1	4	4	13	20	26	25															13
74 1 UC *	4			19		24																14
74 1 UC R	5			20		26																15
74 1 UC A	5			22		26																16
74 2 UC U									35	39				34				12				31
74 2 UC A							31															
74 15 UC A						39																
75 3 UC U									40	35		36		33		26		10				29
75 6 UC U		27					36															
75 7 UC R						26																
75 7 UC A						36																
76 2 UC U									34	38		38		35				13				33
76 7 UC R						28																
76 7 UC A						38																
76 15 UC A						52																
77 2 UC U									37	38				34				13				31
77 7 UC R						30																
77 7 UC A						40																
77 15 UC A						47																
78 2 UC U									33	36				34				12				30
78 2 UC A							34															
78 7 UC R						29																
78 7 UC A						39																

Table 28.4M *(continued from p. 698, continues on p. 702)*
Prevalence of smoking, males

Frequency / Product / Source / Year	12	13	14	15	16	17	18	19	20-24	25-29	30-34	35-39	40-44	45-49	50-54	55-59	60-64	65-69	70-74	75-79	80+	All ages
79 1 UC *	2			13		17																10
79 1 UC R	3			14		19																11
79 1 UC A	3			15		20																11
79 2 UC U									38	44				40				21				38
79 2 UC A							30															
79 7 UC R						22																
79 7 UC A						31																
79 8 UC R										36		51		35		31						40
79 8 A A										37		53		38		36						43
79 15 UC A						42																
80 2 UC U									40	43		43		41				18				38
80 2 UC A							25															
80 7 UC R						18																
80 7 UC A						26																
81 7 UC R						18																
81 7 UC A						26																
82 7 UC R						18																
82 7 UC A						27																
82 9 UC R											33	34	32	29	27	25	21	19	15	11	8	25
82 12 UC U							34															
82 15 UC A						36																
83 2 UC U									37	40				36				22				36
83 2 UC A							23															
83 7 UC R						19																
83 7 UC A						28																
84 7 UC R						16																
84 7 UC A						26																
85 2 UC U									31	38		38		33				20				33
85 2 UC A							20															
85 4 UC A					16				33		37		38		35		27		16			31
85 4 A U									40													
85 7 UC R						17																
85 7 UC A						27																
85 15 UC A						28																
86 3 UC U							24			34		37		31				17				30
86 7 UC R						17																
86 7 UC A						28																
87 2 UC U									31	36				33				17				32
87 2 UC A							22															
87 7 UC R						16																
87 7 UC A						27																
88 2 UC U							26			36				31				21		11		31
88 2 UC A							20															
88 7 UC A						28																
88 15 UC A						28																
89 7 UC A						28																
89 16 UC R	1	2	6	12	13	18	29															12
89 16 UC A	2	5	10	16	19	24	35															16
90 2 UC U							27			33				29				18		8		28
90 2 UC A							22															
90 7 UC A						29																
90 15 UC A						29																
90 17 UC R			8																			
90 17 UC A			18																			

Table 28.4F (continued from p. 699, continues on p. 703)

Table 28.4F Prevalence of smoking, females

Frequency Product Source Year	12	13	14	15	16	17	18	19	20-24	25-29	30-34	35-39	40-44	45-49	50-54	55-59	60-64	65-69	70-74	75-79	80+	All ages
79 1 UC *	4			11		24																12
79 1 UC R	4			12		26																13
79 1 UC A	4			12		27																13
79 2 UC U									34	35				31				13				29
79 2 UC A							34															
79 7 UC R						28																
79 7 UC A						37																
79 8 UC R										34		45		33		30						37
79 8 A A										34		45		34		30						37
79 15 UC A						42																
80 2 UC U									33	32		35		31				17				30
80 2 UC A							28															
80 7 UC R						24																
80 7 UC A						34																
81 7 UC R						22																
81 7 UC A						32																
82 7 UC R						24																
82 7 UC A						33																
82 9 UC R											26	27	25	25	23	22	19	16	12	8	4	21
82 12 UC U							29															
82 15 UC A						37																
83 2 UC U									37	33				31				13				29
83 2 UC A							31															
83 7 UC R						23																
83 7 UC A						33																
84 7 UC R						21																
84 7 UC A						32																
85 2 UC U									32	32		32		30				14				28
85 2 UC A							25															
85 4 UC A					15				30		29		31		27		22		10			25
85 4 A U									27													
85 7 UC R						21																
85 7 UC A						32																
85 15 UC A						27																
86 3 UC U						22				29		29		25				12				24
86 7 UC R						20																
86 7 UC A						31																
87 2 UC U									28	31				29				14				27
87 2 UC A							21															
87 7 UC R						20																
87 7 UC A						31																
88 2 UC U							26			30				28				17		7		26
88 2 UC A							23															
88 7 UC A						29																
88 15 UC A						33																
89 7 UC A						29																
89 16 UC R	1	4	9	11	14	18	21															11
89 16 UC A	3	6	11	16	19	25	26															15
90 2 UC U							23			27				25				16		6		23
90 2 UC A							18															
90 7 UC A						29																
90 15 UC A						20																
90 17 UC R			4																			
90 17 UC A			17																			

Table 28.4M *(continued from p. 700)* Prevalence of smoking, males

Frequency / Product / Source / Year	12	13	14	15	16	17	18	19	20-24	25-29	30-34	35-39	40-44	45-49	50-54	55-59	60-64	65-69	70-74	75-79	80+	All ages
91 2 UC U							24			33			29					18		9		28
91 2 UC A							22															
91 7 UC A						29																
91 15 UC A						27																
91 18 UC R			13																			
91 18 UC A			28																			
92 2 UC A							28			33			29					16				29
92 7 UC A						29																
92 18 UC A	11			26	31	35	40															
93 2 UC A							29			31			29					14				28
93 4 UC A									28		32		30		27		21		11			27
93 7 UC A						31																
93 18 UC R			10	12	15	19																14
93 18 UC A			27	26	31	35																30
94 2 UC A							30			32			28					13				28
94 7 UC A						33																
94 15 UC A	20						37			35		31										32
95 2 UC A							28			31			27					14				27
95 7 UC A						35																
95 15 UC A	21						38			37		30										31
95 18 UC R			9	14	20	22																16
95 18 UC A			32	31	36	42																35

Source: see *Notes on sources of survey data*, p. 714
Product: MC = manufactured cigarettes
TC = total cigarettes (including hand-rolled)
UC = cigarettes (type unspecified)
A = all products

Frequency: A = all smokers (including occasional)
R = regular or daily smokers
All ages: relevant to ages used and as given in original source
U = unspecified
* = refer to *Notes on sources of survey data*, p. 714

Table 28.4F *(continued from p. 701)*
Prevalence of smoking, females

Frequency / Product / Source / Year	Age group 12	13	14	15	16	17	18	19	20-24	25-29	30-34	35-39	40-44	45-49	50-54	55-59	60-64	65-69	70-74	75-79	80+	All ages
91 2 UC U							22			28				25				15		8		24
91 2 UC A							21															
91 7 UC A						28																
91 15 UC A						27																
91 18 UC R			12																			
91 18 UC A			27																			
92 2 UC A							25			29				26				12				25
92 7 UC A						26																
92 18 UC A	12			22	25	32	34															
93 2 UC A							23			27				23				11				23
93 4 UC A									24		26		24		23		17		9			22
93 7 UC A						29																
93 18 UC R			8	13	16	17																14
93 18 UC A			29	30	31	34																31
94 2 UC A							25			28				23				11				23
94 7 UC A						29																
94 15 UC A	18						32			30		25										26
95 2 UC A							22			27				24				12				23
95 7 UC A						32																
95 15 UC A	20						33			32		25										27
95 18 UC R			10	13	19	20																16
95 18 UC A			30	35	36	34																34

Source: see *Notes on sources of survey data*, p. 714
Product: MC = manufactured cigarettes
TC = total cigarettes (including hand-rolled)
UC = cigarettes (type unspecified)
A = all products

Frequency: A = all smokers (including occasional)
R = regular or daily smokers
All ages: relevant to ages used and as given in original source
U = unspecified
* = refer to *Notes on sources of survey data*, p. 714

Table 28.5M Number of cigarettes smoked per smoker per day, males: some selected American surveys by age, 1929-1991

<table>
<tr><th rowspan="2">Product
Source
Year</th><th colspan="21">Age group</th><th rowspan="2">All ages</th></tr>
<tr><th>12</th><th>13</th><th>14</th><th>15</th><th>16</th><th>17</th><th>18</th><th>19</th><th>20-24</th><th>25-29</th><th>30-34</th><th>35-39</th><th>40-44</th><th>45-49</th><th>50-54</th><th>55-59</th><th>60-64</th><th>65-69</th><th>70-74</th><th>75-79</th><th>80+</th></tr>
<tr><td>29 19 UC</td><td colspan="3"></td><td colspan="18">7.2</td><td></td></tr>
<tr><td>47 10 UCE*</td><td colspan="8"></td><td colspan="2">28</td><td colspan="2">29</td><td colspan="2">30</td><td colspan="2">29</td><td colspan="2">28</td><td colspan="3">25</td><td></td></tr>
<tr><td>55 4 UCE</td><td colspan="6"></td><td colspan="3">16</td><td colspan="2">18</td><td colspan="2">19</td><td colspan="2">19</td><td colspan="2">17</td><td colspan="4">14</td><td>18</td></tr>
<tr><td>58 13 UCE</td><td colspan="2"></td><td>6.7</td><td>7.9</td><td>9.4</td><td>11</td><td colspan="15"></td><td>8.9</td></tr>
<tr><td>59 9 UC</td><td colspan="10"></td><td>22</td><td>23</td><td>23</td><td>24</td><td>23</td><td>22</td><td>20</td><td>18</td><td>16</td><td>15</td><td>13</td><td></td></tr>
<tr><td>59 14 UCE*</td><td>4.0</td><td>5.5</td><td>7.2</td><td>9.0</td><td>12</td><td>13</td><td colspan="15"></td><td>9.9</td></tr>
<tr><td>64 3 UCE</td><td colspan="8"></td><td colspan="13">22</td><td></td></tr>
<tr><td>65 2 UCE</td><td colspan="8"></td><td>18</td><td colspan="2">20</td><td colspan="2">21</td><td colspan="4">21</td><td colspan="4">16</td><td>20</td></tr>
<tr><td>66 4 UCE</td><td colspan="6"></td><td colspan="3">17</td><td colspan="2">19</td><td colspan="2">20</td><td colspan="2">20</td><td colspan="2">19</td><td colspan="4">15</td><td>19</td></tr>
<tr><td>67 4 UCE</td><td colspan="5"></td><td colspan="4">16</td><td colspan="4">20</td><td colspan="4">20</td><td colspan="4">15</td><td>19</td></tr>
<tr><td>68 1 UCE</td><td>2.5</td><td>3.8</td><td>13</td><td>11</td><td>12</td><td>14</td><td>16</td><td colspan="14"></td><td>14</td></tr>
<tr><td>68 4 UCE</td><td colspan="5"></td><td colspan="4">16</td><td colspan="4">20</td><td colspan="4">20</td><td colspan="4">16</td><td>19</td></tr>
<tr><td>70 1 UCE</td><td>8.3</td><td>12</td><td>12</td><td>9.5</td><td>14</td><td>16</td><td>16</td><td colspan="14"></td><td>14</td></tr>
<tr><td>70 3 UC</td><td colspan="8"></td><td>21</td><td colspan="2">21</td><td colspan="2">23</td><td colspan="2">24</td><td colspan="2">22</td><td colspan="4">17</td><td>22</td></tr>
<tr><td>72 1 UCE</td><td>14</td><td>9.0</td><td>10</td><td>14</td><td>14</td><td>17</td><td>18</td><td colspan="14"></td><td>16</td></tr>
<tr><td>74 1 UCE</td><td colspan="3">12</td><td colspan="2">16</td><td colspan="2">18</td><td colspan="14"></td><td>17</td></tr>
<tr><td>75 3 UC</td><td colspan="8"></td><td>19</td><td colspan="2">22</td><td colspan="2">23</td><td colspan="2">25</td><td colspan="2">25</td><td colspan="4">20</td><td>23</td></tr>
<tr><td>75 6 UCE</td><td colspan="21"></td><td></td></tr>
<tr><td>76 2 UCE</td><td colspan="8"></td><td>19</td><td colspan="2">21</td><td colspan="2">23</td><td colspan="4">23</td><td colspan="4">18</td><td>21</td></tr>
<tr><td>79 1 UCE</td><td colspan="3">13</td><td colspan="2">14</td><td colspan="2">17</td><td colspan="14"></td><td>15</td></tr>
<tr><td>79 8 UC</td><td colspan="7"></td><td colspan="14">27</td><td></td></tr>
<tr><td>80 2 UC</td><td colspan="8"></td><td>19</td><td colspan="2">22</td><td colspan="2">26</td><td colspan="2">27</td><td colspan="2">23</td><td colspan="4">21</td><td>23</td></tr>
<tr><td>82 9 UC</td><td colspan="10"></td><td>23</td><td>26</td><td>27</td><td>27</td><td>27</td><td>26</td><td>24</td><td>22</td><td>20</td><td>18</td><td>15</td><td></td></tr>
<tr><td>85 2 UC</td><td colspan="6"></td><td colspan="3">17</td><td colspan="2">20</td><td colspan="2">24</td><td colspan="2">25</td><td colspan="2">24</td><td colspan="4">20</td><td>22</td></tr>
<tr><td>88 2 UC</td><td colspan="6"></td><td colspan="3">19</td><td colspan="4">23</td><td colspan="4">25</td><td colspan="2">21</td><td colspan="2">16</td><td>23</td></tr>
<tr><td>91 2 UC</td><td colspan="6"></td><td colspan="15">22</td><td></td></tr>
</table>

Source: see *Notes on sources of survey data*, p. 714

Product: MC = manufactured cigarettes
TC = total cigarettes (including hand-rolled)
UC = cigarettes (type unspecified)
A = all products
U = unspecified

Product (cont): E indicates mean estimated from percentage distribution (see also *Consumption category estimation*, p. xxxiv, and Appendix III, p. 789)

All ages: relevant to ages used and as given in original source

* = refer to *Notes on sources of survey data*, p. 714

Table 28.5F Number of cigarettes smoked per smoker per day, females: some selected American surveys by age, 1929-1991

<table>
<tr><th rowspan="2">Product
Source
Year</th><th colspan="21">Age group</th><th rowspan="2">All ages</th></tr>
<tr><th>12</th><th>13</th><th>14</th><th>15</th><th>16</th><th>17</th><th>18</th><th>19</th><th>20-24</th><th>25-29</th><th>30-34</th><th>35-39</th><th>40-44</th><th>45-49</th><th>50-54</th><th>55-59</th><th>60-64</th><th>65-69</th><th>70-74</th><th>75-79</th><th>80+</th></tr>
<tr><td>29 19 UC</td><td colspan="3"></td><td colspan="18">2.4</td><td></td></tr>
<tr><td>47 10 UCE*</td><td colspan="8"></td><td colspan="2">22</td><td colspan="2">22</td><td colspan="2">23</td><td colspan="2">21</td><td colspan="2">19</td><td colspan="3">18</td><td></td></tr>
<tr><td>55 4 UCE</td><td colspan="6"></td><td colspan="3">12</td><td colspan="2">13</td><td colspan="2">13</td><td colspan="2">13</td><td colspan="2">12</td><td colspan="4">9.4</td><td>13</td></tr>
<tr><td>58 13 UCE</td><td colspan="2"></td><td>4.8</td><td>6.6</td><td>7.2</td><td>7.0</td><td colspan="15"></td><td>6.8</td></tr>
<tr><td>59 9 UC</td><td colspan="10"></td><td>16</td><td>16</td><td>16</td><td>16</td><td>15</td><td>15</td><td>14</td><td>13</td><td>12</td><td>11</td><td>8.5</td><td></td></tr>
<tr><td>59 14 UCE*</td><td>4.6</td><td>5.4</td><td>5.2</td><td>5.3</td><td>6.5</td><td>8.4</td><td colspan="15"></td><td>6.8</td></tr>
<tr><td>64 3 UCE</td><td colspan="8"></td><td colspan="13">17</td><td></td></tr>
<tr><td>65 2 UCE</td><td colspan="8"></td><td>15</td><td colspan="2">16</td><td colspan="2">17</td><td colspan="4">16</td><td colspan="4">13</td><td>16</td></tr>
<tr><td>66 4 UCE</td><td colspan="6"></td><td colspan="3">14</td><td colspan="2">16</td><td colspan="2">16</td><td colspan="2">16</td><td colspan="2">15</td><td colspan="4">13</td><td>16</td></tr>
<tr><td>67 4 UCE</td><td colspan="5"></td><td colspan="4">14</td><td colspan="4">16</td><td colspan="4">16</td><td colspan="4">13</td><td>15</td></tr>
<tr><td>68 1 UCE</td><td>0.0</td><td>10</td><td>4.6</td><td>12</td><td>12</td><td>11</td><td>12</td><td colspan="14"></td><td>12</td></tr>
<tr><td>68 4 UCE</td><td colspan="5"></td><td colspan="4">14</td><td colspan="4">16</td><td colspan="4">16</td><td colspan="4">13</td><td>16</td></tr>
<tr><td>70 1 UCE</td><td>2.5</td><td>18</td><td>9.2</td><td>12</td><td>13</td><td>13</td><td>13</td><td colspan="14"></td><td>12</td></tr>
<tr><td>70 3 UC</td><td colspan="8"></td><td>16</td><td colspan="2">18</td><td colspan="2">19</td><td colspan="2">18</td><td colspan="2">17</td><td colspan="4">14</td><td>18</td></tr>
<tr><td>72 1 UCE</td><td>0.0</td><td>7.0</td><td>13</td><td>11</td><td>10</td><td>12</td><td>15</td><td colspan="14"></td><td>12</td></tr>
<tr><td>74 1 UCE</td><td colspan="3">7.2</td><td colspan="2">12</td><td colspan="2">14</td><td colspan="14"></td><td>13</td></tr>
<tr><td>75 3 UC</td><td colspan="8"></td><td>19</td><td colspan="2">19</td><td colspan="2">20</td><td colspan="2">20</td><td colspan="2">19</td><td colspan="4">16</td><td>19</td></tr>
<tr><td>75 6 UCE</td><td colspan="6"></td><td colspan="5">18</td><td colspan="10"></td><td></td></tr>
<tr><td>76 2 UCE</td><td colspan="8"></td><td>16</td><td colspan="2">18</td><td colspan="2">18</td><td colspan="4">18</td><td colspan="4">15</td><td>18</td></tr>
<tr><td>79 1 UCE</td><td colspan="3">8.6</td><td colspan="2">12</td><td colspan="2">13</td><td colspan="14"></td><td>13</td></tr>
<tr><td>79 8 UC</td><td colspan="11"></td><td colspan="6">18</td><td colspan="4"></td><td></td></tr>
<tr><td>80 2 UC</td><td colspan="8"></td><td>18</td><td colspan="2">19</td><td colspan="2">23</td><td colspan="2">21</td><td colspan="2">20</td><td colspan="4">16</td><td>20</td></tr>
<tr><td>82 9 UC</td><td colspan="10"></td><td>20</td><td>21</td><td>21</td><td>21</td><td>20</td><td>20</td><td>19</td><td>18</td><td>17</td><td>16</td><td>14</td><td></td></tr>
<tr><td>85 2 UC</td><td colspan="6"></td><td colspan="3">15</td><td colspan="2">18</td><td colspan="2">20</td><td colspan="2">20</td><td colspan="2">18</td><td colspan="4">16</td><td>18</td></tr>
<tr><td>88 2 UC</td><td colspan="6"></td><td colspan="3">17</td><td colspan="4">20</td><td colspan="4">21</td><td colspan="2">18</td><td colspan="2">15</td><td>20</td></tr>
<tr><td>91 2 UC</td><td colspan="6"></td><td colspan="15">18</td><td></td></tr>
</table>

Source: see *Notes on sources of survey data*, p. 714

Product: MC = manufactured cigarettes
TC = total cigarettes (including hand-rolled)
UC = cigarettes (type unspecified)
A = all products
U = unspecified

Product (cont): E indicates mean estimated from percentage distribution (see also *Consumption category estimation*, p. xxxiv, and Appendix III, p. 789)

All ages: relevant to ages used and as given in original source

* = refer to *Notes on sources of survey data*, p. 714

Table 28.6M Number of cigarettes smoked per person per day, males: some selected American surveys by age, 1947-1988, with percentage total sales

Product Source Year	Age group																					All ages	% Total sales
	12	13	14	15	16	17	18	19	20-24	25-29	30-34	35-39	40-44	45-49	50-54	55-59	60-64	65-69	70-74	75-79	80+		
47 10 UC *									19		18		18		15		9.7		2.8				114%T
55 4 UC							7.5			11		11		10		7.1		3.1				8.9	60%T
58 13 UC			0.7	1.5	2.4	3.1																1.8	**
59 9 UC											13	14	13	13	12	10	7.7	5.8	4.1	2.6	1.6		**
59 14 UC *	0.3	0.8	1.5	3.4	5.3	5.8																2.6	**
64 3 UC									12														74%T
65 2 UC									10	12		12		11				4.7				10	69%T
66 4 UC							8.0			11		11		11		8.7		3.6				9.3	62%T
67 4 UC						7.0				11				9.8				3.9				9.0	61%T
68 1 UC	0.0	0.0	0.6	1.2	2.1	2.8	4.9															1.6	**
68 4 UC						6.6				11				9.4				4.0				8.7	61%T
70 1 UC	0.1	0.3	0.7	1.0	2.2	3.7	5.7															2.0	**
70 3 UC									10	9.8		11		10		8.2		3.9				9.3	65%T
72 1 UC	0.0	0.3	0.6	1.6	2.0	4.0	5.2															1.9	**
74 1 UC	0.4			2.5		5.1																2.4	**
75 3 UC									7.8	9.7		11		10		8.4		4.9				9.0	64%T
75 6 UC																							**
76 2 UC									8.5	10		11		9.4				4.1				8.9	65%T
79 1 UC	0.3			1.7		3.0																1.5	**
79 8 UC *												11											**
80 2 UC									7.5	9.1		10		9.6				3.6				8.3	63%T
82 9 UC											7.6	8.7	8.5	7.8	7.3	6.5	5.2	4.1	3.0	2.0	1.1		**
85 2 UC							5.3			7.8		9.1		8.2		8.0		4.0				7.1	66%T
88 2 UC							4.7			8.5				7.9				4.4		1.9		7.1	72%T

Table 28.7M Number of cigarettes smoked per person per day, sales-adjusted, males: some selected American surveys[1] by age, 1947-1988, with percentage total sales

Product Source Year	Age group																					All ages	% Total sales
	12	13	14	15	16	17	18	19	20-24	25-29	30-34	35-39	40-44	45-49	50-54	55-59	60-64	65-69	70-74	75-79	80+		
47 10 UC *									17		16		16		13		8.5		2.4				114%T
55 4 UC							12			18		19		17		12		5.2				15	60%T
64 3 UC									16														74%T
65 2 UC									15	18		18		15				6.8				15	69%T
66 4 UC							13			18		18		17		14		5.8				15	62%T
67 4 UC						11				18				16				6.4				15	61%T
68 4 UC						11				18				15				6.5				14	61%T
70 3 UC									16	15		17		16		13		6.0				14	65%T
75 3 UC									12	15		17		16		13		7.7				14	64%T
76 2 UC									13	16		17		14				6.3				14	65%T
80 2 UC									12	15		16		15				5.8				13	63%T
85 2 UC							8.0			12		14		12		12		6.0				11	66%T
88 2 UC							6.6			12				11				6.2		2.7		9.9	72%T

1 Based on those surveys in Table 28.6 with data for both sexes and age range at least 21-64 (see *Cigarette consumption per person*, p. xxxv)

Source: see *Notes on sources of survey data*, p. 714
All ages: relevant to ages used and as given in original source
% Total sales: estimated % of total sales of M = manufactured or T = total cigarette consumption implied by survey, sexes combined, used as adjustment factor in Table 28.7
** = cannot be calculated
--- = adjusted by original author

Product: MC = manufactured cigarettes
TC = total cigarettes (including hand-rolled)
UC = cigarettes (type unspecified)
A = all products
U = unspecified
* = refer to *Notes on sources of survey data*, p. 714

Table 28.6F Number of cigarettes smoked per person per day, females: some selected American surveys by age, 1947-1988, with percentage total sales

<table>
<tr><th rowspan="2">Product
Source
Year</th><th colspan="21">Age group</th><th rowspan="2">All ages</th><th rowspan="2">% Total sales</th></tr>
<tr><th>12</th><th>13</th><th>14</th><th>15</th><th>16</th><th>17</th><th>18</th><th>19</th><th>20-24</th><th>25-29</th><th>30-34</th><th>35-39</th><th>40-44</th><th>45-49</th><th>50-54</th><th>55-59</th><th>60-64</th><th>65-69</th><th>70-74</th><th>75-79</th><th>80+</th></tr>
<tr><td>47 10 UC *</td><td colspan="8"></td><td colspan="2">8.9</td><td colspan="2">9.2</td><td colspan="2">5.9</td><td colspan="2">3.3</td><td colspan="2">2.3</td><td colspan="3">0.5</td><td></td><td>114%T</td></tr>
<tr><td>55 4 UC</td><td colspan="6"></td><td colspan="3">3.3</td><td colspan="2">4.6</td><td colspan="2">4.0</td><td colspan="2">2.8</td><td colspan="2">1.2</td><td colspan="4">0.3</td><td>3.0</td><td>60%T</td></tr>
<tr><td>58 13 UC</td><td colspan="2"></td><td>0.2</td><td>0.5</td><td>0.8</td><td>1.4</td><td colspan="15"></td><td>0.7</td><td>**</td></tr>
<tr><td>59 9 UC</td><td colspan="10"></td><td>6.9</td><td>6.7</td><td>6.3</td><td>5.7</td><td>4.5</td><td>3.1</td><td>2.0</td><td>1.4</td><td>0.9</td><td>0.6</td><td>0.2</td><td></td><td>**</td></tr>
<tr><td>59 14 UC *</td><td>0.1</td><td>0.2</td><td>0.6</td><td>1.5</td><td>2.7</td><td>4.6</td><td colspan="15"></td><td>1.4</td><td>**</td></tr>
<tr><td>64 3 UC</td><td colspan="8"></td><td colspan="13">5.4</td><td></td><td>74%T</td></tr>
<tr><td>65 2 UC</td><td colspan="8"></td><td>6.2</td><td colspan="2">7.2</td><td colspan="2">7.4</td><td colspan="4">5.1</td><td colspan="4">1.3</td><td>5.4</td><td>69%T</td></tr>
<tr><td>66 4 UC</td><td colspan="6"></td><td colspan="3">4.9</td><td colspan="2">6.8</td><td colspan="2">6.6</td><td colspan="2">5.9</td><td colspan="2">3.3</td><td colspan="4">1.0</td><td>4.9</td><td>62%T</td></tr>
<tr><td>67 4 UC</td><td colspan="5"></td><td colspan="4">4.4</td><td colspan="4">6.6</td><td colspan="4">4.9</td><td colspan="4">1.1</td><td>4.8</td><td>61%T</td></tr>
<tr><td>68 1 UC</td><td>0.0</td><td>0.1</td><td>0.0</td><td>0.7</td><td>0.9</td><td>1.3</td><td>2.1</td><td colspan="14"></td><td>0.7</td><td>**</td></tr>
<tr><td>68 4 UC</td><td colspan="5"></td><td colspan="4">4.1</td><td colspan="4">6.6</td><td colspan="4">4.8</td><td colspan="4">1.3</td><td>4.7</td><td>61%T</td></tr>
<tr><td>70 1 UC</td><td>0.0</td><td>0.1</td><td>0.4</td><td>1.0</td><td>1.6</td><td>1.7</td><td>2.9</td><td colspan="14"></td><td>1.1</td><td>**</td></tr>
<tr><td>70 3 UC</td><td colspan="8"></td><td>5.2</td><td colspan="2">7.3</td><td colspan="2">7.2</td><td colspan="2">6.6</td><td colspan="2">4.1</td><td colspan="4">1.4</td><td>5.5</td><td>65%T</td></tr>
<tr><td>72 1 UC</td><td>0.0</td><td>0.2</td><td>0.3</td><td>1.3</td><td>1.4</td><td>2.8</td><td>3.2</td><td colspan="14"></td><td>1.4</td><td>**</td></tr>
<tr><td>74 1 UC</td><td colspan="3">0.3</td><td colspan="2">2.3</td><td colspan="2">3.4</td><td colspan="14"></td><td>1.8</td><td>**</td></tr>
<tr><td>75 3 UC</td><td colspan="8"></td><td>7.4</td><td colspan="2">6.5</td><td colspan="2">7.3</td><td colspan="2">6.7</td><td colspan="2">4.9</td><td colspan="4">1.6</td><td>5.5</td><td>64%T</td></tr>
<tr><td>75 6 UC</td><td colspan="6"></td><td colspan="5">7</td><td colspan="10"></td><td></td><td>**</td></tr>
<tr><td>76 2 UC</td><td colspan="8"></td><td>5.4</td><td colspan="2">6.8</td><td colspan="2">6.9</td><td colspan="4">6.3</td><td colspan="4">2.0</td><td>5.8</td><td>65%T</td></tr>
<tr><td>79 1 UC</td><td colspan="3">0.3</td><td colspan="2">1.4</td><td colspan="2">3.3</td><td colspan="14"></td><td>1.5</td><td>**</td></tr>
<tr><td>79 8 UC *</td><td colspan="11"></td><td colspan="6">6.6</td><td colspan="4"></td><td></td><td>**</td></tr>
<tr><td>80 2 UC</td><td colspan="8"></td><td>5.4</td><td colspan="2">5.9</td><td colspan="2">5.1</td><td colspan="4">5.8</td><td colspan="4">2.6</td><td>5.5</td><td>63%T</td></tr>
<tr><td>82 9 UC</td><td colspan="10"></td><td>5.2</td><td>5.7</td><td>5.2</td><td>5.1</td><td>4.7</td><td>4.3</td><td>3.5</td><td>2.8</td><td>1.9</td><td>1.3</td><td>0.6</td><td></td><td>**</td></tr>
<tr><td>85 2 UC</td><td colspan="6"></td><td colspan="3">4.9</td><td colspan="2">5.8</td><td colspan="2">6.3</td><td colspan="2">6.0</td><td colspan="2">5.4</td><td colspan="4">2.2</td><td>5.1</td><td>66%T</td></tr>
<tr><td>88 2 UC</td><td colspan="6"></td><td colspan="3">4.4</td><td colspan="4">5.9</td><td colspan="4">5.8</td><td colspan="2">3.1</td><td colspan="2">1.1</td><td>5.0</td><td>72%T</td></tr>
</table>

Table 28.7F Number of cigarettes smoked per person per day, sales-adjusted, females: some selected American surveys[1] by age, 1947-1988, with percentage total sales

<table>
<tr><th rowspan="2">Product
Source
Year</th><th colspan="21">Age group</th><th rowspan="2">All ages</th><th rowspan="2">% Total sales</th></tr>
<tr><th>12</th><th>13</th><th>14</th><th>15</th><th>16</th><th>17</th><th>18</th><th>19</th><th>20-24</th><th>25-29</th><th>30-34</th><th>35-39</th><th>40-44</th><th>45-49</th><th>50-54</th><th>55-59</th><th>60-64</th><th>65-69</th><th>70-74</th><th>75-79</th><th>80+</th></tr>
<tr><td>47 10 UC *</td><td colspan="8"></td><td colspan="2">7.8</td><td colspan="2">8.0</td><td colspan="2">5.2</td><td colspan="2">2.9</td><td colspan="2">2.0</td><td colspan="3">0.4</td><td></td><td>114%T</td></tr>
<tr><td>55 4 UC</td><td colspan="6"></td><td colspan="3">5.5</td><td colspan="2">7.7</td><td colspan="2">6.7</td><td colspan="2">4.7</td><td colspan="2">2.0</td><td colspan="4">0.5</td><td>5.0</td><td>60%T</td></tr>
<tr><td>64 3 UC</td><td colspan="8"></td><td colspan="13">7.3</td><td></td><td>74%T</td></tr>
<tr><td>65 2 UC</td><td colspan="8"></td><td>9.0</td><td colspan="2">10</td><td colspan="2">11</td><td colspan="4">7.4</td><td colspan="4">1.9</td><td>7.8</td><td>69%T</td></tr>
<tr><td>66 4 UC</td><td colspan="6"></td><td colspan="3">7.9</td><td colspan="2">11</td><td colspan="2">11</td><td colspan="2">9.6</td><td colspan="2">5.4</td><td colspan="4">1.6</td><td>7.9</td><td>62%T</td></tr>
<tr><td>67 4 UC</td><td colspan="5"></td><td colspan="4">7.2</td><td colspan="4">11</td><td colspan="4">8.0</td><td colspan="4">1.8</td><td>7.8</td><td>61%T</td></tr>
<tr><td>68 4 UC</td><td colspan="5"></td><td colspan="4">6.7</td><td colspan="4">11</td><td colspan="4">7.8</td><td colspan="4">2.1</td><td>7.7</td><td>61%T</td></tr>
<tr><td>70 3 UC</td><td colspan="8"></td><td>8.0</td><td colspan="2">11</td><td colspan="2">11</td><td colspan="2">10</td><td colspan="2">6.3</td><td colspan="4">2.2</td><td>8.5</td><td>65%T</td></tr>
<tr><td>75 3 UC</td><td colspan="8"></td><td>12</td><td colspan="2">10</td><td colspan="2">11</td><td colspan="2">10</td><td colspan="2">7.7</td><td colspan="4">2.5</td><td>8.6</td><td>64%T</td></tr>
<tr><td>76 2 UC</td><td colspan="8"></td><td>8.3</td><td colspan="2">10</td><td colspan="2">11</td><td colspan="4">9.7</td><td colspan="4">3.1</td><td>8.9</td><td>65%T</td></tr>
<tr><td>80 2 UC</td><td colspan="8"></td><td>8.6</td><td colspan="2">9.4</td><td colspan="2">8.2</td><td colspan="4">9.3</td><td colspan="4">4.2</td><td>8.8</td><td>63%T</td></tr>
<tr><td>85 2 UC</td><td colspan="6"></td><td colspan="3">7.4</td><td colspan="2">8.7</td><td colspan="2">9.5</td><td colspan="2">9.0</td><td colspan="2">8.1</td><td colspan="4">3.3</td><td>7.7</td><td>66%T</td></tr>
<tr><td>88 2 UC</td><td colspan="6"></td><td colspan="3">6.2</td><td colspan="4">8.3</td><td colspan="4">8.1</td><td colspan="2">4.3</td><td colspan="2">1.5</td><td>7.0</td><td>72%T</td></tr>
</table>

1 Based on those surveys in Table 28.6 with data for both sexes and age range at least 21-64 (see *Cigarette consumption per person*, p. xxxv)

Source: see *Notes on sources of survey data*, p. 714
All ages: relevant to ages used and as given in original source
% Total sales: estimated % of total sales of M = manufactured or T = total cigarette consumption implied by survey, sexes combined, used as adjustment factor in Table 28.7
** = cannot be calculated
--- = adjusted by original author

Product: MC = manufactured cigarettes
TC = total cigarettes (including hand-rolled)
UC = cigarettes (type unspecified)
A = all products
U = unspecified
* = refer to *Notes on sources of survey data*, p. 714

Table 28.8 Estimated[1] prevalence of smoking and estimated[1] number of cigarettes per person per day (unadjusted and sales-adjusted): summary of Tables 28.4, 28.6 and 28.7, 1935-1995.
Males and females aged 15 years and over

Year	Source[2]	Product[3]	Prevalence[4]						Number of cigarettes						
									Unadjusted[7]			Sales-adjusted[8]			
			Manufactured cigarettes		Total cigarettes[5]		All products[6]		Number/ person/day		Total sales %	Manufactured cigarettes number/ person/day		Total cigarettes[9] number/ person/day	
			M	F	M	F	M	F	M	F		M	F	M	F
1935	11	*UC*			50	17									
1944	5	*UC*			46	34								(8.5	5.1)
1947	10	*UC+A*			52	27	70	27	14.7	5.8	114			12.8	5.1
1949	5	*UC*			52	32								(12.5	6.1)
1955	4	UC			48	23			8.5	2.8	60			14.1	4.7
	4	**UC**			52	26									
1964	3	*UC*			51	30			10.6	5.1	74			14.4	6.9
1965	2	*UC*			50	32			9.8	5.1	69			14.1	7.4
1966	3	*UC*			50	32								(14.3	7.4)
	4	UC			47	30			8.7	4.7	62			14.1	7.6
	4	**UC**			47	31									
1967	4	*UC*			46	30			8.6	4.6	61			14.0	7.5
1968	4	*UC*			44	29			8.3	4.6	61			13.6	7.4
1970	2	*UC*			42	30								(13.2	7.6)
	3	*UC*			40	29			8.5	5.0	65			13.1	7.8
1974	2	*UC*			41	31								(13.3	8.1)
1975	3	*UC*			37	29			8.3	5.2	64			12.9	8.2
1976	2	*UC*			40	31			8.3	5.3	65			12.8	8.1
1977	2	*UC*			39	31								(12.5	8.0)
1978	2	*UC*			37	30								(12.3	7.9)
1979	2	*UC*			37	29								(12.3	7.8)
1980	2	*UC*			37	29			7.7	4.8	63			12.4	7.6
1982	12	*UC*			33	28								(11.6	8.0)
1983	2	*UC*			34	28								(11.0	7.4)
1985	2	*UC*			32	27			6.9	4.9	66			10.3	7.3
	4	**UC**+*A*			31	24	38	26						(10.8	6.9)
1986	3	*UC*			29	23								(10.5	6.7)
1987	2	*UC*			31	26								(10.0	6.8)
1988	2	*UC*			30	25			6.8	4.8	72			9.5	6.7
1990	2	*UC*			28	22								(9.1	5.9)

Table 28.8 *(continued)*

Year	Source[2]	Product[3]	Prevalence[4]						Number of cigarettes							
									Unadjusted[7]			Sales-adjusted[8]			
			Manufactured cigarettes		Total cigarettes[5]		All products[6]		Number/ person/day		Total sales %	Manufactured cigarettes number/ person/day		Total cigarettes[9] number/ person/day	
			M	F	M	F	M	F	M	F		M	F	M	F
1991	2	*UC*			27	23								(8.6	5.8)
1992	2	**UC**			28	24								(8.3	5.7)
1993	2	**UC**			27	22								(8.1	5.3)
	4	**UC**			26	21								(8.1	5.3)
1994	2	**UC**			27	22								(8.0	5.3)
	15	**UC**			32	26								(8.0	5.3)
1995	2	**UC**			26	22								(7.9	5.3)
	15	**UC**			31	27								(7.8	5.4)

1 Surveys covering an age range of at least 21-64 are included. Any gaps in the data for ages 15-20 and 65 years and over are filled in by assumed extensions to the age distribution, given in *Notes on sources of survey data*, p. 714. Method: see *Summary of adult smoking*, p. xxxvi
2 See *Notes on sources of survey data*, p. 714
3 Product: MC = manufactured cigarettes, TC = total cigarettes (including hand-rolled), UC = cigarettes (type unspecified), A = all products, U = unspecified. Frequency of smoking is indicated by: regular or daily smokers in normal type, all smokers (including occasional) in bold, unspecified in italics
4 From Table 28.4
5 This column includes prevalence of smoking classified as UC = cigarettes (type unspecified)
6 This column includes prevalence of smoking classified as U = unspecified product
7 From Table 28.6
8 From Table 28.7, except data in parentheses, which are derived from the prevalence of smoking from Table 28.4 as described in *Summary of adult smoking*, p. xxxvi
9 Number of cigarettes classified as UC = cigarettes (type unspecified) has been adjusted to total cigarette sales and included in this column. For 1944 and 1947, adjustment to sales of total cigarettes uses hand-rolled estimate for 1949

Figure 28.3 Estimated prevalence of smoking of (i) cigarettes and (ii) all tobacco products: by year of survey, 1947-1995.
Males and females aged 15 years and over. *Source:* see Table 28.8

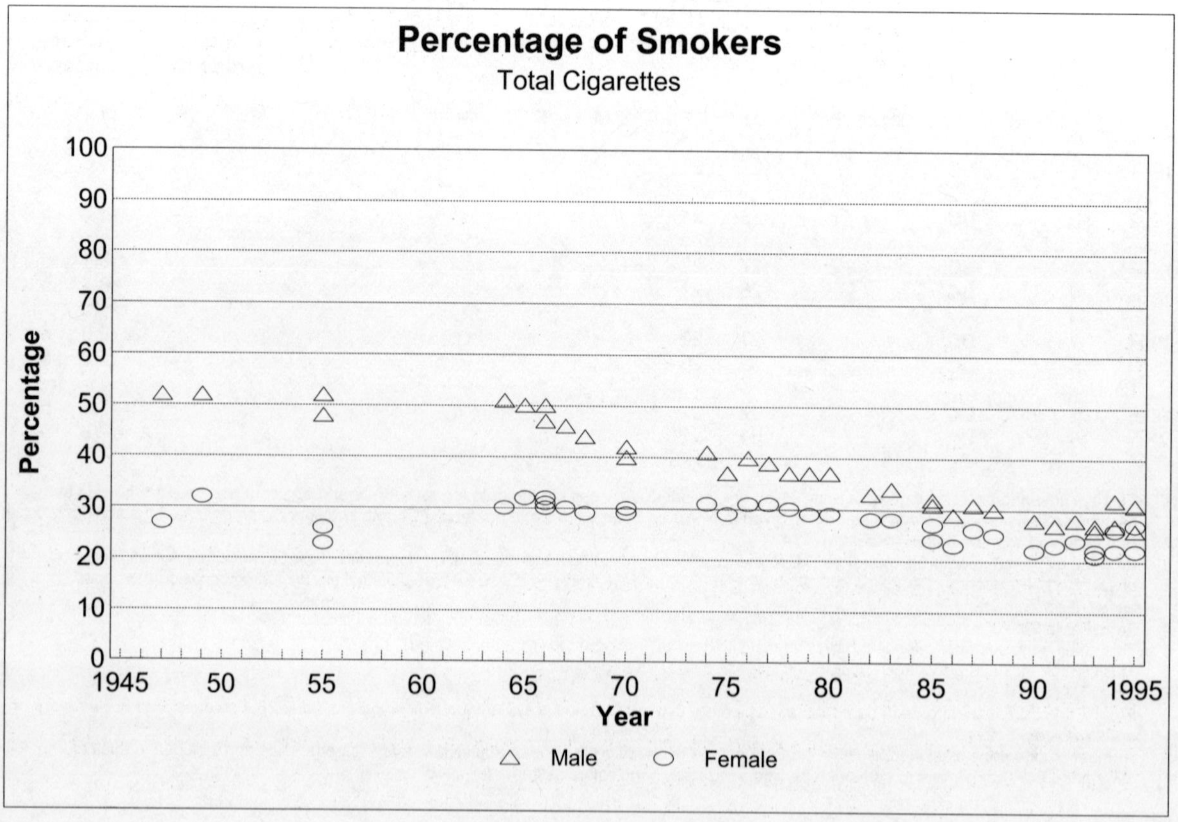

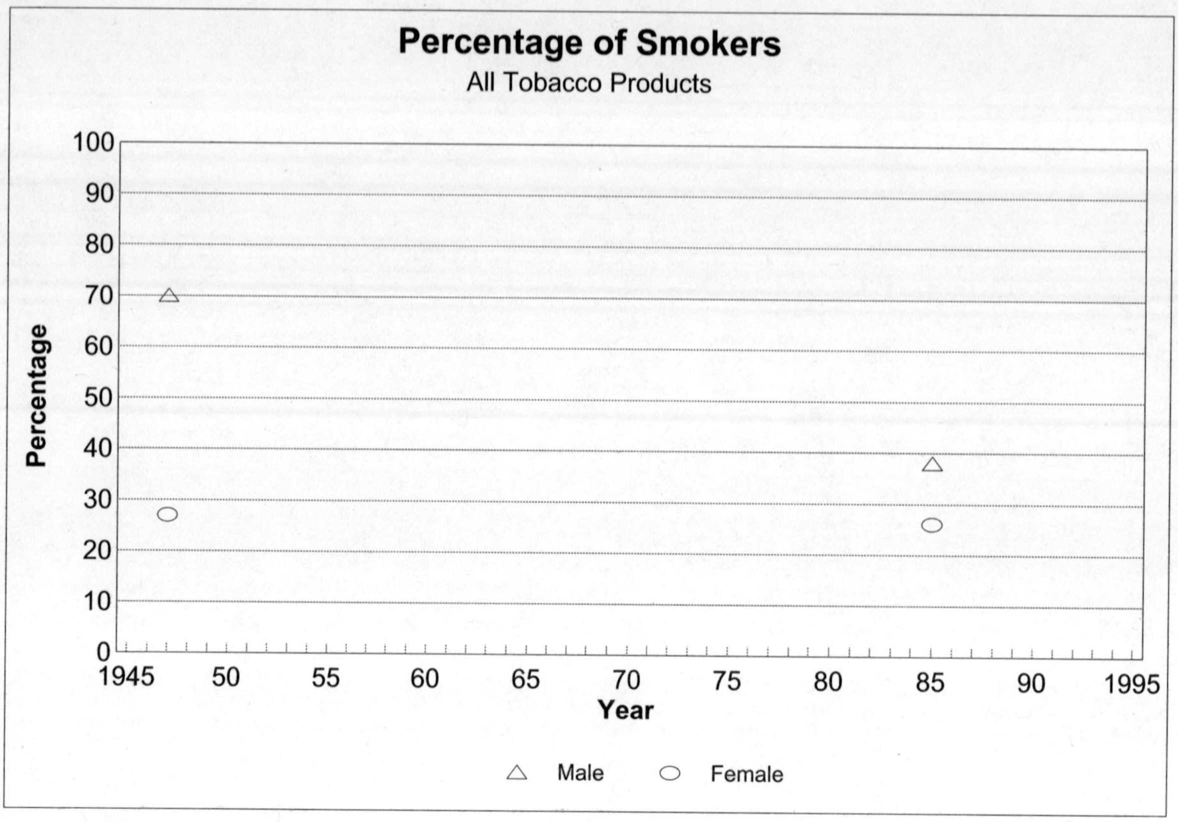

Figure 28.4 Estimated number of cigarettes smoked per person per day, sales-adjusted, 1947-1995.
Males and females aged 15 years and over. *Source:* see Table 28.8

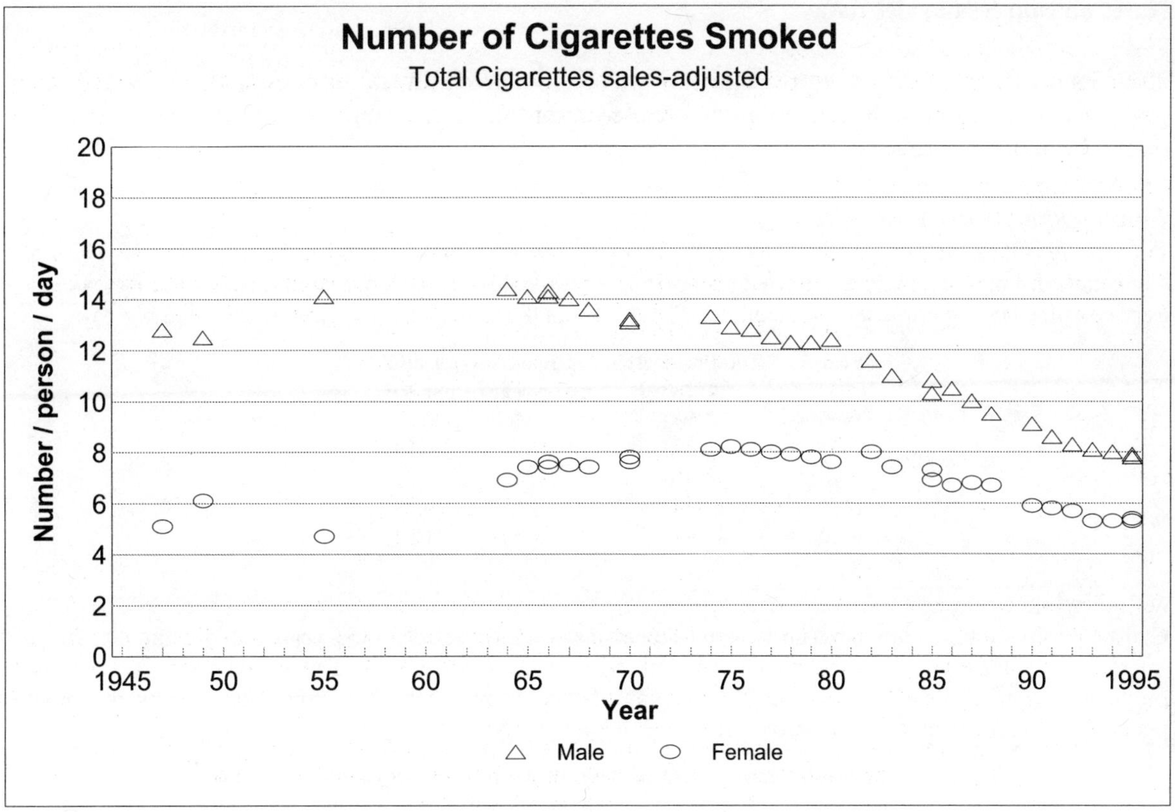

Notes on sources of sales data

The data presented in the tables and figures were obtained from several sources, details of which are given below, together with estimations and related assumptions. Full citations of the sources are given on p. 719 under *References*.

Consumption data before 1920

Giovino *et al* (1994)

Cigarette consumption, given as total and per adult (18+ years old) per year, quoting the Economic Research Service of the US Department of Agriculture (USDA). From these we derived cigarettes per adult per day:

Year	Total cigarettes (millions)	Cigarettes per adult	
		per year	per day
1900	2 500	54	0.15
1905	3 600	70	0.19
1910	8 600	151	0.41
1915	17 900	285	0.78
1920	44 600	665	1.82

Milmore and Conover (1956)

Consumption of tobacco products (unstemmed-processing weight) per adult (15+ years old) quoting the US Internal Revenue Service and the Agricultural Marketing Service of the USDA. The weight of tobacco in finished products is approximately 25% less than the unstemmed-processing weight. The original data are given in pounds per adult per year. From these we derived grams per adult per day:

Year	Consumption per adult per day, unstemmed-processing weight, grams					
	Cigarettes	Cigars	Smoking tobacco	Chewing tobacco	Snuff	Total
1880	0.06	1.69	0.91	3.92	0.15	6.72
1885	0.12	2.00	1.17	4.75	0.21	8.25
1890	0.22	2.21	1.39	4.96	0.27	9.06
1895	0.31	1.94	1.49	4.69	0.26	8.69
1900	0.20	2.47	1.77	4.42	0.37	9.23
1905	0.24	2.87	2.71	4.42	0.46	10.70
1910	0.51	2.72	2.70	4.16	0.58	10.68
1915	1.02	2.70	2.65	3.53	0.55	10.44
1920	2.35	3.05	1.86	2.93	0.58	10.77
1925	3.68	2.47	2.00	2.45	0.56	11.16

Rigdon and Kirchoff (1952) also give figures for per capita consumption of tax-paid tobacco products (1900-1950)

Consumption data for 1920-1974

RP6

Data by weight, originally given to nearest 100 000 pounds, have been converted to tonnes and given to the nearest 10 tonnes (100 000 lbs = 45.359 tonnes). Where weight conversion factors have been quoted in RP6, the weights have been re-calculated without rounding and then converted to tonnes.

Notes as given in RP6

(a) Details of the number of cigarettes and cigars and of the weight of tobacco consumed were obtained from the following sources:

1920-35 *1st Annual Report on Tobacco Statistics*, May 1937.

1936-73 *Annual Report on Tobacco Statistics*, May 1937.

These are published by the United States Department of Agriculture.

(b) Cigarettes were converted from number to weight using a factor of 2.205 lbs.per 1 000 up to 1951. Since that date allowance has been made for the increasing consumption of 'king' size, 'long' size, and filter-tipped cigarettes. Cigars were converted at a rate of 18.6 lbs. per 1 000 up to 1957 and at 18 lbs. per 1 000 from 1958-1963. From 1964 onwards the conversion factors used for large and little cigars were 17.5 lbs per 1 000 and

2.5 lbs per 1 000 respectively.

Consumption data for 1974 onwards (Tables 28.1.2 and 28.2), or 1969 onwards (Table 28.1.4)
USDA
The weights of cigarettes and large cigars in each year (Table 28.1.2) were derived from USDA tables giving the number and weight smoked per capita. The average weight of small cigars (defined as using less than 3 pounds of tobacco per 1 000, i.e. less than 1.36 g per cigar) was not available and has been estimated as 1.3 g. Data by weight, originally given to nearest 100 000 pounds, have been converted to tonnes and given to the nearest 10 tonnes (100 000 lbs = 45.359 tonnes).

The classification of smokeless products changed at the start of 1982, removing fine-cut from the chewing tobacco category and reclassifying it as moist snuff. In 1981 there were 15.1 million pounds (6 850 tonnes) taxable removals of fine-cut. This change in classification therefore accounts for most, but not all, of the redistribution of smokeless volumes from 1981 to 1982.

Smokeless tobacco has two main forms: chewing tobacco and snuff. Chewing tobacco is available in loose leaf form (formerly called scrap), in a pressed rectangle called a plug, or in a twist or roll. These are actively chewed. Snuff may be dry snuff (also called scotch snuff) which is dry, powdered tobacco, or moist snuff which is moist tobacco in fine particles or strips. Snuff is used by placing a pinch of tobacco between the cheek and the gum. During the 1980s moist snuff began to be marketed packaged in small pouches resembling tea bags (Shelton (1982), Gritz *et al* (1985), Tilashalski *et al* (1994)). Moist snuff is the only form of smokeless tobacco which is growing in sales volume. All other types have a shrinking market.

Plain/Filter cigarette consumption
USDA
Represents the proportion of production rather than of consumption of filtered cigarettes.

Tar and nicotine yield of cigarettes
1954-1967 US Surgeon General (1981)
1968-1995 Federal Trade Commission (1998)
There is no standard for assessing yield of smokeless tobacco products. Tilashalski *et al* (1994) measured the nicotine content of a range of smokeless products, as a percentage of the dry weight of the product. Dry weight was chosen as the moisture content of the different products varies considerably (moist snuff generally around 50%, chewing tobacco around 20% moisture). Moist snuff contained about 3% nicotine (except for one brand which contained 0.6%) and chewing tobacco contained 0.77-1.67% nicotine.

Estimates of hand-rolled cigarette consumption for 1949 and 1951-1967
We have taken as our estimate of hand-rolled cigarette consumption 23% of pipe and hand-rolling tobacco sales, at 0.83 g per cigarette
This method of estimation was based on USDA estimates for other years (see below). The smoking of hand-rolled cigarettes appears to have been relatively unimportant since the Second World War. Hammond (1958) comments that the decline in the use of hand-rolled cigarettes probably contributed to the apparent rise in manufactured cigarette consumption between 1935 and 1955. No data on pipe and hand-rolling tobacco separate from chewing tobacco are available before 1949.

Estimates of hand-rolled cigarette consumption for 1950
US Surgeon General (1983), quoting USDA

Estimates of hand-rolled cigarette consumption for 1968 onwards
USDA
These estimates are based on shipments of cigarette papers and tubes. The figures show that the percentage of pipe and hand-rolling tobacco used in hand-rolled cigarettes varied between 15% (1977) and 39% (1995) (see Table 28.1.4), and the weight of tobacco per hand-rolled cigarette varied between 0.84 g (1968) and 0.60 g (1990).

Notes on sources of survey data

Each source of survey data—either an individual survey or a series of surveys repeated over a number of years—is cited by a source number. This number is shown in the tables and corresponds to the source numbers given below, where details of the source publication and of the survey methodology are given. Full citations of the sources are given on p. 719 under *References*.

Source number

1 **USDHEW (United States Department of Health, Education and Welfare) and Health Services and Mental Health Administration (1972, 1974), Green *et al* (1979)**

a. National Teenage Tobacco Surveys. Telephone surveys (1968 survey included 10% personal interviews in non-telephone households). Sample size (1968) 4 931, (1970) 2 640, (1972) 2 790, (1974) 2 553, and (1979) 2 639

b. Smokers: smoked regularly but less than one cigarette a week. Regular smokers: smoked one or more cigarettes a week. Smokers marked frequency *: smoked cigarettes daily

c. Consumption category estimation based on 1-4, 5-9, and 10+ cigarettes/smoker/day

2 **US Surgeon General (1983, 1988, 1994), Fiore *et al* (1989), Novotny *et al* (1990), Harris (1983), Anonymous (1987, 1991a, 1992a, 1993, 1994a, 1994b, 1994c, 1996, 1997)**

a. National Health Interview Surveys. Nationally representative sample of the US non-institutionalized civilian population aged 18+. Before 1974, face-to-face interviews with one adult per household, giving proxy reports for other household members. Since 1974, smoking information taken from self-reports only, using telephone follow-up for household members not interviewed personally. Response rate before 1974 around 96%, but decreased to 90% when limited to self-reports. Data were adjusted for non-response and weighted (by the original authors) to provide national estimates.

Year	Sample size	Response rate (%)
1974	22 052	—
1976	20 978	—
1977	—	—
1978	10 571	—
1979	21 832	—
1980	9 553	—
1983	20 963	—
1985	31 082	—
1987	44 000	—
1988	44 000	—
1990	41 000	83
1991	43 732	88
1992	24 040	87
1993	20 860	81
1994	19 738	80
1995	17 213	81

b. Current smokers: smoked 100 cigarettes and (before 1992) answered affirmatively to question 'Do you smoke cigarettes now?' or (1992 onwards) reported now smoking every day or some days. According to Anonymous (1994a), the inclusion of some-day smoking increases the prevalence estimate by about 1.0%

c. Prevalence of use of other tobacco products was estimated as (Giovino *et al* (1994)):

Year	Cigar smoking		Pipe smoking		Smokeless tobacco	
	Males	Females	Males	Females	Males	Females
1970	16.3	0.2	13.1	0.1	5.2	1.8
1987	5.3	0.1	3.4	0.1	6.1	0.6
1991	3.5	0.1	2.0	0.0	5.6	0.6

d. Consumption category estimation based on: (1965 and 1976) <15, 15-24, and 25+ cigarettes/smoker/day. Cigarettes per smokers (1988) not restricted to regular smokers

e. Assumed extension to age distribution for percentage smokers, age 15-19: males (1965) 30%, (1974-1980) 25%, (1983-1987) 20% and females (1965) 20%, (1974-1980) 25%, (1983-1987) 20%. For age 15-16: (1970 only) males 15% and females 12%. For age 15-17: males and females (1988-1995) 15%. Number of cigarettes/person/day. age 15-19: males (1965) 5.0, (1976) 4.0, (1980) 3.0 and females (1965, 1976) 3.0, (1980) 2.5. For age 15-17: (1985, 1988) males 1.5 and females 2.0

3 **Waingrow *et al* (1968), USDHEW (1973), USDHEW and Public Health Service (1976), US Surgeon General (1983), Anonymous (1987)**

a. Adult Use of Tobacco Surveys.
In 1964 and 1966: primarily in-person household interviews. Sample size (1964) 5 794, (1966) 5 768; response rate 76% and 72% respectively
In 1970: 91% telephone and 9% personal interviews. Sample size 5 200
In 1975: 7% personal interviews. Sample size 12 000
In 1986, 100% telephone interviews, results adjusted to compensate for (inter alia) exclusion of non-telephone households. Representative of non-institutionalized civilian population. Sample size 13 031, response rate 74%

b. Data from 1966 taken from charts

c. Consumption category estimation based on 0-4, 5-14, 15-24, 25-34, 35-44, 45-54, 55-64, and 65+ cigarettes/smoker/day (1964 only)

d. Assumed extension to age distribution for percentage smokers, age 15-20: males (1964, 1966, 1970) 30%, (1975) 25% and females (1964, 1966, 1970) 20%, (1975) 25%. For age 15-16: (1986) males and females 12%. Number of cigarettes/person/day: males (1964, 1970, 1975) 5.0 and females 3.0

4 **USDHEW and Public Health Service (1969), Ahmed and Gleeson (1970), Marcus *et al* (1989), Shopland *et al* (1992, 1996)**

a. Tobacco Use Supplements to Current Population Survey. Representative of civilian non-institutionalized population. 1955 data originally in Haenszel *et al* (1956), later version with minor changes used

	Households	Response rate (%)	Individuals	Proxy interviews (%)	
				Males	Females
1955	21 000	96	45 000	42	17
1966	35 000	96	69 000	65	25
1985	62500	96	114000	—	—
1993	—	95/88[1]	266988	18	18

[1] Represents response rates for core questions and tobacco use supplement respectively

b. Smokers: had smoked at least 100 cigarettes in their lifetime and (1985) smoked at the time of the survey or (1993) smoked every day or some days

c. Product code A (1985 only) includes users of smokeless tobacco. For males, the percentages using each product (including users of more than one product) are snuff 1.8%, chewing tobacco 4.0%, cigars 2.1%, and pipes 2.4%

d. Consumption category estimation based on: (1966) 1-9, 10-20, 21-40, and 41+ cigarettes/smoker/day; (1967 and 1968) <11, 11-20, 21-40, and 41+ cigarettes/smoker/day

e. Assumed extension to age distribution for percentage smokers, age 15-17: males (1955, 1966) 20% and females (1955) 10%, (1966) 15%. Number of cigarettes/person/day: males (1955) 2.0, (1966) 3.0 and females (1955) 1.0, (1966) 2.0. For age 15-16: (1967, 1968) males 15% and females 10%. For age 15: (UC) (1985) males and females 10%. For age 15-19: (A) (1985) males and females 20%

5 **Anonymous (1987), quoting Gallup Poll**

a. Assumed extension to age distribution for percentage smokers, age 15-17: males 20% and females 10%

6 Clark (1976)

a. Sample size 826, drawn from national probability sample of 3 000 households. Year unknown

b. Consumption category estimation based on <1, 1, and 2+ packs per day (assume 1-19, 20, and 21+ cigarettes/smoker/day)

7 US Surgeon General (1989) quoting Johnston *et al* (1987), US Surgeon General (1994), Johnston *et al* (2000)

a. Monitoring the Future surveys among high school seniors, sponsored by the National Institute on Drug Abuse. National samples of high school seniors, but not representative since they do not include high school drop-outs. Sample size (1975) 9 400, (1976-1992) 15 091-18 448, response rate 66-80%

b. Regular smokers: smoked daily. All smokers: smoked any cigarette in last 30 days

8 WHO (1989), WHO MONICA Project (1988)

a. Regional survey forming part of WHO MONICA Project:

Region	Population size	Sample size	Participation rate %	Sample used*		Date
				Males	Females	
Stanford	84 600	1 402	69	698	803	May 1979-Apr 1980

* 'Sample used' includes age 25-34, all other figures are for age 35-64 only

b. *All ages* column relates only to age 35-64 and is standardized to world population

c. Regular cigarette smokers: smoked cigarettes daily. All smokers: smoked cigarettes daily or occasionally, or smoked 1 g pipe tobacco or 1 cigar per week. Cigarettes per smoker refers to regular and occasional cigarette smokers

d. Calculation for cigarettes per person based on % regular cigarette smokers and cigarettes per regular or occasional cigarette smoker, so may underestimate

9 Hammond and Garfinkel (1961, 1964), Thun *et al* (1997)

a. American Cancer Society Cancer Prevention Studies (Million Person Studies) conducted in 25 states, 1959-1960 and 1982-1986. Families with at least one member aged over 45 enrolled by volunteers. Not representative, as sample comprised 97% whites, and over-represented married and better educated persons

b. Entries marked * in Table 28.4 represent analyses of a sub-set of the study (43 068 subjects). The category A A includes a few subjects who smoked, but with smoking pattern uncertain, and a few women who smoked pipes or cigars only

c. Data for 1982 derived by combining prevalence data presented separately for white people and black people. The results are not adjusted for 'unclassifiable' subjects—these accounted for between 1.9% (white men aged 30-34) and 23.4% (black women aged 80-84)

d. Cigarettes per smoker and per person are based on regular cigarette smokers

e. Consumption category estimation based on 1-9, 10-19, 20, 21-39, 40, and 41+ cigarettes/smoker/day

10 Hamtoft and Lindhardt (1955)

a. No original reference, results taken from graph. Survey in Columbus, Ohio. Sample size 2 500, whites only. Results also available (not shown) for blacks, for certain age groups for all tobacco products—they are always higher than the figures for whites

b. Probably same survey described by Mills and Porter (1950), control group of a study of mouth and respiratory cancer. A comparable study in Cincinnati , restricted to white women aged 20-29, showed 41% cigarette smokers

c. Consumption category estimation based on two categories, 1-20 and 21+ cigarettes/smoker/day, and resulting figures should be regarded with caution

d. Assumed extension to age distribution for percentage smokers, age 15-19: males 30% and females 15%. Number of cigarettes/person/day: males 5.0 and females 2.0

e. Assumed no female smoker of other products

11 Rigdon and Kirchoff (1952), quoting Fortune Magazine (1935)

a. Survey conducted by *Fortune Magazine*. Age range and product uncertain

b. Assumed extension to age distribution for percentage smokers, age 15-19: males 30% and females 10%

12 Remington *et al* (1985)

a. Behavioral Risk Factor Surveys, 1981-1983. Sample size 22 236, response rate 80%. Telephone interviews in 28 states
b. Assumed extension to age distribution for percentage smokers, age 15-17: males and females 15%

13 Horn *et al* (1959)

a. Survey by American Cancer Society of schools in and around Portland, Oregon. Sample size (boys) 11 060, (girls) 10 920
b. Smokers: have smoked more than a few times and smoke currently. Regular smokers: smoke at least once a week
c. Consumption category estimation based on 1-4, 5-9, 10-19 and 20+ cigarettes/smoker/day

14 Salber *et al* (1961)

a. A survey of students in public high schools in Newton, Massachusetts. Approximate ages corresponding to school grades. Sample size: (boys) 3 449, (girls) 3 361, response rate 92%
b. Smokers: had smoked at least 10 cigarettes and considered themselves to be smokers
c. Consumption category estimation based on <1 pack/week, 1-4 packs/week and 5+ packs/week (1-<3, 3-10 and 11+ cigarettes/smoker/day assumed). This includes occasional smokers in the 1-<3 cigarettes/smokers/day category and uses a low starting point for the heaviest smoking group and so the resulting figures should be treated with caution

15 US Surgeon General (1994), Office of Applied Studies (1996)

a. National Household Surveys on Drug Abuse conducted by the National Institute on Drug Abuse and Substance Abuse and Mental Health Services Administration (SAMHSA). Response rate average 80%. Data weighted to provide national estimates. Sample size (1994) 17 809, (1995) 17 747
b. Smokers: used cigarettes in the 30 days preceding the survey

16 Anonymous (1991b)

a. Teenage Attitudes and Practices Survey (TAPS), which, in 1989, focussed on tobacco use. Telephone survey of those living in households. Sample size 9 965, response rate 82%. This used a modified version of the National Teenage Tobacco Survey. Data adjusted to provide national estimates. Among 17-18-year-olds, the prevalence of smoking during the previous week was substantially higher among those who had dropped out of school (43.3%) than among non-dropouts (17.1%)
b. Smokers: smoked cigarettes in the 30 days preceding the survey. Regular smokers: smoked cigarettes in the 7 days preceding the survey

17 Hearn *et al* (1991)

a. Survey conducted in 10 Minneapolis schools using a standardized questionnaire. Sample size (males) 237, (females) 202. Response rate 88%. Age range not stated, but average age 15.0 years. Year not stated. Included for comparison with data for USSR from the same source (see Chapter 29, source 41)
b. Smokers: smoked at least a few cigarettes per month. Regular smokers: smoked at least a partial pack of cigarettes a week

18 Anonymous (1992b), Kann *et al* (1995, 1996), Escobedo *et al* (1997)

a. Youth Risk Behavior Surveillance System. Nationally representative surveys of high school students in grades 9-12 in public and private schools. Approximate ages corresponding to school grades.

Year	Sample size	Response rate (%)
1990	11 631	—
1991	12 272	—
1992	10 645	74
1993	16 296	70
1995	10 904	60

b. Smokers: smoked cigarettes on one or more of the 30 days preceding the survey. Regular smokers: smoked cigarettes on 20 or more of the 30 days preceding the survey

c. Prevalence of use of smokeless tobacco was 10.1% in 1990 (Lewis *et al* (1999))
d. A comparison of those who attended school and those who did not gave prevalence of current smoking in 1992 as: (school attenders) 20.4%, (not attending school) 33.7% (Anonymous (1994d))

19 Chollat-Traquet (1992)

a. No original source

References

Ahmed P.I. and Gleeson G.A. (1970). *Changes in cigarette smoking habits. Between 1955 and 1966,* 59. US Department of Health, Education and Welfare. Public Health Service, Rockville, Maryland. (Vital and Health Statistics. Data from the National Health Survey.) 1000-Series 10-No. 59.

Anonymous (1987). Cigarette smoking in the Unites States, 1986. *MMWR Morb Mortal Wkly Rep,* **36**, 581-5.

Anonymous (1991a). Cigarette smoking among adults—United States, 1988. *MMWR Morb Mortal Wkly Rep,* **40**, 757-65.

Anonymous (1991b). Cigarette smoking among youth—United States, 1989. *MMWR Morb Mortal Wkly Rep,* **40**, 712-5.

Anonymous (1992a). Cigarette smoking among adults—United States, 1990. *MMWR Morb Mortal Wkly Rep,* **41**, 354-62.

Anonymous (1992b). Tobacco, alcohol, and other drug use among high school students—United States, 1991. *MMWR Morb Mortal Wkly Rep,* **41**, 698-703.

Anonymous (1993). Cigarette smoking among adults—United States, 1991 (published erratum appears in *MMWR Morb Mortal Wkly Rep* 1993, **42**, 255). *MMWR Morb Mortal Wkly Rep,* **42**, 230-3.

Anonymous (1994a). Cigarette smoking among adults—United States, 1992, and changes in the definition of current cigarette smoking. *MMWR Morb Mortal Wkly Rep,* **43**, 342-6.

Anonymous (1994c). Cigarette smoking among adults—United States, 1993. *MMWR Morb Mortal Wkly Rep,* **43**, 925-30.

Anonymous (1994b). Erratum: Vol. 43, No. 19. *MMWR Morb Mortal Wkly Rep,* **43**, 801-3.

Anonymous (1994d). Health risk behaviors among adolescents who do and do not attend school—United States, 1992. *MMWR Morb Mortal Wkly Rep,* **43**, 129-32.

Anonymous (1996). Cigarette smoking among adults—United States, 1994. *MMWR Morb Mortal Wkly Rep,* **45**, 588-90.

Anonymous (1997). Cigarette smoking among adults—United States, 1995. *MMWR Morb Mortal Wkly Rep,* **46**, 1217-20. ftp://ftp.cdc.gov/pub/Publications/mmwr/wk/mm4651.pdf.

Beese D.H. (ed) (1968). *Tobacco consumption in various countries,* 2nd edition. Tobacco Research Council, London. Research Paper 6.

Beese D.H. (ed) (1972). *Tobacco consumption in various countries,* 3rd edition. Tobacco Research Council, London. Research Paper 6.

Chollat-Traquet C. (1992). *Women and tobacco* . WHO, Geneva.

Clark R. (1976). Cigarette smoking among teen-age girls and young women: Summary of the findings of a survey conducted for the American Cancer Society. 39-46. UICC Technical Report Series 24.

Escobedo L.G., Reddy M. and DuRant R.H. (1997). Relationship between cigarette smoking and health risk and problem behaviors among US adolescents. *Arch Pediatr Adolesc Med,* **151**, 66-71.

Federal Trade Commission (1998). *Federal trade commission report of 'tar,' nicotine, and carbon monoxide of the smoke of 1249 varieties of domestic cigarettes for the year 1995.* http://www.ftc.gov/os/1998/9801/t%26ntxt.htm.

Fiore M.C., Novotny T.E., Pierce J.P., Hatziandreu E.J., Patel K.M. and Davis R.M. (1989). Trends in cigarette smoking in the United States. The changing influence of gender and race. *JAMA,* **261**, 49-55.

Giovino G.A., Schooley M.W., Zhu B.-P., Chrismon J.H., *et al* (1994). Surveillance for selected tobacco-use behaviors—United States, 1900-1994. *MMWR Morb Mortal Wkly Rep,* **43(SS-3)**, 1-43.

Green D.E., Roberts Harris P., Berry M.F., Timpane M. and Tucker M.S. (1979). *Teenage smoking: immediate and long term patterns*. The National Institute of Education, USDHEW, Washington DC.

Gritz E.R., Ksir C. and McCarthy W.J. (1985). Smokeless tobacco use in the United States: past and future trends. *Annals of Behavioural Medicine,* **7**, 24-7.

Haenszel W., Shimkin M.B. and Miller H.P. (1956). *Tobacco smoking patterns in the United States*. United States Public Health Service, Washington DC. Public Health Monograph No.45. Public Health Service Publication No. 463.

Hammond E.C. and Garfinkel L. (1961). Smoking habits of men and women. *J Natl Cancer Inst,* **27**, 419-42.

Hammond E.C. and Garfinkel L. (1964). Changes in cigarette smoking. *J Natl Cancer Inst,* **33**, 49-64.

Hamtoft H. and Lindhardt M. (1955). Tobacco consumption in Denmark. I. The Danish national morbidity survey of 1950, communication no. 8. *Dan Med Bull,* **2**, 213-20.

Harris J.E. (1983). Cigarette smoking among successive birth cohorts of men and women in the United States during 1900-80. *J Natl Cancer Inst,* **71**, 473-9.

Hearn M.D., Prokhorov A.V., Murray D.M., Alexandrov A.A. and Luepker R.V. (1991). Comparison of smoking prevalence in school students sampled from the United States of America and the Union of Soviet Socialist Republics. *Int J Epidemiol,* **20**, 413-5.

Horn D., Courts F.A., Taylor R.M. and Solomon E.S. (1959). Cigarette smoking among high school students. *Am J Public Health,* **49**, 1497-511.

Johnston L.D., O'Malley P.M. and Bachman J.G. (1987). *National trends in drug use and related factors among high school students and young adults, 1975-1986.* US Department of Health and Human Services (USDHHS), Public Health Service, Alcohol, Drug Abuse, and Mental Health Administration, National Institute on Drug Abuse. DHHS Publ No (ADM) 87-1535.[§]

Johnston L.D., O'Malley P.M. and Bachman J.G. (2000). *Monitoring the future, overview of key findings 1999.* National Institute on Drug Abuse, USDHHS. NIH Publication No. 00-4690. http://www.monitoringthefuture.org/.

Kann L., Warren C.W., Harris W.A., Collins J.L., *et al* (1995). Youth risk behavior surveillance—United States, 1993. *MMWR Morb Mortal Wkly Rep,* **44**, 1-56.

Kann L., Warren C.W., Harris W.A., Collins J.L., *et al* (1996). Youth risk behavior surveillance—United States, 1995. *MMWR Morb Mortal Wkly Rep,* **45**, 1-85.

Lee P.N. (ed) (1975). *Tobacco consumption in various countries,* 4th edition. Tobacco Research Council, London. Research Paper 6.

Lewis P.C., Harrell J.S., Deng S. and Bradley C. (1999). Smokeless tobacco use in adolescents: the Cardiovascular Health in Children (CHIC II) study. *J Sch Health,* **69**, 320-5.

Marcus A.C., Shopland D.R., Crane L.A. and Lynn W.R. (1989). Prevalence of cigarette smoking in the United States: Estimates from the 1985 Current Population Survey. *J Natl Cancer Inst,* **81**, 409-14.

Mills C.A. and Porter M.M. (1950). Tobacco smoking habits and cancer of the mouth and respiratory system. *Cancer Res,* **10**, 539-42.

Milmore B.K. and Conover A.G. (1956). Tobacco consumption in the United States, 1880 to 1955. In: Haenszel W., Shimkin M. and Miller H.P. (eds) *Tobacco smoking patterns in the United States*. U.S. Public Health Service, Washington D. C.; 107-11. Public Health Monograph No.45. Public Health Service Publication No. 463.

Novotny T.E., Fiore M.C., Hatziandreu E.J., Giovino G.A., Mills S.L. and Pierce J.P. (1990). Trends in smoking by age and sex, United States, 1974-1987: the implications for disease impact. *Prev Med,* **19**, 552-61.

Office of Applied Studies (1996). *National household survey on drug abuse advance report #18.* http://www.samhsa.gov/oas/nhsda/ar18ttoc.htm.

Remington P.L., Forman M.R., Gentry E.M., Marks J.S., Hogelin G.C. and Trowbridge F.L. (1985). Current smoking trends in the United States. The 1981-1983 behavioral risk factor surveys. *JAMA,* **253**, 2975-8.

Rigdon R.H. and Kirchoff H. (1952). A consideration of some of the theories relative to the etiology and incidence of lung cancer. *Texas Reports on Biology and Medicine,* **10**, 76-91.

RP6, See Beese (ed) (1968), Beese (ed) (1972), Lee (ed) (1975)

Salber E.J., Goldman E., Buka M. and Welsh B. (1961). Smoking habits of high-school students in Newton, Massachusetts. *N Engl J Med,* **265**, 969-74.

Shelton A. (1982). Smokeless sales continue to climb. *Tobacco Reporter,* **109**, 42-4.

Shopland D.R., Hartman A.M., Gibson J.T., Mueller M.D., Kessler L.G. and Lynn W.R. (1996). Cigarette smoking among US adults by state and region: estimates from the current population survey. *J Natl Cancer Inst,* **88**, 1748-58.

Shopland D.R., Niemcryk S.J. and Marconi K.M. (1992). Geographic and gender variations in total tobacco use. *Am J Public Health,* **82**, 103-6.

Thun M.J., Day-Lally C., Myers D.G., Calle E.E., *et al* (1997). Trends in tobacco smoking and mortality from cigarette use in cancer prevention studies I (1959 through 1965) and II 1982 through 1988. In: Burns D., Garfinkel L. and Samet J.M. (eds) *Changes in cigarette-related disease risks and their implications for prevention and control*. USDHHS, NIH, NCI; 305-82. Smoking and Tobacco Control, Monograph 8. NIH Publication Number 97-4213.

Tilashalski K., Rodu B. and Mayfield C. (1994). Assessing the nicotine content of smokeless tobacco products. *J Am Dent Assoc,* **125**, 590, 592, 594.

US Surgeon General (1981). *The health consequences of smoking. The changing cigarette: a report of the Surgeon General*. USDHHS, Public Health Serv. DHHS Publication No (PHS) 81-50156.

US Surgeon General (1983). *The health consequences of smoking. Cardiovascular disease. A report of the Surgeon General*. USDHHS, Public Health Serv, Rockville, Maryland. DHHS Publication No (PHS) 84-50204.

US Surgeon General (1988). *The health consequences of smoking: nicotine addiction. A report of the Surgeon General, 1988*. USDHHS, Atlanta, Georgia. DHHS Publication No (CDC) 88-8406.

US Surgeon General (1989). *Reducing the health consequences of smoking. 25 years of progress. A report of the Surgeon General*. US Public Health Service, Rockville, Maryland. DHHS (CDC) 89-8411.

US Surgeon General (1994). *Preventing tobacco use among young people: a report of the Surgeon General.* USDHHS, Atlanta, Georgia, USA.

USDHEW (1974). *Patterns and prevalence of teen-age cigarette smoking: 1968, 1970, 1972, and 1974*. Center for Disease Control, Bethesda, Maryland. DHEW Publication No (CDC) 75-8701.

USDHEW (1973). *Adult use of tobacco 1970*. USDHEW, USA.

USDHEW and Health Services and Mental Health Administration (1972). *Patterns and prevalence of teen-age cigarette smoking: 1968, 1970, and 1972*. Center for Disease Control, Bethesda, Maryland. DHEW publ. no. (HSM) 73-8701.

USDHEW and Public Health Service (1969). Cigarette smoking status—June 1966, August 1967, and August 1968. *Monthly Vital Statistics Report,* **18 Suppl**, 1-3.

USDHEW and Public Health Service (1976). *Adult use of tobacco—1975*. Centre for Disease Control. National Institutes of Health, Atlanta, Georgia; Bethesda, Maryland.

Waingrow S.M., Horn D. and Ikard F.F. (1968). Dosage patterns of cigarette smoking in American adults. *Am J Public Health,* **58**, 54-70.

WHO (1989). The WHO MONICA project: a worldwide monitoring system for cardiovascular diseases. In: *World health statistics annual 1989*. WHO, Geneva; 25-149.

WHO MONICA Project (1988). Geographical variation in the major risk factors of coronary heart disease in men and women aged 35-64 years. *World Health Stat Q,* **41**, 115-40.

§ Original paper not obtained, but information taken as quoted by another author

Sales data

See Tables 29.1-29.3.

Comprehensive sales data for the 1920s and 1930s are available only for Latvia. At that time papyrosi, a type of cigarette with a hollow paper tube filled only half or a third with tobacco, accounted for about 50% of all tobacco sales, with most of the remainder as smoking tobacco. Sales of conventional style cigarettes were negligible. A similar situation prevailed in Estonia and Lithuania (Hutson (1937)).

From 1960, data are available for the USSR as a whole, for cigarettes only. By that time, papyrosi accounted for 75% of cigarettes, the proportion continuing to decline to below 40% by 1980. Filter cigarettes did not come into use until the mid-1960s, and even by 1980 accounted for only 30% of conventional cigarettes. Between 1960 and the early 1970s the consumption of manufactured cigarettes per adult increased from 4 to 6 cigarettes per day. It remained at that level until the mid-1980s, then decreased to 4 cigarettes per day by 1994. Expressed in terms of the weight of tobacco smoked in cigarettes, and taking into account the changes in cigarette type, we estimate that this is equivalent to an increase from 3 to 5 g per day, then a fall to 4 g per day. Although few data are available, consumption of products other than cigarettes is believed to have been low in this period.

Assessment of sales since the late 1980s is further complicated by large-scale cigarette smuggling (see *Notes on sources of sales data,* p. 745).

Survey data

See Tables 29.4-29.8

Relatively little survey data exist representative of any of the republics, and none for the USSR as a whole. Much of the adult data presented here is drawn from epidemiological studies and is based in specific regions or cities. It is difficult to draw conclusions about trends over time from these disparate sources. Estimates of the prevalence of smoking among those aged 15 years or over are generally in the range of 40-70% for men and 5-20% for women. However, there were some exceptions. Surveys in the Caucasus region in the early 1960s showed a higher prevalence, 70-80%, among men, as did a survey in industrial areas of Russia (source 36). Surveys in the Central Asian region mostly showed a very low prevalence, 0.5-3%, among women. School-based surveys all show that more teenage boys than girls smoked.

Comparison of survey and sales data suggested that one recent survey in Russia (source 50) under-stated consumption by 8%. (We also estimate that an earlier survey under-stated by about 20%, but this estimate should be regarded with caution since the survey data related only to Moscow and the sales data to a later year.) Since 1975, the estimated number of cigarettes smoked per person per day (sales-adjusted) has been 7-10 for men and 1-3 for women, except in the Central Asian region where the estimated number for women is generally less than 1.

Table 29.1.1 Total annual sales of tobacco products, Latvia, 1921-1935

Year	Papyrosi tonnes	Cigars [1] tonnes	Smoking tobacco tonnes	Total tonnes
1921	260	6	150	415
1922	359	8	244	611
1923	447	11	512	971
1924	496	10	659	1164
1925	508	13	523	1044
1926	554	13	538	1104
1927	531	13	551	1095
1928	551	15	651	651
1929	589	17	757	1363
1930	605	17	606	1227
1931	570	14	546	1130
1932	482	10	434	926
1933	500	10	441	951
1934	530	11	443	984
1935	523	12	451	987

1 Including cigarillos, and cigarettes, the annual consumption of which amounted to 0.5-1.5 tonnes

Source: see *Notes on sources of sales data*, p. 745

Table 29.1.2 Total annual sales of cigarettes for individual republics, 1988-1995

	Cigarettes (millions)							
	1988	1989	1990	1991	1992	1993	1994	1995
Armenia	10095	9731	10100	8500	4627	5305		
Azerbaijan	8785	8350	7608	8997	6689	2050	6000	6000
Belarus	12539	12353	12323	13550	13540	13540		
Estonia	1965	1933	1912	2100	2097	2097		
Georgia	9337	9226	9211	9482	6250	8082		
Kazakhstan	20390	19272	16259	15289	15289	20305	15250	
Kyrgyzstan	5091	4823	4883	4884	5100	5816	4000	4000
Latvia	3320	3265	3224	3324	3329	3329		
Lithuania	4545	4479	4435	4882	4881	4881		
Moldova	9658	10232	7582	7600	7500	4900	4800	4800
Russia	200946	190274	196400	195608	184200	184800	177000	211000
Tajikistan	6261	6180	5600	5140	3450	6000		
Turkmenistan	5067	4917	5116	5480	5551	5551		
Ukraine	92627	88318	81074	84507	78808	78808		
Uzbekistan	9737	9918	8977	11400	10700	18600	16900	17000
Total	400363	383271	374704	380743	352011	364064		

Source: see *Notes on sources of sales data*, p. 745

Table 29.1.3 Manufactured cigarettes (i) percentage of production (excluding papyrosi) as filter cigarettes, and (ii) percentage of production (including papyrosi) as filter cigarettes, 1960-1982

Year	% Filter excluding papyrosi	% Filter including papyrosi
1960	0.0	0.0
1961	0.0	0.0
1962	0.9	0.2
1963	1.1	0.3
1964	1.2	0.3
1965	4.5	1.3
1966	6.9	2.3
1967	9.5	3.7
1968	16.9	7.5
1969	20.8	9.6
1970	22.0	10.1
1971	23.4	10.9
1972	23.9	11.5
1973	23.5	11.9
1974	26.1	13.9
1975	29.0	16.1
1976	28.4	16.5
1977	27.3	16.5
1978	29.1	18.5
1979	30.8	20.6
1980	30.6	20.9
1981	30.5	21.0
1982	30.3	21.3

Source : see *Notes on sources of sales data*, p. 745

Table 29.1.4 Manufactured cigarettes, percentage of production as filter cigarettes, for individual republics, 1993-1996

% Filter				
	1993	**1994**	**1995**	**1996**
Azerbaijan	43	42	0	0
Kazakhstan			95	97
Kyrgyzstan		30	30	
Moldova	30	26	25	21
Russia	73	73	71	67
Ukraine		3 - 5		
Uzbekistan		0	3	39

Source : see *Notes on sources of sales data*, p. 745

Table 29.2 Consumption of (i) cigarettes and (ii) all tobacco products, 1960-1994 sales-based data, including estimated hand-rolled cigarette consumption. Males and females aged 15 years and over

Year	Manufactured cigarettes		Hand-rolled cigarettes		Total cigarettes		All tobacco products	
	Total annual in millions	Number/ adult/day	Total annual in millions	Number/ adult/day	Total annual in millions	Number/ adult/day	Total annual in tonnes	Grams/ adult/day
1960	248003	3.9					168642	2.7
1961	252131	4.0					171449	2.7
1962	234697	3.7					159594	2.5
1963	264393	4.2					179787	2.8
1964	298420	4.7					199941	3.2
1965	335754	5.3					224955	3.6
1966	331785	5.2					222296	3.5
1967	313959	4.9					210353	3.3
1968	315119	4.8					226886	3.5
1969	340469	5.2					245138	3.7
1970	365191	5.5					262938	4.0
1971	395579	5.9					304596	4.5
1972	399893	5.9					307918	4.5
1973	409081	6.0					314992	4.6
1974	417180	6.0					337916	4.9
1975	419532	6.0					339821	4.9
1976	429866	6.1					348191	5.0
1977	437008	6.2					353976	5.0
1978	430828	6.0					366204	5.1
1979	416666	5.8					354166	4.9
1980	421186	5.8					358008	4.9
1981	434829	5.9					378301	5.2
1982	425012	5.8					369760	5.0
1983	440172	5.9					382950	5.1
1984	448122	6.0					389866	5.2
1985	448100	5.9					389847	5.2
1986	451299	5.9					392630	5.2
1987	428410	5.6					372717	4.9
1988	418455	5.4					364056	4.7
1989	398956	5.1					347092	4.5
1990	378000	4.8					328860	4.2
1991	383743	4.9					333856	4.2
1992	361063	4.5					314125	4.0
1993	327882	4.1					285257	3.6
1994	352550	4.4					306719	3.9

Source : see *Notes on sources of sales data,* p. 745

Figure 29.1 Daily consumption of (i) manufactured and total number of cigarettes, and (ii) all tobacco products, 1960-1994.
Males and females aged 15 years and over. *Source:* see Table 29.2

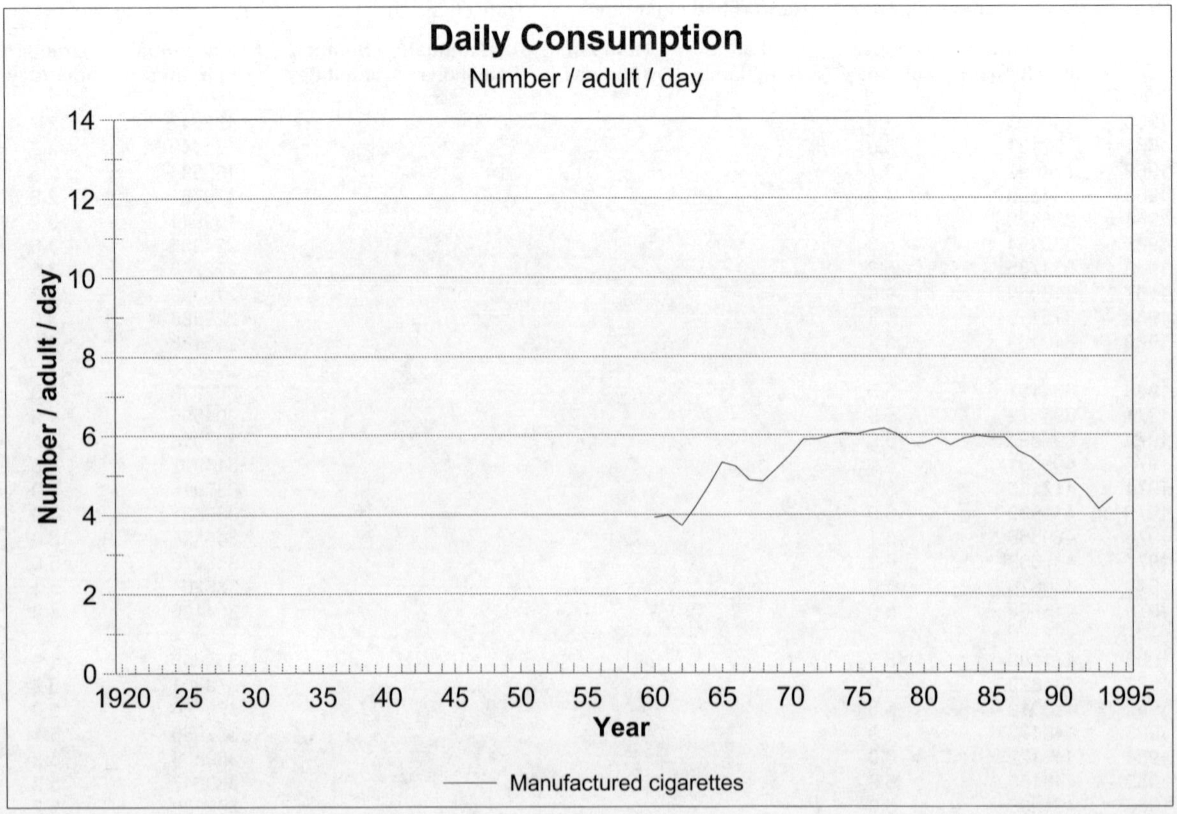

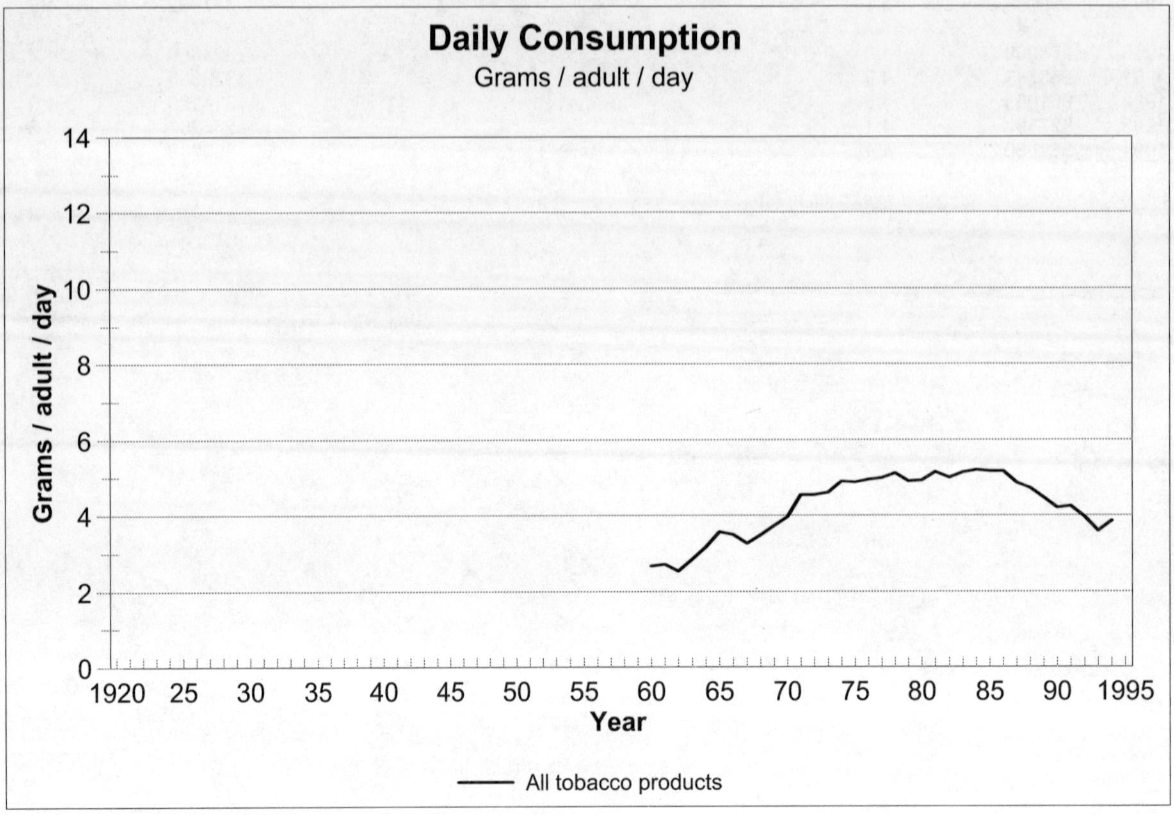

Table 29.3 Percentage sales of tobacco in different forms (by weight), Latvia, selected years 1925-1935

Year	Papyrosi (%)	Cigars(%)	Smoking tobacco(%)
1925	48.7	1.2	50.1
1935	53.0	1.2	45.7

Source : calculated from Tables 29.1.1

Figure 29.2 Percentage sales of tobacco in different forms (by weight), Latvia, selected years 1925-1935
Source: see Table 29.3

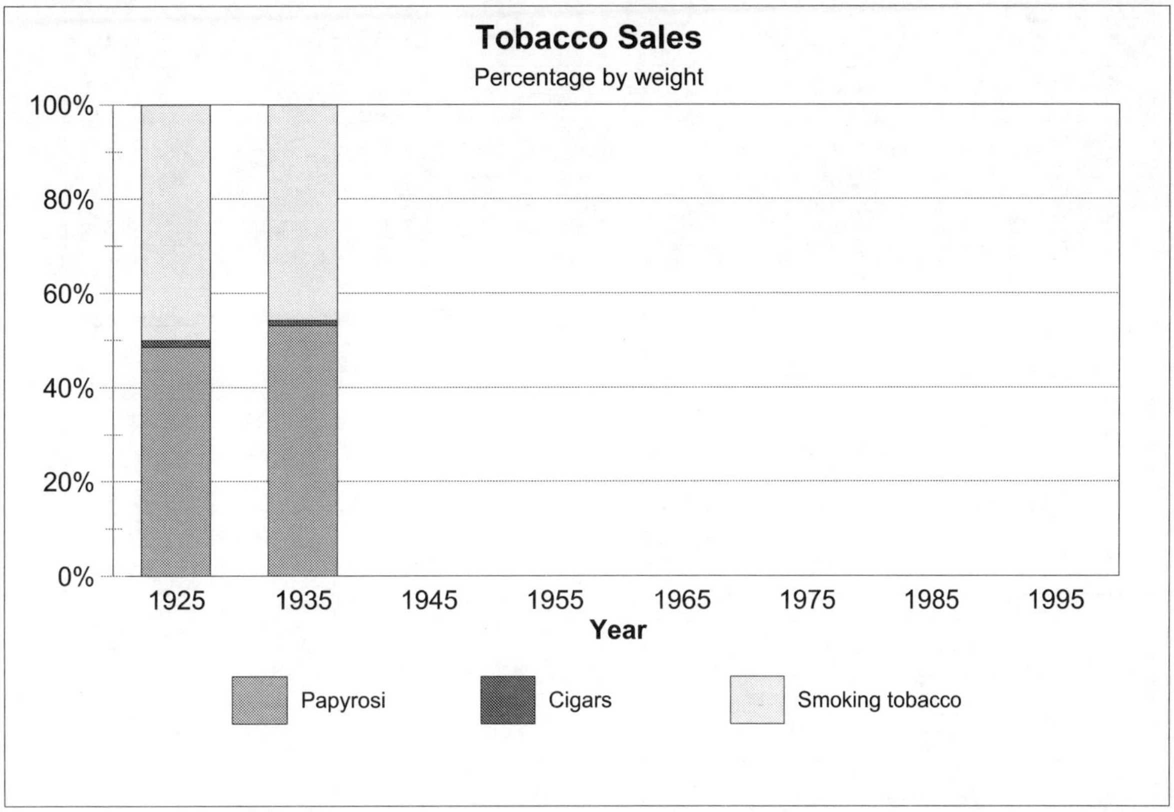

Table 29.4M Prevalence of smoking, males: some selected surveys for USSR and successor republics by age, 1973-1995
(continues on p. 732)

Russia

Frequency Product Source Year	12	13	14	15	16	17	18	19	20-24	25-29	30-34	35-39	40-44	45-49	50-54	55-59	60-64	65-69	70-74	75-79	80+	All ages
75 27 UC U					25				60		63		46		39		36		20			44
75 28 U U				60																		
78 1 UC R													51	49	48	41						48
79 29 U U									60		63		48		45							54
81 30 UC R	10		30																			
81 31 U U	13	38	18	69			66															54
83 29 U U									62		57		48		45							53
84 32 U R	6																					
84 32 U A	15																					
85 7 UC R												52		47		38						46
85 7 A A												57		49		39						49
85 8 UC R												55		50		37						48
85 8 A A												60		51		38						50
85 9 UC R										66		57		57		44						53
85 9 A A										66		58		58		44						54
85 33 U U					46																	
85 34 UC *	2	3	8	17	14	37																
85 34 UC R	7	7	12	23	21	44																
85 34 UC A	14	16	22	35	33	53																
85 35 U U				53																		
86 10 UC R										69		66		60		47						59
86 10 A A										69		66		60		48						59
86 29 U U									60		53		51		39							49
86 36 U U				79																		
86 37 U R	12																					
89 12 U U	44																					
89 32 U R				42																		
89 32 U A				45																		
90 41 UC R			17																			
90 41 UC A			22																			
91 37 U R	22																					
91 38 U U																						
91 42 TC R									64		57		45		48							55
92 39 U U				69																		
92 43 U R										77		61		68		57						65
92 44 U R		40																				
92 45 U U	61																					
93 15 UC R		13		19																		
93 40 U U				42																		
93 44 U U		49																				
93 46 UC A		39																				
93 46 UC R		24																				
93 47 UC R									69													
93 48 U U				67																		
93 49 U U										65												46
94 32 U R				25																		
94 32 U A				34																		
95 34 UC R	9	18	23	38	46	51	52															20
95 34 UC A	30																					
95 50 UC U			19		49		51		64	73		67		63		52		40		18		59
95 50 A U			19		49		52		65	74		67		63		53		40		19		59
95 51 U U	44									59												
95 52 U A		24																				
95 53 U U				66																		

Table 29.4F Prevalence of smoking, females: some selected surveys for USSR and successor republics by age, 1973-1995
(continues on p. 733)

Russia

<table>
<tr><th rowspan="2">Frequency
Product
Source
Year</th><th colspan="21">Age group</th><th rowspan="2">All ages</th></tr>
<tr><th>12</th><th>13</th><th>14</th><th>15</th><th>16</th><th>17</th><th>18</th><th>19</th><th>20-24</th><th>25-29</th><th>30-34</th><th>35-39</th><th>40-44</th><th>45-49</th><th>50-54</th><th>55-59</th><th>60-64</th><th>65-69</th><th>70-74</th><th>75-79</th><th>80+</th></tr>
<tr><td>75 27 UC U</td><td colspan="4"></td><td colspan="4">7</td><td colspan="2">17</td><td colspan="2">19</td><td colspan="2">8</td><td colspan="2">6</td><td colspan="2">11</td><td colspan="3">6</td><td>10</td></tr>
<tr><td>75 28 U U</td><td colspan="3"></td><td colspan="18">9</td><td></td></tr>
<tr><td>78 1 UC R</td><td colspan="21"></td><td></td></tr>
<tr><td>79 29 U U</td><td colspan="8"></td><td colspan="2">17</td><td colspan="2">19</td><td colspan="2">9</td><td colspan="2">9</td><td colspan="5"></td><td>13</td></tr>
<tr><td>81 30 UC R</td><td colspan="21"></td><td></td></tr>
<tr><td>81 31 U U</td><td>0</td><td>4</td><td>4</td><td>17</td><td colspan="2"></td><td colspan="15">8</td><td>6</td></tr>
<tr><td>83 29 U U</td><td colspan="8"></td><td colspan="2">17</td><td colspan="2">19</td><td colspan="2">10</td><td colspan="2">9</td><td colspan="5"></td><td>14</td></tr>
<tr><td>84 32 U R</td><td colspan="21"></td><td></td></tr>
<tr><td>84 32 U A</td><td colspan="21"></td><td></td></tr>
<tr><td>85 7 UC R</td><td colspan="11"></td><td colspan="2">13</td><td colspan="2">6</td><td colspan="2">6</td><td colspan="4"></td><td>9</td></tr>
<tr><td>85 7 A A</td><td colspan="11"></td><td colspan="2">17</td><td colspan="2">8</td><td colspan="2">7</td><td colspan="4"></td><td>10</td></tr>
<tr><td>85 8 UC R</td><td colspan="11"></td><td colspan="2">19</td><td colspan="2">8</td><td colspan="2">7</td><td colspan="4"></td><td>12</td></tr>
<tr><td>85 8 A A</td><td colspan="11"></td><td colspan="2">22</td><td colspan="2">10</td><td colspan="2">8</td><td colspan="4"></td><td>14</td></tr>
<tr><td>85 9 UC R</td><td colspan="9"></td><td colspan="2">3</td><td colspan="2">3</td><td colspan="2">2</td><td colspan="2">3</td><td colspan="4"></td><td>3</td></tr>
<tr><td>85 9 A A</td><td colspan="9"></td><td colspan="2">6</td><td colspan="2">4</td><td colspan="2">2</td><td colspan="2">3</td><td colspan="4"></td><td>3</td></tr>
<tr><td>85 33 U U</td><td colspan="4"></td><td>30</td><td colspan="16"></td><td></td></tr>
<tr><td>85 34 UC *</td><td>0</td><td>0</td><td>1</td><td>5</td><td>4</td><td>12</td><td colspan="15"></td><td></td></tr>
<tr><td>85 34 UC R</td><td>0</td><td>1</td><td>4</td><td>8</td><td>8</td><td>18</td><td colspan="15"></td><td></td></tr>
<tr><td>85 34 UC A</td><td>1</td><td>4</td><td>6</td><td>14</td><td>18</td><td>28</td><td colspan="15"></td><td></td></tr>
<tr><td>85 35 U U</td><td colspan="3"></td><td colspan="18">10</td><td></td></tr>
<tr><td>86 10 UC R</td><td colspan="9"></td><td colspan="2">4</td><td colspan="2">5</td><td colspan="2">2</td><td colspan="2">3</td><td colspan="4"></td><td>3</td></tr>
<tr><td>86 10 A A</td><td colspan="9"></td><td colspan="2">4</td><td colspan="2">6</td><td colspan="2">2</td><td colspan="2">3</td><td colspan="4"></td><td>4</td></tr>
<tr><td>86 29 U U</td><td colspan="8"></td><td colspan="2">11</td><td colspan="2">15</td><td colspan="2">9</td><td colspan="2">3</td><td colspan="5"></td><td>9</td></tr>
<tr><td>86 36 U U</td><td colspan="3"></td><td colspan="18">14</td><td></td></tr>
<tr><td>86 37 U R</td><td colspan="5">3</td><td colspan="16"></td><td></td></tr>
<tr><td>89 12 U U</td><td colspan="3"></td><td colspan="18">10</td><td></td></tr>
<tr><td>89 32 U R</td><td colspan="3"></td><td colspan="3">13</td><td colspan="15"></td><td></td></tr>
<tr><td>89 32 U A</td><td colspan="3"></td><td colspan="3">19</td><td colspan="15"></td><td></td></tr>
<tr><td>90 41 UC R</td><td colspan="2"></td><td>2</td><td colspan="18"></td><td></td></tr>
<tr><td>90 41 UC A</td><td colspan="2"></td><td>6</td><td colspan="18"></td><td></td></tr>
<tr><td>91 37 U R</td><td colspan="5">7</td><td colspan="16"></td><td></td></tr>
<tr><td>91 38 U U</td><td colspan="3"></td><td colspan="18">25</td><td></td></tr>
<tr><td>91 42 TC R</td><td colspan="21"></td><td></td></tr>
<tr><td>92 39 U U</td><td colspan="3"></td><td colspan="18">8</td><td></td></tr>
<tr><td>92 43 U R</td><td colspan="9"></td><td colspan="2">20</td><td colspan="2">13</td><td colspan="2">6</td><td colspan="2">3</td><td colspan="4"></td><td>11</td></tr>
<tr><td>92 44 U R</td><td></td><td colspan="4">25</td><td colspan="16"></td><td></td></tr>
<tr><td>92 45 U U</td><td colspan="3"></td><td colspan="18">17</td><td></td></tr>
<tr><td>93 15 UC R</td><td></td><td>5</td><td></td><td>10</td><td colspan="17"></td><td></td></tr>
<tr><td>93 40 U U</td><td colspan="3"></td><td colspan="3">24</td><td colspan="15"></td><td></td></tr>
<tr><td>93 44 U U</td><td></td><td colspan="4">38</td><td colspan="16"></td><td></td></tr>
<tr><td>93 46 UC A</td><td></td><td colspan="3">12</td><td colspan="17"></td><td></td></tr>
<tr><td>93 46 UC R</td><td></td><td colspan="3">3</td><td colspan="17"></td><td></td></tr>
<tr><td>93 47 UC R</td><td colspan="8"></td><td colspan="8">6</td><td colspan="5"></td><td></td></tr>
<tr><td>93 48 U U</td><td colspan="3"></td><td colspan="18">30</td><td></td></tr>
<tr><td>93 49 U U</td><td colspan="9"></td><td colspan="2">19</td><td colspan="6"></td><td colspan="4"></td><td>12</td></tr>
<tr><td>94 32 U R</td><td colspan="21"></td><td></td></tr>
<tr><td>94 32 U A</td><td colspan="21"></td><td></td></tr>
<tr><td>95 34 UC R</td><td>2</td><td>1</td><td>12</td><td>21</td><td>31</td><td>32</td><td>43</td><td colspan="14"></td><td>12</td></tr>
<tr><td>95 34 UC A</td><td colspan="7">18</td><td colspan="14"></td><td></td></tr>
<tr><td>95 50 UC U</td><td colspan="2"></td><td colspan="2">8</td><td colspan="2">7</td><td colspan="2">18</td><td>19</td><td colspan="2">17</td><td colspan="2">11</td><td colspan="2">9</td><td colspan="2">2</td><td colspan="2">2</td><td colspan="2">1</td><td>9</td></tr>
<tr><td>95 50 A U</td><td colspan="2"></td><td colspan="2">8</td><td colspan="2">7</td><td colspan="2">18</td><td>19</td><td colspan="2">17</td><td colspan="2">11</td><td colspan="2">9</td><td colspan="2">2</td><td colspan="2">2</td><td colspan="2">1</td><td>9</td></tr>
<tr><td>95 51 U U</td><td colspan="3"></td><td colspan="5">13</td><td></td><td colspan="9">18</td><td colspan="3"></td><td></td></tr>
<tr><td>95 52 U A</td><td></td><td colspan="3">31</td><td colspan="17"></td><td></td></tr>
<tr><td>95 53 U U</td><td colspan="21"></td><td></td></tr>
</table>

Table 29.4M *(continued from p. 730, continues on p. 734)*
Prevalence of smoking, males

Estonia

<table>
<tr><td rowspan="2">Frequency
Product
Source
Year</td><td colspan="21">Age group</td><td rowspan="2">All ages</td></tr>
<tr><td>12</td><td>13</td><td>14</td><td>15</td><td>16</td><td>17</td><td>18</td><td>19</td><td>20-24</td><td>25-29</td><td>30-34</td><td>35-39</td><td>40-44</td><td>45-49</td><td>50-54</td><td>55-59</td><td>60-64</td><td>65-69</td><td>70-74</td><td>75-79</td><td>80+</td></tr>
<tr><td>81 54 U U</td><td>9</td><td>12</td><td>19</td><td>20</td><td>28</td><td>37</td><td colspan="15"></td><td></td></tr>
<tr><td>90 55 U R</td><td colspan="6"></td><td colspan="15">45</td><td></td></tr>
<tr><td>90 56 U U</td><td colspan="6"></td><td colspan="3">52</td><td colspan="12"></td><td></td></tr>
<tr><td>91 57 U R</td><td colspan="3"></td><td>10</td><td colspan="17"></td><td></td></tr>
<tr><td>91 57 U A</td><td colspan="3"></td><td>17</td><td colspan="17"></td><td></td></tr>
<tr><td>91 58 UC R</td><td colspan="2"></td><td colspan="2">19</td><td colspan="17"></td><td></td></tr>
<tr><td>91 58 UC A</td><td colspan="2"></td><td colspan="2">24</td><td colspan="17"></td><td></td></tr>
<tr><td>92 13 U U</td><td colspan="3"></td><td colspan="18">49</td><td></td></tr>
<tr><td>92 59 U R</td><td colspan="9"></td><td colspan="2">56</td><td colspan="2">58</td><td colspan="2">47</td><td colspan="2">37</td><td colspan="4"></td><td></td></tr>
<tr><td>93 58 UC R</td><td colspan="2"></td><td colspan="2">28</td><td colspan="17"></td><td></td></tr>
<tr><td>93 58 UC A</td><td colspan="2"></td><td colspan="2">40</td><td colspan="17"></td><td></td></tr>
<tr><td>94 16 UC R</td><td></td><td colspan="2">6</td><td>22</td><td colspan="17"></td><td></td></tr>
<tr><td>94 60 U R</td><td colspan="4"></td><td colspan="17">52</td><td></td></tr>
<tr><td>95 19 UC R</td><td colspan="3"></td><td colspan="2">26</td><td colspan="16"></td><td></td></tr>
<tr><td>95 19 UC A</td><td colspan="3"></td><td colspan="2">37</td><td colspan="16"></td><td></td></tr>
<tr><td>95 58 UC R</td><td colspan="2"></td><td colspan="2">24</td><td colspan="17"></td><td></td></tr>
<tr><td>95 58 UC A</td><td colspan="2"></td><td colspan="2">32</td><td colspan="17"></td><td></td></tr>
<tr><td>95 61 U U</td><td></td><td colspan="6">31</td><td colspan="14"></td><td></td></tr>
</table>

Latvia

<table>
<tr><td rowspan="2">Frequency
Product
Source
Year</td><td colspan="21">Age group</td><td rowspan="2">All ages</td></tr>
<tr><td>12</td><td>13</td><td>14</td><td>15</td><td>16</td><td>17</td><td>18</td><td>19</td><td>20-24</td><td>25-29</td><td>30-34</td><td>35-39</td><td>40-44</td><td>45-49</td><td>50-54</td><td>55-59</td><td>60-64</td><td>65-69</td><td>70-74</td><td>75-79</td><td>80+</td></tr>
<tr><td>90 17 UC A</td><td></td><td>21</td><td></td><td>31</td><td colspan="17"></td><td></td></tr>
<tr><td>93 17 UC R</td><td></td><td>13</td><td></td><td>33</td><td colspan="17"></td><td></td></tr>
<tr><td>93 62 U R</td><td colspan="3"></td><td colspan="18">67</td><td></td></tr>
<tr><td>95 20 UC R</td><td colspan="3"></td><td colspan="2">26</td><td colspan="16"></td><td></td></tr>
<tr><td>95 20 UC A</td><td colspan="3"></td><td colspan="2">39</td><td colspan="16"></td><td></td></tr>
</table>

Lithuania

<table>
<tr><td rowspan="2">Frequency
Product
Source
Year</td><td colspan="21">Age group</td><td rowspan="2">All ages</td></tr>
<tr><td>12</td><td>13</td><td>14</td><td>15</td><td>16</td><td>17</td><td>18</td><td>19</td><td>20-24</td><td>25-29</td><td>30-34</td><td>35-39</td><td>40-44</td><td>45-49</td><td>50-54</td><td>55-59</td><td>60-64</td><td>65-69</td><td>70-74</td><td>75-79</td><td>80+</td></tr>
<tr><td>73 63 UC R</td><td colspan="13"></td><td colspan="3">48</td><td colspan="5"></td><td></td></tr>
<tr><td>78 2 UC R</td><td colspan="12"></td><td>47</td><td>43</td><td>43</td><td>38</td><td colspan="5"></td><td>43</td></tr>
<tr><td>81 64 UC *</td><td colspan="7">12</td><td colspan="14"></td><td></td></tr>
<tr><td>81 64 UC R</td><td colspan="7">21</td><td colspan="14"></td><td></td></tr>
<tr><td>81 64 UC A</td><td colspan="7">26</td><td colspan="14"></td><td></td></tr>
<tr><td>82 64 UC *</td><td colspan="7">10</td><td colspan="14"></td><td></td></tr>
<tr><td>82 64 UC R</td><td colspan="7">18</td><td colspan="14"></td><td></td></tr>
<tr><td>82 64 UC A</td><td colspan="7">24</td><td colspan="14"></td><td></td></tr>
<tr><td>83 65 U U</td><td colspan="21"></td><td></td></tr>
<tr><td>84 11 UC R</td><td colspan="9"></td><td colspan="2">47</td><td colspan="2">31</td><td colspan="2">35</td><td colspan="6"></td><td>38</td></tr>
<tr><td>84 11 A A</td><td colspan="11"></td><td colspan="2">51</td><td colspan="2">33</td><td colspan="2">40</td><td colspan="4"></td><td>42</td></tr>
<tr><td>85 64 UC *</td><td colspan="7">6</td><td colspan="14"></td><td></td></tr>
<tr><td>85 64 UC R</td><td colspan="7">12</td><td colspan="14"></td><td></td></tr>
<tr><td>85 64 UC A</td><td colspan="7">17</td><td colspan="14"></td><td></td></tr>
<tr><td>85 66 U U</td><td colspan="3"></td><td>15</td><td colspan="17"></td><td></td></tr>
<tr><td>92 14 U U</td><td colspan="3"></td><td colspan="18">52</td><td></td></tr>
<tr><td>93 65 U U</td><td colspan="21"></td><td></td></tr>
<tr><td>93 67 UC R</td><td colspan="11"></td><td colspan="6">35</td><td colspan="4"></td><td></td></tr>
<tr><td>94 18 UC R</td><td></td><td colspan="2">3</td><td>15</td><td colspan="17"></td><td></td></tr>
<tr><td>95 21 UC R</td><td colspan="3"></td><td colspan="2">22</td><td colspan="16"></td><td></td></tr>
<tr><td>95 21 UC A</td><td colspan="3"></td><td colspan="2">34</td><td colspan="16"></td><td></td></tr>
<tr><td>95 67 UC R</td><td colspan="17"></td><td colspan="3">16</td><td></td><td></td></tr>
</table>

Table 29.4F *(continued from p. 731, continues on p. 735)*
Prevalence of smoking, females

Estonia

<table>
<tr><th rowspan="2">Frequency
Product
Source
Year</th><th colspan="21">Age group</th><th rowspan="2">All ages</th></tr>
<tr><th>12</th><th>13</th><th>14</th><th>15</th><th>16</th><th>17</th><th>18</th><th>19</th><th>20-24</th><th>25-29</th><th>30-34</th><th>35-39</th><th>40-44</th><th>45-49</th><th>50-54</th><th>55-59</th><th>60-64</th><th>65-69</th><th>70-74</th><th>75-79</th><th>80+</th></tr>
<tr><td>81 54 U U</td><td>1</td><td>1</td><td>2</td><td>4</td><td>6</td><td>13</td><td colspan="15"></td><td></td></tr>
<tr><td>90 55 U R</td><td colspan="6"></td><td colspan="15">15</td><td></td></tr>
<tr><td>90 56 U U</td><td colspan="6"></td><td colspan="3">28</td><td colspan="12"></td><td></td></tr>
<tr><td>91 57 U R</td><td colspan="3"></td><td>2</td><td colspan="17"></td><td></td></tr>
<tr><td>91 57 U A</td><td colspan="3"></td><td>4</td><td colspan="17"></td><td></td></tr>
<tr><td>91 58 UC R</td><td colspan="2"></td><td colspan="2">4</td><td colspan="17"></td><td></td></tr>
<tr><td>91 58 UC A</td><td colspan="2"></td><td colspan="2">11</td><td colspan="17"></td><td></td></tr>
<tr><td>92 13 U U</td><td colspan="3"></td><td colspan="18">20</td><td></td></tr>
<tr><td>92 59 U R</td><td colspan="9"></td><td colspan="2">30</td><td colspan="2">21</td><td colspan="2">17</td><td colspan="2">7</td><td colspan="4"></td><td></td></tr>
<tr><td>93 58 UC R</td><td colspan="2"></td><td colspan="2">14</td><td colspan="17"></td><td></td></tr>
<tr><td>93 58 UC A</td><td colspan="2"></td><td colspan="2">28</td><td colspan="17"></td><td></td></tr>
<tr><td>94 16 UC R</td><td></td><td>1</td><td></td><td>6</td><td colspan="17"></td><td></td></tr>
<tr><td>94 60 U R</td><td colspan="4"></td><td colspan="17">24</td><td></td></tr>
<tr><td>95 19 UC R</td><td colspan="3"></td><td colspan="2">13</td><td colspan="16"></td><td></td></tr>
<tr><td>95 19 UC A</td><td colspan="3"></td><td colspan="2">22</td><td colspan="16"></td><td></td></tr>
<tr><td>95 58 UC R</td><td colspan="2"></td><td colspan="2">17</td><td colspan="17"></td><td></td></tr>
<tr><td>95 58 UC A</td><td colspan="2"></td><td colspan="2">23</td><td colspan="17"></td><td></td></tr>
<tr><td>95 61 U U</td><td></td><td colspan="6">22</td><td colspan="14"></td><td></td></tr>
</table>

Latvia

<table>
<tr><th rowspan="2">Frequency
Product
Source
Year</th><th colspan="21">Age group</th><th rowspan="2">All ages</th></tr>
<tr><th>12</th><th>13</th><th>14</th><th>15</th><th>16</th><th>17</th><th>18</th><th>19</th><th>20-24</th><th>25-29</th><th>30-34</th><th>35-39</th><th>40-44</th><th>45-49</th><th>50-54</th><th>55-59</th><th>60-64</th><th>65-69</th><th>70-74</th><th>75-79</th><th>80+</th></tr>
<tr><td>90 17 UC A</td><td></td><td>8</td><td></td><td>14</td><td colspan="17"></td><td></td></tr>
<tr><td>93 17 UC R</td><td></td><td>3</td><td></td><td>14</td><td colspan="17"></td><td></td></tr>
<tr><td>93 62 U R</td><td colspan="3"></td><td colspan="18">12</td><td></td></tr>
<tr><td>95 20 UC R</td><td colspan="3"></td><td colspan="2">13</td><td colspan="16"></td><td></td></tr>
<tr><td>95 20 UC A</td><td colspan="3"></td><td colspan="2">26</td><td colspan="16"></td><td></td></tr>
</table>

Lithuania

<table>
<tr><th rowspan="2">Frequency
Product
Source
Year</th><th colspan="21">Age group</th><th rowspan="2">All ages</th></tr>
<tr><th>12</th><th>13</th><th>14</th><th>15</th><th>16</th><th>17</th><th>18</th><th>19</th><th>20-24</th><th>25-29</th><th>30-34</th><th>35-39</th><th>40-44</th><th>45-49</th><th>50-54</th><th>55-59</th><th>60-64</th><th>65-69</th><th>70-74</th><th>75-79</th><th>80+</th></tr>
<tr><td>73 63 UC R</td><td colspan="21"></td><td></td></tr>
<tr><td>78 2 UC R</td><td colspan="21"></td><td></td></tr>
<tr><td>81 64 UC *</td><td colspan="7">2</td><td colspan="14"></td><td></td></tr>
<tr><td>81 64 UC R</td><td colspan="7">5</td><td colspan="14"></td><td></td></tr>
<tr><td>81 64 UC A</td><td colspan="7">8</td><td colspan="14"></td><td></td></tr>
<tr><td>82 64 UC *</td><td colspan="7">2</td><td colspan="14"></td><td></td></tr>
<tr><td>82 64 UC R</td><td colspan="7">4</td><td colspan="14"></td><td></td></tr>
<tr><td>82 64 UC A</td><td colspan="7">8</td><td colspan="14"></td><td></td></tr>
<tr><td>83 65 U U</td><td colspan="9"></td><td>8</td><td colspan="11"></td><td></td></tr>
<tr><td>84 11 UC R</td><td colspan="9"></td><td colspan="2">4</td><td colspan="2">4</td><td colspan="2">4</td><td colspan="6"></td><td>4</td></tr>
<tr><td>84 11 A A</td><td colspan="11"></td><td colspan="2">5</td><td colspan="2">6</td><td colspan="2">4</td><td colspan="4"></td><td>5</td></tr>
<tr><td>85 64 UC *</td><td colspan="7">1</td><td colspan="14"></td><td></td></tr>
<tr><td>85 64 UC R</td><td colspan="7">3</td><td colspan="14"></td><td></td></tr>
<tr><td>85 64 UC A</td><td colspan="7">5</td><td colspan="14"></td><td></td></tr>
<tr><td>85 66 U U</td><td colspan="3"></td><td>0</td><td colspan="17"></td><td></td></tr>
<tr><td>92 14 U U</td><td colspan="3"></td><td colspan="18">10</td><td></td></tr>
<tr><td>93 65 U U</td><td colspan="9"></td><td>18</td><td colspan="11"></td><td></td></tr>
<tr><td>93 67 UC R</td><td colspan="11"></td><td colspan="6">5</td><td colspan="4"></td><td></td></tr>
<tr><td>94 18 UC R</td><td></td><td>0</td><td></td><td>4</td><td colspan="17"></td><td></td></tr>
<tr><td>95 21 UC R</td><td colspan="3"></td><td colspan="2">8</td><td colspan="16"></td><td></td></tr>
<tr><td>95 21 UC A</td><td colspan="3"></td><td colspan="2">18</td><td colspan="16"></td><td></td></tr>
<tr><td>95 67 UC R</td><td colspan="17"></td><td colspan="3">2</td><td></td><td></td></tr>
</table>

Table 29.4M *(continued from p. 732)* Prevalence of smoking, males

Ukraine, Belorussia, Moldova

Frequency / Product / Source / Year	12	13	14	15	16	17	18	19	20-24	25-29	30-34	35-39	40-44	45-49	50-54	55-59	60-64	65-69	70-74	75-79	80+	All ages
81 3 UC R													52									
81 4 UC R													34									
81 68 U U									54													
90 69 U U																						
93 68 U U									49													
95 22 UC R				38																		
95 22 UC A				51																		
95 23 U U				60																		
95 24 U U				46																		
95 69 U U																						

Armenia, Azerbaijan, Georgia

Frequency / Product / Source / Year	12	13	14	15	16	17	18	19	20-24	25-29	30-34	35-39	40-44	45-49	50-54	55-59	60-64	65-69	70-74	75-79	80+	All ages
60 70 UC U				78																		
60 71 UC U				79																		
63 72 UC U				69																		
94 73 U U			56																			
94 74 U U	32																					
95 75 U U													57									

Central Asia

Frequency / Product / Source / Year	12	13	14	15	16	17	18	19	20-24	25-29	30-34	35-39	40-44	45-49	50-54	55-59	60-64	65-69	70-74	75-79	80+	All ages
78 76 U U													52									
79 77 U U									72		48											
81 5 UC R													56									
81 6 UC R													48									
81 78 U U													56	51	50	44						51
89 79 UC A				23					50								35					40
89 80 UC A									69								36					50
91 81 U U				27																		
93 82 U U									60		53											49
95 25 U U				54																		
95 26 U U				47																		

Multiple/unspecified region

Frequency / Product / Source / Year	12	13	14	15	16	17	18	19	20-24	25-29	30-34	35-39	40-44	45-49	50-54	55-59	60-64	65-69	70-74	75-79	80+	All ages
77 83 U U				49																		
81 84 U U									78	72	72	67	71	67	55							65
81 85 U U	11			46																		
84 86 U U				48																		

Source: see *Notes on sources of survey data*, p. 746

Product:
MC = manufactured cigarettes
TC = total cigarettes (including hand-rolled)
UC = cigarettes (type unspecified)
A = all products

Frequency:
A = all smokers (including occasional)
R = regular or daily smokers

All ages: relevant to ages used and as given in original source

U = unspecified

* = refer to *Notes on sources of survey data*, p. 746

Table 29.4F (continued from p. 733)
Prevalence of smoking, females

Ukraine, Belorussia, Moldova

<table>
<tr><th rowspan="2">Frequency
Product
Source
Year</th><th colspan="21">Age group</th><th rowspan="2">All ages</th></tr>
<tr><th>12</th><th>13</th><th>14</th><th>15</th><th>16</th><th>17</th><th>18</th><th>19</th><th>20-24</th><th>25-29</th><th>30-34</th><th>35-39</th><th>40-44</th><th>45-49</th><th>50-54</th><th>55-59</th><th>60-64</th><th>65-69</th><th>70-74</th><th>75-79</th><th>80+</th></tr>
<tr><td>81 3 UC R</td><td></td><td></td><td></td><td></td><td></td><td></td><td></td><td></td><td></td><td></td><td></td><td></td><td></td><td></td><td></td><td></td><td></td><td></td><td></td><td></td><td></td><td></td></tr>
<tr><td>81 4 UC R</td><td></td><td></td><td></td><td></td><td></td><td></td><td></td><td></td><td></td><td></td><td></td><td></td><td></td><td></td><td></td><td></td><td></td><td></td><td></td><td></td><td></td><td></td></tr>
<tr><td>81 68 U U</td><td></td><td></td><td></td><td></td><td></td><td></td><td></td><td></td><td colspan="8">5</td><td></td><td></td><td></td><td></td><td></td><td></td></tr>
<tr><td>90 69 U U</td><td></td><td></td><td></td><td colspan="18">5</td><td></td></tr>
<tr><td>93 68 U U</td><td></td><td></td><td></td><td></td><td></td><td></td><td></td><td></td><td colspan="8">11</td><td></td><td></td><td></td><td></td><td></td><td></td></tr>
<tr><td>95 22 UC R</td><td></td><td></td><td></td><td colspan="2">14</td><td></td><td></td><td></td><td></td><td></td><td></td><td></td><td></td><td></td><td></td><td></td><td></td><td></td><td></td><td></td><td></td><td></td></tr>
<tr><td>95 22 UC A</td><td></td><td></td><td></td><td colspan="2">28</td><td></td><td></td><td></td><td></td><td></td><td></td><td></td><td></td><td></td><td></td><td></td><td></td><td></td><td></td><td></td><td></td><td></td></tr>
<tr><td>95 23 U U</td><td></td><td></td><td></td><td colspan="18">12</td><td></td></tr>
<tr><td>95 24 U U</td><td></td><td></td><td></td><td colspan="18">7</td><td></td></tr>
<tr><td>95 69 U U</td><td></td><td></td><td></td><td colspan="18">21</td><td></td></tr>
</table>

Armenia, Azerbaijan, Georgia

<table>
<tr><th rowspan="2">Frequency
Product
Source
Year</th><th colspan="21">Age group</th><th rowspan="2">All ages</th></tr>
<tr><th>12</th><th>13</th><th>14</th><th>15</th><th>16</th><th>17</th><th>18</th><th>19</th><th>20-24</th><th>25-29</th><th>30-34</th><th>35-39</th><th>40-44</th><th>45-49</th><th>50-54</th><th>55-59</th><th>60-64</th><th>65-69</th><th>70-74</th><th>75-79</th><th>80+</th></tr>
<tr><td>60 70 UC U</td><td></td><td></td><td></td><td colspan="18">7</td><td></td></tr>
<tr><td>60 71 UC U</td><td></td><td></td><td></td><td colspan="18">8</td><td></td></tr>
<tr><td>63 72 UC U</td><td></td><td></td><td></td><td colspan="18">5</td><td></td></tr>
<tr><td>94 73 U U</td><td></td><td></td><td colspan="3">21</td><td></td><td></td><td></td><td></td><td></td><td></td><td></td><td></td><td></td><td></td><td></td><td></td><td></td><td></td><td></td><td></td></tr>
<tr><td>94 74 U U</td><td colspan="5">8</td><td></td><td></td><td></td><td></td><td></td><td></td><td></td><td></td><td></td><td></td><td></td><td></td><td></td><td></td><td></td><td></td></tr>
<tr><td>95 75 U U</td><td></td><td></td><td></td><td></td><td></td><td></td><td></td><td></td><td></td><td></td><td></td><td></td><td colspan="5">13</td><td></td><td></td><td></td><td></td><td></td></tr>
</table>

Central Asia

<table>
<tr><th rowspan="2">Frequency
Product
Source
Year</th><th colspan="21">Age group</th><th rowspan="2">All ages</th></tr>
<tr><th>12</th><th>13</th><th>14</th><th>15</th><th>16</th><th>17</th><th>18</th><th>19</th><th>20-24</th><th>25-29</th><th>30-34</th><th>35-39</th><th>40-44</th><th>45-49</th><th>50-54</th><th>55-59</th><th>60-64</th><th>65-69</th><th>70-74</th><th>75-79</th><th>80+</th></tr>
<tr><td>78 76 U U</td><td></td><td></td><td></td><td></td><td></td><td></td><td></td><td></td><td></td><td></td><td></td><td></td><td></td><td></td><td></td><td></td><td></td><td></td><td></td><td></td><td></td><td></td></tr>
<tr><td>79 77 U U</td><td></td><td></td><td></td><td></td><td></td><td></td><td></td><td></td><td colspan="2">15</td><td></td><td></td><td></td><td></td><td></td><td></td><td></td><td></td><td></td><td></td><td></td><td></td></tr>
<tr><td>81 5 UC R</td><td></td><td></td><td></td><td></td><td></td><td></td><td></td><td></td><td></td><td></td><td></td><td></td><td></td><td></td><td></td><td></td><td></td><td></td><td></td><td></td><td></td><td></td></tr>
<tr><td>81 6 UC R</td><td></td><td></td><td></td><td></td><td></td><td></td><td></td><td></td><td></td><td></td><td></td><td></td><td></td><td></td><td></td><td></td><td></td><td></td><td></td><td></td><td></td><td></td></tr>
<tr><td>81 78 U U</td><td></td><td></td><td></td><td></td><td></td><td></td><td></td><td></td><td></td><td></td><td></td><td></td><td></td><td></td><td></td><td></td><td></td><td></td><td></td><td></td><td></td><td></td></tr>
<tr><td>89 79 UC A</td><td></td><td></td><td></td><td colspan="5">1</td><td></td><td></td><td></td><td></td><td></td><td></td><td></td><td></td><td></td><td></td><td></td><td></td><td></td><td>1</td></tr>
<tr><td>89 80 UC A</td><td></td><td></td><td></td><td colspan="18">3</td><td></td></tr>
<tr><td>91 81 U U</td><td></td><td></td><td></td><td colspan="18">1</td><td></td></tr>
<tr><td>93 82 U U</td><td></td><td></td><td></td><td></td><td></td><td></td><td></td><td></td><td colspan="2">11</td><td colspan="2">15</td><td></td><td></td><td></td><td></td><td></td><td></td><td></td><td></td><td></td><td>9</td></tr>
<tr><td>95 25 U U</td><td></td><td></td><td></td><td colspan="18">17</td><td></td></tr>
<tr><td>95 26 U U</td><td></td><td></td><td></td><td colspan="18">2</td><td></td></tr>
</table>

Multiple/unspecified region

<table>
<tr><th rowspan="2">Frequency
Product
Source
Year</th><th colspan="21">Age group</th><th rowspan="2">All ages</th></tr>
<tr><th>12</th><th>13</th><th>14</th><th>15</th><th>16</th><th>17</th><th>18</th><th>19</th><th>20-24</th><th>25-29</th><th>30-34</th><th>35-39</th><th>40-44</th><th>45-49</th><th>50-54</th><th>55-59</th><th>60-64</th><th>65-69</th><th>70-74</th><th>75-79</th><th>80+</th></tr>
<tr><td>77 83 U U</td><td></td><td></td><td></td><td colspan="18">18</td><td></td></tr>
<tr><td>81 84 U U</td><td></td><td></td><td></td><td></td><td></td><td></td><td></td><td></td><td>15</td><td>5</td><td>5</td><td>2</td><td>4</td><td>8</td><td colspan="7">3</td><td>11</td></tr>
<tr><td>81 85 U U</td><td>3</td><td></td><td></td><td>8</td><td></td><td></td><td></td><td></td><td></td><td></td><td></td><td></td><td></td><td></td><td></td><td></td><td></td><td></td><td></td><td></td><td></td><td></td></tr>
<tr><td>84 86 U U</td><td></td><td></td><td></td><td colspan="18">11</td><td></td></tr>
</table>

Source: see *Notes on sources of survey data*, p. 746
Product: MC = manufactured cigarettes
TC = total cigarettes (including hand-rolled)
UC = cigarettes (type unspecified)
A = all products

Frequency: A = all smokers (including occasional)
R = regular or daily smokers
All ages: relevant to ages used and as given in original source
U = unspecified
* = refer to *Notes on sources of survey data*, p. 746

Table 29.5M Number of cigarettes smoked per smoker per day, males: some selected surveys for USSR and successor republics by age, 1973-1995

Russia

<table>
<tr><th rowspan="2">Product
Source
Year</th><th colspan="21">Age group</th><th rowspan="2">All ages</th></tr>
<tr><th>12</th><th>13</th><th>14</th><th>15</th><th>16</th><th>17</th><th>18</th><th>19</th><th>20-24</th><th>25-29</th><th>30-34</th><th>35-39</th><th>40-44</th><th>45-49</th><th>50-54</th><th>55-59</th><th>60-64</th><th>65-69</th><th>70-74</th><th>75-79</th><th>80+</th></tr>
<tr><td>75 27 UC</td><td></td><td></td><td></td><td></td><td colspan="4">9.3</td><td colspan="2">15</td><td colspan="2">16</td><td colspan="2">18</td><td colspan="2">17</td><td colspan="2">17</td><td colspan="3">14</td><td>17</td></tr>
<tr><td>85 7 UC</td><td></td><td></td><td></td><td></td><td></td><td></td><td></td><td></td><td></td><td></td><td></td><td colspan="6">18</td><td></td><td></td><td></td><td></td><td></td></tr>
<tr><td>85 8 UC</td><td></td><td></td><td></td><td></td><td></td><td></td><td></td><td></td><td></td><td></td><td></td><td colspan="6">17</td><td></td><td></td><td></td><td></td><td></td></tr>
<tr><td>85 9 UC</td><td></td><td></td><td></td><td></td><td></td><td></td><td></td><td></td><td></td><td></td><td></td><td colspan="6">17</td><td></td><td></td><td></td><td></td><td></td></tr>
<tr><td>85 34 UC</td><td>0.8</td><td>2.5</td><td>2.6</td><td>4.0</td><td>4.0</td><td>5.3</td><td></td><td></td><td></td><td></td><td></td><td></td><td></td><td></td><td></td><td></td><td></td><td></td><td></td><td></td><td></td><td></td></tr>
<tr><td>86 10 UC</td><td></td><td></td><td></td><td></td><td></td><td></td><td></td><td></td><td></td><td></td><td></td><td colspan="6">17</td><td></td><td></td><td></td><td></td><td></td></tr>
<tr><td>92 43 UC</td><td></td><td></td><td></td><td></td><td></td><td></td><td></td><td></td><td></td><td colspan="8">17</td><td></td><td></td><td></td><td></td><td></td></tr>
<tr><td>95 50 UC</td><td></td><td></td><td colspan="2">6.8</td><td colspan="2">8.4</td><td colspan="2">12</td><td>13</td><td colspan="2">15</td><td colspan="2">16</td><td colspan="2">17</td><td colspan="2">16</td><td colspan="4">14</td><td>15</td></tr>
<tr><td>95 52 UCE</td><td></td><td colspan="3">8</td><td></td><td></td><td></td><td></td><td></td><td></td><td></td><td></td><td></td><td></td><td></td><td></td><td></td><td></td><td></td><td></td><td></td><td></td></tr>
</table>

Estonia

<table>
<tr><th rowspan="2">Product
Source
Year</th><th colspan="21">Age group</th><th rowspan="2">All ages</th></tr>
<tr><th>12</th><th>13</th><th>14</th><th>15</th><th>16</th><th>17</th><th>18</th><th>19</th><th>20-24</th><th>25-29</th><th>30-34</th><th>35-39</th><th>40-44</th><th>45-49</th><th>50-54</th><th>55-59</th><th>60-64</th><th>65-69</th><th>70-74</th><th>75-79</th><th>80+</th></tr>
<tr><td>93 58 UC</td><td></td><td></td><td colspan="2">2.6</td><td></td><td></td><td></td><td></td><td></td><td></td><td></td><td></td><td></td><td></td><td></td><td></td><td></td><td></td><td></td><td></td><td></td><td></td></tr>
<tr><td>95 19 UCE</td><td></td><td></td><td></td><td colspan="2">9.5</td><td></td><td></td><td></td><td></td><td></td><td></td><td></td><td></td><td></td><td></td><td></td><td></td><td></td><td></td><td></td><td></td><td></td></tr>
<tr><td>95 58 UC</td><td></td><td></td><td colspan="2">5.2</td><td></td><td></td><td></td><td></td><td></td><td></td><td></td><td></td><td></td><td></td><td></td><td></td><td></td><td></td><td></td><td></td><td></td><td></td></tr>
</table>

Latvia

<table>
<tr><th rowspan="2">Product
Source
Year</th><th colspan="21">Age group</th><th rowspan="2">All ages</th></tr>
<tr><th>12</th><th>13</th><th>14</th><th>15</th><th>16</th><th>17</th><th>18</th><th>19</th><th>20-24</th><th>25-29</th><th>30-34</th><th>35-39</th><th>40-44</th><th>45-49</th><th>50-54</th><th>55-59</th><th>60-64</th><th>65-69</th><th>70-74</th><th>75-79</th><th>80+</th></tr>
<tr><td>95 20 UCE</td><td></td><td></td><td></td><td colspan="2">8.2</td><td></td><td></td><td></td><td></td><td></td><td></td><td></td><td></td><td></td><td></td><td></td><td></td><td></td><td></td><td></td><td></td><td></td></tr>
</table>

Lithuania

<table>
<tr><th rowspan="2">Product
Source
Year</th><th colspan="21">Age group</th><th rowspan="2">All ages</th></tr>
<tr><th>12</th><th>13</th><th>14</th><th>15</th><th>16</th><th>17</th><th>18</th><th>19</th><th>20-24</th><th>25-29</th><th>30-34</th><th>35-39</th><th>40-44</th><th>45-49</th><th>50-54</th><th>55-59</th><th>60-64</th><th>65-69</th><th>70-74</th><th>75-79</th><th>80+</th></tr>
<tr><td>73 63 UCE</td><td></td><td></td><td></td><td></td><td></td><td></td><td></td><td></td><td></td><td></td><td></td><td></td><td></td><td colspan="3">18</td><td></td><td></td><td></td><td></td><td></td><td></td></tr>
<tr><td>84 11 UC</td><td></td><td></td><td></td><td></td><td></td><td></td><td></td><td></td><td></td><td></td><td></td><td colspan="6">13</td><td></td><td></td><td></td><td></td><td></td></tr>
<tr><td>93 67 UC</td><td></td><td></td><td></td><td></td><td></td><td></td><td></td><td></td><td></td><td></td><td></td><td colspan="6">15</td><td></td><td></td><td></td><td></td><td></td></tr>
<tr><td>95 21 UCE</td><td></td><td></td><td></td><td colspan="2">8.9</td><td></td><td></td><td></td><td></td><td></td><td></td><td></td><td></td><td></td><td></td><td></td><td></td><td></td><td></td><td></td><td></td><td></td></tr>
<tr><td>95 67 UC</td><td></td><td></td><td></td><td></td><td></td><td></td><td></td><td></td><td></td><td></td><td></td><td></td><td></td><td></td><td></td><td></td><td></td><td colspan="3">9.0</td><td></td><td></td></tr>
</table>

Ukraine, Belorussia, Moldova

<table>
<tr><th rowspan="2">Product
Source
Year</th><th colspan="21">Age group</th><th rowspan="2">All ages</th></tr>
<tr><th>12</th><th>13</th><th>14</th><th>15</th><th>16</th><th>17</th><th>18</th><th>19</th><th>20-24</th><th>25-29</th><th>30-34</th><th>35-39</th><th>40-44</th><th>45-49</th><th>50-54</th><th>55-59</th><th>60-64</th><th>65-69</th><th>70-74</th><th>75-79</th><th>80+</th></tr>
<tr><td>90 69 UC</td><td></td><td></td><td></td><td></td><td></td><td></td><td></td><td></td><td></td><td></td><td></td><td></td><td></td><td></td><td></td><td></td><td></td><td></td><td></td><td></td><td></td><td></td></tr>
<tr><td>95 22 UCE</td><td></td><td></td><td></td><td colspan="2">9.4</td><td></td><td></td><td></td><td></td><td></td><td></td><td></td><td></td><td></td><td></td><td></td><td></td><td></td><td></td><td></td><td></td><td></td></tr>
<tr><td>95 69 UC</td><td></td><td></td><td></td><td></td><td></td><td></td><td></td><td></td><td></td><td></td><td></td><td></td><td></td><td></td><td></td><td></td><td></td><td></td><td></td><td></td><td></td><td></td></tr>
</table>

No data for other regions

Source: see *Notes on sources of survey data*, p. 746

Product:
MC = manufactured cigarettes
TC = total cigarettes (including hand-rolled)
UC = cigarettes (type unspecified)
A = all products
U = unspecified

Product (cont): E indicates mean estimated from percentage distribution (see also *Consumption category estimation*, p. xxxiv, and Appendix III, p. 789)

All ages: relevant to ages used and as given in original source

* = refer to *Notes on sources of survey data*, p. 746

Table 29.5F Number of cigarettes smoked per smoker per day, females: some selected surveys for USSR and successor republics by age, 1973-1995

Russia

<table>
<tr><th rowspan="2">Product Source Year</th><th colspan="21">Age group</th><th rowspan="2">All ages</th></tr>
<tr><th>12</th><th>13</th><th>14</th><th>15</th><th>16</th><th>17</th><th>18</th><th>19</th><th>20-24</th><th>25-29</th><th>30-34</th><th>35-39</th><th>40-44</th><th>45-49</th><th>50-54</th><th>55-59</th><th>60-64</th><th>65-69</th><th>70-74</th><th>75-79</th><th>80+</th></tr>
<tr><td>75 27 UC</td><td colspan="4"></td><td colspan="4">6.1</td><td colspan="2">6.1</td><td colspan="2">12</td><td colspan="2">15</td><td colspan="2">10</td><td colspan="2">12</td><td colspan="3">12</td><td>11</td></tr>
<tr><td>85 7 UC</td><td colspan="11"></td><td colspan="6">9.0</td><td colspan="4"></td><td></td></tr>
<tr><td>85 8 UC</td><td colspan="11"></td><td colspan="6">9.0</td><td colspan="4"></td><td></td></tr>
<tr><td>85 9 UC</td><td colspan="11"></td><td colspan="6">10</td><td colspan="4"></td><td></td></tr>
<tr><td>85 34 UC</td><td>0.4</td><td>0.5</td><td>0.9</td><td>1.9</td><td>2.1</td><td>2.6</td><td colspan="15"></td><td></td></tr>
<tr><td>86 10 UC</td><td colspan="11"></td><td colspan="6">7.0</td><td colspan="4"></td><td></td></tr>
<tr><td>92 43 UC</td><td colspan="9"></td><td colspan="8">9</td><td colspan="4"></td><td></td></tr>
<tr><td>95 50 UC</td><td colspan="2"></td><td colspan="2">6.1</td><td colspan="2">5.8</td><td colspan="2">4.9</td><td>6.9</td><td colspan="2">9.0</td><td colspan="2">10</td><td colspan="2">8.4</td><td colspan="2">8.1</td><td colspan="4">9.4</td><td>8.5</td></tr>
<tr><td>95 52 UCE</td><td></td><td colspan="3">8</td><td colspan="17"></td><td></td></tr>
</table>

Estonia

<table>
<tr><th rowspan="2">Product Source Year</th><th colspan="21">Age group</th><th rowspan="2">All ages</th></tr>
<tr><th>12</th><th>13</th><th>14</th><th>15</th><th>16</th><th>17</th><th>18</th><th>19</th><th>20-24</th><th>25-29</th><th>30-34</th><th>35-39</th><th>40-44</th><th>45-49</th><th>50-54</th><th>55-59</th><th>60-64</th><th>65-69</th><th>70-74</th><th>75-79</th><th>80+</th></tr>
<tr><td>93 58 UC</td><td colspan="2"></td><td colspan="2">1.4</td><td colspan="17"></td><td></td></tr>
<tr><td>95 19 UCE</td><td colspan="3"></td><td colspan="2">7.7</td><td colspan="16"></td><td></td></tr>
<tr><td>95 58 UC</td><td colspan="2"></td><td colspan="2">3.1</td><td colspan="17"></td><td></td></tr>
</table>

Latvia

<table>
<tr><th rowspan="2">Product Source Year</th><th colspan="21">Age group</th><th rowspan="2">All ages</th></tr>
<tr><th>12</th><th>13</th><th>14</th><th>15</th><th>16</th><th>17</th><th>18</th><th>19</th><th>20-24</th><th>25-29</th><th>30-34</th><th>35-39</th><th>40-44</th><th>45-49</th><th>50-54</th><th>55-59</th><th>60-64</th><th>65-69</th><th>70-74</th><th>75-79</th><th>80+</th></tr>
<tr><td>95 20 UCE</td><td colspan="3"></td><td colspan="2">6.2</td><td colspan="16"></td><td></td></tr>
</table>

Lithuania

<table>
<tr><th rowspan="2">Product Source Year</th><th colspan="21">Age group</th><th rowspan="2">All ages</th></tr>
<tr><th>12</th><th>13</th><th>14</th><th>15</th><th>16</th><th>17</th><th>18</th><th>19</th><th>20-24</th><th>25-29</th><th>30-34</th><th>35-39</th><th>40-44</th><th>45-49</th><th>50-54</th><th>55-59</th><th>60-64</th><th>65-69</th><th>70-74</th><th>75-79</th><th>80+</th></tr>
<tr><td>73 63 UCE</td><td colspan="21"></td><td></td></tr>
<tr><td>84 11 UC</td><td colspan="11"></td><td colspan="6">8.0</td><td colspan="4"></td><td></td></tr>
<tr><td>93 67 UC</td><td colspan="11"></td><td colspan="6">8.1</td><td colspan="4"></td><td></td></tr>
<tr><td>95 21 UCE</td><td colspan="3"></td><td colspan="2">4.8</td><td colspan="16"></td><td></td></tr>
<tr><td>95 67 UC</td><td colspan="17"></td><td colspan="3">9.7</td><td></td><td></td></tr>
</table>

Ukraine, Belorussia, Moldova

<table>
<tr><th rowspan="2">Product Source Year</th><th colspan="21">Age group</th><th rowspan="2">All ages</th></tr>
<tr><th>12</th><th>13</th><th>14</th><th>15</th><th>16</th><th>17</th><th>18</th><th>19</th><th>20-24</th><th>25-29</th><th>30-34</th><th>35-39</th><th>40-44</th><th>45-49</th><th>50-54</th><th>55-59</th><th>60-64</th><th>65-69</th><th>70-74</th><th>75-79</th><th>80+</th></tr>
<tr><td>90 69 UC</td><td colspan="3"></td><td colspan="18">6.2</td><td></td></tr>
<tr><td>95 22 UCE</td><td colspan="3"></td><td colspan="2">7.0</td><td colspan="16"></td><td></td></tr>
<tr><td>95 69 UC</td><td colspan="3"></td><td colspan="18">8.5</td><td></td></tr>
</table>

No data for other regions

Source: see *Notes on sources of survey data*, p. 746

Product:
- MC = manufactured cigarettes
- TC = total cigarettes (including hand-rolled)
- UC = cigarettes (type unspecified)
- A = all products
- U = unspecified

Product (cont): E indicates mean estimated from percentage distribution (see also *Consumption category estimation*, p. xxxiv, and Appendix III, p. 789)

All ages: relevant to ages used and as given in original source

* = refer to *Notes on sources of survey data*, p. 746

Table 29.6M Number of cigarettes smoked per person per day, males: some selected surveys for USSR and successor republics by age, 1973-1995, with percentage total sales

Russia

<table>
<tr><th rowspan="2">Product Source Year</th><th colspan="21">Age group</th><th rowspan="2">All ages</th><th rowspan="2">% Total sales</th></tr>
<tr><th>12</th><th>13</th><th>14</th><th>15</th><th>16</th><th>17</th><th>18</th><th>19</th><th>20-24</th><th>25-29</th><th>30-34</th><th>35-39</th><th>40-44</th><th>45-49</th><th>50-54</th><th>55-59</th><th>60-64</th><th>65-69</th><th>70-74</th><th>75-79</th><th>80+</th></tr>
<tr><td>75 27 UC</td><td colspan="4"></td><td colspan="4">2.3</td><td colspan="2">9.2</td><td colspan="2">10</td><td colspan="2">8.4</td><td colspan="2">6.7</td><td colspan="2">6.1</td><td colspan="3">2.8</td><td>7.3</td><td>78%M</td></tr>
<tr><td>85 7 UC *</td><td colspan="11"></td><td colspan="6">8.3</td><td colspan="4"></td><td></td><td>**</td></tr>
<tr><td>85 8 UC *</td><td colspan="11"></td><td colspan="6">8.2</td><td colspan="4"></td><td></td><td>**</td></tr>
<tr><td>85 9 UC *</td><td colspan="11"></td><td colspan="6">9.1</td><td colspan="4"></td><td></td><td>**</td></tr>
<tr><td>85 34 UC</td><td>0.1</td><td>0.2</td><td>0.3</td><td>0.9</td><td>0.8</td><td>2.3</td><td colspan="15"></td><td></td><td>**</td></tr>
<tr><td>86 10 UC *</td><td colspan="11"></td><td colspan="6">10</td><td colspan="4"></td><td></td><td>**</td></tr>
<tr><td>92 43 UC</td><td colspan="9"></td><td colspan="8">11</td><td colspan="4"></td><td></td><td>**</td></tr>
<tr><td>95 50 UC</td><td colspan="2"></td><td colspan="2">1.3</td><td colspan="2">4.1</td><td colspan="2">6.3</td><td>8.4</td><td colspan="2">11</td><td colspan="2">11</td><td colspan="2">11</td><td colspan="2">8.2</td><td colspan="4">4.7</td><td>8.9</td><td>92%M</td></tr>
<tr><td>95 52 UC</td><td></td><td colspan="3">2</td><td colspan="17"></td><td></td><td>**</td></tr>
</table>

Estonia

<table>
<tr><th rowspan="2">Product Source Year</th><th colspan="21">Age group</th><th rowspan="2">All ages</th><th rowspan="2">% Total sales</th></tr>
<tr><th>12</th><th>13</th><th>14</th><th>15</th><th>16</th><th>17</th><th>18</th><th>19</th><th>20-24</th><th>25-29</th><th>30-34</th><th>35-39</th><th>40-44</th><th>45-49</th><th>50-54</th><th>55-59</th><th>60-64</th><th>65-69</th><th>70-74</th><th>75-79</th><th>80+</th></tr>
<tr><td>93 58 UC</td><td colspan="2"></td><td colspan="2">0.7</td><td colspan="17"></td><td></td><td>**</td></tr>
<tr><td>95 19 UC</td><td colspan="3"></td><td colspan="2">2.5</td><td colspan="16"></td><td></td><td>**</td></tr>
<tr><td>95 58 UC</td><td colspan="2"></td><td colspan="2">1.3</td><td colspan="17"></td><td></td><td>**</td></tr>
</table>

Latvia

<table>
<tr><th rowspan="2">Product Source Year</th><th colspan="21">Age group</th><th rowspan="2">All ages</th><th rowspan="2">% Total sales</th></tr>
<tr><th>12</th><th>13</th><th>14</th><th>15</th><th>16</th><th>17</th><th>18</th><th>19</th><th>20-24</th><th>25-29</th><th>30-34</th><th>35-39</th><th>40-44</th><th>45-49</th><th>50-54</th><th>55-59</th><th>60-64</th><th>65-69</th><th>70-74</th><th>75-79</th><th>80+</th></tr>
<tr><td>95 20 UC</td><td colspan="3"></td><td colspan="2">2.1</td><td colspan="16"></td><td></td><td>**</td></tr>
</table>

Lithuania

<table>
<tr><th rowspan="2">Product Source Year</th><th colspan="21">Age group</th><th rowspan="2">All ages</th><th rowspan="2">% Total sales</th></tr>
<tr><th>12</th><th>13</th><th>14</th><th>15</th><th>16</th><th>17</th><th>18</th><th>19</th><th>20-24</th><th>25-29</th><th>30-34</th><th>35-39</th><th>40-44</th><th>45-49</th><th>50-54</th><th>55-59</th><th>60-64</th><th>65-69</th><th>70-74</th><th>75-79</th><th>80+</th></tr>
<tr><td>73 63 UC</td><td colspan="13"></td><td colspan="3">8.7</td><td colspan="5"></td><td></td><td>**</td></tr>
<tr><td>84 11 UC *</td><td colspan="11"></td><td colspan="6">5.0</td><td colspan="4"></td><td></td><td>**</td></tr>
<tr><td>93 67 UC</td><td colspan="11"></td><td colspan="6">5.2</td><td colspan="4"></td><td></td><td>**</td></tr>
<tr><td>95 21 UC</td><td colspan="3"></td><td colspan="2">1.9</td><td colspan="16"></td><td></td><td>**</td></tr>
<tr><td>95 67 UC</td><td colspan="17"></td><td colspan="3">1.5</td><td></td><td></td><td>**</td></tr>
</table>

Ukraine, Belorussia, Moldova

<table>
<tr><th rowspan="2">Product Source Year</th><th colspan="21">Age group</th><th rowspan="2">All ages</th><th rowspan="2">% Total sales</th></tr>
<tr><th>12</th><th>13</th><th>14</th><th>15</th><th>16</th><th>17</th><th>18</th><th>19</th><th>20-24</th><th>25-29</th><th>30-34</th><th>35-39</th><th>40-44</th><th>45-49</th><th>50-54</th><th>55-59</th><th>60-64</th><th>65-69</th><th>70-74</th><th>75-79</th><th>80+</th></tr>
<tr><td>90 69 UC</td><td colspan="21"></td><td></td><td>**</td></tr>
<tr><td>95 22 UC</td><td colspan="3"></td><td colspan="2">3.6</td><td colspan="16"></td><td></td><td>**</td></tr>
<tr><td>95 69 UC</td><td colspan="21"></td><td></td><td>**</td></tr>
</table>

No data for other regions

Source: see *Notes on sources of survey data*, p. 746
Product: MC = manufactured cigarettes
TC = total cigarettes (including hand-rolled)
UC = cigarettes (type unspecified)
A = all products
U = unspecified

All ages: relevant to ages used and as given in original source
% Total sales: estimated % of total sales of M = manufactured or T = total cigarette consumption implied by survey, sexes combined
** = cannot be calculated
--- = adjusted by original author
* = refer to *Notes on sources of survey data*, p. 746

Table 29.6F Number of cigarettes smoked per person per day, females: some selected surveys for USSR and successor republics by age, 1973-1995, with percentage total sales

Russia

<table>
<tr><th rowspan="2">Product Source Year</th><th colspan="21">Age group</th><th rowspan="2">All ages</th><th rowspan="2">% Total sales</th></tr>
<tr><th>12</th><th>13</th><th>14</th><th>15</th><th>16</th><th>17</th><th>18</th><th>19</th><th>20-24</th><th>25-29</th><th>30-34</th><th>35-39</th><th>40-44</th><th>45-49</th><th>50-54</th><th>55-59</th><th>60-64</th><th>65-69</th><th>70-74</th><th>75-79</th><th>80+</th></tr>
<tr><td>75 27 UC</td><td colspan="4"></td><td colspan="4">0.5</td><td colspan="2">1.0</td><td colspan="2">2.2</td><td colspan="2">1.2</td><td colspan="2">0.7</td><td colspan="2">1.3</td><td colspan="3">0.7</td><td>1.1</td><td>78%M</td></tr>
<tr><td>85 7 UC *</td><td colspan="11"></td><td colspan="6">0.8</td><td colspan="4"></td><td></td><td>**</td></tr>
<tr><td>85 8 UC *</td><td colspan="11"></td><td colspan="6">1.1</td><td colspan="4"></td><td></td><td>**</td></tr>
<tr><td>85 9 UC *</td><td colspan="11"></td><td colspan="6">0.3</td><td colspan="4"></td><td></td><td>**</td></tr>
<tr><td>85 34 UC</td><td>0.0</td><td>0.0</td><td>0.0</td><td>0.1</td><td>0.2</td><td>0.5</td><td colspan="15"></td><td></td><td>**</td></tr>
<tr><td>86 10 UC *</td><td colspan="11"></td><td colspan="6">0.2</td><td colspan="4"></td><td></td><td>**</td></tr>
<tr><td>92 43 UC</td><td colspan="9"></td><td colspan="8">1.0</td><td colspan="4"></td><td></td><td>**</td></tr>
<tr><td>95 50 UC</td><td colspan="2"></td><td colspan="2">0.5</td><td colspan="2">0.4</td><td colspan="2">0.9</td><td>1.3</td><td colspan="2">1.5</td><td colspan="2">1.1</td><td colspan="2">0.7</td><td colspan="2">0.2</td><td colspan="4">0.1</td><td>0.8</td><td>92%M</td></tr>
<tr><td>95 52 UC</td><td></td><td colspan="3">3</td><td colspan="17"></td><td></td><td>**</td></tr>
</table>

Estonia

<table>
<tr><th rowspan="2">Product Source Year</th><th colspan="21">Age group</th><th rowspan="2">All ages</th><th rowspan="2">% Total sales</th></tr>
<tr><th>12</th><th>13</th><th>14</th><th>15</th><th>16</th><th>17</th><th>18</th><th>19</th><th>20-24</th><th>25-29</th><th>30-34</th><th>35-39</th><th>40-44</th><th>45-49</th><th>50-54</th><th>55-59</th><th>60-64</th><th>65-69</th><th>70-74</th><th>75-79</th><th>80+</th></tr>
<tr><td>93 58 UC</td><td colspan="2"></td><td colspan="2">0.2</td><td colspan="17"></td><td></td><td>**</td></tr>
<tr><td>95 19 UC</td><td colspan="3"></td><td colspan="2">1.0</td><td colspan="16"></td><td></td><td>**</td></tr>
<tr><td>95 58 UC</td><td colspan="2"></td><td colspan="2">0.5</td><td colspan="17"></td><td></td><td>**</td></tr>
</table>

Latvia

<table>
<tr><th rowspan="2">Product Source Year</th><th colspan="21">Age group</th><th rowspan="2">All ages</th><th rowspan="2">% Total sales</th></tr>
<tr><th>12</th><th>13</th><th>14</th><th>15</th><th>16</th><th>17</th><th>18</th><th>19</th><th>20-24</th><th>25-29</th><th>30-34</th><th>35-39</th><th>40-44</th><th>45-49</th><th>50-54</th><th>55-59</th><th>60-64</th><th>65-69</th><th>70-74</th><th>75-79</th><th>80+</th></tr>
<tr><td>95 20 UC</td><td colspan="3"></td><td colspan="2">0.8</td><td colspan="16"></td><td></td><td>**</td></tr>
</table>

Lithuania

<table>
<tr><th rowspan="2">Product Source Year</th><th colspan="21">Age group</th><th rowspan="2">All ages</th><th rowspan="2">% Total sales</th></tr>
<tr><th>12</th><th>13</th><th>14</th><th>15</th><th>16</th><th>17</th><th>18</th><th>19</th><th>20-24</th><th>25-29</th><th>30-34</th><th>35-39</th><th>40-44</th><th>45-49</th><th>50-54</th><th>55-59</th><th>60-64</th><th>65-69</th><th>70-74</th><th>75-79</th><th>80+</th></tr>
<tr><td>73 63 UC</td><td colspan="21"></td><td></td><td>**</td></tr>
<tr><td>84 11 UC *</td><td colspan="11"></td><td colspan="6">0.3</td><td colspan="4"></td><td></td><td>**</td></tr>
<tr><td>93 67 UC</td><td colspan="11"></td><td colspan="6">0.4</td><td colspan="4"></td><td></td><td>**</td></tr>
<tr><td>95 21 UC</td><td colspan="3"></td><td colspan="2">0.4</td><td colspan="16"></td><td></td><td>**</td></tr>
<tr><td>95 67 UC</td><td colspan="17"></td><td colspan="3">0.2</td><td></td><td></td><td>**</td></tr>
</table>

Ukraine, Belorussia, Moldova

<table>
<tr><th rowspan="2">Product Source Year</th><th colspan="21">Age group</th><th rowspan="2">All ages</th><th rowspan="2">% Total sales</th></tr>
<tr><th>12</th><th>13</th><th>14</th><th>15</th><th>16</th><th>17</th><th>18</th><th>19</th><th>20-24</th><th>25-29</th><th>30-34</th><th>35-39</th><th>40-44</th><th>45-49</th><th>50-54</th><th>55-59</th><th>60-64</th><th>65-69</th><th>70-74</th><th>75-79</th><th>80+</th></tr>
<tr><td>90 69 UC</td><td colspan="3"></td><td colspan="18">0.3</td><td></td><td>**</td></tr>
<tr><td>95 22 UC</td><td colspan="3"></td><td colspan="2">1.0</td><td colspan="16"></td><td></td><td>**</td></tr>
<tr><td>95 69 UC</td><td colspan="3"></td><td colspan="18">1.7</td><td></td><td>**</td></tr>
</table>

No data for other regions

Source: see *Notes on sources of survey data*, p. 746
Product: MC = manufactured cigarettes
TC = total cigarettes (including hand-rolled)
UC = cigarettes (type unspecified)
A = all products
U = unspecified

All ages: relevant to ages used and as given in original source
% Total sales: estimated % of total sales of M = manufactured or T = total cigarette consumption implied by survey, sexes combined
** = cannot be calculated
--- = adjusted by original author
* = refer to *Notes on sources of survey data*, p. 746

Table 29.7M Number of cigarettes smoked per person per day, sales-adjusted, males: some selected surveys for USSR and successor republics[1] by age, 1975-1995, with percentage total sales

Russia

<table>
<tr><th rowspan="2">Product
Source
Year</th><th colspan="21">Age group</th><th rowspan="2">All ages</th><th rowspan="2">% Total sales</th></tr>
<tr><th>12</th><th>13</th><th>14</th><th>15</th><th>16</th><th>17</th><th>18</th><th>19</th><th>20-24</th><th>25-29</th><th>30-34</th><th>35-39</th><th>40-44</th><th>45-49</th><th>50-54</th><th>55-59</th><th>60-64</th><th>65-69</th><th>70-74</th><th>75-79</th><th>80+</th></tr>
<tr><td>75 27 UC</td><td colspan="8">2.9</td><td colspan="2">12</td><td colspan="2">13</td><td colspan="2">11</td><td colspan="2">8.6</td><td colspan="2">7.8</td><td colspan="3">3.6</td><td>9.3</td><td>78%M</td></tr>
<tr><td>95 50 UC</td><td colspan="2"></td><td colspan="2">1.4</td><td colspan="2">4.5</td><td colspan="2">6.9</td><td>9.1</td><td colspan="2">12</td><td colspan="2">12</td><td colspan="2">12</td><td colspan="2">9.0</td><td colspan="4">5.1</td><td>9.7</td><td>92%M</td></tr>
</table>

Table 29.7F Number of cigarettes smoked per person per day, sales-adjusted, females: some selected surveys for USSR and successor republics[1] by age, 1975-1995, with percentage total sales

Russia

<table>
<tr><th rowspan="2">Product
Source
Year</th><th colspan="21">Age group</th><th rowspan="2">All ages</th><th rowspan="2">% Total sales</th></tr>
<tr><th>12</th><th>13</th><th>14</th><th>15</th><th>16</th><th>17</th><th>18</th><th>19</th><th>20-24</th><th>25-29</th><th>30-34</th><th>35-39</th><th>40-44</th><th>45-49</th><th>50-54</th><th>55-59</th><th>60-64</th><th>65-69</th><th>70-74</th><th>75-79</th><th>80+</th></tr>
<tr><td>75 27 UC</td><td colspan="8">0.6</td><td colspan="2">1.3</td><td colspan="2">2.8</td><td colspan="2">1.6</td><td colspan="2">0.8</td><td colspan="2">1.6</td><td colspan="3">0.9</td><td>1.4</td><td>78%M</td></tr>
<tr><td>95 50 UC</td><td colspan="2"></td><td colspan="2">0.5</td><td colspan="2">0.4</td><td colspan="2">0.9</td><td>1.5</td><td colspan="2">1.7</td><td colspan="2">1.2</td><td colspan="2">0.8</td><td colspan="2">0.2</td><td colspan="4">0.1</td><td>0.8</td><td>92%M</td></tr>
</table>

1 Based on those surveys in Table 29.6 with data for both sexes and age range at least 21-64 (see also *Cigarette consumption per person*, p. xxxv). See also footnote 8 of Table 29.8. No data for other regions

Source: See *Notes on sources of survey data*, p. 746

Product:
- MC = manufactured cigarettes
- TC = total cigarettes (including hand-rolled)
- UC = cigarettes (type unspecified)
- A = all products
- U = unspecified

All ages: relevant to ages used and as given in original source

% Total sales: Adjustment factor used, estimated % of total sales of M = manufactured or T = total cigarette consumption implied by survey, sexes combined

--- = adjusted by original author

* = refer to *Notes on sources of survey data*, p. 746

Table 29.8 Estimated[1] prevalence of smoking and estimated[1] number of cigarettes per person per day (unadjusted and sales-adjusted): summary of Tables 29.4, 29.6 and 29.7, 1963-1995.
Males and females aged 15 years and over

Year	Source[2]	Product[3]	Prevalence[4]						Number of cigarettes						
									Unadjusted[7]			Sales-adjusted[8]			
			Manufactured cigarettes		Total cigarettes[5]		All products[6]		Number/ person/day		Total sales %	Manufactured cigarettes[9] number/ person/day		Total cigarettes number/ person/day	
			M	F	M	F	M	F	M	F		M	F	M	F
Russia															
1975	27	*UC*			47	11			7.1	1.1	78	9.1	1.4		
	28	*U*					60	9				(9.4	1.2)		
1981	31	*U*					54	6				(10.2	0.9)		
1985	35	*U*					53	10				(9.3	1.4)		
1986	36	*U*					79	14				(9.4	1.3)		
1989	12	*U*					44	10				(8.3	1.5)		
1991	38	*U*						25							
1992	39	*U*					69	8				(8.7	0.8)		
	45	*U*					61	17				(7.6	1.7)		
1993	48	*U*					67	30				(6.8	2.4)		
1995	50	*UC+A*			59	9	59	9	9.1	0.8	92	9.9	0.9		
	53	*U*					66								
Estonia															
1990	55	U					44	15				(7.1	1.9)		
1992	13	*U*					49	20				(7.5	2.5)		
1994	60	U					51	24				(7.4	2.7)		
Latvia															
1993	62	U					67	12				(8.4	1.2)		
Lithuania															
1992	14	*U*					52	10				(8.4	1.3)		
Ukraine, Belorussia, Moldova															
1990	69	UC+*U*						5		0.3					
1995	69	UC+*U*						20		1.7					
	23	*U*					60	12				(9.8	1.6)		
	24	*U*					46	7				(7.8	0.9)		
Armenia, Azerbaijan, Georgia															
1960	70	*UC*			78	7									
	71	*UC*			78	8									
1963	72	*UC*			69	5									

Table 29.8 *(continued)*

Year	Source[2]	Product[3]	Prevalence[4]						Number of cigarettes							
									Unadjusted[7]			Sales-adjusted[8]				
			Manufactured cigarettes		Total cigarettes[5]		All products[6]		Number/ person/day		Total sales %	Manufactured cigarettes[9] number/ person/day		Total cigarettes number/ person/day		
			M	F	M	F	M	F	M	F		M	F	M	F	
Central Asia																
1989	79	**UC**			40	1						(4.6	0.1)			
	80	**UC**			50	3										
1991	81	*U*					27	0.5				(13.6	0.2)			
1993	82	*U*					49	9				(7.0	1.0)			
1995	25	*U*					54	17				(5.9	1.5)			
	26	*U*					47	2				(7.1	0.3)			
Multiple/unspecified region																
1977	83	*U*					49	18				(9.7	2.9)			
1981	84	*U*					65	6				(12.0	0.9)			
1984	86	*U*					48	11				(10.8	2.0)			

1 Surveys covering an age range of at least 21-64 are included. Any gaps in the data for ages 15-20 and 65 years and over are filled in by assumed extensions to the age distribution, given in *Notes on sources of survey data*, p. 746. Method: see *Summary of adult smoking*, p. xxxvi
2 See *Notes on sources of survey data*, p. 746
3 Product: MC = manufactured cigarettes, TC = total cigarettes (including hand-rolled), UC = cigarettes (type unspecified), A = all products, U = unspecified. Frequency of smoking is indicated by: regular or daily smokers in normal type, all smokers (including occasional) in bold, unspecified in italics
4 From Table 29.4
5 This column includes prevalence of smoking classified as UC = cigarettes (type unspecified)
6 This column includes prevalence of smoking classified as U = unspecified product
7 From Table 29.6
8 From Table 29.7, except data in parentheses, which are derived from the prevalence of smoking from Table 29.4 as described in *Summary of adult smoking*, p. xxxvi. Adjustment is to sales in the individual republic; except for *Multiple/unspecified* region where adjustment is to USSR sales. Adjustment is to nearest available year. Since the earliest available sales data for the individual republics is 1988, no adjustment has been done for surveys before 1975. Sales per adult in USSR were stable in the period 1975-1988 (see Table 29.2)
9 Number of cigarettes classified as UC = cigarettes (type unspecified) or U = product unspecified has been adjusted to manufactured cigarette sales and included in this column

Figure 29.3 Estimated prevalence of smoking, Russia: by year of survey, 1975-1995. Males and females aged 15 years and over. *Source:* see Table 29.8

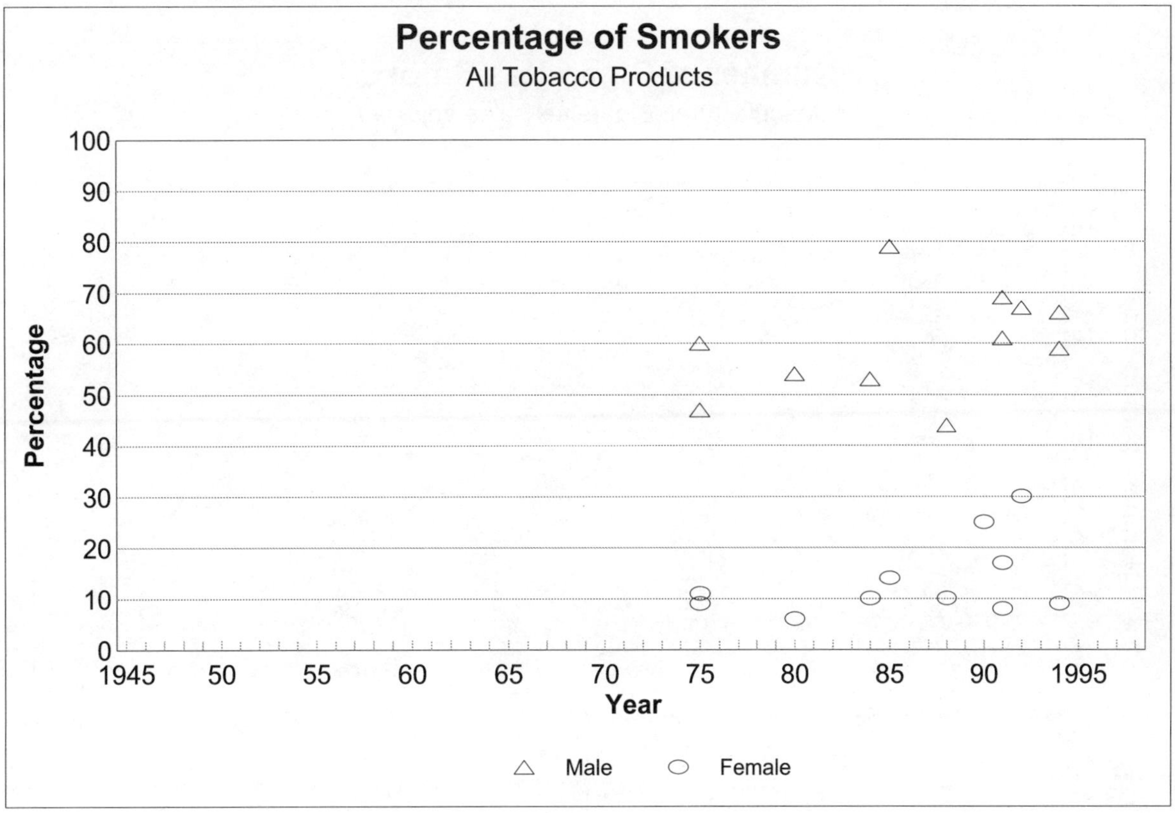

Note : Prevalence data for cigarettes and for all products have been combined here

Figure 29.4 Estimated number of cigarettes smoked per person per day, sales-adjusted, Russia 1975-1995.
Males and females aged 15 years and over. *Source:* see Table 29.8

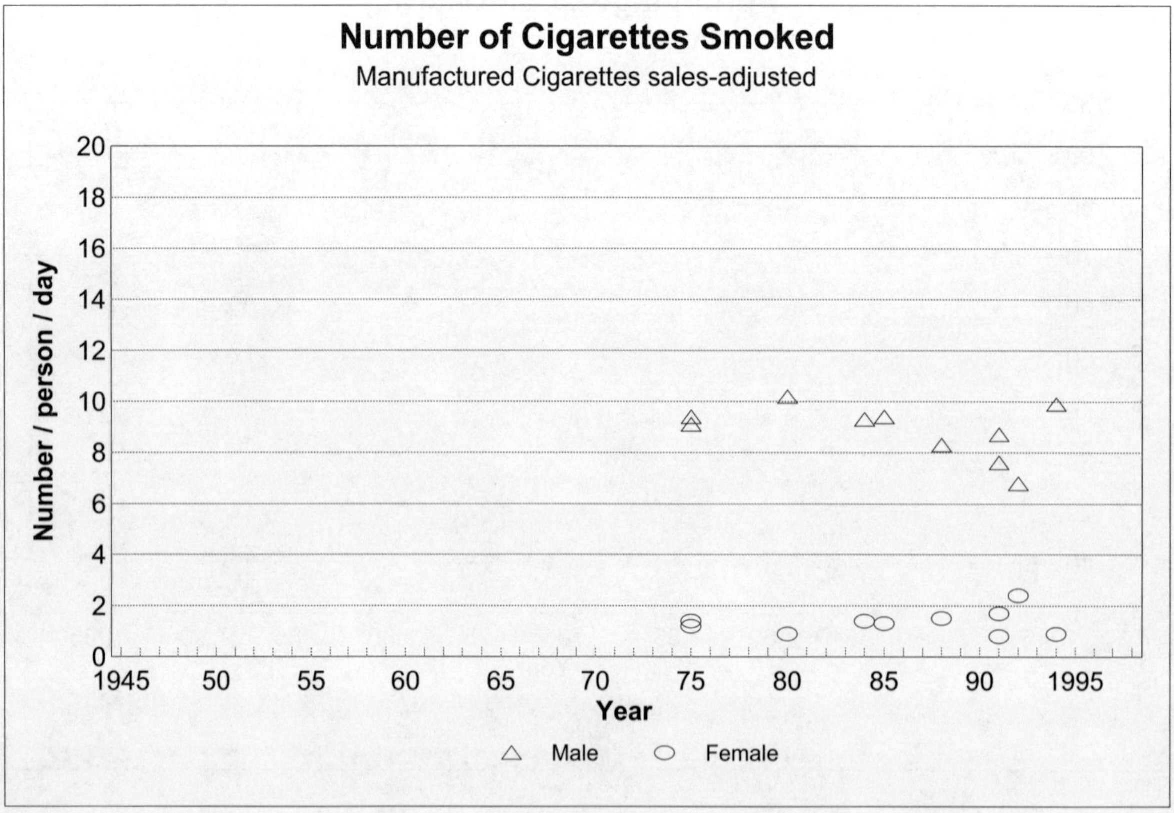

Notes on sources of sales data

The data presented in the tables and figures were obtained from several sources, details of which are given below, together with estimations and related assumptions. Full citations of the sources are given on p. 754 under *References*.

Consumption data for Latvia, 1921-1935

Hutson (1937)

Data, originally given to the nearest 1 000 pounds, have been converted to tonnes and given to the nearest tonne (1 000 lbs = 0.45359 tonnes).

It is also reported that consumption in Lithuania was about 900 tonnes. Papyrosi were the main cigarette type, but conventional cigarettes with light tobacco were also used. Home-grown tobacco was also used in pipes. Production in Estonia was 1 000 million papyrosi and 200 tonnes of smoking tobacco.

Consumption data for USSR and Former Soviet Union (overall), 1960-1994 (Table 29.2)

Zaridze *et al* (1986), United States Department of Agriculture (USDA) Economic Research Service (1996)

Data given for USSR after the break-up of the union represents a total of the data for the individual states of the former Soviet Union, as calculated by the USDA.

Values for cigarettes are the total of western type cigarettes and papyrosi. Papyrosi are traditional Russian cigarettes with a hollow paper tube filled one-third with tobacco (Cooper (1982)). The weights of tobacco are estimated as 0.57 g per papyrosi, 1.13 g per non-filter cigarette and 0.91 g per filter cigarette (USDA (1978)). The approximate percentage of total cigarettes represented by papyrosi is as follows (USDA (1978)):

Year range	Papyrosi (%)
1959-1963	75
1964-1967	72
1968-1970	64
1971-1973	54
1974-1977	44
1978-1980	36

Using these percentages and assuming 30% papyrosi for subsequent years, and assuming an average weight of 1 g per western type cigarette and 0.57 g per papyrosi, we derived the following estimates of the average weight of a cigarette, for conversion from numbers of cigarettes to weights:

Year range	Average weight of a cigarette, g
1959-1963	0.68
1964-1967	0.69
1968-1970	0.72
1971-1973	0.77
1974-1977	0.81
1978-1980	0.85
1981-1995	0.87

Other tobacco products are no longer smoked in any quantity. For example, Russian consumption of makhorka (dark tobacco) for rolling fell from 3 100 tonnes (less than 2% of total tobacco consumption) in 1988 to 364 tonnes in 1993 (Anonymous (1994)). As no other data are available, other products have not been included in the tables, and the column 'All tobacco products' in Table 29.2 represents the estimated weight of cigarettes.

Consumption data for individual republics for 1988 onwards (Table 29.1.2)

USDA Foreign Agricultural Service (1993) and subsequent USDA data

Data are given for all the successor republics for which data are available.

Cigarette smuggling has become a significant problem in recent years in former Soviet Union countries. According to the Russian State Customs Committee, in 1996-1997 up to 80% of imported cigarettes on the Russian market were of contraband provenance (BBC Monitoring International Reports (2000)). The federal tax police service estimate that in 1999 illegal turnover varied between 20% and 40%, depending on region

Anonymous (2000). In Estonia tax banderoles were introduced in 1995 to address smuggling which was said to account for 80% of the cigarettes in the country (Glogan (1995)). In Kyrgyzstan in 1997, illegal imports were said to account for 90% of total cigarette imports (Razgulyaev (1997)).

However, consumption in some republics has reduced sharply due to production shortages and lack of money among the population. According to Horne (1993), demand for cigarettes in Russia in 1993 was much higher than the volume available, potentially being twice that available. The average person could not afford international brands. Consumption in Azerbaijan is said to have declined due to deep recession and sharp declines in consumer purchasing power. Only Moldova exported any cigarettes during 1988-1993 (USDA Foreign Agricultural Service (1993)).

Plain/Filter cigarette consumption

USDA (1978), Zaridze *et al* (1986), USDA Economic Research Service (1996), Anonymous (1994)
Except for the data for Ukraine, these represent the percentage of production rather than of consumption. This measure becomes less representative for recent years when increasing importation of western brands has taken place.

Tar yield of cigarettes

In the 1980s, smoke analysis of 39 brands of cigarettes from factories in the USSR found that tar levels were in the range 19-29 mg per cigarette and nicotine levels 1.0-1.8 mg per cigarette (Zaridze *et al* (1986)).

Franceschi and Naett (1995) state that in Moldova cigarettes are considered high quality when they do not have more than 25 mg tar and 1.3 mg nicotine; and that the average cigarette in Lithuania has 30 mg tar.

The tar yield per cigarette is limited in Uzbekistan to 12 mg, and in Lithuania to 20 mg from 1998, 15 mg from 2000 and 12 mg from 2007; nicotine yield is limited in Uzbekistan to 1.0 mg (Harkin *et al* (1997)).

Estimates of hand-rolled cigarette consumption

No estimates of hand-rolled cigarette consumption in the USSR have been made. However, based on sales of makhora (see above) and assuming 1 g per cigarette, consumption was 0.06 cigarettes per adult per day in Russia in 1988, and reduced still further in later years.

Notes on sources of survey data

Each source of survey data—either an individual survey or a series of surveys repeated over a number of years—is cited by a source number. This number is shown in the tables and corresponds to the source numbers given below, where details of the source publication and of the survey methodology are given. Full citations of the sources are given on p. 754 under *References*. Tables 29-4-29.8 are subdivided into regions, with the final section containing results based on multiple or unspecified regions. Source numbers 1-26 are used for sources for which results are presented in more than one region.

Source number

1-6 Burenkov and Glasunov (1982)

a. Records of the programme for the multifactorial prophylaxis of ischemic heart disease of the All-Union Cardiological Scientific Centre. Year unknown.
1 Moscow; **2** Kaunas, Lithuania; **3** Minsk, Belorussia; **4** Kharkov, Ukraine; **5** Tashkent, Uzbekistan; **6** Frunze, Kirgizia

b. The Moscow and Kaunas studies were also reported by Oleinikov *et al* (1983), Zaridze *et al* (1986). Random samples of the non-institutionalized male population.

		Sample size	**Response rate (%)**
1	Moscow	3 966	66
2	Kaunas	5 482	69

7-11 WHO (1989), WHO MONICA Project (1988)

a. Regional surveys forming part of WHO MONICA project:

	Region	Population size	Sample size	Participation rate (%)	Sample used: Males	Sample used: Females	Date
7	Moscow (intervention)	227 600	3 598	67	1 163	1 234	Jan 1984-Oct 1986
8	Moscow (control)	88 300	1 825	78	770	645	Feb 1984-Feb 1986
9	Novosibirsk (intervention)	46 400	1 720	73	801*	822*	Mar 1985-Jan 1986
10	Novosibirsk (control)	144 000	3 045	69	1 403*	1 417*	Oct 1985-Mar 1986
11	Kaunas	138 200	2 086	69	728	735	Jan 1983–Mar 1985

* Novosibirsk 'sample used' includes age 25-34; all other figures are for age 35-64 only

b. *All ages* column relates only to age 35-64 and is standardized to world population

c. Regular cigarette smokers: smoked cigarettes daily. All smokers: smoked cigarettes daily or occasionally, or smoked 1 g pipe tobacco or 1 cigar per week. Cigarettes per smoker refers to regular and occasional cigarette smokers

d. Calculation for cigarettes per person based on % regular cigarette smokers and cigarettes per regular or occasional cigarette smoker, so may underestimate

12-14 Piha *et al* (1993) quoting WHO

a. No original sources. Age group not stated. Some results may be based on regional studies, with small sample sizes and variable definitions of smoking.
12 Russia; **13** Estonia; **14** Lithuania

b. It was also reported that the prevalence of smoking in Latvia was 35% for sexes combined

15-18 Kalnins *et al* (1995), King and Coles (1992), King *et al* (1996)

a. Part of the HBSC (Health Behaviour in School-Aged Children) Study, a collaborative cross-national research study sponsored by the WHO. School classes or schools were randomly selected, targeting age groups 11 (not presented here), 13 and 15. The target sample size was 1 300 in each age group

b. For Latvia 1990 the sample size was (males) 1 293, (females) 1 715.
For the 1993-94 surveys:

	15 Russia (St Petersburg region)		**16** Estonia		**17** Latvia		**18** Lithuania	
Target age	**Mean age**	**Sample size**	**Mean age**	**Sample size**	**Mean age**	**Sample size**	**Mean age**	**Sample size**
13	13.1	1 294	13.3	1 167	13.7	1 248	13.3	1 886
15	15	1 354	15.3	1 179	15.7	1 263	15.2	1 759

c. Regular smokers: smoke once a week or more

19-22 Hibell *et al* (1997)

a. Nationally representative surveys in Estonia, Latvia, Lithuania and Ukraine forming part of ESPAD (European School Survey Project on Alcohol and Other Drugs). Target was pupils born in 1979, thus age 15-16 at time of survey in March/April 1995 (except Latvia, May 1995). Anonymous questionnaire completed and sealed in envelope by pupil, in class. Teachers present, but discouraged from walking round the classroom, (except Ukraine, where teachers were usually absent, but school administration sometimes present).

		% target group still in school	Sample size: Males	Sample size: Females	Response rate (%): Males	Response rate (%): Females
19	**Estonia**	90	1 438	1 680	82	84
20	**Latvia**	—	2 179		—	
21	**Lithuania**	96	1 502	1 694	88	90
22	**Ukraine**	70	3 332	3 861	93	

b. Results for Latvia are not fully comparable with other countries due to a high level of non-participating classes and some methodological differences. Results for Ukraine should be treated with caution due to a high level of inconsistency, and high truancy rates

c. Regular smokers: smoked 1 or more cigarettes per day in last 30 days. All smokers: smoked in last 30 days

d. Consumption category estimation based on 1-5, 6-10, 11-20, 21+ cigarettes/smoker/day

23-26 Ioffina *et al* (1999) quoting Seenev (1996)

a. Years not stated. Age groups not stated (adult).
23 Ukraine; **24** Moldavia; **25** Kazakhstan; **26** Tashkent, Uzbekistan

27 Oleinikov *et al* (1981)

a. Postal questionnaire in Moscow. Response rate for households 60%. Sample size (households) 966, (males) 1 236, (females) 1 440

b. Year given by Zaridze *et al* (1986)

c. Assumed extension to age distribution for percentage smokers, age 15: males 20% and females 5%. Number of cigarettes/person/day: males 1.0 and females 0.1

28 Loransky (1977)

a. Survey by Central Institute for Scientific Research in Health Education of the USSR Ministry of Health. Results presented are for Moscow. Age group not stated

b. Results for other regions not available, but were described as showing that smoking varied by region, and that the prevalence of smoking among women was 3.5 to 11 times lower than among men

29 Chazova *et al* (1989)

a. Study carried out within the framework of the Study on Multifactorial Prevention of CHD in a district of Moscow. Representative sample

30 Burenkov and Glasunov (1982)

a. Study by All-Union Cardiologial Scientific Centre, in a district of Moscow. Year not stated

31 Shevtshuk and Tarasova (1983)

a. Survey in Lipetsk. Sample size (males) 813, (females) 716

b. Results shown in Table 29.4 are for schoolchildren in grades 7-10, and adults. The following prevalence results for students are also given:

	Males	Females
Primary technical college	56	5.2
Secondary technical college	56	5.9
University	51	5

32 Denisova (2000)

a. Survey in Novosibirsk (western Siberia), with interview and physical examination. Sample studied in 1984-1985 at age 10-14, (males) 660, (females) 658. Same children studied again in 1989-1990 at age 15-17, (males) 317, (females) 345. A new sample was studied in 1994, (males) 319, (females) 300

b. Regular smokers: (1984-1985) smoked weekly, (1989-1990 and 1994) smoked daily. All smokers: (1984-1985 and 1989-1990) undefined, (1994) smoked weekly

33 Geizerova and Masironi (1988)

a. Moscow. No original source

34 Prokhorov *et al* (1988), Chazova *et al* (1989), Prokhorov and Alexandrov (1992), Alexandrov *et al* (2000)

a. Study in secondary schools in Cheremushkinskii district of Moscow. Nine schools selected randomly, none refusing to participate. Approximate ages corresponding to school grades 5-10/11
b. Results presented for 1985 are from anonymous self-completion questionnaires administered in class under supervision of a researcher. Sample size 5 584. Results (not presented here) using 'expert assessment' (see also source 64) were very similar
c. Results for 1995 are based on 'expert assessment'. Sample size (student experts) 220, (total) 3 062
d. Smokers marked as frequency *: smoked at least 1 cigarette per day. Regular smokers: smoked at least 1 cigarette per week. All smokers: includes occasional smokers who have smoked at least 1 cigarette in the last 3 months

35 WHO (1997) quoting Ministry of Health

a. Based on surveys conducted predominantly in the large cities such as Moscow or St Petersburg. Age group not stated

36-40 Hurt (1995) quoting Prokhorov (1993), Tchachenko and Riazantsev (1993)

a. Various studies in Russia
   36 Industrial areas. Age group not stated
   37 Location not stated. Regular smokers: smoked daily
   38 St Petersburg. Age group not stated
   39 Siberia. Age group not stated
   40 Moscow

41 Hearn *et al* (1991)

a. Survey conducted in 4 Moscow schools using standardized questionnaire. Age range not stated, but average age 14.5 years. Year not stated. Sample size (males) 251, (females) 244. Response rate 96%
b. Regular smokers: smoked at least a partial pack of cigarettes a week. All smokers: smoked at least a few cigarettes per month

42 Elgarov *et al* (1992)

a. Random sample of the non-organized population of the region of Nalchik (southern Russia). Year not stated. Sample size (males) 2 562, response rate 70%
b. Results presented are combined from blue and white collar workers—prevalence was higher among blue collar workers at all ages

43 Puska *et al* (1993)

a. Representative survey in Pitkäranta, Republic of Karelia (in the northwestern part of Russia) into prevalence of cardiovascular risk factors. Self-completion questionnaire completed at examination centre. Sample size (males) 500, (females) 500. Response rate (males) 77%, (females) 92%
b. Smokers: smoked regularly for at least a year and had smoked in the last month

44 WHO (1997)

a. Moscow. No original source

45 Morochenko (1993)

a. Russia. No original source. Year not stated

46 Elgarov and Elgarova (1994)

a. Survey of schoolchildren in Nalchik (southern Russia). Approximate ages corresponding to school grades 8-10. Year not stated. Sample size (males) 2 613, (females) 1 985, response rate 86%
b. Regular smokers: smoked 1 or more cigarette per week

47 **Trubacheva *et al* (1994)**

a. Study of coronary atherosclerosis risk factors in two small towns in Western Siberia. Year not stated. Sample size (males) 6 260, (females) 4 576

b. Results presented here are average of the two towns. Smoking prevalence was lower in the second town which had a migrant population

48 **WHO (1996)**

a. Russia. No original source

49 **Bilitchenko and Kharlova (1996)**

a. Moscow. No original source

b. Results in *All ages* column in Table 29.4 relate to age 25-65

50 **Carolina Population Center (1998) and personal communication**

a. Russian Longitudinal Monitoring Survey, round 6. Nationally representative survey, targeting 4 000 households. Personal interviews with all adult household members. Children's questionnaires were answered by an adult. Response rate (households) 80%, (adults) 97%

b. Only 17 men and 2 women were recorded as being smokers other than cigarette smokers

51 **Levshin *et al* (1997, 2000)**

a. Survey of general population in Moscow during 1995-1997. Total sample size 3 000 (including samples of physicians and teachers, results not presented here)

52 **Torabi and Crowe (2000)**

a. Survey in urban and rural schools in the district of St Petersburg. Approximate age group corresponding to 7th-9th grades. Year not stated. Sample size 1 118

b. Smokers: had smoked in last 30 days

c. It is also reported that 3.7% of the students had ever used smokeless tobacco

d. Consumption category estimation based on 1-5, 6-10, 11-20, 21+ cigarettes/smoker/day. The total over these categories is virtually the same as the prevalence given for smokers in last month

53 **Volkova *et al* (2000)**

a. Survey in the Ural region. No original source. Year and age not stated

b. It was also reported that the prevalence of smoking among women was 8-12%

54 **Raudsepp *et al* (1988)**

a. Estonia. Study of pupils at 4th-11th grades. Results presented here are for approximate ages corresponding to 6th-11th grades, sample size (males) 5 365, (females) 6 623

55 **Aareleid *et al* (1994) quoting Lipand *et al* (1992)**

a. Health behaviour survey in Estonia

b. Assumed extension to age distribution for percentage smokers, age 15-17: males 30% and females 10%

56 **WHO (1997)**

a. Estonia. No original source

57 **WHO (1997)**

a. Estonia. No original source

b. Regular smokers: smoked daily

58 Nurk *et al* (1999) and personal communication

a. Cross-sectional surveys at 17 secondary schools in Tallinn, Estonia. Conducted by the CINDI (Countrywide Integrated Noncommunicable Diseases Intervention Programme) Children's Programme team from the Estonian Institute of Cardiology. Confidential questionnaire completed in class with teachers absent. Estonian and Russian students attend separate schools and completed the questionnaire in their mother tongue. Age corresponding to school grade 9.

Year	Sample size		% Estonian
	Males	Females	
1991-1992	609	595	56
1993-1994	509	529	49
1995-1996	450	493	54

b. Regular smokers: smoked once a week. All smokers: smoked in last 3 months

c. Consumption per smoker based on average number smoked per week by regular smokers

59 Puska (1995) quoting Lipand *et al* (1993)

a. National postal survey on health behaviour in Estonia. Sample size (males) 451, (females) 497. Response rate (males) 60%, (females) 66%

60 WHO (1997)

a. Estonia. Nationwide survey. No original source

b. A further 7.9% of adults (sexes combined) were occasional smokers

c. Assumed extension to age distribution for percentage smokers, age 15: males 20% and females 10%

61 Pärna (1999)

a. Study in randomly selected schools in Tallinn, including 10 Estonian- and 7 Russian-speaking schools. Anonymous questionnaires completed in class. Approximate ages corresponding to school grades 8, 10 and 12. Sample size (Estonian) 1 269, (Russian) 901

62 WHO (1997)

a. Latvia. No original source

b. Regular smokers: have smoked for at least a year

63 Bosma *et al* (1994)

a. Kaunas-Rotterdam Intervention Study (KRIS). Baseline cardiovascular screening survey representing various socio-economic strata of the Kaunas male urban population. Sample size 2 452, response rate 69%

b. Consumption category estimation based on 1-9, 10-19, 20+ cigarettes/smoker/day

64 Goshtautas *et al* (1988)

a. Survey of schoolchildren in Kaunus, using method of 'expert assessment', where two student leaders from each class reported the smoking prevalence of their classmates.

	Sample size	
	Males	Females
1981	13 436	14 656
1982	13 521	14 766
1985	13 890	15 608

b. The Moscow part of this study also used self assessment, which is reported as source 34

c. Smokers marked as frequency *: smoked at least 1 cigarette per day. Regular smokers: smoked at least 1 cigarette per week. All smokers: includes occasional smokers who have smoked at least 1 cigarette per month

65 WHO (1997)

a. Lithuania. No original source

66 Geizerova and Masironi (1988)

a. Lithuanian-SSR. No original source
b. Prevalence among girls is given as 'low' in a table, but as 'none' in text

67 Domarkiene *et al* (1999)

a. Surveys in Kaunas, carried out according to the WHO-MONICA protocol.

Year	Age	Sample size	
		Males	Females
1993	35-64	611	628
1995	65-80	476	327

b. Regular smokers: smoked 1+ cigarettes per day

68 Gorbas *et al* (1994)

a. Two epidemiological surveys carried out in Ukraine at an interval of 12 years, but years not stated. Representative of the non-organized population. Sample sizes 2 191, 1 901

69 Kvasha *et al* (1997)

a. Epidemiological study, representative of the female population of Ukraine. Sample size 2 259
b. Year not stated, but results are presented in terms of changes over 5 years
c. 99% of smoking women are reported to be urban citizens

70-72 Zaridze *et al* (1986) quoting Orlovski (1977)

	Location	Sample size	
		Males	Females
70	Armenia	792	893
71	Georgia	544	694
72	Azerbaidjan	695	1 384

73 WHO (1997)

a. Youth in Yerevan, Armenia. No original source

74 WHO (1997), Davidiants (1997)

a. Epidemiological study using random sample in Yerevan, Armenia. Youngest age included is 10. Sample size 245

75 Grim *et al* (1997)

a. 2-stage cluster sample in Tbilisi, Georgia, carried out in 5 days. Year not stated. Sample size 300

76 WHO (1997)

a. Kyrgystan. No original source
b. Tobacco users

77 WHO (1997)

a. Bishkek, Kyrgystan. No original source
b. It is also reported that approximately 50-60% of boys and 2-4% of girls aged 14-16 use tobacco. Smoking by women may be under-reported for cultural reasons

78 Makhmudov and Adilova (1988)

a. Control group from a smoking control study in Tashkent, Uzbekistan. Year not stated. Sample size (males only) 1 590
b. Results presented as source 5 correspond to the active intervention part of this study, sample size 1 982

79-80 WHO (1997)
a. Uzbekistan. No original source. Overall age group not stated. Results shown as source **79** relate to Uzbek population, **80** to other nationalities
b. Smokers: smoked 1+ cigarettes per week

81 WHO (1997)
a. Survey in 1990-1992 in Dashkhovuz, Turkmenistan. No original source. Age group not stated (adults)

82 WHO (1997)
a. Quoting a report published in 1994 (no details). Uzbekistan. Year not stated. Overall age group not stated

83 Adriaanse *et al* (1986)
a. Regional sample, but location not stated. Age not stated

84 Loransky *et al* (1983)
a. Quoting Research Institute of Sanitary Education (USSR Ministry of Health). Survey in 8 towns (Zelinograd (Moscow), Kiev, Erevan, Lipetsk, Ufa, Daugavlpils, Stavropol, Tula). Total sample size (males) 688, (females) 999, sample in each town varies from 87-284
b. Only combined results for all towns are presented here, but prevalence varied from 51% to 78% for men, and from 2% to 24% for women. Age-specific results taken from graph
c. Assumed extension to age distribution for percentage smokers, age 15-19: males 50% and females 10%

85 Loransky *et al* (1983)
a. Survey in 11 towns (Moscow, Zelinograd, Dmitrov, Lipetsk, Ufa, Daugavpils, Essentuki, Chabarovsk, Sukhumi, Vilnius, Kaunas). Approximate ages corresponding to school grades 7 and 10. Sample size overall (males) 1 424, (females) 1 395 in grades 4-10

86 Crofton (1990) quoting Director General of WHO (1988)
a. USSR. Year not stated, probably 1981-1986. Age not stated (adults)

Additional information (not presented in tables)

Denisova (2000) reports a survey in Chukota (far north of Russia), conducted in 1990 under expedition conditions in coastal and tundra settlements. Representative sample, age 15-17. Sample size (males) 165, (females) 157. The prevalence of smoking among girls was 23% among natives and 13% among non-natives. Among boys, both native and non-native, it was 40-41%

Zaridze *et al* (1986) quoting Orlovski (1977) reports a study in 1957 in the Buryat ASSR (in the east of USSR). Sample size (ethnic Buryat) 541, (other) 903. 81% of Buryat women and 10% of other women were cigarette smokers

For Armenia, A. Bazarjian, director of the Armenian National Institute of Health Care's anti-smoking program, reported that 50-56% of teenage boys and 20-25% of girls smoke regularly. The majority smoke 15-20 cigarettes per day. Year not stated. Quoted by Snark News Agency (2000)

For Estonia, Volozh *et al* (1995) reports that in a number of epidemiological risk factor surveys by the Division of Preventive Cardiology of the Estonian Institute of Cardiology, carried out over 14 years and involving 12 000 examinees, 50-54% of men and 17-20% of women were regular smokers

In Georgia, according to WHO (1997), smoking was rare among women before about 1980. In the mid-1990s, the prevalence of smoking among young people (age 17-30) was 40-50% for males, and about 40% for females

References

Aareleid T., Leinsalu M., Rahu M. and Baburin A. (1994). Lung cancer in Estonia in 1968-87: time trends and public health implications. *Eur J Cancer Prev,* **3**, 419-25.

Adriaanse H., van Reek J. and van Zutphen W.M. (1986). Rookgewoonten van atrsen wereldwijd; een overzicht van 100 onderzoekinge naar tabaksgebruik onder artsen in 31 landen in de periode 1951-1985 (Worldwide physicians' smoking habits; a review of 100 surveys into physicians' tobacco consumption in 31 countries in the period 1951-1985. *Ned Tijdschr Geneeskd,* **130**, 2224-9.

Alexandrov A.A., Alexandrova V.Yu. and Ivanova E.I. (2000). Prevalence of smoking among Moscow schoolchildren and approaches to prevention. In: Lu R., Mackay J., Niu S. and Peto R. (eds) *Tobacco: The Growing Epidemic. Proceedings of the Tenth World Conference on Tobacco or Health, 24-28 August 1997, Beijing, China.* Springer-Verlag, London; 266-8.

Anonymous (1994). East keeps tobacco firms alight. *European* **Nov 4-10**:25.

Anonymous (2000). Russia to impose licensing on tobacco manufacturing on August 1. *Novecon* **Jul 10** :

BBC Monitoring International Reports (2000). Russia 'has its problems with controlling tobacco trade'. *BBC Monitoring International Reports*

Bilitchenko T.N. and Kharlova N.V. (1996). Smoking prevention politics in Russia [Abstract]. Conference on global lung health and the 1996 annual meeting of the International Union Against Tubercluosis and Lung Disease (IUATLD) Paris, France 2-5 October 1996. *Tuber Lung Dis,* **77(Suppl 2)**, 42.

Bosma H., Appels A., Sturmans F., Grabauskas V. and Gostautas A. (1994). Differences in mortality and coronary heart disease between Lithuania and the Netherlands: results from the WHO Kaunas-Rotterdam Intervention Study (KRIS). *Int J Epidemiol,* **23**, 12-9.

Burenkov S.P. and Glasunov I.S. (1982). USSR: the preventive approach in public health. *World Health Forum,* **3**, 54-7.

Carolina Population Center (1998). *Russia longitudinal monitoring survey.* http://www.cpc.unc.edu/projects/rlms/.

Chazova L.V., Prokhorova I.N., Prokhorov A.V., Ivanov V.M., Alexandrov A.A. and Sarsenova S.I. (1989). Smoking and some measures of its control. *Ter Arkh,* **1**, 40-3.

Cooper R. (1982). Smoking in the Soviet Union. *BMJ,* **285**, 549-51.

Crofton J. (1990). Tobacco and the Third World. *Thorax,* **45**, 164-9.

Davidiants V. (1997). Prevalence of smoking in Armenia. In: *Tobacco: the growing epidemic. Abstract book, 10th World Conference on Tobacco or Health, Beijing, China, 24-28 August 1997.* 96 (OS 253)

Denisova D. (2000). Prevalence and trends of cigarette smoking among children and adolescents in Siberia. In: Lu R., Mackay J., Niu S. and Peto R. (eds) *Tobacco: The Growing Epidemic. Proceedings of the Tenth World Conference on Tobacco or Health, 24-28 August 1997, Beijing, China.* Springer-Verlag, London; 270-1.

Director General of WHO (1988). *Tobacco or health. Report to the Forty-first World Health Assembly.* WHO, Geneva.[§]

Domarkiene S., Tamosiunas A. and Reklaitiene R. (1999). Smoking habits in Kaunas population [Abstract]. *Nicotine & Tobacco Research,* **1**, 191.

Elgarov A.A. and Elgarova L.V. (1994). Otnoshenie shkol'nikov Nal'chika k vrednym privychkam (Attitude of Nalchik schoolchildren to harmful habits). *Ter Arkh,* **66**, 45-8.

Elgarov A.A., Zhasminova V.G., Konstantinov V.V., Sokolova M.A. and Khuzhokova M.M. (1992). Chastota ishemicheskoi bolezni serdtsa i faktorov ee riska u muzhchin 20-54 let-rabotnikof fizicheskogo i umstvennogo truda (The incidence of coronary heart disease and its risk factors in men aged 20-54 years, blue and white collars). *Ter Arkh,* **64**, 100-3.

Franceschi S. and Naett C. (1995). Trends in smoking in Europe. *Eur J Cancer Prev,* **4**, 271-84.

Geizerova H. and Masironi R. (1988). Cigarette smoking in children and adolescents: world review. In: Aoki M., Hisamichi S. and Tominaga S. (eds) *Smoking and health 1987. Proceedings of the 6th World Conference on Smoking and Health, Tokyo, 9-12 November 1987.* Elsevier Science Publishers B.V. (Biomedical Division), Amsterdam; 601-5. International Congress Series No. 780.

Glogan T. (1995). Baltic tobacco industries struggle to develop. *Tobacco Journal International,* **4**, 54-8.

Gorbas I.M., Smirnova I.P., Kvasha E.A., Davidenko N.V. and Koblyanskaya A.V. (1994). Dynamics of the epidemiological situation coronary heart disease and risk factors within the urban population of Ukraine [Abstract]. *Eur Heart J,* **15(Suppl)**, 373.

Goshtautas A., Prokhorov A., Alexandrov A. and Grigaitite Y. (1988). Comparative data on smoking prevalence among school-children in Moscow and Kaunas. *Kardiology,* **4**, 51-4.

Grim C.E., Grim C.M., Kipshidze N., Kipshidze N.N. and Petersen J. (1997). CVD risk factors in Eastern Europe: a rapid survey of the capital of the Republic of Georgia [Abstract]. *Am J Hypertens,* **10**, 211A.

Harkin A.M., Anderson P. and Goos C. (1997). *Smoking, drinking and drug taking in the European Region.* Alcohol, Drugs and Tobacco Programme, WHO Regional Office for Europe, Copenhagen.

Hearn M.D., Prokhorov A.V., Murray D.M., Alexandrov A.A. and Luepker R.V. (1991). Comparison of smoking prevalence in school students sampled from the United States of America and the Union of Soviet Socialist Republics. *Int J Epidemiol,* **20**, 413-5.

Hibell B., Andersson B., Bjarnason T., Kokkevi A., Morgan M. and Narusk A. (1997). *The 1995 ESPAD report. The European school survey project on alcohol and other drugs. Alcohol and other drug use among students in 26 European countries*. The Swedish Council for Information on Alcohol and Other Drugs. Council of Europe (Pompidou Group).

Horne B. (1993). A cigarette market of many faces in Russia. *Tobacco Journal International,* **6**, 25-8.

Hurt R.D. (1995). Smoking in Russia: what do Stalin and western tobacco companies have in common? *Mayo Clin Proc,* **70**, 1007-11.

Hutson J.B. (1937). *Consumption and production of tobacco in Europe*. USDA, Washington DC. Technical bulletin No. 587.

Ioffina O.B., Kharchenko V.I. and Akopian A.S. (1999). Rol' i znachenie tabakokureniia v zabolevaemosti i smertnosti ot boleznei sistemy krovoobrashcheniia v sovremennoi Rossii. (Role of tobacco smoking on cardiovascular morbidity and mortality in today's Russia). *Ter Arkh,* **71**, 69-73.

Kalnins I., Ranka I., Glazunova J., Platkaja I., *et al* (1995). Health for all young people in Europe: the World Health Organization cross-national study on health behaviour in school-aged children (HBSC) in Latvia. *Journal of Baltic Studies,* **26**, 221-42.

King A., Wold B., Tudor-Smith C. and Harel Y. (1996). *The health of youth, a cross-national survey*. WHO Regional Publications, Europe, Copenhagen. European Series No. 69.

King A.J.C. and Coles B. (1992). *The health of Canada's youth. Views and behaviours of 11-, 13- and 15-year-olds from 11 countries*. Health and Welfare Canada, Ottawa.

Kvasha E., Smirnova I., Corbas I. and Davidenko N. (1997). Smoking problem among the Ukraine female population. In: *Tobacco: the growing epidemic. Abstract book, 10th World Conference on Tobacco or Health, Beijing, China, 24-28 August 1997.* 142 (PO 46)

Levshin V., Drojachih V., Fedichkina T. and Slepchenko N. (2000). Epidemiology of smoking and some determinants of smoking behaviour. In: Lu R., Mackay J., Niu S. and Peto R. (eds) *Tobacco: The Growing Epidemic. Proceedings of the Tenth World Conference on Tobacco or Health, 24-28 August 1997, Beijing, China*. Springer-Verlag, London; 52-4.

Levshin V., Drojachih V., Fedishkina TJ. and Slepchenko N. (1997). Smoking epidemiology and some determinants of smoking behavior. In: *Tobacco: the growing epidemic. Abstract book, 10th World Conference on Tobacco or Health, Beijing, China, 24-28 August 1997.* 33 (OS3)

Lipand A., Kasmel A., Kivilo M., Tasa E., *et al* (1992). *Health behaviour among Estonian adult population, Spring 1990.* National Public Health Institute, Helsinki. B1/1992.§

Lipand A., Kasmel A., Tasa E., Puska P. and Berg M.-A. (1993). *Eesti täiskasvanud elanikkonna terviseuurimus 1992.a. kevadel. (Health behaviour among Estonian adult population spring 1992).* National Public Health Institute, Helsinki. B3/1993.§

Loransky D.N. (1977). Smoking control programs in the USSR. In: Steinfeld J., Griffiths W., Ball K. and Taylor R.M. (eds) *Health consequences, education, cessation activities, and social action, Volume II. Proceedings of the Third World Conference on Smoking and Health, New York City, June 2-5, 1975.* US Department of Health, Education and Welfare, USA; 791-3. DHEW Publication No (NIH) 77-1413.

Loransky D.N., Popova E.B., Chakimova L.S. and Shevtshuk A.G. (1983). State of the smoking problem. *Sovetskoe Zdravookhranenie,* **6**, 33-8.

Makhmudov B.Kh. and Adilova M.S. (1988). Smoking prevalence and control among non-organized population in Tashkent. *Meditsinskii Zhurnal Uzbekistana,* **12**, 44-7.

Morochenko D. (1993). Russian and western manufacturers look for ways of integrating. *Izvestiia* **Sept 24**:B4.

Nurk E., Mittelmark M.B., Suurorg L., Tur I. and Luiga E. (1999). Trends in tobacco use among Estonian and Russian youth in Tallinn. *Scandinavian Journal of Public Health,* **27**, 301-5.

Oleinikov S.P., Chazova L.V., Glazunov I.S., Deev A.D., *et al* (1983). Tobacco smoking and some socio-demographic characteristics (data of cooperative studies in Moscow and Kaunas). *Ter Arkh,* **1**, 57-61.

Oleinikov S.P., Glazunov E.S. and Chazova L.V. (1981). Smoking among men and women of various age groups. *Ter Arkh,* **2**, 111-5.

Orlovski L.V. (1977). Importance of education in the anti-smoking campaign. In: *Proceedings of the meeting of the USSR Academy of Medical Sciences commission on the problem of medical education*., Archangelsk; 122-30.§

Pärna K. (1999). Passive smoking among adolescents in Estonia. *Hum Exp Toxicol,* **18**, 229-332.

Piha T., Besselink E. and Lopez A.D. (1993). Tobacco or health. *World Health Stat Q,* **46**, 188-94.

Prokhorov A.V. (1993). *Smoking in Russia.* WHO Regional Office for Europe, Copenhagen.§

Prokhorov A.V. and Alexandrov A.A. (1992). Tobacco smoking in Moscow school students. *British Journal of Addiction,* **87**, 1469-76.

Prokhorov A.V., Alexandrov A.A., Isakova G.L., Boobnov U.E., *et al* (1988). Smoking prevalence among 5th to 10th grade students. *Sovetskoe Zdravookhranenie,* **4**, 38-42.

Puska P. (1995). Health promotion challenges for countries of the former Soviet Union: results from collaboration between Estonia, Russian Karelia and Finland. *Health Promotion International,* **10**, 219-28.

Puska P., Matilainen T., Jousilahti P., Korhonen H., *et al* (1993). Cardiovascular risk factors in the Republic of Karelia, Russia, and in North Karelia, Finland. *Int J Epidemiol,* **22**, 1048-55.

Raudsepp J., Rahu M. and Propst S. (1988). Õpilaste suitsetamislevimus Eestis 1981. aastal. *Noukogude Eesti Tervishoid,* **1**, 17-20.

Razgulyaev Y. (1997). Regulation government of Kirgizia to reduce tobacco excise. *Business World* **29**:3.

Seenev V. (1996). *Trud,* **6 Sept**, 16.§

Shevtshuk A.G. and Tarasova R.N. (1983). Ob organizatsii sanitarno-prosvetitelnoy raboti v borbe c kureniem. (Organization of an anti-smoking campaign). *Zdravookhranenie Rossiiskoi Federatsii,* **5**, 27-8.

Snark News Agency (2000). 50% of Armenia's population 'smoke regularly'. *Snark News Agency* **Feb 16**.

Tchachenko G.B. and Riazantsev V.K. (1993). *Description of the situation in the Russian Federation.* WHO Regional Office for Europe, Copenhagen.§

Torabi M.R. and Crowe J.W. (2000). Patterns of tobacco use among Russian students. In: Lu R., Mackay J., Niu S. and Peto R. (eds) *Tobacco: The Growing Epidemic. Proceedings of the Tenth World Conference on Tobacco or Health, 24-28 August 1997, Beijing, China.* Springer-Verlag, London; 268-70.

Trubacheva I.A., Levitsky E.F. and Perminova O.A. (1994). Epidemiology of risk factors for coronary atherosclerosis in populations of small towns of Western Siberia [Abstract]. *Atherosclerosis,* **109**, 20-1.

USDA (1978). *Market prospects for tobacco in the Soviet Union. Foreign agriculture circular.* USDA, Washington DC. FT4-4.

USDA Economic Research Service (1996). *Tobacco statistics.* Albert R. Mann Library, Cornell University, Ithaca, New York. ERS 94012. (With supplementary material from Tobacco Annual Reports.). http://usda.mannlib.cornell.edu/data-sets/specialty/94012.

USDA Foreign Agricultural Service (1993). 1993 leaf and cigarette situation: former Soviet Union. *World Tobacco Situation,* **Circular Series FT5-93, May 1993**, 32-7.

Volkova E.G., Karasikova T.B., Levashov S.U., Tkachenko G.B., *et al* (2000). Population attitudes to smoking in Chelyabinsk region, Russian Federation. In: Lu R., Mackay J., Niu S. and Peto R. (eds) *Tobacco: The Growing Epidemic. Proceedings of the Tenth World Conference on Tobacco or Health, 24-28 August 1997, Beijing, China.* Springer-Verlag, London; 62-3.

Volozh O., Kalyuste T. and Solodkaya E. (1995). Smoking and mortality in middle-aged men. In: Slama K. (ed) *Tobacco and Health, Ninth World Conference on Tobacco and Health, Paris, Oct 10-14 1994.* Plenum Press, New York and London; 515-8.

WHO (1989). The WHO MONICA project: a worldwide monitoring system for cardiovascular diseases. In: *World health statistics annual 1989.* WHO, Geneva; 25-149.

WHO MONICA Project (1988). Geographical variation in the major risk factors of coronary heart disease in men and women aged 35-64 years. *World Health Stat Q,* **41**, 115-40.

WHO (1996). *The tobacco epidemic: a global public health emergency.* WHO. Fact sheet No. 118.

WHO (1997). *Tobacco or health: A global status report.* WHO, Geneva. www.cdc.gov/nccdphp/osh/who/whoampro.htm.

Zaridze D.G., Dvoirin V.V., Kobljakov V.A. and Pisklov V.P. (1986). Smoking patterns in the USSR. In: Zaridze D.G. and Peto R. (eds) *Tobacco: a major international health hazard. Proceedings of an international meeting organized by the IARC and co-sponsored by the All-Union Cancer Research Centre of the Academy of Medical Sciences of the USSR, held in Moscow, 4-6 June 1985.* IARC, Lyon; 75-86. IARC Scientific Publications No. 74.

§ Original paper not obtained, but information taken as quoted by another author

Yugoslavia 30

Sales data

See Tables 30.1-30.3.

Consumption of manufactured cigarettes per adult was about 1 cigarette per day in the 1920s and 1930s. By 1960 it had increased to 4, and continued to increase to a peak of nearly 10 in 1979, then levelled at 8-9 cigarettes per day through the 1980s. The proportion of cigarettes which were filtered rose rapidly from 13% in 1966 to 88% in 1972. There is little reliable information on consumption in the 1990s, due to the political situation and to high levels of smuggling. Some data for the successor republics are presented in Table 30.1.2.

Data on consumption of other tobacco products are available for only a few years. Between 1922 and 1935, consumption of all tobacco products combined per adult fell from 3 g to 2 g per day. This was largely due to a halving of the consumption of smoking tobacco. As a proportion of all tobacco, smoking tobacco fell from over 70% to 35%, while cigarettes increased from about 20% to 60%. Small amounts of cigars and chewing tobacco were used, while snuff consumption was negligible.

Survey data

See Tables 30.4-30.8

Few nationally based surveys are available, either for the former Yugoslavia or the successor republics. Most estimates of the prevalence of smoking among men aged 15 years and over were around 50%; among women, they were around 10-15% in 1969-1972 and around 30% in 1985-1995. A recent series of surveys in Slovenia (source 33) were an exception, with prevalence in 1994, for example, 35% among men and 23% among women. One survey in Bosnia and Hercegovina in 1969 (source 9) found that smoking prevalence increased with increased age for both men and women, but this unusual pattern was not seen in the few other surveys which gave age-specific results.

Most surveys of smoking among teenagers were conducted on a local basis in Croatia. In a series of surveys among pupils in Zagreb (source 8) the prevalence of smoking decreased among boys while increasing among girls between 1966 and 1984, then decreased for both sexes, with a particularly sharp decline between 1989 and 1991. The prevalence among pupils in Croatia was higher than in Slovenia when surveyed in 1995 (sources 37-38).

Comparison of sales and survey data was possible in one case, where consumption in Croatia, scaled up to the whole Yugoslav population, under-reported by about 10%. Between 1969 and 1995, the estimated number of cigarettes smoked per person per day (sales-adjusted) was about 10-11 for men, and increased from about 2 to 5 for women.

Table 30.1.1 Total annual sales of tobacco products, 1922 -1935

Year	Cigarettes		Cigars tonnes	Smoking tobacco tonnes	Chewing tobacco tonnes	Snuff tonnes	All tobacco products tonnes
	tonnes	millions					
1922	2034	2034	157	6742	113	0	9046
1923	2188	2188	198	6078	163	0	8627
1924	2688	2688	219	5573	151	4	8635
1925	2866	2866	222	5691	130	6	8915
1926	3137	3137	208	6404	106	7	9862
1927	3463	3463	213	6453	45	6	10180
1928	3760	3760	213	6387	38	5	10403
1929	3997	3997	206	6012	34	3	10252
1930	5069	5069	210	4765	32	3	10079
1931	5463	5463	199	3731	30	4	9427
1932	4991	4991	249	2402	31	5	7678
1933	4815	4815	313	2384	27	6	7545
1934	4620	4620	313	2484	25	6	7448
1935	4529	4529	285	2498	21	6	7339

Source : see *Notes on sources of sales data*, p. 771

Table 30.1.2 Total annual sales of cigarettes, successor republics, 1993 -1995

	Cigarettes (millions)		
	1993	1994	1995
Bosnia Hercegovina	9000		
Croatia	10800	10900	
Macedonia	4000		
Serbia / Montenegro	22000	22700	22650
Slovenia	4500		

Source : see *Notes on sources of sales data*, p. 771

Table 30.1.3 Manufactured cigarettes, percentage of total sales as filter cigarettes, 1960-1984

Year	% Filter
1966	12.8
1967	20.4
1968	40.1
1969	62.2
1970	71.3
1971	79.5
1972	88.4
1984	97

Source : see *Notes on sources of sales data*, p. 771

Table 30.2 Consumption of (i) cigarettes and (ii) all tobacco products, 1922-1993 sales-based data, including estimated hand-rolled cigarette consumption. Males and females aged 15 years and over

Year	Manufactured cigarettes		Hand-rolled cigarettes		Total cigarettes		All tobacco products	
	Total annual in millions	Number/ adult/day	Total annual in millions	Number/ adult/day	Total annual in millions	Number/ adult/day	Total annual in tonnes	Grams/ adult/day
1922	2034	0.7					9046	3.1
1923	2188	0.7					8627	2.9
1924	2688	0.9					8635	2.9
1925	2866	1.0					8915	3.0
1926	3137	1.0					9862	3.1
1927	3463	1.1					10180	3.2
1928	3760	1.2					10403	3.3
1929	3997	1.3					10252	3.3
1930	5069	1.6					10079	3.2
1931	5463	1.6					9427	2.8
1932	4991	1.5					7678	2.3
1933	4815	1.4					7545	2.2
1934	4620	1.4					7448	2.2
1935	4529	1.3					7339	2.2
1960	20122	4.3						
1961	22806	4.8						
1962	22456	4.7						
1963	23211	4.8						
1964	23656	4.8						
1965	26114	5.2						
1966	28786	5.7						
1967	28967	5.6						
1968	30905	5.9						
1969	33229	6.2						
1970	33876	6.2						
1971	35275	6.4						
1972	35837	6.4						
1973	36364	6.4						
1974	40655	7.1						
1975	40553	7.0						
1976	41657	7.1						
1977	46782	7.9						
1978	52982	8.8						
1979	59151	9.7						
1980	54869	8.9						
1981	50027	8.1						
1982	49614	7.9						
1983	55975	8.9						
1984	53357	8.4						
1985	55419	8.6						
1986	57100	8.8						
1987	55304	8.5						
1988	59100	8.9						
1989	56630	8.5						
1990	57078	8.5						
1991	52700	8.0						
1992	45000	6.8						
1993	50300	7.6						

Source : see *Notes on sources of sales data*, p. 771

Figure 30.1 Daily consumption of (i) manufactured cigarettes and (ii) all tobacco products, 1922-1993.
Males and females aged 15 years and over. *Source:* see Table 30.2

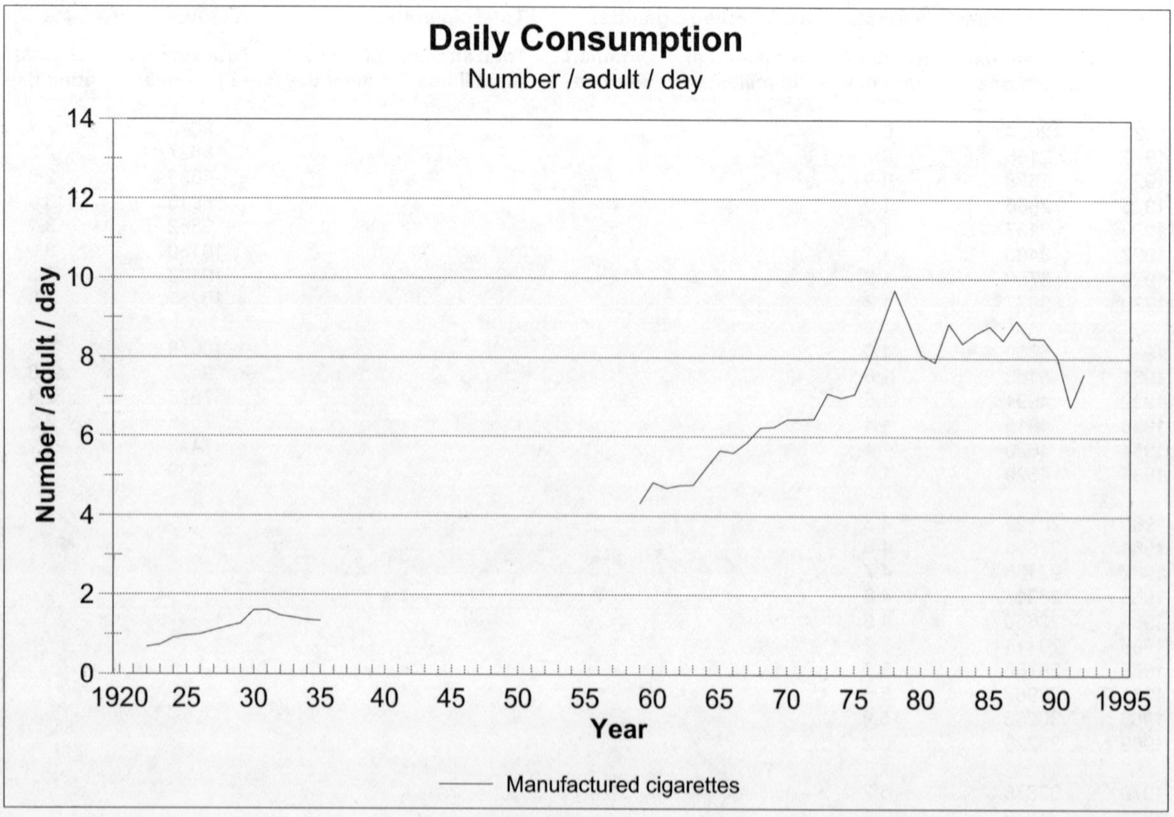

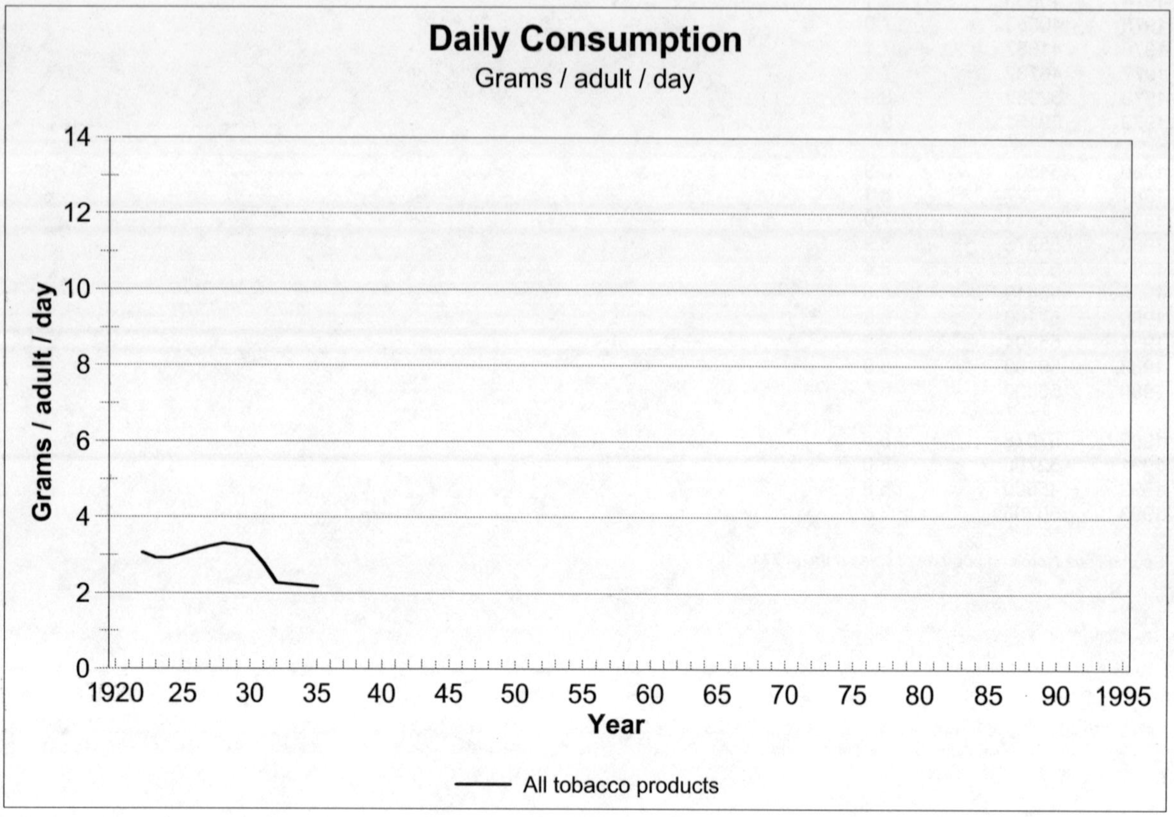

Table 30.3 Percentage sales of tobacco in different forms (by weight), selected years 1925-1935

Year	Cigarettes (%)	Cigars (%)	Smoking tobacco (%)	Chewing tobacco and snuff (%)
1925	32.1	2.5	63.8	1.5
1935	61.7	3.9	34.0	0.3

Source : calculated from Table 30.1.1

Figure 30.2 Percentage sales of tobacco in different forms (by weight), selected years 1925-1935
Source: see Table 30.3

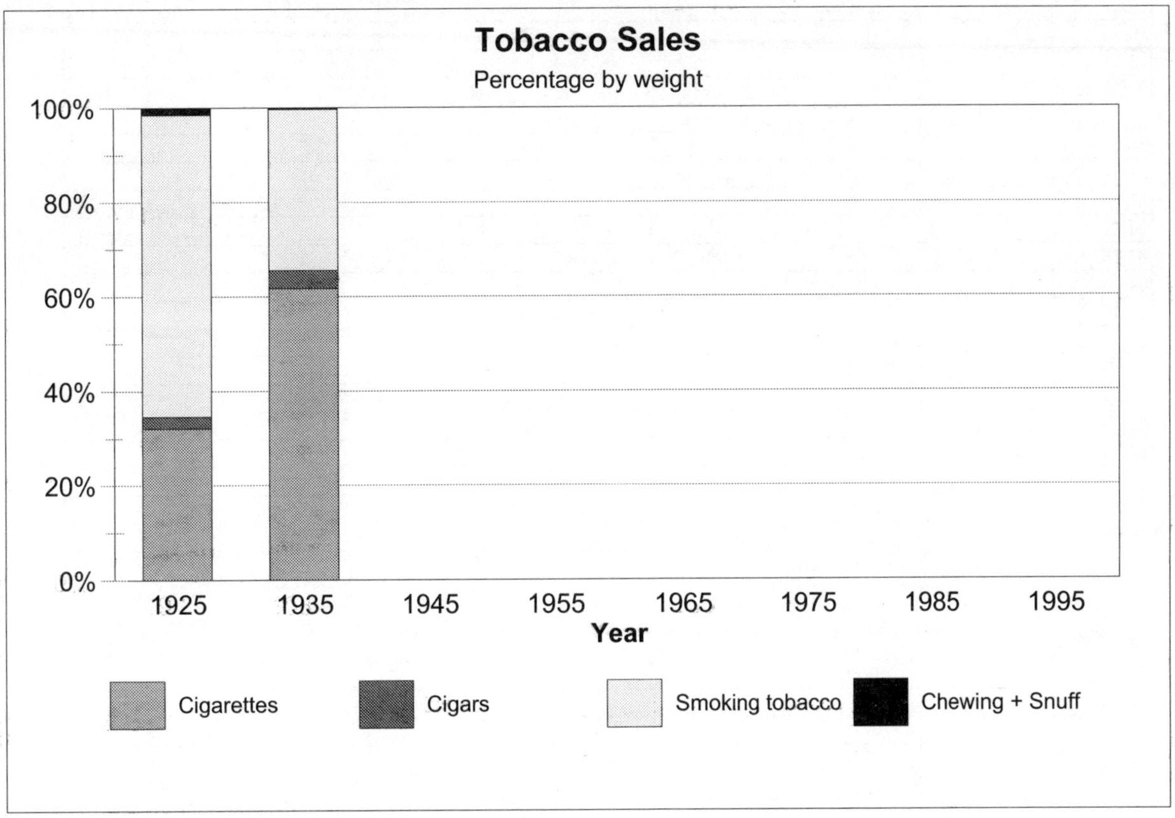

Table 30.4M Prevalence of smoking, males: some selected Yugoslav surveys by age, 1958-1995

Year / Source / Product / Frequency	12	13	14	15	16	17	18	19	20-24	25-29	30-34	35-39	40-44	45-49	50-54	55-59	60-64	65-69	70-74	75-79	80+	All ages
58 1 UC R													54	58	63	56						58
58 2 UC R													58	56	67	60						60
62 3 UC R													49	48	51	46						48
63 4 UC R													62	63	67	59						63
64 5 UC R													50	46	38	32						43
64 6 UC U												70										
64 7 UC U												59										
66 8 U R				29	44	45	46															41
69 9 UC U				28						50		64		66		66						
69 9 A U				28						51		66		72		73						60
70 10 U U				57																		
72 11 UC R												52										
72 12 UC R									55		58		60		54							57
73 8 U R	4	4	16	28	36	45	52															39
74 13 U U				46																		
75 14 U R				17	19	28	54															
79 15 U R				13	20	34	53															
80 27 U U										70												
83 28 U U						38																
84 8 U R				21	26	35	38															29
84 16 U R				20																		
84 17 U R				4	6	24	10															
84 18 U R				3	6	20	11															
84 29 UC R										71		58		47		37						49
84 29 A A										74		60		48		40						51
84 30 MC R				56																		
85 19 U R				7	24																	
85 27 U U				52																		
86 20 U R				27	30	29	52															
86 21 U R				10	18	22	36															
86 22 U R				15	15	15	21															
86 23 U R				9	19	32	38															
86 24 U R					19																	
86 31 UC U			51																			
87 32 U U													46									
88 33 U R				42																		
89 8 U R				14	20	35	40															27
89 25 U R				23	34	23	36															
89 34 U U											54											
90 27 U U										61												
91 8 U R	1	1	4	7	10	15	23															15
91 26 U R				22	24	26	31															
94 33 U R				35																		
94 35 UC R	14	16	21	26	16																	15
95 36 U U				45																		
95 37 UC R				25																		
95 37 UC A				34																		
95 38 UC R				16																		
95 38 UC A				19																		

Source: see *Notes on sources of survey data*, p. 772

Product: MC = manufactured cigarettes
TC = total cigarettes (including hand-rolled)
UC = cigarettes (type unspecified)
A = all products

Frequency: A = all smokers (including occasional)
R = regular or daily smokers

All ages: relevant to ages used and as given in original source

U = unspecified

* = refer to *Notes on sources of survey data*, p. 772

Table 30.4F Prevalence of smoking, females: some selected Yugoslav surveys by age, 1958-1995

Year	Source	Product	Frequency	12	13	14	15	16	17	18	19	20-24	25-29	30-34	35-39	40-44	45-49	50-54	55-59	60-64	65-69	70-74	75-79	80+	All ages
58	1	UC	R																						
58	2	UC	R																						
62	3	UC	R																						
63	4	UC	R																						
64	5	UC	R																						
64	6	UC	U																						
64	7	UC	U																						
66	8	U	R				3	12	10	22															11
69	9	UC	U				3						9		15		26		28						
69	9	A	U				3						9		15		26		28						13
70	10	U	U				10																		
72	11	UC	R													15									
72	12	UC	R									12		11		10		7							10
73	8	U	R	0	1	4	13	16	21	30															20
74	13	U	U				23																		
75	14	U	R				0	6	25	38															
79	15	U	R				3	7	8	7															
80	27	U	U										48												
83	28	U	U						44																
84	8	U	R				10	20	27	34															20
84	16	U	R				19																		
84	17	U	R				5	7	22	26															
84	18	U	R				6	2	14	30															
84	29	UC	R										50		38		24		18						28
84	29	A	A										56		42		26		21						31
84	30	MC	R																						
85	19	U	R				3	12																	
85	27	U	U				31																		
86	20	U	R				19	26	32	47															
86	21	U	R				10	27	19	44															
86	22	U	R				8	12	12	10															
86	23	U	R				7	16	23	34															
86	24	U	R					8																	
86	31	UC	U			44																			
87	32	U	U													12									
88	33	U	R				27																		
89	8	U	R				7	15	22	37															19
89	25	U	R				9	12	21	27															
89	34	U	U										48												
90	27	U	U										40												
91	8	U	R	0	0	2	4	10	12	21															12
91	26	U	R				4	10	13	25															
94	33	U	R				23																		
94	35	UC	U																						
95	36	U	U				30																		
95	37	UC	R				19																		
95	37	UC	A				28																		
95	38	UC	R				15																		
95	38	UC	A				20																		

Source: see *Notes on sources of survey data*, p. 772

Product:
- MC = manufactured cigarettes
- TC = total cigarettes (including hand-rolled)
- UC = cigarettes (type unspecified)
- A = all products

Frequency:
- A = all smokers (including occasional)
- R = regular or daily smokers

All ages: relevant to ages used and as given in original source

U = unspecified

* = refer to *Notes on sources of survey data*, p. 772

Table 30.5M Number of cigarettes smoked per smoker per day, males: some selected Yugoslav surveys by age, 1958-1995

<table>
<tr><th rowspan="2">Product Source Year</th><th colspan="21">Age group</th><th rowspan="2">All ages</th></tr>
<tr><th>12</th><th>13</th><th>14</th><th>15</th><th>16</th><th>17</th><th>18</th><th>19</th><th>20-24</th><th>25-29</th><th>30-34</th><th>35-39</th><th>40-44</th><th>45-49</th><th>50-54</th><th>55-59</th><th>60-64</th><th>65-69</th><th>70-74</th><th>75-79</th><th>80+</th></tr>
<tr><td>58 1 UCE</td><td colspan="12"></td><td>16</td><td>17</td><td>17</td><td>18</td><td colspan="5"></td><td>17</td></tr>
<tr><td>58 2 UCE</td><td colspan="12"></td><td>16</td><td>15</td><td>16</td><td>16</td><td colspan="5"></td><td>16</td></tr>
<tr><td>62 3 UCE</td><td colspan="12"></td><td>16</td><td>17</td><td>14</td><td>14</td><td colspan="5"></td><td>15</td></tr>
<tr><td>63 4 UCE</td><td colspan="12"></td><td>16</td><td>17</td><td>16</td><td>16</td><td colspan="5"></td><td>16</td></tr>
<tr><td>64 5 UCE</td><td colspan="12"></td><td>20</td><td>18</td><td>19</td><td>20</td><td colspan="5"></td><td>19</td></tr>
<tr><td>69 9 AE*</td><td colspan="13"></td><td colspan="2">18</td><td colspan="2">18</td><td colspan="4"></td><td></td></tr>
<tr><td>72 11 UCE</td><td colspan="12"></td><td colspan="4">22</td><td colspan="5"></td><td></td></tr>
<tr><td>72 12 UCE*</td><td colspan="8"></td><td colspan="2">20</td><td colspan="2">20</td><td colspan="2">20</td><td colspan="3">20</td><td colspan="4"></td><td>20</td></tr>
<tr><td>84 29 UC</td><td colspan="11"></td><td colspan="6">24</td><td colspan="4"></td><td></td></tr>
<tr><td>86 31 UC</td><td colspan="2"></td><td colspan="5">9.9</td><td colspan="14"></td><td></td></tr>
<tr><td>87 32 UCE*</td><td colspan="12"></td><td colspan="9">18</td><td></td></tr>
<tr><td>94 35 UC</td><td colspan="5">2.6</td><td colspan="16"></td><td></td></tr>
<tr><td>95 37 UCE</td><td colspan="3"></td><td colspan="2">13</td><td colspan="16"></td><td></td></tr>
<tr><td>95 38 UCE</td><td colspan="3"></td><td colspan="2">11</td><td colspan="16"></td><td></td></tr>
</table>

Table 30.6M Number of cigarettes smoked per person per day, males: some selected Yugoslav surveys by age, 1958-1995, with percentage total sales

<table>
<tr><th rowspan="2">Product Source Year</th><th colspan="21">Age group</th><th rowspan="2">All ages</th><th rowspan="2">% Total sales</th></tr>
<tr><th>12</th><th>13</th><th>14</th><th>15</th><th>16</th><th>17</th><th>18</th><th>19</th><th>20-24</th><th>25-29</th><th>30-34</th><th>35-39</th><th>40-44</th><th>45-49</th><th>50-54</th><th>55-59</th><th>60-64</th><th>65-69</th><th>70-74</th><th>75-79</th><th>80+</th></tr>
<tr><td>58 1 UC</td><td colspan="12"></td><td>8.3</td><td>9.8</td><td>10</td><td>10</td><td colspan="5"></td><td>9.9</td><td>**</td></tr>
<tr><td>58 2 UC</td><td colspan="12"></td><td>9.5</td><td>8.5</td><td>10</td><td>9.3</td><td colspan="5"></td><td>9.5</td><td>**</td></tr>
<tr><td>62 3 UC</td><td colspan="12"></td><td>7.6</td><td>8.0</td><td>7.3</td><td>6.4</td><td colspan="5"></td><td>8.0</td><td>**</td></tr>
<tr><td>63 4 UC</td><td colspan="12"></td><td>9.8</td><td>11</td><td>11</td><td>9.2</td><td colspan="5"></td><td>12</td><td>**</td></tr>
<tr><td>64 5 UC</td><td colspan="12"></td><td>9.9</td><td>8.2</td><td>7.1</td><td>6.4</td><td colspan="5"></td><td>10</td><td>**</td></tr>
<tr><td>69 9 A</td><td colspan="13"></td><td colspan="2">13</td><td colspan="2">13</td><td colspan="4"></td><td></td><td>**</td></tr>
<tr><td>72 11 UC</td><td colspan="12"></td><td colspan="4">12</td><td colspan="5"></td><td></td><td>**</td></tr>
<tr><td>72 12 UC *</td><td colspan="8"></td><td colspan="2">11</td><td colspan="2">12</td><td colspan="2">12</td><td colspan="3">11</td><td colspan="4"></td><td>11</td><td>89%m</td></tr>
<tr><td>84 29 UC *</td><td colspan="11"></td><td colspan="6">12</td><td colspan="4"></td><td></td><td>**</td></tr>
<tr><td>86 31 UC</td><td colspan="2"></td><td colspan="5">5.1</td><td colspan="14"></td><td></td><td>**</td></tr>
<tr><td>87 32 UC *</td><td colspan="12"></td><td colspan="9">8.1</td><td></td><td>**</td></tr>
<tr><td>94 35 UC</td><td colspan="5">0.4</td><td colspan="16"></td><td></td><td>**</td></tr>
<tr><td>95 37 UC</td><td colspan="3"></td><td colspan="2">3.2</td><td colspan="16"></td><td></td><td>**</td></tr>
<tr><td>95 38 UC</td><td colspan="3"></td><td colspan="2">1.7</td><td colspan="16"></td><td></td><td>**</td></tr>
</table>

Table 30.7M Number of cigarettes smoked per person per day, sales-adjusted, males: selected Yugoslav survey[1] by age, 1972, with percentage total sales

<table>
<tr><th rowspan="2">Product Source Year</th><th colspan="21">Age group</th><th rowspan="2">All ages</th><th rowspan="2">% Total sales</th></tr>
<tr><th>12</th><th>13</th><th>14</th><th>15</th><th>16</th><th>17</th><th>18</th><th>19</th><th>20-24</th><th>25-29</th><th>30-34</th><th>35-39</th><th>40-44</th><th>45-49</th><th>50-54</th><th>55-59</th><th>60-64</th><th>65-69</th><th>70-74</th><th>75-79</th><th>80+</th></tr>
<tr><td>72 12 UC *</td><td colspan="8"></td><td colspan="2">12</td><td colspan="2">13</td><td colspan="2">14</td><td colspan="3">12</td><td colspan="4"></td><td>13</td><td>89%m</td></tr>
</table>

1 Based on those surveys in Table 30.6 with data for both sexes and age range at least 21-64 (see *Cigarette consumption per person*, p. xxxv)

Source: see *Notes on sources of survey data*, p. 772
All ages: relevant to ages used and as given in original source
% Total sales: estimated % of total sales of M = manufactured or T = total cigarette consumption implied by survey, sexes combined, used as adjustment factor in Table 30.7
** = cannot be calculated
--- = adjusted by original author
* = refer to *Notes on sources of survey data*, p. 772

Product:
MC = manufactured cigarettes
TC = total cigarettes (including hand-rolled)
UC = cigarettes (type unspecified)
A = all products
U = unspecified
E indicates mean estimated from percentage distribution (see also *Consumption category estimation*, p. xxxiv, and Appendix III, p. 789)

Table 30.5F Number of cigarettes smoked per smoker per day, females: some selected Yugoslav surveys by age, 1958-1995

<table>
<tr><th rowspan="2">Product
Source
Year</th><th colspan="21">Age group</th><th rowspan="2">All ages</th></tr>
<tr><th>12</th><th>13</th><th>14</th><th>15</th><th>16</th><th>17</th><th>18</th><th>19</th><th>20-24</th><th>25-29</th><th>30-34</th><th>35-39</th><th>40-44</th><th>45-49</th><th>50-54</th><th>55-59</th><th>60-64</th><th>65-69</th><th>70-74</th><th>75-79</th><th>80+</th></tr>
<tr><td>58 1 UCE</td><td colspan="21"></td><td></td></tr>
<tr><td>58 2 UCE</td><td colspan="21"></td><td></td></tr>
<tr><td>62 3 UCE</td><td colspan="21"></td><td></td></tr>
<tr><td>63 4 UCE</td><td colspan="21"></td><td></td></tr>
<tr><td>64 5 UCE</td><td colspan="21"></td><td></td></tr>
<tr><td>69 9 AE*</td><td colspan="13"></td><td colspan="2">12</td><td colspan="2">13</td><td colspan="4"></td><td></td></tr>
<tr><td>72 11 UCE</td><td colspan="11"></td><td colspan="5">16</td><td colspan="5"></td><td></td></tr>
<tr><td>72 12 UCE*</td><td colspan="8"></td><td colspan="2">13</td><td colspan="2">15</td><td colspan="2">15</td><td colspan="3">16</td><td colspan="4"></td><td>15</td></tr>
<tr><td>84 29 UC</td><td colspan="11"></td><td colspan="6">15</td><td colspan="4"></td><td></td></tr>
<tr><td>86 31 UC</td><td colspan="2"></td><td colspan="6">6.8</td><td colspan="13"></td><td></td></tr>
<tr><td>87 32 UCE*</td><td colspan="12"></td><td colspan="9">14</td><td></td></tr>
<tr><td>94 35 UC</td><td colspan="21"></td><td></td></tr>
<tr><td>95 37 UCE</td><td colspan="3"></td><td colspan="2">11</td><td colspan="16"></td><td></td></tr>
<tr><td>95 38 UCE</td><td colspan="3"></td><td colspan="2">8.8</td><td colspan="16"></td><td></td></tr>
</table>

Table 30.6F Number of cigarettes smoked per person per day, females: some selected Yugoslav surveys by age, 1958-1995, with percentage total sales

<table>
<tr><th rowspan="2">Product
Source
Year</th><th colspan="21">Age group</th><th rowspan="2">All ages</th><th rowspan="2">% Total sales</th></tr>
<tr><th>12</th><th>13</th><th>14</th><th>15</th><th>16</th><th>17</th><th>18</th><th>19</th><th>20-24</th><th>25-29</th><th>30-34</th><th>35-39</th><th>40-44</th><th>45-49</th><th>50-54</th><th>55-59</th><th>60-64</th><th>65-69</th><th>70-74</th><th>75-79</th><th>80+</th></tr>
<tr><td>58 1 UC</td><td colspan="21"></td><td></td><td>**</td></tr>
<tr><td>58 2 UC</td><td colspan="21"></td><td></td><td>**</td></tr>
<tr><td>62 3 UC</td><td colspan="21"></td><td></td><td>**</td></tr>
<tr><td>63 4 UC</td><td colspan="21"></td><td></td><td>**</td></tr>
<tr><td>64 5 UC</td><td colspan="21"></td><td></td><td>**</td></tr>
<tr><td>69 9 A</td><td colspan="13"></td><td colspan="2">3.0</td><td colspan="2">3.5</td><td colspan="4"></td><td></td><td>**</td></tr>
<tr><td>72 11 UC</td><td colspan="11"></td><td colspan="5">2.3</td><td colspan="5"></td><td></td><td>**</td></tr>
<tr><td>72 12 UC *</td><td colspan="8"></td><td colspan="2">1.6</td><td colspan="2">1.6</td><td colspan="2">1.5</td><td colspan="3">1.1</td><td colspan="4"></td><td>1.5</td><td>89%m</td></tr>
<tr><td>84 29 UC *</td><td colspan="11"></td><td colspan="6">4.2</td><td colspan="4"></td><td></td><td>**</td></tr>
<tr><td>86 31 UC</td><td colspan="2"></td><td colspan="6">3.0</td><td colspan="13"></td><td></td><td>**</td></tr>
<tr><td>87 32 UC *</td><td colspan="12"></td><td colspan="9">1.6</td><td></td><td>**</td></tr>
<tr><td>94 35 UC</td><td colspan="21"></td><td></td><td>**</td></tr>
<tr><td>95 37 UC</td><td colspan="3"></td><td colspan="2">2.0</td><td colspan="16"></td><td></td><td>**</td></tr>
<tr><td>95 38 UC</td><td colspan="3"></td><td colspan="2">1.3</td><td colspan="16"></td><td></td><td>**</td></tr>
</table>

Table 30.7F Number of cigarettes smoked per person per day, sales-adjusted, females: selected Yugoslav survey[1] by age, 1972, with percentage total sales

<table>
<tr><th rowspan="2">Product
Source
Year</th><th colspan="21">Age group</th><th rowspan="2">All ages</th><th rowspan="2">% Total sales</th></tr>
<tr><th>12</th><th>13</th><th>14</th><th>15</th><th>16</th><th>17</th><th>18</th><th>19</th><th>20-24</th><th>25-29</th><th>30-34</th><th>35-39</th><th>40-44</th><th>45-49</th><th>50-54</th><th>55-59</th><th>60-64</th><th>65-69</th><th>70-74</th><th>75-79</th><th>80+</th></tr>
<tr><td>72 12 UC *</td><td colspan="8"></td><td colspan="2">1.8</td><td colspan="2">1.9</td><td colspan="2">1.7</td><td colspan="3">1.2</td><td colspan="4"></td><td>1.6</td><td>89%m</td></tr>
</table>

1 Based on those surveys in Table 30.6 with data for both sexes and age range at least 21-64 (see *Cigarette consumption per person*, p. xxxv)

Source: see *Notes on sources of survey data*, p. 772
All ages: relevant to ages used and as given in original source
% Total sales: estimated % of total sales of M = manufactured or T = total cigarette consumption implied by survey, sexes combined, used as adjustment factor in Table 30.7
** = cannot be calculated
--- = adjusted by original author
* = refer to *Notes on sources of survey data*, p. 772

Product: MC = manufactured cigarettes
TC = total cigarettes (including hand-rolled)
UC = cigarettes (type unspecified)
A = all products
U = unspecified
E indicates mean estimated from percentage distribution (see also *Consumption category estimation*, p. xxxiv, and Appendix III, p. 789)

Table 30.8 Estimated[1] prevalence of smoking and estimated[1] number of cigarettes per person per day (unadjusted and sales-adjusted): summary of Tables 30.4, 30.6 and 30.7, 1969-1995.
Males and females aged 15 years and over

Year	Source[2]	Product[3]	Prevalence[4]						Number of cigarettes						
									Unadjusted[7]			Sales-adjusted[8]			
			Manufactured cigarettes		Total cigarettes[5]		All products[6]		Number/ person/day		Total sales %	Manufactured cigarettes[9] number/ person/day		Total cigarettes number/ person/day	
			M	F	M	F	M	F	M	F		M	F	M	F
1969	9	*UC*+A			50	15	53	15				(10.3	2.4)		
1970	10	*U*					57	10				(11.3	1.6)		
1972	12	UC			53	11			10.2	1.6	89	11.4	1.8		
1984	30	MC	56												
1985	27	*U*					52	31				(11.8	5.6)		
1988	33	U					42	27				(11.8	6.2)		
1994	33	U					35	23				(10.1	5.3)		
1995	36	*U*					45	30				(9.9	5.3)		

1 Surveys covering an age range of at least 21-64 are included. Any gaps in the data for ages 15-20 and 65 years and over are filled in by assumed extensions to the age distribution, given in *Notes on sources of survey data*, p. 772. Method: see *Summary of adult smoking*, p. xxxvi
2 See *Notes on sources of survey data*, p. 772
3 Product: MC = manufactured cigarettes, TC = total cigarettes (including hand-rolled), UC = cigarettes (type unspecified), A = all products, U = unspecified. Frequency of smoking is indicated by: regular or daily smokers in normal type, all smokers (including occasional) in bold, unspecified in italics
4 From Table 30.4
5 This column includes prevalence of smoking classified as UC = cigarettes (type unspecified)
6 This column includes prevalence of smoking classified as U = unspecified product
7 From Table 30.6
8 From Table 30.7, except data in parentheses, which are derived from the prevalence of smoking from Table 30.4 as described in *Summary of adult smoking*, p. xxxvi
9 Number of cigarettes classified as UC = cigarettes (type unspecified) or U = product unspecified has been adjusted to manufactured cigarette sales and included in this column. Before 1990, adjustment is to sales in the former Yugoslavia; for 1994, adjustment is to 1993 sales in Slovenia; for 1995, adjustment is to sales in Serbia and Montenegro

Figure 30.3 Estimated prevalence of smoking of (i) cigarettes and (ii) all tobacco products: by year of survey, 1969-1995.
Males and females aged 15 years and over. *Source:* see Table 30.8

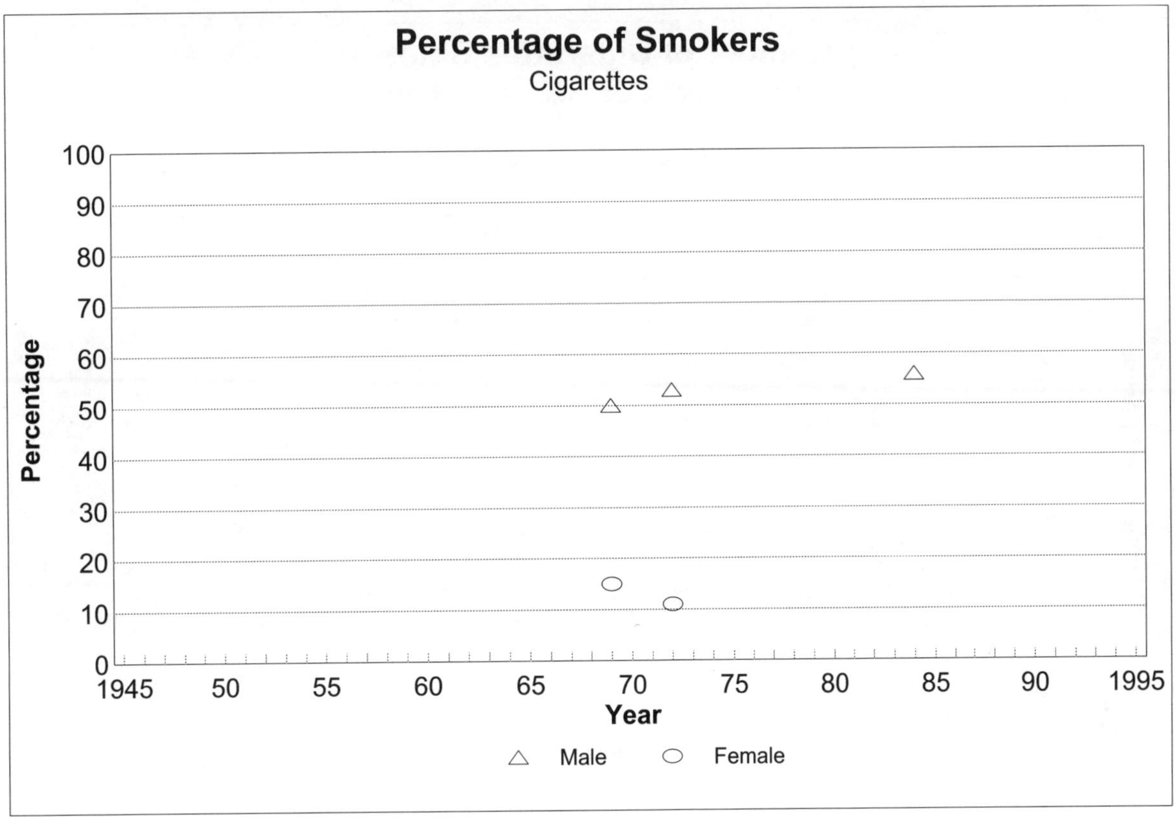

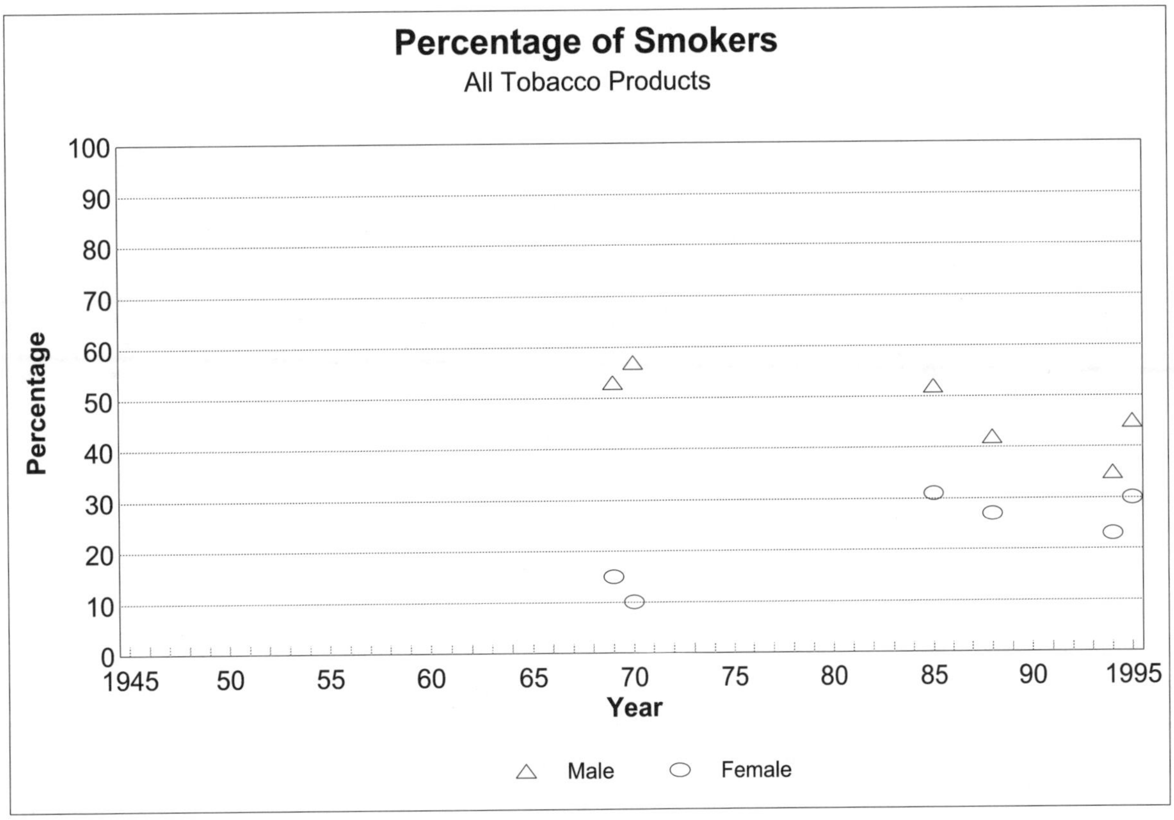

Figure 30.4 Estimated number of cigarettes smoked per person per day, sales-adjusted, 1969-1995.
Males and females aged 15 years and over. *Source:* see Table 30.8

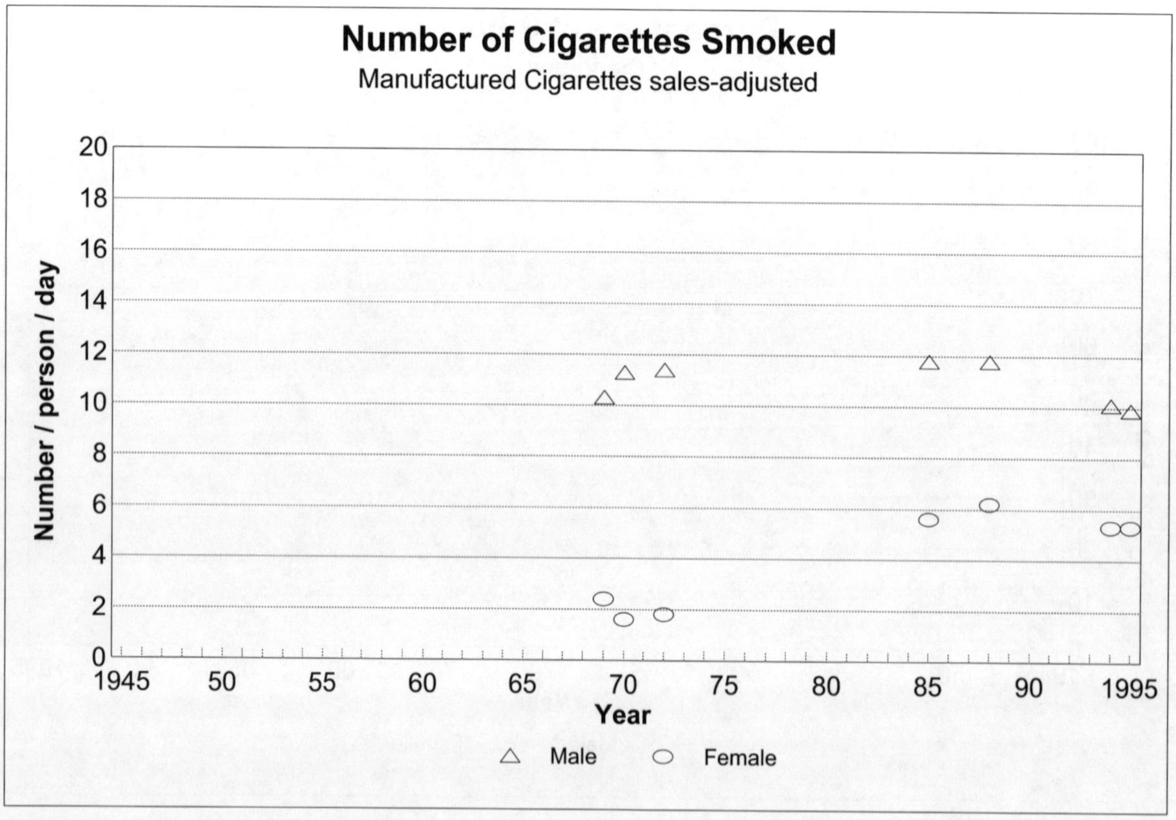

Notes on sources of sales data

The data presented in the tables and figures were obtained from several sources, details of which are given below, together with estimations and related assumptions. Full citations of the sources are given on p. 776 under *References*.

Consumption data

1922-1935 Hutson (1937) *(Table 30.1.1)*

Data were originally given to the nearest 1 000 pounds. They have been converted to tonnes (1 000 lbs = 0.45359 tonnes) and given to the nearest tonne. For conversion from weights to numbers we assumed an average cigarette weight of 1 g.

1960-1995 United States Department of Agriculture (USDA) Economic Research Service (1996), Franceschi and Naett (1995) quoting USDA, Beljo (1995a) *(Tables 31.1.2 and 30.2)*

Consumption data are not available for the years after the breakup of Yugoslavia for most of the successor republics. All the data given for the successor republics are unofficial estimates. The situation was complicated by UN trade embargos, continuing conflict between republics, inflation and cross-border smuggling.

Macedonia experienced an additional trade embargo by Greece which prevented Macedonia using its nearest port, Salonika, for exports. Before the breakup, the republic's production constituted 40-50% of total Yugoslavian production and more than 70% of its production was sold in other parts of Yugoslavia. Macedonian cigarette consumption in 1994 was in the range 3 500-4 000 million pieces, though an exact figure could not be calculated because of extensive smuggling and duty-free sales. For 1996 it is estimated that around 43% of consumption was marketed illegally. (Beljo (1995b), USDA Economic Research Service (1996)).

For the Serbia-Montenegro federation it is estimated that almost 100% of imported cigarettes were smuggled, amounting to 13 000 million cigarettes in 1995 and 13 500 in 1996. UN sanctions, which included restrictions on cigarette imports, were in place from June 1992 until November 1995. (USDA Economic Research Service (1996)).

Smuggled cigarettes were estimated to account for around 40% of the market in Bosnia in 1996 (USDA Economic Research Service (1996)).

Zatonski (1991) stated that most cigarettes smoked in Yugoslavia (around 1990) were king-size.

Alternative estimates of consumption of cigarettes by Krstič (1991) are shown here. They are based on production plus import minus exports. Comparison with the USDA series suggests an average cigarette weight of about 1 g.

	Cigarette consumption (tonnes)
1980	49 304
1981	45 332
1982	45 354
1983	57 683
1984	54 968
1985	55 154
1986	53 294
1987	55 221
1988	58 779
1989	56 133
1990	57 377

Due to lack of any data on sales of other products, we have not included estimates of the consumption of all tobacco products in Table 30.2 for 1960 onwards.

Plain/Filter cigarette consumption

1966-1972 Maxwell (successive years)

1984 Boddewyn (1986)

For 1993-1995 the percentage of production which was of filter cigarettes for the Serbia-Montenegro federation was around 98% (USDA Economic Research Service (1996)).

Tar yield of cigarettes
In 1990, the limits on yields in Yugoslavia were 30 mg of tar and 1.7 mg of nicotine per cigarette (Zatonski (1991)). Around 1995 Croatia had a limit of 15 mg tar per cigarette and Slovenia was drafting a law for a limit of 15 mg of tar per cigarette (Harkin *et al* (1997)).

Estimates of hand-rolled cigarette consumption
No information on smoking of hand-rolled cigarettes is available.

Notes on sources of survey data

Each source of survey data—either an individual survey or a series of surveys repeated over a number of years—is cited by a source number. This number is shown in the tables and corresponds to the source numbers given below, where details of the source publication and of the survey methodology are given. Full citations of the sources are given on p. 776 under *References*.

Source number

1-5 Keys *et al* (1966), Djordjević *et al* (1970)

a. Baseline of Seven Countries Study on cardiovascular disease. Interview including smoking questions before medical examinations.

	Location	Description	Sample size	Response rate (%)
1	Velika Krsna, central Serbia	Farming village	522	97
2	Zrenjanin, central Serbia	Employees at a food-processing plant in a market town	516	'substantially all'
3	Belgrade	All men of the faculty of the University of Belgrade	538	80
4	Dalmatia	Coastal farming villages	727	98
5	Dalj, Slavonia	Large farming village	749	92

b. Occupational groups included in this report because there are few other studies at this time, and for comparability with groups in other countries with same methodology

c. Pipe and cigar consumption is stated to be very uncommon in Serbia, especially away from Belgrade

d. Consumption category estimation based on 1-9, 10-19, 20 or more cigarettes/smoker/day, except *All ages* cigarettes per person data for the three Serbian cohorts which were given directly by Nedeljkovic *et al* (1993). Values estimated by our method would have been slightly lower

e. There is a discrepancy between the two sources on the sample size for Velika Krsna

6-7 Kozarević *et al* (1976)

a. Baseline of Yugoslavia Cardiovascular Disease Study, 1964-1965. All men living in 2 communities and born 1903-1928 were invited for examination, and subjects with definite or possible myocardial infarction were excluded. The communities were Tuzla, a town and surrounding villages in an industrial and mining area in Bosnia, and Remetinic, a suburb of the Croatian capital Zagreb.

		Initial response rate (%)	Eventual sample size
6	Tuzla	94	6 416
7	Remetinic	92	4 618

b. The mean number of cigarettes per day is stated to be 14.9 (both areas combined) but it is unclear whether this is per smoker or per person

8 Prebeg *et al* (1993)

a. Surveys conducted in schools in Zagreb, Croatia, by the Andrija Štampar School of Public Health.

	Sample size		
	Primary	Secondary	
		Boys	Girls
1966	—	476	562
1973	2 112	1 491	2 752
1984	—	1 642	1 800
1989	—	1 463	1 710
1991	2 103	1 366	1 386

Sample sizes shown for Primary schools in 1973 and 1991 include age 11

b. Approximate ages corresponding to school grades. Results shown in *All ages* column for 1973 and 1991 are for Secondary schools only (age 15-18)

c. Regular smokers: smoked daily

d. Insufficient detail was presented to calculate cigarettes per smoker: the percentage of smokers smoking more than 10 cigarettes per day was 30-50% among boys, compared with 20% among girls in 1966 and 30% in other years

9 Smajkic *et al* (1972)

a. Study in 5 districts of Bosnia and Hercegovina. Sample size 6 222

b. Corrected for apparent misprints in Table II

c. Consumption category estimation based on 1-4, 5-15 (assume 5-14), and 15-24 grams/smoker/day, assuming that there were no smokers of 25+ grams. It is unclear whether ex-smokers are included

d. Assumed extension to age distribution for percentage smokers, age 65+: males (cigarettes) 40%, (all products) 50%; females 20%

10 WHO (1997)

a. Nationwide survey in Croatia. No original source. Age group not stated

11 Mimica *et al* (1978)

a. Questionnaire study in a sample population from six communities in Socialist Republic of Croatia (Zabreb-Centar, Zagreb-Črnomerec, Virovitica, Split, Omiš and Vis). Part of a study of respiratory and cardiovascular diseases. Sample size (males) 1 575, (females) 1 690

b. Consumption category estimation based on 1-10, 11-20, 21-30, >30 cigarettes/smoker/day

12 Kulčar *et al* (1974)

a. Estimates based on an epidemiological study on psychosis in 1969-1972 and a representative sample of the population of Croatia. Sample size 23 754

b. Consumption category estimation based on two categories, 1-10 and 11+ cigarettes/smoker/day, and resulting figures should be regarded with caution

c. Assumed extension to age distribution for percentage smokers, age 15-19: males 40%, females 20%. For age 65+: males 40%, females 5%. Number of cigarettes/person/day, age 15-19: males 5.0, females 3.0. For age 65+: males 8.0, females 1.0

13 Jakovljevic (1977)

a. Quoting postgraduate study by A. Markovic. Year not stated

b. Study in 7 general and vocational secondary schools in Belgrade. Sample size 1 896

14-26 Prebeg *et al* (1993)

a. Series of single surveys throughout Croatia. Organized by the Andrija Štampar School of Public Health and conducted by school physicians as an introductory part of the anti-smoking program. There were some differences between the questionnaires used, but definitions of smoking were identical.

	Year	Location	Sample size	
			Males	Females
14	1975	Krapina	298	155
15	1979	Županja	657	684
16	1984	Pula	404	467
17	1984	Rijeka	291	410
18	1984	Duga Resa	115	305
19	1985	Dubrovnik	167	160
20	1986	Zadar	620	1 033
21	1986	Varaždin	363	278
22	1986	Požega	194	390
23	1986	Vinkovci	458	545
24	1986	Osijek	486	461
25	1989	Poreč	265	498
26	1991	Čakovec	387	425

b. Approximate ages corresponding to school grades
c. Regular smokers: smoked daily

27 WHO (1997)

a. National surveys (relating to former Yugoslavia), no further details. Age group not stated for 1985

28 Geizerova and Masironi (1988)

a. No original source

29 WHO (1989), WHO MONICA Project (1988)

a. Regional survey forming part of WHO MONICA project:

Region	Population size	Sample size	Participation rate (%)	Sample used*		Date
				Males	Females	
Novi Sad	99 000	1 448	82	781	733	Sep 1984-Dec 1984

* 'Sample used' includes age 25-34; all other figures are for age 35-64 only

b. *All ages* column relates only to age 35-64 and is standardized to world population
c. Regular cigarette smokers: smoked cigarettes daily. All smokers: smoked cigarettes daily or occasionally, or smoked 1 g pipe tobacco or 1 cigar per week. Cigarettes per smoker refers to regular and occasional cigarette smokers
d. Calculation for cigarettes per person based on % regular cigarette smokers and cigarettes per regular or occasional cigarette smoker, so may underestimate

30 Mackay (1994)

a. No original source. Age group not stated
b. Female prevalence is also reported as 10-36%

31 Grubši*f*-Greblo *et al* (1989)

a. Study of glue sniffing in three secondary schools in Rijeka, Croatia. Sample size (males) 1 119, (females) 1 135

32 Burany *et al* (1992a, 1992b)

a. Multiphase oncologic population screening in Mali Idos, Croatia, a rural area. Sample size 5 555, response rate 91%
b. Based on recall of age of starting to smoke, smoking among women started in the 1960s
c. Consumption category estimation based on two categories, 1-20 and 21+ cigarettes/smoker/day, and resulting figures should be regarded with caution

33 Rehar (2000)

a. Surveys, most recently supported by the Ministry of Health, of the adult population of Slovenia

34 WHO (1997)

a. Slovenia

b. No original source. Age groups shown are those with the highest prevalence

35 Žuškin *et al* (1995)

a. School boys in Zagreb and surrounding area, Croatia. Year not stated.

Age	Sample size
9-11	900
12	436
13	492
14	444
15	416
16	88
Total	2 776

b. Results in *All ages* column in Table 30.4, and in Tables 30.5-6 relate to age 9-16. The prevalence of smoking for ages 12-16 was 19%

c. Regular smokers: smoked 1+ cigarettes per day

d. Cigarettes per smoker calculated from distribution of numbers of cigarettes, given graphically

36 Legetic *et al* (2000) quoting Federal Commission on Addictive Diseases

a. Year unknown. Age group not stated (adults)

b. The results for females shown in Table 30.4 are taken from the published abstract (1997). In the published paper, the prevalence is reported as 25-30%

37-38 Hibell *et al* (1997)

a. Nationally representative surveys in Croatia and Slovenia forming part of ESPAD (European School Survey Project on Alcohol and Other Drugs). Target was pupils born in 1979, thus age 15-16 at time of surveys in April 1995. Approximately 90% of this group still in school in Croatia (not stated for Slovenia). Anonymous questionnaire completed and sealed in envelope by pupil, in class. Teachers or school counsellors present, but discouraged from walking round the classroom.

		Sample size		Response rate (%)	
		Males	**Females**	**Males**	**Females**
37	Croatia	1 518	1 297	91	92
38	Slovenia	1 543	1 763	91	92

b. Regular smokers: smoked 1 or more cigarettes per day in last 30 days. All smokers: smoked in last 30 days

c. Consumption category estimation based on 1-5, 6-10, 11-20, 21+ cigarettes/smoker/day

References

Boddewyn J.J. (ed) (1986). *Tobacco advertising bans and consumption in 16 countries*. International Advertising Association, New York.

Beljo J. (1995a). Cigarette consumption stable in Croatia. *Tobacco Journal International,* **Jul/Aug**, 60-1.

Beljo J. (1995b). New markets still proving elusive for Macedonia. *Tobacco Journal International,* **5**, 32 and 34.

Burany B., Szabo E., Mikov M., Popovic S. and Babcsanyi S. (1992a). Prilog proucavanju pusenja. I. Pusacko iskusto, broj popusenih cigareta (Smoking. I. Smoking habits, number of cigarettes smoked). *Med Pregl,* **45**, 369-72.

Burany B., Szabo E., Mikov M., Popovic S. and Babcsanyi S. (1992b). Prilog proucavanju pusenja. II. Duzina pusackog stanza i faktori od uticaja no pusenje kao drustvenu pojavu. (Smoking. II. Duration of smoking and factors affecting smoking as a social phenomenon). *Med Pregl,* **45**, 451-4.

Djordjević B.S., Balog B., Božinović Lj., Josipović V., *et al* (1970). Three cohorts of men followed five years in Serbia. *Circulation,* **XLI and XLII (Suppl I)**, 123-37.

Franceschi S. and Naett C. (1995). Trends in smoking in Europe. *Eur J Cancer Prev,* **4**, 271-84.

Geizerova H. and Masironi R. (1988). Cigarette smoking in children and adolescents: world review. In: Aoki M., Hisamichi S. and Tominaga S. (eds) *Smoking and health 1987. Proceedings of the 6th World Conference on Smoking and Health, Tokyo, 9-12 November 1987*. Elsevier Science Publishers B.V. (Biomedical Division), Amsterdam; 601-5. International Congress Series No. 780.

Grubšić-Greblo H., Jonjić A. and Vukelić M. (1989). Pojava udisanja para ljepila kod učenika srednjih škola (Manifestations of glue sniffing in secondary school students). *Arh Hig Rada Toksikol,* **40**, 313-8.

Harkin A.M., Anderson P. and Goos C. (1997). *Smoking, drinking and drug taking in the European Region.* Alcohol, Drugs and Tobacco Programme, WHO Regional Office for Europe, Copenhagen.

Hibell B., Andersson B., Bjarnason T., Kokkevi A., Morgan M. and Narusk A. (1997). *The 1995 ESPAD report. The European school survey project on alcohol and other drugs. Alcohol and other drug use among students in 26 European countries*. The Swedish Council for Information on Alcohol and Other Drugs. Council of Europe (Pompidou Group).

Hutson J.B. (1937). *Consumption and production of tobacco in Europe*. USDA, Washington DC. Technical bulletin No. 587.

Jakovljevic D. (1977). Anti-smoking program in Yugoslavia. In: Steinfeld J., Griffiths W., Ball K. and Taylor R.M. (eds) *Health consequences, education, cessation activities, and social action, Volume II. Proceedings of the Third World Conference on Smoking and Health, New York City, June 2-5, 1975*. US Department of Health, Education and Welfare, USA; 795-8. DHEW Publication No (NIH) 77-1413.

Keys A., Aravanis C., Blackburn H.W., van Buchem F.S.P., *et al* (1966). Epidemiological studies related to coronary heart disease: characteristics of men aged 40-59 in seven countries. *Acta Medica Scandinavica,* **Suppl 460**, 8-392.

Kozarević D., Pirc B., Dawber T.R., Gordon T., Zukel W.J. and Vojvodić N. (1976). The Yugoslavia cardiovascular disease study. I. The incidence of coronary heart disease by area. *Journal of Chronic Diseases,* **29**, 405-14.

Krstič N. (1991). The obstacles to an active cigarette price policy in the Republic of Slovenia and Yugoslavia (1980-1990). *Journal of Smoking-Related Disorders,* **2**, 191-202.

Kulčar Ž., Kovačić L. and Bedeniĉ B. (1974). Rasprostranjenost pušenja u stanovništvu SR Hrvatske (Smoking in the population of Croatia). *Lijec Vjesn,* **96**, 467-72.

Legetic B., Planojevic M. and Jakovljevic D. (2000). Yugoslavia: Smoking prevention and control, with special reference to the Novi Sad MONICA project. In: Lu R., Mackay J., Niu S. and Peto R. (eds) *Tobacco: The Growing Epidemic. Proceedings of the Tenth World Conference on Tobacco or Health, 24-28 August 1997, Beijing, China.* Springer-Verlag, London; 505-7.

Mackay J.L. (1994). The fight against tobacco in developing countries. *Tuber Lung Dis,* **75**, 8-24.

Maxwell J.C.Jr. (successive years). How the brands ranked. Maxwell International Estimates. *World Tobacco.*

Mimica M., Šarič M. and Malinar M. (1978). Naša ispitivanja o navici pušenja (A study of the smoking habit). *Arh Hig Rada Toksikol,* **29**, 209-18.

Nedeljkovic S., Ostojic M.C., Grujic M.Z., Josipovic V., *et al* (1993). Coronary heart disease deaths in 25 years. The experience in the three Serbian cohorts of the Seven Countries Study. *Acta Cardiol,* **48**, 11-24.

Prebeg Z., Počekaj A., Lešić M. and Vragović-Košutić A. (1993). Trends in adolescent smoking in Croatia. *Croat Med J,* **34**, 251-6.

Rehar V. (2000). Slovenia: United in non-smoking: New thinking, model and philosophy. In: Lu R., Mackay J., Niu S. and Peto R. (eds) *Tobacco: the growing epidemic. Proceedings of the Tenth World Conference on Tobacco or Health, Beijing, 24-28 August 1997.* Springer-Verlag, London; 485-8.

Smajkic A., Zarakovic G. and Cerkez F. (1972). Navike pušenja kod stanovništva u pet opština u Bosni i Hercegovini (Smoking habits among the population of 5 districts in Bosnia and Hercegovina). *Med Arh,* **26**, 35-8.

USDA Economic Research Service (1996). *Tobacco statistics.* Albert R. Mann Library, Cornell University, Ithaca, New York. ERS 94012. (With supplementary material from Tobacco Annual Reports.). http://usda.mannlib.cornell.edu/data-sets/specialty/94012.

WHO (1989). The WHO MONICA project: a worldwide monitoring system for cardiovascular diseases. In: *World health statistics annual 1989.* WHO, Geneva; 25-149.

WHO MONICA Project (1988). Geographical variation in the major risk factors of coronary heart disease in men and women aged 35-64 years. *World Health Stat Q,* **41**, 115-40.

WHO (1997). *Tobacco or health: A global status report.* WHO, Geneva. www.cdc.gov/nccdphp/osh/who/whoampro.htm.

Zatonski W. (1991). Country reports. *World Smoking and Health,* **16**, 12-21.

Žuškin E., Smolej-Narančić N., Mustajbegović J. and Budak A. (1995). Navika pušenja u školske djece. (Smoking habit in schoolchildren). *Lijec Vjesn,* **117**, 278-81.

Appendix I

Estimated size of adult population

Males and females aged 15 years and over, thousands, selected years 1920 to 1995

Year	Australia			Austria			Belgium		
	Males	Females	Total	Males	Females	Total	Males	Females	Total
1920			3600						
1925			4100			4900			5900
1930			4600			5100			6200
1935			4900			5200			6300
1940			5300			5300			6500
1945	2781	2708	5600			5300			6600
1950	3013	2990	6003	2414	2942	5357	3338	3495	6833
1955	3291	3237	6528	2435	2958	5393	3375	3561	6936
1960	3604	3568	7171	2489	3005	5494	3360	3592	6951
1965	3994	3987	7981	2529	3037	5566	3483	3708	7191
1970	4444	4457	8902	2543	3038	5581	3552	3809	7361
1975	4968	5012	9980	2647	3121	5768	3685	3939	7624
1980	5423	5496	10919	2762	3203	5965	3798	4058	7856
1985	5958	6082	12040	2880	3300	6180	3866	4144	8010
1990	6585	6725	13310	3019	3363	6382	3945	4216	8161
1995	6998	7180	14178	3179	3456	6635			

Year	Bulgaria			Canada			Czechoslovakia [1]		
	Males	Females	Total	Males	Females	Total	Males	Females	Total
1920			34621			57000			
1925			37929			62000	4669	5185	9854
1930			40929			70000	4898	5404	10301
1935						76000			
1940						82000	5732	6164	11896
1945						86000	4412	4801	9213
1950				48728	47526	96254	4407	4811	9218
1955				53228	52371	105599	4543	4952	9495
1960	28816	29350	58166	59752	58632	118384	4758	5177	9936
1965	30962	31419	62381	65308	65264	130572	5076	5496	10572
1970	32516	33002	65518	73850	74883	148733	5287	5726	11013
1975	33675	34344	68019	82819	84529	167348	5441	5904	11345
1980	34078	34920	68998	90677	93683	184360	5563	6035	11598
1985	34937	35982	70919	97431	101614	199045	5615	6103	11718
1990	34932	36603	71535	102556	107685	210241	5806	6293	12099
1995	33446	35565	69011	115998	120168	236166			

Year	Czech Republic			Slovakia			Denmark		
	Males	Females	Total	Males	Females	Total	Males	Females	Total
1920									2200
1925									2400
1930									2600
1935									2800
1940									2900
1945									3000
1950							1548	1606	3154
1955							1599	1661	3259
1960							1680	1746	3426
1965							1780	1847	3627
1970							1858	1923	3781
1975	3646	3955	7601	1796	1948	3744	1918	1991	3909
1980	3727	4043	7771	1836	1992	3827	1982	2073	4055
1985	3762	4089	7851	1853	2014	3867	2037	2134	4171
1990	3899	4241	8139	1916	2077	3993	2085	2180	4264
1995	4036	4374	8410	1994	2160	4153	2115	2206	4321

Year	Finland			France			Germany (Unified/West)		
	Males	Females	Total	Males	Females	Total	Males	Females	Total
1920			2100			28000			
1925			2300			29000			47100
1930			2500			31000			48800
1935			2600			31200			50600
1940			2700			30400			
1945			2800			30900			
1950	1309	1511	2820	15288	17044	32331	16613	19846	36459
1955	1368	1567	2935	15560	17247	32807	18037	21224	39261
1960	1446	1636	3083	16028	17610	33638	19241	22558	41800
1965	1572	1752	3325	17376	18898	36274	21204	24496	45700
1970	1647	1826	3472	18589	20019	38608	21660	24932	46592
1975	1748	1926	3674	19596	20936	40532	22692	25851	48543
1980	1815	1994	3809	20405	21766	42172	23673	26693	50366
1985	1887	2064	3951	21124	22776	43900	24462	27329	51792
1990	1927	2096	4023	21984	23728	45712	25643	27990	53633
1995	1990	2146	4136	22711	24484	47195	32925	35473	68397

Year	Germany (East)			Greece			Hungary [1]		
	Males	Females	Total	Males	Females	Total	Males	Females	Total
1920						3300	2626	2877	5503
1925						4000	2754	2996	5750
1930						4300	2950	3178	6129
1935						4600	3109	3327	6436
1940						4900	3230	3448	6678
1945						5000			
1950	6018	8168	14187	2571	2816	5388	3312	3698	7010
1955	6090	8076	14165	2811	3066	5876	3463	3834	7297
1960	5901	7705	13606	2941	3213	6154	3526	3931	7456
1965	5683	7281	12964	3034	3331	6365	3694	4092	7786
1970	5809	7265	13074	3184	3442	6626	3905	4281	8186
1975	5955	7249	13204	3318	3568	6886	4011	4387	8398
1980	6160	7287	13447	3597	3846	7443	3980	4383	8362
1985	6228	7210	13438	3815	4044	7860	3969	4391	8360
1990	6082	6886	12968	3996	4204	8200	3906	4362	8268
1995				4254	4439	8693	3946	4430	8376

Year	Iceland [2]			Ireland			Israel [3]		
	Males	Females	Total	Males	Females	Total	Males	Females	Total
1920			64			2200			
1925			67			2100			
1930			72			2100			
1935			80			2100			
1940			90			2200			
1945			90			2100			
1950	49	50	99	1075	1042	2118	399	377	776
1955	52	53	105	1035	1016	2050	521	512	1033
1960	57	57	114	979	978	1957	612	607	1219
1965	63	63	126	988	991	1979	765	763	1527
1970	69	68	138	1009	1015	2024	878	884	1762
1975	76	76	152	1067	1080	2147	1148	1173	2320
1980	83	82	165	1178	1187	2366	1277	1314	2590
1985	89	89	178	1240	1265	2506	1404	1450	2854
1990	95	96	191	1258	1288	2546	1573	1629	3202
1995	101	102	202	1337	1386	2724	1906	2001	3906

Year	Italy			Japan			Netherlands		
	Males	Females	Total	Males	Females	Total	Males	Females	Total
1920						35200			
1925			26100			37500			5000
1930			27500			40400			5500
1935			29000			43300			5900
1940			30100			45600			
1945			32100			47300			
1950	16697	18103	34800	25865	27902	53767	3523	3628	7150
1955	17596	18855	36451	28682	30795	59477	3706	3830	7536
1960	18237	19525	37763	31542	33810	65352	3956	4088	8044
1965	18981	20392	39373	35430	37679	73109	4355	4466	8820
1970	19546	21044	40590	38001	40473	78474	4687	4794	9481
1975	20412	21979	42391	40945	43320	84264	5033	5170	10203
1980	21432	23087	44519	43442	46040	89482	5405	5585	10991
1985	22111	24004	46115	45816	48529	94345	5726	5947	11672
1990	23137	25022	48159	48763	51556	100319	5995	6230	12225
1995	23415	25317	48732	50747	53685	104432	6192	6424	12616

Year	New Zealand			Norway			Poland [2]		
	Males	Females	Total	Males	Females	Total	Males	Females	Total
1920			800						
1925			1000						20892
1930			1100			2000			
1935			1100			2200			
1940			1200			2300			
1945			1200			2400			
1950	681	681	1362	1212	1261	2474	8137	9392	17529
1955	734	736	1470	1255	1295	2550	8797	10041	18838
1960	796	800	1596	1310	1347	2657	9255	10413	19668
1965	887	894	1781	1382	1419	2801	10289	11431	21720
1970	949	970	1920	1442	1487	2928	11313	12442	23755
1975	1071	1090	2161	1502	1552	3054	12451	13569	26021
1980	1128	1153	2281	1561	1619	3180	12917	14022	26939
1985	1215	1256	2471	1628	1694	3322	13282	14422	27704
1990	1274	1328	2602	1686	1752	3438	13681	14862	28543
1995	1342	1408	2750	1720	1790	3510	14277	15512	29790

Year	Portugal			Romania [1, 2]			Spain		
	Males	Females	Total	Males	Females	Total	Males	Females	Total
1920						11063			
1925						11939			
1930						12281			16200
1935						12948			17100
1940			5300						18000
1945			5600						18800
1950	2782	3146	5928				9627	10692	20319
1955	2939	3314	6254	5987	6565	12552	10069	11088	21157
1960	2935	3362	6298	6350	6897	13247	10450	11541	21991
1965	2997	3480	6477	6743	7255	13998	10844	12214	23058
1970	2844	3316	6159	7258	7742	15001	11653	12692	24345
1975	3124	3721	6845	7716	8168	15884	12232	13305	25537
1980	3383	3940	7323	7926	8354	16280	13383	14399	27782
1985	3618	4027	7645	8348	8774	17122	14322	15275	29597
1990	3738	4138	7876	8655	9083	17738	15158	16123	31280
1995	3873	4280	8152	8752	9285	18037	15841	16850	32691

Year	Sweden			Switzerland			UK		
	Males	Females	Total	Males	Females	Total	Males	Females	Total
1920			4200				15845	17672	33517
1925			4400				15748	17545	33293
1930			4600				16313	18269	34582
1935			4900			3200	17057	19030	36087
1940			5100			3300	17191	19863	37054
1945			5200			3400	15477	20378	35855
1950	2660	2722	5382	1706	1899	3604	18539	20509	39048
1955	2735	2802	5537	1793	1988	3781	18528	20724	39252
1960	2872	2934	5805	1927	2121	4048	19010	21141	40151
1965	3029	3085	6114	2133	2311	4444	19952	21821	41773
1970	3155	3211	6366	2272	2446	4718	20216	22119	42334
1975	3205	3292	6498	2368	2559	4927	20508	22364	42872
1980	3283	3399	6682	2439	2640	5079	21154	22963	44117
1985	3347	3487	6834	2568	2761	5329	21981	23741	45721
1990	3440	3583	7024	2691	2874	5565	22414	24077	46491
1995	3507	3656	7163	2784	2979	5763	22901	24343	47244

Year	USA			USSR (see also below)			Yugoslavia [1] (see also below)		
	Males	Females	Total	Males	Females	Total	Males	Females	Total
1920			72700						
1925			79900				3891	4204	8094
1930			87100				4169	4452	8621
1935			92900				4477	4780	9257
1940			99000						
1945			79900						
1950			104500				5289	5957	11246
1955	54222	55993	110215				5799	6412	12211
1960	56268	59325	115593			172875	6115	6672	12787
1965	59973	63564	123537			172875	6575	7126	13701
1970	64622	69288	133910			182100	7168	7690	14858
1975	69567	75697	145264			190725	7695	8184	15878
1980	77130	83973	161103			199125	8190	8677	16868
1985	84183	91735	175918	93962	112452	206414	8596	9017	17613
1990	89572	97228	186800	98496	115718	214214	8999	9423	18422
1995	93670	101188	194857	101014	117604	218618	3993	4317	8310

USSR successor republics, 1990	Males	Females	Total
Armenia	1190	1326	2515
Azerbaijan	2278	2506	4785
Belarus	3605	4282	7888
Estonia	557	664	1220
Georgia	1894	2191	4085
Kazakhstan	5492	6056	11549
Kyrgystan	1325	1434	2759
Latvia	948	1142	2091
Lithuania	1342	1556	2897
Moldova	1463	1685	3148
Russia	52318	62198	114517
Tajikistan	1544	1604	3148
Turkmenistan	1083	1150	2233
Ukraine	18357	22385	40742
Uzbekistan	5913	6253	12166

Yugoslavia, successor republics, 1992 [4]	Males	Females	Total
Bosnia	1681	1720	3401
Croatia	1837	2008	3846
Macedonia	712	720	1432
Montenegro	219	230	449
Serbia	3617	3846	7463
Slovenia	767	837	1604

Source: unless otherwise stated, data before 1950 are taken from Lee P.N. (ed) (1975). *Tobacco consumption in various countries,* 4th edition. Tobacco Research Council, London. Research Paper 6 (RP6)
and data for 1950 onwards are taken from WHO.

1 For data before 1950, based on 5-year periods, Alderson M. (1981). *International Mortality Statistics*. Macmillian, London.
2 For data before 1950 (before 1930 for Iceland, before 1935 for Romania), estimated from total population given by http://www.library.uu.nl/wesp/populstat/
3 Up to 1974, Jewish population only, thereafter total population. The Jewish population was 89% of the total population in 1975
4 US Census Bureau International Data Base (IDB), http://www.census.gov/

The following source notes were given in RP6:

Canada	1920-24 *The Canadian Year-Book.* 1925-57 *Canadian Statistical Review*, 1957 and 1958. 1958-1973 Statistics Canada, Census Division.
Finland	Central Statistical Office of Finland
Germany	1926-39 *Bevolkerung und Wirtschaft*, 1871-1957, published by the Western Germany Federal Statistics office, Wiesbasen. 1949-63 *United Nations Demographic Yearbook.* *1964-73 Statistiches Jahrbuch für die Bundesrepublik Deutschland*, published by the Western Germany Federal Statistics office, Wiesbaden.
Netherlands	1923-52 *Bevolking van Nederlqnd*; *Leeftijd en Geslacht*, 1953-73 *Maandstatistiek van Bevolking* and *Statistisch Zakboek*, all published by the Netherlands Central Bureau of Statistics.
Norway	Central Bureau of Statistics Norway.
Switzerland	Annuaire Statistique de la Suisse
USA	1920-45 *Historical Statistics of the United States*, 1789-1945, published by the United States Department of Commerce. 1946-72 *United Nations Monthly Bulletin of Statistics* and *United Nations Demographic Yearbook.*

Appendix II

Comparisons of manufactured and hand-rolled cigarettes and differences in the way they are smoked

In the UK in the past, most manufactured cigarettes were 70 mm in length and filled wholly with tobacco. Today, the vast majority have filters, and they are also available in longer lengths (e.g. 85 mm and 100 mm). Generally, the longer the cigarette, the longer is the filter. Although few direct data are available on the average weight of tobacco in cigarettes, comparison of the total sales by number and by weight (see Tables 27.1.1 and 27.1.2) suggests that the weight had remained at about 1.0 g from 1920 to 1960, but then decreased to 0.7 g in 1975 and rose again to 0.8 g by 1985.

Fine-cut tobacco purchased for use in hand-rolled cigarettes was usually taxed and priced at a rate lower per cigarette than the tobacco in manufactured cigarettes, and the smoker who made his own cigarettes generally did so at least in part to economize, even when the two types of cigarettes contained the same amount of tobacco. However, he economized further by putting less tobacco, and sometimes very much less, into each cigarette. Estimates of 0.8 g per cigarette in the 1930s, falling to 0.5 g in the early 1980s, have been used by the TAC (Tobacco Advisory Council), based on sales of tobacco and consumer survey findings.

Another motive for smoking hand-rolled cigarettes is the availability of stronger blends of tobacco. With the phasing out in recent decades of the brands of manufactured cigarettes with the highest tar delivery, a smoker determined to have a full-flavoured cigarette can only obtain one by making his own.

The tobacco used for hand-rolled cigarettes contains more moisture than that in manufactured cigarettes. This is essential; otherwise the tobacco would be too brittle to handle satisfactorily when it is made into cigarettes. The higher moisture content has two consequences. First, the tobacco has a stronger flavour than it would have had at a lower moisture content. Second, the hand-rolled cigarette is liable to go out when it is placed in any ashtray between puffs, encouraging the smoker to take more frequent puffs or to hold the cigarette longer in his mouth.

Another difference between the ways in which hand-rolled and manufactured cigarettes are smoked is that the former are frequently smoked down to a short butt length. The length to which a manufactured cigarette can be smoked is limited by the length of the filter.

Many of these considerations also apply to other countries.

Data on the average weight of tobacco in manufactured cigarettes are rarely given directly. Comparable data for sales of manufactured cigarettes by both weight and number are available for only a few countries and limited years. The weight of tobacco per cigarette, given directly or estimated from these data since 1950, is summarized as follows:

	Estimated weight of tobacco per manufactured cigarette (g)							
	1950	1960	1970	1975	1980	1985	1990	1995
Australia					0.82	0.79	0.74	
Canada	1.46	1.28	0.95	0.89	0.83	0.81	0.77	0.71
Denmark	1.25	1.24	1.27					
Finland								
Russian-type	0.45	0.44	0.40					
Other	1.08	0.92	0.99					
Overall	0.79	0.79	0.97					
Germany	1.10	1.08	0.98					
Greece	1.14	1.14	1.14	1.14	1.14	1.00	1.00	1.00
Ireland	1.00	1.00	0.86		0.80	0.84		
Japan		1.00	1.00					
New Zealand		1.10					0.84	0.76
Norway	1.20	1.09	1.09					
Sweden	1.11	1.04	0.81		0.70	0.68		
UK	0.97	0.98	0.76		0.80	0.83		
USA	1.30			0.85	0.80	0.79	0.79	0.76

This shows a generally decreasing tobacco content for most countries. A recent increase is seen in Ireland and the UK. The pattern in Finland is influenced by the decreasing sales of Russian-type cigarettes with low tobacco content. A similar effect with decreasing papyrosi sales is seen in USSR (see *Notes on sources of sales data,* p. 745).

A tax differential between manufactured and hand-rolled cigarettes exists in several countries. Lower cost is an important motive for the smoking of hand-rolled cigarettes as can be seen in Germany[1] and Norway[2].

Few data are available on the average tobacco content of hand-rolled cigarettes (or of the extent of use of filters, tubes, or manual cigarette makers). The average tobacco content of a hand-rolled cigarette has been assumed to be 1.25 g in Flemish-speaking Belgium[3] and the Netherlands[4], and 1.0 g by other sources in the Netherlands[5,6], Germany[7], and Canada[8]. Rickert et al.[9] in Canada, in an experiment testing 13 popular brands of fine-cut tobacco, made up cigarettes by manually inserting the tobacco into filter tubes using a manual filter cigarette maker. The average weight of cigarettes was 1.4 g. Dymond[10] gives the average weight of a hand-rolled cigarette as 0.8 g in Finland, 0.76 g in France, 0.778 g in Germany, 0.78 g in Netherlands, 0.9 g in Norway and 0.49 g in UK; and gives the moisture content of fine-cut tobacco as usually 16-18% and sometimes as high as 22% (much higher than that of manufactured cigarettes). Mørck et al.[2] estimated that 10% of hand-rolled cigarettes in Norway and 87% in Denmark were filter cigarettes.

References

1. Junge B, Tiefelsdorf M, Arab-Kohlmeier L. Tabakkonsum in der Bundesrepublik Deutschland. Strukturveränderungen in drei Jahrzehnten. *Pravention* 1989;**2**:35-40.

2. Mørck HI, Linde J, Agner E, Hein HO, Gyntelberg F, Nielsen PE. Tobaksforbrug og rygevaner i Norden 1920-1980. (Tobacco consumption and smoking habits in the Nordic countries). *Nord Med* 1982;**97**:134-46.

3. Joossens L. *Les comportements et les attitudes de la population Flamande face à la consommation du tabac*. Brussels: CRIOC; 1981.

4. de Haas JH. Rookpatroon in Nederland. Gaan mannen minder roken? *Hart Bull* 1973;**4**:77-86.

5. de Haas JH, de Haas-Posthuma JH. *Zo rookt Nederland. Evolutie van het landelijk rookpatroon in Nederland naar sexe en leeftijd, in samenhang met welstand. (Smoking habits in the Netherlands. Evolution of the national smoking pattern in the Netherlands according to sex and age, in conjunction with level of prosperity).* 's-Gravenhage: Stichting Volksgezondheid en Roken; 1980.

6. Stichting Volksgezondheid en Roken (Foundation for Smoking and Health). *Jaarverslag (Annual report).* 's-Gravenhage: Stichting Volksgezondheid en Roken; successive years.

7. Todd GF. *Cigarette Data Collection : A record of six cigarette smoking parameters in 20 countries.* Internal report. 1986.

8. Millar WJ. *Smoking behaviour of Canadians 1981.* Canada: Health and Welfare Canada; 1983.

9. Rickert WS, Robinson JC, Bray DF, Rogers B, Collishaw NE. Characterization of tobacco products: A comparative study of the tar, nicotine, and carbon monoxide yields of cigars, manufactured cigarettes, and cigarettes made from fine-cut tobacco. *Prev Med* 1985;**14**:226-33.

10. Dymond HF. A survey of roll-your-own tobacco use and practice and considerations for the analysis of smoking articles made from it. *Tob Sci* 1996;**40**:82-6.

Appendix III

Consumption category estimation

The method used in this report to estimate the means of consumption categories of numbers of cigarettes smoked per day was introduced by Todd in 1986[1] This was a modification of an earlier method given by Todd in 1978[2].

The 1978 method used a standard distribution based on detailed frequency distributions of male and female cigarette smokers that had applied in the UK. This distribution separated those who smoked a number of cigarettes ending with five or zero from those who smoked a number in the intervening categories. The standard distribution was modified when detailed distributions from the New Zealand Censuses of 1976 and 1981 became available. By combining the two censuses, data on over 700 000 male and 600 000 female smokers were available in 11 consumption categories (1-4, 5-9, ..., 45-49, and 50+). This enabled better distributions to be constructed for those smoking larger numbers of cigarettes.

The 1986 standard distribution is given below:

1986 standard distribution

Consumption category	Male smokers	Female smokers	Assumed mean of consumption category
	%	%	
1-4	7	10	2.5
5	4	5	5
6-9	6	10	7.5
10	13	17	10
11-14	7	8	12.5
15	8	11	15
16-19	4	4	17.5
20	25	20	20
21-24	6	5	22.5
25	4	3	25
26-29	2	1	27.5
30	5	2	30
31-34	1	1	32.5
35	1	0	35
36-39	0	0	37.5
40	4	2	40
41-44	0	0	
45	0	0	
46-49	0	0	
50	2	1	50
51-59	0	0	
60	1	0	60
61+	0	0	
	100	100	

Use of the standard distribution assumes that, for the country, age, and sex group in question, the shape of the distribution within each consumption category (e.g. 16-24) was the same as in the standard distribution. This procedure seems reasonable where consumption categories are small, e.g. 1-5, 6-10, 11-20. 21-30, and 31+. Its validity where few consumption categories were used, e.g. 10-14 and 15+, is less certain. On rare occasions when consumption categories used non-standard dividing points (e.g. 8-12) we split the standard category by assuming a uniform distribution over the standard category.

References

1. Todd GF. *Cigarette Data Collection : A record of six cigarette smoking parameters in 20 countries.* Internal report. 1986.

2. Todd GF. Cigarette consumption per adult of each sex in various countries. *J Epidemiol Community Health* 1978;**32**:289-93.

Appendix IV

Estimation of prevalence of smoking by standardized age groups

The age-specific data on prevalence of smoking, presented in Table 4 for each country, are often difficult to interpret owing to the different age groups used. Data presented according to a set of standard age groups would be more useful, for instance for comparison with mortality trends, which are commonly presented by 5-year age groups. For the purpose of facilitating interpretation of the data, this appendix describes a method with two objectives:

(i) to estimate the prevalence in each of the standard narrower age groups that it contains from the prevalence given by a survey for a broad age group

(ii) to extrapolate the prevalence to cover the whole age range from a survey covering a large proportion of the adult age range.

The method is described briefly here. A full description is available on request from the authors.

We defined 23 standard age groups, corresponding to single years of age from 12 to 20, 21-24, five year age groups from 25-29 to 80-84, and 85+. We defined *n* as the number of age groups for which a survey presents results. Each surveyed age group, *j*, corresponds to one or more standard age groups, and the first and last of these corresponding groups are denoted a_j and b_j. We defined the prevalence of smoking in the surveyed age group as X_j and the population based on the WHO European Standard population as P_j. Hence the number of smokers was calculated as X_jP_j. We then defined the statistics Q_j and R_j by the formulae

$$Q_j = \frac{\sum_{k=1}^{j} P_k}{\sum_{k=1}^{n} P_k}$$

and

$$R_j = \frac{\sum_{k=1}^{j} (X_kP_k)}{\sum_{k=1}^{n} (X_kP_k)}$$

so that Q_j represents the proportion of the population in age group *j* or less, and R_j represents the proportion of all smokers in age group *j* or less.

The statistic R_j is independent of the overall prevalence of smoking in the population and was considered suitable for combining age-specific results from different sources. The values of R_j were plotted against Q_j for all surveys that met certain criteria:

(i) included in the first edition of this book, i.e. for 22 countries and up to 1985,

(ii) had age boundaries which corresponded to age boundaries of standard age groups, and (iii) covered the full adult age range (15 years and over) with at least two age groups. It was found that the shape of these curves was affected by a number of factors, namely sex, time period, and also type of tobacco product for males and country for females. A smooth curve was fitted to each subgroup of surveys defined by these factors, with values R_i^* at the points corresponding to all the standard age groups. The slopes between these points, denoted by w_i for standard age group i, were calculated by

$$w_i = \frac{R_i^* - R_{i-1}^*}{Q_i - Q_{i-1}}$$

and are given in Table A4.1.

The values of w_i could then be used as weights to allow objectives (i) and (ii) to be achieved. First, the prevalence in standard age group i, denoted by x_i where i was within the original age range of the survey (i.e. $a_1 \le i \le b_n$), was estimated by

$$x_i = \frac{X_j w_i \left(\sum_{k=a_j}^{b_j} p_k\right)}{\sum_{k=a_j}^{b_j} (p_k w_k)} \qquad \text{where } j \text{ satisfies } a_j \le i \le b_j$$

Second, where i lay outside the surveyed age range (i.e. $i < a_1$ or $i > b_n$), the estimate of the extrapolated prevalence, denoted by y_i , was

$$y_i = \frac{w_i \sum_{k=a_L}^{b_L} (X_k P_k)}{\sum_{k=a_L}^{b_L} (W_k P_k)} \qquad \text{where } L = 1 \text{ for } i < a_1 \text{ and } L = n \text{ for } i > b_n$$

This method was applied to all surveys in Table 4 (of the first edition) of each country, with the extrapolating estimates y_i only being carried out if certain minimum age range criteria were met. Two further simple averaging processes were performed, firstly to convert to 5-year age groups for ages 15-19 and 20-24, and secondly to combine surveys within 5-year time periods according to product groupings appropriate for each country. Any gaps between the first and last periods surveyed were estimated by a simple linear interpolation within each age group. Although there were some problems due to misfit of the selected R^* curves to certain individual surveys or to combining surveys with different definitions or methodologies, particularly with surveys of teenagers, the results generally appeared plausible.

A similar approach was followed for the 'cigarette consumption per adult, sales-adjusted' data from Table 7 of each country. As previously, a number of factors affected the shape of the curves, but here it was not possible to allocate effects clearly to country and decade. Moreover the estimation was based on surveys from relatively few country/decade settings but was required to be applied more widely. For each sex, five basic shapes of curve were identified, and the weights are shown in Tables A4.2. The method was applied to all surveys in Table 6 for each country, assuming a sales-adjustment factor of 80% for those surveys which did not meet the criteria for calculation of a factor. The allocations of the weights to the countries are shown in Table A4.3.

The resulting tables of prevalence and consumption estimates by standard age groups and time periods are available from the authors on request. Tables A4.4 and A4.5 give the estimates for Sweden as an example. It is intended to extend this work up to 1995 and to all countries covered by this edition, and the results will also be available in due course.

Because this appendix presents our method of interpreting available data, its results have not been included in the main part of this volume, which is essentially a source of original data. Nevertheless the tables in the following pages constitute a useful attempt to provide statistics in a standard format.

Table A4.1 Weights by standard age group—prevalence

	Age group 12	13	14	15	16	17	18	19	20	21-24	25-29	30-34	35-39	40-44	45-49	50-54	55-59	50-64	65-69	70-74	75-79	80-84	85+
Males																							
Pre-1960 all products	14.2	28.4	43.8	54.5	62.5	67.3	69.0	69.0	93.5	110.1	111.1	111.8	112.7	113.0	109.8	106.3	99.7	96.3	86.5	79.3	71.2	71.2	71.2
1960+ all products	12.7	25.5	39.2	48.8	56.0	60.2	76.6	111.2	102.1	104.2	103.6	110.5	110.3	107.8	108.3	107.2	105.0	98.0	94.2	85.6	77.2	69.1	69.1
Pre-1960 cigarettes	11.8	23.6	36.3	45.1	51.8	55.7	100.2	117.6	115.3	115.3	123.7	122.1	125.5	116.4	115.0	108.6	89.5	80.7	63.2	52.0	41.7	35.0	26.9
1960+ cigarettes	13.0	26.1	40.1	49.9	57.3	61.6	85.4	85.4	105.9	117.7	120.1	115.9	111.1	110.2	109.5	103.9	102.0	89.6	81.3	66.1	59.3	52.8	46.5
Females																							
1960s group 1	21.0	42.0	70.7	85.8	97.5	102.4	153.3	256.0	192.1	147.2	129.1	123.1	130.1	115.8	105.3	85.0	59.2	56.5	34.0	31.2	11.7	11.7	11.7
1970s group 1	24.9	49.9	84.1	102.0	115.9	121.9	167.2	117.7	165.5	150.8	144.4	128.9	115.1	102.0	97.3	84.1	72.8	52.2	44.7	31.1	27.9	17.8	17.8
1980s group 1	17.4	34.9	58.8	71.3	81.0	85.2	102.7	116.6	143.3	158.3	149.7	125.1	122.2	110.3	109.9	81.4	78.3	58.6	55.9	33.0	29.1	19.7	19.7
1940s/1950s USA, Denmark	12.8	25.6	43.2	52.4	59.5	62.5	135.2	157.9	147.8	147.8	154.7	148.0	144.3	131.3	93.1	84.0	62.4	41.9	31.8	17.2	15.1	15.1	15.1
1960s group 2	10.8	21.7	36.6	44.4	50.5	53.0	77.5	77.5	104.5	122.6	131.4	130.4	127.9	125.2	112.5	109.7	90.4	80.8	55.9	43.0	24.9	19.0	15.3
1970s group 2	15.5	31.0	52.3	63.5	72.1	75.8	101.5	107.7	118.6	124.6	124.3	117.6	116.5	115.8	117.1	105.2	95.2	71.3	62.9	48.4	46.5	32.0	22.6
1980s group 2	14.8	29.7	50.0	60.7	68.9	72.4	94.3	97.1	116.4	124.9	124.7	116.3	112.9	108.3	105.7	101.3	102.2	84.3	76.8	55.7	56.0	40.1	40.1
1970s Japan				34.1	34.1	34.1	34.1	47.7	61.2	74.8	78.1	81.4	92.4	100.0	116.2	124.8	132.5	131.5	130.5	130.5	130.5	130.5	130.5
1980s Japan				59.1	59.1	59.1	59.1	80.4	101.6	122.9	117.6	112.2	104.8	102.7	97.2	93.8	93.0	95.9	99.1	99.1	99.1	99.1	99.1

Notes

'All products' includes unspecified product
'Cigarettes' include total, manufactured, or unspecified cigarette type

Group 1 includes Austria, Belgium, Finland, France, Germany, Greece, Italy, Netherlands, Norway, Portugal, Spain, Sweden, Switzerland
Group 2 includes Australia, Canada, Denmark, Ireland, Israel, New Zealand, UK, USA

Table A4.2 Weights by standard age group—cigarettes per person

	Age group 12	13	14	15	16	17	18	19	20	21-24	25-29	30-34	35-39	40-44	45-49	50-54	55-59	50-64	65-69	70-74	75-79	80-84	85+
Males																							
Main	5.4	10.8	20.2	27.0	37.6	59.2	78.6	85.3	97.5	109.4	115.0	119.1	120.2	121.2	119.2	114.4	105.1	89.4	74.4	57.6	42.4	28.2	22.9
High	6.3	12.7	23.8	31.7	42.6	64.8	76.2	98.8	109.9	125.3	131.4	130.3	126.3	119.2	112.4	103.3	85.8	75.1	58.2	51.2	41.5	42.3	42.3
Flat	5.6	11.2	21.0	28.0	39.1	61.4	81.6	95.3	97.8	109.5	113.3	113.3	113.3	113.3	113.3	112.0	107.3	100.5	89.2	69.0	50.8	33.8	27.5
Very High	8.0	16.1	30.1	40.1	56.0	88.0	116.9	138.9	144.6	150.3	152.5	154.8	145.9	134.7	106.9	90.2	57.3	39.4	15.7	10.0	3.3	2.2	1.8
Low	5.5	11.0	20.7	27.5	38.4	60.4	80.2	90.3	89.2	88.2	90.6	93.0	100.5	105.7	115.2	119.6	121.8	119.4	112.4	107.2	89.5	70.0	46.5
Females																							
Main	2.7	6.8	17.6	27.0	56.3	74.1	83.8	83.8	102.3	124.3	131.6	128.7	127.2	124.8	121.8	111.3	94.0	70.3	49.5	33.6	22.6	15.0	12.5
High	3.2	8.1	21.1	32.5	67.6	89.0	112.8	112.8	126.0	138.5	138.7	132.2	131.1	123.1	117.9	96.7	80.3	56.2	43.9	26.4	21.2	15.2	15.1
Very High	3.8	9.7	25.1	38.6	80.4	105.8	134.4	140.5	163.0	177.2	168.3	155.2	134.8	144.0	87.4	71.4	52.4	40.2	30.8	22.4	17.1	11.3	11.3
Low	2.6	6.5	16.8	25.8	53.8	70.8	89.9	89.4	99.8	111.9	114.0	116.7	119.8	120.5	119.8	116.0	108.3	91.8	68.3	47.2	31.8	22.8	15.6
Very Low	1.1	2.6	6.8	10.5	21.9	28.8	36.6	42.2	52.2	62.3	65.8	69.2	90.0	107.3	129.8	135.0	150.6	151.9	146.9	121.4	103.8	91.6	87.6

Note
See Table A4.3 for allocation of country/decade to weighting set

Table A4.3 Allocations to weighting set for cigarettes per person

	Males					Females				
	1940s	**1950s**	**1960s**	**1970s**	**1980s**	**1940s**	**1950s**	**1960s**	**1970s**	**1980s**
Australia		main	**main**	**main**			main	**main**	**main**	
Austria				flat	**flat**				main	**main**
Belgium					**high**					**very high**
Canada			**main**	**main**	**main**			**main**	**main**	**main**
Denmark	**very high**	high	**high**	**main**		**very high**	high	**high**	**main**	
Finland			high	**high**	**high**			very high	**very high**	**very high**
France			high	**high**	**high**			very high	very high	**very high**
Germany		main	main	main			very high	very high	very high	
Greece		**very low**			flat					
Ireland			**flat**	**flat**	**flat**			**low**	**low**	**low**
Israel			high	**high**	**high**				**main**	**main**
Italy	main	main	main	main	main	very high	very high	very high	very high	**very high**
Japan			flat	**flat**	**flat**			very low	**very low**	**low**
Netherlands		main		**main**	main		high		**high**	high
New Zealand				**main**	**main**				**main**	**main**
Norway				**main**	**main**				**high**	**main**
Portugal										
Spain				main	main				very high	very high
Sweden			**high**					**very high**	very high	
Switzerland				**high**	**high**				**very high**	**very high**
UK	**main**	**main**	**main**	**main**	**main**	**main**	**main**	**main**	**main**	**low**
USA	**high**	**main**	**main**	**main**	**main**	**very high**	**very high**	**main**	**main**	**low**

Note 1: Bold type indicates country/decades with surveys contributing to the estimation of weights. Normal type indicates other country/decades for which weights were required

Note 2: Sets do not have the same definitions for males as for females

Table A4.4 Estimated prevalence of smoking by 5-year age groups and 5-year periods, Sweden

Years	n1	n2	Age group 15-19	20-24	25-29	30-34	35-39	40-44	45-49	50-54	55-59	60-64	65-69	70-74	75-79	80-84	85+
Males - A																	
1946-1950	1	0	32.1	53.1	55.3	55.6	56.1	56.2	54.6	52.9	49.6	47.9	43.1	39.5	35.4	35.4	35.4
1951-1955	0	15	33.4	54.8	55.9	57.3	56.9	56.5	55.5	53.5	50.9	48.6	44.8	37.2	33.4	32.3	32.3
1956-1960	0	15	34.7	56.5	56.5	59.1	57.7	56.8	56.5	54.1	52.2	49.3	46.4	34.8	31.3	29.3	29.3
1961-1965	2	0	36.0	58.2	57.0	60.8	58.5	57.2	57.4	54.7	53.6	50.0	48.1	32.5	29.3	26.2	26.2
1966-1970	1	0	38.3	56.4	56.3	60.0	59.9	58.5	58.8	58.2	57.0	53.2	51.1	46.5	41.9	37.5	37.5
1971-1975	6-10	0	40.2	56.4	56.3	60.0	59.9	58.6	58.8	58.2	57.0	53.2	51.2	46.5	41.9	37.5	37.5
1976-1980	8-12	0	29.4	43.4	45.0	48.1	47.2	46.2	46.1	45.6	44.5	41.5	39.8	35.7	30.5	27.3	27.3
1981-1985	3-5	0	25.0	32.4	35.9	38.3	38.6	37.7	36.8	36.4	34.1	31.8	29.4	26.7	22.2	19.9	19.9
Males - TC/MC																	
1961-1965	2	0	29.5	56.9	52.0	50.2	46.9	46.5	46.2	40.8	40.0	35.2	31.9	19.2	17.3	15.3	13.5
1966-1970	3	0	25.9	44.0	45.8	44.2	42.4	42.0	41.8	38.0	37.3	32.5	29.5	16.2	14.6	12.9	11.4
1971-1975	8	0	28.5	44.4	46.1	43.0	41.2	40.2	39.9	37.7	37.0	32.8	29.8	17.8	16.0	14.3	12.5
1976-1980	6	0	19.6	33.1	34.5	37.3	35.8	35.5	35.2	30.2	29.7	26.0	23.6	16.5	14.8	13.2	11.6
1981-1985	5	0	16.0	27.1	31.3	32.9	34.7	34.5	34.3	30.2	28.9	25.3	23.0	18.0	16.1	14.3	12.6
Females - A																	
1946-1950	1	0	12.0	13.5	11.1	10.6	11.2	10.0	9.1	7.3	5.1	4.9	2.9	2.7	1.0	1.0	1.0
1951-1955	0	15	18.9	22.2	20.3	19.3	18.5	16.5	15.0	11.3	7.9	7.5	4.5	2.8	1.1	1.1	1.1
1956-1960	0	15	25.8	30.9	29.4	28.1	25.7	22.9	20.8	15.2	10.6	10.1	6.1	3.0	1.1	1.1	1.1
1961-1965	2	0	32.8	39.6	38.6	36.8	33.0	29.4	26.7	19.2	13.4	12.8	7.7	3.1	1.2	1.2	1.2
1966-1970	2	0	48.2	54.2	44.8	42.8	45.2	44.3	39.7	32.8	29.1	19.4	11.6	10.7	4.0	4.0	4.0
1971-1975	6-10	0	51.4	56.1	52.7	47.1	42.0	37.2	35.5	30.7	26.6	19.1	16.3	11.4	10.2	6.5	6.5
1976-1980	8-12	0	41.3	49.4	47.3	41.7	37.5	33.4	32.2	26.9	24.2	17.5	15.0	9.8	8.2	5.3	5.3
1981-1985	3-5	0	24.5	45.0	45.9	38.3	40.1	36.2	38.5	28.5	27.5	20.6	17.9	10.6	9.4	6.4	6.4
Females - TC/MC																	
1961-1965	2	0	32.7	39.5	38.4	36.7	32.8	29.2	26.5	19.0	13.3	12.7	7.6	3.1	1.2	1.2	1.2
1966-1970	3	0	41.4	46.4	40.3	37.4	37.2	33.1	30.6	24.9	18.9	14.9	10.4	5.6	3.1	2.5	2.5
1971-1975	8	0	43.8	50.1	47.2	41.7	37.2	33.3	31.8	26.9	23.3	16.4	14.1	6.9	6.2	4.0	4.0
1976-1980	6	0	35.1	43.9	41.6	40.0	36.7	32.7	31.6	27.0	24.1	17.5	15.5	6.0	5.3	3.5	3.5
1981-1985	5	0	25.8	43.8	42.2	37.0	35.9	32.4	34.0	26.7	25.1	18.8	18.0	7.7	6.8	4.6	4.6

n_1 = number of surveys averaged within period, may vary between age groups
n_2 = number of age groups based on interperiod interpolation only
A = prevalence of smoking of all tobacco products
TC/MC = estimates taken to apply to smoking either total or manufactured
Source: Estimated from Tables 19.4.1/2, pp.379-382 of first edition, equivalent to Table 25.4, pp. 602-607 of this edition

Table A4.5 Estimated cigarettes per person, sales-adjusted, by 5-year age groups and 5-year periods, Sweden

Years	n1	n2	Age group 15-19	20-24	25-29	30-34	35-39	40-44	45-49	50-54	55-59	60-64	65-69	70-74	75-79	80-84	85+
Males																	
1961-1965	1	0	2.7	6.2	8.2	8.1	7.2	6.8	6.4	4.9	4.1	3.6	2.8	1.7	1.4	1.4	1.4
1966-1970	1	0	2.7	5.3	5.7	5.6	5.5	5.2	4.9	3.8	3.2	2.5	1.9	1.3	1.0	1.0	1.0
1971-1975	1	0	3.5	6.3	6.8	6.0	5.8	5.2	5.0	4.5	3.8	3.3	2.6	2.3	1.8	1.9	1.9
Females																	
1961-1965	1	0	2.3	4.9	4.5	4.1	4.3	3.6	2.8	1.7	1.3	1.0	0.7	1.0	0.7	0.5	0.5
1966-1970	1	0	3.3	5.6	5.5	5.0	4.4	3.7	2.8	2.2	1.6	0.9	0.7	0.2	0.1	0.1	0.1
1971-1975	1	0	4.1	6.7	6.4	5.1	4.4	4.0	3.1	2.5	1.8	1.4	1.1	0.8	0.6	0.4	0.4

n_1 = number of surveys averaged within period, may vary between age groups
n_2 = number of age groups based on inter-period interpolation only

Source: Estimated from Tables 19.6 and 19.7, pp. 386-387 of first edition, equivalent to Tables 25.6 and 25.7 pp. 610-611 of this edition

Appendix V

Estimating past smoking habits by an indirect method, with application to Great Britain

Nationally-based surveys of smoking habits are now carried out regularly in many countries. However, such surveys existed in relatively few countries before 1970, as has been demonstrated in the chapters of this book. Several researchers have therefore attempted to estimate the prevalence of smoking for earlier periods indirectly, using data on past smoking habits recalled in a recent survey. Based on current age, smoking status (never/ former/ current), age of starting to smoke and, for former smokers, age of stopping, each subject's smoking status can be derived for each year throughout life, thus allowing estimation of the prevalence of smoking by calendar year. A list of references to such attempts, relevant to the countries in this book, is given below.

We have carried out such an analysis for Great Britain and compared direct and indirect estimates back to 1948. The results are described briefly in this Appendix, a fuller description, including a discussion of a number of sources of potential bias in the indirect estimates, being available on request.

Two surveys were used as sources of indirect data.

(1) The 1984-1985 Health and Lifestyle Study (HALS) (Cox *et al* (1987)) of 9 003 subjects aged 18+, was chosen because it was large, representative of the British population, and enquired in moderate detail about smoking. Questions related to manufactured and hand-rolled cigarettes combined, with less detailed information available for pipe and cigar smoking.

(2) The 1978-1981 Alderson Hospital In-Patient Study (AHIP) (Alderson *et al* (1985)) was chosen because it used an exceptionally detailed questionnaire on manufactured cigarette (MC) smoking history. The 4 950 subjects selected for study were aged 35-74 and hospitalized in England with non-smoking-associated diseases. Questions related to regular smoking, separately for MC, hand-rolled cigarettes, pipes and cigars. Detailed questions on the amounts of MC smoked at up to 10 time points since age 16 allowed for estimates on the level of smoking to be calculated.

Direct estimates were obtained from surveys conducted by the Tobacco Advisory Council (TAC) and predecessor organizations (see Chapter 27, survey source 1).

Table A5.1 presents estimates of prevalence of smoking from the three sources, for selected years. The age groups presented are those most commonly used by TAC. The average difference over the period 1948-1975 between the direct and indirect estimates is also shown. There is generally a good correspondence between the three sets of estimates, with the same time trends evident at all age groups for both sexes, except that the AHIP estimates fall more steeply in the final 5 years than do the other sources (an effect which may be associated with ill health, even though the subjects' diseases were not smoking associated). For the central age groups (about age 20-60) the HALS and AHIP estimates for cigarette smoking are generally a little higher than TAC for males, but lower for females. For older male smokers of all products TAC estimates are consistently highest.

Table A5.2 presents the average MC smoked per MC smoker from two sources, for selected years. AHIP estimates are almost always higher than TAC estimates except after 1975. However both sources show the male consumption to be higher than the female consumption by a factor of 1.5 to 2, with consumption rising with time in each sex and age group. Similar age patterns are seen at each year for both sources, with the amount smoked increasing up to age 25 and little variation between ages 25 and 60. The AHIP estimates decline less at age 60+ than do the TAC estimates, which may in part be an artefact of the different age distributions.

Tables A5.3-A5.5 show the estimates from the two indirect sources by sex and birth cohort going back to 1920.

In the fuller version of this appendix (available on request) we discuss potential sources of bias in indirect estimates, including choice of subjects, definitions of smoking, quit periods, missing data, and inaccurate reporting. We demonstrate that bias due to differential mortality between smokers and nonsmokers (only survivors being able to contribute to the survey) should be minor if attention is limited to subjects aged under 70 at interview. The high level of agreement between the prevalence estimates suggests that most of the sources of potential bias have not in fact had a large influence. Indeed it is surprising that the differences in the definitions of 'cigarette' smoking (with hand-rolled cigarettes included only for HALS) has not had a noticeable impact on the estimated cigarette smoking prevalence for older men. Conversely, none of the factors discussed explains why estimates of the level of smoking are higher based on indirect rather than on direct methods.

For both prevalence and level of smoking, the indirect estimates show patterns similar to the direct estimates in respect of sex, age, cohort and time. Indirect estimates therefore represent a useful approach when direct estimates are not available.

References

Alderson M.R., Lee P.N. and Wang R. (1985). Risks of lung cancer, chronic bronchitis, ischaemic heart disease, and stroke in relation to type of cigarette smoked. *J Epidemiol Community Health,* **39**, 286-93.

Cox B.D., Blaxter M., Buckle A.L.J., Fenner N.P., *et al* (1987). *The health and lifestyle survey. Preliminary report of a nationwide survey of the physical and mental health, attitudes and lifestyle of a random sample of 9 003 British adults.* Health Promotion Research Trust, London.

Published papers presenting indirect estimates or similar analyses

Berrino F., Merletti F., Zubiri A., Del Moral A., *et al* (1988). A comparative study of smoking, drinking and dietary habits in population samples in France, Italy, Spain and Switzerland. II. Tobacco smoking. *Rev Epidemiol Sante Publique,* **36**, 166-76.

Birkett N.J. (1997). Trends in smoking by birth cohort for births between 1940 and 1975: a reconstructed cohort analysis of the 1990 Ontario health survey. *Prev Med,* **26**, 534-41.

Brenner H. (1993). A birth cohort analysis of the smoking epidemic in West Germany. *J Epidemiol Community Health,* **47**, 54-8.

Burns D.M., Lee L., Shen L.Z., Gilpin E., *et al* (1997). Cigarette smoking behavior in the United States. In: Burns D., Garfinkel L. and Samet J.M. (eds) *Changes in cigarette-related disease risks and their implications for prevention and control.* USDHHS, NIH, NCI; 13-112. (Smoking and Tobacco Control, Monograph 8.) NIH Publication Number 97-4213.

Degenhardt L., Lynskey M. and Hall W. (2000). Cohort trends in the age of initiation of drug use in Australia. *Australian and New Zealand Journal of Public Health,* **24**, 421-6.

Durston B. and Jamrozik K. (eds) (1990). *Tobacco & health 1990. The global war. Proceedings of the Seventh World Conference on Tobacco and Health, Perth, Western Australia, 1-5 April 1990.* Organising Committee of the Seventh World Conference on Tobacco and Health, 189 Royal Street, East Perth, Western Australia 6004.

Escobedo L.G. and Peddicord J.P. (1996). Smoking prevalence in US birth cohorts: the influence of gender and education. *Am J Public Health,* **86**, 231-6.

Escobedo L.G. and Peddicord J.P. (1997). Long-term trends in cigarette smoking among young U.S. adults. *Addict Behav,* **22**, 427-30.

Escobedo L.G. and Remington P.L. (1989). Birth cohort analysis of prevalence of cigarette smoking among

Hispanics in the United States. *JAMA,* **261**, 66-9.

Ferrence R.G. (1988). Sex differences in cigarette smoking in Canada, 1900-1978: a reconstructed cohort study. *Can J Public Health,* **79**, 160-5.

Gilpin E.A., Lee L., Evans N. and Pierce J.P. (1994). Smoking initiation rates in adults and minors: United States, 1944-1988. *Am J Epidemiol,* **140**, 535-43.

Harris J.E. (1983). Cigarette smoking among successive birth cohorts of men and women in the United States during 1900-80. *J Natl Cancer Inst,* **71**, 473-9.

Heuer C. and Becker N. (1999). Smoking prevalence and lung cancer mortality in Germany. *J Epidemiol Biostat,* **4**, 45-52.

Hyndman J., Hobbs M., Jamrozik K., Hockey R. and Parsons R. (1990). A retrospective cohort study of smoking habits in Australia. In: Durston B. and Jamrozik K. (eds) *Tobacco and health 1990. The global war. Proceedings of the 7th world conference on tobacco and health, Perth, Western Australia, 1st-5th April 1990.* Organising committee of the Seventh World Conference on Tobacco and Health, 189 Royal Street, East Perth, Western Australia 6004; 264-7.

Jensen O.M. (1975). Lung cancer and smoking in Danish women. *Int J Cancer,* **15**, 954-61.

Johnson R.A. and Gerstein D.R. (1998). Initiation of use of alcohol, cigarettes, marijuana, cocaine, and other substances in US birth cohorts since 1919. *Am J Public Health,* **88**, 27-33.

La Vecchia C., Decarli A. and Pagano R. (1986). Prevalence of cigarette smoking among subsequent cohorts of Italian males and females. *Prev Med,* **15**, 606-13.

Laaksonen M., Uutela A., Vartiainen E. and Jousilahti P. (1997). Development of smoking by birth cohort in Eastern Finland 1972-92. In: *10th World Conference on Tobacco or Health, Beijing, China, 24-28 August 1997.* 46 (OS 54)

Launoy G., Milan Cl., Milan Ch., Coudray B., *et al* (1995). Evolution of tobacco consumption by men in France between 1930 and 1990. In: Slama K. (ed) *Tobacco and Health, Ninth World Conference on Tobacco and Health, Paris, Oct 10-14 1994.* Plenum Press, New York and London; 711-3.

Nordlund L.A. (1998). Trends in smoking habits and lung cancer in Sweden. *Eur J Cancer Prev,* **7**, 109-16.

Pelletier F., Marcil-Gratton N. and Légaré J. (1996). A cohort approach to tobacco use and mortality: the case of Quebec. *Prev Med,* **25**, 730-40.

Rønneberg A., Hafstad A. and Lund K.E. (1994a). Røykevaner siden 1910 blant norske menn og kvinner født etter 1890 (Smoking habits since 1910 among Norwegian men and women born after 1890). *Tidsskr Nor Laegeforen,* **114**, 1623-6.

Rønneberg A., Lund K.E. and Hafstad A. (1994b). Lifetime smoking habits among Norwegian men and women born between 1890 and 1974. *Int J Epidemiol,* **23**, 267-76.

Tolley H.D., Crane L. and Shipley N. (1991). Smoking prevalence and lung cancer death rates. In: *Strategies to control tobacco use in the United States: a blueprint for public health action in the 1990's.* US Dept Health & Human Services, Public Health Service, NIH, Bethesda, Md; 73-126. Smoking and Tobacco Control Monograph 1. NIH publication 92-3316.

Weinkam J.J. and Sterling T.D. (1990). Age related changes in age of starting to smoke. *J Clin Epidemiol,* **43**, 133-40.

Table A5.1 Prevalence of smoking at selected years from different sources

Sex	Age group[2]		1950 TAC	1950 HALS	1950 AHIP	1960 TAC	1960 HALS	1960 AHIP	1970 TAC	1970 HALS	1970 AHIP	Average difference[1] 1948-1975 HALS-TAC	Average difference[1] 1948-1975 AHIP-TAC
Males	16-19	%C	51	44	49	65	56	49	55	53		-1.9	-4.13
		%A	52	45	52	65	56	52	56	53		-3.2	-2.73
	20-24	%C	68	73	71	67	60	63	58	61		2.1	2.44
		%A	71	74	76	70	61	69	65	62		-1.1	3.24
	25-34	%C	70	77	72	64	69	68	60	64	60	6.5	4
		%A	79	81	81	73	72	75	70	67	65	0.5	1.6
	35-59	%C	66	70	64	64	67	62	55	58	57	4.2	0.6
		%A	81	78	76	78	74	76	71	65	70	-4.3	-1.7
	60+	%C				46	45		46	47	39	0.65	-4.26
		%A				69	64		68	60	57	-8.55	-7.66
Females	16-19	%C	36	26	29	45	34	36	52	42		-5.7	-1.83
	20-24	%C	48	46	55	48	45	45	54	51		-1.9	0.14
	25-34	%C	53	47	53	53	50	53	51	48	51	-2.4	0.6
	35-59	%C	38	34	38	47	41	46	50	45	48	-6.5	-2
	60+	%C				22	16		26	21	27	-5.85	0.66

%C - Prevalence of MC smoking (TAC and AHIP) or cigarette smoking (HALS)
%A - Prevalence of smoking any product
[1] Calculated from estimates as whole numbers, no greater precision being available for TAC
[2] For the indirect estimates, the base is all subjects falling within the age group at that year, but these subjects may come from a more limited age range. Estimates based on less than 20 subjects have been omitted. For instance, in 1970, the AHIP subjects were aged 24-68, so that the group headed 60+ actually contains subjects 60-68, and the age group 20-24 has been omitted as it contained only 4 male and 2 female 24-years olds.
[3] 1948-1963
[4] 1948-1968
[5] 1960-1975
[6] 1965-1975

Table A5.2 Average number of MC smoked per smoker at selected years from different sources

Sex	Age group[1]	1950 TAC	1950 AHIP	1960 TAC	1960 AHIP	1970 TAC	1970 AHIP
Males	16-19	9.7	14.6	13	15.7		
	20-24	14.1	19.1	17.9	18.1		
	25-29	19.9	17.7	19.6	19.6	19.5	24.9
	30-34			18.6	23.2	19.9	22.4
	35-49			21.2	21.9	20.8	24.3
	50-59			21	21.3	19.9	22.9
	60+					15.8	21.1
Females	16-19	5.2	10	7.3	10.3		
	20-24	7.8	10.6	9.6	12.3		
	25-29	7.4	11.8	9.5	14	14.5	15.3
	30-34			11.9	13	13.7	15.3
	35-49			12.2	13.9	14.7	15.7
	50-59			10.7	12.4	14.2	15.3
	60+					10.1	13.9

[1] See footnote 2 to table A5.1

Table A5.3 HALS Study. Prevalence (%) of smoking at selected years, by sex and birth cohort

Year of birth	Year 1920	1925	1930	1935	1940	1945	1950	1955	1960	1965	1970	1975	1980	1985
Male - cigarette smoking														
1890-1899	47	47	47	47	47	40	40	40	40	33	13	13	13	7
1900-1909	33	62	75	76	75	73	68	65	61	55	48	38	29	19
1910-1919	1*	13	41	63	75	76	74	69	64	60	53	48	38	28
1920-1929			1	11	40	71	76	76	73	70	61	53	46	32
1930-1939					1	10	31	58	63	63	57	52	46	36
1940-1949							1	9	36	63	66	58	49	40
1950-1959									1	10	36	53	50	39
1960-1969											1	11	35	36
Male - smoking of any product														
1890-1899	73	67	67	67	67	60	60	60	53	47	33	33	33	20
1900-1909	35	67	80	81	82	81	77	75	71	65	60	50	42	31
1910-1919	1	13	42	65	77	81	79	75	71	69	64	60	49	37
1920-1929			1	12	41	73	79	79	77	74	67	59	54	40
1930-1939					2	11	32	60	65	66	62	58	53	44
1940-1949							1	9	36	64	69	63	55	46
1950-1959									1	10	36	54	51	41
1960-1969											1	11	35	36
Female - cigarette smoking														
1890-1899	15	19	19	19	19	23	21	21	17	15	13	13	13	8
1900-1909	3	10	19	23	28	29	30	28	26	24	20	17	14	10
1910-1919	0	1	8	23	34	38	39	39	39	39	36	32	26	21
1920-1929			0	2	19	46	51	53	52	52	50	49	44	36
1930-1939					0	3	16	36	47	48	48	46	43	34
1940-1949							0	2	19	44	49	45	39	33
1950-1959									0	4	28	46	45	35
1960-1969											0	9	35	36

* This group of smokers comprises 2 subjects born in 1910 and starting at ages 8 and 9, 1 subject born in 1911 starting at age 7 and 2 subjects born in 1912 starting at ages 6 and 8.

Table A5.4 AHIP Study. Prevalence (%) of smoking at selected years, by sex and birth cohort

Year of birth	Year 1920	1925	1930	1935	1940	1945	1950	1955	1960	1965	1970	1975	1980[1]
Male - MC smoking													
1900-1909	13	48	63	66	67	67	64	59	53	45	38	30	16
1910-1919	0	7	33	55	65	68	64	63	60	55	50	43	28
1920-1929			1	8	39	69	74	72	69	65	60	51	39
1930-1939					1	8	36	60	66	64	61	53	43
1940-1949							2	13	54	64	63	48	39
Male - smoking of any product													
1900-1909	14	53	72	77	78	80	77	77	72	56	47	47	32
1910-1919	0	7	36	61	74	77	75	75	73	70	65	57	40
1920-1929			1	9	43	76	82	81	79	76	72	67	51
1930-1939					1	8	38	64	72	71	69	64	53
1940-1949							2	14	57	69	69	57	50
Females - MC smoking													
1900-1909	1	9	17	20	25	30	31	30	30	29	24	19	13
1910-1919	0	1	8	26	37	45	45	45	45	45	41	35	23
1920-1929			0	3	22	47	55	57	57	56	54	49	37
1930-1939					0	4	22	43	47	46	49	45	39
1940-1949							1	1	34	50	52	47	35

[1] Estimates for 1980 are generally based on fewer subjects as they exclude subjects hospitalized before 1980

Table A5.5 AHIP Study. Average number of MC per smoker at selected years, by sex and birth cohort

Year of birth	Year 1920	1925	1930	1935	1940	1945	1950	1955	1960	1965	1970	1975	1980
Male													
1900-1909	9.2	12.0	16.4	17.6					21.2	20.7	21.5	20.3	17.7
1910-1919		7.9	11.7	15.1	17.7	18.7			22.1	22.2	22.2	21.1	18.8
1920-1929				10.4	12.9	17.1	20.0	20.4	22.1	23.5	24.1	25.1	23
1930-1939						12.1	13.9	17.5	19.7	23.5	24.4	25.5	24.6
1940-1949								10.4	15.1	19.2	23.6	25.0	24.1
Female													
1900-1909	5.9	7.0	9.2	10.0					12.8	14.1	14.4	13.3	12.4
1910-1919		5.3	7.3	8.6	10.5	12.1			13.8	14.7	15.0	15.0	14.1
1920-1929				7.8	9.5	10.9	11.3	11.1	13.5	14.8	15.3	16.3	15.9
1930-1939						6.8	9.6	12.0	13.4	15.5	16.2	17.9	16.8
1940-1949								7.6	9.8	13.8	15.7	18.7	17.5